Modern System of Ophthalmology (MSO) Series

Disorders of
Cornea and
Ocular Surface

Modern System of Ophthalmology (MSO) Series

Disorders of
Cornea and
Ocular Surface

Editor-in-Chief

AK Khurana MS, FAICO, CTO (London)
Professor, Department of Ophthalmology
SGT Medical College Hospital and Research Institute, Budhera, Gurugram
Former Senior Professor and Head, Regional Institute of Ophthalmology
Pt. BD Sharma Postgraduate Institute of Medical Sciences, Rohtak, Haryana

Editors

Namrata Sharma MD
Professor of Ophthalmology
Cornea, Cataract and Refractive Surgery Services
RP Center for Ophthalmic Sciences
AIIMS, New Delhi

Aruj K Khurana
DNB (Sankara Nethralaya, Chennai), FICO, FUR
Assistant Professor, Department of Ophthalmology
World College of Medical Sciences and Research
Jhajjar

Rajesh Sinha MD
Professor of Ophthalmology
Cornea, Cataract and Refractive Surgery Services
RP Center for Ophthalmic Sciences
AIIMS, New Delhi

Bhawna Khurana MS, DNB, FICO, FRCS
Fellow Orbit, Oculoplasty and Oncology from
Narayana Nethralaya, Bengaluru
Former Assistant Professor, SGRRIMHS and
Shri Mahant Indiresh Hospital, Dehradun

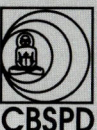

CBSPD

CBS Publishers & Distributors Pvt Ltd

New Delhi • Bengaluru • Chennai • Kochi • Kolkata • Lucknow • Mumbai
Hyderabad • Jharkhand • Nagpur • Patna • Pune • Uttarakhand

Modern System of Ophthalmology (MSO) Series

Disorders of
Cornea and
Ocular Surface

ISBN: 978-93-88902-67-0

Copyright © AK Khurana

First Edition 2020
Reprint **2025**

Published by **Satish Kumar Jain** and produced by **Varun Jain** for
CBS Publishers & Distributors Pvt Ltd
4819/XI Prahlad Street, 24 Ansari Road, Daryaganj, New Delhi 110 002, India.
Ph: 011-23266838, 23289259   Website: www.cbspd.com
                                    e-mail: delhi@cbspd.com

Corporate Office: 204 FIE, Industrial Area, Patparganj, Delhi 110 092
Ph: 011-4934 4934   Fax: 011-4934 4935   e-mail: publishing@cbspd.com;
                                               publicity@cbspd.com

Branches

- **Bengaluru:** Seema House 2975, 17th Cross, KR Road, Banasankari 2nd Stage, Bengaluru 560 070, Karnataka, India
  Ph: +91-80-26771678/79   Fax: +91-80-26771680   e-mail: bangalore@cbspd.com
- **Chennai:** 7, Subbaraya Street, Shenoy Nagar, Chennai 600 030, Tamil Nadu, India
  Ph: +91-44-26680620, 26681266   Fax: +91-44-42032115   e-mail: chennai@cbspd.com
- **Kochi:** 42/1325, 1326, Power House Road, Opp KSEB, Power House, Ernakulam Kochi 682 018, Kerala, India
  Ph: +91-484-4059061-65,67   e-mail: kochi@cbspd.com
- **Kolkata:** 147, Hind Ceramics Compound, 1st Floor, Nilgunj Road, Belghoria, Kolkata-700056, West Bengal, India
  Ph: +033-25633055, 033-25633056   e-mail: kolkata@cbspd.com
- **Lucknow:** Basement, Khushnuma Complex, 7 Meerabai Marg (Behind Jawahar Bhawan), Lucknow-226001, UP, India
  Ph: +0522-4000032   e-mail: tiwari.lucknow@cbspd.com
- **Mumbai:** PWD Shed, Gala no 25/26, Ramchandra Bhatt Marg, Next to JJ Hospital Gate no. 2, Opp. Union Bank of India, Noorbaug, Mumbai-400009, Maharashtra, India
  Ph: 022-66661880/89   e-mail: mumbai@cbspd.com

Representatives

- Hyderabad   0-9885175004   • Jharkhand   0-9811541605   • Nagpur   0-8692091830
- Patna   0-9334159340   • Pune   0-9664372571   • Uttarakhand 0-9716462459iv

Printed at Magic International, Noida, UP, India

List of Contributors

AK Khurana MS, FAICO, CTO (London)
Professor, Department of Ophthalmology
SGT Medical College Hospital and Research
Institute, Budhera, Gurugram

Namrata Sharma MD
Professor, Cornea, Cataract and Refractive
Surgery Services, RP Center for Ophthalmic
Sciences, AIIMS, New Delhi

Rajesh Sinha MD
Professor, Cornea, Cataract and Refractive
Surgery Services, RP Center for Ophthalmic
Sciences, AIIMS, New Delhi

Aruj K Khurana DNB, FICO (UK)
Assistant Professor
Department of Ophthalmology
World College of Medical Sciences and
Research, Jhajjar

Bhawna P Khurana MS, DNB, FICO (UK), FRCS
Fellow Orbit, Oculoplasty and Oncology from
Narayana Nethralaya, Bengaluru
Former Assistant Professor, SGRRIMHS and
Shri Mahant Indiresh Hospital, Dehradun

Indu Khurana MD
Dean Academics
World College of Medical Sciences and
Research, Gurawar, Jhajjar

Neha Adhlakha MS
Assistant Professor
Department of Ophthalmology
Shaheed Hasan Khan Mewati Government
Medical College, Mewat, Haryana

Sameera Irfan FRCS
Consultant Ophthalmologist
En Vision, Lahore, Pakistan

Urmil Chawla MS, DNB
Professor, Department of Ophthalmology
RIO, PGIMS, Rohtak

Poonam Kishore MS
Professor, Cornea Unit
Department of Ophthalmology
KGMU, Lucknow

Arun Sharma MS
Associate Professor, Cornea Unit
Department of Ophthalmology
KGMU, Lucknow

Surbhi Agarwal MS (Ophth)
PG Candidate
Department of Ophthalmology
KGMU, Lucknow

Srujna D MS
Associate Professor
Department of Ophthalmology
Armed Forces Medical College, Pune

Rachna Meel MD
Associate Professor
RP Center for Ophthalmic Sciences
AIIMS, New Delhi

Pallavi Sugandhi MS
Cornea and Refractive Surgery Services
Eye7 Chaudhary Eye Centre

Rinky Agarwal MD
RP Center for Ophthalmic Sciences
AIIMS, New Delhi

Praful K Maharana MD
Assistant Professor
RP Center for Ophthalmic Sciences
AIIMS, New Delhi

Pranita Sahay MS
RP Center for Ophthalmic Sciences
AIIMS, New Delhi

Ritu Nagpal MS
Healing Touch Eye Centre
Vikaspuri, New Delhi

Mansi Tripathi MS
RP Center for Ophthalmic Sciences
AIIMS, New Delhi

Noopur Gupta MS, DNB, PhD
Associate Professor
Cornea, Cataract and Refractive Surgery
Services, RP Center for Ophthalmic Sciences
AIIMS, New Delhi

Ritika Mukhija MD, FICO
Senior Resident, RP Center for Ophthalmic
Sciences, AIIMS, New Delhi

Ritika Sachdev MS
Additional Director
Medical Services Centre for Sight Group of
Eye Hospitals, New Delhi

Radhika Tandan MD
Professor, Cornea, Cataract and Refractive
Surgery Services, RP Center for Ophthalmic
Sciences, AIIMS, New Delhi

Darshan Kansara MS
Consultant, Sudarshan Eye Hospital and
Cornea Laser Centre

Sridevi Nair
RP Center for Ophthalmic Sciences
AIIMS, New Delhi

VS Sangwan
Director Research and Consultant
Cornea and Ocular surface Services
Shroff Charity Eye Hospital
Daryaganj, New Delhi

Aastha Singh
Cornea and Ocular Surface Services
Shroff Charity Eye Hospital
Daryaganj, New Delhi

Tanuj Sharma
Cornea and Ocular Surface Services
Shroff Charity Eye Hospital
Daryaganj, New Delhi

Nikunj V Patel
Cornea and Ocular Surface Services
Shroff Charity Eye Hospital
Daryaganj, New Delhi

Arpna Gandhi
Cornea and Ocular Surface Services
Shroff Charity Eye Hospital
Daryaganj, New Delhi

Devashish Mandal
Cornea and Ocular Surface Services
Shroff Charity Eye Hospital
Daryaganj, New Delhi

Sandeep Gupta
RP Center for Ophthalmic Sciences
AIIMS, New Delhi

Harkrishanan Vannadil
Eyeris Eye Care, Hyderabad

Geetha Iyer
Department of Cornea
Sankara Nethralaya
18 College Road, Chennai

Srikant Gupta
Former Professor
Department of Ophthalmology
Institute of Medical Sciences
BHU, Varanasi

Shweta Agarwal
Department of Cornea
Sankara Nethralaya
18 College Road, Chennai

Bhaskaran Sriniwasan
Department of Cornea
Sankara Nethralaya
18 College Road, Chennai

Farin Rajmohmad Sheikh
RP Center for Ophthalmic Sciences
AIIMS, New Delhi

Foreword

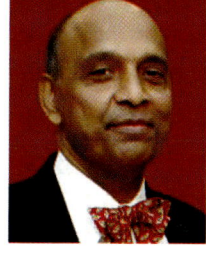

Education on different aspects of corneal disorders and their management needs significant improvement in many residency training programmes in India and the developing world. The availability of appropriate tools of education to correct this malady is a major requirement in our system.

The book *Disorders of Cornea and Ocular Surface* intended for this group of ophthalmologists in training is one such effort. In fact, this can also be a good resource for many practicing comprehensive ophthalmologists to enhance their knowledge of current understanding in the care of corneal disorders. The book is written in a way that it meets the demands of all these groups encompassing comprehensive review as well as practical tips. Various contributing authors deserve appreciation.

My compliments to Drs AK Khurana, Namrata Sharma and Rajesh Sinha for this valuable addition to the education materials in ophthalmology.

My best wishes for the success of this book.

Gullapalli N Rao
LV Prasad Eye Institute

Preface

Modern System of Ophthalmology (MSO) series comprises separate volumes on different subspecialities of ophthalmology. Each volume is planned with a very specific aim to cater to the needs of postgraduate students in ophthalmology.

Salient Features of MSO Series

- Each volume is edited by different editors, yet the layout and organization has been kept identical.
- Editors of different volumes are masters in their subspeciality with an uncanny knack of picking up the right perspectives.
- Text matter is designed to meet the needs of residents in ophthalmology with a comprehensive coverage in a concise manner. Text is complete and up-to-date with recent advances incorporated.
- Text is organized in such a way that the students can easily understand, retain and reproduce it. Various levels of headings, subheadings, bold face and italics given in the text will be helpful for a quick revision of the subject.
- A brief list of chapter contents given in the beginning of each chapter provides a clear layout of the text.
- Text has been profusely illustrated with high quality coloured photographs and computer drawn colour diagrams which provide vivid details.
- Exposition of the text is such that an average postgraduate student will find it easy to glean through and assimilate the facts for longer retention.

Disorders of Cornea and Ocular Surface This volume of MSO series covers comprehensively the disorders of cornea and ocular surface, which form the formidable and a sizeable portion of the day-to-day ophthalmic practice. Over the years, cornea has emerged as one of the most important subspecialities of ophthalmology. Consequently, a lot of books and manuals are available on this subject. However, the text matter in most of such books is in much more details than the requirement of postgraduate students and general ophthalmologists and are thus practically meant for fellows in the speciality of cornea and the cornea specialists. Keeping in view the above, in this volume of MSO, an effort has been made to include only the essential text and practical tips for the benefit of the trainee ophthalmologists and general ophthalmologists. Undoubtedly, the fellows of the speciality of cornea will also find it as an handy manuscript for their needs.

Text Matter of this volume, which provides an up-to-date coverage with incorporated recent advances on disorders of cornea and ocular surface, has been organised into eight sections:

Section I   Anatomy and Physiology of Cornea and Ocular Surface
Section II   Clinical Evaluation and Investigative Techniques for Cornea and Ocular Surface
Section III   Developmental Anomalies and Metabolic Disorders of Conjunctiva and Cornea
Section IV   Diseases of Conjunctiva and Ocular Surface
Section V   Inflammatory Diseases of Cornea
Section VI   Non-inflammatory Diseases of Cornea
Section VII   Surgical Procedures for Ocular Surface and Cornea
Section VIII   Corneal Blindness and Eye Banking

Editorial Team of this volume comprises ophthalmologists dedicated to the subspeciality of cornea and/or to academics and book writing in ophthalmology. The editor of this volume, Dr Namrata Sharma, presently Professor, Department of Ophthalmology, Cornea, Cataract and Refractive Surgery Services at RP Center for Ophthalmic Sciences, AIIMS, New Delhi, has vast clinical and research experience in the speciality. She has extensively published research papers and has also authored and co-authored nine books in the subject of diseases of cornea. Another editor Dr Rajesh Sinha is also presently Professor, Department of Ophthalmology, Cornea, Cataract and Refractive Surgery Services at RP Center for Ophthalmic Sciences, AIIMS, New Delhi. He has published three textbooks and four educational manuals. Another editor Dr Aruj K Khurana, currently working as an Assistant Professor, Department of Ophthalmology, World College of Medical Sciences and Research, Jhajjar, has been trained at Sankara Nethralaya, Chennai, and Narayana Nethralaya, Bengaluru. He is consultant, Vitreo-Retina specialist. However, because of his interest in writing, he is deeply associated with each volume of MSO series. Dr Bhawna P Khurana is trained at Guru Nanak Eye Centre, MAMC, New Delhi, in strabismology and paediatric ophthalmology, and at Narayana Nethralaya, Bengaluru, in orbit, oculoplasty and ocular oncology. She has worked in the Department of Ophthalmology at AIIMS, Rishikesh, and as an Assistant Professor, Ophthalmology at SGRRIMHS and associated Shri Mahant Indiresh Hospital, Dehradun.

Acknowledgement needs to be made to all those who have been instrumental in making this volume a reality. The generous help received, especially from Dr Urmil Chawla, Professor, RIO, PGIMS, Rohtak, Dr Neha Adhlakha, Assistant Professor, Department of Ophthalmology, Shaheed Hasan Khan, Mewati Government Medical College, Nuh, Mewat, and all the contributors of this volume is duly acknowledged. Thanks are also due to Prof PK Shinghal, Head, and all other faculty members and residents of Department of Ophthalmology, SGT Medical College, Budhera, Gurugram, for their co-operation. I want to put on record the remarkable assistance rendered by Dr Aruj Kumar Khurana and Dr Bhawna P Khurana in compiling the whole MSO series.

I also thank Sh Manmohan Chawla, Managing Trustee, Ms Madhupreet Chawla, Chairperson, Sh Ram Bahadur Rai, Chancellor, Prof Shyam Lal Singla, Pro-Chancellor, Dr Gurpreet Singh Tuteja, Pro Vice-Chancellor, Prof Sansar Sharma, Dean, FHMS, and Mr. Khanna, HR Manager, SGT University, for providing an atmosphere conducive to such activities.

The affection and moral support received from my daughter Dr Arushi and son-in-law Dr Gurukripa, Fellows at Mayo Clinic, Rochester, MN, USA, and my wife Prof Indu Khurana, Academic Dean, World College of Medical Sciences and Research, Gurawar, Jhajjar, made my task untiring.

The enthusiastic co-operation received from Mr SK Jain CMD, Mr YN Arjuna Senior Vice President—Publishing, Editorial and Publicity, and Mrs Ritu Chawla GM, Production; CBS Publishers & Distributors, New Delhi, needs special acknowledgement. Mr Sanju and Mr Neeraj, graphic artists, Mr Ananda Mohanty, Proof Reader and Mr Dharmvir, DTP Operator and Proof Reader need special mention because of their efforts to provide considerable beauty to this volume. In spite of the best efforts, a venture like this is unlikely to be error-free. Constructive criticism and suggestions from the readers are invited for further improvement in this volume.

AK Khurana
Editor-in-Chief

Contents

Section IV: DISEASES OF CONJUNCTIVA AND OCULAR SURFACE

Section V: INFLAMMATORY DISEASES OF CORNEA

Section VI: NON-INFLAMMATORY DISEASES OF CORNEA

Section VII: SURGICAL PROCEDURES FOR OCULAR SURFACE AND CORNEA

Section VIII: CORNEAL BLINDNESS AND EYE BANKING

Section
I

Anatomy and Physiology of Cornea and Ocular Surface

Anatomy and Physiology of Conjunctiva and Ocular Surface

Chapter Outline

OCULAR SURFACE
- Components of ocular surface

CONJUNCTIVA
- Gross anatomy

- Microscopic structure of conjunctiva
- Conjunctival glands
- Accessory conjunctival structures
- Vessels and nerves of conjunctiva

OCULAR SURFACE

COMPONENTS OF OCULAR SURFACE

Ocular surface, the term introduced by Thoft in 1978, refers to an integrated functional unit consisting of following structures (Fig. 1.1):
- *Epithelial lining* of the lid margins, conjunctiva, and cornea;
- *Eyelid glands* such as meibomian glands, glands of Moll and Zeis;
- *Ocular mucosal adnexa* (i.e. lacrimal gland, and the lacrimal drainage system); and
- *The tear film*.

These structures are not only interconnected through a continuous epithelium but share the same vascular, nervous, immune and hormonal control systems for their proper functioning. If one of these structures is not functioning properly, the functioning of other components is also affected and gradually the whole ocular surface is compromised.

Anatomy and physiology of ocular surface thus can be described under following heads:
- *Anatomy and physiology of conjunctiva*, described in the following text in this chapter.
- *Anatomy and physiology of corneal epithelium*, which is described in Chapter 2.

- *Anatomy and physiology of tear film*, which is described in Chapter 14: Tear Film and Dry Eye Disease.
- *Anatomy and physiology of meibomian glands*, which is described in Chapter 18: Blepharitis and Meibomian Gland Dysfunction.

CONJUNCTIVA

GROSS ANATOMY

The conjunctiva is a translucent mucous membrane which lines the posterior surface of the *eyelids* and *anterior aspect* of the eyeball. The name conjunctiva (conjoin: to join) has been given to this mucous membrane owing to the fact that it joins the eyeball to the lids. It stretches from the lid margin to the limbus and encloses a complex space called conjunctival sac which is open in front at the palpebral fissure.

Parts of conjunctiva

Conjunctiva can be divided into following parts (Fig. 1.1):
- *Palpebral conjunctiva:* Marginal, tarsal and orbital
- *Bulbar conjunctiva:* Scleral and limbal
- *Conjunctival fornix:* Superior, inferior, lateral and medial.

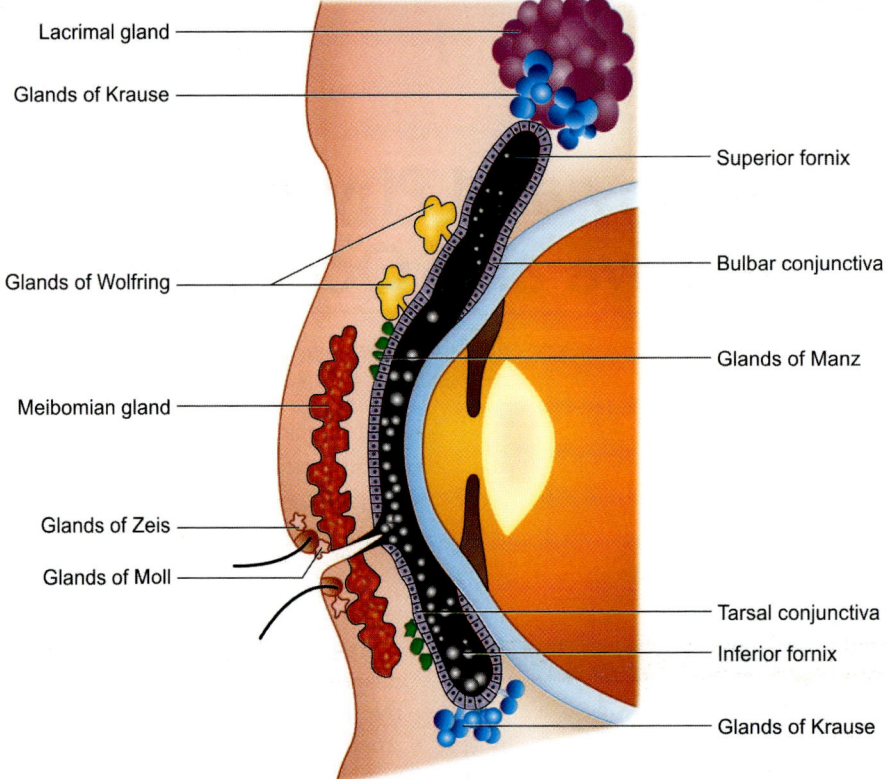

Fig. 1.1: *Ocular surface, parts of conjunctiva and conjunctival glands*

1. Palpebral conjunctiva

Palpebral conjunctiva is stratified squamous epithelium. It lines the lids and can be sub-divided into marginal, tarsal and orbital conjunctivae.

i. *Marginal conjunctiva* extends from the lid margin to about 2 mm on the back of the lid up to a shallow groove—the *sulcus subtarsalis*. It is actually a transitional zone between skin and the conjunctiva proper. At the sulcus subtarsalis, the perforating vessels pass through the tarsus to supply the conjunctiva. This sulcus is a common site for lodgement of a conjunctival foreign body.

ii. *Tarsal conjunctiva* is thin, transparent and highly vascular. It is firmly adherent to the whole tarsal plate in the upper lid. In the lower lid, it is adherent only to half width of the tarsus. The tarsal glands are seen through it as yellow streaks. Tarsal conjunctiva is a common site for the follicular and papillary reactions.

iii. *Orbital part* of palpebral conjunctiva lies loose between the tarsal plate and fornix. Orbital conjunctiva of the upper lid is loose and lies over the Müller's muscle.

2. Bulbar conjunctiva

Bulbar conjunctiva is stratified columnar epithelium. It is thin, transparent and lies loose over the underlying structures and thus can be moved easily. It attaches firmly 1 mm posterior to sclerocorneal limbus. It is separated from the anterior sclera by episcleral tissue and Tenon's capsule. Subconjunctival vessels and the anterior ciliary arteries forming the pericorneal plexus can be seen in the loose tissue under the bulbar conjunctiva. A 3 mm ridge of bulbar conjunctiva around the cornea is called *limbal conjunctiva*. In the area of limbus, the conjunctiva, Tenon's capsule and the episcleral tissue are fused into a dense tissue which is strongly adherent to the underlying corneoscleral junction. It is the perferred site for obtaining a firm hold (fixation) of the eyeball with the forceps during ocular surgery.

3. Conjunctival fornix

Conjunctival fornix is a continuous circular cul-de-sac, which is broken only on the medial side by caruncle and the plica semilunaris (Fig. 1.2). Conjunctival fornix joins the bulbar conjunctiva with the palpebral conjunctiva. It can be subdivided into superior, inferior, medial and lateral fornices.

i. *Superior fornix.* It extends from slightly above the upper border of the tarsal plate to a distance about 10 mm from the upper limbus and is thus located at the level of superior orbital margin. The extension of the fascial sheath of the levator and superior rectus muscles is attached to the conjunctiva in the upper part of the superior fornix. It helps in maintaining the recess of the superior fornix in the movements of the upper lid. In the subconjunctival tissue of the superior fornix are present glands of Krause and Müller's muscle. A knife passed through the superior fornix, enters the fibrous tissue between the levator and superior rectus muscles. A foreign body lodged in the superior fornix can be seen after double eversion of the upper lid.

ii. *Inferior fornix.* It extends from slightly below the lower border of the lower tarsal plate to a distance about 8 mm from the lower limbus and is located near the inferior orbital margin. The extension of the fascial sheath of the inferior rectus and inferior oblique muscles is attached to the conjunctival fold in the lower fornix. It helps in maintaining the recess of the inferior fornix during movements of the lower lid. Glands of Krause are lodged in the sub-conjunctival tissue of the lower fornix. A knife passed through the lower fornix will enter the fibrous tissue between the inferior rectus and inferior palpebral muscle and on further push it hits the aponeurotic expansion from the inferior rectus and inferior oblique muscles.

iii. *Lateral fornix.* It is a small cul-de-sac which extends to just behind the equator of the eyeball and is about 14 mm from the lateral limbus and about 5 mm from the lateral canthus.

iv. *Medial fornix.* It is a shallow cul-de-sac in which lie the caruncle and plica semilunaris dipped in the pool of tears called the 'lacus lacrimalis' or 'tear-lake'.

MICROSCOPIC STRUCTURE OF CONJUNCTIVA

Histologically, conjunctiva consists of three layers, namely (1) epithelium, (2) adenoid layer, and (3) fibrous layer (Fig. 1.3).

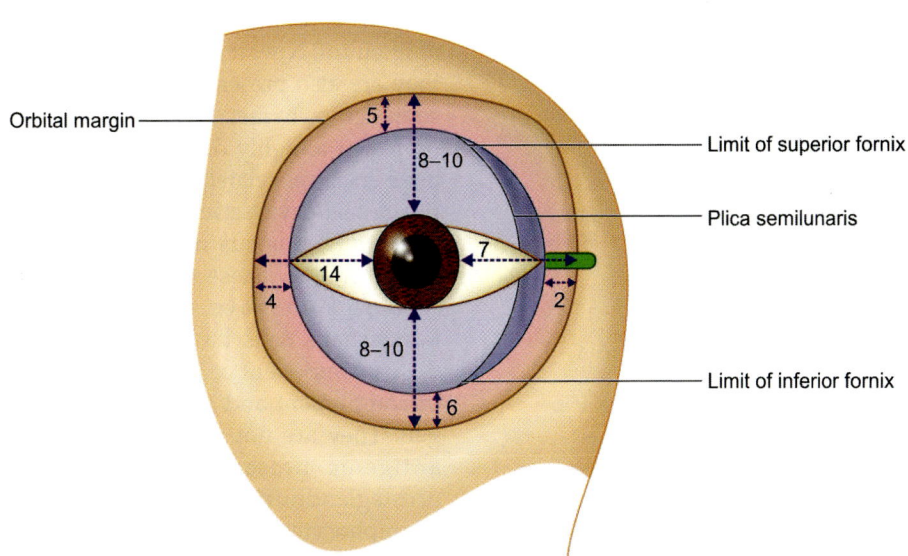

Fig. 1.2: *Conjunctival fornices*

1. Epithelium

■ *Layers of epithelial cells* in conjunctiva vary from region-to-region and its different parts are as follows (Fig. 1.3B):

• *Marginal conjunctiva is* 5-layered non-keratinised stratified squamous type of epithelium. The most superficial layer is of squamous cells, intermediate 3 layers of polyhedral cells and deepest layer of cylindrical cells. Goblet cells, absent at mucocutaneous junction, begin to appear in this part of conjunctival epithelium.

• *Tarsal conjunctiva* has two-layered epithelium, superficial layer of cylindrical cells and a deep layer of cubical cells in the upper lid. While the lower tarsal conjunctiva is composed of 3–4 layers of cells which from deep to superficial are layers of cubical cells, polygonal cells, elongated wedge-shaped cells and the cone-shaped cells.

• *Fornix and bulbar conjunctiva* has three-layered epithelium, a superficial layer of cylindrical cells, middle layer of polyhedral cells and a deep layer of cuboidal cells.

• *Limbal conjunctiva* is again many-layered (8 to 10) stratified squamous epithelium. Most superficial layers are one to two layers of squamous cells. Intermediate several layers are of polygonal cells and basal layer is of small cylindrical or cubical cells. The limbal epithelium forms the papillae of the limbal palisades of Vogt. The epithelium of pallisade zone provides the germinative zone for the corneal epithelium.

■ *Goblet cells* are present in between the epithelial cells in all the regions of conjunctiva, particularly aggregated in the tarsal conjunctival crypts (Henle's crypts) and on the bulbar conjunctiva nasal to the limbus (Maaz's glands).

■ *Melanocytes* are found in the conjunctiva at limbus, fornix, caruncle and at the site of entry of anterior ciliary vessels.

■ *Langerhans cells* were originally described in humans as dendritic cells in the basal corneal epithelium. Now it has been demonstrated that they are also present in almost all parts of the conjunctiva. In fact, Langerhans cells appear to represent a highly differentiated cell line from bone marrow related to the monocyte-macrophage-histiocyte series, which are present in the epidermis, mucous membranes, thymus and lymph nodes. These cells stain positively for ATPase and have no desmosomes. The Langerhans cells have surface receptors for the Fc component of IgG, the third component of compliment and surface HLA-DR (Ia) antigen. They are not phagocytic but function in antigenic presentation, lymphokine and prostaglandin production, and stimulation of T lymphocytes. They are reported to be involved in allograft rejection of the cornea, and in contact hypersensitivity of the skin.

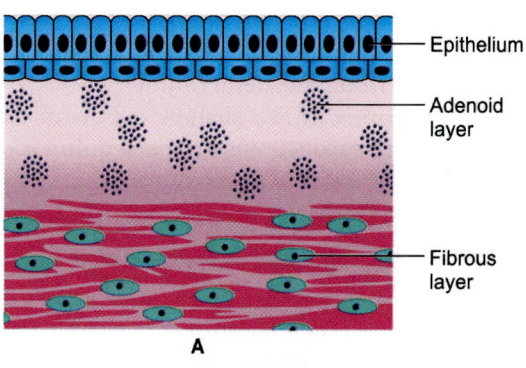

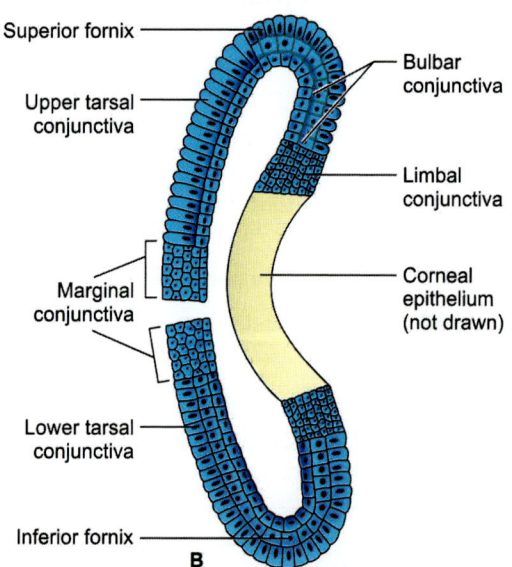

Fig. 1.3: *Microscopic structure of conjunctiva showing three layers (A); and arrangement of epithelial cells in different regions of conjunctiva (B)*

Conjunctival stem cells

Conjunctival stem cells, thought to be present predominantly in forniceal conjunctiva, account for the self-renewing property of conjunctiva. These cells are intrinsically distinct from the limbal stem cells and have distinctly separate lineage than the limbal stem cell. Unlike limbal stem cells, the conjunctival stem cells are bipotent and produce both goblet and non-goblet epithelial cells.

Conjunctiva-associated lymphoid tissue

Conjunctiva-associated lymphoid tissue (CALT) is similar to mucosa-associated lymphoid tissue (MALT) present in the gut and bronchi, and plays a significant role in antigen uptake and processing. The specialized epithelial cells of MALT, called M-cells, engulf and deliver antigens to neighbouring antigen-processing cells (APCs). Thus, the CALT plays a key role in local active immunity and in developing immune tolerance. In addition to conjunctiva, MALT-like tissue is also present in lacrimal gland, tear film and cornea.

2. Adenoid layer

It is also called lymphoid layer and consists of fine connective tissue reticulum in the meshes of which lie lymphocytes. This layer is most developed in the fornices and ends at the subtarsal fold. It is not present since birth but develops after 2–3 months of life. For this reason, conjunctival inflammation in an infant does not produce follicular reaction.

3. Fibrous layer

It consists of a meshwork of collagenous and elastic fibres. It is thicker than the adenoid layer, except in the region of tarsal conjunctiva, where it is very thin. This layer contains vessels and nerves of conjunctiva. It blends with the underlying Tenon's capsule in the region of bulbar conjunctiva. The adenoid layer and the fibrous layer are collectively known as the *substantia propria* of the conjunctiva.

CONJUNCTIVAL GLANDS

The conjunctiva contains two types of glands: The mucin secretory glands (goblet cells, crypts of Henle, glands of Manz), and the accessory lacrimal glands (glands of Krause and glands of Wolfring) (Fig. 1.1).

The mucin glands

1. *Goblet cells.* These are unicellular mucous glands located abundantly within the epithelium of all the regions of the conjunctiva except the marginal mucocutaneous junction and limbal conjunctiva. The goblet cells are round or oval in shape with an eccentric flattened nucleus near the base of the cell. It contains a prominent Golgi apparatus with numerous mucus pockets in the cytoplasm. The goblet cells are formed from the deepest cells (basal layer) of the conjunctiva and migrate towards the surface. These cells are destroyed after discharging their content, the mucin. The density of goblet cells is high in children and young adults. They are more numerous on the nasal side, particularly in the bulbar conjunctiva and inferior fornix (Fig. 1.4).

The mucin secreted by goblet cells lubricates and protects the epithelial cells of the conjunctiva and the cornea and ensures the tear film stability by lowering the surface tension.

The absence of tear fluid has no effect on the desiccation, but destruction of the goblet cells as in epithelial xerosis (hypovitaminosis A) and parenchymatous xerosis, leads to desiccation of

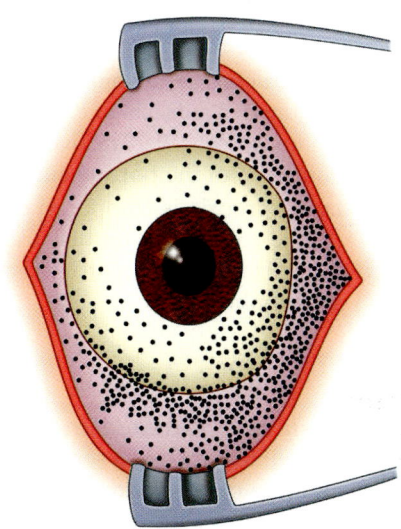

Fig. 1.4: *Goblet cell density (black dots) in different parts of conjunctiva*

the conjunctiva. The number of goblet cells is greatly increased in the inflammatory conditions.

2. *Henle's glands*. Crypts of Henle are not true glands but folds of the mucous membrane present in the palpebral conjunctiva between the tarsal plates and the fornices. These are tubular structures with lumina of 15–30 μm which contains a few goblet cells. These resemble Lieberkühn's crypts in the large intestine.

3. *Glands of Manz*. These are found in the limbal conjunctiva in animals like pig, calf or ox. Their existence in human beings is controversial.

Accessory lacrimal glands

These include:

1. Glands of Krause
2. Glands of Wolfring
3. Intraorbital glands
4. Glands in the caruncle and plica semilunaris

ACCESSORY CONJUNCTIVAL STRUCTURES

Plica semilunaris

It is a pinkish crescentric fold of the conjunctiva, present in the medial canthus. Its lateral free border is concave which becomes less prominent on abduction but forms a cul-de-sac about 2 mm in depth when the eyeball is adducted. It is a vestigial structure in human beings and represents the nictitating membrane (the third eyelid) of the lower animals.

■ ***Microscopic structure.*** The epithelium of this part of the conjunctiva consists of 8 to 10 layers of cells with many goblet cells. The deepest layer is cylindrical instead of the normal cubical.

The substantia propria is composed of loose connective tissue containing numerous blood vessels, a lobule of fat, a few non-striated muscle fibres and melanophores.

Caruncle

The caruncle is a small (5 mm × 3 mm), soft, ovoid, pinkish mass situated in the inner canthus, just medial to the plica semilunaris. In reality, it is a piece of modified skin (a part of the margin of the lower lid which gets cut off due to development of the inferior canaliculi) and so is covered with stratified squamous epithelium and contains sweat glands, sebaceous glands and hair follicles. It differs from the skin by the presence of accessory lacrimal glands of Krause, presence of plenty of goblet cells and absence of keratinisation in the epithelium. The connective tissue underlying the caruncle is in contact with the septum orbitale and the medial check ligament.

- *Blood supply* is through the superior medial palpebral artery.
- *Lymphatics* drain into submandibular lymph glands.
- *Nerve supply* is from the inferior trochlear nerve.

VESSELS AND NERVES OF CONJUNCTIVA

Arterial supply of conjunctiva

Arteries supplying the conjunctiva (Fig. 1.5) are derived from three sources:

1. Marginal arterial arcade
2. Peripheral arterial arcade, and
3. Anterior ciliary arteries.

1. Marginal arterial arcade

It is formed by anastomosis of medial and lateral palpebral arteries and lies in the submuscular plane in front of the tarsal plate, 2 mm away from the lid margin, in each lid. The perforating branches from the marginal arterial arcade pierce the tarsus at the sulcus subtarsalis to reach the conjunctiva, where they divide into marginal and tarsal branches. The tarsal branches anastomose with the branches from the peripheral arcade.

2. Peripheral arterial arcade

It is situated at the upper border of the tarsus in the upper lid. Its perforating branches pierce the palpebral muscle to reach the conjunctiva and sends off descending and ascending branches.

The descending branches supply the tarsal conjunctiva and anastomose with the branches of the marginal arterial arcade at the level of sulcus subtarsalis.

The ascending branches pass upwards and then bend round the superior fornix to descend under the bulbar conjunctiva as *posterior conjunctival arteries*. At about 4 mm from the limbus, the posterior conjunctival arteries anastomose with the anterior conjunctival arteries (branches of

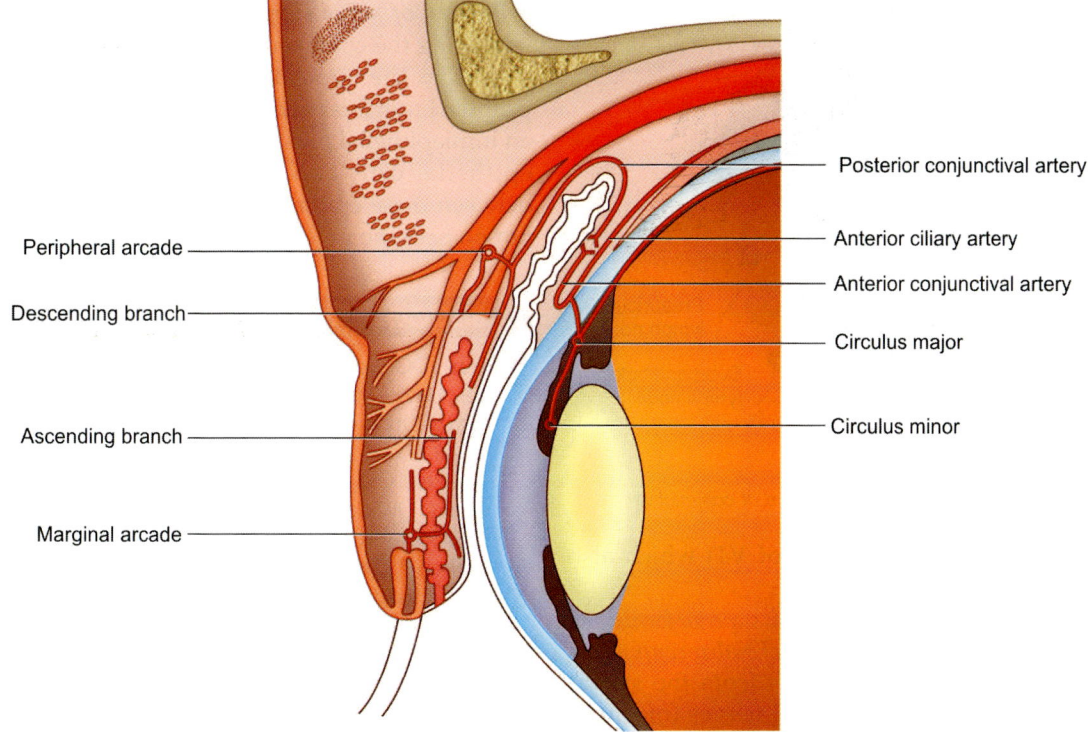

Fig. 1.5: *Blood supply of conjunctiva*

anterior ciliary arteries) forming the pericorneal plexus. The posterior conjunctival vessels move with the movement of the bulbar conjunctiva. In conjunctivitis, there is hyperaemia of the superficial conjunctival vessels derived from the posterior conjunctival vessels.

3. Anterior ciliary arteries

These are branches of muscular arteries (total 7—2 from each rectus muscle except 1 from the lateral rectus). These arteries give off *anterior conjunctival arteries* just before piercing the sclera at about 4 mm from the limbus.

The anterior conjunctival arteries move forward towards the limbus at a plane deeper than the posterior conjunctival arteries. These anastomose with each other forming a series of arcades parallel to the corneal margin and also form the pericorneal plexus.

To summarize

- *The palpebral conjunctiva and fornices are* supplied by branches from the marginal and peripheral arcades of the eyelids.

- *Bulbar conjunctiva* is supplied by posterior and anterior conjunctival arteries.

Venous drainage of conjunctiva

The veins from the conjunctiva drain into the venous plexus of eyelids which in turn drain into the superior or inferior ophthalmic veins.

A circumcorneal zone of veins about 5–6 mm from the limbus drain into the anterior ciliary veins.

Lymphatics of the conjunctiva

Conjunctival lymphatics are arranged in two layers: A superficial and a deep. Lymphatics from the lateral side drain into *preauricular lymph nodes* and those from the medial side into the *submandibular lymph nodes* (Fig. 1.6).

Nerve supply of conjunctiva

- *Distribution of nerve supply of conjunctiva* is as below:

- *Bulbar conjunctiva, in its anterior two-thirds circumcorneal zone*, is supplied by the branches

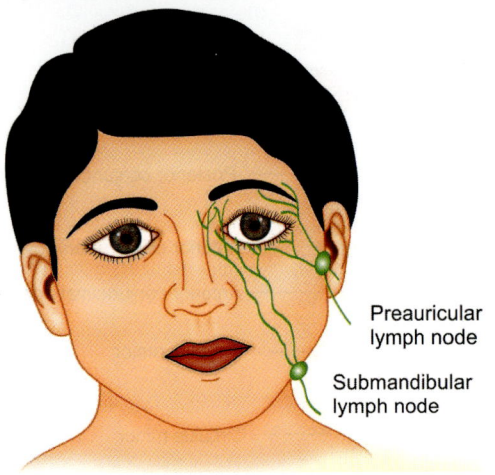

Preauricular lymph node

Submandibular lymph node

Fig. 1.6: *Lymphatic drainage of conjunctiva*

■ *Pattern of nerve supply.* The nerve branches supplying the conjunctiva form a subepithelial plexus in the superficial part of substantia propria. From this plexus, the fibres pass to form an intraepithelial plexus around the base of the epithelial cells and send free nerve fibrils between these epithelial cells. These nerves do not possess the myelin sheath.

from *long ciliary nerves* (of V1) which also supply the cornea.

- *Superior plapebral conjunctiva, superior fornix and superior peripheral one-third of bulbar conjunctiva* are supplied by branches from the supra-trochlear and supraorbital nerves (of infra-trochlear nerve (branch of nasociliary nerve), frontal nerve and lacrimal nerves (of V1).
- *Lateral inferior palpebral conjunctiva, lateral fornix and lateral part of inferior peripheral one-third of bulbar conjunctiva* are supplied by branches from the lacrimal nerve (of V1).
- *Nasal inferior palpebral conjunctiva, nasal fornix and nasal half of peripheral one-third of bulbar conjunctiva* are supplied by branches of infraorbital nerve (of V2).

BIBLIOGRAPHY

1. Puro DG. Role of ion channels in the functional response of conjunctival goblet cells to dry eye. Am J Physiol, Cell Physiol 2018; 315(2): C236–C246.
2. Ruskell GL. Innervation of the conjunctiva. Trans Ophthalmol Soc UK. 1985; 104 (Pt 4): 390–95.
3. Steven P, Gebert A. Conjunctiva-associated lymphoid tissue–current knowledge, animal models and experimental prospects. Ophthalmic Res 2009; 42(1): 2–8.
4. Takahashi Y, Watanabe A, Matsuda H, Nakamura Y, Nakano T, Asamoto K, Ikeda H, Kakizaki H. Anatomy of secretory glands in the eyelid and conjunctiva: a photographic review. Ophthalmic Plast Reconstr Surg 2013; 29(3): 215–19.
5. Wolosin JM, Budak MT, Akinci MA. Ocular surface epithelial and stem cell development. Int J Dev Biol 2004; 48(8–9): 981–91.
6. Wotherspoon AC, Hardman-Lea S, Isaacson PG. Mucosa-associated lymphoid tissue (MALT) in the human conjunctiva. J Pathol 1994; 174(1): 33–37.

Chapter

2

Anatomy and Physiology of Cornea

ANATOMY OF CORNEA

The cornea is a transparent, avascular, watch-glass-like structure. It forms anterior one-sixth of the outer fibrous coat of the eyeball.

DIMENSIONS

- *Anterior surface* of cornea is elliptical with an average horizontal diameter of 11.75 mm and vertical diameter of 11 mm.
- *Posterior surface* of cornea is circular with an average diameter of 11.5 mm.
- *Thickness* of cornea in the centre is about 0.52 mm; while at the periphery, it is 0.67 mm.
- *Radius of curvature:* The central 5 mm area of the cornea forms the powerful refracting surface of the eye. The anterior and posterior radii of curvature of the central part of cornea are 7.8 mm and 6.5 mm, respectively.
- *Refractive power* of the anterior surface of cornea is about +48 D and that of its posterior surface is about –5 D. Thus, the net refractive power of cornea is about +43 D which is three-fourths of the total refractive power of the eye (60 dioptres).
- *Refractive index* of the cornea is 1.37.

HISTOLOGY

Histologically, originally the cornea was considered to consist of five distinct layers, from anterior to posterior, these are: Epithelium, Bowman's membrane, substantia propria (corneal stroma), Descemet's membrane and endothelium. However, recently a new layer between the corneal stroma and Descemet's membrane named Dua's layer (pre-Descemet's membrane) has been discovered, and thus now, the cornea is considered to consist of six layers (Fig. 2.1).

1. Epithelium

Corneal epithelium is of stratified squamous non-keratinized type and becomes continuous with epithelium of the bulbar conjunctiva at the limbus. It is about 50–90 μm thick, represents 10% of corneal thickness and consists of

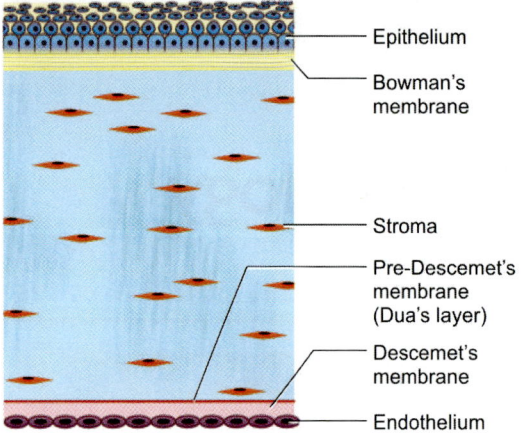

Fig. 2.1: *Microscopic structure of cornea*

Epithelium

Bowman's membrane

Stroma

Pre-Descemet's membrane (Dua's layer)

Descemet's membrane

Endothelium

5–7 layers of cells. The deepest (basal) layer is made up of columnar cells, next mid-epithelial 2–3 layers of wing or umbrella cells and the most superficial two layers are of flattened cells. The corneal epithelium sheds at a regular interval and is replaced by growth from its basal cells. It is estimated that the entire epithelium is replaced in a period of 6–8 days via mitotic activity of basal cells. Some important features of various layers of epithelium are described below.

Basal layer

Basal layer (Fig. 2.2) comprises tall columnar polygonal-shaped cells arranged in a palisade-like manner on a basement membrane. Basal cells have a width of 12 μm and density of approximately 6000 cells/mm². It forms the germinal layer of the epithelium and undergoes mitosis to produce daughter cells which continuously migrate anteriorly into the wing cell layer. The basal cell has an oval nucleus and its cytoplasm contains a few organelles. Some intermediate filaments, microtubules, free ribosomes, rough-surfaced endoplasmic reticulum and occasional Golgi apparatus are seen. The mitochondria are small and a few, suggesting low aerobic oxidation and more dependence on the pentose shunt for metabolism.

The basal cells are firmly joined laterally to the other basal cells and anteriorly to the wing

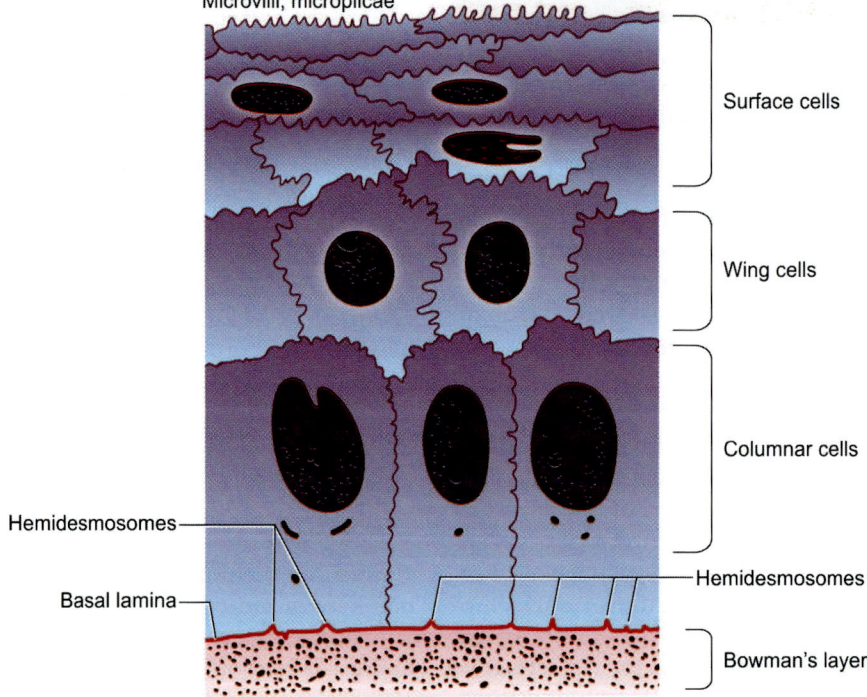

Microvilli, microplicae

Surface cells

Wing cells

Columnar cells

Hemidesmosomes

Basal lamina

Hemidesmosomes

Bowman's layer

Fig. 2.2: *Microscopic structure of corneal epithelium*

cells by desmosomes and *zonula occludens*. These tight intercellular junctions account for the epithelium's transparency as well as its resistance to the flow of water, electrolytes and glucose, along with inhibiting pathological entrance, i.e. its barrier function.

■ *Limbal stem cells.* The basal cells of the limbal area constitute the so-called limbal stem cells. Epithelial stem cells are the undifferentiated pluripotent stem cells found in the limbal basal epithelium of palisades of Vogt. They are the source of new corneal epithelium. These slow-cycling stem cells divide and give rise to a progeny of daughter cells (*transient amplifying cells*) which amplify, proliferate continuously, migrate centripetally and serve to maintain the corneal epithelium.

Diffuse damage to the limbal stem cells (e.g. in chemical burns, Stevens-Johnson syndrome, pemphigoid, trachoma) leads to chronic epithelial surface defects and invasion of conjunctival epithelium onto the cornea.

■ *Non-epithelial cells* also appear within the corneal epithelial layer especially in the peripheral cornea. These cells include wandering histiocytes, macrophages, lymphocyte, and pigmented melanocyte. Antigen presenting Langerhans cells are formed peripherally and move centrally with age or in response to keratitis.

■ *Basal lamina.* The basement membrane of the basal cells is PAS positive structure. It is extracellular secretory product of basal epithelial cells. Posteriorly, it blends indistinctly into Bowman's membrane. Anteriorly, firm adhesions are formed between it and the basal cells by the filaments extending from the latter called *adhesion complex*, made up of hemidesmosomes and type VII collagen fibrils. In fact, the basement membrane is of utmost importance in epithelial cell adhesions. When abnormal, it is associated with recurrent erosions and epithelial defects.

Applied aspects of anchoring/adhesion complex
• Holds epithelium to basement membrane and its stroma, so its defect as seen in epider-molysis bullosa, can lead to bullae formation.

• Reduplication of basement membrane as seen with ageing or in diabetes mellitus leads to abnormal epithelial adhesions and increased predisposition to epithelial erosions.

Wing cells

Wing cells form 2–3 layers of the polyhedral-shaped cells. Their nuclei are flattened parallel to the surface and cytoplasmic organelles decrease as compared to the basal cells. They are attached with the basal cells posteriorly and other wing cells laterally and anteriorly, via tight junctions.

Flattened cells

Flattened cells constitute two most superficial cell layers. Superficial cells represent the highest level of differentiation and are chronologically the oldest epithelial cells. These cells are long (45 mm) and thin (4 mm) with flattened nuclei. The desmosomal attachment and maculae occludentes are more numerous in these cells. Further, zonulae occludentes seen in the lateral cell walls are also found in this layer. The anterior cell wall of the most superficial cells has many microvilli (each 0.5 mm in height) which play an important role in the tear film stability. The microvilli contain glycocalyx which is associated with tear film. An important feature of the superficial cell layer is the presence of junctional complexes formed with laterally adjacent cells which maintain the barrier function of the epithelium. A clinical test to determine whether the barrier is intact uses dyes such as fluorescein.

Functions of epithelium

• It is extraordinary regular in thickness with smooth wet apical surface for serving as major refractive surface of the eye.
• It serves as a major surface to respond to wound healing.
• It helps in providing barrier to fluid loss and pathological entrance to the organisms.

2. Bowman's membrane (layer)

This layer consists of acellular mass of condensed collagen fibrils. It is about 8–14 μm in thickness and binds the corneal stroma anteriorly with basement membrane of the epithelium. It is not a true elastic membrane but simply a condensed superficial part of the stroma.

Bowman's layer is secreted during embryogenesis by the anterior stromal keratocytes and epithelium. It is composed of randomly packed type I and type V collagen fibres that are enmeshed in a matrix consisting of proteoglycans and glycoproteins.

It shows considerable resistance to infection and injury. Unlike Descemet's membrane once destroyed, it does not regenerate.

■ *Function of Bowman's membrane.* It acts as a smooth base for epithelium uniformity thus helps in refraction.

3. Stroma (substantia propria)

This layer is about 0.5 mm in thickness and constitutes most of the cornea (90% of total thickness). It consists of collagen fibrils (lamellae) and cells embedded in hydrated matrix of proteoglycans (ground substance).

Corneal lamellae

The lamellae consist of fibrils with a macroperiodicity (640Å) typical of collagen. The stroma's collagen types are I, III, V and VI. Among the various subtypes, type I predominates. Type VII forms the anchoring fibril of the epithelium. The corneal lamellae are arranged in many layers (200–250). In each layer, they are not only parallel to each other but also to the corneal plane and become continuous with the scleral lamellae at the limbus. They vary in disposition according to the area of the cornea. They have oblique orientation in the anterior one-third of the stroma. In the posterior two-thirds of the stroma, the alternating layers of lamellae are at right angles to each other.

Studies, using X-ray diffraction techniques, have shown that the parallel arrangement of the central corneal fibrils extends to the periphery where the fibrils adopt a concentric configuration to form a 'weave' at the limbus. This imparts considerable strength to the peripheral cornea and permits it to maintain its curvature and thus its optical properties. Previous studies have shown that the corneal fibrils, running in two preferred orientations in the central cornea, bend as they approach the peripheral cornea to run circumferentially and form the peripheral collagen ring.

The parallel arrangement of lamellae in the cornea allows an easy intralamellar dissection during superficial keratectomy and lamellar keratoplasty. The peculiar arrangement of lamellae has also been implicated in the corneal transparency.

Stromal cells

The cells present among the lamellae are keratocytes, wandering macrophages, histiocytes and a few lymphocytes.

■ *Corneal keratocytes* about 2.4 million in number constitute 2–4% of the volume of the stroma in humans. The keratocytes are fibroblasts which are found throughout the stroma, between, and occasionally extending into the lamellae. The keratocytes have a flattened cell body, a large eccentric nucleus and long branching processes which form contact with other cells in the same layer, but do not form a syncytium. It is believed that these cells produce ground substance and collagen fibrils during embryogenesis and after injury.

■ *Wandering cells* of the stroma migrate from the marginal loops of the corneal blood vessels to the site of injury.

Ground substance of stroma

Ground substance of cornea consists of hydrated matrix of proteoglycans that run along and between the collagen fibrils. The primary glycosaminoglycans of stroma are keratin sulphate and chondroitin sulphate in the ratio of 3:1. Maximum concentration of keratin sulphate occurs in the centre and that of chondroitin sulphate in the periphery. The glycosaminoglycan components (e.g. keratin sulphate) of the ground substance are highly charged and account for the swelling property of the stroma. The keratocytes which lie between the corneal lamellae synthesize both the collagen and proteoglycans.

Functions of stroma

It acts as a window to the right passage and meshes with surrounding scleral connective tissue to form a rigid frame for maintaing IOP.

4. Pre-Descemet's membrane

Pre-Descemet's membrane, also known as *Dua's layer,* has been discovered in 2013 by Dr. Harminder Dua, an ophthalmologist of Indian origin working in Great Britain. Located anterior to Descemet membrane, it is about 15 mm thick acellular structure which is very strong and impervious to air. Dua's layer (DL) primarily composed of collagen type 1. Collagens 4 and 6 are also present (more in DL compared to corneal stroma). Collagen 5 is also present (weakly positive in both DL and stroma). Proteoglycans present are lumican, mimecan and decorin (intensity equal in DL and stroma). CD34 negative, which proves lack of keratocytes in DL. Unlike DM, DL does not extend to the periphery.

5. Descemet's membrane (posterior elastic lamina)

It is a strong homogenous layer which is separated from the stroma by pre-Descemet's membrane. It represents the basement membrane of the corneal endothelium from which it is produced. Though elasticity is one of its physical characteristics, it is made up of collagen and glycoprotein with no elastic fibres visible by electron microscopy. Its thickness varies with age, being 3 μm at birth and 10–12 μm in young adults. It is very resistant to chemical agents, trauma, infection and pathological processes. Even when whole of the stroma is sloughed off, the Descemet's membrane can maintain the integrity of the eyeball for long. Further, unlike Bowman's membrane, when destroyed it can regenerate. Normally, it remains in a state of tension and when torn it curls inwards on itself. In the periphery, it appears to end at the anterior limit of the trabecular meshwork as Schwalbe's line (ring).

On electron microscopy, Descemet's membrane can be divided into two distinct regions: An anterior one-third having a vertically banded pattern and the posterior two-thirds appearing amorphous and granular. The posterior surface of the Descemet's membrane, at the periphery, shows rounded wart-like excrescences called *Hassall-Henle bodies,* which increase with advancing age. Similar central excrescences, known as guttatae, are seen with advancing age in Fuchs' dystrophy.

6. Endothelium

- *Consists of a single layer of flat polygonal (mainly hexagonal) cells,* which on slit-lamp biomicroscopy appear as a mosaic on Descemet's membrane.
- *Cell density of endothelium* is around 6000 cells/mm² at birth. In the human adults, these cells have hardly any ability to divide. The cell count falls by about 26% in the first year and a further 26% is lost over the next 11 years. Therefore, with increasing age, the number of cells is reduced to about 2400–3000 cells/mm² in young adults. The defect left by the dying cells is filled by enlargement (polymegathism) of the remaining cells. Hence, these cells vary in diameter from 18 to 20 micron early in life to 40 micron or more in the aged.
- *There is a considerable functional reserve* for the endothelium. Therefore, corneal decompensation occurs only after more than 75% of the adult age cells are lost (i.e. when the endothelial cell count becomes less than 500 cells/mm²).
- *Endothelial cells are best evaluated* by specular microscopy.
- *Endothelial cells are attached to the Descemet's membrane* by hemidesmosomes and laterally to each other by tight interdigitating junctional complexes. The desmosomal linkages and zonulae occludentes are continuous around the entire cell, and thus close the intercellular space from the anterior chamber. This linkage is calcium-dependent and plays an important role in maintaining the barrier function of endothelium.
- *Endothelium also contains an active pump mechanism* and is involved in active secretion and protein synthesis.
- *High metabolic activity and energy production* for *the above process* by the endothelial cells is

evidenced by the presence of abundant mitochondria, free ribosomes, rough- and smooth-surfaced endoplasmic reticulum and Golgi complexes in the cytoplasm of the cells. In the eye, next to photoreceptors, the endothelial cells contain the highest number of mitochondria.

BLOOD SUPPLY AND NERVE SUPPLY

Blood supply of the cornea

The cornea is an avascular structure. Small loops derived from the anterior ciliary vessels invade its periphery for about 1 mm and provide nourishment. Actually, these loops are not in the cornea but in the subconjunctival tissue which overlaps the cornea.

Nerve supply of the cornea

The cornea has a rich supply of sensory nerve endings derived mainly from the long ciliary nerves which are branches of the nasociliary nerve (a branch of ophthalmic division of the trigeminal nerve). The long ciliary nerves after arising from the nasociliary nerve enter the eyeball around the optic nerve along with the short ciliary nerves and run forward in the suprachoroidal space. A short distance from the limbus, these nerves pierce the sclera to leave the eyeball, divide dichotomously and connect with each other and the conjunctival nerves to form *a pericorneal plexus of the nerves*. About 60–80 myelinated trunks from the pericorneal plexus enter the cornea at various levels, viz. sclera (the principal regions), episclera and conjunctiva. After having gone for 1–2 mm in the stroma, the corneal nerves lose their myelin sheath, branch dichotomously and form a *stromal plexus*. Although, some nerves end in mid-stroma, most pass anteriorly and form a *subepithelial plexus*. The fibres from here penetrate the pores in Bowman's membrane, lose their Schwann's sheath, divide into filaments under the basal layer of epithelium which extend between the cells of all the layers of epithelium, and form *intraepithelial plexus*. The nerves end in the epithelium as fine-beaded filaments (Box 2.1).

Thus, the cornea has an extensive innervational density which is highest near the centre

---

Box 2.1   *Pattern of corneal innervation*

Myelinated and non-myelinated axons distribute radially around periphery of cornea
↓
Enter substantia propria of stroma in radial manner and branch dichotomously (loose myelin sheath)
↓
Preterminal fibres form a plexus in mid-stroma
↓
Subepithelial plexus formed
↓
Intraepithelial plexus formed where the axons are devoid of Schwann cells

---

Box 2.2 *Physiological variations in corneal sensation*

- Most sensitive at apex, least at superior limbus.
- Sensitivity lowest in morning and highest in evening.
- Sensitivity decreases with age

---

and gradually decreases towards the periphery. However, there are no nerves in the central posterior part of the cornea, Descemet's membrane and endothelium (Box 2.2).

PHYSIOLOGY OF CORNEA

INTRODUCTION

Functions of cornea

The two primary physiologic functions of the cornea are:

1. *To act as a powerful refracting lens of fixed focus* that transmits light in an orderly fashion for proper image formation, and
2. *To protect the intraocular contents.*

In addition, the cornea also plays an important role in:

- Absorption of topically applied drugs, and
- Wound repair after anterior segment surgery or trauma.

Cornea performs these functions by maintaining its transparency and replacement of its tissues.

BIOCHEMICAL AND PHYSIOLOGICAL PROCESSES CONCERNED WITH THE FUNCTIONING OF THE CORNEA

- Biochemical composition of cornea
- Metabolism of cornea
- Corneal transparency
- Cell turnover and wound healing in the cornea

BIOCHEMICAL COMPOSITION OF CORNEA

Biochemical composition of cornea is heterogenous owing to differences in cellularity and morphology of its different layers, namely epithelium, Bowman's membrane, stroma, pre-Descemet's membrane, Descemet's membrane and endothelium.

Under normal conditions, biochemically cornea consists of approximately 80% water and 20% solids (19.8% organic matter and 0.2% inorganic salts). However, hydration of cornea is quite variable, since exposure of the cornea in the living animals allows sufficient evaporation to reduce corneal hydration.

EPITHELIUM

Corneal epithelium constitutes 10% of the total wet weight of the cornea. Its essential biochemical components are as follows:

- *Water* represents 70% of the wet weight.
- *Protein* synthesis in epithelium is five times higher than the stroma and about 2 times higher than the endothelium and Descemet's membrane.
- *Lipids* (phospholipids and cholesterol) are mainly present in the cell membranes and constitute about 5.4% of the dry weight of the epithelium. *Enzymes* necessary for glycolysis, Krebs cycle and Na^+, K^+ activated ATPase are present in high levels in the epithelium.
- The epithelium contains *ATP* (2000 mmol/kg wet weight), *glycogen* (10 mg/g), *glutathione* (75 to 180 mg/g) and *ascorbic acid* (47 to 94 mg/100 g).
- *Acetylcholine* (ACh) and cholinesterases are also present in high levels in epithelium. Perhaps these play a role in cation transport as well as in trophic nerve function.
- *Electrolytes.* Epithelium contains high concentration of K^+ (142 mEq/L H_2O) and low concentration of Na^+ (75 mEq/L H_2O) and Cl^- (30 mEq/L H_2O) as compared to the stroma (Table 2.1).

Table 2.1: *Electrolyte composition (in mEq/L H_2O) of rabbit cornea, plasma, aqueous humour and tears*

	Na^+	K^+	Cl^-
Cornea			
Whole cornea	156	28	97
Stroma	172	21	108
Epithelium	75	142	30
Aqueous humour	143.5	5.2	108
Plasma	151	5.2	109
Tears	149	12	131

STROMA

Stroma constitutes main bulk (90% of total thickness) of the cornea. It contains 75 to 80% water (wet weight). Remaining solids (20 to 25%) include mainly extracellular collagen, other soluble proteins, mucopolysaccharides (chondroitin, keratan, and *dermatan* sulphates) and salts (Table 2.2).

Differences in the biochemical composition of anterior and posterior stroma

- *Anterior stroma has less water* (3.04 gm H_2O dry weight) as compared to posterior stroma (3.85 gm H_2O dry weight). This is due to atmospheric drying and increased amount of dermatan sulphate which has less water sorptive capacity.
- *Less glucose*, 3.89 µm/gm H_2O in anterior stroma as compared to posterior stroma (4.93 µm/gm H_2O).
- *More dermatan sulphate and less keratan sulphate* in anterior stroma.

Table 2.2: *Biochemical composition of stroma*

Substance	%
Water	78
Collagen	15
Other proteins	5
Keratan sulphate	0.7
Chondroitin sulphate	0.3
Salts	1

Collagen

Collagen fibrils (lamellae), embedded in hydrated matrix of proteoglycans, essentially constitute the corneal stroma. These present the typical 64–66 nm periodicity of the collagen.

Collagen constitutes approximately 70% of dry weight of human cornea. Type I collagen is the predominant type, although collagen types III, V (10–20%), VI (15.1%), VII, XII and XIV have also been found in normal adult cornea. The diameter of corneal collagen fibrils (35 nm) and spacing between these fibrils (55 nm) is remarkably constant. There appears to be an inverse correlation between the number of carbohydrate units and the fibril diameter of collagen. The corneal collagen, like the collagen from other structures such as skin and tendons, has a high glycine, proline and hydroxyproline content. The mature collagen is a helix composed of two alpha chains (molecular weight 80,000) and one beta chain (molecular weight 160,000). The corneal collagen is dissolved by proteolytic enzymes such as collagenase, which has important implication in corneal ulceration.

In boiling water or acids, the corneal collagen is converted into gelatin, which accounts for the acid corneal burns being less serious than the alkali burns.

Soluble proteins

These constitute 5% of wet weight of stroma (and 25% of dry weight of the tissue) and include albumin, immunoglobulins, and glycoproteins. The high levels of antibody proteins (immunoglobulins G, A and M), present in the cornea have immunologic implications. The corneal immunoglobulins are probably derived from the serum and diffuse into the centre from the limbus.

Proteoglycans

Proteoglycans are a family of glycosylated proteins that contain at least one glycosaminoglycan chain covalently bonded to a protein core. Glycosaminoglycans (GAGs) or the so-called acid-mucopolysaccharides represent 4 to 4.5% of the dry weight of the cornea.

■ *Cornea contains three major GAG fractions,* namely:
• *Keratan sulphate* (50%),
• *Chondroitin sulphate* A (25%), and
• *Chondroitin* (25%), present exclusively in the cornea).

■ *GAGs are present in the interfibrillar space of the corneal stroma* and account for the *'stromal swelling pressure'* (normal—60 mm Hg), i.e. its tendency to imbibe water and thus plays an important role in the maintenance of the corneal hydration level and transparency as they have water sorptive capacity.

■ *An abnormal accumulation of GAG occurs in the corneal stroma* of the patients affected by the inborn errors of GAG metabolism known as *mucopolysaccharidosis.*

Enzymes

Glycolytic and Krebs cycle enzymes are present in the stromal keratocytes. However, the enzymatic activity of the corneal stroma is very low when compared with that of the epithelium, on weight basis. The adenosine triphosphate (ATP) content of the stroma is also low (10 to 15 mmol/kg wet tissue).

Matrix metalloproteinases

Matrix metalloproteinases (MMPs) are calcium-dependent zinc containing endoproteinase family of enzymes that breakdown components of extracellular matrix. In the cornea, they help maintain the normal framework and have a crucial role in remodelling after injury. MMPs are secreted as proenzymes by infiltrating inflammatory cells or by cells resident in the tissue. They are then activated by cleavage of a peptide from their N-terminal end. All MMPs require a metal cofactor. The MMPs of cornea have different substrates:
• MMP-1 (collagenase I) is active against collagen types I, II, and III.
• MMP-2 (gelatinase A) and MMP-9 (gelatinase B) are active against collagen types IV, V, and VII as well as gelatins and fibronectin.
• MMP-3 (stromelysin I) breaks down proteoglycans and fibronectin.
• MMPs 7, 8, 9, 11 are other substrates.

Note. Only MMP-2 has been detected in normal cornea, the other MMPs mentioned above are found in the cornea only after injury. MMPs 1, 2 and 3 are products of stromal cells, whereas MMP-9 is produced by the corneal epithelium which is most importantly involved in the corneal inflammation.

Proteinase inhibitor of cornea

Proteinase inhibitors of cornea are mainly synthesized by resident cells of cornea; and some are derived from tears, aqueous humour, and limbal blood vessels. These include:

- α_1 proteinase inhibitor,
- α_1 antichymotrypsin,
- α_2 macroglobulin,
- Plasminogen activator inhibitors 1 and 2, and
- Tissue inhibitor of metalloproteinases

■ *Functions* Proteinase inhibitors of the cornea play a key role in corneal protection by restricting damage during corneal inflammation, ulceration and wound healing.

Electrolytes

Concentration of Na^+ is high and that of K^+ is low in the stroma as compared to the epithelium. Concentration of electrolytes in the cornea and three fluids surrounding it (viz. plasma, aqueous and tear) is shown in Table 2.1. In the stroma, the sum of diffusible cations, sodium and potassium (172 + 21 = 193 mEq/L H_2O) is in excess of the diffusible anion chloride (108 mEq/L H_2O). Part of the anions may be provided by bicarbonate ions (25 to 35 mEq/L H_2O) and remaining by the acidic GAG (acting as anions) and the corneal collagen molecules.

PRE-DESCEMET'S MEMBRANE AND DESCEMET'S MEMBRANE

These layers are made up of collagen (73%) and glycoproteins. The collagen differs from typical connective tissue collagen in that it lacks typical 640-A banded collagen fibrils and have a high content of hydroxyproline, glycine and hydroxyglycine. Unlike stroma, the Descemet's membrane does not contain GAG. The collagen of Descemet's membrane is insoluble (except in strong alkali or acids), and extremely resistant to chemical and enzymatic (collagenase) action than the corneal stromal collagen. This accounts for the resistance offered by Descemet's membrane to trauma, chemical agents, infection and a barrier to perforation in deep corneal ulcers.

ENDOTHELIUM

Owing to delicate nature of this single cell-layered structure, it has not been possible to analyse its biochemical composition without inducing artifactual changes. However, the histochemical examination of the endothelium has shown the presence of enzymes needed for glycolysis and Krebs cycle.

■ METABOLISM OF CORNEA

The cornea, among other activities, requires energy for maintenance of its transparency and dehydration. Energy in the form of ATP is generated by the breakdown of glucose. The most actively metabolising layers of the cornea are epithelium and endothelium, the former being ten times thicker than the latter, requires a proportionately larger supply of metabolic substrates. The sources of nutrients required for the corneal metabolism and the metabolic pathway involved are described below briefly.

SOURCES OF NUTRIENTS

1. Oxygen

- *Epithelium* derives oxygen mainly from atmosphere through the tear film (an active process) as well as through the limbal capillaries. A tight-fitting contact lens made of non-oxygen-permeable material such as polymethyl methacrylate (PMMA) interferes with oxygen uptake of epithelium and causes intracellular oedema, a decrease in epithelial glycogen and an increase in lactic acid. This confirms the fact that atmosphere is the main source of oxygen for the epithelium. Epithelium consumes oxygen ten times greater than stroma. The oxygen required by the epithelium is about one-tenth of that available from the atmosphere when the eyes are open and about one-fourth of that available from the palpebral conjunctiva when the eyes are closed.
- *Endothelium* derives most of its required oxygen from the aqueous humour, which has an oxygen tension of about 40 mm Hg.

- *Mean total corneal oxygen consumption* (QO$_2$) of the human cornea is approximately 9.5 ml O$_2$ cm^{-2} hr^{-1}. Mean QO$_2$ for epithelium and endothelium is 5 to 6 and that of stroma alone is 0.44.
- *Minimum oxygen tension for normal corneal hydration* ranges between 11 and 19 mm Hg. Below this critical range, the cornea will hydrate and swell.

2. Glucose

The respiratory quotient (RQ) for the cornea is 1.0, indicating that glucose metabolism is the prime energy source. It is now confirmed that the aqueous humour is the main source of glucose supply not only for the endothelium but also for the corneal stroma as well as the epithelium. A negligible amount of glucose also enters the cornea from the tear film and by diffusion from the perilimbal capillaries. It has been estimated that the minimal requirements of epithelial glucose consumption are 50–60 mg/cm^2/hr. In the absence of an exogenous supply of glucose or when the tissue needs additional energy (especially after injury or surgical wounds), the glycogen stored in the corneal epithelium is broken down to glucose at a rate of 25 mg/hr/cornea. It has been assumed that perhaps fatty acids might also be used by the epithelium and stroma after prolonged periods of glucose deprivation.

3. Amino acids

A continuous supply of the amino acids is required to allow synthesis of proteins needed for the constant shedding and replacement (by mitosis) of the epithelial cells of the cornea. It appears that like glucose, amino acids are also supplied from the aqueous humour, principally by passive diffusion. Amino acids in quantities sufficient for the synthesis of about 10 mg/hour of proteins by the epithelial cells can enter by diffusion. An additional active transport of amino acids has not been totally ruled out.

METABOLIC PATHWAYS IN CORNEA

Following pathways of glucose metabolism are present in the cornea (Fig. 2.3).

1. Glycolysis

In normal conditions, all the glucose consumed by the cornea can be accounted for by either respiratory or glycolytic activity. Histochemical studies have shown that many enzymes of the Embden-Meyerhof pathway of glycolysis and the tricarboxylic acid (Krebs) cycle are present in all of the cells of cornea.

Rate of glucose consumption by the whole cornea is approximately 100 mg/hr/cm^2 with 90% being consumed by the epithelium. Through glycolysis, glucose is broken down to lactic acid

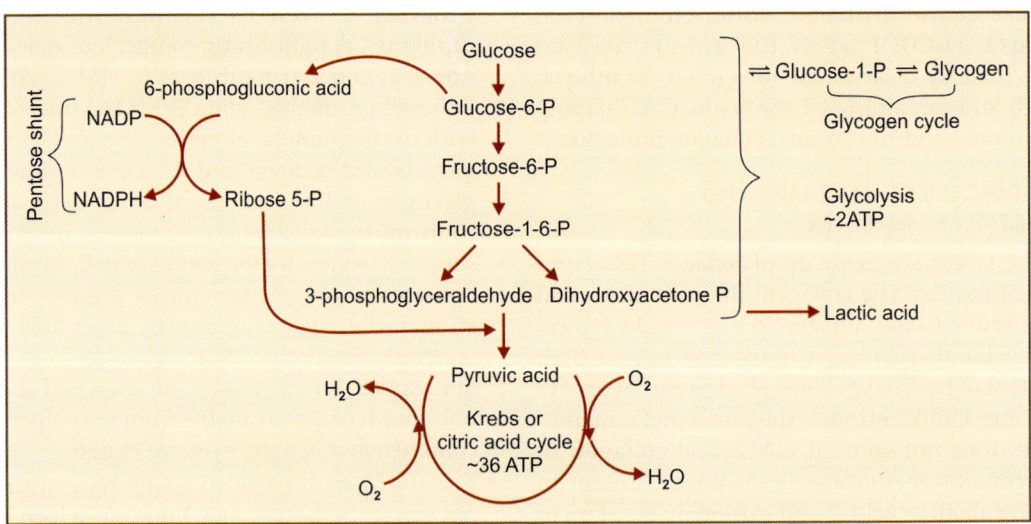

Fig. 2.3: *Pathways of glucose metabolism in cornea*

producing energy in the form of 2 molecules of ATP/molecule of glucose broken down. While, through Krebs or citric acid cycle, 36 ATP molecules are produced per molecule of glucose oxidized (Fig. 2.3).

Corneal glucose utilization studies indicate that 88% of the total glucose consumed is metabolized no further than lactic acid, leaving 12% to be oxidized by the cellular respiratory systems. This high activity of glycolysis in comparison to the limited activity of tricarboxyl acid cycle, leads to accumulation of lactate even in aerobic condition. It is likely that the lactate is eliminated from the cornea by diffusion through the epithelium.

2. Hexose monophosphate/pentose shunt

In the corneal epithelium and endothelium, glucose is also metabolised through the hexose monophosphate shunt (pentose shunt), but without a net gain in ATP. The purpose of glucose metabolism through the pentose shunt is the production of NADPH which is utilized in the biosynthesis of lipids by corneal epithelium. The ribose produced by the pentose shunt may be used to build the nucleic acids— DNA and RNA.

3. Krebs cycle

It is a complex cycle which yields H_2O, CO_2 and 36 molecules of ATP/cycle of oxidation of pyruvic acid (Fig. 2.3).

■ CORNEAL TRANSPARENCY

The main physiologic function of the cornea is to act as a major refracting medium, so that a clear retinal image is formed. Maintenance of corneal transparency of high degree is a prerequisite to perform this function.

Normal corneal transparency is the result of anatomical and physical factors:
- *Anatomical factors* include uniform and regular arrangement of the corneal epithelium, a peculiar arrangement of the corneal lamellae and corneal avascularity.
- *Physiological factor is* relative state of corneal dehydration.

Note. Therefore, almost any process which upsets the anatomy or physiology of the cornea will cause loss of transparency to some degree.

FACTORS AFFECTING CORNEAL TRANSPARENCY

1. Corneal epithelium and tear film

Normal epithelium is transparent due to the homogenicity of its refractive index. The basal cells are firmly joined laterally to the other basal cells and anteriorly to the wing cells by desmosomes and maculae occludentes. These tight intercellular junctions account for the epithelium's transparency as well as its resistance to the flow of water, electrolytes and glucose, i.e. its barrier function. Normal precorneal tear film plays an important role in maintaining the transparency of epithelium. Therefore, conditions associated with tear film abnormalities and/or corneal epithelial abnormalities may result in loss of corneal transparency.

2. Arrangement of stromal lamellae

Following theories have been put forward to explain the role of a peculiar arrangement of the stromal lamellae in corneal transparency. These are:

i. *Maurice theory.* Maurice in 1957 proposed that the cornea is transparent because the uniform collagen fibrils are arranged in a regular lattice so that scattered light is destroyed by the mutual interference. He stated that as long as the fibrils are regularly arranged in a lattice, having less diameter (275–300Å) and separated by less than a wavelength of light (4000 to 7000Å), the cornea will remain transparent (Fig. 2.4). Loss of transparency will result, if this regular arrangement is altered by stromal oedema or mechanical stress (Fig. 2.5). So, whenever the distance between these collagen fibrils is increased, it can lead to bullae formation as in pseudophakic bullous keratopathy (PBK).

Absence of lattice arrangement of fibrils on electron microscopy reported by some workers is a point against the Maurice theory.

ii. *Theory of Goldman et al.* Goldman *et al* in 1968 after applying diffraction theory to the problem concluded that the lattice arrangement is not a necessary condition for stromal

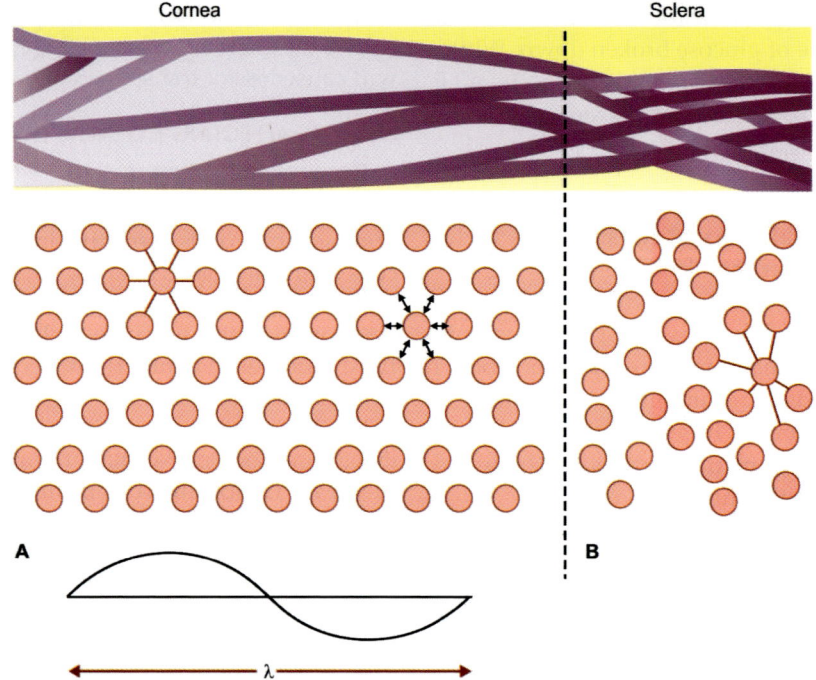

Fig. 2.4: *Cross-sectional view showing regular arrangement of the corneal fibrils as basis of corneal transparency (Maurice theory) (A); vis-à-vis irregular arrangement of sclera fibres (B)*

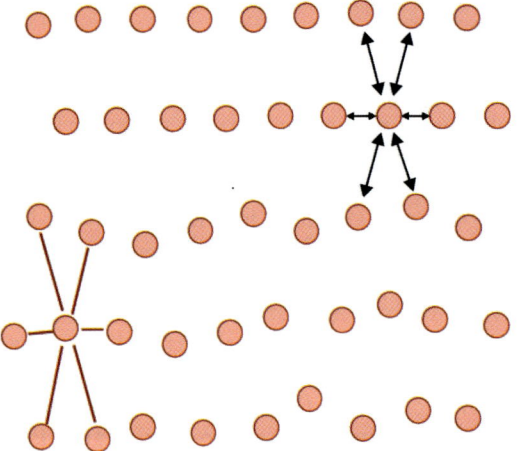

Fig. 2.5: *Cross-sectional view showing irregular arrangement of corneal fibrils as basis of loss of the corneal transparency (Maurice theory)*

transparency. Rather they postulated that the cornea is transparent because the fibrils are small in relationship to the light and do not interfere with light transmission unless they are larger than one-half a wavelength of light (2000Å). In confirmation of their theory, they found *'lakes'*—

areas devoid of collagen with dimensions greater than 2000Å, in swollen non-transparent human corneas. Similar 'lakes' can be found surrounding keratocytes in oedematous human corneas.

iii. *Expression of corneal crystallins in keratocytes* is a further structural adaptation to minimize light scatter.

Note. However, theory of Maurice as well as that of Goldman *et al* fail to explain the occurrence of rapid clouding of cornea associated with acute rise in intraocular pressure and the rapid clearing of the cornea with reduction of intraocular pressure.

3. Corneal vascularization

The cornea is avascular except for small loops which invade the periphery for about 1 mm. However, various disease processes of the cornea may be associated with corneal vascularization. The purpose of this process is to bring the defence mechanisms into play against the noxious agents. It facilitates nutrition, transport of systemic antibiotics and drugs. Progressive vascularization, however, is a harmful process—as it interferes with the functional properties of the cornea, especially its transparency.

Pathogenesis of corneal vascularization

The factors that keep the normal cornea avascular are unknown and so is the pathogenesis of corneal vascularization. However, various theories which have been proposed largely agree on the role of chemical and mechanical factors in producing corneal vascularization.

i. *Chemical theory.* There may be presence of vasostimulatory factor (VSF) or the breaking down (destruction) of previously existing vasoinhibitory factor (VIF).

- *Role of vasoinhibitory factor (VIF).* The idea that avascularity of the cornea might be due to the presence of a VIF preventing vascular invasion was put forward by Meyer and Chafre. They postulated that the sulphate ester of hyaluronic acid (stromal glycosaminoglycan) acts as VIF. However, other workers after experimental studies have discarded this view.
- *Role of vasostimulatory factor (VSF).* Campbell and Michaelson 1949, using experimental corneal burns, postulated the release of VSF at the site of lesion which diffuses through the stroma to the limbus and stimulates new vessel growth from the limbal plexus. The exact nature of VSF is unknown, but it is thought to be a low molecular weight amine. It has also been postulated that corneal hypoxia also induces neovascularization by activation of VSF.

ii. *Mechanical theory.* Cogan postulated that blood vessels cannot invade normal cornea because of its compact structural nature and that loosening of the compactness of corneal tissue due to oedema was mandatory for neovascularization. This mechanical theory was agreed to by many workers. However, Langham doubted the adequacy of oedema alone being responsible for the vascularization. Clinically also it has been seen that in Fuchs' dystrophy and aphakic bullous keratopathy, it is rare for the vascularization to occur even when the oedema extends to limbus.

iii. *Combined mechanical and chemical theory.* Maurice *et al* have demonstrated that both release of some vasostimulatory factor (VSF) and structural loosening of compact corneal stroma by oedema are necessary for the neovascularization to occur.

iv. *Role of leucocytes.* Some workers have postulated that corneal vascularization is a manifestation of inflammatory response and that leucocytes perform an essential role in stimulating corneal vascular growth. However, other investigators could not confirm this.

Types of corneal vascularization

Normal corneal vascularization according to depth of involvement may be:

- *Superficial vascularization*: Vessels originate from superficial limbal plexus. Superficial vessels are usually arranged in arborizing pattern, present below the epithelial layer and their continuity can be traced with the conjunctival vessels. They are dark red in colour and they branch dichotomously.
- *Deep vascularization*: Vessels are derived from anterior ciliary arteries. Deep vessels are usually straight, lie in the stroma, not anastomosing and their continuity cannot be traced beyond the limbus. They are pink in colour.
- *Retrocorneal pannus*: It is seen in syphilitic cause of interstitial keratitis.

4. Corneal hydration

The normal cornea maintains itself in a state of relative dehydration, which is essential for the corneal transparency. The water content of normal cornea is approximately 80%, which is the highest water content of any connective tissue in the body. It is kept constant by a balance of factors which draw water in the cornea (e.g. swelling pressure of the stromal matrix and intraocular pressure) and the factors which prevent the flow of water in the cornea (viz. the mechanical barrier action of epithelium which constitutes a relatively impermeable membrane) and those which draw water out of the cornea (e.g. active pumping action of the corneal endothelium). Disturbance of any of these factors leads to corneal oedema, wherein its hydration becomes above 80%, central thickness increases and transparency reduces. Since the cornea swells only in the direction of thickness, therefore, corneal thickness and hydration are linearly related. Clinically, corneal thickness is measured using a corneal pachymeter and from it an idea of corneal hydration is made.

Factors affecting corneal hydration

i. Stromal swelling pressure. Swelling pressure (SP) is the 'keystone' of corneal biophysics. It is a pressure (60 mm Hg) exerted by the glyco-saminoglycans (GAGs) of the corneal stroma which act like a sponge. The electrostatic repulsion of the anionic charges on the GAG molecule expands the tissue, sucking in the fluid with equal but negative pressure called imbibition pressure (IP). The values of imbibition pressure are equal to swelling pressure *in vitro* (i.e. in excised corneal tissue) but *in vivo* IP is reduced by the values equivalent to intraocular pressure (IOP), i.e. IP = IOP–SP or IP = 17–60 = –43 mm Hg. The cornea thus has a swelling pressure and a metabolic pump (the endothelium) designed to maintain it as described below. The swelling pressure generates a level of interfibrillar tension and may be the biophysical mechanism whereby the fibrils are maintained in their normal arrangement. In addition, the swelling pressure may reciprocally activate chloride channels.

ii. Barrier function of epithelium and endo-thelium. Both the epithelium and endothelium function as barriers to excessive flow of water and diffusion of electrolytes into the stroma due to their semipermeable nature. The corneal epithelium offers twice the resistance to water flow as does the endothelium and is thus practically a perfect semipermeable membrane for small solutes such as sodium chloride and urea when they are used to produce hypertonicity of the solution bathing the cornea. While, in the case of endothelium, these solutes diffuse across the layer, while water is extracted osmotically. The barrier function of the endothelium is calcium dependent. Corneal transparency is decreased and corneal thickness is increased when the corneal endothelium is damaged and to a lesser extent when the epithelium is damaged.

iii. Hydration control by active pump mechanisms. It is now established that the corneal endothelium plays a predominant role in controlling fluid transport due to several enzyme pump systems present in it. The pump mechanisms are active processes, requiring energy and are thus dependent upon the metabolic activity of cornea (cyclic AMP does not seem to be involved). The enzyme pump systems which collectively regulate fluid and ionic transport across the cell layer are as follows (Fig. 2.6).

- *Na^+/K^+–ATPase pump system* present in the endothelium is several folds more active than its counterpart in the epithelium. The enzyme Na^+/K^+ activated ATPase mediates the active extrusion of the Na^+ from the tissue. Oubain, a specific ATPase inhibitor, when applied topically to the eye or injected into the anterior chamber, blocks endothelial fluid transport and results in corneal overhydration.

- *A bicarbonate-dependent ATPase* has also been reported in endothelial cells; depletion of bicarbonate from incubation/perfusion medium induces swelling. The enzyme seems to be present in mitochondria and not on the plasma membrane. Enzyme inhibition by thiocyanate is paralleled by inhibition of fluid transport.

- *Carbonic anhydrase enzyme* has also been implicated in the regulation of fluid transport, since carbonic anhydrase inhibitors decrease the flow of fluid from stroma to aqueous humour. The enzyme has been localized almost exclusively in the corneal endothelium and, as in most tissues, produces bicarbonate (HCO_3) ions and hydrogen (H^+) ions.

- *Na^+/H^+ pump* has also been postulated at the lateral plasma membrane surface. From the above, it is quite clear that a complex series of metabolically dependent reactions occur in the endothelium and epithelium to maintain proper fluid/ionic balance and deturgescence in the cornea. Besides these systems, passive ion movement also occurs, in that K^+, Cl^- and HCO_3^- ions diffuse into the aqueous humour. In the contralateral direction, Na^+, Cl^- and HCO_3^- passively diffuse from the aqueous into the cornea.

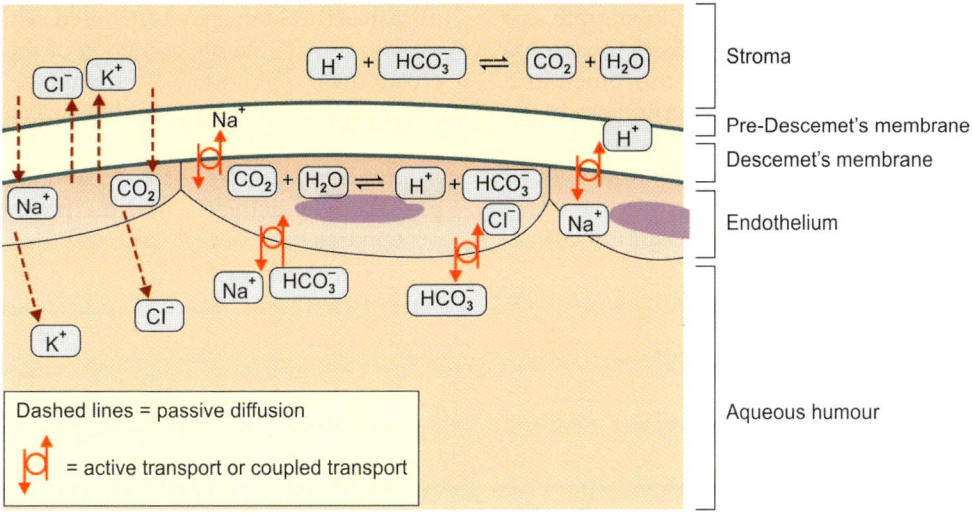

Fig. 2.6: *Endothelial active pump mechanisms controlling the corneal hydration*

iv. *Evaporation of water from the corneal surface.* The evaporation of water from the precorneal tear film would concentrate this fluid and increase its osmolarity relative to the cornea. The hypertonicity of the tear film could draw water from the cornea. However, this loss of fluid is readily replaced by aqueous and, therefore, figures little in corneal dehydration.

v. *Intraocular pressure.* It has been shown that when the intraocular pressure (IOP) exceeds the swelling pressure of the corneal stroma, epithelial oedema will occur. This correlates well with the occurrence of clinically detectable (on slit-lamp examination) corneal oedema when the IOP is raised above 50 mm Hg. However, when swelling pressure is low, corneal oedema can occur even with normal IOP as seen in endothelial dystrophy.

5. Cellular factors affecting transparency

Corneal fibroblasts (keratocytes) are important in maintaining transparency, as they are the source of stromal collagens and proteoglycans. Although most of the changes that occur in the assembly of the matrix are post-transitional, the enzymes that induce these changes are present in keratocytes in which these genes have been specifically induced. (Specific enzyme defects are associated with corneal opacification as in the mucopolysaccharidoses.)

- *Collagen turnover in early postnatal life* is about 24 to 50 hours but there is a little information on adult collagen metabolism. For both collagen and GAGs, studies on cultured keratocytes have not been very informative since these cells produce a range of GAGs not found *in vivo.* In contrast, organ cultures of cornea produce a panel of GAGs more akin to that found *in vivo.* The preferential production of KS-PG to CS/DS-PG in corneal cells from different species has been attributed to relatively hypoxic conditions and to anaerobic glycolysis, which favour the former in rabbit cornea, the development of transparency correlates with dramatic increase in concentration of KS-PG in the early postnatal period.
- *Corneal crystallins,* i.e. water-soluble protein of keratocytes (transketolase and aldehyde dehydrogenase class IA1), also contribute to corneal transparency at the cellular level.

■ CELL TURNOVER AND WOUND HEALING IN THE CORNEA

EPITHELIUM

Corneal epithelium heals by sequence of three processes: Migration, mitosis and differentiation. The epithelium is constantly being regenerated by mitotic activity in the basal layer of cells. However, after epithelial debridement, the initial response of epithelium is to migrate as a flattened sheet of single cells across the stroma to close the defect. Hemidesmosomes and intercellular contacts then reform and gradually the single layer is restored to its six-layered architecture by mitotic activity in the peripheral basal cells.

- *Migration of the epithelial cells occurs in a predictable manner* as sheets of cells that produce geometric patterns as the advancing sheets meet in the centre. Migration of cells begins after 5–6 hours of injury and occurs at a rate of 60–80 μm/hr. Migration of epithelial cells is achieved by marked cytoskeletal and cell shape changes involving redistribution of actin–myosin fibrils. Changes in actin distribution in the cell are preceded by changes in actin-binding proteins such as fodrin and E-cadherin, which are under genetic regulation via growth factors. Vinoclin protein is also increased which promote interaction of contractile protein actin with adhesion proteins like talin and integrin.

- *Migration of the cells is also dependent on matrix-induced intracellular signaling* via components such as fibronectin/fibrin, laminin and collagen peptides through cell surface integrins. The role of fibronectin/fibrin in corneal epithelial resurfacing is unclear since these proteins do not appear to be essential for migration *in vitro*. However, it has been suggested that they facilitate healing where the normal basement membrane and, in particular, its laminin component has been lost, but are not essential for wound healing. The clinical application of fibronectin/fibrin to non-healing corneal ulcers has, however, been disappointing. It is also noticed that cell migration requires increased Ca^{2+}, cyclic AMP, cyclic GMP and increased acetylcholine levels.

- *Adhesion of epithelium to the basement membrane and Bowman's layer* is normally achieved via hemidesmosomes, the lamina densa and the anchoring type VII collagen fibrils. However, while hemidesmosomes form during the early stages of pre-epithelialization (18 hours), many days elapse before anchoring fibrils reappear, and many months pass before full

ultrastructural integrity is restored. This may explain in part the phenomenon of recurrent erosion where there has been damage to the superficial stromal layers of the cornea.

- *Proteolytic activity in repairing epithelial defects is also important*—both urokinase type plasminogen activator and matrix metalloproteinases have been implicated.

- *Most of the mitotic activity in the epithelium takes place at the limbus* where stem cells undergo several rounds of division to repopulate the entire corneal surface. However, attempts to promote wound healing using growth-promoting agents such as epidermal growth factor and retinoic acid have not met with great success.

- *Conjunctival cells, limbal stem cells, and normal corneal epithelial cells* can be distinguished by their cytokeratin profile and by the types of protein present in their junctional complexes.

STROMA

Incisional wounds of the cornea that involve the stroma may be accidental or intentional. The immediate effect is to cause wound gape and imbibition of water from tears by the GAGs (*see* above). This causes localized opacification (light scatter) and initiates a series of events in the cornea directed to closing the wound. These include deposition of fibrin within the wound, rapid epithelialization of the wound incision, and activation of the keratocytes to divide and synthesize collagen and GAGs. During the early phase of corneal wound healing, there is loss of specialization in the keratocytes such that they revert to a fibroblast-like function and lay down collagen and GAGs found in any typical wound, e.g. hyaluronic acid, types I and III collagens, and matrix glycoproteins. In addition, the size and arrangement of the fibrils are not regular, further contributing to the corneal opacity. In extensive wounds, this opacification remains permanently, however, in smaller, well-defined wounds there is an attempt by the cornea to restore clarity by producing normal corneal matrix components.

Since the corneal curvature is a function of tension in its circumferential fibres, restoration of the normal curvature will not be achieved unless the edges of the wound are apposed by surgical reconstruction. This is the basis of refractive corneal surgery where partial thickness wounds are intentionally left to heal in a gaping configuration; limited incisions in the periphery of the cornea alter its refractive power, the degree of which can be precisely determined by the number and depth of incisions. More recently, there has been an explosion of interest in the use argon-Fl and ultraviolet laser energy to produce precise customized incisions in the stroma by 'ablating' the tissues. Ablation is thought to be caused by photon-photon interactions derived from thermal reactions or directly by photoablation, whereby molecular disintegration is induced. Further developments in refractive surgery include laser *in situ* keratomileusis (LASIK) in which the surface of the cornea is reconfigured by raising a corneal flap, laser ablation of the exposed stromal bed and restoring the corneal flap without sutures. Both these and conventional surgical corneal incisions are fully epithelialized in the normal manner, with epithelial migration into the depths of the wound sometimes producing excessive layer of cells.

ENDOTHELIUM

The corneal endothelium does not normally undergo mitosis in humans even after direct injury as in a perforating corneal wound. Endothelial defects are repaired by migration and enlargement of surrounding cells. With age, there is a decline in the number of endothelial cells with an increase in their size and variable morphology. The response to direct wounding is to undergo 'cell slide', as occurs in the epithelium in the early stages of migration. If sufficient numbers of endothelial cells are lost, the cell layer cannot perform its pumping action and the cornea imbibes water (decompensates) and becomes opaque.

VASCULARIZATION

Vascularization of the cornea occurs when vessels from the conjunctiva or the deep episcleral plexus invade the periphery of the cornea during healing of the wound or corneal ulcers. When corneal epithelial or stromal defects fail to close promptly, often as a result of infection or during the severe inflammatory response of chemical injury such as acid and alkali corneal burns, the continued release of proteolytic enzymes causes degradation of the stroma and increases the risk of spontaneous perforation. Matrix metalloproteinases, such as matrilysin and stromelysin and MMP-9 as well as plasminogen activators (uPA and tPA) are released both by the incoming leucocytes and the resident epithelial and stromal cells. Cytokines, such as interleukin 1 (IL-1), IL-6, and IL-8, tumour necrosis factor α (TNF-α) and TGF-β, macrophage inflammatory proteins (MIP) la and b, and granulocytes-macrophage colony-stimulating factor (GM-CSF), liberated from the inflammatory and local cells stimulate further ingress of inflammatory cells and initiate a vascularization response. Vessels advance across the cornea to the site of injury or infection and contribute to the eventual opaque 'leucoma' of the healed cornea. Inhibitors of angiogenesis are also released during the process such as angiostatin and Kl-5, which are proteolytic fragments of plasminogen itself.

CORNEAL PHYSIOLOGY: APPLIED ASPECTS

Important applied aspects to be considered in relation to corneal physiology are:
- Drug permeability across cornea, and
- Effects of contact lens wear on corneal physiology.

DRUG PERMEABILITY ACROSS THE CORNEA

Topically instilled medications largely penetrate intraocularly through the cornea. Many factors which affect the drug penetration through the cornea are as follows.

1. Lipid and water solubility of the drug

The corneal epithelium and endothelium being lipophilic are crossed readily by the non-polar (lipid-soluble) drug. The stroma being hydrophilic is easily crossed by polar (water-soluble) compounds. Therefore, a drug should be amphipathic, that is, have both lipid and water solubility to readily penetrate across the cornea.

2. Molecular size, weight and concentration of the drug

As discussed above, the lipid-soluble molecules can cross the corneal epithelium easily irrespective of their molecular size, while water-soluble molecules with the molecular size less than 4 A only can filter through the pores which exist in the cell membrane.

It has been reported that the substances with molecular weights of less than 100 can pass readily through the cell membrane and those with more than 500 cannot.

It has also been reported that when the substances with large molecular size are used in high concentration, then a small amount of drug can cross the cornea following laws of mass action. The rate of penetration through the cornea of the drug such as pilocarpine, homatropine, atropine and steroids depends upon their concentration in the solution.

3. Ionic form of the drugs

The drugs intended for topical use in eye must have capacity to exist in both ionized and non-ionized form for a better penetration through the cornea since only non-ionized drugs can penetrate through the epithelium and the ionized drugs can pass through the stroma. True electrolytes or non-electrolytes cannot penetrate these various barriers. Therefore, fluorescein, a negatively charged ion, cannot penetrate the intact epithelium and this property forms the basis of fluorescein dye test.

A typical model of the drug existing both in non-ionized and ionized form for penetration through cornea has been proposed by Kinsey for homatropine. As shown in Fig. 2.7, in the tear film, ionized homatropine (R_3NH^+) converts into non-ionized free base (R_3N) which readily crosses cornea through the epithelium and gets ionized (R_3NH^+) in the stroma. Near the endothelium, it again becomes non-ionized (R_3N), crosses it and in the aqueous humour becomes ionized (R_3NH^+).

4. pH of the solution

pH may affect the penetration of the solutes by its effect on the electrical charges and stability of solutions. The pH of the solution may be varied from 4 to 10 without affecting the permeability of the epithelium, but solution outside this range increases the permeability.

5. Tonicity of the solution

Hypotonic solutions (those below 0.9% of sodium chloride) increase the permeability of the epithelium considerably.

6. Surface active agents

Agents that reduce surface tension, increase corneal wetting and, therefore, present more

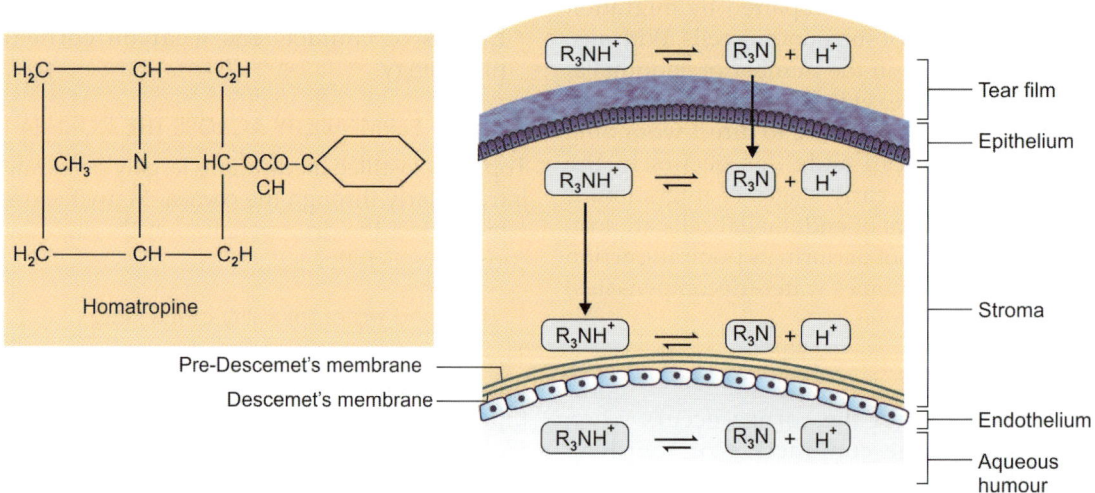

Fig. 2.7: *A model of drug (homatropine) existing in both ionized and non-ionized from for penetration through the cornea (after Kinsey)*

drug for absorption. Benzalkonium chloride used as preservative also acts as wetting agent and thus increases the drug absorption.

7. Pro-drug form

Pro-drug forms are lipophilic and after absorption through epithelium are converted into proper drug which can easily pass through stroma. For example, dipivefrin is pro-drug which is converted into epinephrine after its absorption into the eye. Dipivefrin is more lipophilic than epinephrine and thus its corneal penetration is increased 17 times.

■ EFFECTS OF CONTACT LENS WEAR ON CORNEAL PHYSIOLOGY

Contact lenses predominantly affect the function of the epithelium. This layer receives its oxygen from tears and its glucose from the circulation via the aqueous and the limbal vessels. Contact lenses reduce the direct availability of oxygen to the epithelium, thus shifting the balance from aerobic to anaerobic metabolism. Lactate levels in the cornea are doubled with contact lens wear and carbon dioxide production is increased. The induced acidosis has a direct effect on stromal hydration by impairing stromal deturgescence mechanism (see below).

Hard (rigid) contact lenses are usually made from polymethylmethacrylate (PMMA) and have the greatest effect on corneal function; in addition to restricting oxygen availability, hard lenses deplete glycogen stores, even though the level of glucose availability is not reduced. It has been suggested that hard lens-induced inhibition of aerobic enzymes such as hexo-kinase reduces direct glucose utilization by the cornea. Prolonged wear of hard contact lenses is, therefore, not possible owing to the damaging effect on corneal transparency induced by the disturbed metabolism.

Soft contact lenses are made from polymers of HEMA, poly-HEMA vinylpyrrolidones, silicone, or other similar materials, and permit extended wear of lens owing to their permeability to oxygen and carbon dioxide. However, there is still some degree of lactate accumulation with soft lenses and prolonged use appears to affect the function of the endothelium. Manufacturers of contact lenses are continually producing newer biomimetic type lenses with increased water content (up to 59%) in attempts to support normal corneal physiology (hydrogel lenses).

Gas permeable rigid lens, which combines the reduced toxicity of PMMA with high gas transfer capability, is a popular compromise in contact lens type.

DK value of contact lenses. The wide variety of lens types and materials have led to their being characterized on the basis of their oxygen flux defined as the DK value,

$$\text{Oxygen flux} = DK/L \times DP$$

where D is the diffusion coefficient, K is the solubility and L is the thickness of lens material. DP is the change in the partial pressure of oxygen across the material. HEMA and PMMA have a low oxygen flux, while hydrogels and silicones have a high flux.

Both the thickness of the lens and the DK value determine its suitability for use in term of its gas permeability. The actual amount of oxygen that reaches the cornea is the most important factor in the design of a contact lens and most practioners describe contact lenses in terms of their equivalent oxygen performance (EOP).

Contact lenses may have deleterious effects on the epithelium, causing:

- Thinning, reduction in the hemidesmosome density and the number of anchoring fibrils, and reduced adhesion of the epithelium to the basement membrane. This may be a direct effect of low oxygen transmitting lenses on basal epithelial cell proliferation. This is especially true of extended wear hydrogel lenses.

- In severe cases, excessive use of contact lenses produces epithelial oedema and keratopathy in the form of punctate epithelial erosions.

- Rigid contact lenses also produce tear film instability by causing damage to the epithelium in the mucin layer in particular.

- They also cause limbal redness, epithelial microcytes formation and endothelium polymegethism.

BIBLIOGRAPHY

1. Ehlers N, Hjortdal J. Corneal thickness: measurement and implication. Exp Eye Res 2004; 78: 543–48.
2. Ehlers N, Hjortdal J. The cornea, epithelium and stroma. In: J Fischbarg (Ed.). Advances in Organ Biology, Vol. 10. Amsterdam: Elsevier, 2005; 83–112.
3. Hansen, FK. Clinical study of normal human central corneal thickness. Acta Ophthalmol Scand 1971; 49: 82–89.
4. Jacobsen IA, Jensen OA, Prause JU. Structure and composition of Bowman's membrane. Study by frozen resin cracking. Acta Ophthalmol (Copenh) 1984; 62: 39–53.
5. Nishida T. Cornea. In: JH Krachmer, MJ Mannis, EJ Holland (Eds). Cornea, 2nd edn. Philadelphia, PA: Elsevier, Mosby. 2005; 3–26.
6. Olsen T, Ehlers N. The thickness of the human cornea as determined by a specular method. Acta Ophthalmol Scand 1984; 62: 859–71.
7. Reinstein DZ, Archer TJ, Gobbe M, Silverman RH, Coleman DJ. Epithelial thickness in the normal cornea: three-dimensional display with Artemis very high-frequency digital ultrasound. J Refract Surg 2008; 24: 571–81.

Section
II

Clinical Evaluation and Investigative Techniques for Cornea and Ocular Surface

3

Clinical Evaluation and Investigations for Corneal Diseases

CLINICAL EVALUATION

PRESENTING SYMPTOMS OF CORNEAL DISEASES

Knowledge of the clinical features is an important step in the management of corneal diseases. A proper diagnosis and treatment cannot be done without an accurate assessment of the clinical features. Common symptoms of corneal diseases are pain, decreased vision, discharge, lacrimation, redness, photophobia and blepharospasm.

PAIN

- Pain is the commonest symptom of the inflammatory lesions of the cornea due to its rich innervation.
- Pain in corneal diseases occurs due to direct stimulation of the sensory nerves in the cornea or as the consequence of inflammation or ciliary spasm.
- Direct stimulation of the corneal nerves causes pain which is severe in intensity and sharp in nature while corneal inflammation produces severe pain but of a dull aching or throbbing nature.
- The severity of pain may range from minimal discomfort to an excruciating pain.
- The type of causative organism and the depth of the ulceration influence the severity of pain. In general, superficial ulcers are more painful than deep corneal ulcers. This is due to the rich sensory nerve supply presents in the superficial part of the cornea.
- A small dendrite of herpes simplex or a *Candida* species cause minimal pain and may only be associated with foreign body sensation. In contrast, a patient with *Acanthamoeba keratitis* presents with an excruciating pain,

during corneal epithelial involvement due to radial keratoneuritis. The pain is usually out of proportion to the objective clinical findings, the alleviation of which may require strong analgesics and narcotics.

- A sudden relief in pain, in a case of progressing corneal ulcer may be indicative of the perforation of ulcer.

DECREASED VISUAL ACUITY

- Visual loss is a common symptom in patients with corneal disease and occurs most commonly due to loss of transparency of the cornea.
- Acute loss of vision is due to acute inflammatory conditions of the cornea and is associated with other symptoms of inflammation, pain and vascular injection.
- Gradual loss of vision is more likely to be associated with a slowly evolving corneal pathology.
- Most cases of corneal ulcer report with a history of sudden decrease in vision. The extent of decrease in vision depends on the duration, severity, location of the lesion and involvement of other ocular structures.
- Central corneal ulcers, particularly those caused by organisms like Pseudomonas, *Staphylococcus aureus* and *Fusarium* species are invariably associated with significant loss of visual acuity.
- Other factors that can reduce visual acuity include the presence of an associated pupillary membrane, hypopyon, cataract, glaucoma and endophthalmitis.
- The vision may not be severely reduced in cases which have small, peripheral ulcers, such as those caused by herpes simplex and non-coagulase Staphylococcus.
- In *Acanthamoeba keratitis*, vision may not be significantly reduced during the initial stages, when the corneal epithelium alone is involved. Later, as the infection spreads deeper into the corneal stroma, visual acuity is severely reduced.

DISCHARGE

- Almost all cases of corneal ulcers present with a complaint of discharge from the affected eye.

The type of the discharge may be watery, mucoid, mucopurulent or frankly purulent.

- A watery discharge usually occurs due to a viral ulcer or a small bacterial ulcer or else it may also be due to reflex tearing.
- However, microbial keratitis caused by *Pseudomonas* and *Gonococcus* species is associated with a mucopurulent discharge.
- Corneal ulcers caused due to Pseudomonas are particularly associated with a greenish-yellowish discharge.
- A membranous discharge is seen with keratitis caused by *Corynebacterium diphtheriae*.

LACRIMATION

Lacrimation occurs as a result of lacrimatory reflex mediated by fifth nerve (afferent) and secretomotor fibres of the seventh nerve (efferent). Fifth nerve ending in cornea is stimulated in corneal frame, inflammation and if infections.

Redness: Redness of eyes occurs due to congestion of circumcorneal vessels.

PHOTOPHOBIA

- Term applied to the discomfort experienced on the exposure to bright light due to stimulation of nerve endings.
- Severe photophobia only accompanies denudation of the epithelium, but many inflammatory diseases are accompanied by some iridocyclitis, and spasm of the sphincter of the iris and the ciliary muscle.

BLEPHAROSPASM

- It is caused by corneal irritation due to the stimulation of the terminal fibres of the corneal nerves.
- This blepharospasm is not completely abolished in the dark, but is greatly diminished by thorough anaesthetisation. It is thus a reflex predominantly involving the trigeminal nerve.

EXAMINATION OF CORNEA

SYSTEMATIC APPROACH FOR CORNEAL EXAMINATION

Examination of cornea should be done under following headings: Shape, size, surface, curvature, thickness, vascularization, transparency, and sensation.

SHAPE

- The anterior surface of the normal cornea is horizontally elliptical with an average horizontal diameter of 11.7 mm and vertical diameter of 11 mm.
- In hypotony, the vertical diameter becomes less and the cornea looks more elliptical.
- In phthisis, the cornea looks quadrilateral in shape.
- In extreme degrees of microphthalmos, the cornea becomes very small and irregular.
- Keratoglobus is an ectatic condition in which cornea becomes thin and bulges out like a globe.
- Keratoconus is an ectatic condition in which cornea becomes cone shaped.
- Cornea plana, i.e. flat curvature of cornea which may occur in patients with severe hypotony.

SIZE

The anterior surface of normal cornea is elliptical with an average horizontal diameter of 11.7 mm and vertical diameter of 11 mm. The best method to determine the corneal diameter is by corneal callipers under local anaesthesia in adults and general anaesthesia in children. Diameter should be measured both vertically and horizontally in both the eyes.

Abnormalities of corneal size can be:

Causes of decreased corneal size are: Microphthalmos, microcornea, phthisis bulbi, atrophic bulbi, and nanophthalmos.

Microcornea, when the anterior horizontal diameter is less than 10 mm. It may occur isolated or as a part of microphthalmos.

Megalocornea is labelled when the horizontal diameter is more than 13 mm. Common **causes** of increased corneal size are congenital megalocornea, buphthalmos, macrophthalmos (keratoglobus).

SURFACE

Smoothness of the corneal surface is disturbed due to abrasions, ulceration, ectatic scars and facets. Changes in smoothness of surface can be detected by slit-lamp biomicroscopy, window reflex test and Placido's disc.

Placido's keratoscopic disc is a disc painted with alternating black and white circles. It may be used to assess the smoothness and curvature of the corneal surface. Normally, on looking through the hole in the centre of disc, a uniform sharp image of the circles is seen on the cornea. Irregularities in the corneal surface cause distortion of the circles (Fig. 3.1A to C).

Window reflex test. Patient is seated facing a window. Image of the window formed on the normal cornea in uniform and sharp. In irregular corneal surface the image of window formed in distorted.

CURVATURE

Normally cornea is more curved than the sclera hence it bulges beyond the limbus. The average corneal curvature is 8 mm. Curvature is slightly more in the central 3 mm, which is called *the optical zone.* Curvature of the central zone is best measured by *the keratometer,* while the peripheral

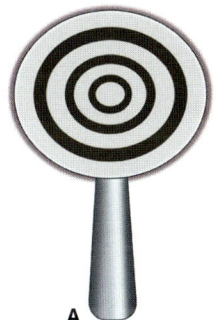 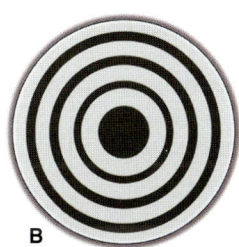 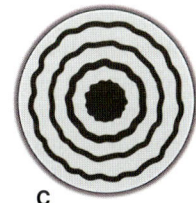

Fig. 3.1: *A, Placido disc; B, Placido disc reflex from normal cornea; C, Placido disc reflex from irregular corneal surface*

cornea is measured by *the photokeratoscope* and *topography*. Cornea is more curved vertically due to pressure of the lids. Increased curvature results in physiological myopic astigmatism of 0.5 D in horizontal axis. This is called with the rule astigmatism.

Corneal curvature is increased in: Keratoconus, buphthalmos, keratoglobus, and pellucid degeneration.

Corneal curvature is decreased in: Microcornea, microphthalmos, cornea plana, phthisis bulbi, hypotony, perforation of globe, and postsurgical tight suture.

Corneal curvature is irregular in: Pterygium, keratoconus, keratectasia, corneal staphyloma, pellucid degeneration of cornea, ciliary staphyloma, limbal growth and postsurgical following: Keratoplasty, glaucoma surgery, and retinal detachment surgery.

THICKNESS

Normal cornea does not have uniform thickness. It is thicker (0.9 mm) on the periphery and thinnest in the centre (0.6 mm). This is due to difference in corneal curvature of the two surfaces. Posterior surface is more curved than the anterior surface. Corneal thickness is measured by pachymeter. Corneal thickness is increased due to oedema of either stroma or epithelium or both.

Causes of thickened cornea are: Disciform keratitis, endothelial decompensation, epithelial oedema, corneal leucoma, and hydrops of cornea.

Causes of thin cornea are: Keratoconus, keratectasia, buphthalmos, pellucid degeneration, Mooren's ulcer, and Terrien's degeneration.

CORNEAL VASCULARIZATION

Normal cornea is avascular except for small capillary loops which are present in the periphery for about 1 mm. In pathological states, it can be invaded by vessels as a defence mechanism against the disease or injury. When vessels are present, an exact note of their position, whether superficial or deep and their distribution whether localised, general, or peripheral should be made.

Superficial corneal vascularization. In it, the vessels are arranged usually in an arborising pattern, present below the epithelial layer and their continuity can be traced with the conjunctival vessels (Fig. 3.2A).

Deep vascularization. In it, the vessels are generally derived from anterior ciliary arteries and lie in the corneal stroma. These vessels are usually straight, not anastomosing and their continuity cannot be traced beyond the limbus. Deep vessels may be arranged as terminal loops (Fig. 3.2B), brush (Fig. 3.2C), parasol, umbel (Fig. 3.2D), network or interstitial arcade.

Differences between superficial and deep vascularization of cornea are given in Table 3.1.

Causes of superficial corneal vascularization are: Trachoma, leprosy, phlycten, spring catarrh, riboflavin deficiency, Mooren's ulcer, indolent corneal ulcer, and vascularization of leucoma.

Causes of deep corneal vascularization are: Interstitial keratitis, disciform keratitis, alkali burn, and sclerosing keratitis.

Pannus

When extensive superficial vascularization is associated with white cuff of cellular infiltration, it is termed *pannus* (Fig. 3.3). In *progressive pannus*, corneal infiltration is ahead of vessels while in *regressive pannus,* it lags behind.

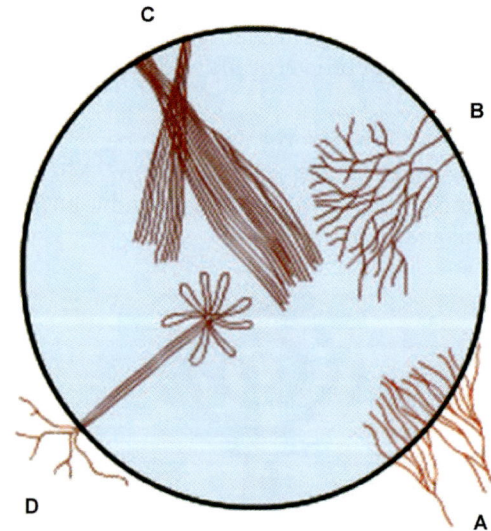

Fig. 3.2: *Corneal vascularization. (A) Superficial; (B) Deep corneal vascularization—terminal loops; (C) Deep corneal vascularization—brush; (D) Deep corneal vascularization—umbel*

Table 3.1: *Differences between superficial and deep corneal vascularization*

Superficial corneal vascularization	Deep corneal vascularization
Corneal vessels can be traced over the limbus onto the conjunctiva	Corneal vessels abruptly end at the limbus
Vessels are bright red and well-defined	Vessels are ill-defined and cause only a diffuse red blush
Superficial vessels branch in an arborescent manner	Deep vessels run parallel to each other in a radial fashion
Superficial vessels raise the epithelium and make the corneal surface irregular	Deep vessels do not disturb the corneal surface

Causes of pannus include:

- Chlamydia inclusion conjunctivitis and trachoma
- Tight contact lens wear
- Ocular rosacea
- Phlycten
- Superior limbic keratoconjunctivitis
- Staphylococcal hypersensitivity
- Vernal keratoconjunctivitis
- Chemical burn
- Aniridia
- Leprosy.

TRANSPARENCY

To maintain its optical property cornea has to be transparent, and most of the diseases of cornea cause a loss of this transparency. Transparency of cornea is lost in corneal oedema, opacity, ulceration, dystrophies, degenerations, vascularization and due to deposits in the cornea.

Corneal opacity

Corneal opacity can be stationary or progressive. They may vary in shape, size, number and

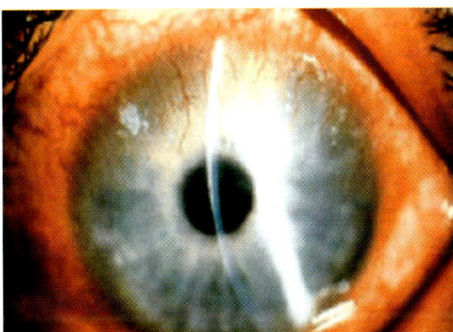

Fig. 3.3: *Pannus*

depth. They may be unilateral or bilateral. Most of the opacities are painless but some of them may be associated with pain due to non-corneal causes.

Examination for corneal opacity is best done with the help of a slit-lamp. Note the number, site, size, shape, density (nebular, macular or leucomatous) and surface of the opacity.

Position. Position of a corneal opacity is noted in relation to the limbus, pupil and meridian (face of clock).

Number. Number of corneal opacities may vary from single to multiple.

Shape. Corneal opacities may assume various shapes according to position, depth and pathology.

- *Dendritic pattern* is seen in herpes simplex and herpes zoster.
- *Dome-shaped opacity* with base at the limbus, occurs following healing of phlycten.
- *Tongue-shaped opacity* is produced by sclerosing keratitis and epithelial down growth.
- *Arc on the periphery* is typical of arcus senilis.

Grading of opacity

All corneal opacities are white in colour. Their shades vary according to depth. Opacities of epithelium and superficial stroma are the faintest; those involving full thickness are the densest. Depending on the density, corneal opacity is graded as nebula, macula and leucoma.

Nebular corneal opacity. It is a faint opacity which results due to superficial scars involving Bowman's layer and superficial stroma. A thin, diffuse nebula covering the pupillary area interferes more with vision than the localised leucoma away from pupillary area (Fig. 3.4A).

Macular corneal opacity. It is a semi-dense opacity produced when scarring involves about half of the corneal stroma (Fig. 3.4B).

Leucomatous corneal opacity. It is a dense white opacity which results due to scarring of more than half of the stroma (Fig. 3.4C).

Adherent leucoma. It results when healing occurs after perforation of cornea with incarceration of iris (Fig. 3.4D).

Corneal opacity at birth

Causes of corneal opacity at birth can be remembered with the mnemonic **STUMPED.**

Sclerocornea

Trauma (birth trauma)

Ulcer

Mucopolysaccharidosis

Peter's anomaly

Endothelial dystrophy, stromal dystrophy

Dermoid

Other causes are:
- Congenital glaucoma
- Interstitial keratitis
- Rubella keratitis.

CORNEAL SENSATIONS

Cornea is a highly sensitive structure. Sensitivity of the cornea is a protective mechanism. The ophthalmic branch of the fifth cranial nerve (trigeminal) carries sensory fibres for the cornea. If the cornea senses stimulation (ranging from mild irritation to intense pain), then the eyelid will close, providing protection to the cornea and distribution of tears. As the corneal sensitivity is decreased, then the blinking/ tearing mechanism will decrease, leaving the corneal epithelium exposed to dehydration. Anesthetic corneas may develop a characteristic interpalpebral horizontal band of punctate epithelial staining. Untreated, this may progress to an epithelial defect and subsequent stromal loss (neurotrophic ulcer). Ocular sensitivity is greatest in the central cornea except in elderly patients, in whom the peripheral cornea is the most sensitive. Sensitivity drops rapidly as distance from the limbus increases. The temporal limbus is significantly more sensitive than the inferior limbus.

To test the corneal sensations, patient is asked to look ahead; the examiner touches the corneal surface with a fine twisted cotton (which is brought from the side to avoid menace reflex) and observes the blinking response (Fig. 3.5).

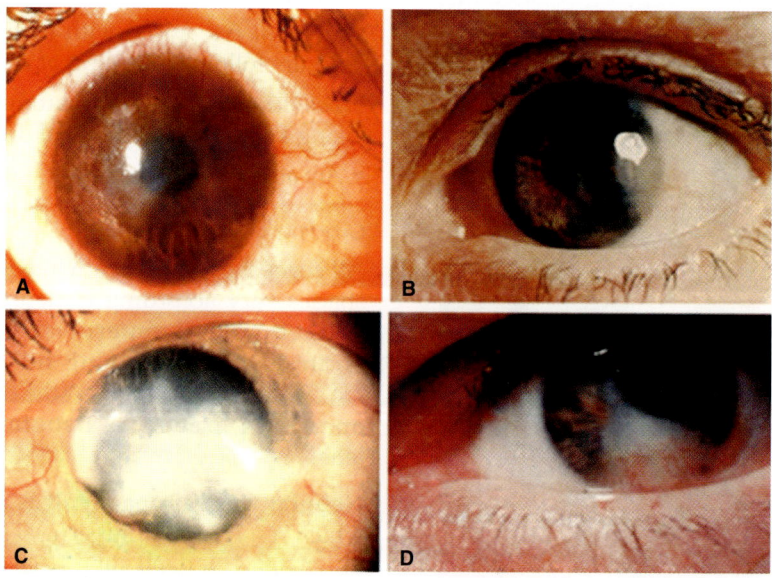

Fig. 3.4: *Corneal opacity. A, Nebular; B, Macular; C, Leucomatous; D, Adherent leucoma*

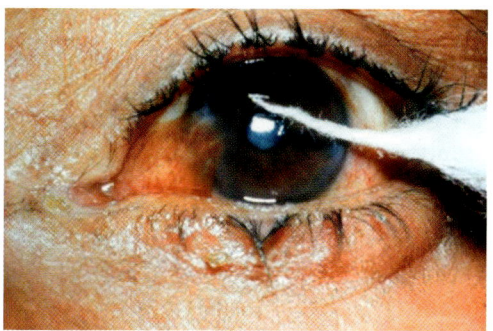

Fig. 3.5: *Testing of the corneal sensations with cotton wisp*

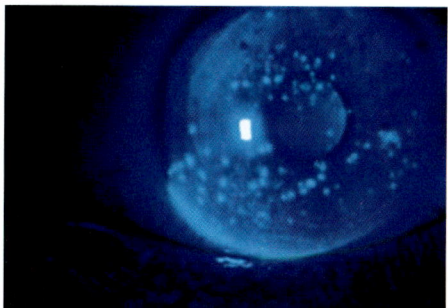

Fig. 3.6: *Punctate epithelial keratitis*

Normally, there is a brisk reflex closure of lids. Always compare the effect with that on the opposite side. The exact quantitative measurement of the corneal sensations is made with the help of an aesthesiometer.

Causes of reduced corneal sensations

- Herpes simplex keratitis
- Herpes zoster ophthalmicus
- Hansen disease (leprosy)
- Surgical trauma (PK, LASIK, large limbal incisions, ablation of the trigeminal ganglion)
- Topical medications (anaesthetics, NSAIDs, β-blockers, and carbonic anhydrase inhibitors)
- Cocaine abuse
- Aneurysms
- Tumours (acoustic neuroma, neurofibroma, or angioma)
- Cerebrovascular events
- Multiple sclerosis
- Hereditary causes. Familial dysautonomia (Riley-Day syndrome).

SIGNS OF COMMON CORNEAL DISEASES

Superficial keratitis

Punctate epithelial keratitis (PEK). Granular, swollen epithelial cells with focal intraepithelial infiltrates. They are visible unstained but stain well with rose bengal and variably with fluorescein (Fig. 3.6).

Causes: Adenoviral, molluscum contagiosum, early herpes simplex and herpes zoster, microsporidial and systemic viral infections (e.g. measles, varicella, rubella) and Thygeson superficial punctate keratitis.

Superficial punctate keratitis. Corneal epithelial defect with dot-like morphology (Fig. 3.7).

Punctate epithelial erosions (PEE): Tiny depressed grey-white epithelial defects that stain brightly with fluorescein and poorly with rose bengal (Fig. 3.8).

- *Superior erosions* are caused by tarsal foreign bodies, concretions, superior limbic keratopathy, vernal catarrh, floppy eyelid syndrome and mechanically induced keratoconjunctivitis.

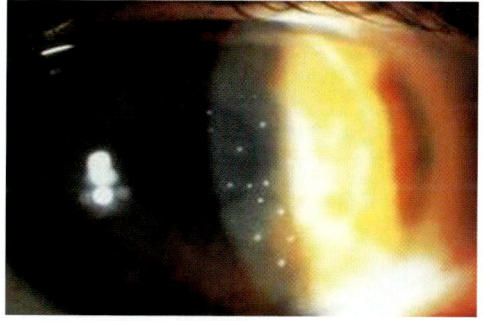

Fig. 3.7: *Superficial punctate keratitis*

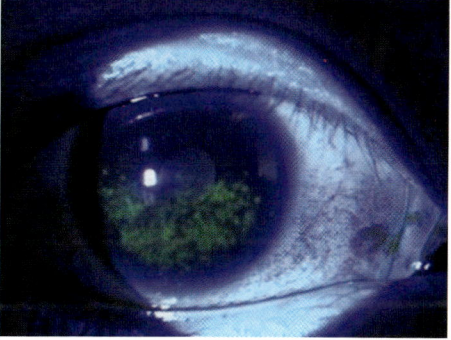

Fig. 3.8: *Punctate epithelial erosions*

- *Erosion of interpalpebral cornea* is caused by exposure to ultraviolet light, as in exposure to welding, snow blindness, and by neuro-paralytic keratitis.
- *Inferior erosions.* Chronic blepharitis, lago-phthalmos, eye drop toxicity, self-induced, aberrant eyelashes and entropion.
- *Central erosions.* Prolonged contact lens wear.
- *Diffuse erosions.* Some cases of viral and bacterial conjunctivitis, and toxicity to drops.

Subepithelial infiltrates. Tiny subsurface foci of non-staining inflammatory infiltrates (Fig. 3.9).

Causes include severe or prolonged adenoviral keratoconjunctivitis, herpes zoster keratitis, adult inclusion conjunctivitis, marginal keratitis, rosacea and Thygeson superficial punctate keratitis.

Punctate subepithelial keratitis is a feature of (Fig. 3.10):
- Adenovirus
- Epstein-Barr virus infection
- Reiter disease
- Corneal graft rejection.

Corneal ulcer

In ulcer, there is a breach in the continuity of the corneal epithelium, corneal ulcers present as greyish-white irregular areas surrounded by infiltration and having a margin and a floor. The ulcer stains brightly with fluorescein (Fig. 3.11) and the edges stain better than the floor.

Dendritc corneal ulcer: Linear branch-shaped epithelial lesions (Fig. 3.12):
- Herpes simplex dendritic ulcer (true dendrite)
- Herpes zoster
- Acanthamoeba
- Epithelial rejection line
- Healing epithelial defects
- Use of soft contact lens
- Tyrosinemia II.

Corneal oedema

- Appears like empty spaces in the epithelium that may be converted into actual bullae, which are 1–2 mm in size (Fig. 3.13).
- Bullae are vesicle-like structures laden with fluid, which on rupture produce severe pain.

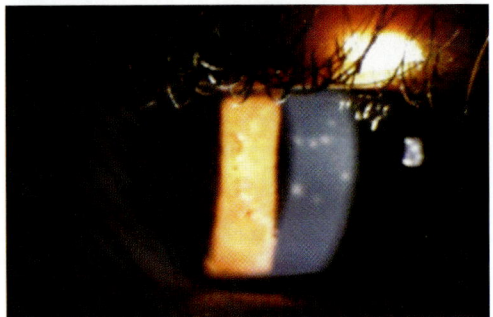

Fig. 3.9: *Subepithelial infiltrates*

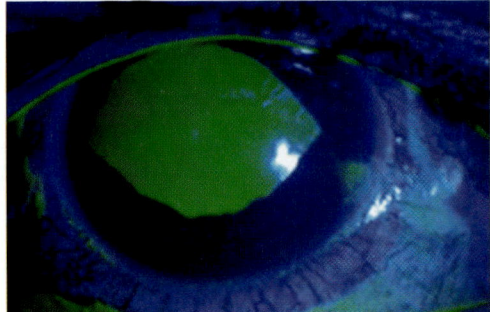

Fig. 3.11: *Corneal ulcer stained with fluorescein*

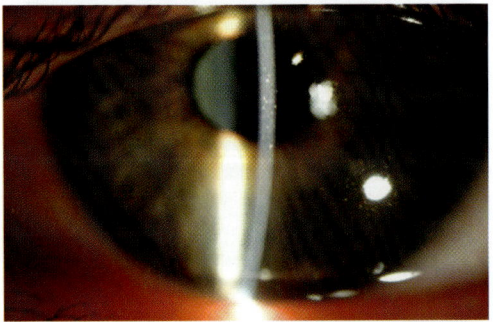

Fig. 3.10: *Punctate subepithelial keratitis*

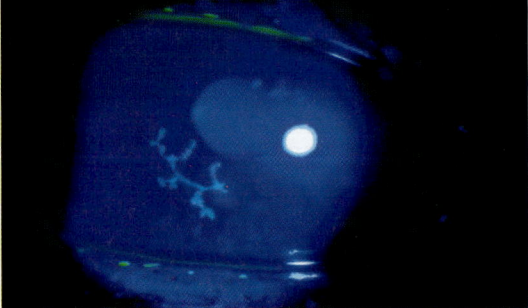

Fig. 3.12: *Corneal dendrites*

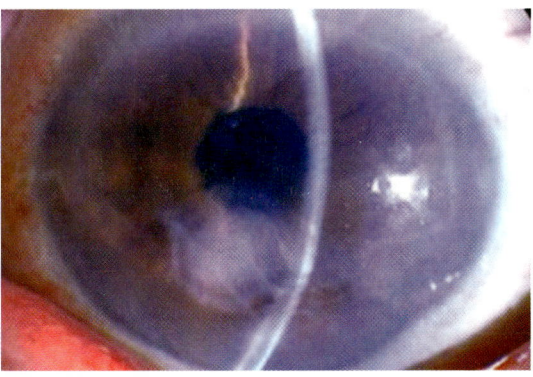

Fig. 3.13: *Corneal oedema*

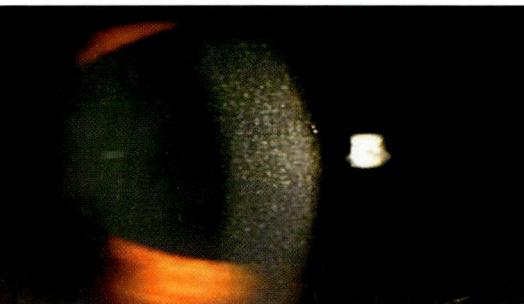

Fig. 3.15: *Corneal crystals*

They are found in acute congestive glaucoma, endothelial decompensation, trauma, following IOL implantation, vitreous touching the endothelium following ICC extraction, Fuchs' endothelial dystrophy, long-standing interstitial keratitis and keratoconus.

Noninflammatory stromal oedema (Fig. 3.14):
- Post-cataract surgery—bullous keratopathy
- Hydrops of keratoconus/keratoglobus
- Fuchs' endothelial dystrophy
- Acute angle closure glaucoma
- Corneal graft rejection
- Blunt anterior segment trauma
- Congenital hereditary endothelial dystrophy.

Corneal crystals

Aggregation of material in the corneal substance is seen in (Fig. 3.15):
- Schnyder crystalline keratopathy
- Cystinosis

- Multiple myeloma
- Gout
- Uraemia
- Hypergammaglobulinaemia
- Drugs (indomethacin)
- Lecithin cholesterol acyltransferase deficiency
- Tangier disease
- Chrysiasis.

Deposition of iron occurs in the intraepithelial layer

- *Rust ring.* Residual rust following metallic foreign body
- *Hudson-Stahli line.* Irregular line in inter-palpebral area in normal cornea (age related)
- *Ferry line.* Deposition of iron at advancing edge of filtering bleb
- *Stocker line.* Accumulation of iron just in front of the head of pterygium (Fig. 3.16)
- *Fleischer ring.* Circular yellow-brown ring at the base of cone in keratoconus
- *Dalgleish line.* Congenital spherocytosis.

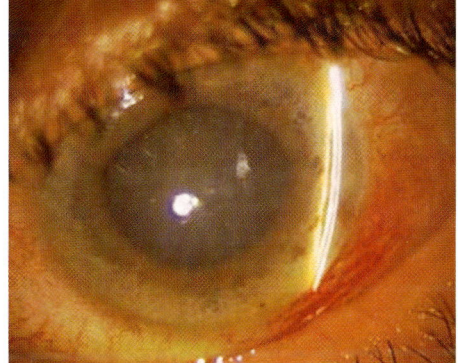

Fig. 3.14: *Non-inflammatory stromal oedema*

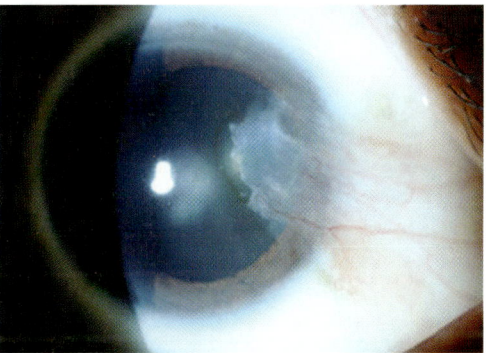

Fig. 3.16: *Stocker's line in pterygium*

Corneal filaments

Strands of mucus admixed with epithelium, attached at one end to the corneal surface, that stain well with rose bengal (Fig. 3.17). The unattached end moves with each blink. Filaments are seen in:

- Keratoconjunctivitis sicca
- Superior limbic keratoconjunctivitis
- Recurrent erosions
- Exposure keratitis
- Eye patching.

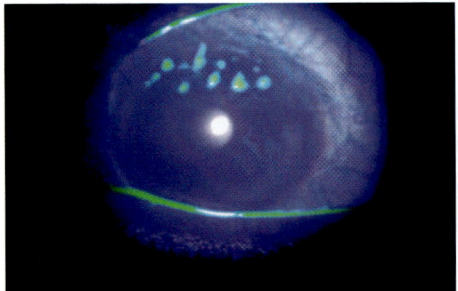

Fig. 3.17: *Corneal filaments*

Enlarged corneal nerves

Prominent corneal nerves are seen in (Fig. 3.18):
- Multiple endocrine neoplasia type IIb
- Keratoconus
- Neurofibromatosis type 1
- Refsum disease
- Congenital glaucoma.

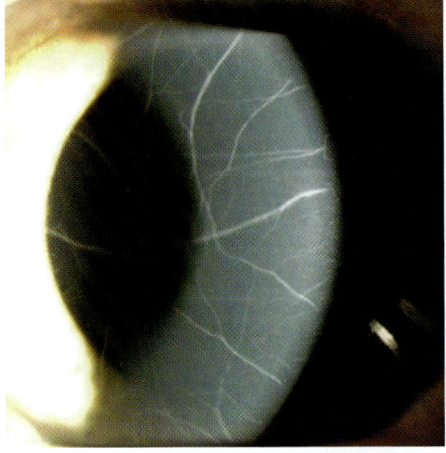

Fig. 3.18: *Enlarged corneal nerves*

- Leprosy
- Primary amyloidosis
- Hereditary icthyosis
- Idiopathic
- Acanthamoeba keratitis
- Failed corneal graft.

Whorl keratopathy

Arrangement of yellow golden deposits in whorl pattern (also called Cat-Whisker's keratopathy is seen in (Fig. 3.19):
- Amiodarone
- Atovaquone
- Chloroquine
- Chlorpromazine
- Indomethacin
- Fabry disease.

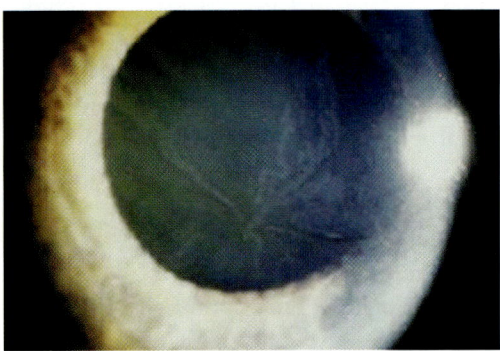

Fig. 3.19: *Whorl keratopathy*

Band keratopathy

Peripheral interpalpebral calcification leaving an area of clear limbus (Fig. 3.20).

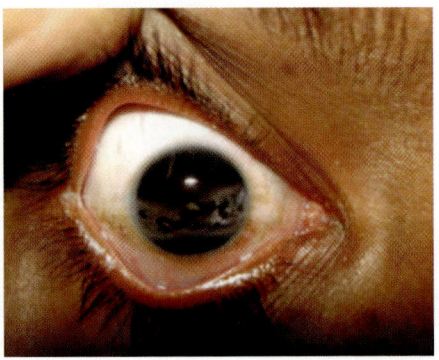

Fig. 3.20: *Band keratopathy*

Ocular causes are:
- Chronic iridocyclitis
- Phthisis bulbi
- Silicone oil in anterior chamber.

Metabolic causes are:
- Increased calcium and phosphorous product
- Gout
- Chronic renal failure
- Hereditary icthyosis.

Nummular keratitis

Large multiple coin lesions surrounded by halo of stromal haze (Fig. 3.21)
- Herpes zoster ophthalmicus
- Epstein-Barr virus infection
- Lyme disease
- Onchocerciasis
- Brucellosis.

Interstitial keratitis (Fig. 3.22)
- Herpes simplex/herpes zoster
- Mumps
- Syphilis
- Tuberculosis
- Leprosy
- Lyme disease
- Cogan syndrome.

Encroachment from conjunctiva over cornea
- Pterygium (Fig. 3.23)
- Dermoid

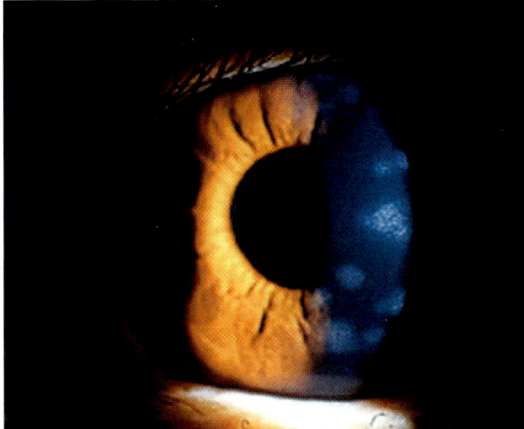

Fig. 3.21: *Nummular keratitis*

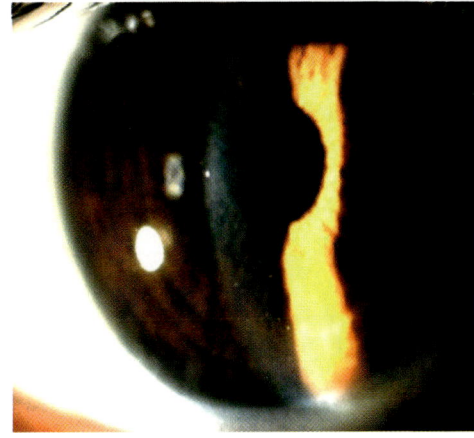

Fig. 3.22: *Interstitial keratitis*

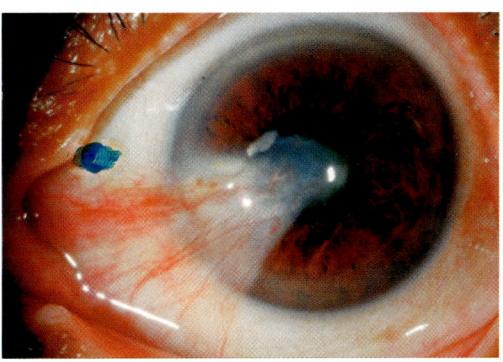

Fig. 3.23: *Pterygium*

- Phlyctenular keratoconjunctivitis
- Large glaucoma bleb.

SLIT-LAMP EXAMINATION TECHNIQUES FOR CORNEA

Slit-lamp examination is an essential technique for examining the cornea. Normal cornea has structures which refract and scatter light. Pathological processes tend to produce irregularities which are even more obvious.

- *Direct illumination*
  - Diffuse illumination
  - Focal illumination
- *Indirect illumination*
  - Sclerotic scatter
  - Retroillumination
- *Specular reflection.*

Diffuse broad-beam illumination

The wide beam provides diffuse illumination such as would be obtained from the illumination provided by a penlight or muscle light. It is used to perform a general inspection of the anterior segment and adnexal structures under magnification (Fig. 3.24).

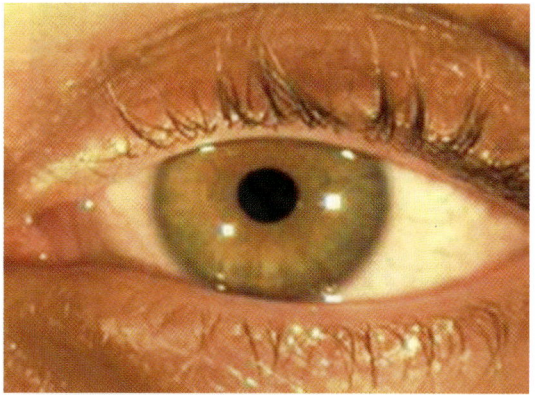

Fig. 3.24: *Diffuse broad-beam illumination*

Applications
- Examination of sclera
- Assessment of the tear film (qualitative and quantitative)
- General observation of the surfaces of cornea and lens
- General survey of anterior segment
- Staining pattern of the ocular surface
- Assessment of contact lenses fitting.

Focal illumination

Direct focal illumination or 'slit-beam' illumination provides an optical section or parallelopiped view from light angled (not coaxial) through tissue with a bright, thin beam with lower magnification to visualise anterior chamber (AC) depth and higher magnification to visualise corneal depth and pathology (Fig. 3.25).

Applications
- To determine the depth or elevation of a defect of the cornea, conjunctiva.
- To detect changes in corneal and conjunctival thickness.
- To examine epithelial surface pathologies like intraepithelial cysts and bullae.
- To assess depths of foreign bodies, scars and opacities.

Indirect illumination

This mode of illumination enhances contrast during visualisation of defects at various levels of the cornea. Indirect modes of illumination are retroillumination and sclerotic scatter.

Retroillumination
- It is the technique of visualising structures against an illuminated background.
- The beam of light, directed at a location more posterior than the object of interest, is reflected and viewed in its return pathway toward the examiner.

There are two types of retroillumination:

a. *Direct retroillumination* caused by direct reflection at surfaces such as the iris, crystalline lens or the fundus (Fig. 3.26).

b. *Indirect retroillumination* caused by diffuse reflection in the medium, i.e. at all scattering media and surfaces in the anterior and posterior segments (Fig. 3.27).

The common findings include:

Cornea: Vascularizations, microcysts, vacuoles, oedema, deposits like amyloid, particles in tear film, defect or folds in the Descemet's membranes, keratic precipitates.

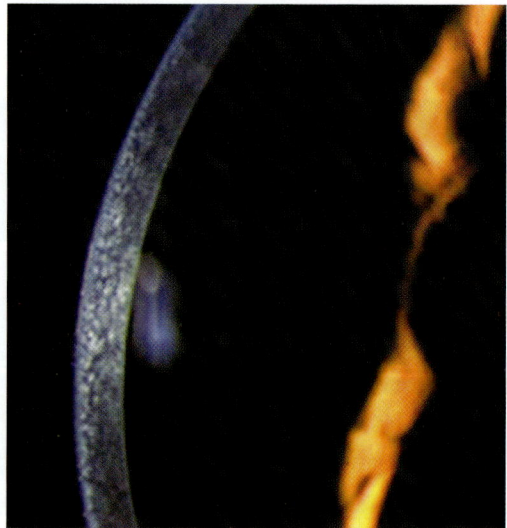

Fig. 3.25: *Focal illumination*

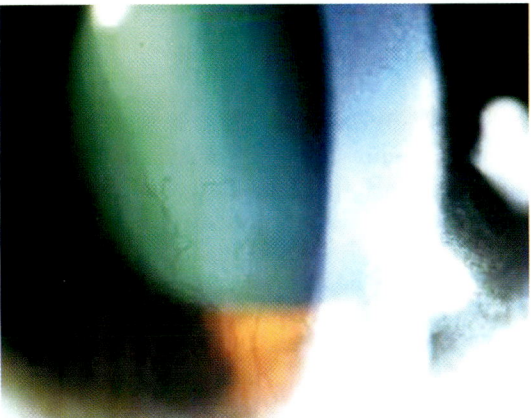

Fig. 3.26: *Direct retroillumination*

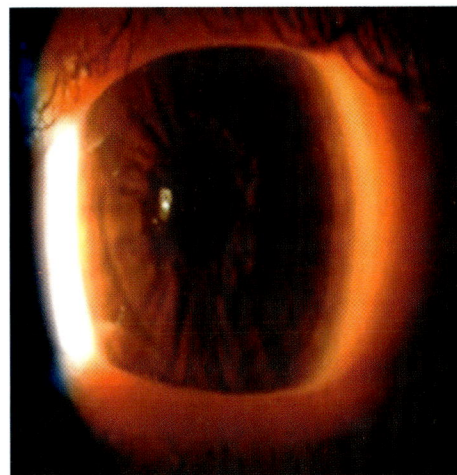

Fig. 3.28: *Sclerotic scatter*

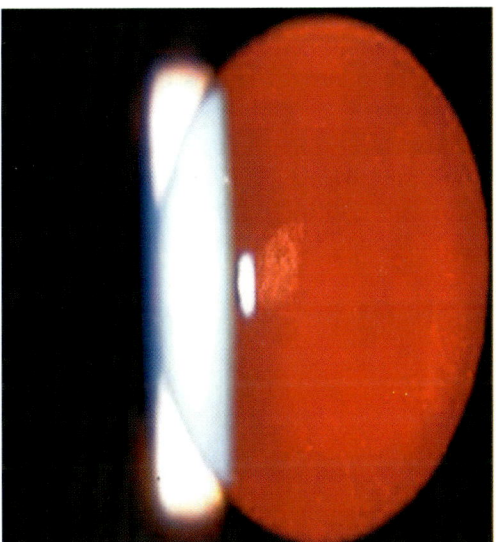

Fig. 3.27: *Indirect retroillumination*

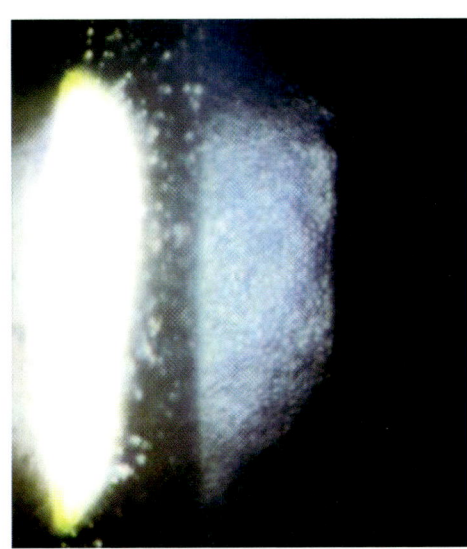

Fig. 3.29: *Specular reflection*

Sclerotic scatter

- Sclerotic scatter is used to detect subtle epithelial or stromal irregularities (Fig. 3.28).
- It is performed by directing the light beam tangentially towards the limbus until the entire limbal circumference appears to glow.

Specular reflection

- Specular reflection is derived from the German word *Spiegel* or 'mirror-like' reflection in contrast to scattered light.
- It is used to evaluate the corneal endothelium (Fig. 3.29).

- It relies on the difference in refractive indices between the two media producing reflection at the interface.

Applications

- To evaluate the endothelial cells for size and shape.
- To identify the irregularities in the Descemet's membrane, e.g. guttata in early diagnosis of Fuchs' endothelial dystrophy.
- Pigment deposits and keratic precipitates on the endothelium.

DIAGNOSTIC DYES USED IN CORNEAL DISEASES

FLUORESCEIN DYE

- The fluorescein molecule emits green light (520 nm) when it is excited by cobalt blue filter (490 nm).
- Nontoxic to corneal epithelium and is taken up in areas in which disruption of cell-cell junctions exist or epithelium is absent completely.
- It is useful in the documentation of corneal epithelial defects resulting from abrasion or active herpetic infection (Fig. 3.30).
- The observed patterns can often provide clues toward determining the etiology of disease. For example, exposure keratopathy typically results in fluorescein uptake in the interpalpebral space, whereas a toxic keratopathy (such as after chemical exposure) most often results in diffuse uptake across the entire cornea.
- True staining should be distinguished from pooling, in which the fluorescein collects in depressions on the ocular surface but is not taken up because of the presence of an intact epithelium.
- 'Negative' staining can also occur and refers to the pattern of fluorescein collection around elevated lesions on the surface of the eye.
- In the Seidel test, fluorescein is also used to demonstrate wound leakage by providing a fluorescent background through which streams of aqueous are revealed.

ROSE BENGAL

- Unlike fluorescein, rose bengal exhibits toxicity *in vitro*, but is considered safe for clinical applications. It is a derivative of the fluorescein molecule and stains devitalised epithelial cells and healthy epithelial cells when they are not protected by a healthy layer of mucin (Fig. 3.31).
- Accordingly, severe tear film abnormalities result in rose bengal, but not fluorescein, staining.
- The two dyes may be used consecutively to provide a more complete assessment of the integrity of the ocular surface. As with fluorescein, rose bengal comes concentrated on paper strips.
- Unlike fluorescein, however, it is nonfluorescent, and so can be viewed in direct light, and is irritating to the patient, usually requiring application of topical anaesthetic.

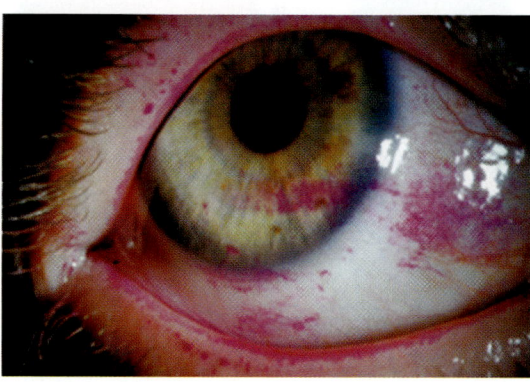

Fig. 3.31: *Rose bengal staining*

LISSAMINE GREEN

- Lissamine green offers many of the same applications as rose bengal, and its patterns of distribution are observed and recorded with white light (Fig. 3.32).
- It similarly stains with rose bengal (dead and degenerated cells as well as disrupted cell-cell junctions) but produces much less irritation.

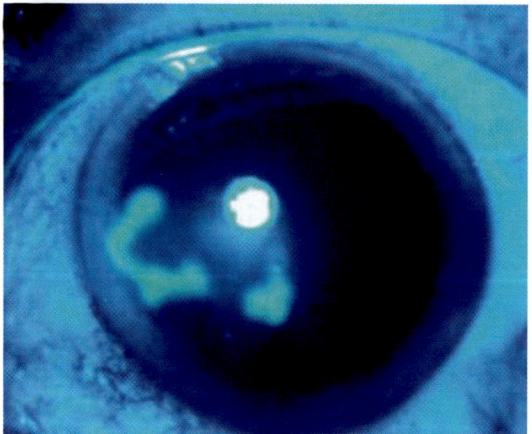

Fig. 3.30: *Fluorescein dye staining*

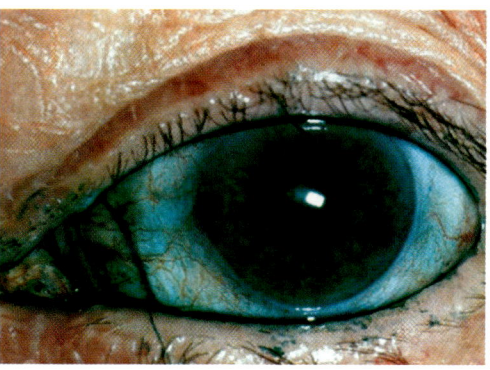

Fig. 3.32: *Lissamine green staining*

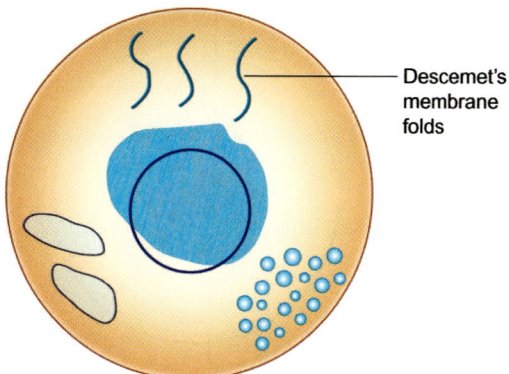

Fig. 3.33B: *Wavy lines to document Descemet's membrane folds*

CORNEAL DRAWING WITH COLOUR CODING

Clinical signs should be illustrated with a colour-coded labelled diagram, including lesion dimensions, is particularly useful to facilitate monitoring.

Documentation of corneal signs

Black
- Limbus
- Scars
- Degenerations/deposits/guttate
- Foreign bodies
- Sutures
- Contact lens
- Band keratopathy.

Blue
- Fine blue circles for epithelial oedema (Fig. 3.33A)

- Wavy lines to document Descemet's membrane folds (Fig. 3.33B)
- Blue shading for stromal oedema.

Brown
- Pigmentation—iron or melanin
- Pupil and iris
- Peripheral anterior synechiae.

Red
- Blood vessels are added in red. Superficial vessels are wavy lines that begin outside the limbus and deep vessels are straight lines that begin at the limbus (Fig. 3.34).
- Filaments
- Rose bengal staining
- Haemorrhages
- Hyphaema.

Yellow
- Infiltrate (Fig. 3.35)
- Hypopyon (Fig. 3.36)

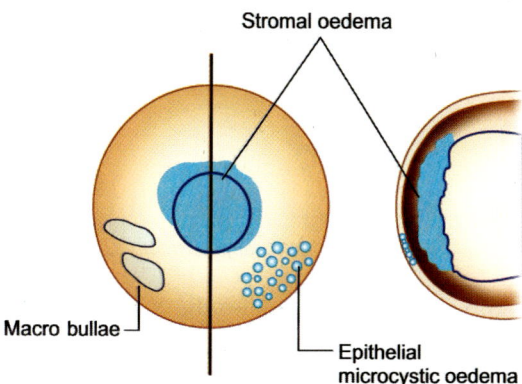

Fig. 3.33A: *Blue circles for epithelial oedema*

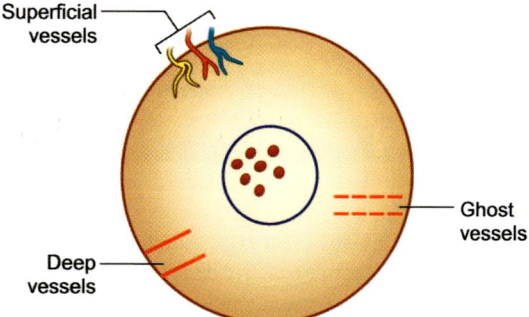

Fig. 3.34: *Red colour to document blood vessels*

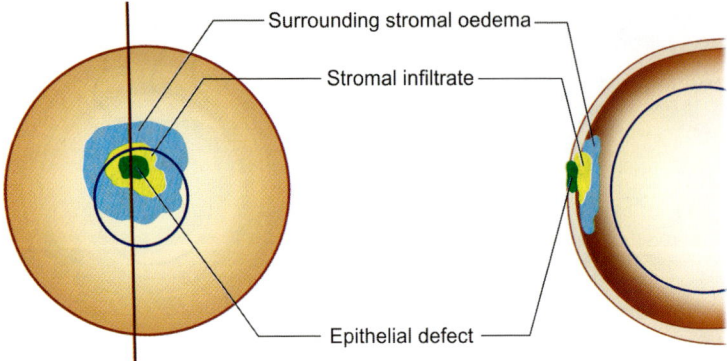

Fig. 3.35: *Yellow colour to document corneal infiltrate*

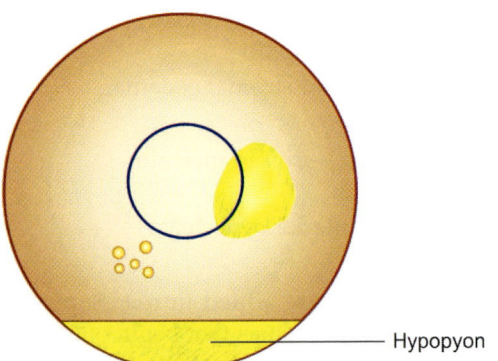

Fig. 3.36: *Yellow colour to document corneal hypopyon*

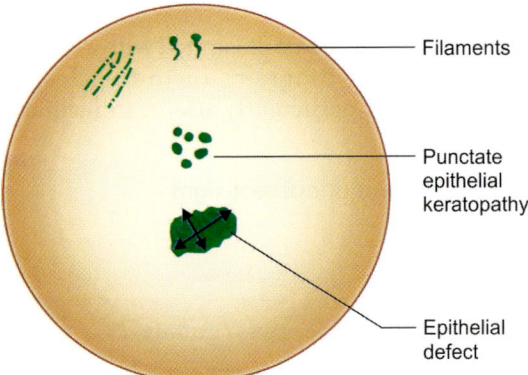

Fig. 3.37: *Green colour to document filaments and epithelial defect*

- Keratic precipitates
- Nuclear sclerosis.

Green
- Fluorescein stain
- Superficial punctate keratitis (SPK)
- Epithelial defect (Fig. 3.37)
- Filaments
- Vitreous.

INVESTIGATIVE TECHNIQUES FOR CORNEAL DISEASES

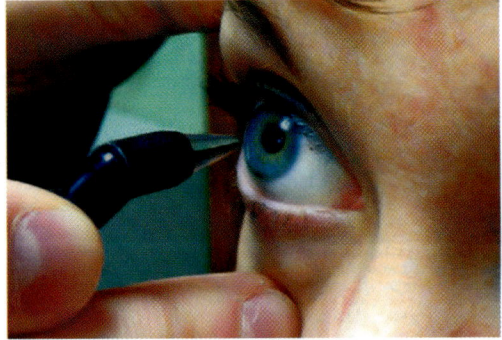

Fig. 3.38: *Corneal pachymetry*

PACHYMETRY

Pachymetry (Greek words: *Pachos* = thick + *metry* = to measure) is the term used for the measurement of corneal thickness (Fig. 3.38). It is an important indicator of the health status of the cornea especially of corneal endothelial pump function. It estimates the corneal barrier and endothelial pump function. It also measures the corneal rigidity and consequently has an impact on the accuracy of intraocular pressure (IOP) measurement by applanation tonometry.

The normal corneal thickness varies from central to peripheral limbus. It ranges from 0.7 to 0.9 mm at the limbus and varies between 0.49 and 0.56 mm at the centre. The central corneal thickness (CCT) reading of 0.7 mm or more is indicative of endothelial decompensation. The mean CCT as shown by various studies is 0.51–0.52 mm. Peripheral corneal thickness is asymmetric so that temporal cornea is thinnest followed by the inferior cornea.

Applications

Corneal thickness evaluation has an important role in the following clinical situations:

Glaucoma for applying correction factor in actual intraocular pressure (IOP) determination.

Congenital glaucoma to assess the amount of corneal oedema.

Refractive surgeries. (a) Preoperative screening, and (b) treatment plan of keratorefractive procedures like LASIK, astigmatic keratotomy, and previously even prior to radial keratotomy.

Postoperative follow-up of keratoplasty patients to determine endothelial cell function and its recovery and to become alert to early graft decompensation.

Contact lens to assess corneal oedema and in orthokeratology.

Assessing the thinness of the cornea as in corneal disorders like Terrien's and pellucid marginal degenerations, keratoconus, keratoglobus, post-LASIK ectasia.

Other cases of corneal decompensation. For monitoring and evaluating corneal oedema and endothelial function as in herpetic endotheliitis.

Techniques of pachymetry

Techniques for measuring CCT include optical pachymetry, ultrasound pachymetry, confocal microscopy, ultrasound biomicroscopy, optical ray path analysis or scanning slit corneal topography, and optical coherence tomography.

For further details, *see* Chapter 9.

KERATOMETRY

It is also known as ophthalmometry. It is used to measure the radius of curvature of the anterior surface of the cornea (Fig. 3.39). It should be perform to know if there is any change is caused to the eye due to the fit of the contact lens. It is useful in monitoring the changes in the curvature in corneal ectatic disorders. However, unfortunately, if the curvature changes are significant, it is difficult to measure it in advance stages through keratometer. It plays a major role in calculating intraocular lens power and because of its low cost and ease of use it is widely used.

Clinical uses of keratometry

- Objective method for determining curvature of the cornea
- To estimate the amount and direction of corneal astigmatism
- The ocular biometry for the IOL power calculation
- To monitor pre- and post-surgical astigmatism
- Differential diagnosis of axial versus refractive anisometropia
- To diagnose and monitor keratoconus and other corneal diseases.
- For contact lens fitting by base curve selection
- To detect rigid gas permeable lens flexure.

For details of techniques and interpretations of keratometry, *see* Chapter 9.

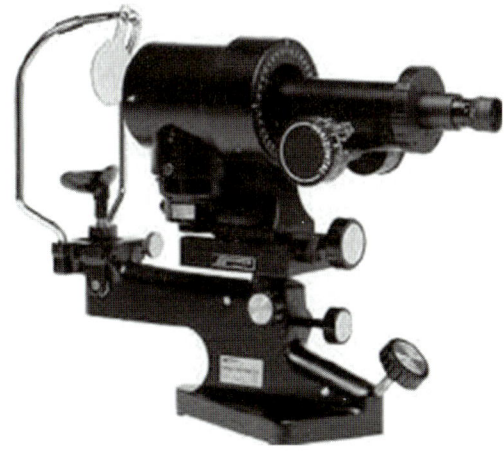

Fig. 3.39: *Keratometer (Bausch and Lomb type)*

CORNEAL TOPOGRAPHY

The cornea is the most important refractive element of the human eye, providing approximately two-thirds of its optical power (Fig. 3.40). Detailed examination of the corneal curvature is an essential part of the work-up before refractive surgery, for fitting of contact lens and for diagnosis and management of ectatic disorders. Keratometry was one of the earliest methods for measuring corneal shape. However, it gives limited information about corneal shape and appreciates only gross amount of astigmatism. These limitations led to the development of more advanced techniques for evaluating corneal shape. Three types of systems are used to measure corneal topography: Placido based, elevation based and interferometric. Recently Scheimpflug imaging has become increasingly popular.

Indications

Common indications for corneal topography in practice are:

I. *Refractive surgery patients*
   - Preoperative assessment
   - Postoperative follow-up
   - For augmentation procedures.
II. *Diagnostic indication*
   - Screening for ocular disease
   - Corneal ectasia
   - Contact lens-induced corneal warpage.

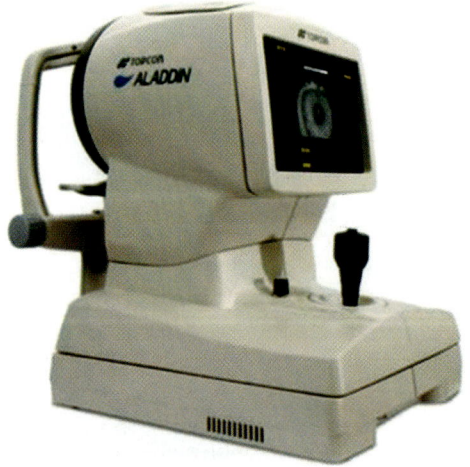

Fig. 3.40: *Corneal topographer*

- Planning surgical incision (cataract, astigmatic keratotomy). Incision location, length, depth
- Contact lens fitting in irregular corneas
- Intraocular lens power calculation in special situations
- Management of astigmatism. Adjustment of incisions or sutures
- Keratoplasty follow-up.

For details of techniques and interpretation of corneal topography, *see* Chapter 10.

CONFOCAL MICROSCOPY

Confocal microscopy is a bioimaging technique which allows non-invasive *in vivo* analysis of corneal microstructure and function (Fig. 3.41). It creates sharp images of a specimen that would otherwise appear blurred when viewed with a conventional microscope. This is achieved by excluding most of light from the specimen that is not from microscope's focal plane. It has been used to investigate numerous corneal diseases: Epithelial changes, stromal degenerative or dystrophic diseases, endothelial pathologies, corneal deposits, infections and traumatic lesions.

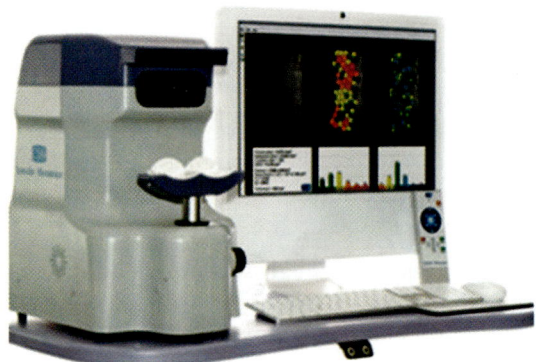

Fig. 3.41: *Confocal microscope*

Confocal microscopes: prototypes

There are three different types that are used clinically in ophthalmology:

1. Tandem scanning confocal microscope
2. Slit scanning confocal microscope
3. Confocal laser scanning microscope.

Confocal microscopy of the normal human cornea

Superficial cells are seen with clear visible cell borders, bright cytoplasm and black nuclei. These cells are characteristically polygonal, usually hexagonal in shape. The intermediate layer of wing cells comprises cells smaller than the superficial cells, with bright cell borders and dark cytoplasm. These cells are fairly uniform in size and shape. The basal epithelial cells are located just above the Bowman's membrane and are seen as a distinct mosaic with light cell boundaries. The basal epithelial cells are the smallest cells in the epithelium. The Bowman's layer appears as a homogenous acellular layer and nerve fibres of the subepithelial nerve plexus are seen as beaded nerve fibres. Keratocyte nuclei are identified as bright reflections in the stroma. The anterior stromal keratocyte nuclei are more abundant and oval compared to the posterior keratocyte nuclei which are less abundant and more oblong in shape. Endothelial cells are visible as bright cell bodies and dark cell boundaries, characteristically hexagonal in shape with fairly uniform appearance in size and shape.

Applications

- *Detection and management of infectious keratitis:* Viral, bacterial, parasitic (Acanthamoeba), and fungal.
- *Detection and management of corneal dystrophies:* Fuchs' endothelial dystrophy, lattice dystrophy, epithelial basement membrane dystrophy, granular dystrophy, and corneal stem cell deficiency.
- *Monitoring contact lens-induced corneal changes*
- *Pre- and post-refractive surgery assessment:* LASIK and LASEK flap evaluations and radial keratotomy.
- *Monitoring corneal grafts* with the capability to distinguish between corneal oedema due to corneal graft rejection (caused by presence of inflammatory cells) and endothelial decomposition (caused by low endothelial cell counts without presence of inflammatory cells).
- *Conjunctival and limbal structures may be monitored* for cysts, inflammation and proliferation of cells. Edges of healing blebs may also be monitored.
- *Endothelial cell counting capabilities.* With for a semiautomated cell count of any layer in the cornea. Monitoring of cell densities anywhere from epithelium to endothelium may be done.
- *Corneal thickness*/flap thickness measurement.

For details of technique and interpretation of confocal micorscopy, *see* Chapter 8.

SPECULAR MICROSCOPY

Specular microscopy is a noninvasive photographic technique that allows to visualise and analyse the corneal endothelium (Fig. 3.42). Using computer-assisted morphometry, modern specular microscopes analyse the size, shape and population of the endothelial cells. The instrument projects light onto the cornea and captures the image that is reflected from the optical interface between the corneal endothelium and the aqueous humour. The reflected image is analysed by the instrument and displayed as a specular photomicrograph. In clinical practice, specular microscopy is the most accurate way to examine the corneal

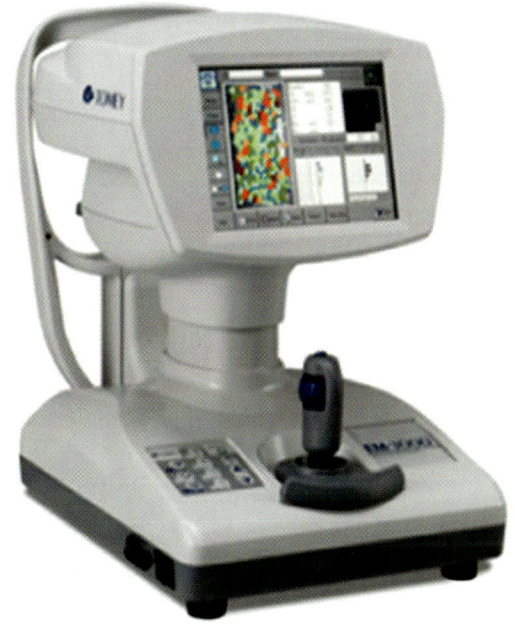

Fig. 3.42: *Specular microscope*

endothelium. The young normal corneal endothelium, as seen by specular microscopy shows a quasi-regular array of hexagonal cells, all having nearly the same size.

Analysis of specular microscopy

Quantitative analysis

Cell density. Means number of cells counted per mm square. Normal endothelial cell density decreases with age, it being 3500 cells/mm² in children and gradually declining to about 2000 cells/mm² in older eyes. An average value for adults is 2400 cells/mm² (1500–3500) with a mean cell size of 150–350 μm. Corneas with low cell density (fewer than 1000 cells/mm²) might not tolerate intraocular surgery.

Coefficient of variation. The mean cell area divided by the standard deviation of mean cell area, normally less than 0.30.

Qualitative analysis

Pleomorphism means asymmetry in cell shape. **Polymegathism** means asymmetry in cell size.

Causes of polymegathism
- Long-term contact lens wear
- Postcataract surgery
- Postpenetrating keratoplasty
- Keratoconus
- Ageing
- Diabetes.

Clinical applications
- Preoperative assessment of the donor cornea
- Corneal oedema
- Corneal degenerations
- Corneal dystrophies
- Ocular inflammation
- Contact lens endotheliopathy
- Early diagnosis of Fuchs' endothelial dystrophy
- Various refractive surgical procedures
- Bullous keratopathy
- Keratoconus
- Recurrent corneal erosions
- Corneal dystrophy
- Corneal ectasia

- Postcorneal transplant
- Glaucoma
- Evaluation of donor corneal endothelium and the effect of preservation (eye banking).

For details, *see* Chapter 8.

ANTERIOR SEGMENT OCT

Anterior segment optical coherence tomography (ASOCT) produces high-resolution, three-dimensional cross-sectional images of the anterior segment that uses low coherence interferometry to achieve axial resolution in the range of 3–20 μm (Fig. 3.43). The principle of OCT is analogous to ultrasound, but it uses light instead of sound. It is a completely non-invasive technique. As it uses interferometry for depth resolution, it can have a long working distance and a wide field of transverse scanning compared to confocal microscopy. Its applications are being expanded and now include pachymetry, corneal topography, ectatic corneal disorders, microbial keratitis, keratoplasty, corneal opacity, intrastromal corneal ring segments, anterior chamber biometry, corneal implants, anterior chamber tumours and refractive surgery.

Applications of anterior segment optical coherence tomography

1. Measuring corneal thickness: Central corneal thickness is important for planning and performing refractive surgery, for assessing corneal diseases as well as monitoring glaucoma progression in patients with ocular hypertension and primary open-angle glaucoma.

2. Corneal topography. For details, *see* Chapter 10.

3. Ectatic corneal disorders. ASOCT is important for diagnosis and management of corneal ectatic disorders like keratoconus, Terrien's

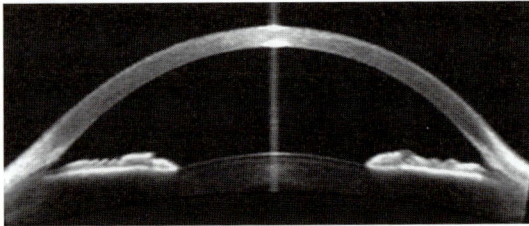

Fig. 3.43: *Anterior segment OCT*

marginal degeneration and pellucid marginal degeneration and their complication, especially in acute hydrops and its monitoring. Although moderate to advanced keratoconus is easily recognized by the characteristic topographic pattern and classic clinical signs, it can be difficult to distinguish subclinical forms of disease from normal corneas, because patients usually present with normal visual acuity, stable topographic patterns and minimal or no clinical signs. In these cases, OCT produces highly reliable pachymetry map, that can detect keratoconus, ectasia and corneal thinning conditions before refractive laser surgeries.

4. Microbial keratitis. OCT can also be used for corneal imaging and assessment, in conjunction with slit-lamp biomicroscopy in cases of microbial keratitis to monitor progression of the disease. OCT can be particularly useful in assessing the depth of corneal ulcers. The affected area of keratitis is represented by the OCT as higher intense regions. In deciding the response of a certain keratitis to treatment, the OCT images can be followed by examining the depth and density of these affected areas. When indicated, the area for corneal biopsy can be ascertained by identifying the densest areas of infiltration. Areas of impending perforation and severe thinning can also be imaged on ASOCT. Decision on performing either lamellar keratoplasty or full-thickness penetrating keratoplasty can be made by examining the depth of infection on the ASOCT images.

5. OCT for corneal transplantation. The anterior segment optical coherence tomography is useful in the preoperative and postoperative evaluation and management of corneal transplant patients. Recent advances in lamellar keratoplasty have made it an attractive alternative to conventional full-thickness penetrating keratoplasty (PKP). These have led to the development of customized component surgery, which involves targeted replacement of diseased corneal tissue while retaining healthy layers. Corneal surgeons have used anterior lamellar keratoplasty techniques, such as deep anterior lamellar keratoplasty (DALK), to manage conditions affecting the anterior layers. Nearly

all corneal stromal can be removed with retention of Descemet's membrane and host endothelium, eliminating the risk of endothelial rejection. In endothelial keratoplasty procedures, such as Descemet's stripping endothelial keratoplasty, the AS-OCT can be used to determine donor graft thickness, graft attachment, positioning, interface issues and donor configuration. Similarly, it is useful to detect presence of a pseudo-AC following deep anterior lamellar keratoplasty in the early postoperative period.

6. Accurate measurement of opacities and rings. AS-OCT scanning allows surgeons to accurately determine the depth of corneal opacities, enabling them to choose the most appropriate treatment: Excimer laser or lamellar or penetrating keratoplasty. Insertion of shallow intrastromal corneal ring segments increases the incidence of epithelial and stromal breakdown and ring extrusion. AS-OCT can assess the depth and position of intracorneal rings to determine the risk of extrusion.

7. Anterior chamber biometry. The accurate measurement of anterior chamber dimensions is important prior to implanting refractive phakic IOLs. The anterior segment optical coherence tomography produces. High-resolution images with accurate and reproducible biometry including AC depth, angle-to-angle width and iris profile, although sulcus to sulcus distance is unable to be accurately measured. This assists preoperatively in choosing the appropriate sized IOL, as well as examining the *in vivo* position of the phakic IOL, that is, its relationship to the endothelium, crystalline lens, trabecular meshwork and iris. This is critical to avoid complications of phakic IOL insertion, such as lens endothelial touch and angle closure glaucoma. The anterior segment optical coherence tomography is able to measure these AC parameters accurately, directly and in all meridians as compared to conventional white-to-white measurements.

8. Corneal implants: The anterior segment optical coherence tomography is able to accurately determine the depth and position of intrastromal ring segments, such as INTACS and

KeraRings. These are crescent-shaped segments of polymethylmethacrylate that have been used for the treatment of post-LASIK corneal ectasias, pellucid marginal degeneration and keratoconus. Implanting intacs at the proper depth is important for good visual outcome and to avoid complications, such as extrusion. Similarly, the AS-OCT can be used to image corneal inlays for the treatment of presbyopia, such as the Presbylens.

9. Anterior segment tumours: Anterior iris pathology can be imaged by AS-OCT and is able to differentiate small cystic from solid lesions. It can image small non-pigmented tumours but cannot penetrate larger tumours, pigmented tumours or tumours involving the ciliary body. Visualisation of the posterior chamber is suboptimal as the infrared light is significantly attenuated by the iris pigment epithelium.

10. Laser-assisted *in situ* keratomileusis and other refractive surgeries. Imaging of the corneal layers with high speed OCT provide useful information relevant to keratorefractive surgery, especially in laser *in situ* keratomileusis (LASIK). Corneal flap thickness is an important parameter in LASIK because it determines the amount of residual stroma available for ablation. By directly measuring corneal flap thickness intraoperatively, it can potentially improve the predictability of LASIK. Owing to superior resolution of morphological features, it can also be used for postoperative assessment of the anatomical correlates of the refractive outcome. It can also provide the comprehensive pachymetry map of the entire cornea and helps in the detection of normal from abnormally thin corneas in which subtractive refractive surgery like LASIK may need to be avoided.

Advantages of AS-OCT

- It is a non-contact method therefore do not cause indentation of the angle by placement of the scleral cup on the eye (which is required to maintain the water bath in UBM). Also, no possibility of corneal abrasion or punctate epithelial erosions (possible with UBM).
- Shorter imaging time (patient set-up in UBM takes longer. Also, only one angle is imaged at a time with the UBM).

- Rapid image acquisition. Eight frames can be captured per second, allowing operator to choose the best centred image.
- Requires less expertise to perform—small learning curve for the operator.
- Target may be used to induce accommodation in the eye being imaged (this is especially useful in the evaluation of accommodative intraocular lenses).
- More comfortable for the patient, due to non-contact technique, upright position and rapid imaging acquisition.

VIDEOKERATOGRAPHY

Keratorefractive surgery has been a powerful stimulus for the development of sophisticated systems for mapping extensible corneal shape (Fig. 3.44). Videokeratography involves system for image capture, surface reconstruction and data output. Image capture involves projection of an image onto the surface of the cornea and capture of the reflected image with a digital video camera. It provides both qualitative and quantitative information about the corneal surface. Surface reconstruction depends on edge detection software and algorithms for calculating corneal shape (usually expressed as dioptric power) from the image analysis. Data output can

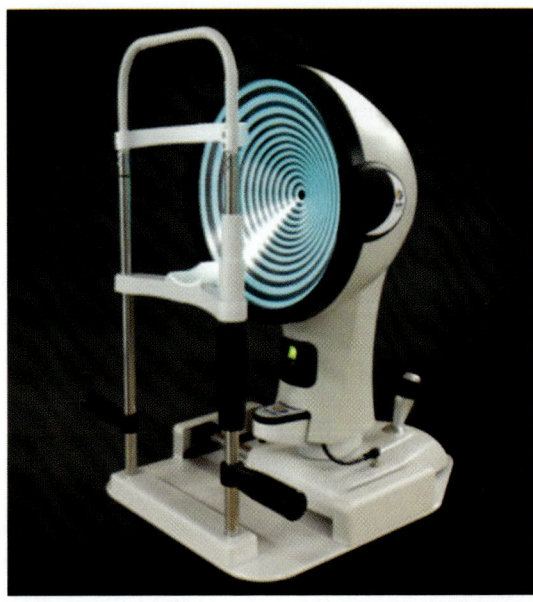

Fig. 3.44: *Videokeratography*

be in several forms, such as data tables, colour-coded curvature maps or wire mesh models. Furthermore, developments in videokeratography have revealed considerable irregular variation within individual corneas and from one person to another. There is a degree of symmetry from one eye to the contralateral eye. Corneal topographical maps have been likened to fingerprints, there being a similarity between apparently normal corneas but also distinct differences. Corneal topography may therefore be considered as another expression of the uniqueness of the individual. Not only are maps of the corneal surface unique to the individual, they vary with time, even in people without any evidence of corneal disease. The shape determined by videokeratography is a measure of optical power, with true physical shape being inferred. In most situations, it is the corneal refractive power which is of interest and progress in videokeratography has developed parallel to keratorefractive surgery. There is a growing movement in refractive surgery which considers minor changes in corneal topography as important limitations on visual potential and amenability to surgery.

Applications for videokeratography

- To screen patients prior to refractive surgery and evaluating them after surgery.
- To screen patients for irregular astigmatism, corneal warpage and keratoconus prior to refractive surgery.
- To evaluate the cornea after cataract surgery and to understand patients visual complaints.
- To direct management after penetrating keratoplasty.
- To plan astigmatic surgery.
- To fit contact lenses in patients with irregular astigmatism.
- To evaluate unexplained visual loss and to determine visual complications from corneal dystrophies, scars, pterygia, recurrent erosions, and chalazia.

CORNEAL AESTHESIOMETRY

Corneal aesthesiometry is important to examine cases involving the lesions of the fifth cranial nerve, cases with ulcerative keratitis and degenerative lesions.

Quantitative methods
- Cochet-Bonnet aesthesiometer
- Non-contact air puff technique
- Larson-Millodot aesthesiometer.

Handheld aesthesiometer (Cochet-Bonnet)

- The handheld aesthesiometer (Cochet-Bonnet) is a device that contains a thin, retractable, nylon monofilament that extends up to 6 cm in length (Fig. 3.45).
- Variable pressure can be applied by the device by adjusting the length. The monofilament ranges from 60 to 5 mm and as the length is decreased, the pressure increases from 11 to 200 mm/gm.
- If the filament is applied perpendicularly to the corneal surface, most patients will feel the nylon thread when it is extended to a full 6 cm.
- If the filament has to be shortened to 4 cm or less, the corneal sensation is inferred to have decreased.
- A value below 2 cm is diagnostic of significant hypoaesthesia.

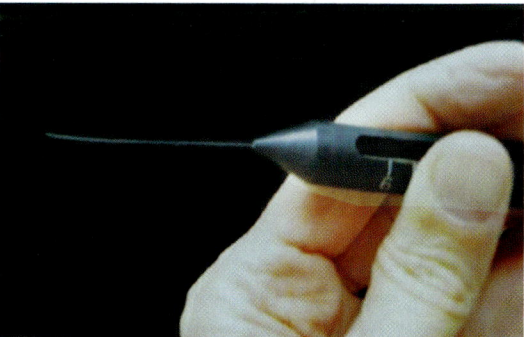

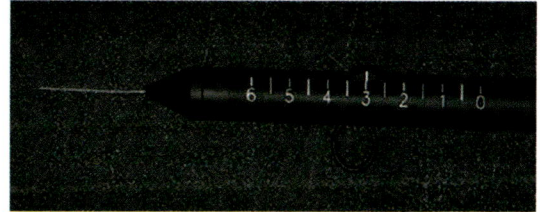

Fig. 3.45: *Cochet-Bonnet aesthesiometer*

Steps for using the handheld aesthesiometer are:

- Extend the filament to full length of 6 cm
- Retract the filament incrementally in 0.5 cm steps until the patient can feel its contact
- Record the length (the shorter the length indicates decreased sensation)
- Compare the fellow cornea
- Repeat steps 1–4 in each quadrant: Superior, temporal, inferior, nasal
- Sterilise the filament and retract back into the device to protect it from damage.

Limitations with this technique are that it is invasive, and can cause epithelial damage thereby producing an increased sensitivity due to the presence of free nerve endings within the corneal epithelium. Thus, the minimum stimulus is also suprathreshold and the range of stimulus intensity is limited. The bending of the thread under its own weight, particularly when the thread is long makes it difficult to make an accurate observation of the end-point. Subject apprehension also compromises the testing.

Non-contact air puff technique

- Uses controlled pulses of pressure of air to stimulate the cornea.
- It measures the corneal nerve threshold by using a composite stimulus consisting of air pressure, tear evaporation and disruption.
- An adjustable valve couples with a pressure sensor to control the output from a compressed air reservoir to within 0.01 mbar.
- The stimulus is applied to the eye through a stimulus jet comprising a brass tube of length 35 mm and diameter of 6 mm with a central 0.5 mm diameter longitudinal bore.
- The settings for stimulus duration that are available include 0.5, 0.9 and 1.5 seconds. A stimulus threshold of 0.9 mm has been recommended as standard setting presuming that a longer duration might result in corneal drying and shorter duration might be too quick for the subject's response.
- A slit-lamp attachment enables positioning the stimulus jet close to the eye examined. A clear plastic centimeter ruler attached to the mount enables setting the testing distance at 1 cm.

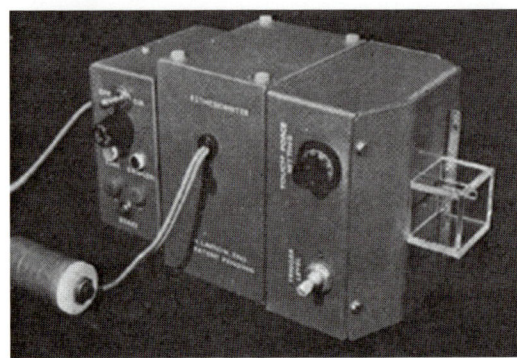

Fig. 3.46: *Larson-Millodot aesthesiometer*

- The stimulus jet is aligned to the center of the cornea.
- Testing is started with the application of suprathreshold stimulus and the patient usually responds describing it at a cold sensation or pressure type of sensation. On approaching the threshold, the stimuli may be difficult to describe.
- Measurements are made in millibars of air pressure required.

Larson-Millodot aesthesiometer

- In Larson-Millodot aesthesiometer (Fig. 3.46), the probe tip is made of fine platinum wire bent doubled so that the tip has known and reproducible dimensions.
- The probe is automatically advanced toward the eye at a constant rate upon the operator's command.
- When the cornea is touched with a force equal to the test force, the probe is retracted quickly and automatically.
- The force applied to the cornea can be set at any value within the range of this instrument and this force will not be exceeded.
- The range of settings for practical purposes is from 1 to 200 mg and any force within these limits can be set with an accuracy of ±5 mg operation.

TECHNIQUES FOR MICROBIOLOGICAL AND CYTOLOGICAL EVALUATION

The key for successful treatment of microbial keratitis relies on prompt and reliable detection of the causative microorganism with timely prescription of specifically targeted effective antimicrobial agent. Figure 3.47 summarises the microbiological evaluation of corneal scraping. The culture method with or without smears for staining is the gold standard for pathogen identification. Ideally, samples should be collected prior to the start of antibiotic treatment. Treatment can be initiated based on the results of smear examination and, if required modified in accordance with the culture and sensitivity results.

Sample collection devices

- Platinum spatula
- Surgical blade no. 15
- Calcium alginate swab.

Generally, the edge of the corneal ulceration rather than the central ulcer crater is the most suitable location for scraping since viable pathogens tend to be found at this point. After scraping, staining of smeared specimen should be performed to provide an early detection of the offending organism and can guide initial antimicrobial treatment.

Laboratory methods

Laboratory method is identification of bacteria, fungus, parasite, non-viral includes:

- Direct microscopy
- Culture and identification
- Molecular methods.

Direct microscopy. Stains used are:

Type of stain	Organisms
Gram stain	Bacteria (mainly), fungus and Acanthamoeba
KOH	Fungus (mainly), Acanthamoeba and Nocardia (Fig. 3.48)
Giemsa	Bacteria, fungi, Chlamydiae, Acanthamoeba
Acid fast	Mycobacterium, Nocardia
Acridine orange	Bacteria, fungi, Acanthamoeba
Calcoflour white	Fungus and Acanthamoeba

Culture and identification of pathogens

Corneal scraping with culture remains the gold standard for the diagnosis of suspected infectious keratitis. PCR may be used as a screening diagnosis test when microbial keratitis is suspected. Culture provides several key advantages including capture for organism identification and antimicrobial agent susceptibility testing.

Culture media: The standard culture media for suspected bacterial keratitis include blood agar, chocolate agar and thioglycolate broth (Fig. 3.49). For isolation of fungi, Sabouraud's dextrose agar (SDA) is commonly selected. Ocular specimens should be incubated in 5–7% CO_2 at 35°–37°C. The incubation period varies according to each species. For aerobic bacteria, the culture media should be kept for at least 7 days before discarding.

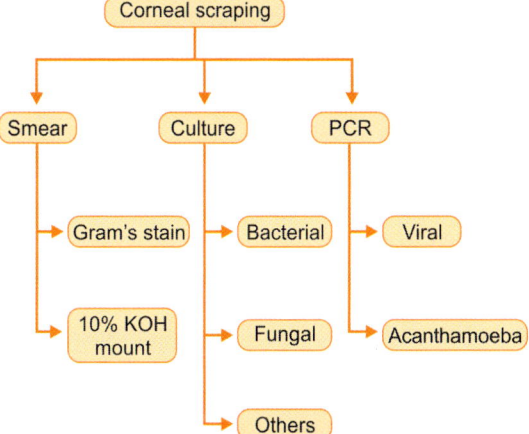

Fig. 3.47: *Microbiological evaluation of corneal scraping*

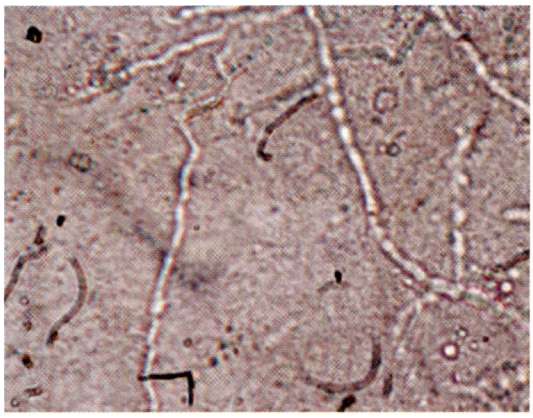

Fig. 3.48: *KOH mount showing hyphae*

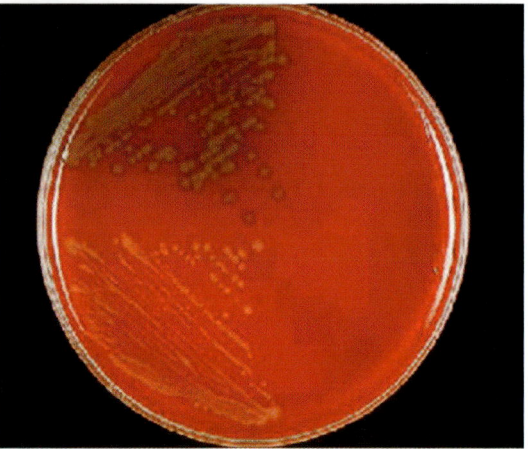

Fig. 3.49: *Blood agar culture plate*

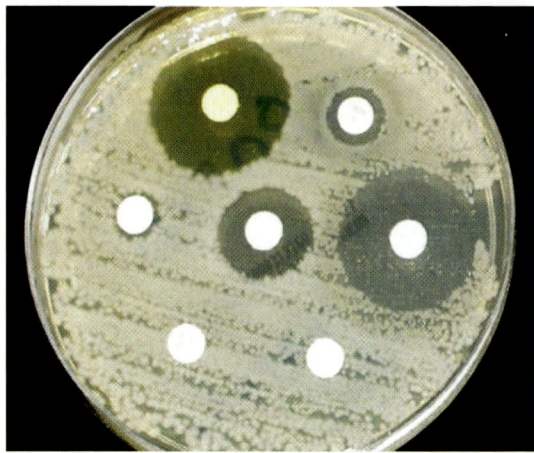

Fig. 3.50: *Antimicrobial susceptibility testing*

Media	Common isolates
Blood agar	Aerobic and facultative anaerobic bacteria
Chocolate agar	Aerobic and facultative anaerobic bacteria
Thioglycollate broth	Aerobic and facultative anaerobic bacteria
SDA	Fungi
Thayer-Martin agar	Pathogenic Neisseria
LJ media	Mycobacterium, Nocardia
Brain heart infusion broth	Fungi
Non-nutrient agar	Acanthamoeba seeded with *E. coli*

Antimicrobial susceptibility testing

Susceptibility testing is performed to determine the most effective antimicrobial agent available. Standard disc diffusion or microdilution techniques are the preferred laboratory methods for antimicrobial susceptibility testing against bacterial ocular isolates (Fig. 7.50). Antimicrobial containing disks are placed on the agar surface inoculated with a pure culture of the organism and antimicrobial susceptibility is determined.

Viral diagnostic testing

Different used methods to identify viral pathogens consist of viral culture, microscopy, antigen detection, nucleic acid detection and serology.

Viral culture followed by direct or indirect immunofluorescent antigen detection remains the gold standard of viral identification. Samples from corneal scrapings are placed on glass slides, then stained with hematoxylin and eosin. Tzanck, Giemsa, or Papanicolaou for light microscopic examination as an alternative option for possible diagnosis. The specimens for viral culture or PCR should be collected onto Dacron swabs and transported to the testing laboratory immediately. In addition, specimens should be kept moist and at 4°C during the transportation.

CORNEAL BIOPSY

Corneal biopsy is a useful procedure in the diagnosis and management of corneal inflammation, infections, degenerations, dystrophies and corneal manifestations of systemic diseases. Usually a partial thickness biopsy should be performed. Full-thickness biopsy should be reserved only for tectonic indications in advanced disease. It is indicated in cases with deep stromal abscess or in case where repeated culture shows negative reports but there is strong suspicion of infection. The cornea is anaesthetised and 0.2 to 0.3 mm trephine is used to outline the area to be biopsied. Usually a depth of about 0.1 to 0.2 mm is dissected out. The tissue is then sent for histopathological as well as microbiological analysis.

Indications

Infectious corneal processes

- Deep suppurative stromal keratitis
- Keratitis with atypical presentation
- Fungal or Acanthamoeba keratitis that does not respond to other treatment
- Culture negative keratitis.

Neoplastic. Conjunctival neoplasms with extension through limbus onto cornea.

Techniques

- Firstly, slit-lamp biomicroscopic examination should be performed. Depth of the infiltrate and overlying corneal thickness should be assessed.
- Keep the patient in supine position under operating microscope.
- Operating eye should be prepared and draped under all aseptic precautions.
- Insert the eye speculum.
- A sponge soaked in proparacaine should be placed on the limbus for 1–2 minutes so as to anaesthesise the eye.
- For a partial-thickness biopsy, trephination is performed with a small diameter punch (2–5 mm). The trephine is placed such that it includes the lesion as well as normal healthy cornea. The blade should be rotated back and forth between the thumb and forefinger.
- After trephination, careful dissection of the tissue is performed with a crescent blade, which is held flat against the cornea to prevent perforation. The corneal button must be grasped gently with the forceps to prevent crushing the tissue.

- After complete excision of the tissue, the biopsy specimen is transferred from the crescent blade to the appropriate transport media.
- Postoperatively, in the case of suspected microbial keratitis, the same antimicrobial regimen is continued.
- An antibiotic ointment may be added for comfort during the day- and at night-time.

Complications

Complications from biopsy include scarring, irregular astigmatism, poor or delayed healing and perforation.

BIBLIOGRAPHY

1. Basic and Clinical Science Course. External disease and cornea (2011–2012 edn.). American Academy of Ophthalmology. 2012.
2. Dua Harminder S, Faraj Lana A, Said Dalia G, Gray Trevor, Lowe James. "Human Corneal Anatomy Redefined". Ophthalmology 2013; 120(9): 1778–85.
3. Facts About the Cornea and Corneal Disease. National Eye Institute. Archived from the original on 2005; 03–27.
4. Huang AJW, Wichiensin P, Yang MC. Bacterial keratitis. Chapter 81. In: Krachmer JH, Mannis MH, Holland EJ: Cornea: Fundamental, Diagnosis and Management, NY, 2005; 1005–33.
5. Maurice, DM. "The structure and transparency of the cornea". J Physiol 1957; 136(2): 263–86.
6. Nottingham J. Practical observations on conical cornea: and on the short sight, and other defects of vision connected with it. London: J. Churchill, 1854.
7. Sachdev MS, Honavar SG, Thakar M. Diagnostic tests for corneal diseases. Indian J Ophthalmol 1994; 42: 89–99.

Chapter

4

Clinical Evaluation of the Ocular Surface

INTRODUCTION

All components of the ocular surface (cornea, the pre-corneal tear film, conjunctiva, lacrimal glands, and the eyelids) act as a single functional unit that not only preserves the quality of refractive surface of an eye, but protects it against injury and harmful effects of changing bodily/environmental conditions. The pre-corneal tear film is the most dynamic structure of this functional unit, and its production and turnover is essential in maintaining the health of the ocular surface.

Any event that disturbs the homeostasis of this functional unit results in a vicious cycle of a gradually worsening ocular surface disease. It may manifest as chronic punctate keratopathy, recurrent corneal erosions, filamentary keratitis, persistent/non-healing epithelial defect, infectious keratitis, non-healing corneal ulcer, bacterial conjunctivitis, culture-negative conjunctivitis, cicatrising conjunctivitis, corneal melting and ocular surface failure. Hence, it is important to assess all components of this functional unit, and to grade the severity of ocular surface disease at the initial presentation, so that an improvement with therapy can be objectively assessed.

OCULAR HISTORY

A detailed history of patient's presenting complaints, duration of symptoms, previous and current therapy, previous ocular disease and its treatment, general health, occupation is important. This will serve as a guide as to what investigations are necessary and what to look for while examining such a patient.

A patient may present with a myriad of symptoms like *ocular discomfort, moist or watery eyes, itching, redness, discharge, glare particularly while driving, floaters, hazy vision, asthenopia, headaches, pain, photophobia; these symptoms gradually worsen to cause severe blepharospasm that visually handicaps the patient. Therefore, any patient that presents with blepharospasm needs to be thoroughly examined for an underlying ocular surface disease.*

Similarly, blurring of vision, asthenopia and headaches are most commonly caused by ametropia or decompensated heterophoria, but they may also be caused by ocular surface disease (OSD).

SPECIFIC TESTS FOR OSD

In order to arrive at a proper diagnosis, to grade the severity of disease and to assess the efficacy of treatment, it is extremely important to quantify the baseline OSD before initiating any oral or topical medication. The therapy for OSD is long term, and specific parameters need to be monitored at each follow-up visit to assess how long the therapy needs to be continued.

Subjectively, symptoms are assessed by questionnaires regarding the patient's symptoms on a standardised form and their severity being graded/scored from 1–4. The patient needs to score the symptoms while sitting in the waiting room. At least 14 such questionnaires are available on the PubMed; the most commonly used and validated is the ocular surface disease index (OSDI) which comprises 32 questions. This form needs to be filled in by the patient at each follow-up visit too, and the clinician compares it with the one filled in at the first visit.

Since ocular surface is not just one structure, an objective assessment of all 6 structures is mandatory to arrive at an accurate clinical diagnosis. There is no single test that is sufficiently specific to permit an absolute diagnosis. All structures need to be examined in a systemic order.

1. GENERAL APPEARANCE OF THE PATIENT

Since OSD can be associated with autoimmune disorders that involve multiple body systems, e.g. rheumatoid arthritis, SLE, polyarteritis nodosa, sarcoidosis, thyroid eye disease, vitiligo, a patient's general symptoms, the therapy being taken and facial/body appearance needs to be assessed.

2. FACIAL APPEARANCE

- Examine the face and look for *brow droop* (Fig. 4.1): The eyebrows should be symmetrical and at the level of supraorbital rim in males while

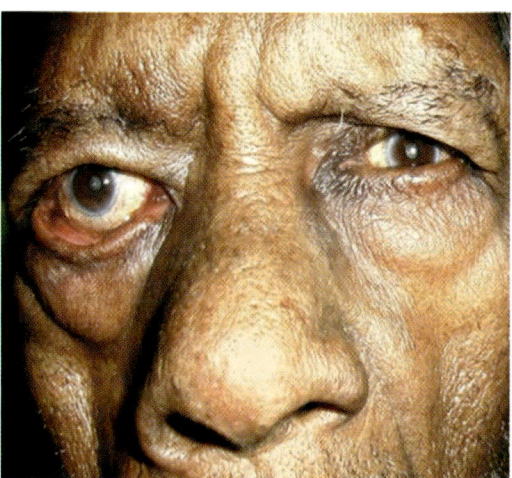

Fig. 4.1: *Right facial palsy with brow droop, dermatochalasis, ectropion lower lid, scleral show*

they are slightly above the supraorbital rim in females. If one eyebrow is kept higher by the patient with furrows on the forehead on that side, it means the patient is trying hard to lift up that eyelid to counteract ptosis.
- Assess the frequency of blinking. Increased frequency of blinking is an important sign of ocular irritation, anxiety, and OSD.
- Look for and try picking up excess skin between the brow and upper lid. This excessive lax skin (dermatochalasis) occurs with old age, frequently rubbing of eyes, following lid oedema. It may give the false impression of a ptosis or entropion of the upper lid.
- Presence of *blepharospasm* (Fig. 4.2) should be noted, whether it is localised to the eyelids, or

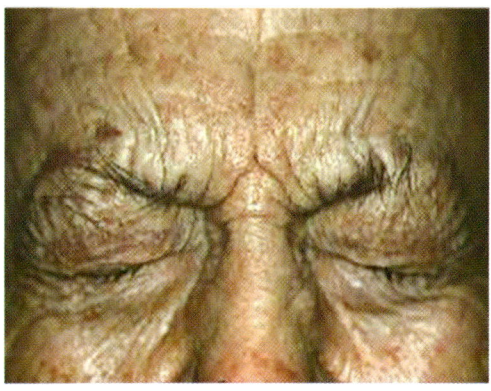

Fig. 4.2: *Severe blepharospasm*

involving the forehead, brow, and facial muscles.

- Presence of acne, rhinophyma, and facial palsy needs to be noted.

3. ASSESSMENT OF POSITION OF EYELIDS

It is important to note the position of both eyelids (Fig. 4.3), the upper lid should cover the upper limbus by 1–2 mm while the lower lid should be at the level of the lower limbus, without any visible sclera (scleral show).

- *Lateral canthal angle* should be 1–2 mm higher than the medial, and both angles should be sharp; any rounding of angles is a sign of lid laxity.
- *Blink dynamics* should be carefully noted while the patient is being examined on the slit-lamp: The upper lid should cover the whole cornea and reach the lower lid when the lids close during a normal blink. (If the upper lid fails to close onto the lower lid, it is unable to moisten the exposed part of the cornea/sclera, and cannot pick up the tear film from the lower meniscus.)

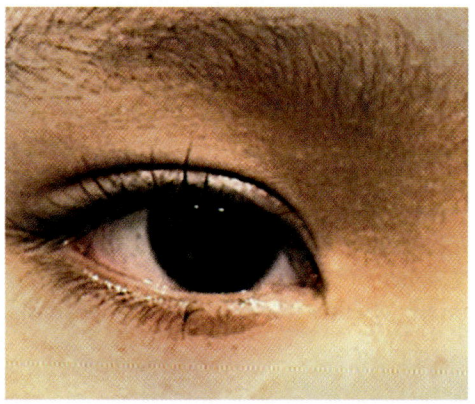

Fig. 4.3: *Upper lid covering upper limbus, lower lid at the level of limbus, lateral canthal angle 2 mm higher than the medial*

4. HORIZONTAL LOWER LID LAXITY

The lower lid skin should be pinched in between examiner's index finger and thumb and the lower lid margin tried to be pulled away from the globe (pull test). Normally, the lower lid margin should be firmly opposed to the globe particularly in young people. With age, as the tissues become lax, the lid loses its tension and

the lower lid margin sags downwards resulting in scleral show (Fig. 4.4).

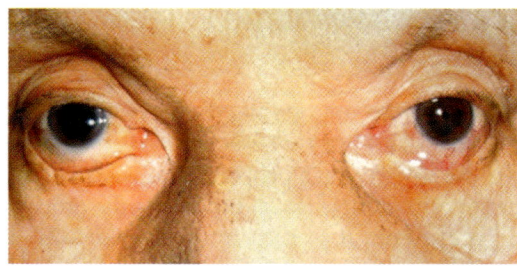

Fig. 4.4: *Lower lid laxity, ectropion, scleral show, punctal eversion*

5. ASSESSMENT OF MEIBOMIAN GLAND DYSFUNCTION

Clinical assessment

i. ***Lid margin*** is assessed for hyperaemia, telangiectasia, blocked meibomian ducts (Fig. 4.5) keratinisation, thickening, foaminess or frothing at the canthal angles and along the lid margin, presence of trichiasis or distichiasis (Fig. 4.6). The presence of scales (Fig. 4.7) along eyelash follicles noted (keeping in mind Demodex infestation).

ii. ***Meibomian duct orifice:*** For plugging (thick meibum), notching (indicating lost/atrophic glands), changes in the orifice position with respect to the mucocutaneous junction, distichiasis (Fig. 4.8).

iii. ***Meibum quality*** is assessed by applying pressure to the eyelid margin and noting the quality of secretion whether clear, opaque, vicid, cheesy.

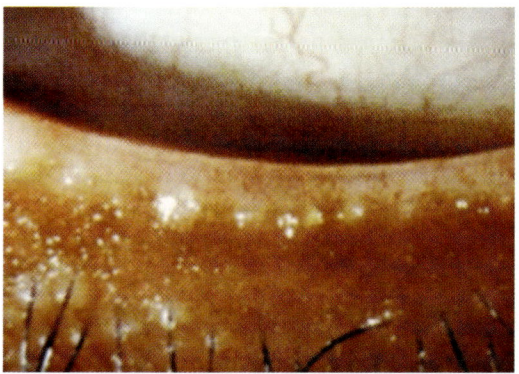

Fig. 4.5: *Blocked meibomian ducts with thick meibum, lid margin telangiectasia*

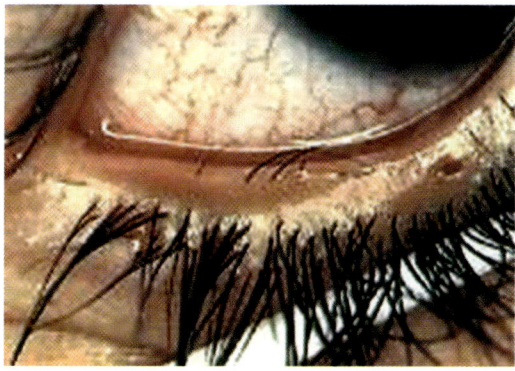

Fig. 4.6: *Distichiasis*

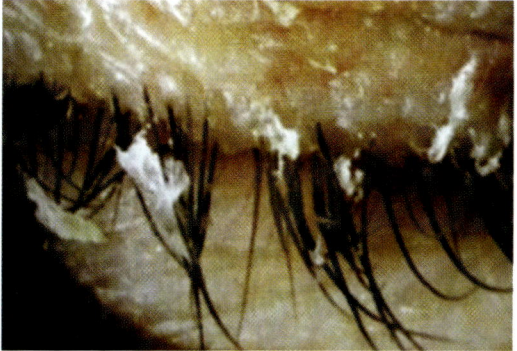

Fig. 4.7: *Scales along eyelashes*

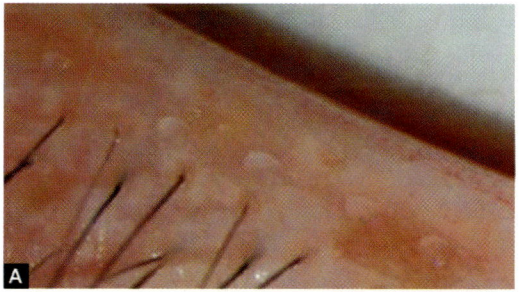

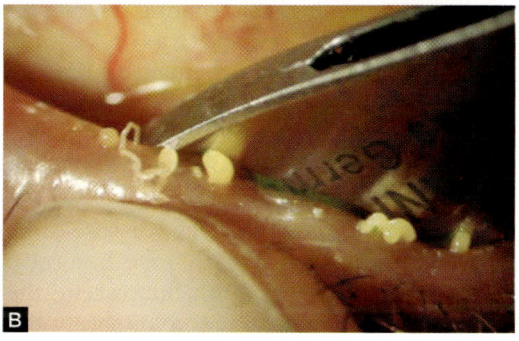

Fig. 4.8: A, *Normal meibum quality; B, Thick, cheesy meibum*

iv. *Meibomian gland expressibility (MGE):* Noting the ease with which it is expressed and its texture. This is a clinical score that helps in assessing the severity of disease at initial presentation, and how it improves with treatment. The number of glands that can be expressed with mild pressure either with a cotton-tipped swab or a commercially available device that is specifically formulated for this purpose. Five glands in the nasal, middle, and lateral thirds of the lower eyelid (total 15 glands) are expressed and scored at each visit. A score of zero indicates a complete blockage of ducts and total absence of meibum. A score of 15 indicates that the glands are expressible throughout the lower eyelid. Patients with MGE score 0–5 are always symptomatic, and those with a score of 7 or more, are usually asymptomatic.

Investigations

i. *Meibography:* Meibomian gland morphology, density, and dropout may be analysed with meibography or meiboscopy to help diagnose meibomian gland dysfunction. Meiboscopy is the visualisation of the meibomian gland via transillumination of the eyelid (can be easily done by viewing an everted lid on the infrared image of an auto-refractometer).

Meibography implies photographic image documentation by commercially available devices like Oculus Keratograph and the Tear Science LipiView. Dynamic meibomian imaging (DMI) from the LipiView device provides a distinct picture of the entire everted inferior tarsal plate, allowing both the clinician and the patient to assess the extent of meibomian gland dysfunction and its characteristic meibomian gland dropout.

ii. *Meibometry:* Lipid on the lower central lid margin is blotted onto a plastic tape, and the amount taken up is read by optical densitometry. This provides an indirect measure of the steady state level of the meibomian lipid.

6. TEAR MENISCUS AND ITS HEIGHT

The normal tear volume is estimated to be about of 8.5 µl, which is distributed as 4.5 µl in the conjunctival cul-de-sac and approximately 2.9 µl in the tear menisci and 1.1 µl as the preocular tear film. This dynamically balanced distribution of tears is critical in formulating a healthy and long-lasting tear film, which protects the ocular surface during eye opening. The tear volume in the conjunctival cul-de-sac replenishes the tear menisci (from which, the tears are picked up at each blink and spread as the precorneal tear film) and this constant, dynamic interaction between the two determines the stability of the tear film, and the tear film turnover.

The height of lower meniscus can easily be measured by narrowing the slit-lamp beam (Fig. 4.9). Normally, it is 1.5–2 mm.

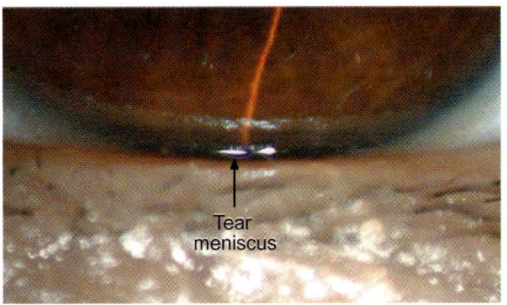

Fig. 4.9: *Assessment of tear meniscus on slit-lamp examination*

Meniscometry (measurement of tear meniscus height, radius and cross-sectional area). A rotatable projection system with a target comprising black and white stripes is projected onto the lower central tear film meniscus. Images are recorded and then transferred to a computer for calculation of the radius of curvature. Several commercially available imaging devices can provide serial quantitative measurements. Non-invasive measurements like optical coherence tomography (OCT) instrument helps to characterise the entire tear film system based on the changes in a single compartment by snapshot measurements.

7. TEAR FILM BREAKUP TIME

Tear film breakup time (TBUT) is determined by measuring the interval between the instillation of a drop of fluorescein and the appearance of black islands or dry spots on the cornea (Fig. 4.10).

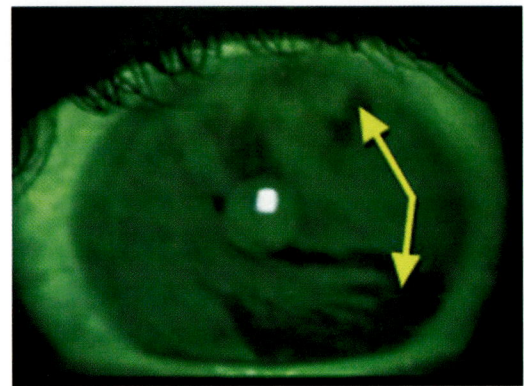

Fig. 4.10: *Dark islands in green fluorescence*

The test is performed prior to the instillation of anaesthetic eye drops (as they are toxic to the corneal epithelium and produce dry spots). A fluorescein strip is moistened with saline and applied to the inferior cul-de-sac. After several blinks, the tear film is examined using a broad-beam of slit-lamp with a blue filter. A healthy corneal and conjunctival surface has a uniform green fluorescence. Time is noted when dark islands or dry spots appear on the cornea prior to the blink. If they appear in less than 10 seconds, it is considered abnormal. The exact site on the cornea is also noted. Several devices can measure the TBUT objectively, including the Oculus Keratograph.

8. EPITHELIAL STAINING

Several dyes like rose bengal, lissamine green, and fluorescein are used to evaluate the state of corneal and conjunctival surface epithelium. Rose bengal and lissamine green stain dead/devitalized epithelial cells as well as healthy cells that have lost their mucin coating. Fluorescein does not stain a dry spot, as it becomes hydrophobic after losing its mucin coating, and it appears as a blue spot in the uniform green fluorescence of the tear film. Fluorescein pools in the areas of epithelial erosions and stains the exposed basement membrane.

Early or mild cases of dry eye disease can be detected more easily with rose bengal or lissamine staining than with fluorescein; they also stain the conjunctiva more intensely than the cornea.

Lissamine green has the combined advantages of fluorescein and rose bengal staining. Like rose bengal, it stains healthy epithelial cells that are not protected by a mucin layer, and like fluorescein, it stains degenerating or dead cells. It avoids the pain, discomfort, and corneal toxicity associated with rose bengal, but is less sensitive and more transient and difficult to appreciate on a slit-lamp examination.

Staining of the cornea in the inter-palpebral or nasal cornea is seen in dry eye disease due to aqueous deficiency (Fig. 4.11A). An inferior limbal staining indicates evaporative dry eye disease due to meibomian gland dysfunction (the toxic meibum damaging the ocular surface) (Fig. 4.11B). Similarly, a linear pattern of inferior conjunctiva and corneal staining by rose bengal or lissamine is characteristic of meibomian gland dysfunction (MGD).

The intensity of staining noted at each clinical visit on a scale of 0–3 in 3 areas: The nasal conjunctiva, temporal and inferior conjunctiva,

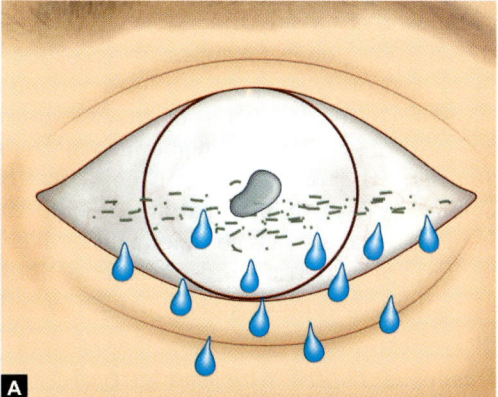

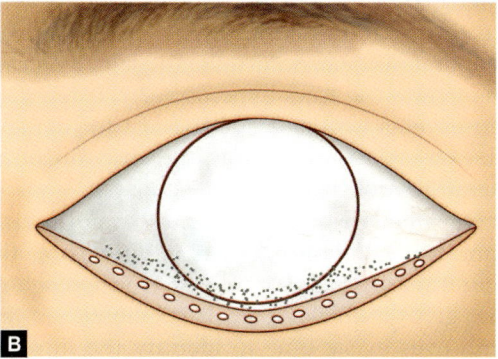

Fig. 4.11: *Corneal staining pattern in: A, Aqueous deficiency dry eye; B, Evaporative dry eye*

and the cornea. The maximum possible score is 9, and a score of 3.5 or higher is considered positive for dry eye disease. This should be recorded in notes.

9. SCHIRMER'S TEST

It is used to test aqueous tear production. The test is performed for both eyes simultaneously and under the same test conditions at each visit, i.e. the same test (either with or without anaesthetic), away from the fan to reduce tear evaporation, away from the vent of an air conditioner, either with eyes open or eyes closed and patient should not talk during the test. It is divided into Schirmer I and Schirmer II test.

Schirmer I test has two branches: Schirmer I test without the anaesthesia and then with the topical anaesthesia.

- *Schirmer I test without anaesthesia* measures the basal tear secretion (which is from the accessory lacrimal glands) as well as the reflex secretion from the main lacrimal gland whose secretory activity is stimulated by the irritating nature of the filter paper. Less than 10 mm of wetting after 5 minutes is diagnostic of ATD. The test is relatively specific, but it is poorly sensitive.

- *Schirmer I test performed after topical anaesthesia* measures only the basal lacrimal secretion. It is highly specific and sensitive for a dry eye disease due to aqueous deficiency. It is performed by instilling a topical anaesthetic and then placing a thin strip of filter paper (5 × 35 mm) in the inferior cul-de-sac in the lateral canthus. The corners of a soft tissue paper may be used to wick all liquid from the inferior fornix by capillary attraction without any wiping or direct irritation before the paper is placed. The patient closes the eyes for 5 minutes, and the amount of wetting in the paper strip is measured.

The normal value is 15 mm or more; less than 5 mm of wetting is abnormal; 5–10 mm is equivocal.

Schirmer II test is used to measure only the reflex tear production which is from the main lacrimal gland. It is performed without instilling any topical anaesthetic into the eyes. The nasal mucosa is irritated with a cotton-tipped applicator, then the filter paper strips are placed at the lateral canthus and the tear production measured. This test may be done, if the initial Schirmer I test yields abnormal results. Wetting of less than 15 mm after 5 minutes is consistent with abnormalities of reflex secretion.

Absence of nasal lacrimal reflex watering, presence of serum autoantibodies, and severe ocular surface disease demonstrated by fluorescein or rose bengal staining strongly favours the diagnosis of SS-associated dry eye disease.

10. ASSESSMENT OF CORNEA

The surface of cornea should be assessed for pannus, vascularisation, mucous plaques (Fig. 4.12), epithelial defects, thinned areas, and central corneal thickness measured. Corneal thickness is reduced in patients with dry eye disease as a result of the hypertonicity of tear film in these patients. Corneal thickness has been shown to increase after treatment with artificial tears, and this may be a useful diagnostic and follow-up criterion for dry eye disease. Visual acuity and corneal topography and keratometry readings have been shown to improve after the use of artificial tears.

11. TEAR FERNING TEST (TFT)

This assesses the quality of tears (electrolyte concentration) and hyperosmolarity. A drop of tear fluid is collected from the lower meniscus and placed onto a microscope slide and allowed

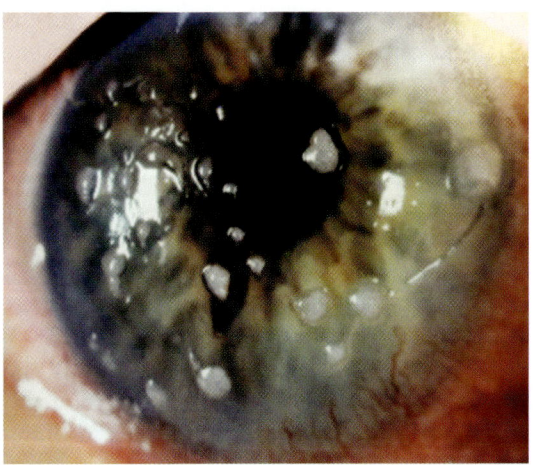

Fig. 4.12: *Mucous plaques on cornea*

to dry by evaporation. Different forms of branching crystallisation patterns can be observed and classified. This test permits the separation of healthy eyes from dry eyes based on ferning patterns.

12. TESTS TO QUANTIFY TEAR COMPONENTS

Additional tests may be performed to quantify each individual tear component.

Lipid component: Lipids may be tested for by collecting meibum, either by squeezing the eyelid margin to express meibum, or by using sterile curettes to suck meibum from the individual gland orifices. Analysis is performed by high pressure liquid chromatography (HPLC) or gas chromatography with mass spectroscopy (GC-MS).

Aqueous component: The aqueous can be tested for the tear film osmolarity, lysozyme, lactoferrin, epidermal growth factor (EGF), aquaporin, lipocalin, and immunoglobulin A (IgA) concentrations with enzyme-linked immunosorbent assay (ELISA) techniques.

Lysozyme accounts for approximately 20–40% of total tear protein. The main disadvantage of its testing is its lack of specificity as large amounts are produced in meibomitis, bacterial conjunctivitis and herpes simplex keratitis. Lactoferrin has antibacterial and antioxidant functions. Its analysis is commercially available through colorimetric solid-phase and ELISA techniques and offers good correlation with other tests.

Measurement of tear film osmolarity: Tear film osmolarity is increased in patients with dry eyes. As the aqueous component of the tearful evaporates, the concentration of salts increases and makes the tears hyperosmolar. It is a very sensitive as well as a specific test for dry eye disease evaluation, staging, and ongoing monitoring of therapeutic response.

The measurement is done by collecting nanolitre (nl) volume of tear fluid from the lateral tear meniscus and tested in a machine that gives a quick result. It is essential to test both eyes every time to identify the intraeye difference of osmolarity; a difference of 8 mOsm/L or more between the two eyes is considered abnormal. If the osmolarity score is 300 mOsm/L or greater in the higher scoring eye, this is abnormal. From 300 to 320 mOsm/L is graded as mild; from 320 to 340 mOsm/L is graded as moderate; and greater than 340 mOsm/L is graded as a severe dry eye disease.

Mucin component: Mucins may be analysed by using impression cytology or brush cytology techniques, in which epithelial and goblet cells are tested for mucin by immunofluorescence, flow cytometry, ELISA, or immunoblotting techniques. When the mucin layer of the tear is decreased, as seen in xerophthalmia or ocular cicatricial pemphigoid, squamous metaplasia and keratinisation of cornea and conjunctiva occurs.

Matrix metalloproteinase 9: The production of MMP-9 for epithelial maintenance may be up-regulated in dry eye disease or contact lens use. MMP-9 on the ocular surface can now be measured by special kits.

The tear turnover rate, defined as the percentage by which the fluorescein concentration in tears decreases per minute after instillation, is also reduced in patients with symptomatic dry eye disease. It is determined by means of fluorophotometry.

BIBLIOGRAPHY

1. Dorota H Szczesna, David Alonso-Caneiro, D Robert Iskander, Scott A Read, Michael J Collins. Predicting dry eye using noninvasive techniques of tear film surface assessment. Cornea 2011; 52(2).
2. Maharaj R. *In vivo* ocular surface osmolarity in a dry eye population. Clin Refrac Optom 2017; 28(1): 3–6.
3. Na Li, Xin-Guo Deng, Mei-Feng He. Comparison of the Schirmer I test with and without topical anesthesia for diagnosing dry eye. Int J Ophthalmol 2012; 5(4): 478–81.
4. Rocha G, Gulliver E, Borovik A, Chan CC. Randomized, masked, *in vitro* comparison of three commercially available tear film osmometers. Clin Ophthalmol 2017; 11: 243–48.
5. Sambursky R, Davitt WF, 3rd, Friedberg M, Tauber S. Prospective, multicenter, clinical evaluation of point-of-care matrix metalloproteinase-9 test for confirming dry eye disease. Cornea 2014; 33(8): 812–18.
6. Wolffsohn JS, Arita R, Chalmers R, et al. TFOS DEWS II Diagnostic Methodology report. Ocul Surf 2017; 15(3): 539–74.

Chapter

5

Microbiological and Pathological Investigations for Corneal Diseases

Chapter Outline

MICROBIOLOGICAL INVESTIGATIONS

Microbial keratitis may be caused by bacteria, fungi, parasites or viruses. A well equipped microbiology laboratory is important for handling and processing of ocular samples, especially corneal samples.

Samples for the microbiological investigations of a suspected microbial keratitis must be collected before initiating antibacterial treatment. Treatment can be initiated based on the results of smears and culture and sensitivity reports.

COLLECTION OF SAMPLES

Samples collected from the infected corneal tissue are valuable for diagnosis of microbial keratitis. Any foreign body on cornea, contact lenses, lens solutions may be collected. Corneal scraping is best done under slit-lamp or operating microscope after instillation of a topical anesthetic. The cornea is first stained by fluorescein. A Kimura spatula (Fig. 5.1) is the

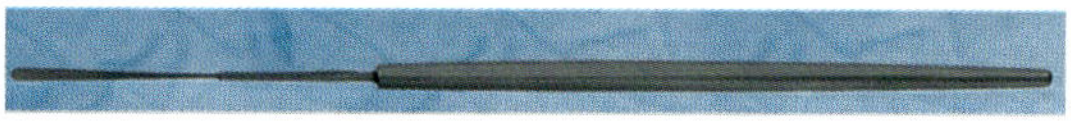

Fig. 5.1: *Kimura spatula*

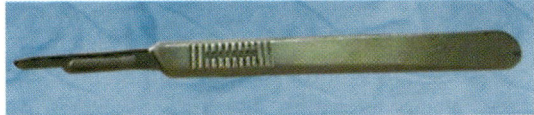

Fig. 5.2: *Bard-Parker 15 No. blade*

best device to collect corneal sample. A 15 No. Bard-Parker knife (Fig. 5.2) may be used, if it is not available. To scrape the cornea, lids are separated by the index finger and thumb of the examiner. The debris and discharge are removed. The patient is asked to keep both eyes open and fix at a distant object. Multiple scrapings are done from the margins and bed of the ulcer. Adherent exudates on the surface of the ulcer may be removed using a sterile cotton swab prior to the collection of scrapings. The blade or spatula is scraped over the surface and peripheral margins of the infiltrated cornea. Each scraping is used to inoculate the media. To prepare a slide, the scraping is spread over slides for staining and wet preparation. The tissue specimen is placed in a sterile Petri dish for sectioning.

TRANSPORTATION OF CORNEAL SAMPLES TO THE LABORATORY

The scrapings are plated directly onto culture media or smeared onto clean glass slides. Corneal biopsy tissue can be transported to microbiology laboratory in a sterile dry Petri dish or in a sterile bottle with sterile saline. Exudates from the anterior chamber may also be directly plated on culture media and smeared on slides.

PROCESSING OF CORNEAL SCRAPINGS

DIRECT SMEAR EXAMINATION METHODS

Different culture media may be used in ocular microbiology laboratory. The choice of media to be inoculated and staining methods for smears, vary according to the type of sample. Corneal scrapings are processed for bacteria, fungi and Acanthamoeba. Processing for viral cultures is done whenever indicated. Inoculated media plates and tubes must be placed in appropriate atmosphere and temperature for appropriate length of time.

CULTURE METHODS

There are three types of culture media: Non-selective (viz. blood, chocolate or nutrient agar), selective, and differential. A selective medium promotes the growth of desired organisms while inhibiting the undesirable organisms. A differential medium provides a visible indication of a physiological property, such as the fermentation of a carbohydrate. For most organisms encountered in ophthalmology, blood and chocolate agar (for bacteria), Sabouraud's agar (for fungi) and thioglycollate and brain heart infusion broth (for bacteria and fungi) should be sufficient.

Blood agar

Blood agar (Fig. 5.3) consists of an agar base, derived from sea weed, with a peptic digest of animal tissue, dextrose and yeast extract. It is an enriched, non-selective medium able to grow most aerobes (except *Neisseria, Haemophilus*, and *Moraxella* species), anaerobes (with vitamin K, cysteine, and hemin supplementation), and fungi. Using this differentiating medium, the degree of hemolysis caused by hemolysins is assessed to differentiate among gram-positive bacteria.

Chocolate agar

Chocolate agar (Fig. 5.4) is composed of sheep blood that provides factors X (hemin) and V (nicotinamide adenine dinucleotide) necessary for growth of *Haemophilus* species, *N. gonorrhoeae, N. meningitidis*, and Moraxella organisms.

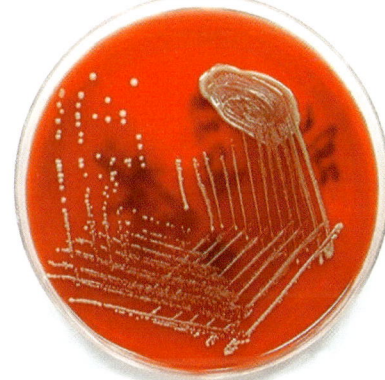

Fig. 5.3: *Blood agar*

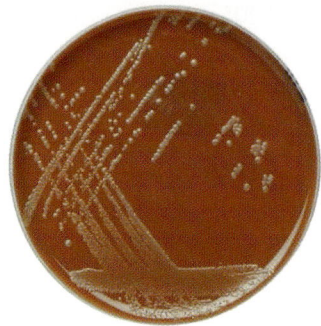

Fig. 5.4: *Chocolate agar*

Brain heart infusion broth

Brain heart infusion (BHI) (Fig. 5.5) is a nutrient-rich medium, and can therefore be used to culture a variety of *fastidious* organisms. It has been used to *culture streptococci, pneumococci* and *meningococci*, which can be otherwise challenging to grow. BHI is made by combining an infusion from boiled *bovine* or *porcine* heart and brain with a variety of other nutrients.

Sabouraud dextrose agar

Sabouraud dextrose agar (SDA) (Fig. 5.6) is used for the isolation, cultivation and maintenance of non-pathogenic and pathogenic species of **fungi** and **yeasts**. SDA was formulated by Sabouraud in 1892 for culturing dermatophytes. The pH is adjusted to approximately 5.6 in order to enhance the growth of fungi, especially **dermatophytes**, and to slightly inhibit bacterial growth in clinical specimens. **Peptone** (enzymatic digest of casein and enzymatic digest of animal tissue) provides the nitrogen and vitamin source required for organism growth in SDA. **Dextrose** is added as the energy and carbon source. **Agar** is the solidifying agent. **Chloramphenicol** and/or **tetracycline** may be added as broad spectrum antimicrobials to inhibit the growth of a wide range of gram-positive and gram-negative bacteria. **Gentamicin** is added to further inhibit the growth of gram-negative bacteria.

Enriched thioglycollate broth

Enriched thioglycollate broth (Fig. 5.7) is a enriched differential medium used primarily to determine the oxygen requirements of micro-organisms. Sodium thioglycollate in the medium consumes oxygen and permits the growth of obligate anaerobes. It allows the differentiation of obligate aerobes, obligate anaerobes, facultative anaerobes and microaerophils.

Löwenstein-Jensen agar

Löwenstein-Jensen agar (Fig. 5.8) is a growth medium especially used for culture of

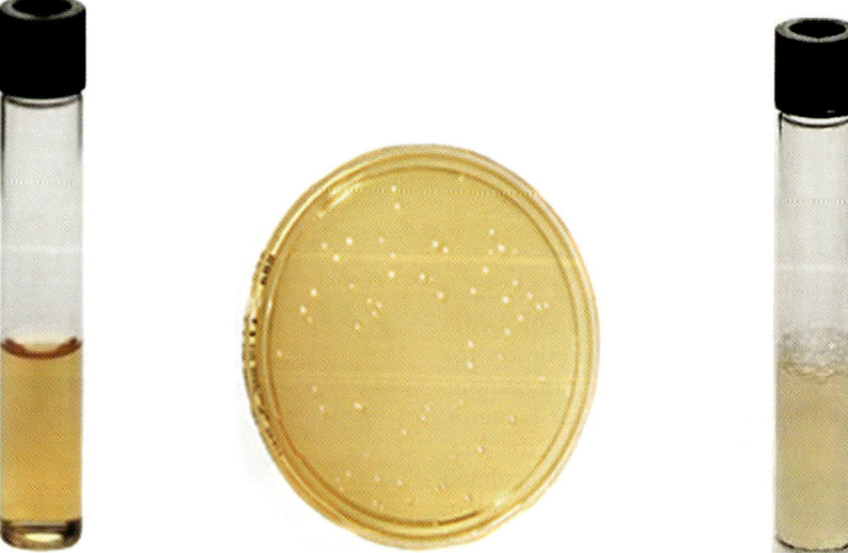

Fig. 5.5: *Brain heart infusion broth*   **Fig. 5.6:** *Sabouraud dextrose agar*   **Fig. 5.7:** *Enriched thioglycollate broth*

Mycobacterium species notably, *Mycobacterium tuberculosis*. When grown on LJ medium, *M. tuberculosis* appears as brown granular colonies. The medium must be incubated for a significant length of time, usually four weeks.

Incubation

Agar plates should be incubated for a minimum of 48 hours at 37°C for bacteria and 32°C for fungi. Cultures for bacteria should be plated out on two agar plates for both aerobic and anaerobic conditions. If a microaerophilic bacterium is suspected, then that growth condition should also be included. Both bacteria and fungi grow better in an atmosphere of 5% carbon dioxide than in air alone. Anaerobic plates should be incubated in an anaerobic cabinet for 7 days or for 14 days if *Propionibacterium acnes* is suspected. Fluid enrichment media should be incubated for 14 days at 37°C and then subcultured.

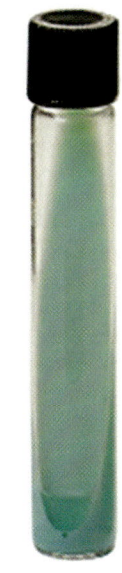

Fig. 5.8: *Löwenstein-Jensen agar*

Acanthamoeba Cultures

Since Acanthamoeba keratitis can mimic fungal, bacterial or viral ulcers, it is recommended that all corneal ulcers be cultured for Acanthamoeba on two non-nutrient agar (NNA) with *E. coli* overlay. The NNA should be incubated at 35°C and 27°–30°C and examined daily under 4X objective to visualize fine serpentine indentation lines with trophozoites on the surface of the medium. The media are incubated for 7–10 days before reported negative. Initially, appearing trophozoites on the medium surface gradually turn into cysts in 7–10 days time. Detailed morphology of trophozoites or cysts can be appreciated by transferring them in a drop of saline on a slide and observing under the microscope (Fig. 5.9).

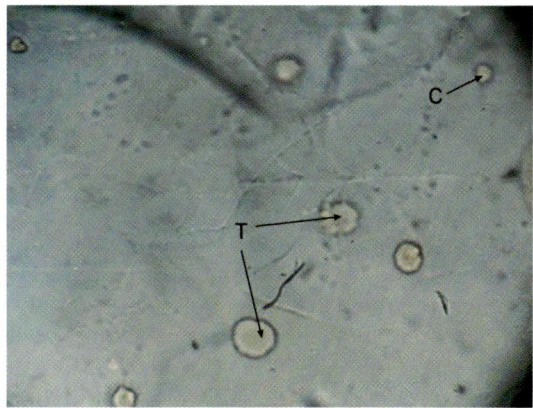

Fig. 5.9: *Acanthamoeba cysts and trophozoites on non-nutrient agar enriched with E. coli*

Viral Cultures

In centres where tissue culture facility is available, virus isolation techniques may be performed. Both conventional and shell vial techniques should be performed. While choosing cell lines, it is advisable to maintain one primary cell line (e.g. primary monkey kidney), one continuous cell line (e.g. Vero, HEp 2, HeLa) and one human diploid cell line (e.g. MRC-5). Most often, as in ocular virology, results can be given by 72 hours using shell vial techniques. Additional cell lines may be maintained for specific pathogens like Chlamydia (e.g. McCoy cells) (Fig. 5.10). Specimens collected during early stages of an infection and inoculating them into cell cultures as soon as possible give best results.

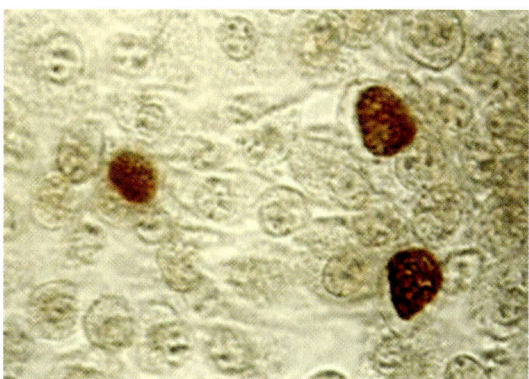

Fig. 5.10: *Chlamydia culture on McCoy cell line*

ANTIMICROBIAL SUSCEPTIBILITY TESTING

Kirby-Bauer disc diffusion (Fig. 5.11) technique remains the most widely used test to determine antimicrobial susceptibility of bacterial isolates. Both the ophthalmologist and the microbiologist should be aware, however, that results of disc diffusion susceptibility tests relate to levels of drug achievable in serum and do not relate directly to the concentration of drug produced in the preocular tear film and ocular tissues by standard routes of administration. Estimation of the minimal inhibitory concentrations (MIC) of antibiotics may provide more useful information to the ophthalmologist than simply labelling an isolate as susceptible or resistant. The panel of agents to be tested should be based on drugs used in an institution or community and the relative susceptibility of the organisms. Stringent quality control measures are critical in achieving reliable antibiotic susceptibility results by disc diffusion method. Density of the inoculum, type of medium, thickness of the medium, duration of incubation, and concentration and potency of the drug in the discs all can affect the zone of inhibition. The value of antifungal susceptibility testing for therapy of ocular fungal infection is yet to be established, however, broth dilution as well as disc diffusion methods have been described.

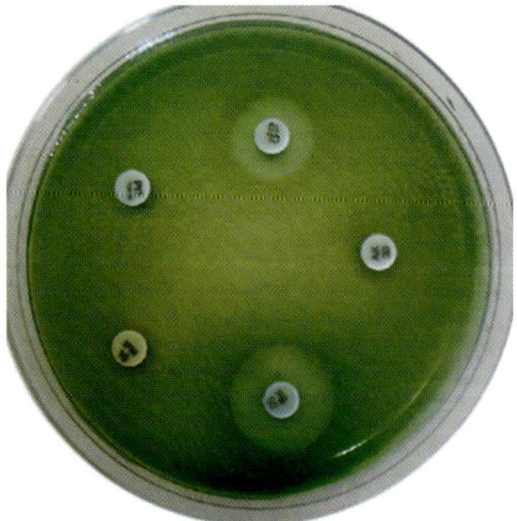

Fig. 5.11: *Kirby-Bauer disc diffusion for antimicrobial susceptibility*

COMMON STAINING PROCEDURES FOR CORNEAL SCRAPINGS IN THE DIAGNOSIS OF KERATITIS

The stains used to identify various organisms include potassium hydroxide wet mount preparation, Gram stain, Giemsa stain and special stains such as Ziehl-Neelsen acid-fast stain, fluorochromatic stains and modified Grocott-Gomori methenamine silver nitrate stain.

POTASSIUM HYDROXIDE WET MOUNT PREPARATION

Potassium hydroxide (KOH) preparation (Fig. 5.12) is used for the rapid detection of fungal elements in clinical specimen, as it clears the specimen making fungal elements more visible during direct microscopic examination. KOH is a strong alkali. When specimen is mixed with 20% w/v KOH, it softens, digests and clears the tissues surrounding the fungi so that the hyphae and conidia (spores) of fungi can be seen under the microscope.

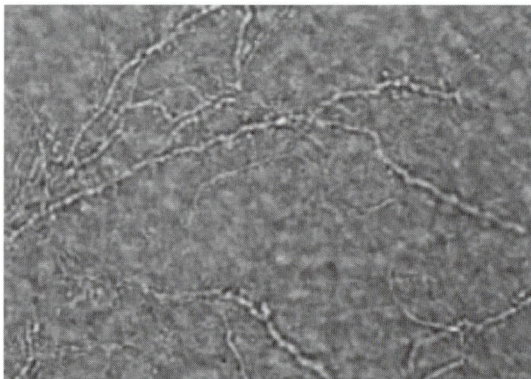

Fig. 5.12: *Potassium hydroxide wet mount preparation*

Procedure of KOH preparation is as below
- Place a drop of KOH solution on a slide.
- Transfer the specimen to the drop of KOH and cover with glass. Place the slide in a Petri dish, or other container with a lid, together with a damp piece of filter paper or cotton wool to prevent the preparation from drying out.
- As soon as the specimen has cleared, examine it microscopically using the 10X and 40X objectives with the condenser iris diaphragm closed sufficiently to give a good contrast. If

too intense a light source is used the contrast will not be adequate and the unstained fungi will not be seen.

GRAM'S STAIN

Gram staining (Fig. 5.13) is the most commonly used differential staining techniques in microbiology, which was introduced by Danish bacteriologist Hans Christian Gram in 1884. This test differentiates the bacteria into gram-positive and gram-negative, which helps in the classification and differentiation of microorganisms.

Reagents used in Gram staining include
- Crystal violet, the primary stain
- Iodine, the mordant
- A decolourizer made of acetone and alcohol (95%)
- Safranin, the counterstain

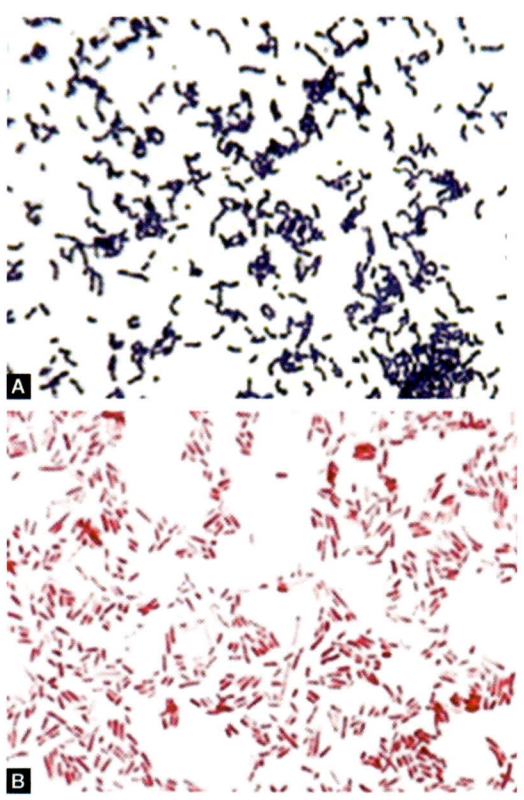

Fig. 5.13: *A, Gram staining showing gram-positive bacteria; B, Gram staining showing gram-negative bacteria*

Procedure of Gram staining is as below
- Take a clean, grease-free slide.
- Prepare the smear of suspension on the clean slide with sample.
- Air dry and heat fix
- Pour crystal violet and keep for about 30 seconds to 1 minute and rinse with water.
- Flood the Gram's iodine for 1 minute and wash with water.
- Then, wash with 95% alcohol or acetone for about 10–20 seconds and rinse with water.
- Add safranin for about 1 minute and wash with water.
- Air dry, blot dry and observe under microscope.

Interpretation is as below:
- Gram-positive: *Blue/purple colour*
- Gram-negative: *Red colour*

Principle of gram staining

When the bacteria is stained with primary stain crystal violet and fixed by the mordant, some of the bacteria are able to retain the primary stain and some are decolourized by alcohol. The cell walls of gram-positive bacteria have a thick layer of protein-sugar complexes called peptidoglycan and lipid content is low. Decolourizing the cell causes this thick cell wall to dehydrate and shrink, which closes the pores in the cell wall and prevents the stain from exiting the cell. So, the ethanol cannot remove the crystal violet-iodine complex that is bound to the thick layer of peptidoglycan of gram-positive bacteria and appears blue or purple in colour.

In case of gram-negative bacteria, cell wall also takes up the CV-iodine complex but due to the thin layer of peptidoglycan and thick outer layer which is formed of lipids, CV-iodine complex gets washed off. When they are exposed to alcohol, decolourizer dissolves the lipids in the cell walls, which allows the CV-iodine complex to leach out of the cells. Then when again stained with safranin, they take the stain and appears red in colour.

GIEMSA STAIN

Giemsa stain (Fig. 5.14) is one of the Romanowsky type stains, which use eosin, methylene

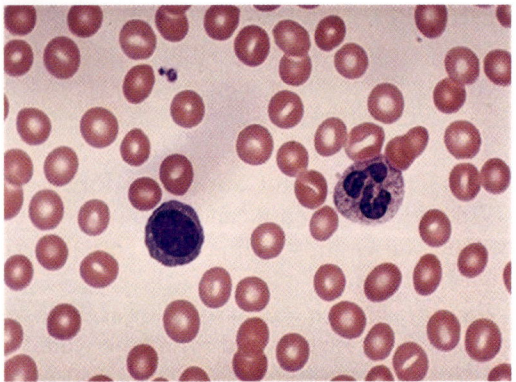

Fig. 5.14: *Giemsa staining*

blue and azure dyes. It stains the DNA in the nuclei of the human cells and cytoplasmic RNA in the lymphocytes. The Giemsa stain is usually used to determine the type of inflammatory cells present. This stain differentiates bacteria from fungi, and also identifies chlamydia inclusion bodies and cysts and trophozoites of Acanthamoeba species. It identifies the normal and inflammatory cells. With Giemsa technique the bacteria appear dark blue in colour. The yeast cells and fungal hyphae absorb the stain and appear purple or blue while the cell walls and the septations do not stain.

Giemsa staining procedure is as below

- Fix slide in a Coplin jar containing methyl alcohol for 5 min.
- Prepare fresh stain solution in a Coplin staining jar.
- Place 2 ml of stock Giemsa stain in the bottom of the Coplin jar
- Add distilled water to within ½ inch of the top (approximately 70 ml)
- Incubate slide in stain at 35°C for 60 min
- Differentiate using two changes of 95% ethyl alcohol
- Rinse in tap water
- Allow to air dry

Principle of Giemsa staining

Giemsa stain is commonly used when there is need to examine the blood smear for the parasites but is a good stain for routine examination of blood smear and used to differentiate nuclear and cytoplasmic morphology of the various cells of the blood like platelets, RBCs, WBCs as well as the parasites. This stain is the most dependable stain for blood parasites, particularly in thick blood smears. It is a type of Romanowsky stains, it contains both the acidic and basic dyes which have the affinity for basic and acidic components of the blood cells respectively. The acidic dye, eosin and azure variably stains the basic components of the cells, i.e. the cytoplasm, granules etc. and the basic dye, methylene blue stains the acidic components, especially the nucleus of the cell. The stain must be diluted for use with water buffered to pH 6.8 or 7.2, depending on the specific technique used.

ZIEHL-NEELSEN STAINING

Ziehl-Neelsen staining (Fig. 5.15) is the differential staining technique which was first developed by Ziehl and later on modified by Neelsen. So, this method is also called **Ziehl-Neelsen staining** technique. Neelsen in 1883 used Ziehl's carbol fuchsin and heat then decolourized with an acid alcohol, and counterstained with methylene blue. This method is used for those microorganisms which are not stained by simple or Gram staining method, particularly the member of genus Mycobacterium, are resistant and can only be visualized by acid-fast staining.

The main aim of this staining is to differentiate bacteria into acid-fast group and non-acid fast group.

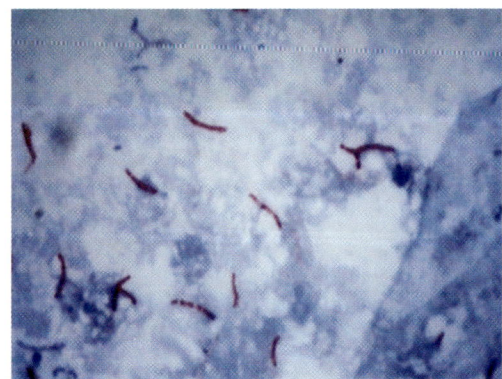

Fig. 5.15: *Ziehl-Neelsen staining*

Procedure of acid-fast stain is as below

- Make a thin smear of the specimen for study and heat fix by passing the slide 3–4 times through the flame of a Bunsen burner or use a slide warmer at 65°–75°C. Do not overheat.
- Place the slide on staining rack and pour carbol fuschin over smear and heat gently underside of the slide by passing a flame under the rack until fumes appear (without boiling). Do not overheat and allow it to stand for 5 minutes.
- Rinse smear with water until no colour appears in the effluent.
- Pour 20% sulphuric acid, wait for one minute and keep on repeating this step until the slide appears light pink in colour (15–20 sec).
- Wash well with clean water.
- Cover the smear with methylene blue or malachite green stain for 1–2 minutes.
- Wash off the stain with clean water.
- Wipe the back of the slide clean and place it in a draining rack for the smear to air-dry (do not blot dry).
- Examine the smear microscopically, using the 100X oil immersion objective.

Principle of acid-fast stain

When the smear is stained with carbol fuchsin, it solubilizes the lipoidal material present in the mycobacterial cell wall but by the application of heat, carbol fuchsin further penetrates through lipoidal wall and enters into cytoplasm. Then after all cell appears red, the smear is decolourized with decolourizing agent (3% HCl in 95% of alcohol) but the acid-fast cells are resistant due to the presence of large amount of lipoidal material in their cell wall which prevents the penetration of decolourizing solution (Table 5.1). The non-acid-fast organisms lack the lipoidal material in their cell wall due to which they are easily decolourized, leaving the cells colourless. Then the smear is stained with counter-stain, methylene blue. Only decolourized cells absorb the counter-stain and take its colour and appears blue while acid-fast cells retain the red colour.

LACTOPHENOL COTTON BLUE PREPARATION

The lactophenol cotton blue (LPCB) wet mount preparation (Fig. 5.16) is the most widely used method of staining and observing fungi and is simple to prepare. The preparation has three components:

- **Phenol:** Kills any live organisms
- **Lactic acid:** It preserves fungal structures
- **Cotton blue:** It stains the chitin in the fungal cell walls.

Lactophenol cotton blue solution is a **mounting medium** and **staining agent** used in the preparation of slides for microscopic examination of fungi. Fungal elements are stained intensely blue.

Preparation of lactophenol cotton blue (LPCB) slide mounts

- Place a drop of 70% alcohol on a microscope slide.
- Immerse the specimen/material in the drop of alcohol.

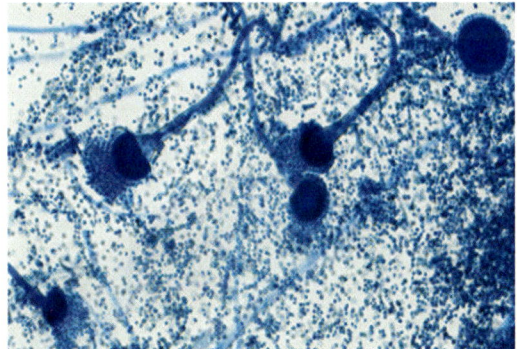

Fig. 5.16: Lactophenol cotton blue preparation

Table 5.1: Principle of acid-fast stain			
Application of	Reagent	Acid-fast	Non-acid-fast
Primary dye	Carbol fuchsin	Red	Red
Decolourizer	Acid alcohol	Red	Colourless
Counter-stain	Methylene blue	Red	Blue

- Add one, or at the most two drops of lacto-phenol cotton blue stain before the alcohol dries out.
- Holding the coverslip between forefinger and thumb, touch one edge of the drop of mountant with the coverslip edge, and lower gently, avoiding air bubbles. The preparation is now ready for examination.

GROCOTT-GOMORI METHENAMINE SILVER NITRATE STAIN

The modified Gomori methenamine silver nitrate stain (GMS stain kit) (Fig. 5.17) is intended for use in the histologic visualization of fungi, basement membrane and some opportunistic organisms such as *Pneumocystis carinii.*

Tissue sample: 5 µm paraffin sections of neutral buffered formalin fixed tissue are suitable. Other fixatives are likely to be satisfactory. A section adhesive is recommended.

Method is as below

- Bring sections to water via xylene and ethanol.
- Oxidise with 5% chromic acid (chromium trioxide) for 60–90 minutes.
- Rinse well with tap water.
- Bleach with sodium bisulphite for 1 minute.
- Rinse well with tap water.
- Rinse with distilled water.
- Treat with methenamine silver solution at 50°C until impregnated (up to 3 hours)
- Wash with distilled water.
- Tone with 0.1% gold chloride solution for 5 minutes.

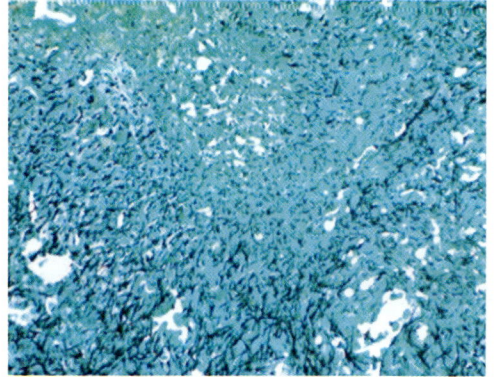

Fig. 5.17: *Grocott-Gomori methenamine silver nitrate stain*

- Rinse with distilled water.
- Fix in 2% sodium thiosulphate for 5 minutes.
- Wash well with running tap water.
- Counterstain with light green, neutral red or a light H and E.
- Rinse with tap water.
- Dehydrate with ethanol, clear with xylene and mount with a resinous medium.

Expected results
- Oxidisable carbohydrates, including glycogen and fungi-black.

PATHOLOGICAL INVESTIGATIONS

CONJUNCTIVAL IMPRESSION CYTOLOGY

Conjunctival impression cytology is a technique used to study ocular surface disorders. It is a simple, non-invasive technique, can be repeated easily, done on OPD (outpatient department) basis and does not require any specialized gadgets. Impression cytology, with cellulose acetate filters, was introduced in 1977 as a minimally invasive conjunctival biopsy. It provides an alternative to conjunctival diagnostic excision biopsy or conjunctival smears made from scrapes taken with a blunt spatula. Applications for impression cytology include diagnosing ocular surface disorders, documenting sequential changes in the conjunctival and corneal surface over time, staging conjunctival squamous metaplasia and monitoring effects of treatment.

METHODS

Cellulose acetate filter paper is used to collect specimen. Cellulose acetate paper is cut in size of 3 × 10 mm with diagonal end. Eye is anesthetized by one drop of paracaine. Palpebral fissure is widened by retracting eyelid with finger and thumb of one hand, with other hand filter paper applied over the bulbar conjunctiva and left for 4–6 seconds. Then filter paper is removed with forceps in a peeling motion. The specimen is then fixed by dipping in a fixative containing glacial acetic acid, formaldehyde and ethyl alcohol in ratio 1:1:20 for 10 minutes. Then it is rinsed in tap water for two minutes. The strip is dipped in 0.05% periodic Schiff reagent for

8 minutes sodium metabisulfite for 2 minutes and in haematoxylin for 30 seconds. The strip is rinsed for 2 minutes with tap water after each step above. Now, 95% ethyl alcohol is applied over strip for 2 minutes. The strip is dehydrated with absolute alcohol. Lastly xylin is applied over filter paper to make it transparent. The stained specimen is mounted over a slide with coverslip and examined under microscope.

Impression cytology of normal corneal surface showing corneal epithelial cells (Fig. 5.18): Normal cells are flat with a prominent nucleus. The nuclear cytoplasmic ratio is low.

The limbal epithelial cells are small, densely packed with a high nuclear cytoplasmic ratio. The limbal zone is clearly demarcated from the adjacent corneal epithelial cells.

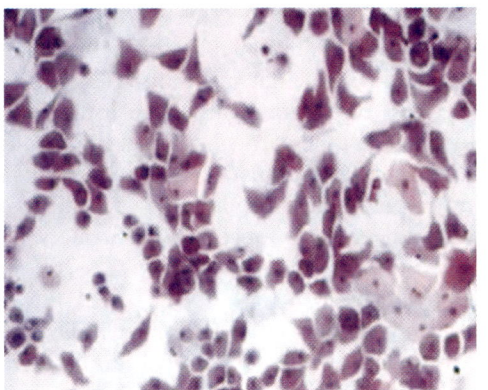

Fig. 5.18: *Impression cytology of normal corneal surface showing corneal epithelial cells*

ANALYSIS

A number of different aspects of the CIC specimen can be evaluated using a microscope for analysis of adherent cells: Goblet cell density and morphology, the nuclear/cytoplasm (N/C) ratio, nuclear morphology and inclusions, colour of the cytoplasm, emergence of keratinisation, epithelial cell morphology, epithelial cell size, presence of inflammatory cells and cell sheet quality.

APPLICATIONS OF CONJUNCTIVAL IMPRESSION CYTOLOGY

It has been used to investigate the normal ocular surface, dry eye effects, effects of chronic conjunctivitis, impact of contact lenses on the ocular surface, vitamin deficiency, limbal deficiency, presence of micro-organisms, effects of therapeutic interventions, ocular surface neoplasia, keratoconus and the effects of systemic diseases like diabetes, renal failure, thyroid disease and anorexia.

Contact lenses

Contact lenses are known to produce changes to the normal structure of the conjunctiva (Fig. 5.19). Squamous metaplasia is a term that is commonly used to describe the changes that occur in CIC specimens as a result of contact lens wear. Squamous metaplasia is defined as "the transformation of pseudostratified ciliated epithelium into stratified squamous epithelium as occurs in certain pathologic conditions" or "reversible change in which one adult cell type is replaced by another cell type". Squamous metaplasia is determined in CIC by the gradual changes that occur in the morphology and density of conjunctival goblet and epithelial cells. Contact lenses result in numerous cellular changes. Various morphologic nuclear changes occur in squamous metaplasia including pyknosis, two or more nuclei and aniso-nucleosis. As a result of contact lens wear, the N/C ratio decreases. Increase in the size of epithelial cells is a common occurrence in contact lens wear. The density of goblet cells decreases. There is greater expression of antigens HLA DR and CD23.

Dry eye and avitaminosis A

The cellular changes seen were increased epithelial cell size and absent or reduced

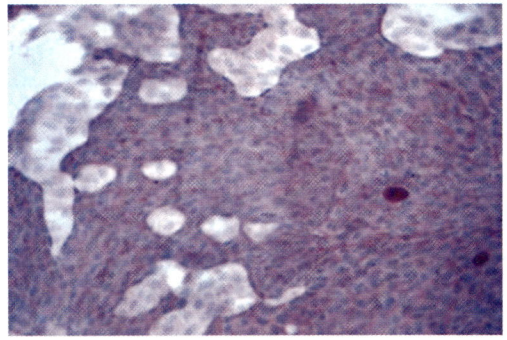

Fig. 5.19: *Conjunctival impression cytology in contact lens wearers*

densities of goblet cells in children suffering from xerophthalmia as a result of avitaminosis A. Snake-like chromatin, other nuclear changes, metaplasia, changes in cell size, decreased N/C ratios, and decreased goblet cell density all occurred in dry eye subjects (Fig. 5.20). Other CIC changes that occur with KCS are: Hyperplasia, hypertrophy, cellular flattening, decreased goblet cell density, snake-like chromatin, and other nuclear changes.

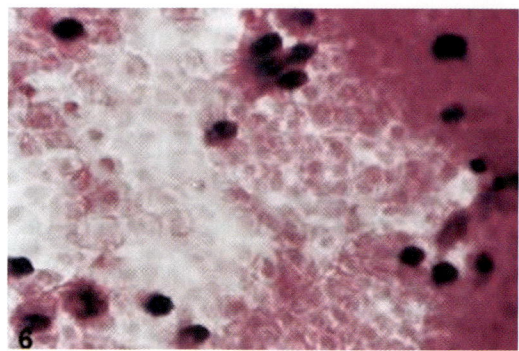

Fig. 5.21: *Conjunctival impression cytology in keratoconus patients*

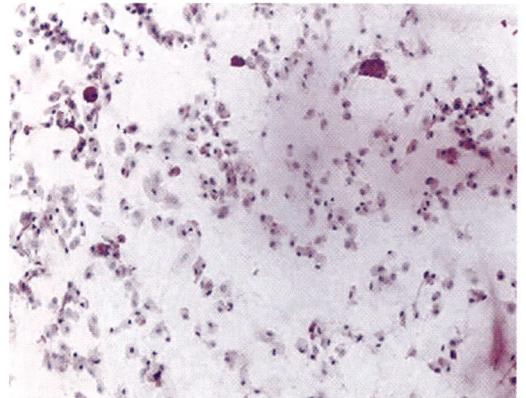

Fig. 5.20: *Conjunctival impression cytology in dry eye patients*

Keratoconus

Fukuchi et al have shown that two lysosomal enzymes, acid esterase and acid phosphatase, are more prominent in the conjunctivas of keratoconic subjects. McMahon et al and Shen et al have also shown that lysosomal enzyme levels are increased in keratoconic conjunctivas making use of CIC. In both reports the feasibility of using CIC (and not surgical biopsy as in Fukuchi et al) for investigating lysosomal enzyme levels in keratoconic conjunctivas was stressed. Goblet cell density decrease and squamous metaplasia were shown to be significantly higher in keratoconic conjunctivas when compared with normal subjects (Fig. 5.21). Both findings were related to the extent of the progression of the keratoconus.

Ocular burns

Ocular burns constitute true ocular emergencies and both thermal and chemical burns represent potentially blinding ocular injuries. It has been recognised that the extent of tissue damage is a prognostic indicator of recovery following ocular surface injury. Recovery of ocular surface burns depends upon the causative agent and the extent of damage to corneal, limbal, and conjunctival tissues at the time of injury. IC has enabled documentation of limbal cell deficiency in patients with ocular burns and other surface disorders by demonstrating the presence of goblet cells on the corneal surface. Limbal stem cell deficiency has also been assessed using immunoperoxidase staining for cytokeratins: K3 for corneal, and K19 for conjunctival phenotype.

Thyroid orbitopathy (TO)

A common complication of TO is DED, which occurs due to increased proptosis and lower lid retraction (and thus exposed ocular surfaces), resulting in incomplete blinking and partial distribution of tears across the ocular surface. This causes enhanced evaporation of tears, hyperosmolarity and resultant ocular surface inflammation. Study by Ismailova et al assessed patients with TO in order to ascertain morphological changes of the ocular surface. Using IC, the authors reported goblet cell loss, extreme desquamation of superficial cells and epithelial keratinisation (Fig. 5.22).

Ocular allergies

Patients with ocular surface allergies have shown evidence of increased eosinophils, which appear to mediate allergic conditions through release of histamine. Study by Aragona P et al showed alteration in the conjunctival epithelium during the course of vernal conjunctivitis as examined by conjunctival impression cytology.

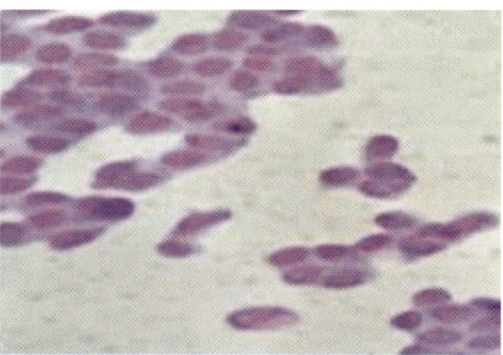

Fig. 5.22: *Conjunctival impression cytology in thyroid orbito-pathy*

The results of impression cytology demonstrated that all cytological parameters were significantly modified in vernal conjunctivitis patients; the earliest alterations were found in the distribution of goblet cells, in the intercellular junctions, in the chromatin morphology and in the degree of keratinisation. The morphometric comparison showed that in vernal conjunctivitis patients the mean number of goblet cells per field was significantly higher. Impression cytology can, therefore, be a simple, non-invasive and cheap method for the study of the ocular surface in vernal conjunctivitis.

CORNEAL BIOPSY

Corneal biopsy may be useful in establishing the diagnosis and prompt institution of appropriate management in progressive keratitis of unknown cause. Inability to obtain a definitive diagnosis in a case of chronic keratitis may be related to previous use of antimicrobials that interfere with standard cultures or by the fastidious growth of unusual pathogens in culture. Corneal biopsy is a useful procedure in the diagnosis and management of corneal inflammation, infections, degenerations, dystrophies and corneal manifestations of systemic diseases. Usually a partial thickness biopsy should be performed. Full-thickness biopsy should be reserved only for tectonic indications in advanced disease. It is indicated in cases with deep stromal abscess or in case where repeated culture shows negative reports but there is strong suspicion of infection. Repeated failed attempts to isolate pathogens from patients with persistent ulceration and chronic inflammation suggest that offending organisms are deep in the cornea and not accessible to scrapings. For these patients corneal biopsy is necessary.

INDICATIONS

Infectious corneal processes
- Deep suppurative stromal keratitis
- Keratitis with atypical presentation
- Fungal or acanthamoebal keratitis that does not respond to other treatment
- Culture negative keratitis

Neoplastic conditions
Conjunctival neoplasms with extension through limbus onto cornea.

TECHNIQUE

Setting: Slit lamp or operating room

Equipment required include:
- Speculum
- Trephine
- Sharp blade (preferably diamond)
- Fine forceps

Procedures are as below:
- Antimicrobials may be discontinued 24 hours prior to the procedure.
- Firstly slit-lamp biomicroscopic examination should be performed. Depth of the infiltrate and overlying corneal thickness should be assessed.
- Keep the patient in supine position under operating microscope.
- Operating eye should be prepared and draped under all aseptic precautions.
- Insert the eye speculum
- A sponge soaked in proparacaine should be placed on the limbus for 1–2 minutes so as to anaesthesise the eye.
- A site away from the visual axis and at the edge of the pathology is chosen. For a partial-thickness biopsy, trephination is performed with a small diameter punch (2–5 mm). The trephine is placed such that it includes the lesion as well as normal healthy cornea. The blade should be rotated back and forth between the thumb and forefinger.

- After trephination, careful dissection of the tissue is performed with a crescent blade, which is held flat against the cornea to prevent perforation. The corneal button must be grasped gently with the forceps to prevent crushing the tissue.
- A femtosecond laser may also be used to obtain the biopsy tissue.
- After complete excision of the tissue, the biopsy specimen is transferred from the crescent blade to the appropriate transport media.
- Infected tissue obtained is cut in half and sent for culture and histology. It is best to alert the pathologist as to the suspected diagnoses and to expect a small specimen.
- Postoperatively, in the case of suspected microbial keratitis, the same antimicrobial regimen is continued.
- An antibiotic ointment may be added for comfort during the day- and at night-time.

FOLLOW-UP AND POSTOPERATIVE CARE

Topical antibiotic and a cycloplegic agent should be prescribed until the epithelium covers the site of biopsy. Patients should be closely followed up and monitored.

Complications: Complications from biopsy include scarring, irregular astigmatism, poor or delayed healing and perforation.

BIBLIOGRAPHY

1. Benson WH, Lanier JD. Comparison of techniques for culturing corneal ulcers. Ophthalmology 1992; 99: 800–4.
2. Cameron N Ly, Jeanette N Pham, Paul R Badenoch, Sydney M Bell, Glenn Hawkins, Dianne L Rafferty and Kathleen A McClellan, Bacteria commonly isolated from keratitis specimens retain antibiotic susceptibility to fluoroquinolones and gentamicin plus cephalothin, Clinical and Experimental Ophthalmology, 2006; 34(1): 44–50.
3. Dart, J. K. G., F. Stapleton, and D. Minassian. Contact lenses and other risk factors in microbial keratitis. Lancet 1991; 338: 650–53.
4. Epley KD, Katz HR, Herling I, Lasky JB. Platinum spatula versus mini-tip culturette in culturing bacterial keratitis. Cornea 1998; 17: 74–78.
5. Khanal B, Deb M, Panda A, Harinder Singh Sethi, Laboratory Diagnosis in Ulcerative Keratitis, Ophthalmic Research 10.1159/000084273, 2005; 37(3): 123–27.
6. McLeod SD, Kolahdouz-Isfahani A, Rosamian K, et al. The role of smears, cultures and anti-biotic sensitivity testing in the management of suspected infectious keratitis. Ophthalmology 1996; 103: 23–28.
7. Verena Prokosch, Zisis Gatzioufas, Solon Thanos, Tobias Stupp. Microbiological findings and predisposing risk factors in corneal ulcers, Graefe's Archive for Clinical and Experimental Ophthalmology 2012; 250(3): 369.

Specular Microscopy and Confocal Microscopy of Cornea

SPECULAR MICROSCOPY

INTRODUCTION

Specular microscopy is a procedure that provides the clinical and morphological study of corneal endothelial cells *in vivo* without disturbing their function. Efforts were made by Vogt, more than 75 years ago, to examine the endothelial cell morphology in the reflected light of the slit-lamp biomicroscope. However, fine rapid movements of the eye and limited magnification preclude the use of this technique for systematic studies of the endothelium. Maurice (1968) introduced the 'specular microscope' for examination of the corneal endothelial cells at high magnification (4003). This instrument used Vogt's reflection principle but separated illuminating and viewing light paths at a fixed angle in a split microscope objective. Laing (1975) adopted specular microscope for clinical use. He replaced the original water immersion lens with a dipping case

objective to applanate the cornea. Baurne et al (1976) simplified the specular microscope for rapid endothelial examination and photography at 2003.

OPTICS

The specular microscope is a reflected light microscope which projects a slit of light onto the cornea and utilizes the light reflected from an optical interface of tissue for image formation (rather than light transmitted through the tissue sample). It is the difference in refractive indices between the endothelial cells and aqueous humour which gives rise to this specular or mirror-like reflection at the flat posterior surface. The reflected light is estimated to be about 0.02% of the incident light. Figure 6.1 shows a drawing of the optics of the visualization of the endothelial mosaic produced by slit-lamp biomicroscopy. Reflected light from the epithelium and stroma obscures the view of the endothelium unless a narrow slit of light is used for illumination. Laing described that specular

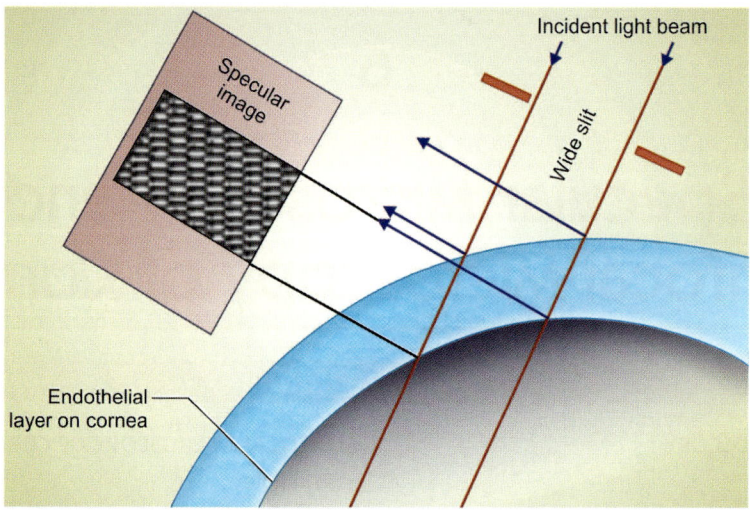

Fig. 6.1: *Schematic drawing of the endothelial layers as seen with slit-lamp microscopy. Note the wide angle between the illuminating beam and the observation path needed to remove the annoying surface reflection and stroma scatter from view of the endothelial mosaic*

microscopy yields an image with three or four distinct zones (Fig. 6.2), depending upon the width of the illuminating slit as:

Zone 1. Epithelium-/lens-coupling fluid

Zone 2. Corneal stroma

Zone 3. Corneal endothelium

Zone 4. Aqueous humour.

The boundary between endothelial region (zone 3) and aqueous region (zone 4) is almost dark and is termed the *dark boundary*. The boundary between endothelium region (zone 3) and stroma (zone 2) is usually bright and is termed the *bright boundary*.

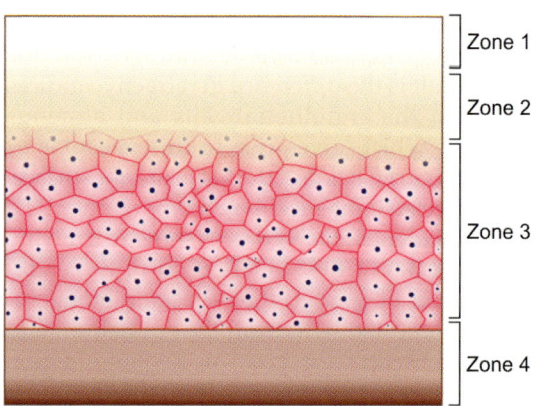

Fig. 6.2: *Specular micrograph of endothelial cells showing four distinct zones*

TYPES OF SPECULAR MICROSCOPES

There are two basic types of clinical specular microscopes.

1. CONTACT SPECULAR MICROSCOPES

Commercially available contact specular microscopes include:

• Keller-Konan, SP-580 (Konan Medical USA, Torrance, CA, USA)

• EM-1000 (Tomey, Erlangen, Germany).

In such types of specular microscopes, a contact lens with a coupling fluid of index of refraction similar to that of cornea is used to eliminate the corneal surface reflection. The corneal thickness in such an arrangement can be thought to also include the contact lens thickness. The reflection from the surface of contact lens replaces that of the corneal surface. However, because of the thickness of contact lens, the surface reflection is moved well over to side (Fig. 6.3).

Such specular microscopes provide good resolution and magnification. But the patients are less comfortable and there is a risk of spread of infection, if strict sterile precautions are not taken. Further, manipulating the cornea with this technique may cause *artefacts*, especially in fragile, diseased cornea.

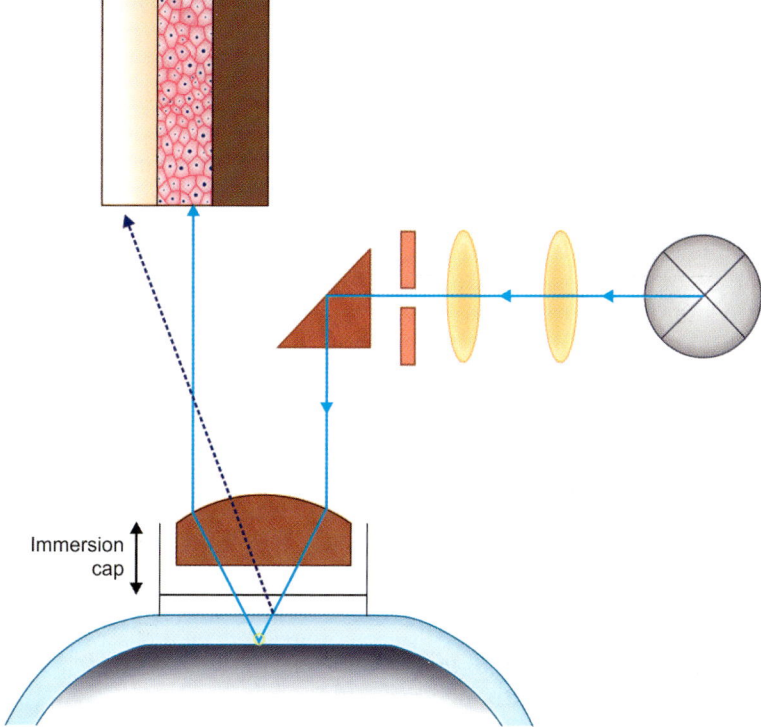

Fig. 6.3: *Optics of contact lens-assisted endothelial specular microscope*

2. NONCONTACT SPECULAR MICROSCOPES

Commercially available noncontact specular microscope includes:

- Automated SM is SP-3000p (Topcon Medical Systems Inc. Paramus, NJ, USA).

In noncontact specular microscopes, the bothersome reflection from the front corneal surface is eliminated by increasing the angle of incidence. As shown in Fig. 6.1, by increasing the angle of incidence, the anterior reflection is moved to the side, covering less of specular reflection from the endothelium. These microscopes have the advantages of greater patient tolerance and acceptability, and there is no risk of trauma to the cornea. However, a broader view is obtained at the expense of resolution and magnification due to uncontrolled eye movements.

WIDE-FIELD SPECULAR MICROSCOPES

A modification to the standard specular microscope has been described with the use of a scanning mirror. In this way, fields of 800 m in diameter have been achieved with no loss in contrast. The technique allows continuous viewing of the 800 m diameter area because of the high speed of mirror oscillation.

Advantages

The wide-field specular microscopes combine the advantages of both the above microscopes.

- Field of view is 10–15 times larger, the resolution is high and image quality is less susceptible to eye movements.
- Endothelial layer topography is more readily evaluated. The relocation of a specified region of the endothelium is relatively easy and the larger field provides more accurate cell counts.
- *Resolution of endothelium* has been further improved by the addition of highly sensitive video cameras and recording systems, as well as a variety of optic improvements such as scanning mirror system.

- Annoying reflections from the incident light have been minimized by the improvements in optics.

PROCEDURE AND METHOD OF ANALYSIS

PROCEDURE

Currently available contact and noncontact wide-field specular microscopes are easy to use with little patient discomfort. The procedure is first explained to the patient to relieve any anxiety. The contact specular microscopy procedure is very similar to that of Goldmann applanation tonometry (Fig. 6.4A). The whole cornea should be systematically scanned to ensure complete evaluation of the endothelial mosaic—centrally, superiorly, inferiorly, nasally and temporally (Fig. 6.4B).

METHODS OF ANALYSIS

For cell analysis, a minimum of 75 cells should be counted. The early processing methods were tedious and time-consuming. The introduction of large-field microscopes has made the process a bit simplified.

Methods of endothelial cell analysis are as follows:

1. *Cell density.* The number of cells in a photographic field are counted to obtain the cell density. The cell count is calculated per square millimetre. The cell density of endothelium is around 3500 cells/mm² in young adults, which decreases with the advancing age (2000 cells/mm²). There is a considerable functional reserve for the endothelium. Corneas with cell count, 1000 cells/mm² poorly tolerate intraocular surgery.
2. *Fixed frame analysis.* In this method, the photograph of endothelial cells is compared with the drawings of endothelial mosaic of known size.
3. *Tracing analysis.* The tracing of the individual cell outlines can be made and subsequently analysed for individual cell areas and other parameters.
4. *Analysis of digested cells.* The cells may be digested after tracing their outlines, using a digesting tablet. The analysis can then be made using a photograph—a negative image on a television screen or a videotaped recording.
5. *Computerised image analysis.* The computerised cell analysis provides the mean cell density, i.e. cells per square millimetre, and frequency distribution of the individual cell sizes, and analyses the polygonality.

QUANTITATIVE AND QUALITATIVE ANALYSIS BY SPECULAR MICROSCOPY

Calculation of cell density (quantitative analysis): To calculate the cell density, a rectangular area can be determined manually. All the cells completely within the border of the rectangle as well as those touching two adjacent borders are marked. However, this technique

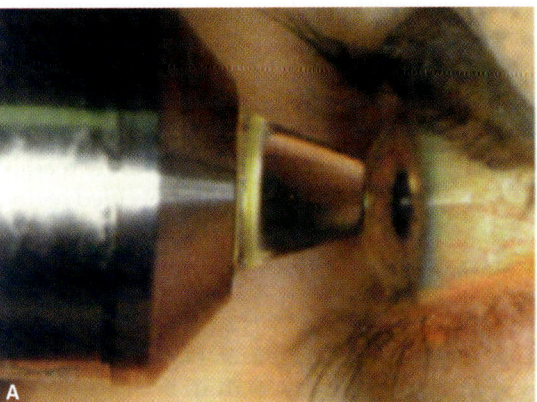
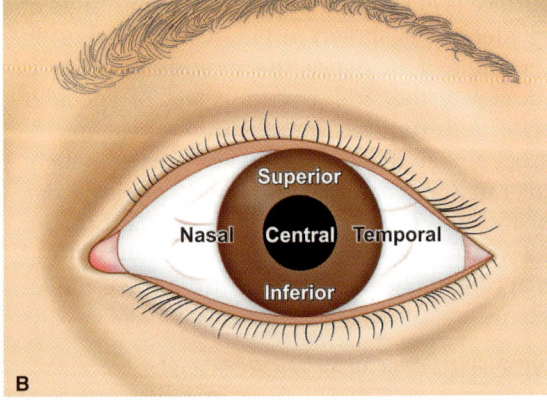

Fig. 6.4: *Procedure of specular microscopy: A, Placement of applanation cone in the centre of cornea with the light shining through the pupil; B, Areas of cornea for systematic scanning of endothelium*

gives only the cell density in cells per square millimetre. The other method is to mark the centre of adjacent cells. This allows automated computation of the mean cell area, maximum cell area (MAX), minimum cell area (MIN), number of cells actually analysed (NUM), mean cell density (CD) and standard deviation of the mean cell area (SD).

Study of cell morphology (qualitative analysis)

Alterations in morphology, such as variations in cell size, i.e. polymegathism and cell shape, i.e. pleomorphism, and asymmetry of the cell population may be more reliable indices of endothelial stress than mean cell density alone.

- *Coefficient of variation*. The degree of uniformity of cell size is determined by measuring the areas of a population of cells and calculating the coefficient of variance, which is the standard deviation of mean cell area divided by the mean cell area, i.e. SD/AVE. The normal endothelium has a coefficient of variance of 0.25. An increase in this value means that the cell size is variable and is known as polymegathism. Cell size varies over a wide range in a number of disorders, and endothelial cells may assume shapes that are substantially different from their usual hexagonal appearance.
- *Percentage of hexagonal cells*. Cell boundaries normally intersect in a manner that results in three angles of intersection, each approximately 608. The endothelial mosaic in healthy young corneas consists of 70–80% hexagonal cells. A decrease in hexagonality with a concomitant increase in the number of cells with more or fewer than six sides is known as pleomorphism.

COMMERCIALLY AVAILABLE SPECULAR MICROSCOPES

KONAN NONCON ROBO SPECULAR MICROSCOPE

It is a computerised noncontact type of specular microscope. It includes an autofocus device to record the specular images readily. There is also an incorporated semi-automated image analysing programme. The software programme has got two analysing modalities for cell density and cell morphology. With Konan Noncon Robo SP8000, it is possible (i) to calculate the individual cell area, with which the coefficient of variance can be deduced as a degree of polymegathism and (ii) to analyse the polygonality, i.e. percentage of hexagonality.

KEELER-KONAN SPECULAR MICROSCOPE

It is a contact type wide-field specular microscope. Its advantages over the noncontact type wide-field specular microscope are:

- It allows more detailed study of corneal endothelium. Different magnification cones can be used to study the endothelial morphology.
- It also allows the study of corneal epithelium, corneal stroma, the crystalline lens epithelial surface, the surface of intraocular lens (IOL) and the posterior capsule. The entire cornea can be examined by moving the cone manually over the corneal surface.

CLINICAL USES OF SPECULAR MICROSCOPY

1. Assessment of changes in the endothelium:
   - With ageing
   - Following surgical procedures such as:
     - Corneal grafting
     - Cataract surgery with or without IOL implantation
     - Newer procedures like excimer laser, LASIK, etc.
   - With associated conditions such as:
     - Glaucoma
     - Uveitis
     - Contact lens wear
     - Trauma—blunt or penetrating
   - With use of intracameral drugs, irrigating solutions and topical medications.
2. Assessment of endothelium in donor corneas and the effect of preservation.
3. Assessment of naturally occurring diseases, degenerations and dystrophies.
4. Assessment of longitudinal effect of surgical procedures.
5. Measurement of corneal thickness, i.e. pachymetry (with contact type only).
6. Assessment of the epithelium of the cornea and the crystalline lens.

CONFOCAL MICROSCOPY OF CORNEA

Clinical confocal microscopy is a new bioimaging technique which enables non-invasive analysis of corneal structure and function. Minsky described the first confocal microscope in 1957. Since then several improvisions have occurred. Bohnke and Masters (1999) have detailed the optical techniques for ocular biomicroscopy and theoretical foundations of confocal microscopy. The most modern confocal microscopes have light source focused onto a small volume within the specimen tissue, and a confocal detector is used to collect the resulting signal to produce an image with enhanced lateral and axial resolution. This new imaging paradigm and its application *in vivo* provide insight into the understanding of the structure and function of the eye.

PRINCIPLE

The principle of the confocal microscope was first described by Minsky. He proposed that both the illumination (condenser) and observation (objective) systems be focused on a single point (have common focal points); hence the name 'confocal' microscopy (Fig. 6.5). This dramatically improved the axial (z) and lateral (x, y) resolution of microscopy by eliminating out focus information, bringing lateral resolution to an order of 1–2 µm and axial resolution to 5–10 µm. This allows for possible magnification of up to 600 times, depending on the numerical aperture of the objective lens used.

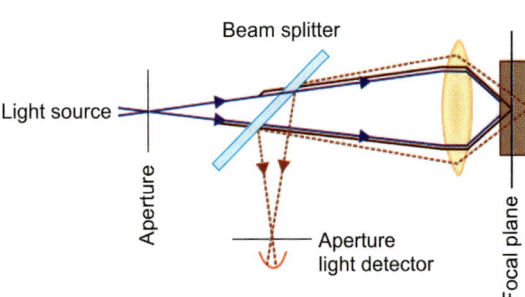

Fig. 6.5: *Diagrammatic representation of the optical principles of the confocal microscope*

As the field of view of the confocal imaging systems is limited, it is necessary to rapidly scan the focal point across the sample and reconstruct the image to allow a real-time on-screen view.

TYPES OF CONFOCAL MICROSCOPE

Depending on the method of scanning, following types of confocal microscopes are known.

1. *Tandem scanning confocal microscope.* Optics of tandem scanning confocal microscope is depicted in Fig. 6.6. In it, thousands of light beams are moved over the fixed object, generating a high scan rate. These parallel beams are generated by a Nipkow wheel—a disc with thousands of pinholes spinning at high-speed. These apertures are arranged in tandem, i.e. as

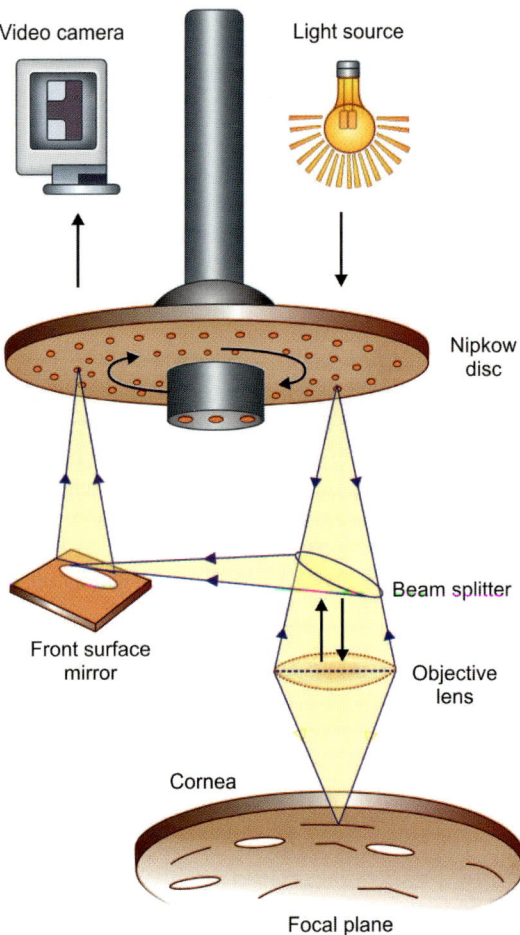

Fig. 6.6: *Optics of tandem scanning confocal microscope*

diametrically opposed pairs. Light passes through one pinhole and is then reflected back through the corresponding pinhole situated opposite. The high-speed rotation of the disc enables the light beam to scan the full field of view many times a second, thus producing a real-time image.

2. *The scanning slit confocal microscope* uses a light source with one-dimensional spot scanning instead of two-dimensional spot scanning.

3. *The confocal laser scanning microscope* uses a laser beam and this generates a mono-chromatic, bright, intense, sharply focused and coherent light. A novel digital confocal laser scanning microscope, recently developed, is a combination of the Heidelberg retina tomo-graphy II (HRT II) and the Rostock cornea module. The laser scanning microscope (LSM) has a computer-controlled hydraulic linear scanning device and a water contact objective and diode laser beam of 670 nm wavelength is used as the light source. The Rostock scanning laser confocal microscope provides reproducible images of high resolution with uniform illumi-nation and precise depth measurements.

CONFOCAL MICROSCOPY OF THE NORMAL HUMAN CORNEA

- *Superficial epithelial cells* are seen with clear visible cell borders, bright cytoplasm and black nuclei. These cells are characteristically polygonal, usually hexagonal in shape (Fig. 6.7A).
- *Intermediate layer of wing cells* comprises cells smaller than the superficial cells, with bright cell borders and dark cytoplasm. These cells are fairly uniform in size and shape (Fig. 6.7B).
- *Basal epithelial cells* are located just above the Bowman's membrane and are seen as a distinct mosaic, with light cell boundaries. The basal epithelial cells are the smallest cells in the epithelium (Fig. 6.7C).
- *Bowman's layer* appears as a homogenous acel-lular layer and nerve fibres of the subepithelial nerve plexus are seen as beaded nerve fibres (Fig. 6.7D).
- *Keratocyte nuclei* are identified as bright reflections in the stroma. The anterior stromal keratocyte nuclei are more abundant and oval compared to the posterior keratocyte nuclei, which were less abundant and more oblong in shape (Fig. 6.7E).
- *Endothelial cells* are visible as bright cell bodies and dark cell boundaries, characteristically hexagonal in shape with fairly uniform appearance in size and shape (Fig. 6.7F).

CONFOCAL MICROSCOPY IN CORNEAL PATHOLOGIES

Confocal microscopy is useful in following corneal pathologies:

1. *Keratoconus.* The characteristic stromal changes seen are multiple 'striae' represented by thin hyporeflective lines oriented vertically, horizontally and obliquely.
2. *Corneal dystrophies,* e.g.
   - *Granular dystrophy.* Characteristic changes are highly reflective, bright, dense struc-tures in the anterior and mid-stroma.
   - *Limbus,* i.e. junction of conjunctiva and cornea is shown in Fig. 6.7G.
   - *Palisades of Vogt* is shown in Fig. 6.7H.
   - *Posterior polymorphous dystrophy* is characterized by multiple round vesicles at the level of Descemet's membrane and endothelium.
   - *Fuchs' endothelial dystrophy.* The cornea guttata appear dark with a bright central reflex. In advanced stage, endothelial cells are seen distorted.
3. *Measurement of flap thickness in LASIK* is obtained by measuring the distance between the high reflective spike from the front surface of the cornea and the low reflective interface.
4. *Intracorneal deposits* that can be seen directly with confocal microscopy include:
   - *Exogenous deposits,* e.g. Acanthamoeba cyst and ova, drug deposits (amiodarone, chloroquine), deposits after contact lens use, refractive surgery and vitreoretinal surgery using silicone oil.
   - *Endogenous deposits* as seen in Wilson's disease, hyperlipidaemia, Fabry's disease, and haemosiderosis.

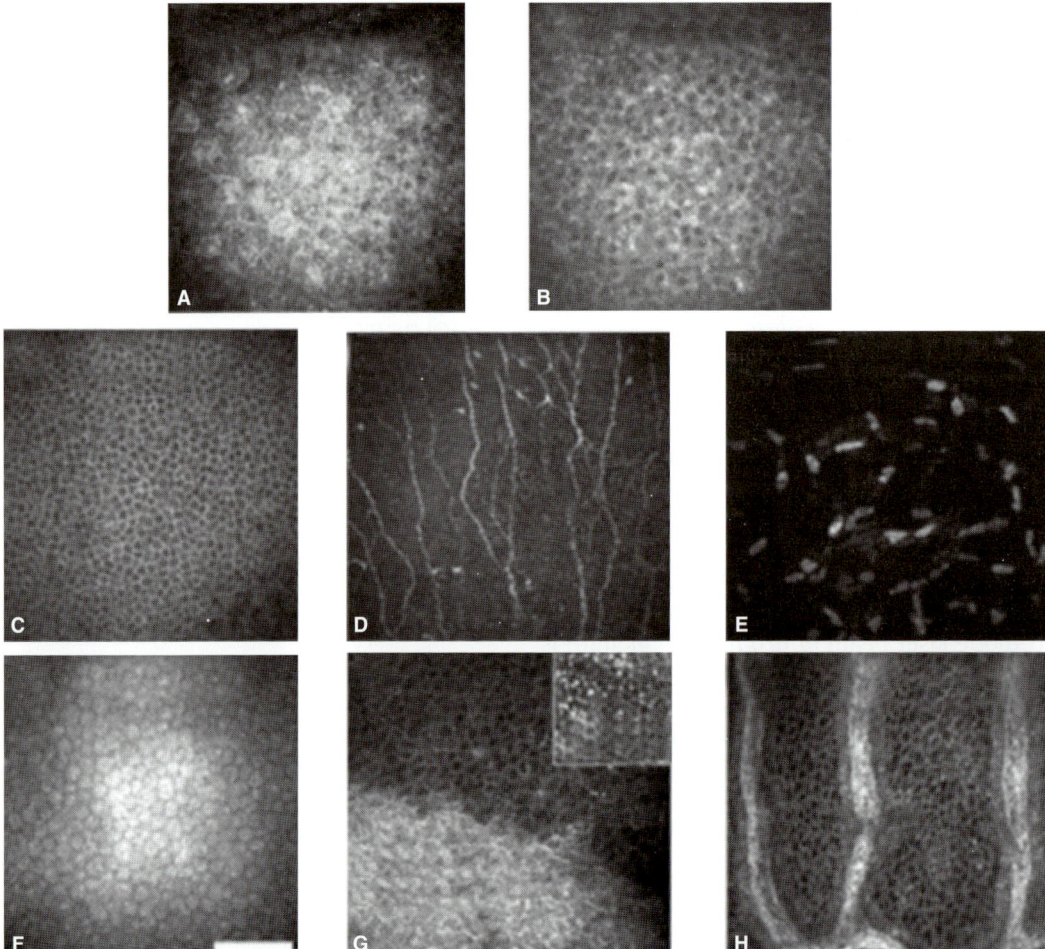

Fig. 6.7: *Confocal microscopy of normal human cornea: A, Superficial epithelial cells are seen with prominent nuclei; B, Wing cells; C, Basal epithelial cells are seen as small cells with high cell density and well-demarcated cell borders; D, Bowman's layer; E, Mid-stroma; F, Endothelium; G, Limbal epithelium, i.e. junction of conjunctiva and cornea; H, Palisades of Vogt*

OTHER CORNEAL ENDOTHELIAL SCANS

CONFOSCAN

Confoscan 4 (Nidek, Inc.) is a fully automatic, fast (takes <12 sec) non-contact endothelial microscope with 20X probe. It has a 5-micron accuracy in confocal pachymetry with Z-ring optics which improves the image stability. It produces high quality imaging through opacities.

HEIDELBERG RETINAL TOMOGRAPH 3 (HRT 3)

Heidelberg retinal tomograph 3 (HRT 3) in conjunction with Rostock cornea module (RCM)

(Heidelberg Engineering, Germany) is a microscope which has a 1 micron resolution. It scans the entire cornea from epithelium to endothelium layer by laser. It uses 670 nm red wavelength diode laser. It offers 400 times magnification with an axial high resolution. This helps in early accurate and rapid diagnosis, expediating initiation of therapy, follow-ups and hence visual outcomes specially in Acanthamoeba keratitis, in fungal keratitis like Aspergillus and Fusarium. Confocal microscopy helps in examining flap-related complications and images of the particles at the interface. It can also aid in assessment of the wound healing following refractive surgery. It also helps in the study of corneal nerve alterations following corneal surgery and in systemic diseases like diabetic neuropathy.

Limitation. It is difficult to visualize bacteria and viruses owing to their size <0.5 micron length.

BIBLIOGRAPHY

1. Amos WB, White JG. How the Confocal Laser Scanning Microscope entered Biological Research. Biology of the Cell 2003; 95(6): 335–42.
2. Binder PS, Akers P, Zavala EY. Endothelial cell density determined by specular microscopy and scanning electron microscopy. Ophthalmology. 1979; 86: 1831–47.
3. Davidovits P, Egger MD. Scanning laser microscope for biological investigations. Applied Optics. 1971; 10(7): 1615–9.
4. Egger MD, Petran M. New reflected-light microscope for viewing unstained brain and ganglion cells. Science 1967 July; 157(786): 305–7.
5. Laing RA, Oak SS, Leibowitz HM. Specialized Microscopy of the Cornea: Specular Microscopy. In: Leibowitz HM, Waring GO (Eds). Corneal Disorders: Clinical Diagnosis and Management, 2nd ed. Philadelphia: WB Saunders Company, 1998: 83–122.
6. Laing RA, Sandstrom MM, Leibowitz HM. Clinical specular microscopy. I. Optical principles. Archives of Ophthalmology 1979; 97: 1714–19.
7. McCarey BE, Edelhauser HF, Lynn MJ. Review of corneal endothelial specular microscopy for FDA clinical trials of refractive procedures, surgical devices, and new intraocular drugs and solutions. Cornea 2008; 27(1): 1–16.
8. Niederer RL, Perumal D, Sherwin T, McGhee CN. Age-related differences in the normal human cornea: a laser scanning *in vivo* confocal microscopy study. Br J Ophthalmol 2007; 91(9): 1165–69.
9. Patel DV, McGhee CN. Contemporary *in vivo* confocal microscopy of the living human cornea using white light and laser scanning techniques: a major review. Clin. Experiment. Ophthalmol 2007; 35(1): 71–88.
10. Sibug ME, Datiles MB, Kashima K, et al. Specular microscopy studies on the corneal endothelium after cessation of contact lens wear. Cornea 1991; 10(5): 395–401.

Chapter

7

Corneal Pachymetry, Hysteresis and Keratometry

CORNEAL PACHYMETRY

INTRODUCTION

The word *'pachos'* means 'thick' in Greek. Corneal thickness measurement is necessary to evaluate the health of cornea and the endothelial pump function. It has been studied extensively in literature and finds extreme importance in today's age of keratorefractive procedures and lamellar corneal transplantation procedures. We have moved from the days of exclusive full thickness transplants to transplanting individual layers of the cornea (DSAEK, DALK, DSEK, DMEK) which rely heavily on measurement of preoperative, intraoperative and postoperative corneal thickness for preoperative decision-making and evaluating postoperative outcomes.

Normal cornea is prolate shaped with the thickness increasing from the center to the periphery. The thickness is 0.7 to 0.9 mm at the limbus and 0.49 to 0.56 mm at the center, the temporal cornea being the thinnest. Studies have shown that the corneal thickness normally increases with the age above 40.

METHODS OF PACHYMETRY

Various instruments have been devised for the measurement of corneal thickness and are referred to as 'pachymeters'. Methods of pachymetry can be divided based on the underlying technique used and based on contact versus noncontact methods.

Based on the technique, pachymetry can be divided as below:

 I. ***Ultrasonic pachymetry***
  - Conventional ultrasonic pachymetry
  - Ultrasound biomicroscopy (UBM).
 II. ***Optical pachymetry***
  - Slit-lamp pachymetry
  - Specular microscopy
  - Optical coherence tomography (OCT)
  - Optical low coherence interferometry
  - Confocal microscopy
  - Laser Doppler interferometry.
 III. ***Optical pachymetry with corneal topographers***
  - Orbscan
  - Pentacam
  - Pachycam.

 IV. ***Pachymetry with ocular response analyzer (ORA)***

Based on contact versus noncontact methods, the pachymeter can be grouped as below:
 I. ***Contact methods*** include:
  - Ultrasonic pachymetry
  - Optical methods such as confocal microscopy.
 II. ***Noncontact methods*** include:
  - Optical biometry with a single Scheimpflug camera (Sirius or Pentacam)
  - Dual Scheimpflug camera (Galilei)
  - Optical coherence tomography (OCT, such as Visante)
  - Online optical coherence pachymetry (Orbscan).

Some of the modern day pachymeters are described briefly.

I. ULTRASOUND-BASED PACHYMETERS

CONVENTIONAL ULTRASOUND-BASED PACHYMETER

Ultrasound (US) pachymetry (Fig. 7.1) introduced by Henderson and Kremer in 1980, is considered to be the gold standard method for pachymetry because of a high degree of reproducibility.

Principle: The high frequency sound waves reflect from the anterior and posterior surfaces and the machine measures the time difference in transit between echoes from the transducer of the probe and the reflected signal received from the surfaces of the cornea.

$$\text{Corneal thickness} = \frac{\text{Transit time} \times \text{Propagation velocity}}{2}$$

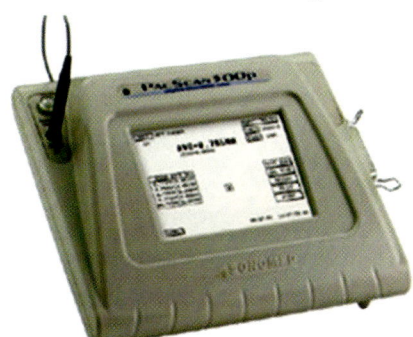

Fig. 7.1: *Ultrasonic pachymeter*

Components

1. *Probe.* The probe handle consists of a piezo-electric crystal which vibrates at 10–20 MHz. The probe tip is narrow 2 mm in diameter to ensure a local contact on central cornea.

2. *Transducer.* The transducer sends ultrasound waves through the probe and receives echoes back form the cornea.

The exact posterior reflection point of sound may be located between Descemet's membrane and the anterior chamber. The ultrasound probe may displace the tear film 7 to 40 microns and therefore underestimate corneal epithelial thickness.

Advantages and disadvantages of ultrasound pachymetry are summarized below.

Advantages
- Fast
- Simple to use
- Minimum observer variation
- Good reproducibility
- Portable
- Intraoperative usage.

Disadvantages
- Contact method
- Need for topical anaesthesia
- Accuracy dependent on location of corneal touch
- Applanation may disturb readings
- Low resolution
- Not accurate in corneal oedema
- Variability of sound velocity in wet and dry tissues.

PACHYMETRY WITH ULTRASOUND BIOMICROSCOPY (UBM)

Ultrasound biomicroscopy (UBM) is a newer technology using high frequency ultrasound to examine the anterior segment of the eye at a higher resolution. Probes may have frequencies of 35 or 50 MHz.

Advantages and disadvantages

Advantages and disadvantages of UBM pachymetry are summarized below:

Advantages include:
- High resolution
- Useful in opaque cornea
- Separate layers of cornea discerned.

Disadvantages include:
- Coupling fluid immersion is discomforting
- Contact method
- No intraoperative usage
- No standardisation.

■ II. OPTICAL PACHYMETRY

SLIT-LAMP PACHYMETRY

Optical pachymetry using the **slit-lamp's pachymeter** attachment (Haag-Streit AG, Koenitz, Switzerland) can be done using a slit-beam projected perpendicular to the cornea.

Instrument description

Optical pachymeter is used with the slit-lamp. It hangs over the objectives of the microscope from a part attached to the microscope body. The left objective is occluded by the pachymeter while the right one has two glass plates with parallel sides placed in front of it. These plates rest one on top of the other, with the junction between them situated so as to horizontally bisect the objective. The upper plate can be rotated while the lower plate is fixed and positioned so that its faces are normal to the axis of microscope.

Optical principle

The optical pachymeter utilises the principle of optical image doubling and is designed to measure the distance between the Purkinje-Sanson images formed by the anterior and posterior corneal surfaces, a value that represents the corneal thickness.

Optics

Working optics of the optical doubling pachymeter depicted in Fig. 7.2 is described below:
- The slit-beam (a in Fig. 7.2) illuminates the patient's cornea.
- The image is viewed through a biomicroscope, half through a glass plate orthogonal to the path of light (b in Fig. 7.2) and half through another glass plate rotated through an angle (c in Fig. 7.2).

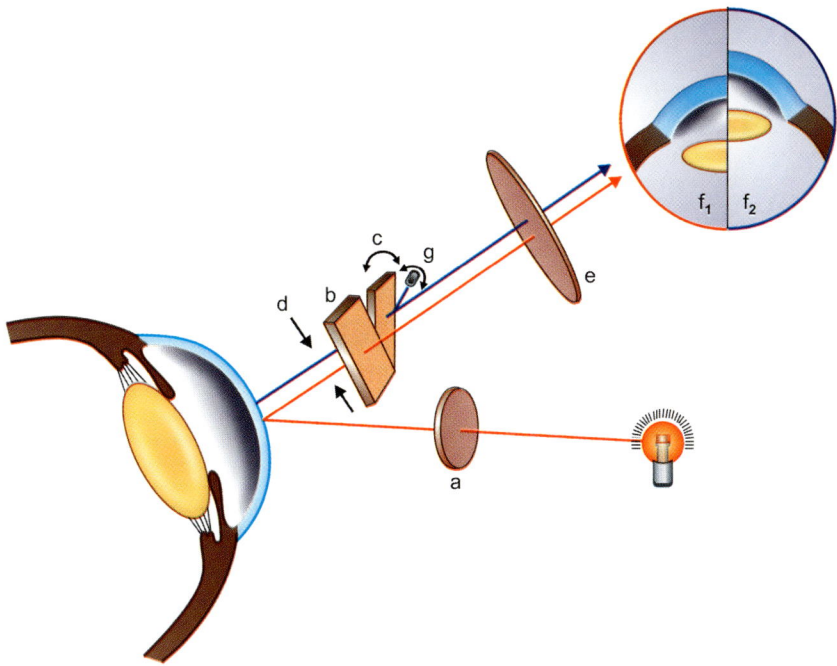

Fig. 7.2: *Optics of the optical pachymeter (for explanation, see text)*

- The beam path through glass plate is displaced laterally for a distance (d in Fig. 7.2) that varies depending upon the angle of rotation.
- Through the eyepiece (e in Fig. 7.2), the observer views a split image. The half of the image (f_1 in Fig. 7.2) comes from the fixed plate and the other half (f_2 in Fig. 7.2) from the rotatable plate.

Measurement of corneal thickness

- To measure the corneal thickness (Fig. 7.3), the observer aligns the endothelial surface of one image with epithelial surface of the other image by carefully adjusting the rotatable plate (d in Fig. 7.2).
- Value of corneal thickness is read off the calibrated scale (g in Fig. 7.2).
- As the apparent thickness of the cornea varies with the angle between the slit-lamp and the microscope, it is essential to set this at some predetermined value before a measurement is made. With the Haag-Streit slit-lamp, this angle should be 40° (Fig. 7.2).
- Thickness can be read from a scale on the instrument which is graded from 0 to 1.2 mm.

- The two methods of measurement are the "just touch" method and the "overlap method" in which the outer surface of the epithelium of the top corneal section is aligned with the inner surface of the endothelium of the bottom section of the cornea.

Disadvantages of slit-lamp optical pachymeter

- Contact procedure
- Lack of repeatability
- Observer bias
- Width of slit-beam variable
- Requires a slit-lamp.

SPECULAR MICROSCOPY PACHYMETRY

Principle

Pachymetry using specular microscopy is based on the focusing of light rays on the front and back surfaces of the cornea and measures the distance between the two surfaces accordingly. Two types of specular microscopes are: Non-contact and contact. Noncontact specular microscopy has been found to give more consistent readings from operator to operator but gives a lower reading than contact methods,

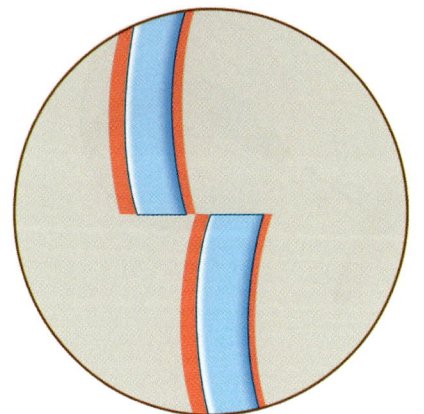

Fig. 7.3: *End point of slit-lamp optical pachymetry*

namely the ultrasound pachymetry or contact specular microscopes.

Advantages and disadvantages

Advantages include:
- Operator independent
- Noninvasive
- Measures the endothelial cell counts also.

Disadvantages include:
- Cannot differentiate central/peripheral corneal readings
- Contact method
- Less reproducible
- Can be only used in clear corneas.

PACHYMETRY WITH ANTERIOR SEGMENT OPTICAL COHERENCE TOMOGRAPHY

The OCT of the anterior segment gives high resolution images of the cornea along with colour coded maps of the corneal thickness.

Advantages of ASOCT pachymeters

- Noncontact
- Noninvasive
- Rapid acquisition
- Measures through corneal opacity
- Can measure layers of cornea separately.

PACHYMETRY WITH PARTIAL COHERENCE INTERFEROMETRY

IOL master 700 (Carl Zeiss Meditec, USA) and Lenstar (Haag-Streit) have revolutionized biometry, i.e. determination of IOL power before cataract surgery. They also measure the corneal thickness by a noncontact method from the anterior and posterior corneal surfaces. This is a rapid method, not requiring local anaesthesia as compared to ultrasonic method.

III. OPTICAL PACHYMETRY WITH CORNEAL TOPOGRAPHERS

PACHYMETRY WITH ORBSCAN II

Principle

Orbscan II (Bausch and Lomb, Rochester, New York, USA) is based on scanning optical slit technology which projects light at a 45° angle and measures the anterior corneal surface elevation/topography and pachymetry. Posterior elevation map is extrapolated from the anterior elevation map and pachymetry data by comparing them with a best fit sphere.

The whole corneal pachymetry can be mapped and the thinnest points defined in a pictorial representation.

Studies have suggested that the scanning slit observes the pachymetry from the air-tear interface of the hydrated corneal epithelium, thereby overestimating the thickness as compared to the US pachymetry with a mean difference of 28 to 54 µm. Hence, an acoustic factor (AF) of 0.92 has been defined to obtain values closer to the US readings. However, Orbscan II with AF of 0.92 underestimates the thickness of thin corneas of normal patients and in keratoconic eyes, post-PRK and post-LASIK eyes. AF of 0.92 has been reported to also overestimate thickness in the thickest of corneas.

Disadvantages of Orbscan II pachymetry

- Scattering from corneal haze and interfaces may interfere with the scanning slit.
- Measurements are adjusted for prolate shape of cornea only.
- Motion artifacts.

PACHYMETRY WITH SCHEIMPFLUG TECHNOLOGY-BASED IMAGING

Principle

Pentacam (Oculus Optikgerate GmbH, Wetzlar, Germany) consists of an automatically rotating

Scheimpflug camera and a slit illumination system which images the entire anterior segment including the cornea, lens and the anterior chamber. 12–50 captures are made by the rotating slit with 500 true elevation points on each slit thereby calculating 2500 height values, which are then used to map a three-dimensional model of the entire anterior eye segment.

Pentacam gives the true anterior and posterior elevation maps and the entire corneal pachymetry is obtained by their difference, which is displayed in a colour map. Thinnest point is also determined.

Advantages of Pentacam pachymetry

- Noncontact
- Noninvasive
- Eye movement correction available
- High quality of images.

Disadvantages Pentacam has been of late shown to give higher readings than the US pachymeter and noncontact specular microscope. However, Pentacam has mostly been shown to be corresponding to the US values in thin corneas.

IV. OPTICAL PACHYMETRY WITH OCULAR RESPONSE ANALYSER

Ocular response analyser (Reichert Ophthalmic Ins., NY, USA) is a new instrument, which measures the biomechanical properties of the cornea, namely corneal hysteresis (CH) along with the central thickness using an in-built 20 MHz US pachymeter.

CLINICAL APPLICATIONS OF CORNEAL PACHYMETRY

I. IN CORNEAL DISORDERS

1. Keratoconus diagnosis and management. Keratoconus (KC) is a bilateral noninflammatory progressive disease of the cornea which causes thinning and ectasia of the cornea with irregular astigmatism and cornel scarring. KC patients have both central and peripheral corneal thinning. Pentacam and other latest tomographic instruments can exactly point out the point of thinnest pachymetry based on which treatment modalities, e.g. CXL, intrastromal ring segments, etc. can be planned. D value is used

to differentiate between healthy and keratoconic corneas with a value of 1.6 SD or more being suspicious, and 2.6 SD or more as definitely keratoconic.

2. Corneal transplant procedures. Preoperative planning of corneal transplant procedures require an accurate pachymetry measurement, especially for lamellar procedures. Further, on follow-up for tracking the postoperative improvement of corneal oedema and the assessment of grafts for endothelial pump function, pachymetry plays an important role.

3. Monitoring endothelial cell function. Endothelial cell loss is related to loss of maintenance of the corneal transparency and normal thickness of the cornea causing stromal oedema. Cornea may be monitored for decompensation using pachymetry in postoperative cases of cataract surgery, penetrating keratoplasty, vitreoretinal surgery, etc.

II. IN GLAUCOMA

1. Glaucoma risk prediction. Ocular hypertension treatment study (OHTS) group has identified thin corneas to be an independent risk factor for the development of open angle glaucoma in people with OHT and this occurrence is also affected by other parameters like age, sex and race. Increased CCT in OHT may lead to recording of a falsely high IOP, whereas patients of low/normal tension glaucoma may have thin CCT leading to falsely low IOP measurement. PITX2 mutation positive Axenfeld-Rieger syndrome patients, pseudoexfoliation syndrome (PXF) cases and primary open angle glaucoma (POAG) cases may have lower pachymetry readings.

2. IOP measurement. Goldmann applanation tonometry (GAT) has been the gold standard for IOP measurement for decades now. However, Goldmann had assumed that the resistance of the cornea to indentation was compensated for the surface tension of the tear film for a corneal thickness of 520 mcm. The principle behind this is the 'Imbert-Fick's law' which assumes the cornea to be a flexible uniform sphere which is infinitely thin. Neither is the cornea regular nor infinitely thin. Hence, measurement of IOP with indentation techniques like Goldmann applanation tonometry, pneumotonometry and non-contact tonometry (NCT) are affected by the thickness of the cornea, viz. underestimating IOP in thinner corneas and overestimating in rigid ones. A correction factor of 0.7 mcm for every 10 mm Hg increase in IOP is applied. Pneumotonometer and NCT are especially susceptible to errors more than GAT, as these procedures require indentation of a larger surface area of the cornea. Dynamic contour tonometry (DCT) is a newer modality which is very less affected by the corneal thickness changes. It measures IOP using a strain gauge which creates a tight-fitting contact on the corneal surface and hence, is not affected by the corneal biomechanical properties.

III. IN REFRACTIVE SURGERY

1. Refractive surgery procedures. Preoperative screening and treatment planning for hyperopia and myopia require accurate pachymetry for procedures like LASIK, PRK and SMILE. Inadequate corneal thickness may require the patient to undergo an intraocular lens implantation instead of a lamellar corneal procedure.

2. Postrefractive ectasias. Thinning and corneal curvatural abnormalities postrefractive surgery may be detected using the latest tomographic instruments for diagnosing postrefractive ectasias and for further management using CXL, intrastromal ring segments, PRK, etc.

█ FACTORS MODIFYING PACHYMETRY

1. *Age.* For the majority of individuals, there is no substantial change in CCT beyond the infant years. However, some reports have found CCT to increase after 40 years of age.

2. *Sex.* Inconclusive reports have been published with males having higher CCT. But generally, sex has not been found to be a modifying factor for pachymetry. Higher contact lens usage among women may falsely lead to increased CCT readings.

3. *Race.* African-American persons have thinner corneas as compared to the white population. Similar trend has been observed in Asian population.

4. *Diurnal variation.* Pachymetry readings have been shown to be thinnest after awakening while thickens during the overnight period. This diurnal cycle in corneal thickness could be affected in women by factors like hormonal changes along the menstrual cycle, pregnancy, or oral contraceptive pills.

5. *Contact lens usage.* PMMA, hydrogel and rigid gas permeable (RGP) contact lenses affect the corneal thickness differently. The period of lens wear also becomes an important determinant. A short-term oedema may get resolved on prompt discontinuation of the lenses. Long-term contact lens wearers may show thinning of the cornea. This may be related to the thinning or instability of the tear film leading to a dry eye, thereby causing increased evaporation and desiccation of cornea. In refractive surgery planning, it has been advised to measure CCT after a minimum period of two weeks following contact lens wear discontinuation.

6. *Post-surgery.* Almost every anterior segment surgery specially cataract surgery, penetrating keratoplasty, etc. may cause postoperative corneal oedema for a week to one month, which returns to normal by 2–3 months. With modern phacoemulsification machines with improved phacodynamics and fluidics, the incidence of corneal oedema and the duration of persistence of this oedema has reduced.

7. *Chronic diseases.* Diabetes has been associated with an increased corneal thickness. Contact lens usage or chronic diseases affecting CCT is mostly within the usual range of variance and hence they do not necessitate the routine use of CCT measurement for monitoring. However, postsurgical causes may require the same.

█ CORNEAL HYSTERESIS

DEFINITION AND FACTS ABOUT CORNEAL HYSTERESIS

- **Corneal hysteresis** is a recently characterized viscoelastic property of the cornea. Cornea contains characteristics of both elastic and viscous materials. Corneal hysteresis reflects the ability of corneal tissue to absorb and dissipate energy during a bidirectional applanation process (where energy is lost as heat during the rapid loading/unloading of the cornea). In other words, corneal hysteresis is a measure of the stiffness or rigidity of the cornea. To better understand corneal hysteresis, consider the memory foam material used to make pillows and mattresses. Applying pressure deforms the material, but upon releasing the pressure, the material returns to its original shape slowly (a visco-elastic response) rather than bouncing back instantly like a stretched rubber band upon release (which is a purely elastic response).

- **Corneal hysteresis is a biomechanical corneal behaviour** and not a static physical property like corneal thickness. Corneal hysteresis is lower in eyes with higher IOP and normalizes after IOP reduction. Then hysteresis is not actually an intrinsic or constant property, but a measurement characterizing how a material or system responds to the loading and unloading of an applied force.

- **Corneal hysteresis measurement is repeatable in individual eyes** and strongly correlated in right and left eyes of the same patient. Corneal hysteresis, however, differs from person to person. It is not strongly correlated with other common metrics such as corneal radius, astigmatism, spherical equivalence (SE), axial length, and IOP measured by GAT. Corneal hysteresis and central corneal thickness (CCT) are moderately correlated in normal corneas and weakly to moderately correlated in corneas with disorder. Corneal hysteresis is lower than normal in patients with corneal disorders such as Fuchs' keratoconus, and glaucoma.

- **African-Americans have lower corneal hysteresis than Hispanics and White**s, but it is unclear whether this is explained by the association between corneal hysteresis and CCT or intergroup differences in corneal hysteresis that are independent of CCT.

- Various investigators have found associations between corneal hysteresis and optic nerve head (ONH) morphology.

CORNEAL HYSTERESIS: RELEVANCE IN GLAUCOMA

- Several studies have compared the biochemical characteristics of eyes with and without glaucoma. It has been repeatedly shown that patients with glaucoma have significantly lower corneal hysteresis and CCT than individuals with normal eyes.

- Corneal hysteresis has been shown to be lower in various types of glaucomatous eyes in comparison to normal eyes; these include POAG, PACG, NTG, and pseudoexfoliative glaucoma.

- Low corneal hysteresis is associated with glaucomatous visual field and optic nerve progression.

- Low-baseline corneal hysteresis is associated with a greater magnitude of IOP reduction following various glaucoma therapies including topical prostaglandin therapy and SLT.

- Corneal hysteresis (but not CCT or IOP) was associated with overall structural glaucomatous progression seen on a retrospective study of serial fundus photographs analyzed using flicker chronoscopy. This finding indicated that corneal hysteresis is directly associated with progressive glaucomatous optic neuropathy.

- Intraocular pressure reduction leads to an increase in corneal hysteresis.

- Biomechanical properties provide valuable information about the risk of glaucoma development and progression and may predict the effectiveness of various glaucoma therapies for individual patients. Although CCT continues to be a valuable tool, clinicians should also consider incorporating hysteresis measurements into practice. In several studies comparing the two variables, corneal hysteresis was more strongly related to progression than CCT. Corneal hysteresis has been the subject of considerable research recently, and with further investigation, its clinical implications for the diagnosis and management of glaucoma will become clearer.

MEASUREMENT OF CORNEAL HYSTERESIS: OCULAR RESPONSE ANALYSER

The ocular response analyser (ORA) measures the corneal hysteresis. The ORA applies an air puff on the anterior surface of the cornea and cause the cornea to deform. It measures the intensity of the reflected infrared light from the deforming corneal surface and reports several indices for diagnosis. It measures the biomechanical properties of the cornea which is useful in comparing LASIK and surface ablation as well as to evaluate the effect of creating a flap on corneal strength. It utilizes a dynamic, bidirectional applanation process and accurately measures the IOP. It takes into account the corneal hydration, connective tissue composition and bioelasticity, and contribute to the response of the corneoscleral shell, to the force applied during the measurement of IOP. It has a built in 20 MHz ultrasound pachymeter that measures CCT.

Advantages
- It is a noncontact procedure
- Superficial anaesthesia is not required
- The technique is speedy and offers high accuracy and repeatability
- It can diagnose corneal ectasia earlier than conventional diagnostic aids.

Disadvantages
- The high cost of equipment
- The doubts in standardization and need for recurrent calibration.

KERATOMETRY

PRINCIPLE OF KERATOMETRY

Keratometry is measurement of curvature of the anterior surface of cornea across a fixed chord length, usually 2–3 mm, which lies within the optical spherical zone of the cornea.

Keratometry is based on the fact that the anterior surface of the cornea acts as a convex mirror and the size of the image formed varies with its curvature. The greater the curvature of cornea, lesser is the image size. Therefore, from the size of the image formed by the anterior surface of cornea (1st Purkinje image), the radius of curvature of cornea can be calculated as below.

In Fig. 7.4, consider an object AB that forms an image A′B′ after reflection at the anterior surface of cornea. Ray AC passing towards centre of curvature C of the cornea is reflected back on itself. Ray AQ is reflected towards QS and seems to meet the ray AC at A′, forming the

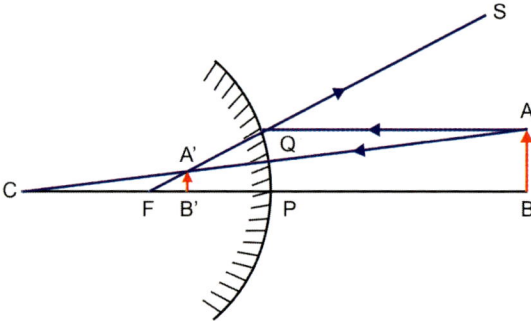

Fig. 7.4: *Principle of keratometry*

image A′B′. Now, if the object AB is at infinity then A′B′ will be very small and situated at the focus F. Therefore, B′P will be focal distance or ½ of radius of curvature of the mirror.

Thus, if $AB = o, A'B' = I, B'P = u$

then $CP = r, \dfrac{r}{2} = u \, 2\, \dfrac{I}{o}$

or $r = \dfrac{2uI}{o}$

The distance BP denoted by u is kept constant for any instrument by using a short focus telescope in order to view the reflected image. From this it is clear that for known object size, measurements of image size will allow us to determine r, the radius of curvature.

The accurate measurement of such an image, however, raises a problem since it is impossible to immobilize the living eye completely while the image is under observation. This has been overcome by devices using the *principle of visible doubling*. In one type of instrument, the image is doubled by refraction through two rotating glass plates which are then adjusted so that the lower edge of one image coincides with the upper edge of the other. If the eye moves during the process, both the images move together, and so difficulties in adjustment are avoided. From the amount of rotation of the glass plate necessary just to double the image, its size can be calculated.

In other types of keratometers, the amount of doubling is fixed but size of external object can be varied. Helmholtz (1854) utilized this principle to devise the first keratometer. He gave the

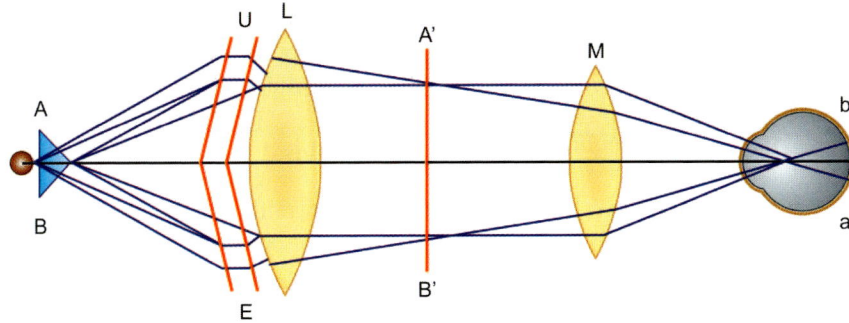

Fig. 7.5: *Optics of Helmholtz keratometer*

name ophthalmometer to it but later on kerato-meter was found to be more appropriate term.

HELMHOLTZ KERATOMETER

Though presently not in use, the Helmholtz keratometer is described here as a tribute to the inventor. Helmholtz keratometer consists of two plates. Each plate displaces the image through half its length and the total displacement gives the size of image. The doubling of image dispenses with the necessity of immobilizing the living eye. If the eye moves during the process, both the images move together and, therefore, difficulties in adjustment are avoided. The glass plates are of known thickness and index of refraction, placed side by side, so that each covers half of the object of a short-distance tele-scope. The axis of telescope coincides with the plane of separation of glass plates. These plates can be inclined one to the other at known angles, and the angle of incidence of light falling on them from a point in front can be varied and measured.

Optics of Helmholtz keratometer

As shown in Fig. 7.5, rays from point O meet the plates at U and E and undergo lateral displacement after refraction. As viewed through L, the two objects appear at A and B. The eyepiece M is so arranged that its principal focus coincides with the images A' and B' and receives parallel rays which come to the focus without accommodation on the retina at a and b. As shown in Fig. 7.6, if the position of plates is such that the two images A and B just touch at O then

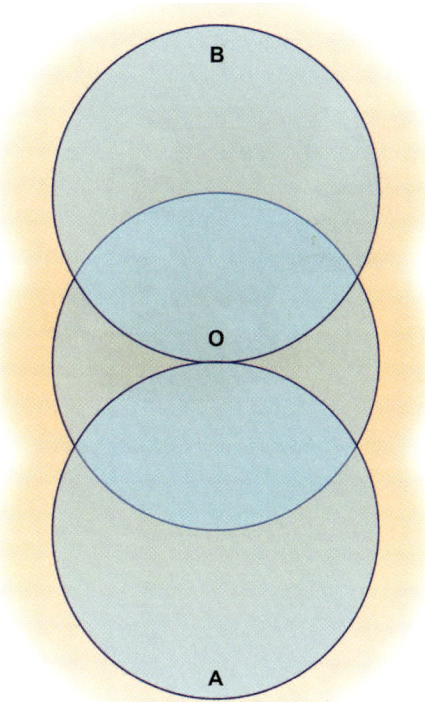

Fig. 7.6: *Measurement of the size of image in Helmholtz keratometer (observer's view)*

each plate has displaced the image through half its length and the total displacement gives the size of the image. The original instrument has undergone several modifications and nowadays several keratometers are in use.

An ideal keratometer must be able to measure the radii in various meridia about the axis of the cornea. Thus, instruments are designed that can be rotated with respect to a particular axis. The objects are called mires. In order to avoid the error due to constant motion of eyes, a doubling device has been introduced.

■ BAUSCH AND LOMB KERATOMETER

Principle

The working of Reichert (Bausch and Lomb) keratometer (Fig. 7.7) is based on the principle of *constant object size and variable image size*.

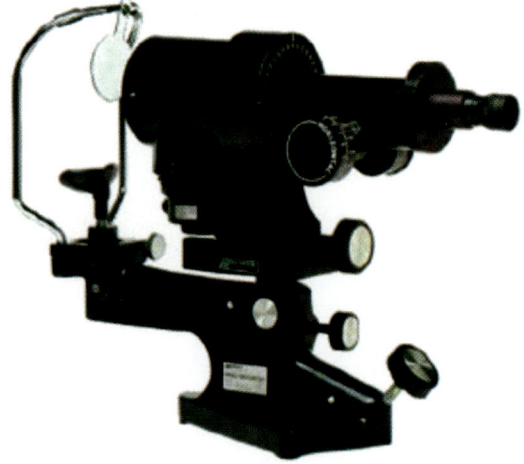

Fig. 7.7: *Bausch and Lomb keratometer*

Optical system and other parts

The functioning of the optical system (Fig. 7.8) and the other parts of this keratometer are as below:

1. **The object** is a circular mire with two plus and two minus signs (Fig. 7.9). As shown in Fig. 7.8, a lamp illuminates the mire by means of a diagonally placed mirror. Light from the mire strikes the patient's cornea and produces a diminished image behind it. This image becomes the object for the remainder of optical system.

2. **The objective lens** focuses the light from the image of the mire (new object) along the central axis.

3. **Diaphragm and doubling prisms**. A four-aperture diaphragm is situated near the objective lens. Beyond the diaphragms are two doubling prisms, one with its base up and other with its base out. The prisms can be moved independently, parallel to the central axis of the instrument. Light passing through the left aperture of diaphragm is made to deviate above the central optical axis by a base-up prism. Light passing through the right aperture is deviated by the base-out prism, placing the second image to the right of the central axis. Light passing through upper and lower apertures does not pass through either prism and an image is

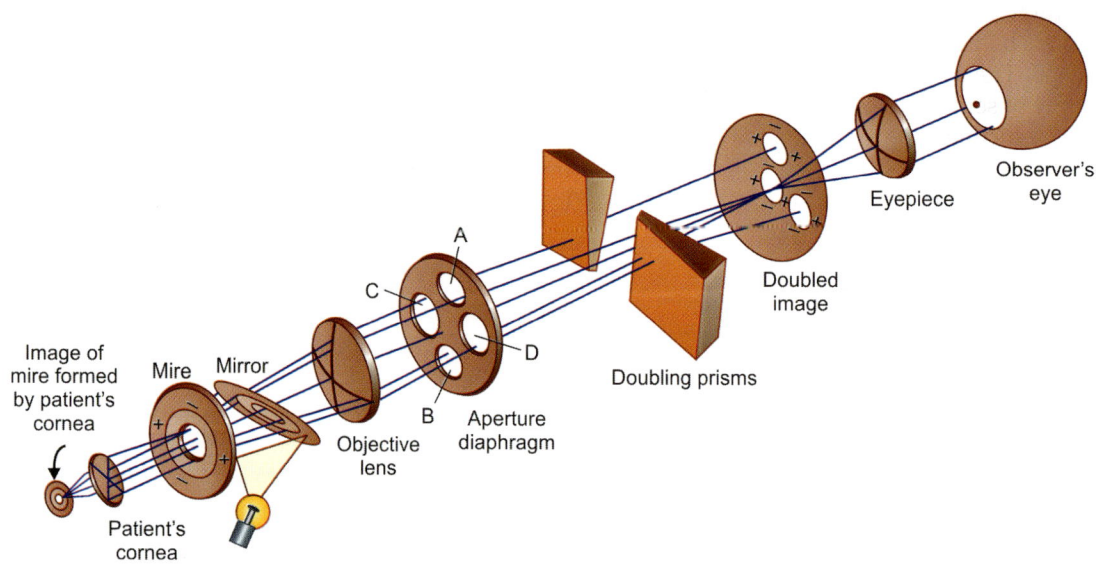

Fig. 7.8: *Optical system of Bausch and Lomb keratometer*

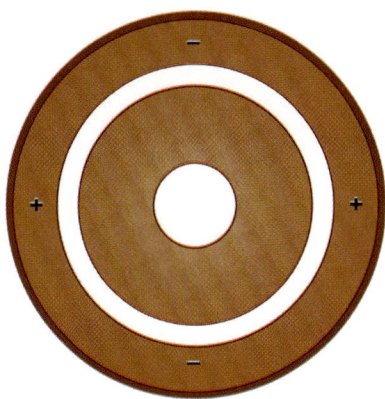

Fig. 7.9: *Configuration of the mires used in Bausch and Lomb keratometer*

produced in the axis. The total area of upper and lower apertures is equal to the area of each of the other two apertures. Thus, brightness of the images is equal. The upper and lower apertures also act as Scheiner's disc, doubling the central image, whenever the instrument is not focused precisely on the central mire image. So, continuous monitoring of correct focus can be done. Thus, the image-doubling mechanism is unique in Bausch and Lomb keratometer, in that double images are produced side by side as well as at 90° from each other. This allows the measurement of the power of cornea in two meridia, without rotating the instrument. Therefore, it is also known as 'one-position keratometer'. The doubling device also moves parallel to the control axis of the instrument so that the amount of separation can be raised.

4. **The eyepiece lens** enables the examiner to observe the magnified view of the doubled image.

Procedure of keratometry

1. **Instrument adjustment.** The instrument is calibrated before use. A white paper is held in front of the objective piece and a black line is focused sharply on it. The keratometer is then calibrated with steel balls. A steel ball of known radius of curvature is placed before the keratometer and its value is set on the scale or dial. The mires are focused by clockwise and anti-clockwise movement of the eyepiece through trial and error. When mires are in focus, the calibration is complete.

2. **Patient adjustment.** The patient is seated in front of the instrument with chin on the chin rest and head against the head rest. The eye that is not being examined is covered with the occluder. Then, the chin is raised or lowered till the patient's pupil and the projective knob are at the same level.

3. **Focusing of mire.** After adjusting the instrument and the patient, the mire is focused in the centre of cornea. Figure 7.9 shows the patient's view of mire and Fig. 7.10A shows the view first seen by the examiner. Note that the central image is doubled, indicating that the instrument is not correctly focused on the corneal image of the mire.

4. **Measurement of corneal curvature**
- *The instrument is correctly focused* on the corneal image so that central image is no longer doubled (Fig. 7.10B).
- *To measure the curvature in horizontal meridian*, the plus signs of the central and left images are superimposed using the horizontal measuring control and the reading is noted (Fig. 7.10C).
- *Then to measure the curvature in the vertical meridian*, the minus signs of the central and upper images are coincided with the help of vertical measuring control and the readings are noted (Fig. 7.10D).
- *Regular astigmatism.* For each eye the difference between horizontal and vertical dioptre readings gives the approximate amount of corneal astigmatism. Normally, horizontal and vertical dioptre readings are 90° apart.
- *In the presence of oblique astigmatism,* the two plus signs will not be aligned (Fig. 7.10E). The entire instrument is then rotated till the two plus signs are aligned (Fig. 7.10F). A scale associated with the instrument rotation indicates, in degrees, one meridian of the oblique astigmatism. Corneal radius of power is then measured in this meridian and in the meridian 90° to it as described above.

Interpreting findings

Spherical cornea is characterized by:
- No difference in the power between two principal meridia
- The mires seen as perfect sphere.

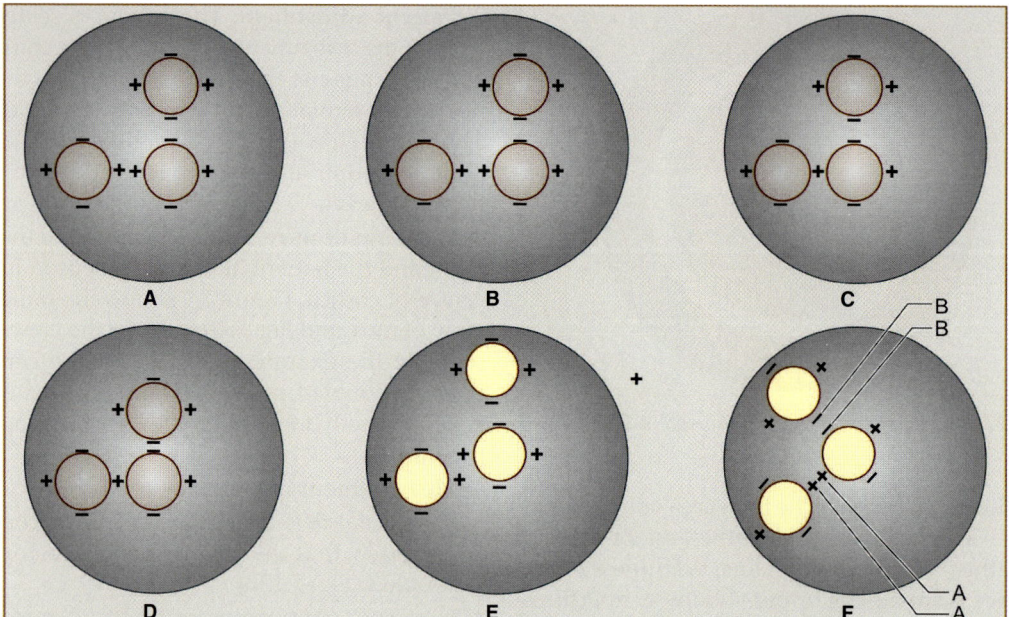

Fig. 7.10: *Examiner's view of the mires. A, When not focussed properly; B, Mires focussed properly but not aligned; C, Alignment of mires when measuring horizontal meridian; D, Vertical alignment of mires; E, Non-aligned mires in oblique astigmatism; F, Alignment of plus signs in oblique astigmatism*

Astigmatism is characterized by:
- Difference in the power between two principal meridia
- Horizontally, oval mires are seen in with-the-rule astigmatism
- Vertically, oval mires are seen in against-the-rule astigmatism
- In oblique astigmatism, the principal meridia are between 30–60° and 120–150°.

Irregular anterior corneal surface is characterized by:
- Irregular mires
- Doubling of mires.

Keratoconus is characterized by:
- Inclination and jumping of mires is seen while attempting to adjust the mires. When an attempt is made to superimpose the plus mires, they will jump above and below each other (*pulsating mires*).
- Minification of mires is seen in advanced keratoconus (K >52 D) due to increased amount of myopia.
- Oval mires are seen due to large astigmatism.

- Irregular, wavy and distorted mires also indicate advanced keratoconus.

JAVAL-SCHIÖTZ KERATOMETER

Principle

The working of Javal-Schiötz keratometer (Fig. 7.11) is based on the principle of *variable object size and constant image size*.

Optical system and other parts

The functioning of optical system (Fig. 7.12) and other parts of this keratometer is as below:

1. **The object** in this system consists of two mires (A and B), mounted on an arc on which they can be moved synchronously (Figs 7.12 and 7.13). Since, the two mires together form the object, the variable size is attained by their movement.

One mire is stepped and has a green filter and other mire is rectangular and has a red filter. The mires are divided horizontally through the centre (Fig. 7.14). The mires are illuminated by small lamps. The image of these mires formed by the patient's cornea (1st Purkinje image) acts

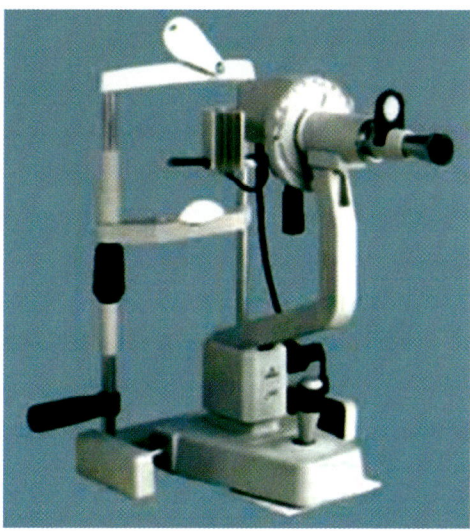

Fig. 7.11: *Javal-Schiötz keratometer*

as *an object for the rest of the optical system* of the keratometer.

2. **Objective lens and doubling prism** form the *doubled image* of the new object (image of the mires formed by cornea). The doubling prism used in this instrument is a Wollaston type. It produces a fixed image doubling by the birefringent (double refracting) characteristic of the material of which it is made.

3. **The eyepiece lens** enables the examiner to observe the magnified view of the doubled image.

Procedure of keratometry

1. **Instrument adjustment.** A white paper is held in front of the objective piece and a black line is focused on it. Then the instrument is calibrated to make it ready for use.

2. **Patient adjustment.** The patient is seated in front of the keratometer with chin on the chin rest and forehead against the forehead rest. The chin rest is adjusted to bring the eye at the level of telescope (T) of the instrument (Fig. 7.13). The eye not being examined is covered with an occluder provided with the instrument.

3. **Adjustment of mires.** The mires are adjusted in such a way that they are focused in the centre of patient's cornea. Figure 7.14 shows the patient's view of mires and Fig. 7.15 shows the view of the doubled mire image as seen by the examiner through the instrument's eyepiece.

4. **Recording of keratometric readings.** Only the central pair of images is used when measurements are made. By changing the separation of mires, the separation of these two images can be changed. When the two control images just meet, the scales associated with the mire separation indicate the correct corneal radius and the dioptric power of the cornea.

The radius of curvature is first found in one meridian. Then the entire optical system is rotated by 90° about its central axis. The measurement of the radius of curvature in the

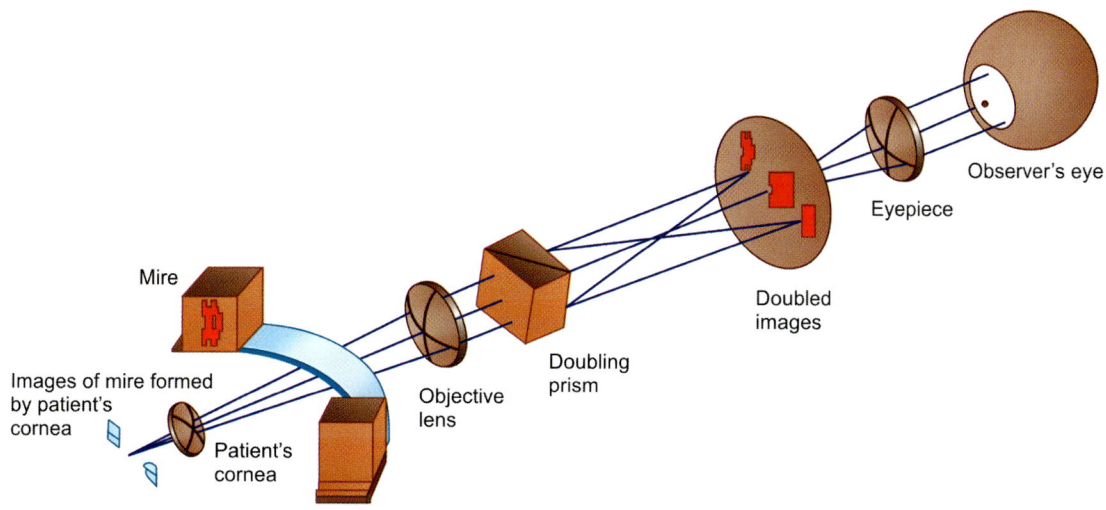

Fig. 7.12: *Optical system of Javal-Schiötz keratometer*

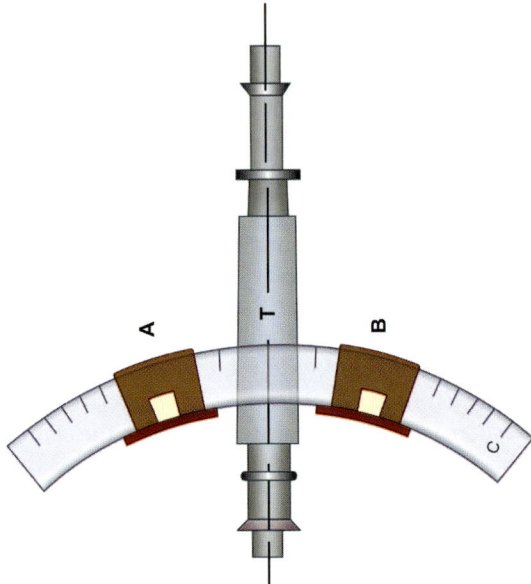

Fig. 7.13: *Basic structure of Javal-Schiötz keratometer showing placement of mires A and B on the arc*

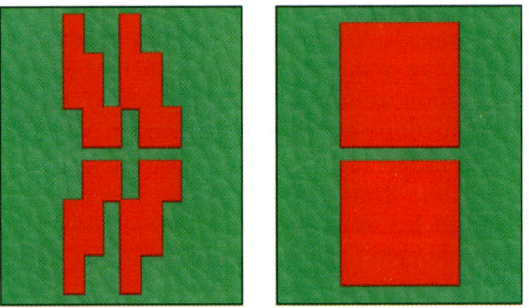

Fig. 7.14: *Patient's view of the mires*

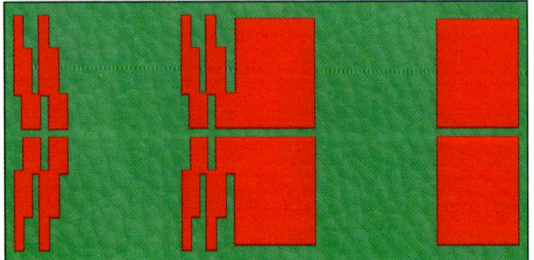

Fig. 7.15: *Examiner's view of doubled mire image*

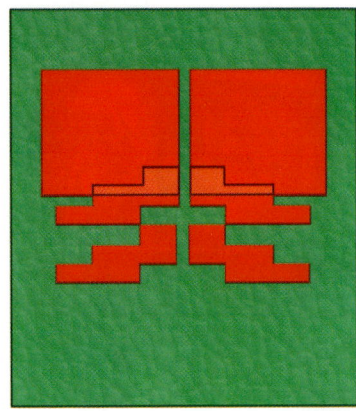

Fig. 7.16: *Overlapping of mires in corneal astigmatism*

may move further apart. Since, the stepped mire (staircase pattern) is green and the rectangular mire is red, the area of overlap appears whitish. Each step of the mire corresponds to 1 D of corneal power and thus, the number of steps overlapped gives the approximate degree of astigmatism.

When *oblique astigmatism* is present and the mires are horizontal, the central bisecting lines of the images are not aligned (Fig. 7.17A). In such cases, the instrument is rotated until the control lines are aligned (Fig. 7.17B). A scale associated with the instrument rotation indicates, in degrees, one meridian of the oblique astigmatism. Corneal radius or power is then measured in this meridian and also in the meridian 90° to it as usual.

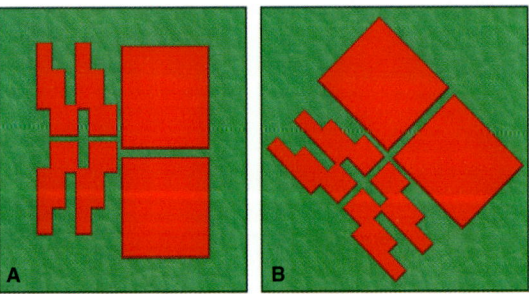

Fig. 7.17: *Appearance of images in oblique astigmatism when mires are horizontal before (A) and after alignment (B)*

SURGICAL/OPERATING KERATOMETER

The surgical keratometer is attached to the operating microscope. It is helpful in monitoring the astigmatism during corneal/limbal surgery.

second meridian which is perpendicular to the first one is then made in the similar way. When the corneal astigmatism is present, there may occur overlapping of the mires (Fig. 7.16) or they

Factors limiting accuracy

The accuracy of surgical keratometer is limited due to the following factors:

- Difficulty in aligning the patient's visual axis and the keratometer's optical axis.
- Keratometers are calibrated for a fixed distance from the anterior cornea. The different microscope objective lenses result in different focal lengths and, therefore, different working distance.
- Air in the anterior chamber results in a second target reflection.
- External pressure on the globe results in a change in the corneal curvature.

AUTOMATED KERATOMETER

Essentially, an autokeratometer is similar to manual keratometer. In it the reflected image of target is focused on to a photodetector which measures image size, and radius of curvature is computed. The target mires are illuminated with infrared light, and an infrared photodetector is used.

Advantages of autokeratometers are the following:

- A compact device
- Very short-time consuming
- Comparatively easy to operate.

Precision of autokeratometry. Almost all the studies have found exceptionally high precision with autokeratometry.

Availability of autokeratometer. Autokeratometers are available alone and more commonly in association with autorefractometers as *auto-kerato-refractometers* (e.g. Nidek ARK 2000-S autokerato-refractometer).

Automated keratometry option is also available in the following equipment:

- The IOL master
- Pentacam
- Orbscan
- Corneal topographer.

Handheld autokeratometers are also available, e.g. palmscan 2000 and Handy Ref K (uses synchro scan technology) (Fig. 7.18).

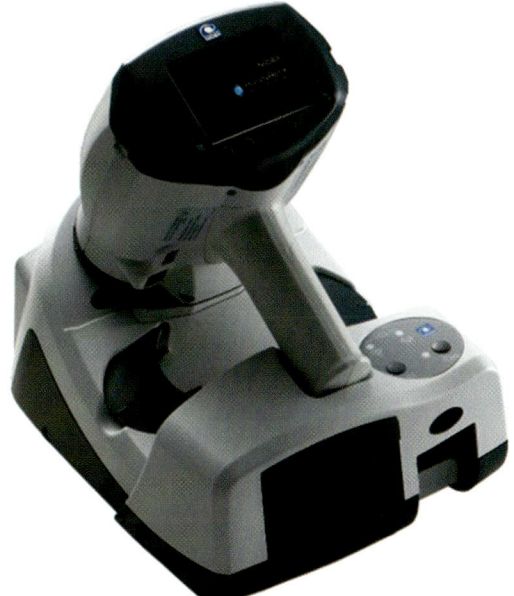

Fig. 7.18: *Handheld autokeratometer*

RELATIONSHIP BETWEEN RADIUS OF CURVATURE AND DIOPTRIC POWER OF CORNEA

The following equation gives the relationship between radius of curvature and dioptric power of the cornea:

$$D = \frac{n-1}{r}$$

where D is dioptric power of the cornea, n is the index of refraction of the cornea and r is the radius of cornea in metres.

Since, the invention of ophthalmometer by Helmholtz, the index of refraction of the cornea has been taken 1.3375 for calibrating the instrument. Therefore,

$$r = \frac{1.3375 - 1}{D} \text{ m}$$

or

$$r = \frac{337.5 - 1}{D} \text{ mm}$$

Usually, the keratometers are calibrated both for radius of curvature and corresponding dioptres. Otherwise, the conversion can also be made by using the above described equation. For a ready reference, conversion table is also available.

Range of keratometer is 36–52 D (6.5–9.38 mm). Its lower limit can be extended up to 30 D (5.6 mm) and upper limit up to 61 D (10.9 mm) by interposing a lens of –1.0 D and 11.25 D, respectively, in front of the objective of telescope.

CLINICAL USES, LIMITATIONS AND SOURCES OF ERROR

CLINICAL USES OF KERATOMETER

The various uses of keratometer in day-to-day ophthalmic practice are as follows:

1. It helps in measurement of *corneal astigmatic* error.
2. It helps to estimate the radius of curvature of the anterior surface of cornea. So, it is of great use in *contact lens fitting*.
3. Keratometer is used to monitor the shape of the cornea in keratoconus and keratoglobus.
4. We may be able *to assess the refractive error* in cases with hazy media (rough estimate on the basis that the normal measurement is 43.5 D—comparison of the two eyes in these cases is useful).
5. Keratometry has gained a special place in *IOL (intraocular lens) power calculation*. The K readings are taken with the help of keratometer and along with axial length, these are utilised to calculate IOL power in SRK (Sanders, Retzlaff and Kraff) formula for IOL power calculation.
6. It is used to monitor pre- and post-surgical astigmatism.
7. It is used for differential diagnosis of axial versus curvatural anisometropia.
8. It is used to detect rigid gas-permeable lens flexure.

LIMITATIONS OF KERATOMETRY

1. The measurements of keratometer are based on a false assumption that the cornea is a symmetrical spherical or spherocylindrical structure, with two principal meridia separated from each other by 90°, whereas the cornea in reality is aspheric.
2. It measures the refractive status of a very small central area of cornea (3–4 mm), ignoring the peripheral corneal zones.

3. It loses its accuracy when measuring very flat (<40 D) or very steep (>50 D) cornea.
4. Finally, small corneal irregularities would preclude the use of keratometer due to irregular astigmatism.
5. Assumed index of refraction in radius to dioptre conversion.
6. One-position instruments assume regular astigmatism.
7. Distance to focal point is approximated by distance to image.
8. The use of para-axial optics to calculate surface power.
9. It cannot describe corneal asphericity.

SOURCES OF ERROR IN KERATOMETRY

- Improper calibration
- Faulty positioning of the patient
- Improper fixation by the patient
- Accommodative fluctuation by examiner
- Localized corneal distortion
- Excessive tearing
- Abnormal lid position
- Improper focusing of the corneal image.

BIBLIOGRAPHY

1. Armitage BS, Schoessler JP. Overnight corneal swelling response in adapted and unadapted extended wear patients. Am J Optom Physiol Opt 1988; 65: 155–61.
2. Brautaset RL, Nilsson M, et al. Central and peripheral corneal thinning in keratoconus. Cornea 2013; 32; 257–61.
3. Cheng AC, Tang E, et al. Correction factor in Orbscan II in the assessment of corneal pachymetry. 2006; 25(10): 1158–61.
4. Correia FF, Ramos I, et al. Topometric and tomographic indices for the diagnosis of keratoconus. Int J of Keratoconus Ectatic Corneal Dis 2012; 1: 92–99.
5. Cox I, Ames K. Effect of eye patching on the overnight corneal swelling response with rigid contact lenses. Optom Vis Sci 1989; 66: 207–8.
6. Douthwaite W, Pardhan S. Comparison of a videokeratoscope and an autokeratometer as predictors of the optimum back surface curves of rigid corneal contact lenses. Ophthalmic Physiol Opt. 1997 Sep; 17(5): 409–13.

7. Elliott DB. Clinical Procedures in Primary Eye Care (3rd edn.). Edinburgh/New York: Butterworth-Heinemann Ltd 2007; 85–90.

8. Friling R, Weinberger D, Kremer I, Avisar R, Sirota L, Snir M. Keratometry measurements in preterm and full term newborn infants. Br J Ophthalmol 2004; 88(1): 8–10.

9. Fujioka M, Nakamura M, et al. Comparison of Pentacam Scheimpflug camera with ultrasound pachymetry and noncontact specular microscopy in measuring central corneal thickness. Curr Eye Res 2007; 32: 89–94.

10. Gutmark R, Guyton DL. Origins of the Keratometer and its Evolving Role in Ophthalmology. Survey of Ophthalmology 2010; 55(5): 481–97.

11. Haque S, Simpson T, et al. Corneal and epithelial thickness in keratoconus: a comparison of ultrasonic pachymetry, Orbscan II, and optical coherence tomography. J Refract Surg 2006; 22(5): 486–93.

12. Hashemi H, Roshani M, et al. Effect of corneal thickness on the agreement between ultrasound and Orbscan II pachymetry. J Cataract Refract Surg 2007; 33(10): 1694–1700.

13. Hoffer KJ. Biometry of 7,500 cataractous eyes. Am J Ophthalmol 1980; 90(3): 360–68.

14. Javaloy J, Vidal MT, et al. Comparison of four corneal pachymetry techniques in corneal refractive surgery. J Refract Surg 2004; 20, 29–34.

15. Khoramnia R, Rabsilber TM, et al. Central and peripheral pachymetry measurements according to age using the Pentacam rotating Scheimpflug camera. J Cataract Refract Surg 2007; 33: 830–36.

16. Lass JH, Gal RL, et al. Cornea Donor Study Investigator Group. Ophthalmology 2008; 115(4): 627–32.

17. Lei Y, Zheng X, et al. Effects of long-term soft contact lens wear on the corneal thickness and corneal epithelial thickness of myopic subjects. Mol Med Rep 2015; 11(3): 2020–26.

18. Mandell RB, Fatt I. Thinning of the human cornea on awakening. Nature 1965; 208: 292–93.

19. Mehrdad Mohammadpour, et al. Central Corneal Thickness Measurement Using Ultrasonic Pachymetry, Rotating Scheimpflug Camera, and Scanning-slit Topography Exclusively in Thin Non-keratoconic Corneas. J Ophthalmic Vis Res 2016; 11(3): 245–51.

20. Noonan CP, Rao GP, Kaye SB, Green JR, Chandna A. Validation of a handheld automated keratometer in adults. J Cataract Refract Surg 1998; 24(3): 411–14.

21. Polse KA. Changes in corneal hydration after discontinuing contact lens wear. Am J Optom Arch Am Acad Optom 1972; 49: 511–16.

22. Saleh Al-Ageel, et al. Comparison of central corneal thickness measurements by Pentacam, noncontact specular microscope, and ultrasound pachymetry in normal and post-LASIK eyes. Saudi J Ophthalmol 2009; 23(3–4): 181–87.

23. Sophia Y Wang, et al. The impact of central corneal thickness on the risk for glaucoma in a large multiethnic population. J Glaucoma 2014; 23(9): 606–12.

24. Suzuki S, Oshika T, et al. Corneal thickness measurements: scanning-slit corneal topography and noncontact specular microscopy versus ultrasonic pachymetry. J Cataract Refract Surg 2003; 29(7): 1313–18.

25. Tam ES, Rootman DS. Comparison of central corneal thickness measurements by specular microscopy, ultrasound pachymetry, and ultrasound biomicroscopy. J Cataract Refract Surg 2003; 29: 179–84.

26. Trivedi RH, Wilson ME, Peterseim MM, Lal G. Axial length and keratometry in eyes with pediatric cataract. Annual American Society of Cataract and Refractive Surgeons Symposium on Cataract, IOL, and Refractive Surgery San Francisco, CA 2003 April; 12–16.

Chapter

8

Corneal Topography and Aberrometry

CORNEAL TOPOGRAPHY

GENERAL CONSIDERATIONS

Corneal topography refers to study of shape of corneal surface. The term corneal topography system (CTS), or videokeratography, implies computerized, video-assisted technique that provides detailed information about the shape of the corneal surface.

Present day technologies allow three-dimensional evaluation with cross-sectional images and are thus referred to as *corneal tomography systems.*

WORKING PRINCIPLES

Present day available corneal topography and tomography systems are based on one or combination of more than one below given working principles:

- Placido-disc principle-based corneal topography/tomography systems
- Slit-scanning principle corneal tomography system (e.g. Orbscan III)
- Scheimpflug imaging principle-based systems (e.g. Pentacam, Sirius, Galilei)
- High speed anterior segment optical coherence tomography (AS-OCT)
- Digital rasterstereography-based topography systems
- Laser halographic interferometry-based topography systems
- Very high frequency (VHF) ultrasound-based system.

COMMONLY USED TOPOGRAPHY/TOMOGRAPHY SYSTEMS

Commonly used corneal topography systems and aberrometry systems are listed in Table 8.1.

Table 8.1: *Commonly used topography system and aberrometry system*

A. CORNEAL TOPOGRAPHY AND TOMOGRAPHY SYSTEMS

I. Placido-Disc-based System

1. EyeSys Desktop (*EyeSys Vision, Inc., US*)	• Placido-ring/cone
2. Tomey TMS-4M (*Tomey Corp, Japan*)	• Placido-disc-based
3. CA-200F Corneal Analyzer (*Topcon Medical Systems, Inc., Japan*)	• Placido-disc-based topography system (with 24 rings measuring over 10,000 data points and eight blue LED lights for fluorescein images to aid in contact lens simulation)
4. AstraMax (*Laser Sight Technology Florial*)	• Placido-disc-based, 3D corneal topography

II. Scheimpflug Rotating Imaging-based Systems

1. Pentacam AXL (*Oculus, Germany*)	• Dual Scheimpflug and Placido-disc imaging
2. Oculyzer (*Wavelight AG, Germany*)	• Dual Scheimpflug and Placido-disc imaging
3. Preciso (*iVIS Technologies, Taranto, Italy*)	• Dual Scheimpflug and Placido-disc imaging
4. Galilei G6 (*Zeimer, Switzerland*)	• Dual Scheimpflug and Placido-disc imaging
5. TMS-5 (*Tomey Corp, Japan*)	• Dual Scheimpflug and Placido-disc imaging
6. Sirius (*CSO, Italy*)	• Dual Scheimpflug and Placido-disc imaging

III. Horizontal Slit Scan-based System

1. Orbscan IIIz (*Bausch and Lomb, Rochester, New York*)	• Dual horizontal slit scan and Placido-disc imaging

IV. Rasterstereography-based System

1. PAR Corneal Topography System (*CTS; Par Vision Systems Corp., New Hartford, NY*)	• Elevation-based systems which project a grid onto the corneal surface after instillation of fluorescein • Distortions in grid patterns are analyzed to determine corneal elevation-based on camera and grid projection angles (rasterstereography)

V. Very High Frequency (VHF) Ultrasound-based System

1. Artemis 3 (*ARC Scan, Colorado*)	I. ARC scanning with very high frequency ultrasound

Contd.

Table 8.1 *Commonly used topography system and aberrometry system (Contd.)*

2. Visante Omni (*Carl Zeiss Meditec, Germany*)	II. Rotating optical coherence tomography and Placido-disc imaging
3. SS1000 Casia (*Tomey Corp, Japan*)	III. Rotating optical coherence tomography
VI. Optical Coherence Tomography-based Systems	
1. RTVue-100 (*Optovue, Inc. Fremont, CA*)	• Spectral domain optical coherence tomography-guided corneal power measurement (both anterior and posterior curvatures)
2. IOL Master 700 (*Carl Zeiss Meditec, Germany*)	• Swept Source OCT Technology with 32-Marker Placido pattern
3. 3D OCT-2000 (5) (*Topcon Medical Systems*)	• Spectral domain OCT
4. Cirrus HD-OCT 5000 (2) (*Carl Zeiss Meditec, Germany*)	• Spectral domain OCT, confocal scanning laser Ophthalmoscope (CSLO)
B. CORNEAL TOPOGRAPHERS WITH ABERROMETERS	
1. KR-1W Wavefront Analyzer (*Topcon Medical Systems*)	• Hartmann-Shack aberrometry • Near-infrared corneal topography
2. i-Trace (*Tracey Technologies, Houston*)	• Ray-tracing aberrometery • Placido-disc corneal topography (sequentially projects 256 near-infrared laser beams into the eye to measure forward aberrations, processing data point by point)
3. Atlas 9000 Corneal Topography System (*Carl Zeiss Meditec, Germany*)	• Placido-disc topography (22-ring) • Patented "Cone-of-Focus" alignment system
4. OPD-Scan III (*Nidek, Gamagori, Japan*)	• Ray-tracing aberrometry • Placido-disc topography (33 Blue mires) • Dynamic skiascopy for aberrometry
5. Wavelight Allegro Oculyzer II (*Alcon, US*)	• Rotating 3D Scheimpflug imaging topography • Tscherning principle aberrometry
6. Cassini TCA (*i-Optics, USA*)	• Placido-disc corneal topography • Ray-tracing aberrometry systems
7. Discovery (*Innovative Visual Systems, US*)	• Placido-disc corneal topography • Hartmann-Shack principle
C. ABERROMETERS	
1. Zywave® II Wavefront Aberrometer (*Bausch and Lomb*)	• Hartmann-Shack principle
2. WASCA Analyzer/Aberrometer (*Carl Zeiss Meditec, Germany*)	• Hartmann-Shack principle
3. LADARWave (*Alcon, US*)	• Hartmann-Shack principle
4. Visx Waves can Wavefront Aberrometer (*Abbott Medical Optics, Inc. (AMO), US*)	• Hartmann-Shack principle
5. Wavelight Allegro Analyzer (*Alcon, US*)	• Tscherning principle
6. Optiwave Refractive Analysis® (ORA) System (*Wavetec, US*)	• Infrared light and Talbot-Moiré interferometry (intraoperative wavefront aberrometer)
7. HOLOS IntraOp Wavefront Aberrometer (*Clarity Medical Systems, Inc., US*)	• Continuous real time intraoperative wavefront aberrometer

PLACIDO-DISC-BASED CORNEAL TOPOGRAPHY SYSTEMS

Placido-disc corneal topography systems were originally limited to evaluation of the anterior corneal surface. Presently many of the Placido-disc-based systems include the imaging of back surface of cornea and direct evaluation of elevational changes of both anterior and posterior corneal surfaces, enabling point-to-point pachymetry. In other words, the corneal topography system, now can be called *corneal tomographs*, as they allow three-dimensional evaluation of corneal tissue. This technique has an excellent accuracy and reproducibility. Most corneal topographers evaluate 8000–10,000 specific points across the entire corneal surface.

PLACIDO-DISC PRINCIPLE

Placido-disc-based corneal topography systems work on the reflection principle. The anterior surface of the cornea acts like a convex mirror and hence, the size of the image formed by it is determined by its curvature. A steeply curved cornea will produce a smaller image while a flatter cornea will produce a larger image of the same object situated at the same distance from the cornea. These devices thus measure the slope and compute the curvature. They have different projection devices that use lighted circular rings of varying sizes and numbers, these rings are reflected by convex cornea and through an opening in the centre of the target, the images are obtained by an acquisition camera.

BASIC UNIT OF CORNEAL TOPOGRAPHY SYSTEMS

The basic unit of a corneal topographic/tomographic system thus primarily consists of:

- A projection device
- Acquisition device (video camera)
- Analytical device (a digital computer attached with a slit-lamp chin rest)

1. Projection device

These systems imply Placido-disc-based projection device. Historically, the Placido-disc-based systems are the first to be developed and thus are the most widely used and understood. Most Placido-disc-based systems project around 8–32 concentric rings on the cornea. The rings are numbered from inside out. A specified ring in different instruments may cover different areas. Therefore, it is important to mention the diameter of the projected ring along with the number. The virtual images of these reflected rings are located anterior to the iris.

2. Video camera

The reflected images of rings projected on to the cornea are captured on charge-coupled device (CCD) camera for video-keratoscope. The image accuracy and precision are—images of rings are digitized and algorithms are used to determine the radius of curvature of innermost ring. Once this is determined then the distance of next ring from this is calculated and used to determine curvature of this ring and so on till peripheral ring is achieved. The cornea between rings is not imaged and no actual data for these points and the apex of cornea which is inside innermost ring is also not measured.

- Dioptric power is calculated from curvature using the formula:

$$Dioptric\ power = \frac{\text{refractive index of cornea} - \text{refractive index of air}}{\text{radius of curvature in metres}}$$

- Measured radius of curvature is of anterior corneal surface, so provides power of anterior surface while cannot measure the true power of posterior corneal surface.

3. Computer

The video camera is hooked up to a computer that generates a 'topographic map' of corneal curvature based on the measured distance between the rings reflected from the cornea. The accuracy of corneal curvature data processing depends a lot on the software-editing features. After analysis, the graphic picture of the patients' topography is displayed in various forms.

LIMITATIONS OF PLACIDO-DISC-BASED TOPOGRAPHY SYSTEMS

Limitations of Placido-disc-based topography systems include the following:

- There is *a lack of standardization between instruments*; it depends on reference axis, alignment, and focus. The corneal apex is the point of maximum curvature on the cornea, whereas the vertex is the point nearest to the camera of the Placido instrument located on the corneal topographer axis (CT axis). Before acquisition, the topographer aligns this axis normal to the cornea. This is possible only in ideal scenario but in patients with positive angle kappa the line of sight does not pass through apex of cornea and the reflected image appears displaced and is shown as asymmetric bow tie in otherwise normal cornea. The effect of decentration is nullified to an extent in elevation based devices.

- *The elevation maps* are derived in Placido devices by using angle of reflection and by making mathematical assumptions, so cannot be as accurate as true elevation maps of slit scan Scheimpflug devices.
- *Intraobserver and interobserver* variability errors, alignment errors, focussing errors or errors of calibration.
- *Central regions* require a higher degree of subpixel resolution in order to detect a 0.25 D change than do peripheral region.
- *Difficulties in determination of the power and location* of the steepest meridian when using artificial tears in postpenetrating keratoplasty eyes.

COMMERCIALLY AVAILABLE PLACIDO-DISC TOPOGRAPHY SYSTEMS

Commercially available corneal topography systems based on Placido-disc principle are listed in Table 8.1. Cardinal features of the some of presently available systems are described briefly.

1. EyeSys Desktop

EyeSys Desktop (Fig. 8.1B) from EyeSys Vision, Inc., US, is a 25-ring videokeratoscopic device with USB 2 connectivity with fast image processing time of 3 seconds and colour-coded contour map plots in addition to a host of other presentation schemes including customized packages. It analyses 9000 data points. The software with the system takes the Stiles-Crawford effect into consideration and allows display of relative brightness of light entering the pupil. This results in more practically useful information. It utilises the technology of EyeSys 2000 corneal analysis system.

EyeVista is the portable available model with similar functions, with which patients confined to a bed or wheelchair can easily be examined and supine patients can be mapped in the operating room under a surgical microscope.

2. TMS-4 Topographic Modelling System

The TMS-4 Topographic Modelling System from Computed Anatomy, Inc. through Tomey Technology, Inc., Cambridge, utilizes 31 projected rings providing 7000 data points. The corneal coverage is 0.02–11.00 mm with an accuracy of 0.10 D. It has a patented laser alignment system for accurate alignment and an exclusive refractive surgery planning programme.

3. AstraMax

AstraMax is a Placido-disc corneal tomography system manufactured by LaserSight Technologies, Inc., Winter Park, Florida (Fig. 8.1C). AstraMax is a new generation 3D corneal topography with enhanced resolution ideally suited for custom cornea-based treatment. AstraMax

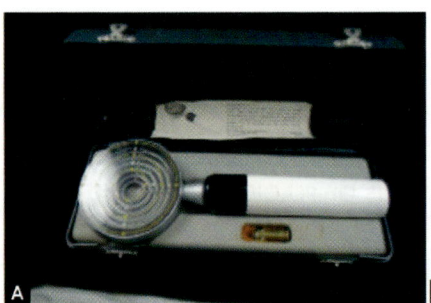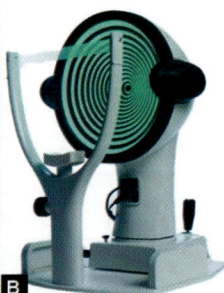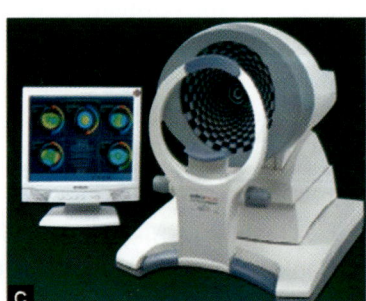

Fig. 8.1: *A, Placido-disc keratoscope (Keeler's); B, Corneal topography system: EyeSys Desktop (EyeSys Vision, Inc.); C, Corneal tomography system (AstraMax)*

is a three-camera imaging system that uses stereo ray-tracing for high precision, patient-specific corneal measurements. Patented polar grid yields critical measurements to measure complex corneal shapes. High definition graphics provide eye simulations and 3D surface modelling.

4. Atlas 9000 corneal topography system

Working principles of Atlas 9000 Corneal Topography System (*Carl Ziess, Germany*) include:

- *Ray-tracing technology* to displays higher order corneal aberrations.
- *Placido-disc technology* with *Cone-of-Focus* alignment system. It has *nonvisible Placido ring illumination* which is comfortable for even the most light-sensitive patients. The 22-ring Placido-disc is optimized to avoid ring cross-over, which allows reliable results for a wide range of patients.

Applications. This system, based on corneal wavefront analysis, is a diagnostic instrument that measures the curvature of the cornea and produces topographical images. It supports many important optometric applications, including contact lens fitting, pathology detection and management and selection of aspheric IOLs.

5. OPD scan III

The OPD III (*Nidek, Japan*) is five-in-one refractive work station which combines:

- *Wavefront aberrometry* gives assessment of visual acuity and quality of vision in addition to traditional refraction and keratometry. Simulation of retinal contrast sensitivity and visual acuity charts enable objective quantification of visual clarity.
- *Corneal topography* provides intuitive maps and numerical data for the corneal surface and provides neural network assisted detection of corneal pathology such as keratoconus suspect, keratoconus and pellucid marginal degeneration.
- *Autorefractometer* provides exceptionally accurate refractions for various pupil diameters including refractions under photopic and mesopic conditions, critical for proper

assessment of both refractive surgery patients and common refractive problems.

- *Autokeratometer* provides conventional keratometry and novel corneal surface descriptors such as APP (average pupil power) and ECCP (effective central corneal power) which aid in the calculation of the correct IOL power for postoperative corneas.
- *Pupillometry* measures photopic and mesopic pupil diameters. Pupil images reveal the shape of photopic and mesopic pupils, which can alter refraction and important surgical data. Identification of the first Purkinje image (corneal light reflex) and pupil centre are provided. The distance between these two landmarks is calculated to assist in centration during refractive surgery and to assess IOL centration.

6. Cassini TCA

Cassini total corneal astigmatism (TCA) (*I-optics, USA*) uses multicoloured LED point-to-point ray-tracing to provide a GPS-like analysis of the cornea along with high resolution images utilized for surgical guidance. There is a total of 679 LEDs; 224 red, 224 green, 224 yellow and 7 white. The unique measuring principle enables highly accurate and repeatable measurements of the total corneal astigmatism. Cassini TCA measures the posterior cornea using second Purkinje reflections and provides a total corneal astigmatism measurement. The multicoloured LED coverage is equal across the entire cornea, leaving no space for central scotoma. The accurate axis and magnitude of astigmatism play a vital part in the correct selection and positioning of a toric IOL.

DISPLAY OF PLACIDO-DISC-BASED CORNEAL TOPOGRAPHIC SYSTEM DATA

The corneal topographic data analysed by the computers can be displayed in the following formats:

- A. Numerical power plots
- B. Keratometry view
- C. Photokeratoscopic view
- D. Profile view
- E. Colour-coded topographic maps.

The most useful form of data presentation is a colour-coded corneal contour map, which will be discussed in detail.

A. NUMERICAL POWER PLOTS

In numerical power plots, the corneal curvature of specific areas is shown in dioptre values (Fig. 8.2). The data are displayed in 10 concentric circular zones with 1 mm interval between each. The numerical values are displayed in colour, which are in agreement with the colour scale being used. The display also shows the average dioptric value of each of the 10 concentric circular zones individually along with the average overall corneal curvature.

B. KERATOMETRIC VIEW

Keratometric view (Fig. 8.3) depicts the keratometric reading in two principal meridia (K_1 and K_2) in three different zones simultaneously. The three zones measured are *central* 3 mm zone (as in a conventional keratometry), *intermediate* 3–5 mm zone and *peripheral* 5–7 mm zone.

It is an important map for assessing the skewing of semi-meridia. The more the keratometric readings in principal meridia deviate from being perpendicular to each other, the more irregular or non-orthogonal corneal astigmatism exists.

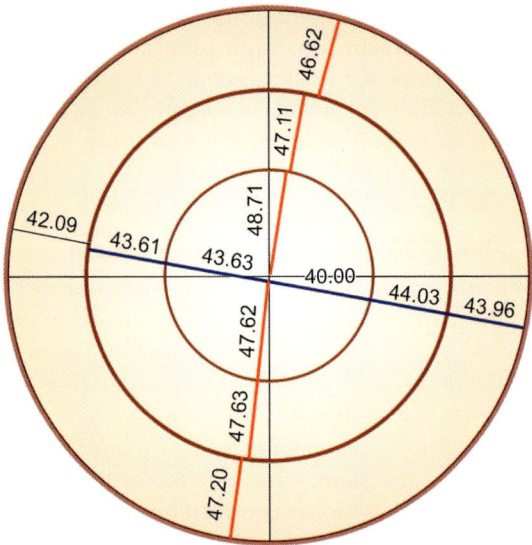

Fig. 8.3: *Keratometric view of the data (Courtesy: Dr Rajib Mukherjee)*

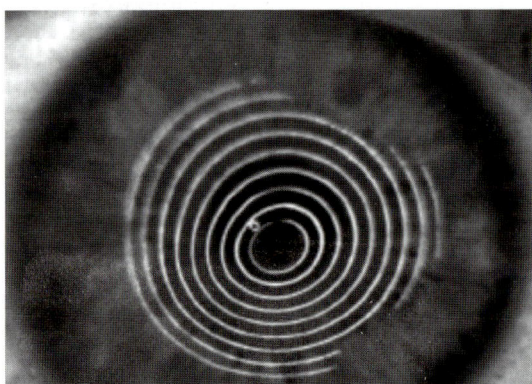

Fig. 8.4: *Photokeratoscopic view showing egging of mires in a patient with keratoconus (Courtesy: Dr Rajib Mukherjee)*

C. PHOTOKERATOSCOPIC VIEW

Photokeratoscopic view (Fig. 8.4) depicts the actual black and white photograph of the Placido rings captured by the video camera. This view helps in confirming the proper patient fixation and in identifying the eye captured. The reflected rings on the cornea are situated more towards the limbus on one side than the other, and on the nasal side the distance between the rings is comparatively narrower.

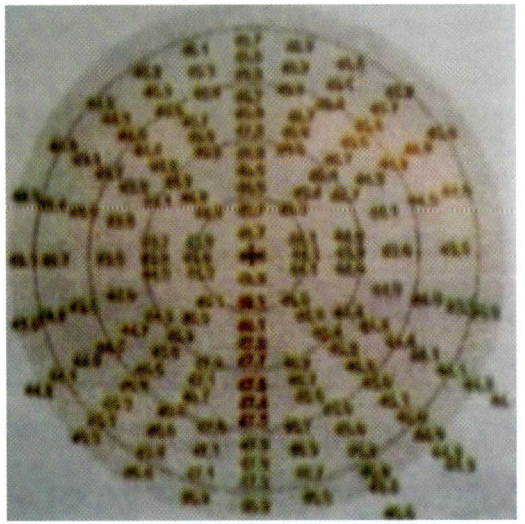

Fig. 8.2: *Numerical power plot (Courtesy: Dr Rajib Mukherjee)*

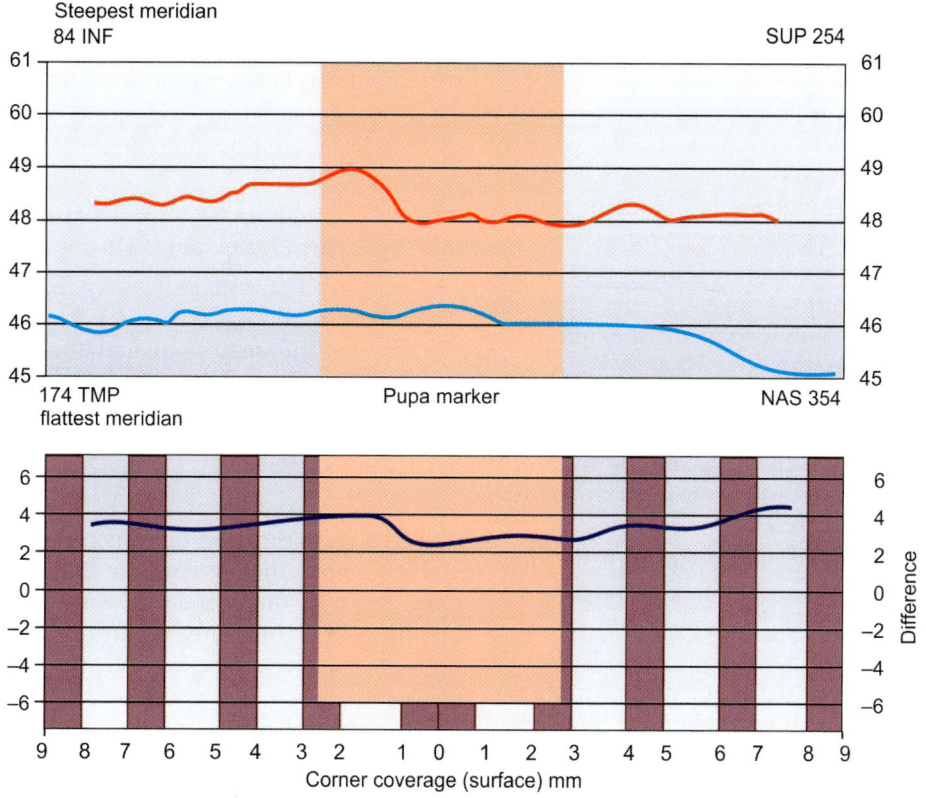

Fig. 8.5: *Profile view (Courtesy: Dr Rajib Mukherjee)*

D. PAR CTS PROFILE VIEW

The profile view (Fig. 8.5) shows the graphical plotting along the XY axis of the steepest and the flattest meridia of the cornea and the difference between the two in dioptres. The display button shows the astigmatic difference (difference plot, or delta map) between the flat and steep meridia. A grey zone in this difference plot denotes the pupillary area. In a symmetrical eye, the tracing across this grey band is a straight line. In the presence of astigmatism, an apparent slag is seen. This slag increases, with the asymmetricity of cornea.

E. COLOUR-CODED TOPOGRAPHIC MAP

Colour-coded contour maps of the cornea are the most useful and most commonly used display formation.

Interpretation of a colour map

While interpreting colour-coded contour maps of the cornea, following parameters should be considered:

1. *Colour codes.* These are used as follows:
- *Hot colours,* i.e. red and its various hues represent the steep portions of cornea.
- *Cool colours,* i.e. blue and its various hues represent the flat portions of cornea.
- So, the colours red–orange–yellow–green–purple–blue denote progressively lessening refractive power.

The colour intensity is relative, meaning that an area of 45D is less red as compared to an area of 46D.

2. *The scale used.* It is very important to know the scale used before interpreting a colour map. The two apparently similar maps may in fact show markedly different cornea depending upon the scale used. The commonly used scales are absolute and normalized scales:

Absolute scale. In it, each colour represents a 1.5D interval between 35 and 50D, whereas above and below this range, colours represent 5D intervals. This scale is useful in routine practice (e.g. preoperative screening).

- *Disadvantage* of absolute scale is that it does not show subtle changes of curvature and thus can miss subtle local changes (e.g. early keratoconus).

   Normalized scale. In it, the cornea is divided into 11 equal colours spanning that eye's total dioptric power. In this scale, more minute topographic details within an individual cornea are appreciated.

- *Advantage* of normalized scale is that it shows more detailed description of the surface than the absolute scale.
- *Disadvantage* of normalized scale is that the colours of two different maps cannot be compared directly and have to be interpreted based on the keratometric values from their different colour scales.

   Note: Figure 8.6 shows a corneal topography map with different scales. Many workers feel that the absolute scale is easier to read and the normalized scale magnifies clinically insignificant information.

3. *Quantitative indices.* As part of the display, quantitative indices are also generated to give extra information. These include the following:

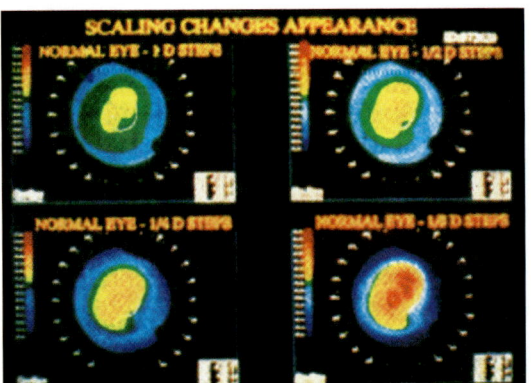

Fig. 8.6: *Scaling change showing apparently different maps of the same cornea (Courtesy: Dr Rajib Mukherjee)*

- Predicted visual acuity based on corneal shape
- Simulated keratometric readings (Sim K)
- Mean keratometry reading
- Surface regularity index (corenal irregularity measurement)
- Surface asymmetry index (shape factor SF)
- Point spread function (PSF)

i. *Simulated keratometric readings.* These characterise corneal curvatures in the central 3 mm area. The steep simulated K reading is the steepest meridian of the cornea in central 3 mm area. The flattest Sim K reading is the flattest meridian of the cornea and is, by definition, 90° apart.

ii. *Surface asymmetry index.* The index of asphericity indicates how much the curvature changes upon movement from the centre to the periphery of the cornea. A normal cornea is prolate (i.e. becomes flatter towards the periphery) and has the asphericity Q of –0.26. A prolate surface has negative Q value and an oblate surface has positive Q value. Most myopic laser vision corrections change the anterior corneal surface from prolate to oblate. A negative SF usually indicates a post-refractive surgery eye with the centre flatter than the periphery. The SFs (e^2) for the general population are as follows:

- Normal 0.13 to 0.35
- Borderline 0.02 to 0.12 and 0.36 to 0.46
- Abnormal –1.0 to 0.01 and 0.47 to 1.0

iii. *Surface regularity index/corneal irregularity measurement (CIM).* It is a number or index which represents the irregularity of the corneal surface. The higher the irregularity index, the more difficult it is to fit the corneal surface with a contact lens. It often can predict irregular astigmatism or visual distortions. Higher CIM values indicate that ocular pathology such as keratoconus or other pathological cases is more probable. The general population exhibits the following distribution ranges:

- Normal 0.03 to 0.68 μm
- Borderline 0.69 to 1.0 μm
- Abnormal 1.1 to 5.0 μm

iv. *Mean toric keratometry.* The mean toric keratometry (TKM) indices use elevation data to compare the toric reference to the actual cornea. The mean apical curvature value helps select the best toric fit using a sphero-cylinder design. This provides the most accurate toric representation of a patient's cornea. Human TKM ranges are as follows:

- Normal 43.10 to 45.90 diopters
- Borderline 41.80 to 43.00 diopters and 46.00 to 47.20 diopters
- Abnormal 36.00 diopters to 41.70 diopters and 47.3 diopters to 60.0 diopters.

Pathfinder corneal analysis. The Atlas Corneal Topographer (Carl Zeiss Meditec, Inc.) uses special software that combines the above indices (CIM, SF and TKM) to determine the probability of irregular corneas. This helps practitioners qualitatively and quantitatively, measure the probability of keratoconus. The pathfinder corneal analysis also helps determine whether a GP or soft toric lens fits poorly on the cornea or should be replaced with a different base curve. It also helps when fitting GP lenses. New keratoconus fitting philosophies use a lens-to-cornea relationship with less central bearing. Trend with Time or Stars technology can monitor corneal disease and determine how corneal shape responds with new contact lens designs.

Corneal topographic patterns in normal corneas

The normal cornea flattens progressively from the centre to the periphery by 2–4D, with the nasal area flattening more than the temporal area. The topographic pattern of the two corneas of an individual often shows mirror-image symmetry, and small variations in patterns are unique for the individual.

Depending upon the corneal curvature, Rabinowitz et al in 1996 described 10 different corneal topographic patterns in normal eyes as seen on colour-coded absolute scale maps (Fig. 8.7). These can be grouped as follows (figures in the parentheses indicate approximate distribution of keratographic patterns):

Regular pattern (Fig. 8.7)
- Round (23%)
- Oval (21%)
- Steepening:
  - Superior steepening
  - Inferior steepening

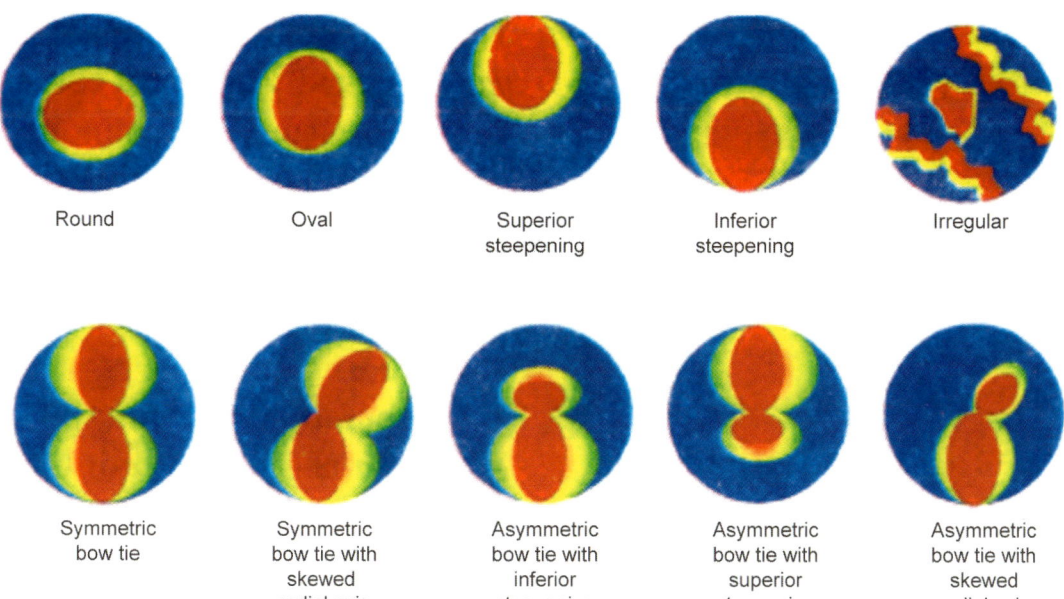

| Round | Oval | Superior steepening | Inferior steepening | Irregular |

| Symmetric bow tie | Symmetric bow tie with skewed radial axis | Asymmetric bow tie with inferior steepening | Asymmetric bow tie with superior steepening | Asymmetric bow tie with skewed radial axis |

Fig. 8.7: *Corneal topographic pattern seen on colour-coded maps in absolute scale (Rabinowitz et al 1996; Courtesy: Dr Rajib Mukherjee)*

Astigmatic patterns (Fig. 8.7)

- *Symmetrical and orthogonal*, i.e. bow tie effect (18%)
  Symmetrical bow tie with non-skewed axis
  Symmetrical bow tie with skewed radial axis
- *Asymmetrical and orthogonal* (31%)
  Asymmetric bow tie with superior steepening
  Asymmetric bow tie with inferior steepening
  Asymmetric bow tie with skewed radial axis
- *Irregular*, i.e. no pattern and non-orthogonal (7%)

Formats for display of data on colour maps

Various formats used for display of data on colour-coded maps are as follows.

1. Corneal power map (sagittal or axial)

The corneal power map (Fig. 8.8) is 24-colour representation of dioptric power at various points on the cornea. The radius of curvature is measured 360 times for each Placido ring image from centre to vertex. The sagittal algorithm averages the data points from first to the next ring and so on. Due to common reference axis, small irregularities may not be visible or smoothened out. They are spherically based and assume that centre of rotation of best fit sphere lies on optical axis. The axial map is more com-monly used to produce a good estimate of overall corneal shape, which appears smooth with a little noise as it provides average of adjacent curvature values.

2. Tangential map

The tangential map (Fig. 8.9) gives better geographical representation of the cornea as compared to the axial/sagittal corneal map. In it, tangents are projected outwards from the centre vertex 360°. Ring curvature is measured along the tangent (ring intersection). This is also known as *instantaneous curvature map*. This is the best indicator of corneal shape but is a poor indicator of corneal power. Therefore, tangential reading must never be used for calculating K values. This map is a very useful tool for accurate diagnosis of corneal ectatic conditions like keratoconus and also accentuates focal abnormalities as more sensitive.

3. Elevation map

Elevation is not measured directly by Placido-based topographers, but certain assumptions allow the construction of elevation maps. Elevation of a point on the corneal surface displays the height of the point on the corneal surface relative to a spherical reference surface. The reference surface in most instruments was

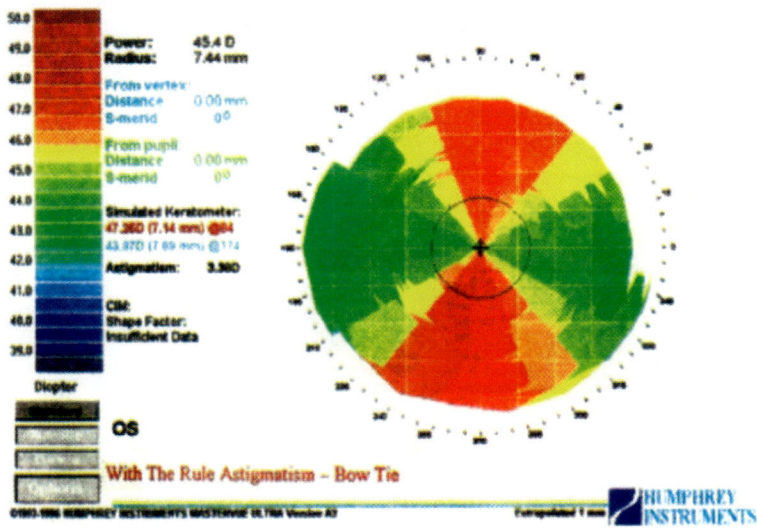

Fig. 8.8: *Corneal power map showing symmetrical 'bow tie pattern' in a patient having with-the-rule astigmatism (Courtesy: Dr Rajib Mukherjee)*

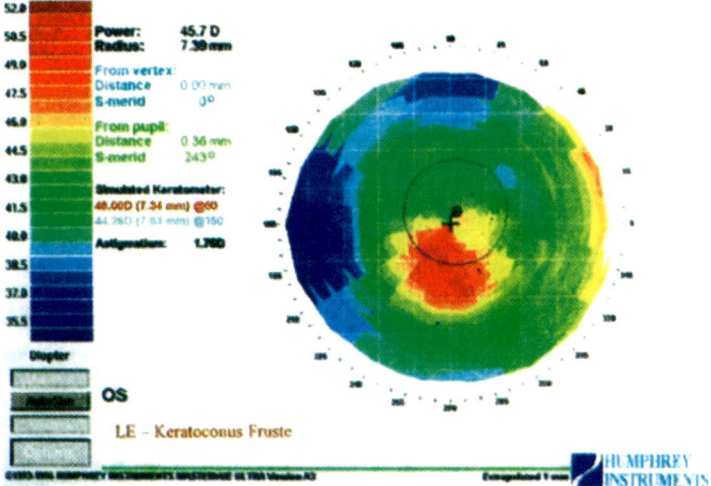

Fig. 8.9: *Tangential map showing inferior steepening in a patient with keratoconus left eye (Courtesy: Dr Rajib Mukherjee)*

chosen to be a sphere. Best mathematical approximation of the actual corneal surface, called best-fit sphere, is calculated by instrument software for every elevation map separately. The same surface may appear different when mapped against different reference surfaces. Consequently, it is difficult to compare directly two elevation maps that likely have slightly different best-fit spheres as reference values, and comparison only can be intuitive. The elevation map (Fig. 8.10) helps in distinguishing localized elevations (steep because of projection) from otherwise steep corneal area. The interpretation

can be confusing, but it is important to remember that 'Red is raised (steep)' and 'Blue is below (flat)'. The hotter colours show areas that are elevated above the reference sphere and cooler colours represent the areas that are depressed under the reference sphere. The elevation measurements are simply difference measurements.

In laser refractive surgery, the refractive power is changed by removing tissue from the corneal surface, and elevation data appear more relevant for calculation of ablation depth and optical zones.

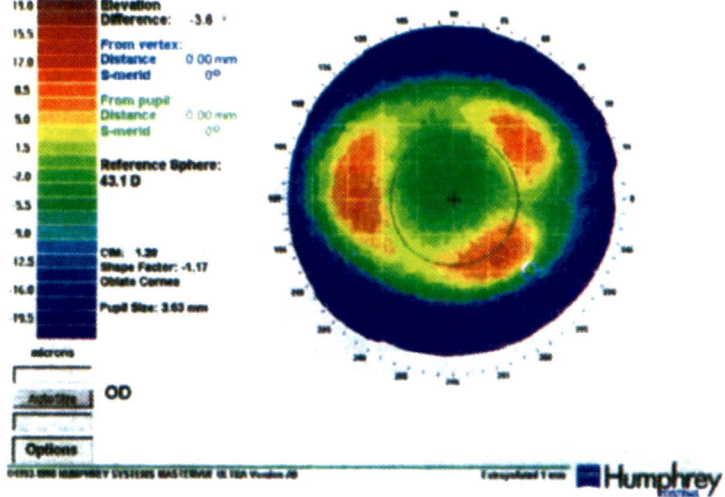

Fig. 8.10: *Elevation map of a post-radial keratotomy (post-RK) patient (Courtesy: Dr Rajib Mukherjee)*

4. Refractive power map

The refractive power map (Fig. 8.11) modified the standard map, taking into account the effects of spherical aberrations. It illustrates how the corneal curvature refracts light in true dioptres of power and not curvature. It uses ray-tracings and Snellen's law of optics to perform the calculations.

In it, the spherical cornea has cooler colours in the centre with increasing hotter colours extending out to the periphery (Fig. 8.11). Thus, in true sense, the refractive map should be called the *asphericity map* of the cornea. This map is very useful for determining the optical zone for rigid gas-permeable lenses and also in performing refractive corneal surgery.

5. Irregularity map

The irregularity map (Fig. 8.12) shows areas on cornea that are hot in colour. It displays the distortion of cornea using previous elevation map results with toric reference instead of a

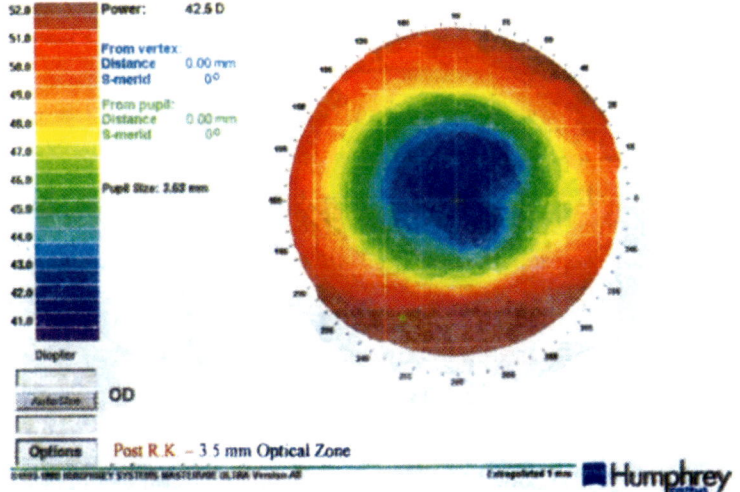

Fig. 8.11: *Refractive power map of a post-RK patient (Courtesy: Dr Rajib Mukherjee)*

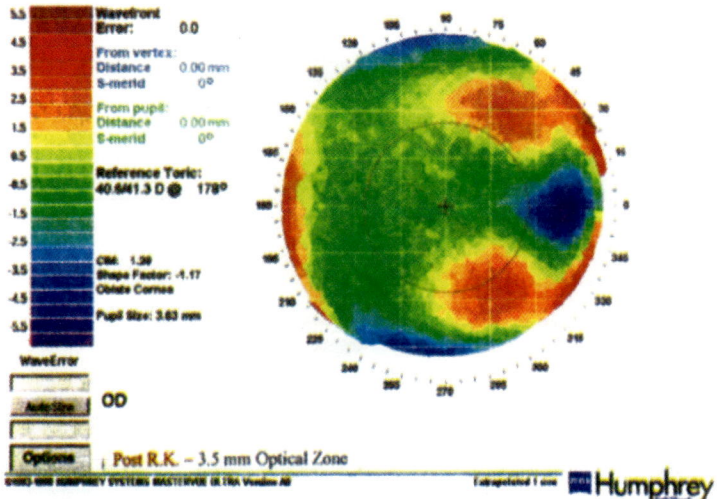

Fig. 8.12: *Irregularity map of a post-RK patient (Courtesy: Dr Rajib Mukherjee)*

reference sphere. The hotter colours represent the higher value of distortion measured in units of wavefront error. The wavefront number can be translated to dioptre of distorted power, known as *spectacle blur.* This map allows the surgeon to quickly assert, if the cornea is causing poor visual acuity. If there is a significant hot colour within the pupil zone, the acuity will be compromised.

6. Trend and time display

In this, changes occurring in topography with time (postoperatively) can be displayed in chronological order (Fig. 8.13).

7. Difference display map

Difference display map (Fig. 8.14) exhibits the comparative difference in two given topographic maps.

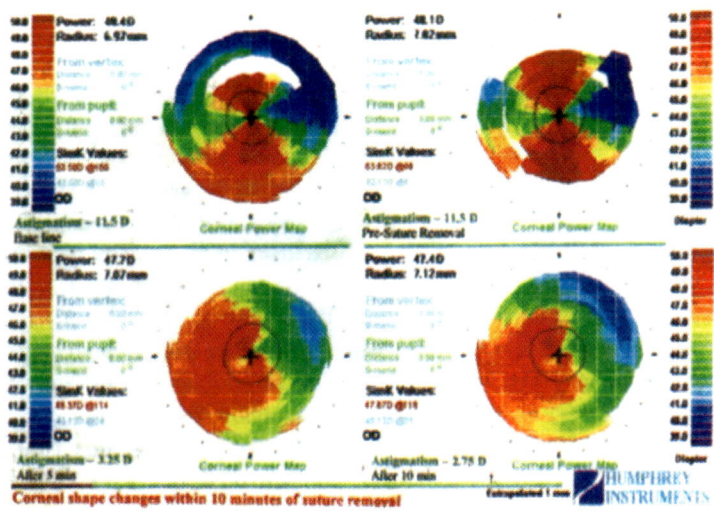

Fig. 8.13: *Trend with time display (Courtesy: Dr Rajib Mukherjee)*

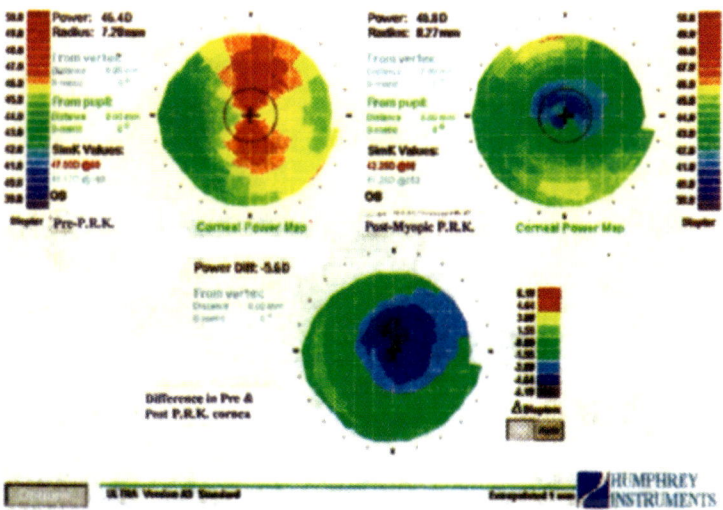

Fig. 8.14: *Difference display map (Courtesy: Dr Rajib Mukherjee)*

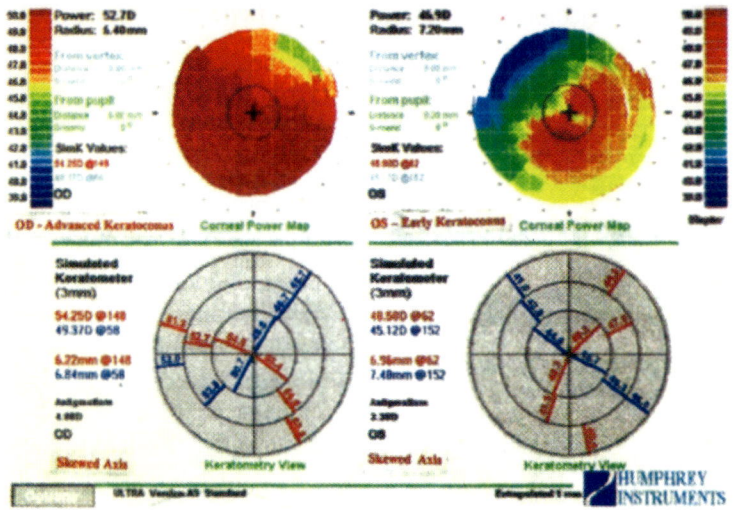

Fig. 8.15: *Right eye/left eye (OD/OS) compare map (Courtesy: Dr Rajib Mukherjee)*

8. Right eye/left eye (OD/OS) compare map
(Fig. 8.15)

Allows comparison of both eyes simultaneously.

SLIT-SCANNING CORNEAL TOMOGRAPHY SYSTEM

Working principle. Slit-imaging' tomography system uses scanning slits that step over the corneal surface to acquire topographic information. This is similar to a slit-lamp in principle. In this principle, an edge point on the corneal surface is triangulated by mathematically intersecting the diffuse reflected edge ray of the camera with the calibrated slit beam surface. Two slits are used, positioned at 45° angles to the right and left of the instrument axis. Twenty slit images are captured from each direction with overlap in a 7 mm diameter central area. Total corneal coverage is up to 10 mm, depending on the individual corneal shape. All images are captured within approximately 1.5 seconds.

In addition to the digital capture of the anterior surface of the cornea, this system is also capable of directly measuring the posterior surface. Thus, corneal thickness (defined by the distance between anterior and posterior surface) can be instantly measured at any point on the cornea.

Commercially available system, based on this principle, the Orbscan listed in Table 8.1 is described here.

ORBSCAN III

Orbscan, introduced in 1995, which was later improved in 1999 to Orbscan II and now in 2014 to Orbscan III (Fig. 8.16). It combines the advantages of slit-scanning technology with an advanced Placido-disc system, i.e. it is actually a hybrid system consisting of a projective (slit-

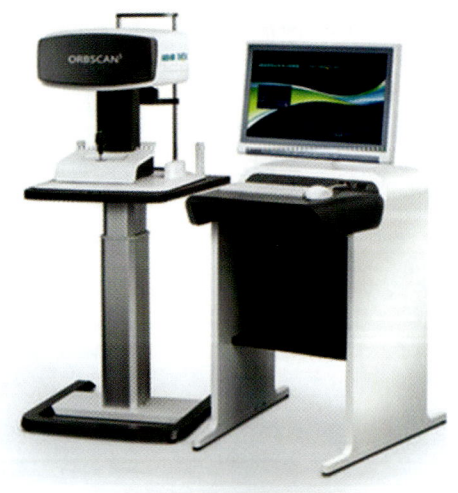

Fig. 8.16: *Orbscan III*

scanning) and reflective (Placido-disc) technique.

The Orbscan III system uses the principle of projection. Forty scanning slit beams (20 from the left and 20 from the right with up to 240 data points per slit) are used to scan the cornea from limbus to limbus and to measure independently the x, y and z locations of several thousand points on each surface. Orbscan III acquires over 23000 data points as compared to 9000 data points Orbscan II in 1.5 seconds to meticulously map the entire corneal surface (11 mm). The images captured are then used to construct the anterior corneal surface, posterior corneal surface, and anterior iris (white to white diameter) and anterior lens surfaces. Data regarding the corneal pachymetry and anterior chamber depth are also displayed. It also provides pre- and postoperative difference map. The advantage of this system is that slit scan imaging is not dependent on spherical assumption. Eye tracking is used to reduce data error resulting from eye movement.

TOPOGRAPHY MAPS WITH ORBSCAN

The computer calculates a hypothetical sphere that matches as close as possible to the actual corneal shape being measured. This is called the best fit sphere (BFS). It then compares the real surface to the hypothetical sphere, showing areas 'above' the surface of the sphere in warm colours, and areas 'below' the surface in cool colours (Fig. 8.17).

Green is 'sea level' (match with a sphere that best matches the cornea). Warmer colours are above 'sea level'. Cooler colours are below 'sea level'. The normal cornea is prolate, meaning that meridional curvature decreases from centre to periphery. The result is a *central hill of warm colour*. Immediately surrounding the central hill is an annular sea of *cool colours* where the cornea dips below the reference surface. In the far periphery, the prolate cornea again rises above the reference surface, producing *peripheral highlands*.

Functions: The Orbscan III provides:
• Anterior and posterior corneal elevation and curvature

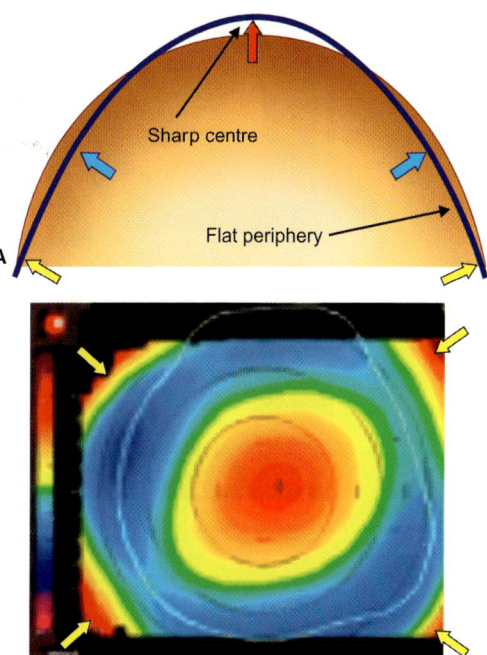

Fig. 8.17: *Orbscan elevation maps. A, In prolate cornea; B, In a cylindrical cornea*

• Full corneal pachymetry
• White to white diameter
• Pre- and postoperative difference maps

Quad map

Quad map refers to the typical Orbscan map which comprises following four different maps, each portraying different information about cornea (Fig. 8.18):
• Anterior elevation map (anterior float)
• Posterior elevation map (posterior float)
• Curvature map (axial keratometry map)
• Pachymetry map.

Anterior elevation map and posterior elevation map

Anterior elevation map, also known as anterior float, and posterior elevation map, also known as posterior float are shown in the top left hand map and top right hand map, respectively, in Fig. 8.18.

As mentioned earlier, slit-scanning provides elevation data, and this can also create a 3D interpretation of the cornea. A 3D interpretation of both elevation maps can be seen in Fig. 8.18.

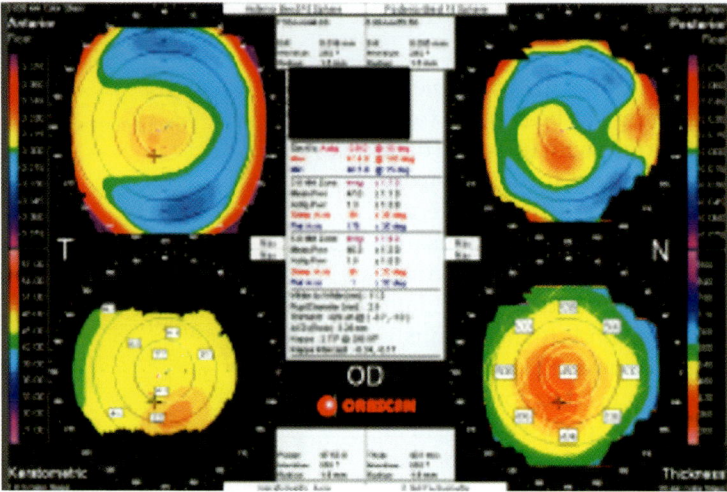

Fig. 8.18: *Orbscan: Quad map*

The meshwork effect indicates how the cornea would appear, if it were entirely spherical and is referred to as the reference sphere. This elevation data can be interpreted usefully in a number of ways.

Curvature map (axial keratometry map)

The axial keratometry map is based on Placido technology. This is similar to maps produced from the majority of commercially available topography systems, and provides detailed keratometric information across the diameter of the cornea.

For LASIK surgery, this information is important for a number of reasons. The 'K' readings are important, because limits of 'K' readings are between certain values; the cornea must be neither too steep nor too flat. It is difficult for the microkeratome (blade designed for flap cutting), to create a good quality corneal flap in LASIK, if either of these extremes is the case, as this can lead to surgical flap complications.

In addition, 'K' readings of more than 48D are an indication of potential keratoconus, particularly where there is decentred inferonasally. Details of the 'K' readings can be found in the stats and data information in the centre of the quad map.

Pachymetry map

This is map four of our quad map in Fig. 8.18. Traditionally, pachymetry has been measured using ultrasound, which provides a reading of corneal thickness from Bowman's membrane to Descemet's membrane. Through slit-scanning technology, Orbscan provides us with a pachymetry reading from the *precorneal tear film to the endothelium,* therefore, slightly thicker readings can be expected. The Orbscan can, however, be calibrated to take this into consideration when comparing readings. The true advantage of the pachymetry map is that it *provides us with thickness information across the cornea from limbus to limbus, not just* in single points as with ultrasound. This once again gives the opportunity to detect areas of weakness, thinning or scarring. Auffarth et al state that the relationship between the highest point on anterior and posterior elevation maps, and the thinnest point (shown by a yellow dot) is an indicator of keratoconus.

SCHEIMPFLUG IMAGING-BASED CORNEAL TOPOGRAPHY SYSTEMS

WORKING PRINCIPLE

Scheimpflug imaging is based on a geometric rule that describes the orientation of the plane of focus of an optical system when the lens plane is not parallel to image plane. In this scenario, an oblique tangent can be drawn from the image, object and lens planes and the point of intersection is Scheimpflug point, where image is in best focus.

COMMERCIALLY AVAILABLE SYSTEMS

Commercially available systems based on the principle are depicted in Table 8.1. Commonly used Scheimpflug imaging-based systems include:

- Pentacam
- Galilei
- Sirius.

PENTACAM

Pentacam, a popular system-based on this principle can obtain 50 images in less than 2 seconds. Each image has 500 true elevation points for a total of 25000 true elevation points for surface of cornea. The Pentacam has 2 cameras, one is for detection and measurement of pupil, helps in fixation and orientation. The second camera is used for visualization of anterior segment. Pentacam is able to image both anterior and posterior surfaces of cornea.

Latest version, Pentacam AXL (Oculus Optik-gerate GmbH, Wetzlar, Germany) is the up-graded Pentacam HR, with axial length measurement which allows surgeons, in addition to other features, to make IOL calculations.

CLINICAL APPLICATIONS OF PENTACAM CORNEAL TOPOGRAPHY

- Measurement of corneal shape
- Measurement of corneal thickness (pachymetry), including relative pachymetry maps.
- Measurement of corneal power.
  - Corneal elevation maps
  - Corneal curvature maps
  - Keratoconus screening
  - Preoperative screening before refractive surgery
  - Corneal wavefront analysis

MEASUREMENT OF CORNEAL SHAPE

Topography includes making a map that describes the elevations and depressions on the surfaces of the cornea similar to the way that a topographic map illustrates the mountains and valleys on a geographic terrain (Fig. 8.19). With the Pentacam, topographic analysis of the corneal front and back surfaces is based on the true elevation measurement from one side of the cornea to the other (limbus to limbus). In addition to the larger area, the Pentacam provides significantly more accurate elevation measurements than other machines. In addition, other Placido-disc-based topographic devices must infer elevation from curvature data. Such inferences can lead to improper medical conclusions.

MEASUREMENT OF CORNEAL THICKNESS (PACHYMETRY)

One of the most important measurements about the cornea besides its shape is the true thickness. Because the Pentacam provides highly accurate information about both the front and back surfaces of the cornea, it is possible to generate 25,000 data points that describe the true thickness of the cornea across its entire breadth and width (Fig. 8.20). This is the ideal as even manual ultrasound pachymetry can only image one single data point making it nearly impossible to provide the amount of thickness detail that can be obtained with the Pentacam.

- *Corneal thickness* is calculated from the top of the epithelium to the anterior surface of the endothelium, excluding the tear film. It is displayed as a color image over its entire area from limbus to limbus.
- The software allows for IOP modification taking into consideration the corneal thickness. This feature is of immense importance for obtaining IOP in post-refractive surgery patients as well as ocular hypertension and glaucoma screening.
- Important parameters like thickness in the center of the pupil, apical corneal thickness and the thinnest location are provided. The distance and position of the thinnest point relative to the apex of the cornea are also available which are useful for early detection of keratoconus.
- *Anterior chamber analysis* includes a calculation of the chamber angle, chamber volume and chamber height and a manual measuring function at any location in the anterior chamber of the eye.

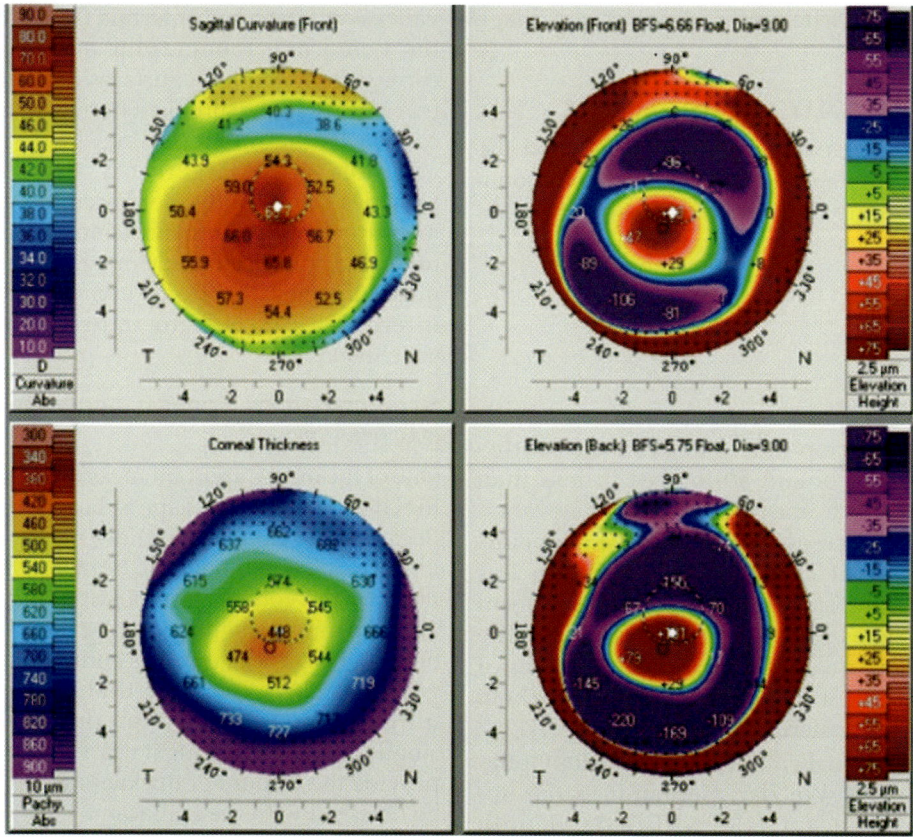

Fig. 8.19: *Pentacam: Corneal topography*

- *It has availability of 2 map and 4 map comparisons and numerical analysis of anterior segment progression* which is useful to compare preoperative and postoperative results in refractive surgeries and also see the long-term progression follow-up in patients undergoing collagen crosslinking.

- The *corneal thickness spatial profile and percentage thickness increase graphs* describe the annular pachymetric increase from the thinnest point. These graphs are available on the Pentacam and have been successfully used.

- *Pachymetric progression indices (PPIs)* are calculated for all hemimeridia over the entire 360° of the cornea, so that the average of all meridians (PPI-Ave) and the *meridian with maximal (PPI-Max) pachymetric increase* are noted.

- *Ambrósio's relational thickness (ART)* is calculated as the ratio between the thinnest point and

PPI. The "ART" concept combines thinnest with the pachymetric distribution, which facilitates the identification of an abnormal cornea despite its thinnest value. The Ambrósio relational thickness (ART) is calculated for the average and maximal progression indices (ART-Ave and ART-Max). The best cut-offs for the diagnosis of keratoconus are 339 for ART-Max and 427 µm for ART-Ave. For detecting ectasia susceptibility, we use 391 µm for ART-Max and 512 µm for ART-Ave. Practically, it is best not to perform LASIK, if ART-Max is lower than 400 µm.

- *Belin/Ambrósio display (BAD)* considers the deviations of normality values for different parameters, so that a value of zero represents the average of the normal population and one represents the value of one SD toward the disease (ectasia) value. A final 'D' is

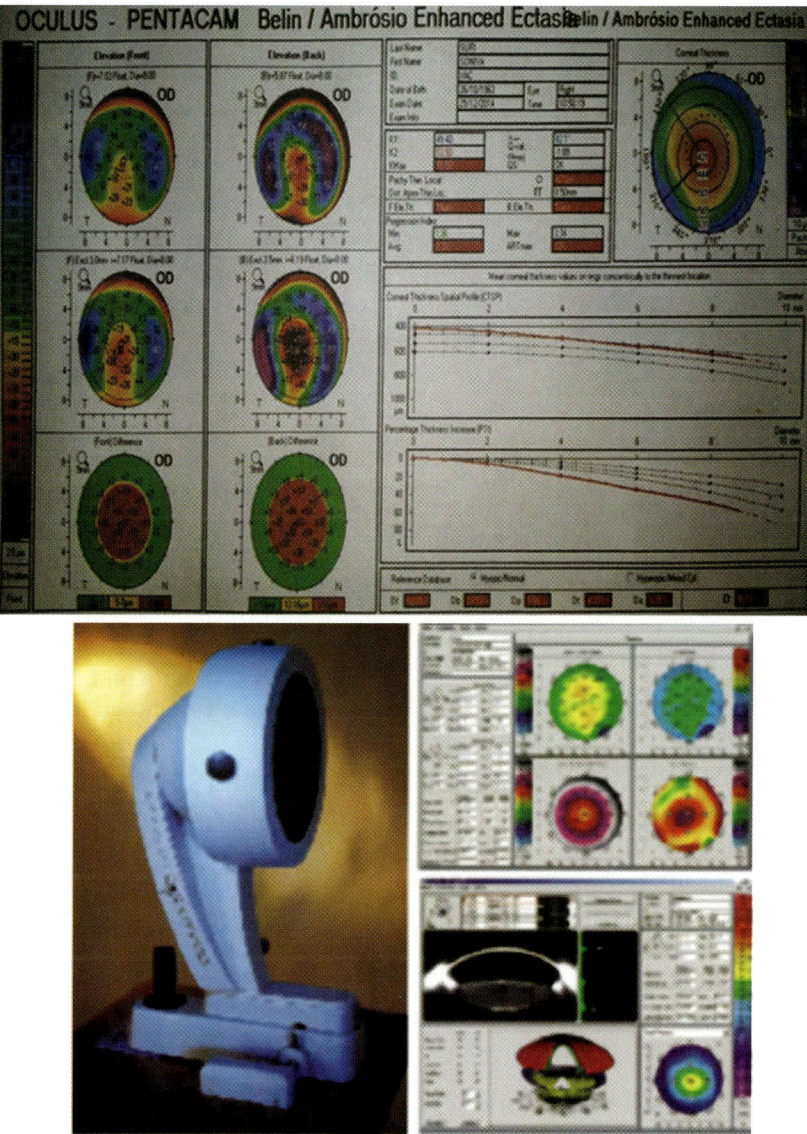

Fig. 8.20: *Pentacam analysis including pachymetry*

calculated based on a regression analysis that weighs differently the parameters.

♦ *Belin/Ambrósio display (BAD) II* software package features an enhanced reference surface that excludes the 3.5 to 4 mm area centred on the thinnest part of the cornea in order to eliminate the ectatic regions or "mountains". The goal of the BAD was to combine elevation based and pachymetric

corneal evaluation in one comprehensive display to give the clinician a global view of the tomographic structure of the cornea.

MEASUREMENT OF CORNEAL POWER

Scheimpflug imaging can also be used to measure corneal power, which is of interest to surgeons performing cataract surgery. This application is especially useful in patients following excimer keratorefractive surgery, in which the relationship between the anterior and posterior surfaces is altered yielding inaccurate keratometry readings required for intraocular lens (IOL) calculation. For example, following myopic LASIK, an overestimation of keratometry readings causes an underestimation of IOL power resulting in hyperopic outcomes. Conversely, following hyperopic PRK, an underestimation of the keratometry readings causes an overestimation of the IOL power resulting in myopic outcomes.

Keratoconus screening

Pentacam is the only technology which gives the direct measurement of elevation data and hence detection of keratoconus. There is an in-built keratoconus screening software which also helps in grading of keratoconus (KK1–4).

Preoperative screening before refractive surgery

Pentacam has facility for preoperative screening before refractive surgery to exclude ectasia and forme fruste. Diagnostic criteria for detecting forme fruste based on magnitude of elevation maps put forth by Michel W. Belin is as follows:

- Normal values for anterior elevation are differences less than +12 µm
  - Between +12 and +15 µm are suspicious
  - Greater than +15 µm indicate keratoconus.
- Normal values for posterior elevation are approximately 5 µm higher than those for anterior elevation.

Corneal wavefront analysis

The anterior and posterior corneal surface is described separately by Zernike polynomials based on the measured elevation data. Together the corneal wavefront analysis and keratoconus detection improve the preoperative screening for patients who are interested in refractive surgery as well as the postoperative progression control.

ADVANTAGES OF PENTACAM

Advantages of Pentacam as corneal topographer include:

- Higher resolution of central cornea
- Measure surface irregularities—keratoconus

- Calculate pachymetry from limbus to limbus
- Wavefront analysis to detect higher order aberrations.

OCULAR COHERENCE TOMOGRAPHY-BASED CORNEAL TOPOGRAPHY

Ocular coherence tomography (OCT) of the cornea is an optical method of cross-sectional scanning based on reflection and scattering of light from the structures within the cornea. *Optical interferometry* is *used to generate a log reactivity prole*. Each peak of the prole corresponds to specific layers of the cornea. Low coherence interferometry achieves axial resolutions from 3 to 20 µm using a noncontact technique. A large area can be imaged in a single scan, and the images have been used to identify the thickness of the corneal epithelium, LASIK flap, intracorneal ring segment depth, and three-dimensional structure of the cornea under normal or pathologic conditions with precision. A sample image is shown in Fig. 8.21A.

COMMERCIALLY AVAILABLE OCT SYSTEMS

Commercially available OCT systems for corneal tomography include (Table 8.1):

- *Visante Omni* (Carl Zeiss Meditec, Germany). It is based on rotating optical coherence tomography and Placido-disc imaging.
- *SS1000 Casia* (Tomey Corp, Japan). It is based on rotating optical coherence tomography.
- *RTVue-100* (Optovue, Fremont, USA). It is based on spectral Domain Optical Coherence Tomography-guided corneal power measurement (both anterior and posterior curvatures).
- *IOL Master 700* (Carl Zeiss Meditec, Germany). It is based On swept Source OCT Technology with 32-Marker Placido pattern.

VERY HIGH FREQUENCY ULTRASOUND CORNEAL TOMOGRAPHY SYSTEMS

Artemis 3 imaging machine (Arescan, Morrison, Colorado) is a very high frequency (VHF) ultrasound biomicroscope which allows corneal tomographic study. VHF ultrasound scans a series of meridia in an arc motion matched to

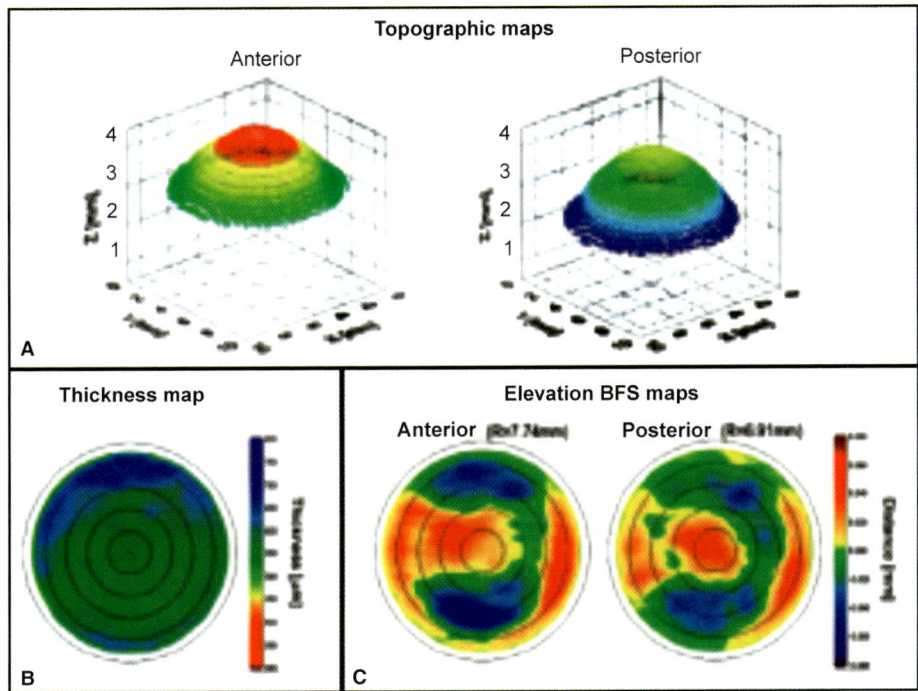

Fig. 8.21A to C: *Corneal topography with anterior segment OCT*

the curvature of the cornea. This allows measurement of the thickness of individual corneal layers over an 8–10 μm zone in three dimensions, as seen in Fig. 8.21B. This technology can produce topographic maps of the individual corneal layers, such as the epithelium, and the stroma. It has been reported that the topographic information can guide free cap replacement based on epithelial irregularities. This system has been shown to measure flap thickness with high reproducibility.

DIGITAL RASTERSTEREOGRAPHY-BASED TOPOGRAPHY SYSTEMS

Rasterstereography-based CTS uses a calibrated grid which is projected to the corneal surface and the diffuse reflection is recorded at two separate known angles. Commercially available *PAR CTS* is based on this technology.

PAR CTS

The PAR CTS from PAR Microsystems, Inc. PAR Vision Systems Corp., New Hartford, New York,

uses close range photogrammetry (rasterphotogrammetry) to measure and produce a corneal topographic map. A grid pattern of horizontal and vertical lines spaced 0.2 mm apart is used.

Corneal rasterphotogrammetry involves imaging of a projected grid onto the cornea. A modified operating room microscope or slit-lamp, as described by Warnick et al can be utilized. PAR Technology (New Hartford, New York) records video images of the projected grid to give a corneal topography map. Sodium fluorescein is added to the tear film and is excited by blue light which causes a grid pattern to become visible on the cornea. This is then imaged by the camera and analysed by a digital image processor using algorithms to give information about corneal topography. The accuracy of the system is 0.3D for a diameter of 7 mm. The contour plots of the cornea appear like keratographs, but actually each line is an isopter, representing areas of equal height on the corneal surface. The advantage of this system over the keratoscopic one is that it includes information across the whole of the cornea and even includes part of the sclera. Furthermore, the projected nature of the test does not allow interference due to corneal surface or stromal defects.

Note. This system is not much in use presently.

LASER HALOGRAPHIC INTERFEROMETRY-BASED TOPOGRAPHY SYSTEMS

Working principle. Laser halographic interferometry-based CTS relies on sophisticated optical techniques of *'light wave interference' fringes as projection device.* The commercially available CTS, the Corneal Lens Analysis System II (CLAS II) unit, is based on this technique.

CLAS II UNIT

It is a non-Placido-disc-based CTS machine which is based on the technology of laser holographic interferometry. The CLAS II applies three-dimensional imaging to the analysis of corneal surface changes. The object and reference beams are not split. Instead they oscillate at the same frequency and remain in phase with each other, thus minimizing the effects of vibration. The CLAS II analyses optical aberrations from reflecting surface by measuring the optical path difference (OPD). This is a measurement of the different path that light takes when it is reflected from a surface.

Note. This system is not much in use presently.

CLINICAL APPLICATIONS AND LIMITATIONS OF CORNEAL TOPOGRAPHY SYSTEMS

CLINICAL APPLICATIONS

1. Role in early diagnosis of corneal diseases

Computer-assisted videokeratography is helpful in diagnosing following conditions in early stages, i.e. before they could have been diagnosed otherwise:

- Keratoconus
- Epithelial dystrophies and other epitheliopathies
- Terrien's marginal degeneration
- Pellucid marginal degeneration.

2. Topography and contact lenses

- Corneal topographic analysis helps in giving a comfortable fit in routine contact lens practice, particularly in rigid contact lens fitting, thus providing maximum possible visual correction.
- It is of unquestioned help in contact lens fitting of difficult cases such as:
  - ◆ Postkeratoplasty
  - ◆ Keratoconus
  - ◆ Postradial keratotomy

  Other conditions with irregular astigmatism.
- It also helps in early diagnosis of contact lens-induced changes in cornea like central irregular astigmatism, corneal warpage and loss of radial symmetry. These changes are usually reversible.
- The practitioner and contact lens manufacturer can use corneal topography to verify contact lens specifications, however, complex they may be.

3. Topography in keratoconus

- One of the most useful applications of corneal topography is the *detection of keratoconus* before the appearance of slit-lamp findings.
- Topography has helped a lot in *understanding the features of keratoconus.* Before the introduction of this technique, keratoconus was described as having two basic shapes: Oral and nipple type. Videokeratography has demonstrated that corneal shape is more complex than was previously described.
- Classically, keratoconus is depicted as a localized area of increased surface power, surrounded by concentric zones of decreased surface power (Fig. 8.22). The area of steepening may occur anywhere on the cornea. Most frequently, initial involvement is seen in inferotemporal quadrant with superior half of the cornea remaining normal at this stage. Thereafter, the steepening spreads nasally, and then eventually to the superotemporal cornea. The superonasal cornea is the last part to be affected.
- *Contact lens fitting in keratoconus,* which otherwise is very difficult, is facilitated by topography studies.

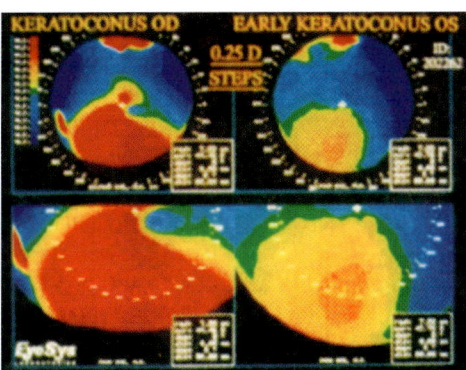

Fig. 8.22: *Corneal topography colour map in a patient with bilateral keratoconus*

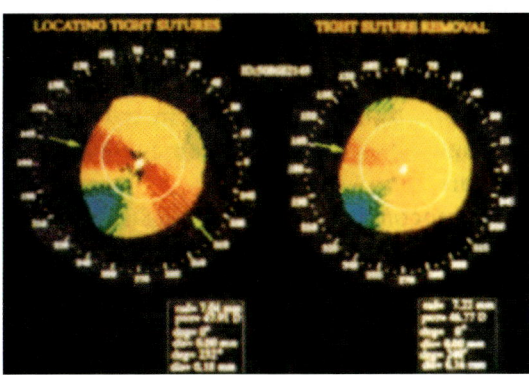

Fig. 8.23: *Corneal topography colour map in a patient with postpenetrating keratoplasty (tight suture at 1658)*

- Videographic analysis of family members of patients with keratoconus has demonstrated a mild form of disease without any overt clinical signs. This was called *forme fruste* by Amsler.

4. Topography in RK

- The role of corneal topography in RK is in evaluating the cornea pre- and postoperatively, i.e. to understand better the mechanics of surgery and, therefore, to further improve the predictability of the procedure in future. *Preoperative topography* reveals that corneas with same central curvature given by keratometer may have markedly different shapes, i.e. prolate, oblate and spherical. *Postoperative topography* reveals flattening of the entire cornea with only relative peripheral steepening.
- ***Repeat RK surgery***, when required, can be better planned with the help of colour-coded maps.
- ***Contact lens fitting post-RK*** can be a problem wherein the keratometric methods would lead to a very flat fit based on central corneal curvature measurements. Corneal topographic methods of contact lens fitting allow peripheral corneal topography evaluation and thus, the prescription of a steeper lens based on these curvatures.

5. Role of topography in postkeratoplasty astigmatism

- *Removal of tight sutures* for control of post-penetrating keratoplasty (PK) astigmatism has been facilitated by the advent of corneal topography (Fig. 8.23).
- *Corneal relaxing incisions* when required to manage post-PK astigmatism are better planned with topographic evaluation. After the advent of topography, the relaxing incision is placed at the steepest corneal meridian at the steepest point and not at the graft–host interface as was advocated earlier.
- If topography reveals excessive corneal flattening due to wound gap (diagnosed by the typical tear drop formation on videokeratographic image), then wound revision and wedge resection may be indicated instead of relaxing incision 90°away.
- *Post-PK contact lens fitting* by corneal topographic analysis has shown better results as compared to lens selection based on keratometric finding.

6. Role of topography in PRK and LASIK

Corneal topography is virtually indispensable for performing photorefractive keratectomy (PRK) and laser-assisted *in situ* keratomileusis (LASIK). Keratorefractive surgery in general has been made more predictable with the use of corneal topography.

- Videokeratography is not only essential for screening candidates for these procedures but it also provides important information about the quality of ablation zone, the diameter of the ablated zone, centration of the ablation and the stability of topographic alterations.

- Differential topographic maps are used to give the desired dioptric change in the corneal power.
- *Decentration of the ablation* zone detected on postoperative topography might explain postoperative halo or glare effect.
- *Irregular ablation zones* (as is seen in central islands) often explain decreased visual acuity and decreased quality of vision after these procedures. Recognition of these abnormal zones has resulted in modification of the procedures to prevent their occurrence.

7. Other applications of topography

- *IOL power calculation* can be done more accurately by employing the corneal topography to measure the necessary K value, instead of using the conventional keratometer.
- *Laser pachymetry* for corneal thickness is possible with *corneal modelling systems*, using a dual beam scanning laser slit-lamp.
- *Corneal topographic analysis* can be stored to show the pre- and postoperative conditions for self-study and patient satisfaction purposes.

LIMITATIONS

Though quite useful and advanced, computerised corneal topography does have some limitations:

1. *Algorithms for power calculation* are based on spherical optical systems, which may lead to qualitative and quantitative erroneous interpretations as the normal cornea is aspheric.
2. The *correlation between corneal curvature and power* (as shown by colour-coded maps) is valid for spheres and elliptical surfaces as long as there are no areas of abrupt transition in corneal curvature. If abrupt transition exists, software directly showing the surface elevation is more accurate than one that back calculates it from dioptric files. In fact, manufacturers have been advised to display colour curvature maps instead of colour dioptric maps.
3. *Data is averaged across meridia*, thus tending to magnify the 'blend' zones rather than show the sharp boundaries, if present, e.g. in pre- and postoperative PRK patients.

4. *The formulae employed* for power calculation are centred on the corneal apex and not on the more relevant line of sight.
5. *Central corneal power is interpolated* from central rings and it may give overestimations in cases of oblate corneas.
6. The *keratometric index of refraction* (1.3375) usually employed underestimates the changes in corneal power after procedures like PRK, as the actual index of refraction of the cornea is 1.376.
7. Videokeratography maps after an unsuccessful PRK may not show a change in corneal topography based on corneal surface, although a change in corneal thickness has taken place.
8. Placido-disc-based computerized videokeratographic instruments have *problems of critical focus* and inability to measure highly irregular corneas.

ABERROMETRY AND WAVEFRONT TECHNOLOGY

ABERRATIONS

Although the human eye is an optical marvel, yet it suffers many deviations from being an ideal optical system. All forms of deviations (refractive errors) are basically aberrations. Aberrations can be grouped as below:

I. *Lower order aberrations* include myopia, hypermetropia and regular astigmatism. These aberrations can be understood without sophisticated analytical methods and surgically can be treated by conventional LASIK. LOA constitutes 85% of aberrations. There are three types of LOA:

- Tilt of prism
- Defocus
- Astigmatic aberration

II. *Higher order aberrations* are subtle deviations from the ideal optical system. These constitute 5% of aberrations of the eye and include spherical aberrations, chromatic aberrations, coma, decentring, oblique aberration and centring.

The higher order aberrations do not lend themselves to easy solutions. Thus, the higher order aberrations limit the potential visual acuity of the eye. It is a well-known fact that the retina has a much higher resolving power and a much better potential visual acuity of about 6/2–6/1.5, but this is greatly reduced by diffraction of light and the aberrations of the eye.

RAY ABERRATIONS VERSUS WAVE ABERRATIONS

There are two ways to analyse aberrations: Ray aberrations and wave aberrations.

RAY ABERRATIONS

Ray aberrometry is based on Snell's law. Ideally, all rays from a single object point converge to a single image point. This ideal is never achieved in practice due to aberrations. In ray aberrometry, an imaginary plane is located near the desired image point and the intersection of each ray with the plane is plotted as a spot diagram (Fig. 8.24). Usually spot diagrams are generated for several planes in front of, at and behind the image, yielding a set of through focus spot diagrams. The advantage of the spot diagram is that it gives an immediate visual representation of the total amount of aberration present and the image quality. However, spot diagrams are more difficult to interpret when several aberrations are present, as is usually the case in most optical systems, including the eye. Therefore, in practice, ray aberrometry is not much popular.

WAVE ABERRATIONS

Wavefront refers to any isochronic surface associated with a specific object point. The term

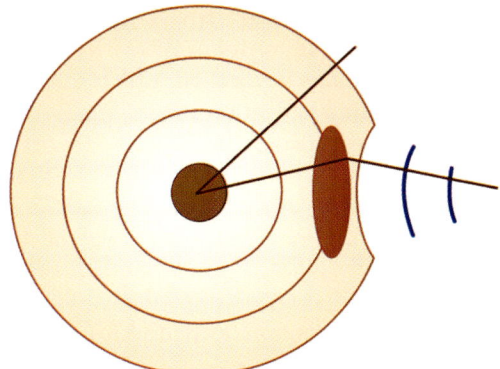

Fig. 8.25: *Diagrammatic depiction of wavefront associated with only one object point. Note that all light from a single object point reaches the wavefront simultaneously. Also note that rays are perpendicular to the wavefront*

isochronic means equal time. Thus, the amount of time required for light to travel from a specified object point to the wavefront is equal for all rays (Fig. 8.25). Note that wavefront is associated with only one object point. Wavefront and rays are two different but closely related ways of representing how light propagates through an optical system. In fact, the rays are perpendicular to the wavefront. Thus, given the shape of the wavefront, the direction of any light ray can be calculated. Conversely, from the direction of light rays, the shape of wavefront can be calculated.

Wave aberrations. In a perfect optical system, there are no distortions induced by the lens system. The ideal wavefront of the perfect optical system thus has spherical shape. The wavefront aberration refers to the OPD between the actual image wavefront and the ideal spherical wavefront. Since the wavefront aberration is the difference between two surfaces, therefore, its surface is usually shaped somewhat like a potato chip.

ZERNIKE'S POLYNOMIALS AND ZERNIKE'S TERMS

The monochromatic aberrations are defined and quantified in terms of what are known as Zernike's polynomials (ZPs), consisting of Zernike's terms (ZT) and associated spot diagrams.

Using the wavefront sensor method, the aberrations up to 10th order of ZP have been

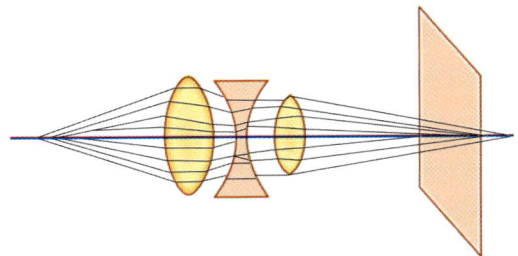

Fig. 8.24: *Ray aberrations and formation of spot diagram in relation to an imaginary plane located near the desired image point*

determined. However, for 3 mm pupils, aberrations up to 4th order of ZP are important and the aberrations beyond 4th order are small and have minimal effect on image quality. For 7.3 mm large pupils, the 5th to 8th order aberrations have substantial contribution to the deterioration of image quality. Zernicke coefficient is an expression of the amount of each individual aberration. Equations are used to calculate ZC for each polynomials.

The most important and commonly encountered 1st to 4th orders of ZP consist of 14 Zernike's terms (ZT).

Zero to 5th order ZPs are as below (Fig. 8.26):
- *0 order ZP* is also called *piston error*. It consists of the term ZT 0. It has no clinical equivalent and is not significant.
- *1st order ZP* is also called *tilt*. The clinical equivalent is prism and it consists of terms ZT 1 and 2.
- *2nd order ZP*. It corresponds to classical *spherocylindrical correction of refractive errors* and consists of ZT 3.4 and 5. ZT 4 equals *spherical correction* that corrects the optical aberration of *defocus*. ZT 3–5 equals *astigmatism*.

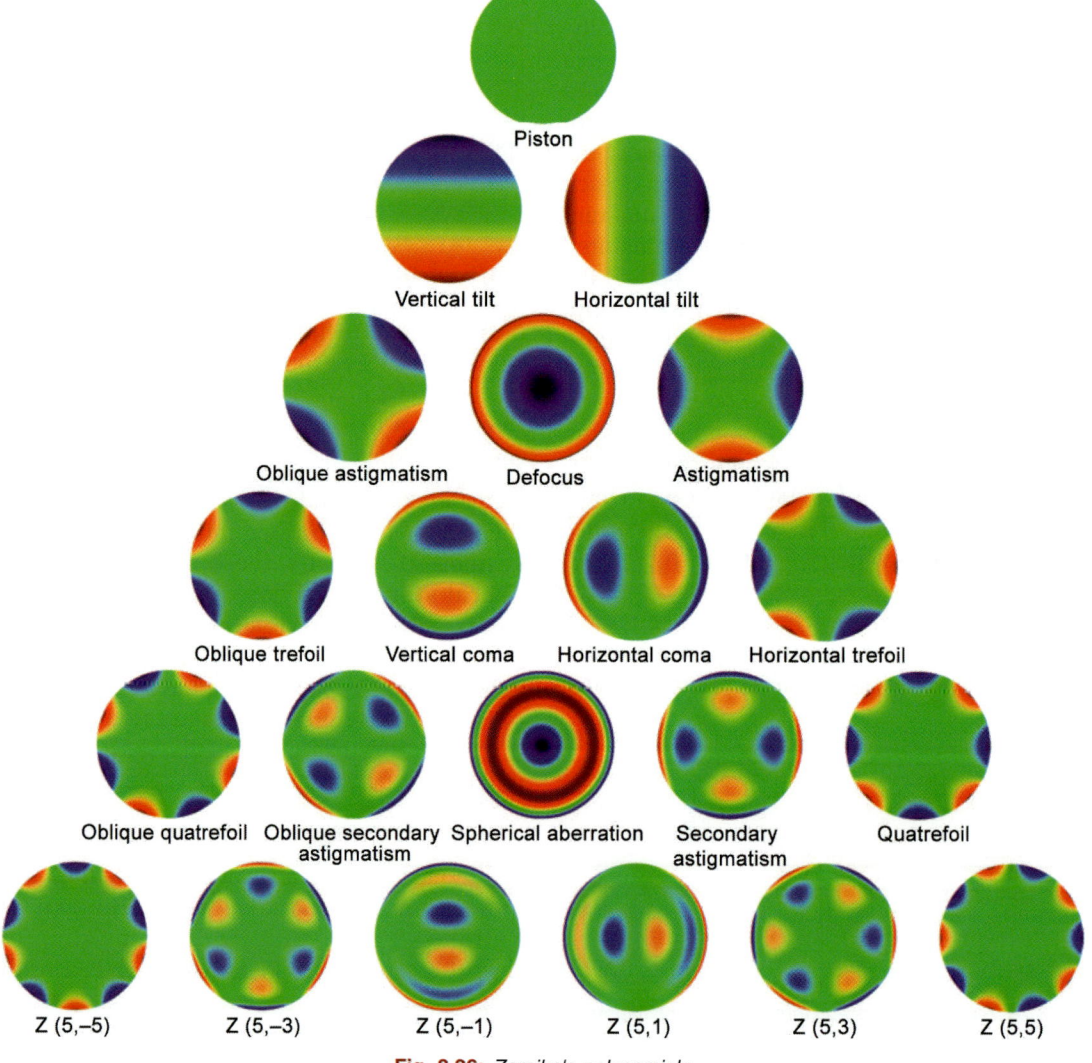

Fig. 8.26: *Zernike's polynomials*

- *3rd order ZP* consists of ZT 6–9. The ZT 6 and 9 correspond to *trefoil* and ZT 7 and 8 correspond to *coma* aberration.
- *4th order ZP* consists of ZT 10–14. ZT 10 and 14 correspond to *quadrupole* and ZT 11, 12 and 13 correspond to *spherical aberrations.*
- *5th order ZP* consists of ZT 15–20 and corresponds to *secondary coma.*

Note. In normal human eyes of young patients, the contribution to higher order aberrations is as below:
- 3rd order ZP – 40%
- 4th order ZP – 25%
- 5th and 6th order ZP – 30%

OCULAR WAVEFRONT

A wavefront is the locus of points characterized by propagation of position of the same phase: A propagation of a line in 1D, a curve in 2D or a surface for a wave in 3D. The understanding of the optical quality of the eye is becoming more accurate with the ability to precisely measure the lower and higher order wave aberrations using ocular wavefront sensing techniques. Reliable measurements of the ocular wave aberration also make it possible to correct these aberrations to improve visual performance.

TOTAL OCULAR WAVEFRONT VERSUS CORNEAL WAVEFRONT

The total ocular wavefront is equal to corneal wavefront plus internal wavefront. Thus, the corneal wavefront is one of the components of the *total ocular wavefront* which can be calculated from the corneal topographic height data, using an algorithm. An algorithm is the calculous procedure used to reconstruct corneal geometry from the calculation of the position of points on the corneal surface relative to axis or a reference sphere.

OPTICAL PATH DIFFERENCE

Optical path difference (OPD) refers to the difference between the corneal wavefront and an ideal wavefront. It is similar to the spherical offset which is the height difference between the cornea and a sphere. The OPD forms the basis of corneal wavefront theories.

In ray-tracing, the Snell's law is applied to the corneal surface to calculate OPD. Rays are traced from the fovea out of the eye. In the time, a ray travels 3 µm in the cornea, it travels for 4 µm in air. Thus, the *rule of 3*, i.e. every 3 µm of distortion from the ideal shape of the cornea will produce a 11 µm difference in the OPD map and a –1 µm difference in the wavefront error map.

CORNEAL WAVEFRONT MAP

Corneal wavefront map created from the corneal topography can be fitted with a ZP decomposition in the same way that total ocular wavefront is measured by aberrometry and fitted with the same polynomial decomposition. Further, the corneal wavefront map can be broken down into and viewed as:
- Zernike's coefficient
- PSF
- Simulated vision chart
- Modulation transfer function (like contrast sensitivity)
- A street where the patient can see a street scene simulated pre- and postoperatively. This is particularly important for the patients undergoing treatment on highly aberrated corneas to realize the meaning of wavefront and how it adds sharpness to the vision.

FACTORS AFFECTING TOTAL OCULAR WAVEFRONT

Total aberrations of the eye as measures by wavefront analyses are affected by following factors:

1. *Age.* Total ocular wavefront varies with age, as the aberrations increase with age due to change in both crystalline lens and the cornea. Note that the aberrations of cornea and crystalline lens neutralize each other in the young people. With the increase in age, this balance is lost and thus aberrations of the eye are increased.

2. *Size of pupil.* The total ocular wavefront map obtained with Hartmann-Shack sensor depends upon the size of the pupil. The pupil becomes small in size with age, which may somewhat offset the increase in aberration occurring with increase in age.

Therefore, the increase in total ocular wavefront aberration with dilatation of the pupil is more significant in the elderly. Aberrations, particularly coma, depend greatly on pupil centration. The change in pupil size with change in illumination due to effect of mydriatics/miotics shifts the pupil centration and thus changes the aberrations.

3. *Accommodation.* Due to changes in the shape, position and alignment of the lens with respect to pupil and cornea during accommodation, there occurs change in the wavefront aberrations.

4. *Chromatic aberration.* Presently used aberrometers are laser based, which can measure aberrations at only one wavelength. Thus, the chromatic aberration, one of the eye's major optical defects, is not measured by the clinically used aberrometers.

5. *Tear film.* Any local change in the tear film affects the ocular aberrations. Such an effect is more prominent in individuals with tear film anomalies, specially the dry eye.

6. *Misalignment of the eyes* during wavefront aberrometry affects the accuracy of measurement. Alignment of the eyes is especially critical for higher order aberrations.

7. *Refractive errors*, especially when large, affect the measurement of higher order aberrations. This is because the lower order aberrations affect the image quality much more than the higher order aberrations.

Note. It is important to note that corneal wavefront in contrast to total ocular wavefront is:

- Relatively stable over time and allows serial measurement
- Not affected by pupil diameter
- Not affected by accommodation.

MEASUREMENT UNIT OF ABERRATIONS

Measurement unit of aberrations is micron, which is a point-wise measure of the amount of light that is advanced or retarded with reference to a plane. The integrated or total amount of distortion from a reference surface is measured with root means square (RMS), commonly used mathematical method for reporting distortions.

- RMSg (gross): Has to be correlated with manifest refraction.
- RMSh (higher): >0.2 μm needs to be evaluated.
- RMSg lower order + higher order aberrations.

WAVEFRONT ABERROMETRY

Aberrometry refers to analysis of optical aberrations. The analysis of higher order aberrations including irregular astigmatism requires advanced technology. Until recently, there was no need to analyse these defects in detail. However, recently aberrometry has become clinically important, since the progress in imaging and refractive surgery may allow the correction of certain aberrations.

Wavefront aberrometry or the so-called wavefront technology is more popular in clinical practice and is in many ways easier than the ray aberrometry. Wavefront aberrometry refers to measurement of aberrations in the optical system of the eye by wavefront analysis. All methods of measuring the aberrations of the human eye evaluate how the light that enters the eye is modified. With each of these approaches, light is imaged onto the retina, and either the image position on the retina or the wavefront as it emerges from the eye is measured.

Commercially available aberrometers, listed in Table 8.1, can be classified into following types and according to operating principle:

    I. Backward/outgoing projection type
- Hartmann-Shack aberrometry

   II. Forward/ingoing projection type
- Tscherning aberroscope
- Ray-tracing aberrometry.

1. HARTMANN-SHACK ABERROMETRY

Hartmann-Shack style aberrometers are currently the most commonly used. In such devices, a single laser beam is projected as a spot on the retina (Fig. 8.27A) and the reflected bundle of rays passes through the optical system of the eye. It is then picked up by an array of small lenslets, which focus these rays into spots on an array of a CCD camera, very much like the compound eye of an insect (Fig. 8.27B). Then the mosaic of spots is used to define the wavefront and analyse its deformation (Fig.

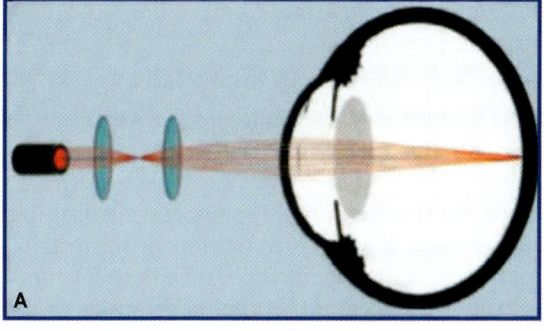
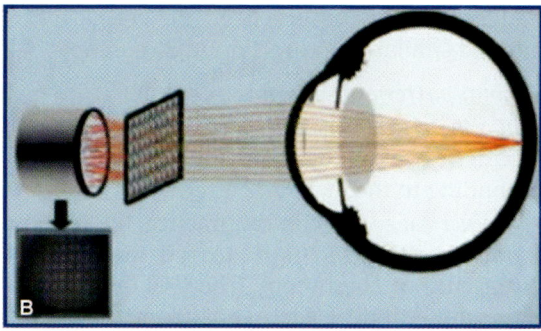

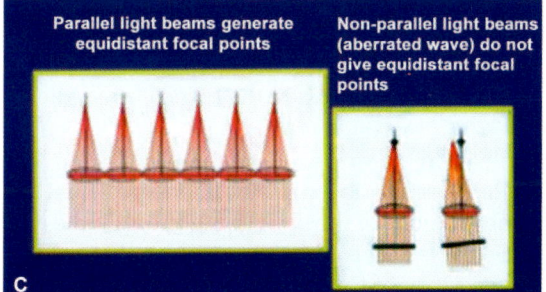
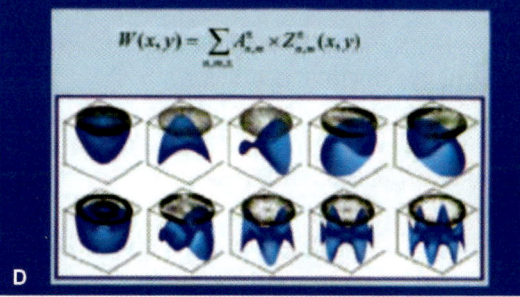

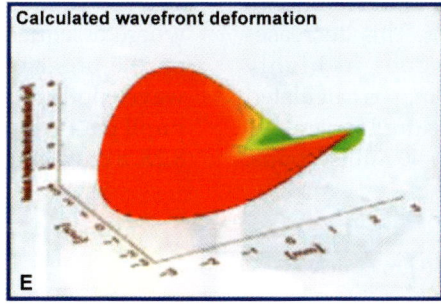

Fig. 8.27: *Optics of wavefront aberrometer. A, A narrow laser beam is focused to the retina to generate a point source; B, Array of small lenses focusing the outcoming light ray from the retina on the charge-coupled device camera; C, Determination of the wavefront deformation by analyzing the direction of the light ray; D, Various shapes of wavefronts represented as a sum of Zernike's polynomials; E, Wavefront pattern of astigmatism polynomials*

8.27C). The position, the pattern and the PSF of each spot are then analysed and a colour-coded picture of the wavefront is generated by the aberrometer. The shape of the wavefront is represented as a sum of ZPs, each describing a certain deformation (Fig. 8.27D). As an example, the wavefront pattern for astigmatism is shown in Fig. 8.27E.

Commercially available aberrometers based on Hartmann-Shack principle include:
- LASER wave (Alcon)
- Zywave 3, as part of Zyoptix Diofnest work station 3, i.e. ZDW 3 (Bausch and Lomb)
- WaveScan WaveFront System (VISX)
- Corneal WaveFront Analyser (Schwind Eyetech Solution)
  - WaveScan WaveFront System (AMO)
  - WaveLight Oculyzer II (ALCON)
  - Alleye Oculyzer.

2. TSCHERNING ABERROSCOPE

Tscherning aberroscope is basically an ingoing retinal imaging aberrometer. In it, a bundle of equidistant light rays is shone on cornea, which is imaged on the retina. A low-light CCD camera linked to a computer is used to analyse the pattern of spots observed on the retina by a method similar to indirect ophthalmoscopy.

Retinal pattern observed is as below:

- *In a theoretically aberration-free eye*, the retinal pattern consists of equidistant spots corresponding to the incident pattern.
- *In a normal eye*, in clinical practice, the retinal pattern observed is distorted due to the presence of aberrations. The CCD measures the deviation of each spot from the ideal equidistant position.

Commercially available aberrometer based on Tscherning principle includes:

- Allergretto (from wavelight).

3. RAY-TRACING ABERROMETRY

In this system, pattern of one ray, rather than all rays at the same time, is analysed. In fact, a point incident on the retina and the location of its conjugate focus is analysed with reference to the ideal conjugate focus point. This decreases the chance of crossing the rays in highly aberrated eyes. The wavefront map is calculated from the many such points measured separately. The total time of scanning is 10–40 milliseconds.

Commercially available device based on Ray-tracing principle is:

- NIDEK OPD Scan III (from Nidek)
- iTrace (Tracey Technologies, USA).

iTRACE SYSTEM

The iTrace system (Tracey Technologies, Houston, Tx) is a combination of ray-tracing aberrometry and Placido's disc corneal topography to measure the total aberrations of the eye. It is a serial, double pass and forward projection type retinal image aberrometer. A topographer is added in the same unit as the aberrometer to measure the corneal aberrations.

Principle of iTrace

- Ray-tracing aberrometry measures forward aberrations of the light going through the eye. So, it is more physiological as the natural trajectory of the light is being analysed.
- The iTrace uses this principle of ray-tracing where a sequential series of infrared beams on the order of 100 microns and a 785 nm wavelength each is projected into the entrance pupil parallel to the eye's line of sight. In Fig. 8.28, a diagram of the ray-tracing technique is

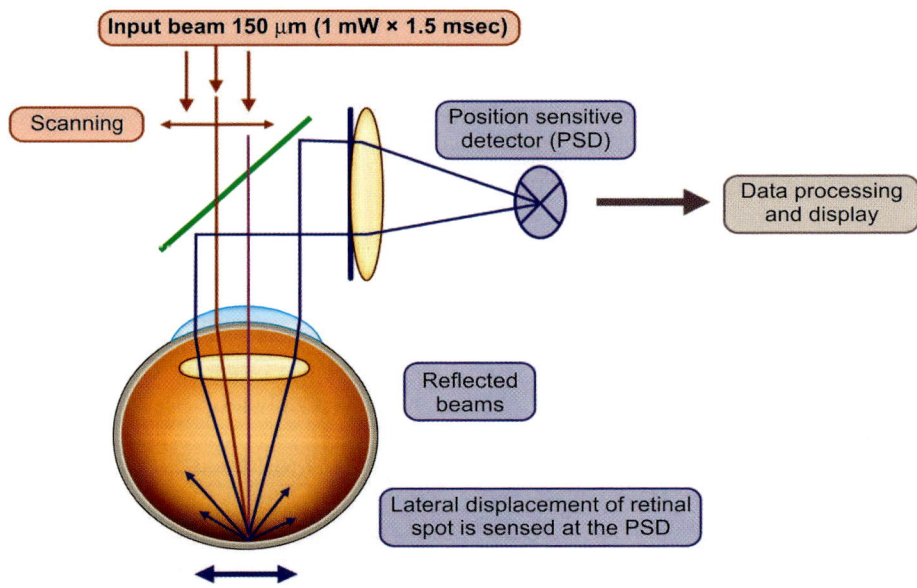

Fig. 8.28: *Diagram of the ray-tracing technique*

shown. It measures the exact location where the laser beam reaches the retina by means of the retroreflected light captured by reference lineal sensors X, Y. Local aberrations in the path of the laser beam through the cornea and the internal structures cause a shift in the location on the retina.

- This process continues until 64 laser beams have been projected through the entrance pupil 4 times each (256 points) at high speed (approximately 250 milliseconds). Each of these points represents the entrance of parallel light rays into the eye, which become refracted by the eye's optical power and eventually focus on the retina. All 256 points would be concentrated at a single point in the center of the macula in an emmetropic eye and reconstruction of the real wavefront error is done.

Data Analysis

1. Wavefront analysis
2. Topographic analysis

I. Wavefront (WF) analysis

This depends upon the concept of retinal spot diagram (RSD), which consists of a set of points projected through the pupil onto the retina. RSD is used to obtain modulation transfer function (MTF) and point spread function (PSF).

PSF shows the image obtained in the retina when the patient sees a point source of light. A sharper and smaller PSF is considered to be better. The MTF is a measure of the transfer of modulation (or contrast) from the subject to the image by an optical system at different spatial frequencies. It measures how accurately it reproduces (or transfers) detail from the object to the image produced by the lens.

Basic data graphs

Basic data graphs include:

1. *Wavefront verification display* shows the RSD with the horizontal and vertical point profile.
2. *Wavefront map* [total and higher order aberrations (HOA)] is a colour-coded map with warm colours showing that the wavefront is in front of the reference plane and cool colours showing retardation.
3. *The root mean square (RMS),* measures the magnitude of aberrations.

4. Total refractive and HOA refractive maps
5. PSF total and HOA PSF
6. Snellen letter total and HOA
7. *Zernike polynomials bar graph*, showing the total, corneal and internal aberrations.

Uses of aberration analysis

1. *In case of high total aberrations,* it helps to decide whether the refractive procedure would be better in cornea or lens.
2. *Before and after cataract surgery* the analysis helps to study the induced or compensated aberrations by the IOL.
3. It also helps to identify which type of IOL will be suitable and to analyse different types of IOL.
4. The contribution of an opacified lens in total ocular aberrations can be measured.
5. *Measurement of angle alpha and angle kappa* to plan for premium IOLs.
6. To evaluate the corneal and total astigmatism.

II. Corneal topographic (CT) analysis

This is based on a Placido-disc format named Vista, which covers up to 10 mm of peripheral cornea. This provides:

1. Standard keratometric readings
2. Refractive power of cornea in central 3 mm
3. Corneal index: Inferosuperior (IS) index
4. Topographic maps, such as:
   - Standard axial map
   - Tangential curvature map
   - Refractive map
   - Elevation map
   - Corneal wavefront map.

Advantages of ray-tracing aberrometry

1. It allows sequential capture of data and there is no confusion since each point is processed separately and sequentially.
2. The pattern of laser beams projected adapts to the pupil size.
3. High accuracy and resolution since each point is measured separately using linear detectors.
4. The x-y scanner can be programmed to analyse any other rectilinear or polar pattern.
5. iTrace is less susceptible to eye motion and tear film artifacts.

INTRAOPERATIVE, REAL-TIME WAVEFRONT-GUIDED ABERROMETRY

These aberrometers have been evolved recently to refine the outcome of laser vision correction and cataract surgery by providing greater diagnostic refractive precision. This core technology, referred to as HOLOS (Clarity Medical Systems, Inc., Pleasanton, CA) is a novel technique for dynamically achieving accurate wavefront images or refractive profiles for real-time, refinement during surgery.

OPERATING PRINCIPLE

- The aberrometer use Talbot Moire's interferometry based on two transmission grids spaced a specific distance apart and rotated relative to each other. The spectacle correction in an aberrated ocular wavefront is determined by using fourier transfer calculation and is represented in the resulting interferogram.

- *Light source (collimated) used is the 830 nm superluminescent diode*, which is launched into the eye and focused on the retina to create the returned wavefront. The collected data on the magnitude and location of the offset error by the quad detector is correlated with the refractive error of the eye. The sequential wavefront aberrometer achieves real-time, high-resolution sampling mainly by the speed at which the mirror rotates and the number and position of samples synchronised to pulses of the light source per revolution (Fig. 8.29).
- *The refractive outcome of the real-time sampling* is seen in an image overlaying a live eye image as viewed through the microscope and is presented as both qualitatively and quantitatively.
- *The qualitative data is seen* as a circle for spherical error, a thin ellipse for astigmatism and a dot for emmetropia.
- *The quantitative data is displayed* as sphere, cylinder and axis at the bottom of the screen.

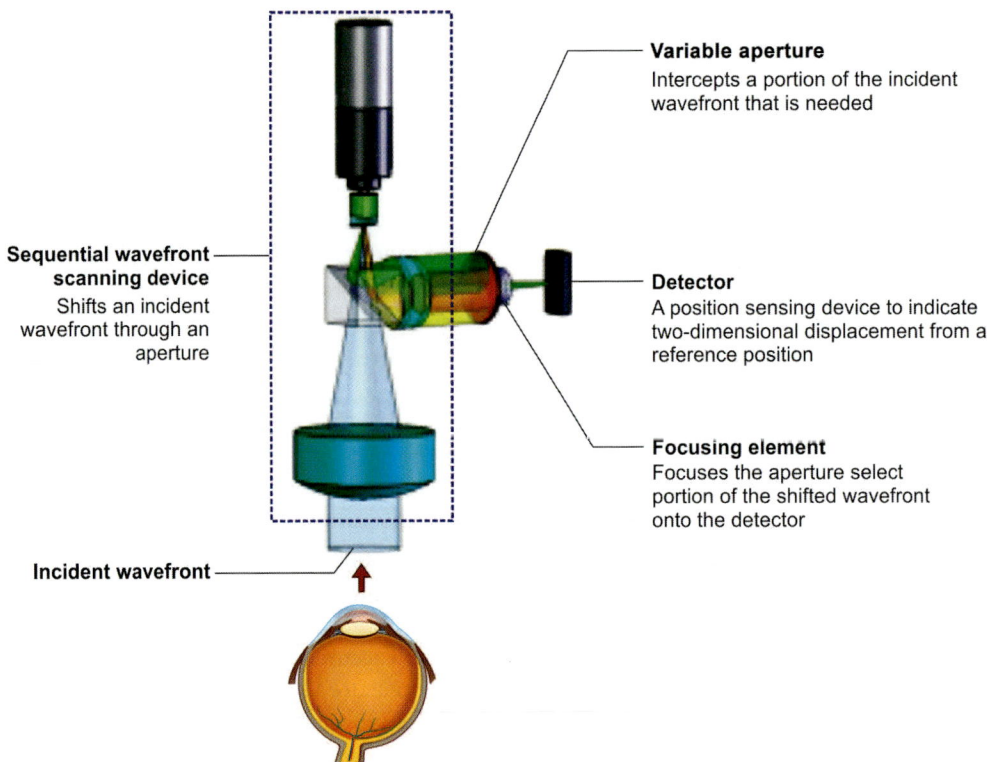

Variable aperture
Intercepts a portion of the incident wavefront that is needed

Sequential wavefront scanning device
Shifts an incident wavefront through an aperture

Detector
A position sensing device to indicate two-dimensional displacement from a reference position

Focusing element
Focuses the aperture select portion of the shifted wavefront onto the detector

Incident wavefront

Fig. 8.29: *Working principle of intraoperative wavefront aberrometry*

CLINICAL APPLICATIONS AND ADVANTAGES

- Identification of the astigmatic axis during surgery instead of the preoperative markings, which can save, time.
- The potential to manage the LRIs by guiding their placement location and using real-time feedback to titrate their length until neutralisation.
- The real-time refraction can also guide the toric IOL rotation until neutralisation.
- The added size and dimensions do not change the surgeon's working distance.
- Provides high quality data regardless of the microscope or room illumination.
- Does not lengthen the surgical time.
- The real-time refractive data is integrated with the surgical video obtained.

CLINICAL APPLICATIONS OF ABERROMETRY

1. *Wavefront-guided refractive surgery* has become very popular nowadays.
2. *Role in early diagnosis of keratoconus.* Wavefront technology is an excellent adjunct to topography in the diagnosis of an early keratoconus. A topographic map showing slight inferior steepening accompanied by significant coma on wavefront analysis could be a cause for great concern. Preliminary research indicates that using a combination of inferior/superior value (derived from topography) and vertical coma (derived from wavefront) best separates early keratoconus from normal.

   Increase of ocular HOA in keratoconic eyes results from an increase in corneal HOA. Coma-like aberrations are dominant compared with spherical-like aberrations in keratoconic eyes. Wavefront analysis will enable us not only to evaluate the quality of vision but also to differentiate keratoconic eyes from normal eyes by analysing characteristics of HOA. Typically, it may show increased values of Zernike's coefficient—C_7 and C_8.

3. *Wavefront-guided LASIK enhancement.* Corneal wavefront-guided enhancements in patients with night vision symptoms and high positive spherical aberrations after myopic laser refractive surgery is effective in improving night vision symptoms, reducing corneal spherical aberrations and decreasing asphericity of cornea.

4. *Intraoperative real-time wavefront-guided aberrometry* quite useful and becoming popular.

BIBLIOGRAPHY

1. Alpins Noel JK, Ong G Stamatelatos. New method of quantifying corneal topographic astigmatism that corresponds with manifest refractive cylinder. Journal of Cataract and Refractive Surgery 2012; 38(11): 1978–88.
2. Aristodemou P, Knox Cartwright NE, Sparrow JM, Johnston RL. Formula choice: Hoffer Q, Holladay 1, or SRK/T and refractive outcomes in 8108 eyes after cataract surgery with biometry by partial coherence interferometry. J Cataract Refract Surg 2011; 37: 63–71.
3. Busin M, Wilmanns I, Spitznas M. Automated corneal topography: computerized analysis of photokeratoscope images. Graefes Arch Clin Exp Ophthalmol 1989; 227(3): 230–6.
4. Byun YS, Chung SH, Park YG, Joo CK. Posterior Corneal Curvature Assessment after Epi-LASIK for Myopia: Comparison of Orbscan II and Pentacam Imaging. Korean J Ophthalmol 2012; 26(1): 6–9.
5. Fung MW, et al. "Corneal Topography and Imaging" (2015). Medscape website. Updated 17 March 2016. Accessed 6 May 2017.
6. Karnowski K, Kaluzny BJ, Szkulmowski M, Gora M, Wojtkowski M. Corneal topography with high-speed swept source OCT in clinical examination. Biomed Opt Express 2011; 12(9): 2709–20.
7. Liu Z, Huang AJ, Pflugfelder SC. Evaluation of corneal thickness and topography in normal eyes using the Orbscan corneal topography system. Br J Ophthalmol 1999; 83(7): 774–8.
8. Unterhorst HA, Rubin A. Ocular aberrations and wavefront aberrometry: A review. Afr Vision Eye Health 2015; 74(1), Art. #21, 6 pages.
9. Wiley WF, Bafna S. Intraoperative aberrometry guided cataract surgery. International Ophthalmology Clinics 2011; 51(2): 119–29.
10. Yesilirmak N, Palioura S, Culbertson W, Yoo SH, Donaldson K. Intraoperative wavefront aberrometry for toric intraocular lens placement in eyes with a history of refractive surgery. Journal of Refractive Surgery 2016; 32(1): 69–70.

Chapter

9

Ultrasound Biomicroscopy of Cornea

ULTRASOUND BIOMICROSCOPY MACHINE

Ultrasound biomicroscope (UBM) is a high frequency ultrasound machine (with 50–100 MHz transducers) used to image ocular structures anterior to the pars plana region of the eye. It produces cross sectional images of anterior segment structures providing a lateral resolution of 50 µm and an axial resolution of 25 µm with a depth of penetration of approximately 4–5 mm. The field of view is 4 × 4 mm and the scan rate is 5 frames/second. The high-resolution cross-sectional images acquired by the ultrasound biomicroscope are akin to an *in vivo* histological section.

PARTS OF UBM

It mainly consists of hard disc, video monitor, mouse, probe, foot switch, CD drive and printer. There are three main components of the hard disc of the UBM machine:

- Transducer
- High-frequency signal processing.
- Precise motion control

TRANSDUCER

UBM incorporates 50–100 MHz polymers transducers which are incorporated in a B-mode clinical scanner. The transducer is mounted on a pulley with the piezoelectric crystal fixed on a large handle. Normal B-scan transducer has oil filled covering with a membrane over the piezoelectric crystals. The penetration of the 50 MHz UBM transducer is poor, hence the transducer has an open crystal and there is no membrane covering the crystal to avoid signal loss. Therefore, excessive contact between the globe and the moving transducers must be avoided to prevent abrasions.

HIGH FREQUENCY SIGNAL PROCESSING

The reflected radio frequency is processed by the signal processing unit. The signal processing unit in UBM is specially designed to handle high frequency signals. In UBM, the movements of the transducer have to be smooth to scan adjacent areas in the anterior segment. During normal B-scan the movement of the transducer is over a wide area covering the entire eyeball. To enable this smooth movement, there is a special motion control device for the transducer.

PRECISE MOTION CONTROL

The UBM uses a speed of sound constant of 1500 m/s to convert time to distance measurements. The UBM machine is equipped with software so that gain, time of gain and delay can be adjusted. The video monitor, on which the real-time image is displayed, can be recorded on videotape for later analysis. Series of eye cups are provided with the machine to create a water bath for the coupling agent. These special cups fit in between the eyelids, keeping them open.

IMAGE ACQUISITION

After instilling 4% lignocaine in the eye, a plastic eye cap is used to gently part the lids and retain a layer of 2% methylcellulose or normal saline as the coupling agent. To maintain a steady fixation and constant accommodation, the patient is asked to fix at with the fellow eye on a ceiling target. The probe is manually moved perpendicular to the structure to be scanned.

NORMAL ANTERIOR SEGMENT STRUCTURES ON UBM IMAGE

Images produced by UBM have a resolution of 40 microns, and are seen similar to those seen on a low power microscope. Cornea is first structure seen on UBM.

CORNEA

All corneal layers can be differentiated in cross section on UBM image (Fig. 9.1).

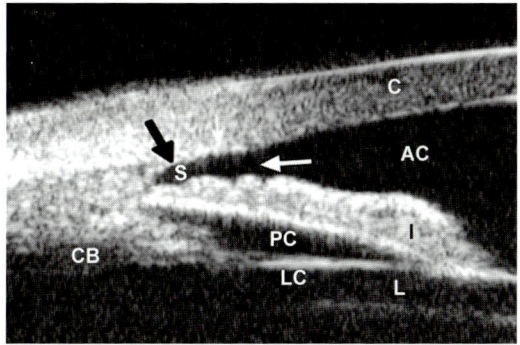

Fig. 9.1: *Ultrasound biomicroscopic appearance of a normal eye. The cornea (C), sclera (S), anterior chamber (AC), posterior chamber (PC), iris (I), ciliary body (CB), lens capsule (LC), and lens (L) can be identified*

- *Epithelium and Bowman's membrane*. The first highly reflective line is the surface of the corneal epithelium. The epithelium can be differentiated from Bowman's membrane, which forms a highly reflective line just below this. The distance between these two lines is the epithelial thickness.

- *Corneal stroma* reveals a low internal reflectivity that is lower than that found in the more irregular collagen distribution of the sclera. This difference allows definition of the corneoscleral junction.

- *Descemet's membrane and endothelium*. The endothelium cannot be differentiated from Descemet's membrane, but together, they form a single highly reflective line at the posterior corneal margin. Greater definition of corneal structure can be achieved with higher frequency transducers.

- *Sclera and cornea–sclera junction*. The normal sclera has relatively high reflectivity compared to the cornea. This high reflectivity allows definition of the corneoscleral junction and usually allows scleral tissue to be differentiated from the less reflective episcleral tissue and the less reflective ciliary body and peripheral choroid. The sclera is generally thickest in the region of the scleral spur. The scleral spur forms an important landmark for orientation and measuring distances in the region. The insertion of muscle tendons into the sclera can be outlined. The sclera can be seen to be significantly thinned below the muscle insertion. Anterior ciliary vessels can be seen penetrating through the scleral tissue near the limbus.

OTHER ANTERIOR SEGMENT STRUCTURES

The AC is seen as an echo poor area between the cornea and the iris. The AC depth can be measured from the posterior surface of the cornea to the anterior capsule. The normal AC depth is 2.5–3.0 mm.

The iris is seen as a flat uniform echogenic area. The iris and ciliary body converge in the iris recess and insert into the scleral spur. The area under the peripheral iris and above the ciliary processes is defined as the ciliary sulcus.

The angle can be studied in a cross-section by orienting the probe in a radial fashion at the limbus. The scleral spur is the most important landmark in the angle on UBM. The scleral spur is seen as small echogenic dot when the line between the sclera and ciliary body is traced to the AC.

Ciliary body can be clearly defined by UBM from the ciliary processes to the para plana. The ciliary processes vary in appearances and configuration. The axial view of the ciliary processes is seen when taking a section of the angle. The individual processes are better seen in a transverse section through the ciliary processes.

The anterior zonular surface can be consistently imaged by UBM. The zonules are seen as a medium reflective line extending from the ciliary processes to the lens surface.

APPLICATIONS AND LIMITATIONS OF UBM

APPLICATIONS OF UBM

CORNEAL OEDEMA

Corneal oedema can occur from many causes, most involving some form of endothelial pathology. Ultrasound biomicroscopy provides a highly accurate method of assessing changes in corneal thickness. In corneal oedema:

- *Epithelial surface echo* is more irregular, and the epithelium shows some internal reflectivity that is not apparent in normal cornea. The distance from the surface echo to the echo from Bowman's membrane is increased (Fig. 9.2).
- *Stromal reflectivity* is generally increased in corneal oedema. This is most likely due to the separation of the corneal lamellae by oedema fluid.
- *Bullae*. In bullous keratopathy can be imaged as a separation of the epithelium from Bowman's membrane.
- *Thickness of the corneal stroma* can be measured independently of epithelial thickness, by measuring the distance from the Bowman's membrane reflection to the reflection from the endothelial surface.

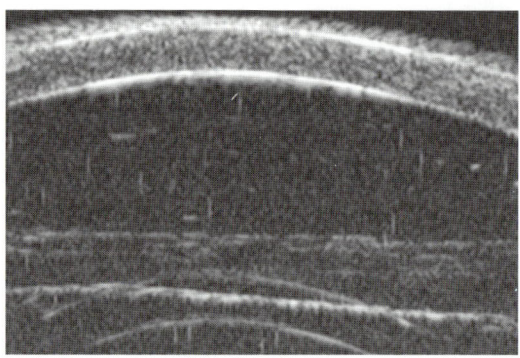

Fig. 9.2: *UBM showing corneal oedema*

CORNEAL OPACITY

Ultrasound biomicroscopy provides some information on the scarring process, allows quantitative assessment of corneal thinning, and provides information on underlying anterior segment changes (Fig. 9.3). Generally the region of a corneal scar shows higher reflectivity than the surrounding normal cornea, probably due to the disruption of the very regular corneal lamellae present in normal corneal structure. If calcification is present, the reflectivity increases to high levels and shadowing.

CORNEAL GRAFTS

Ultrasound biomicroscopy provides method of assessing corneal grafts. Corneal oedema, thickening of corneal stroma and epithelium can be assessed. In addition, aberrations at the graft host junction can be assessed (Fig. 9.4). This area is often difficult to visualise at the slit-lamp because of scarring present due to healing at the suture line and the frequent opacity of the residual host cornea. The graft–host junction is usually identifiable by a change in reflectivity

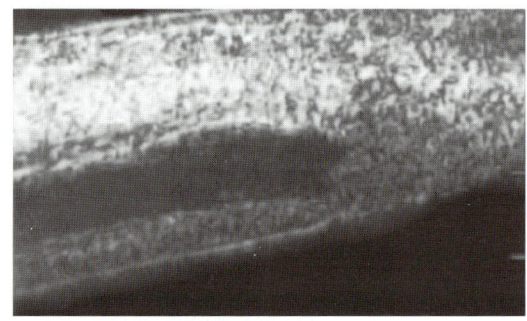

Fig. 9.3: *UBM showing corneal opacification*

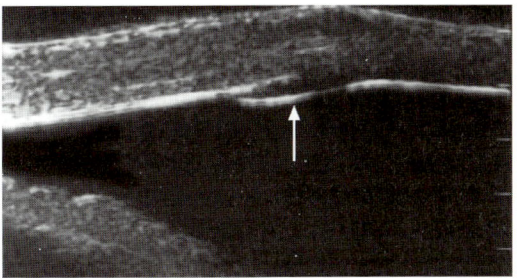

Fig. 9.4: *UBM showing corneal graft*

from the more weakly reflective graft and the more highly reflective pathological host cornea. Aberrations such as a step or irregularity between the host cornea and the graft are easily discernible. Any posterior wound gaping can also be imaged. These capabilities provide a method of determining the accuracy of graft placement.

ANTERIOR SEGMENT FOREIGN BODIES

The presence of an intraocular foreign body (IOFB) is a common complication of ocular trauma. For surgical planning, the localisation of IOFBs has to be accurate. The diagnosis of presence of a foreign body using UBM made based on high reflective echoes causing shadowing or reverberations (Fig. 9.5). UBM, however, provides the precise locations of IOFBs and additional information on damaged structures of anterior segment. However, high reflective echoes produced by IOFBs result in complete shadowing of all structures behind them. Also, glass foreign bodies produce characteristic reverberations posterior to them. Furthermore, shadowing observed with high-

frequency UBM is more prominent than that observed using low-frequency B-scan ultrasound. Nonetheless, the detection of anterior segment foreign bodies and associated ocular damage is best achieved with UBM.

TUMOURS OF ANTERIOR SURFACE OF EYE

Ultrasound biomicroscopy is an important adjunct in the management of anterior segment tumours. It provides a clear image of even the smallest anterior segment lesions. Tumours and tumour-like conditions over the sclera, conjunctiva, and cornea can be easily diagnosed by direct examination. The role of UBM in anterior surface tumours is to assess the depth of the tumour and study the layer of origin of the tumour. Such assessment by UBM helps in treatment planning of tumours. UBM helps to study the amount of infiltration of the cornea and sclera in limbal tumours. The ability to measure these lesions accurately adds the dimension of depth to criteria for demonstrating growth (Fig. 9.6). Generally, a radial cross-section image is obtained through the thickest part of the tumour as determined by careful scanning. This method is reproducible and allows accurate serial measurements. The ability to determine the underlying structure of the tumour allows improved classification and the ability to determine ciliary body involvement.

LIMITATIONS OF UBM

The most important limitation of UBM is depth. UBM cannot visualise structures deeper than 4 mm from the surface. The other limitation of UBM is that it cannot be performed in presence of an open corneal or scleral wound.

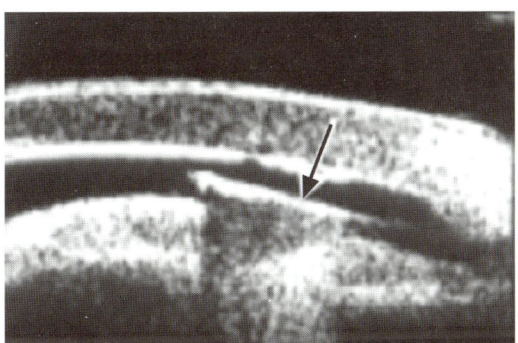

Fig. 9.5: *UBM showing anterior segment foreign body*

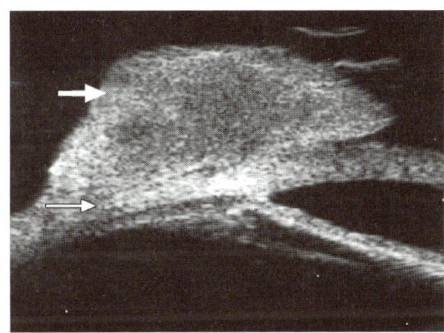

Fig. 9.6: *UBM showing anterior segment tumour*

BIBLIOGRAPHY

1. Berinstein DM, Gentile RC, Sidoti PA, et al. Ultrasound biomicroscopy in anterior ocular trauma. Ophthalmic Surg Lasers 1997; 28: 201–07.
2. Bhatt DC. Ultrasound biomicroscopy: An overview. J Clin Ophthalmol Res 2014; 2: 115-23.
3. Gazzard G, Friedman DS, Devereux JG, Chew P, Seah SK. A prospective ultrasound biomicroscopy evaluation of changes in anterior segment morphology after laser iridotomy in Asian eyes. Ophthalmology 2003; 110: 630-38.
4. Ishikawa H, Schuman JS. Anterior segment imaging: Ultrasound biomiscroscopy. Ophthalmol Clin N Am 2004; 17: 7-20.
5. Lowe RF. Causes of shallow anterior chamber in primary angle closure glaucoma. Am J Ophthalmol 1969; 67: 87-93.
6. Marchini G, Pagliarusco A, Toscano A, et al. Ultrasound biomicroscopic and conventional ultrasonographic study of ocular dimentions in primary angle-closure glaucoma. Ophthalmology 1998; 105: 2091–98.
7. Pavlin CJ, Easterbook M, Hurwitz JJ. Ultrasound biomicroscopy in the assessment of anterior scleral diseases. Am J Ophthalmol 1993; 116: 628–30.
8. Palvin CJ, Harasiwicz K, Foster FS. Utrasound biomicroscopy of anterior segment structures in normal and glaucomatous eyes. Am J Ophthalmol 1992; 113: 381–89.
9. Palvin CJ, Harasiwicz K, Sherar MS, Foster MS. Clinical use of Ultrasound Biomicroscopy. Ophthalmology 1991; 98: 287–95.
10. Pavlin CJ, Mcwhae JA, McGowan HD. Ultrasound biomicroscopy of Anterior segment tumours. Ophthalmology 1992; 99: 1220–28.
11. Sherer Md, Starkoski BG, TaylorWB, Foster FS. A 100 MHz B-scan ultrasound backscatter microscope. Ultrason Imaging 1989; 11: 95–105.
12. Tanuj Dada, Gaurav Kumar, Sanjay Kumar Mishra. Ultrasound Biomicroscopy in Glaucoma: An Update. Journal of Current Glaucoma Practice 2008; 2(3): 17–32.

Anterior Segment Optical Coherence Tomography

ANTERIOR SEGMENT OPTICAL COHERENCE TOMOGRAPHY: GENERAL CONSIDERATIONS

INTRODUCTION

Anterior segment optical coherence tomography (AS-OCT) is a high resolution, three-dimensional, cross-sectional imaging modality that uses principle of low coherence interferometry to achieve axial resolution in the range of 3–20 µm. OCT is similar to ultrasound except that the light is used instead of sound. Anterior segment imaging using OCT was first demonstrated by Izatt et al in 1994 by using light with wavelength of 830 µm.[1,2] OCT performs imaging by measuring the echo time delay and magnitude of backscattered or back reflected light. It is an excellent novice tool for diagnosis and documentation of corneal pathologies, surgeries and response to treatment.[3]

PRINCIPLES OF ANTERIOR SEGMENT OCT

OCT is based on the principle of low coherence interferometry and is similar to ultrasonography in concept except that it uses infrared light instead of sound waves to obtain images. The principle of AS-OCT is based on the measurement of delay in light reflected from various tissue structures. Low coherence infrared light is split by the beam splitter of a Michelson interferometer into two components out of which one is directed to a movable mirror in the reference arm and the other beam passes through the tissue of interest. An optical detector in the final arm of the Michelson interferometer then detects the interference between the reference and tissue signals. The strength of each

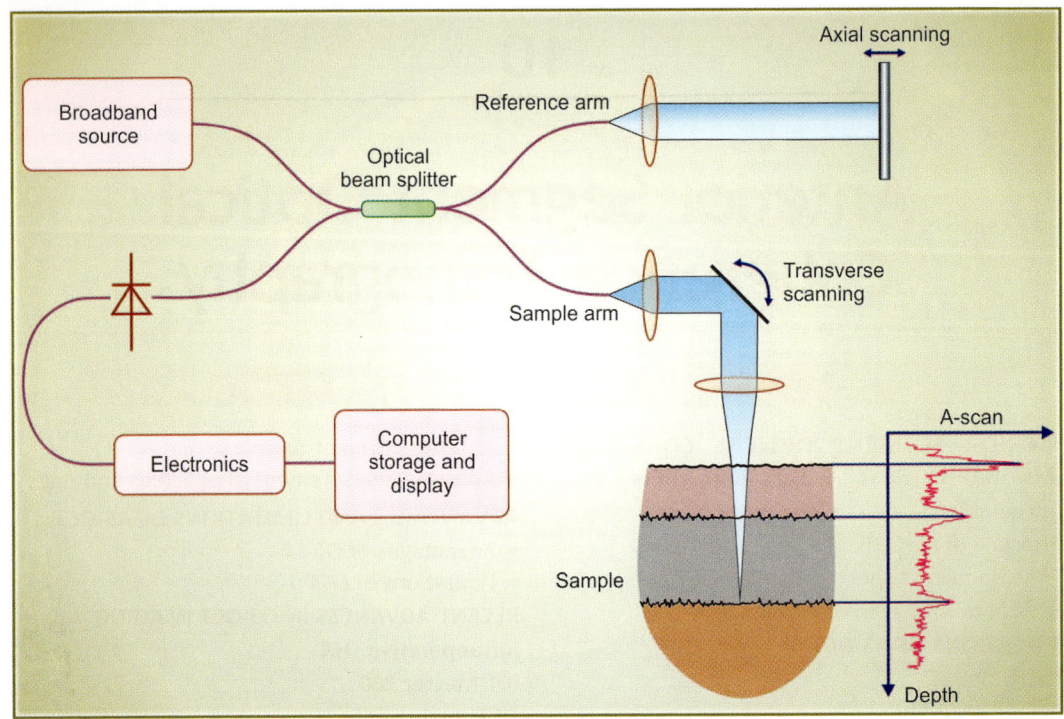

Fig. 10.1: *Flow chart depicting the principle of AS-OCT*

reflected signal is a function of depth in each scan (Fig. 10.1).[4]

TIME DOMAIN VS SPECTRAL DOMAIN OCT

Two OCT platforms have been developed for clinical use: Time domain and spectral (or Fourier) domain.

TIME DOMAIN OCT

Time domain OCT (TD-OCT) utilises a moveable reference mirror. The mirror moves for each A-scan to determine the ocular structure's depth, and this limits the speed at which the image is acquired. On the other hand, Fourier domain OCT (FD-OCT), has a fixed reference mirror to measure the depth information and uses a Fourier transformation algorithm of the spectral interferogram to produce the A-scan, thus resulting in faster acquisition and better image quality.[4]

TD AS-OCT systems include the Visante AS-OCT (Carl Zeiss Meditec, Inc., Dublin, CA) and SL-OCT (Heidelberg Engineering GmbH, Tiergartenstr, Heidelberg, Germany). The Visante OCT which received Food and Drug Administration approval in 2005, is the fastest commercial time domain model, performing rapid 2000 A-scans per second. It uses a wavelength of 1310 nm allowing better tissue penetration and reduced scattering. With the image acquisition of 8 frames/sec, it achieves an axial resolution of 18 μm and a lateral resolution of 60 μm.

FOURIER DOMAIN OCT

FD-OCT is divided into two types: Spectral domain OCT (SD-OCT) and Swept-source OCT (SS-OCT).

Some of commercially approved SD-OCT machines include: RTVue (Optovue, Inc., Fremont, California), Cirrus HD-OCT (Carl Zeiss Meditec, Inc., Dublin, California), Spectralis (Heidelberg Engineering, Inc., Heidelberg, Germany), SOCT Copernicus (Optopol Technology, Zawiercie, Poland) and 3D OCT-1000 (Topcon, Paramus, New Jersey).

RTVue utilises light at 840 nm wavelength and measures all echoes of light simultaneously as compared to sequentially in the case of TD-OCT thus improving sensitivity and imaging speed.

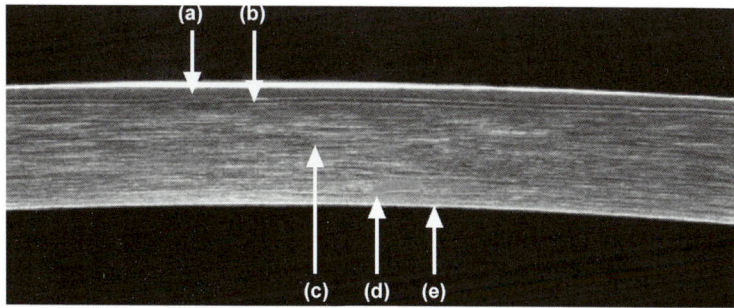

Fig. 10.2: *Horizontal OCT scan of normal cornea. (a) Epithelium; (b) Bowman's layer; (c) Corneal stromal layer; (d) Descemet's membrane; (e) Endothelium*

The scanning speed is 26,000 A-scans per second, 65 times faster than the scanning capability of TD-OCT and resolution is 5 µm. *Spectralis* (Heidelberg Engineering, Inc.) is another SD-OCT that obtains about 40,000 A-scans per second.

HORIZONTAL OCT SCAN OF NORMAL CORNEA

A horizontal OCT examination of healthy cornea shows a highly reflective tear film over epithelium, Bowman's layer, stromal layer, Descemet's membrane and endothelium (Fig. 10.2). AS-OCT is able to assess a wide range of anterior segment (AS) parameters with several uses in different ocular pathologies.

APPLICATIONS OF ANTERIOR SEGMENT OPTICAL COHERENCE TOMOGRAPHY

1. PACHYMETRY

Central corneal thickness is important for planning and performing refractive surgery, for assessing corneal diseases as well as monitoring glaucoma progression in patients with ocular hypertension and primary open angle glaucoma. Non-contact anterior segment OCT (AS-OCT) equipment provide high resolution cross-sectional imaging of the cornea (Fig. 10.3) and allows both central and regional pachymetry as well as sophisticated goniometry of the iridocorneal angle and other anterior segment structures. AS-OCT has advantages over ultrasonic pachymetry in that it is a non-invasive, non-contact technique. Unlike ultrasonic pachymetry, AS-OCT can easily be used to assess regional differences in the cornea and the facility for the patient to fixate on a target allows more accurate identification of the central corneal surface.

2. ECTATIC DISORDERS

AS-OCT has been crucial in diagnosis and management of corneal ectasias like keratoconus, pellucid marginal degeneration and Terrien marginal degeneration. It gives a pachymetry

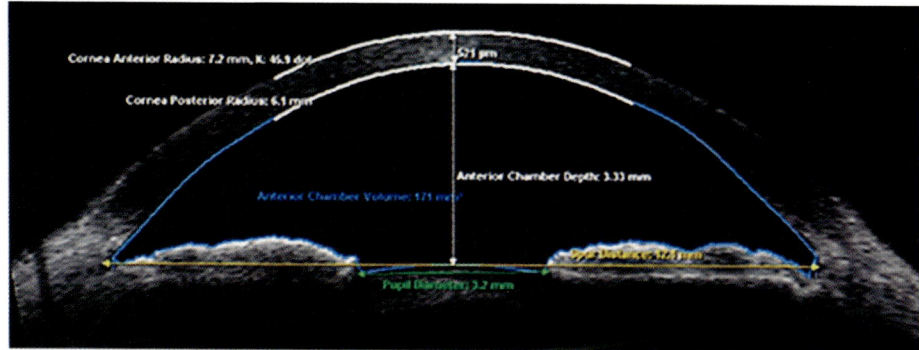

Fig. 10.3: *AS-OCT for measuring central corneal thickness*

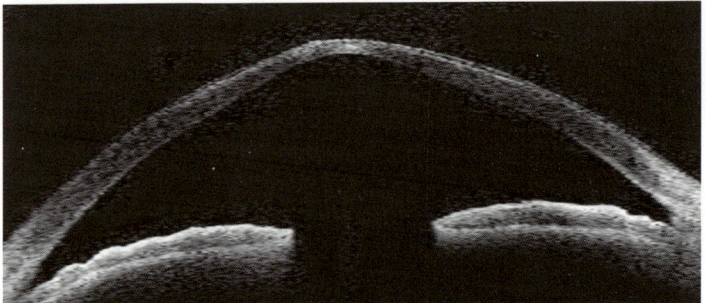

Fig. 10.4: *AS-OCT showing keratoconus*

map, consisting of 10 mm radial lines along eight meridians centred on vertex, which aid in diagnosis of early corneal ectasias with normal visual acuity and minimal clinical signs (Fig. 10.4). It has a higher resolution as compared to other imaging techniques and can also map the thickness of cornea in normal, opacified and postoperative corneas. Although moderate to advanced keratoconus is easily recognised by the characteristic topographic pattern and classic clinical signs, it can be difficult to distinguish subclinical forms of disease from normal corneas, because patients usually present with normal visual acuity, stable topographic patterns and minimal or no clinical signs. In these cases, OCT produces highly reliable pachymetry map, that can detect keratoconus, ectasia and corneal thinning conditions before refractive laser surgeries. Early detection of keratoconus is key to enable access to treatment with corneal collagen cross-linking, thus preventing the development of corneal scarring and possible need for corneal transplantation. Swept-source Fourier domain AS-OCT is found to discriminate normal eyes from subclinical keratoconus. AS-OCT is found useful to find the depth of demarcation following corneal collagen cross-linking.

OCT can diagnose keratoconus by using 4 parameters, based on the central 5 mm diameter region of the pachymetry map (Fig. 10.5):

i. **I–S:** The average thickness of the inferior (I) octant minus the average thickness of the superior (S) octant.

ii. **IT–SN:** The average thickness of the inferotemporal (IT) octant minus the average thickness of the superonasal (SN) octant.

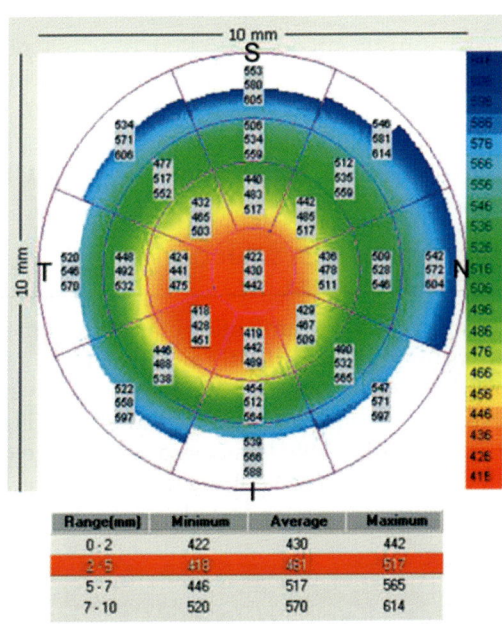

Range(mm)	Minimum	Average	Maximum
0 - 2	422	430	442
2 - 5	418	461	517
5 - 7	446	517	565
7 - 10	520	570	614

Fig. 10.5: *Visante pachymetry map of a keratoconic eye with central thinning. I–S = 442–483 = –41 mm; IT–SN = 428–485 = –57 mm; Min = 422 mm; Min–Max = 422–517 = –99 mm. The pachymetry map was abnormal in two indices (IT–SN and Min); a third index was borderline (Min–Max), in that it fell below keratoconus diagnostic cut-off values*

I=inferior; IT=inforotemporal; Max=maximum; Min=minimum; S=superior; SN=superonasal

iii. **Minimum:** The thinnest corneal thickness

iv. **Minimum–maximum:** The minimum pachymetry minus the maximum pachymetry.

Diagnostic cut-off points for these parameters: Asymmetry that is more negative than –45 mm for I-S or IT–SN indicates keratoconus, as does a minimum thickness of less than 470 mm or a minimum–maximum difference that is more negative than −100 mm. One abnormal para-meter provides reason to suspect keratoconus, and two or more abnormal parameters give a definite diagnosis.

In keratoconus patients, AS-OCT is found useful for qualitative evaluation of the cornea before and after implantation of the intrastromal ring. AS-OCT is found useful to evaluate the Descemet's membrane tear, dimensions of intrastromal clefts, and corneal thickness in acute corneal hydrops of keratoconus (Fig. 10.6). AS-OCT is also useful in assessing the response of treatment following interventions such as injection of sulphur hexafluoride (SF6)/per-fluoropropane (C3F8) gas into the anterior chamber.

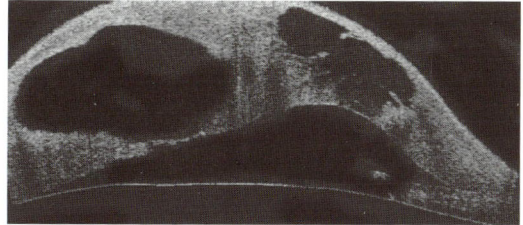

Fig. 10.6: *AS-OCT showing acute hydrops*

3. KERATOPLASTY

AS-OCT is used as an imaging tool for penetrating (PK) as well as lamellar keratoplasty (both anterior lamellar and posterior lamellar keratoplasty).

i. Penetrating keratoplasty

AS-OCT is used to visualise the depth of corneal involvement preoperatively to make a decision of performing a full thickness corneal transplant. Postoperatively, it helps to monitor the graft–host junction apposition, any retained host

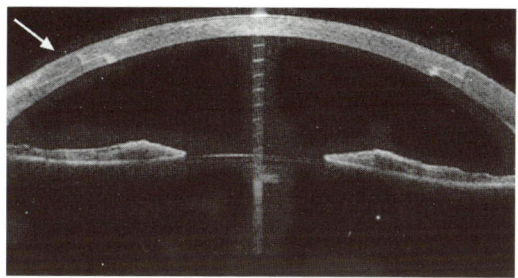

Fig. 10.7: *AS-OCT image of a patient who has undergone femtosecond laser-assisted keratoplasty at 3 months postoperatively showing scarring and good approximation at the interface (mushroom configuration shown with an arrow)*

Descemet's membrane (DM) or double chamber and presence of any DMD due to surgical trauma. In PK with femtosecond laser appli-cations,[5] OCT can identify top hat, mushroom (Fig. 10.7), zigzag-shaped incisions, alignment of donor and host cornea and the depth of the sutures.

ii. Lamellar keratoplasty

AS-OCT has revolutionised the treatment planning and postoperative monitoring of lamellar grafts.

Anterior lamellar corneal transplantation

AS-OCT helps in deciphering the exact depth of corneal involvement by the opacity (Fig. 10.8).[6] This helps in deciding the type of lamellar transplant needed for the patient. In superficial involvement of cornea, a sutureless superficial anterior lamellar keratoplasty (SALK) can be performed wherein a 200 µm depth of corneal opacity can be removed with a microkeratome (Fig. 10.9). In deeper cases of anterior to mid-stromal involvement, an automated lamellar therapeutic keratoplasty (ALTK) can be

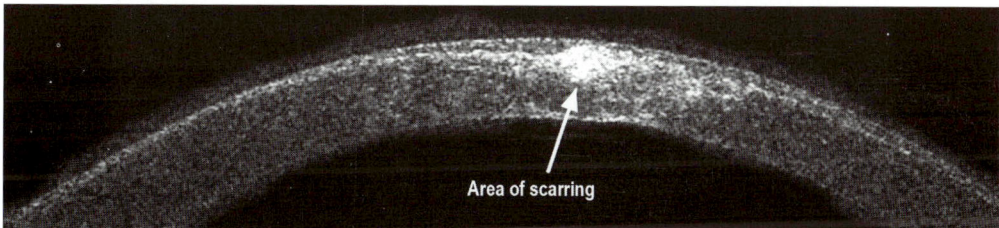

Area of scarring

Fig. 10.8: *AS-OCT scan showing the presence of scarring involving the anterior corneal layers for which an automated lamellar therapeutic keratoplasty can be performed*

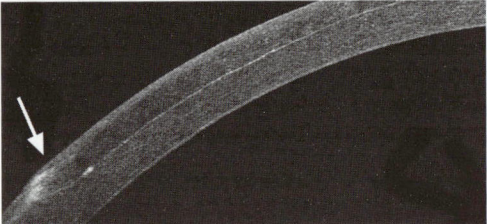

Fig. 10.9: *AS-OCT scan of a sutureless anterior lamellar graft one month postoperatively showing a good graft-host apposition with epithelial remodelling*

performed with sutures. In cases where the opacity reaches up to the posterior stroma without involvement of the DM, a deep anterior lamellar keratoplasty can be performed (Fig. 10.10).

Posterior lamellar corneal transplantation

Posterior lamellar keratoplasty is especially useful in cases of endothelial dysfunction wherein only the replacement of posterior Descemet's endothelial complex can be done. It includes Descemet's stripping automated endothelial keratoplasty (DSAEK)[7] and more recently Descemet's membrane endothelial keratoplasty (DMEK). AS-OCT provides an estimation of graft thickness (Figs 10.11 and 10.12) and monitoring the same in cases of graft rejection or failure. The most common post-operative complication in DSAEK is donor graft detachment. In these cases, early recognition and

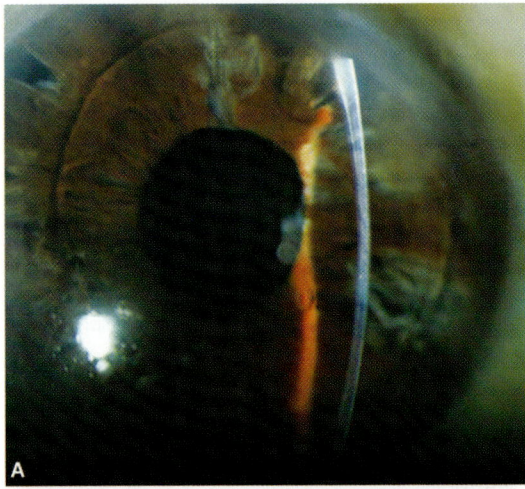

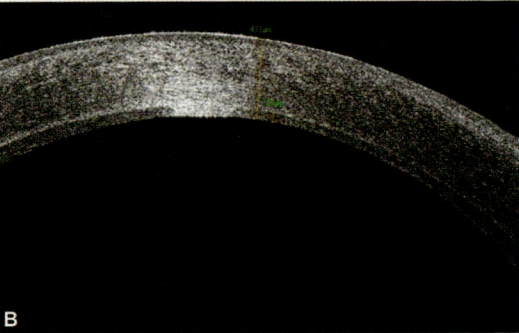

Fig. 10.11: *Clinical photograph (A); and AS-OCT scan (B) of a DSAEK graft on postoperative day 1 showing a well attached and centred graft along with the graft and the host thickness*

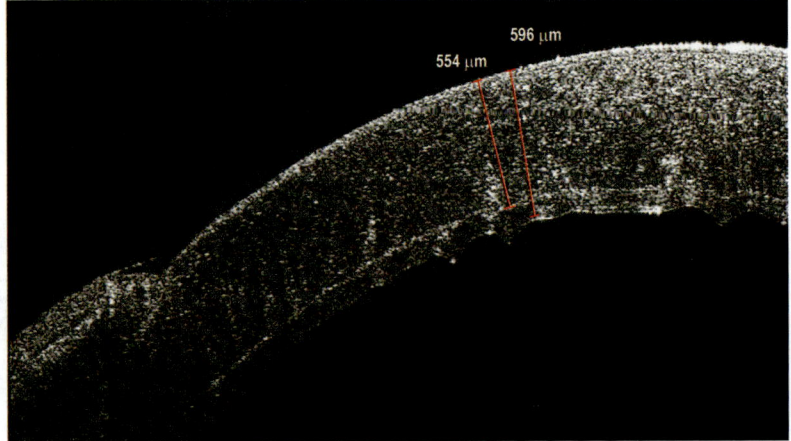

Fig. 10.10: *AS-OCT scan of pre-descemetic deep anterior lamellar keratoplasty showing the graft–host junction with good approximation*

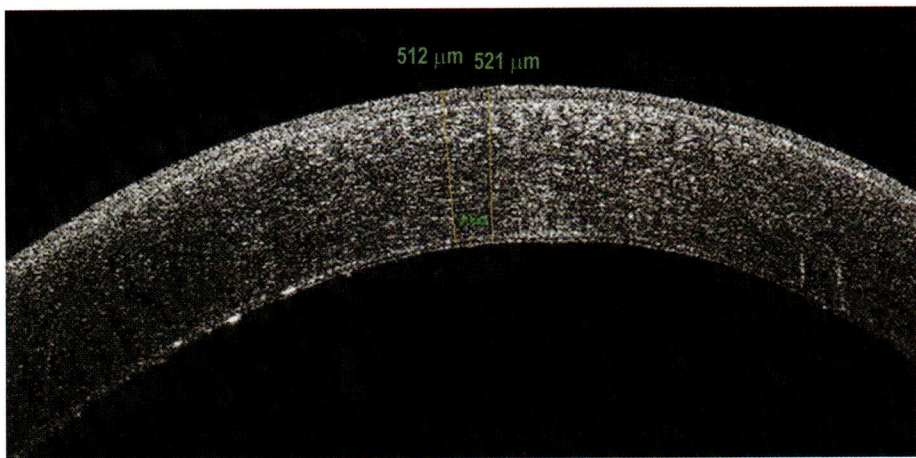

Fig. 10.12: *AS-OCT scan of a well-attached DMEK graft on postoperative day 2 showing a graft thickness of 30 µm with minimal interface haze*

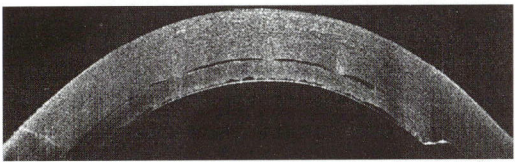

Fig. 10.13: *AS-OCT scan showing interface fluid pockets one day postoperatively following DSAEK*

management is mandatory to avoid graft failure. AS-OCT is used to confirm the presence of interface fluid (Fig. 10.13), localised or total graft dislocation (Fig. 10.14) after DSAEK surgery especially in cloudy corneas with limited anterior chamber involvement.

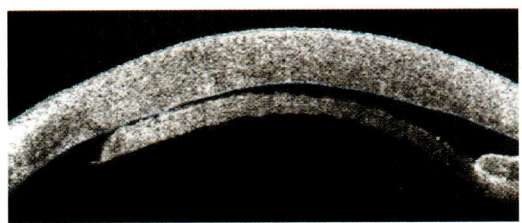

Fig. 10.14: *AS-OCT scan showing graft dislocation in an operated case of DSAEK one day postoperatively*

4. REFRACTIVE SURGERIES

AS-OCT can visualise the LASIK flap in the early postoperative period to evaluate the performance of microkeratome or femtosecond laser being used. It can also visualise the flaps many months or years later.[13] An OCT evaluation of the residual stromal bed and flap can assess the potential safety of performing an enhancement by lifting the flap (Figs 10.15 and 10.16).

a. Phakic IOL

Accurate measurement and biometric analyses of the anterior segment of the eye have become extremely critical, because of the increased use of refractive phakic IOLs.[14] OCT can image the entire AC and yield measurements such as AC depth, angle-to-angle width and iris profile (Fig. 10.17). Postoperatively, AS-OCT is used in the examination of the position of the IOL and can be used to visualise the contact between the refractive implant and the crystalline lens. It gives information about the vaulting which should ideally be between 250 µm and 750 µm (Fig. 10.18).

b. Intrastromal corneal ring segments

High-resolution OCT can image the intrastromal corneal rings,[15] providing a much more accurate depth and position assessment (Fig. 10.19). If the surgeon does not place the intrastromal corneal ring segments deep enough, it may result in severe complications, such as epithelial-stromal breakdown and extrusion. On the other hand, implants that are too deep may carry a high-risk for perforation into the AC. Hence, the OCT scan can help cornea surgeons improve their techniques and avoid depth-related problems earlier.

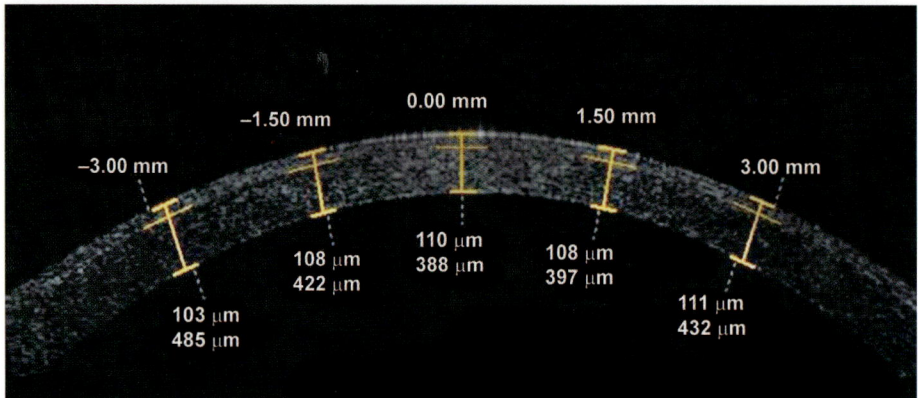

Fig. 10.15: *Optical coherence tomography scan (RTVue) of a femtosecond laser flap, 1 week postoperative, with an adequate residual stromal bed*

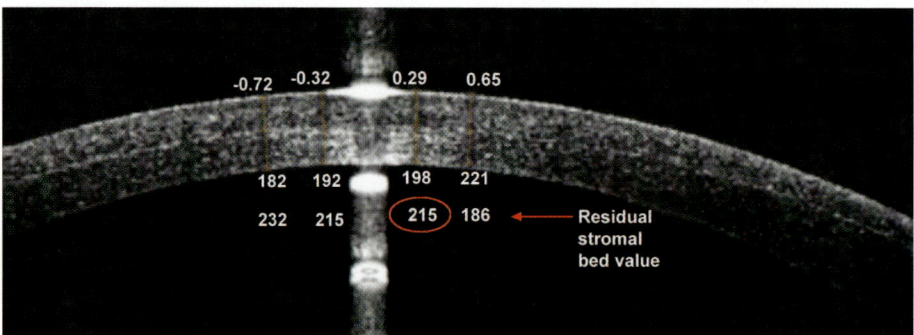

Fig. 10.16: *Optical coherence tomography scan (RTVue) of the cornea post-LASIK with a thick flap and a thin residual stromal bed (<250 mm)*

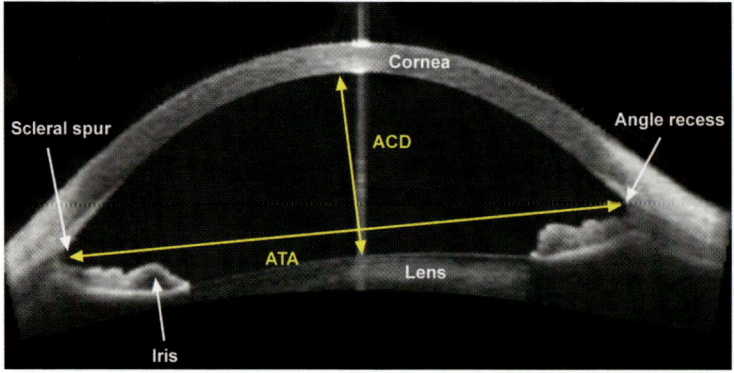

Fig. 10.17: *Visante optical coherence tomography of an anterior chamber measurement in a phakic patient. ACD: Anterior chamber depth; ATA: Angle-to-angle width*

c. AS-OCT in femtosecond laser-assisted cataract surgery

The most recent and exciting advancement in refractive surgery is the development of femtosecond laser-assisted cataract surgery. These systems are capable of performing corneal incisions, continuous curvilinear capsulorhexis, nucleus softening and lens fragmentation. These

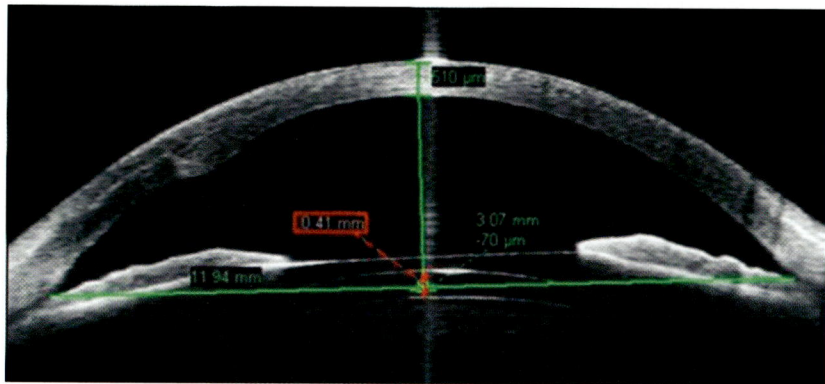

Fig. 10.18: *AS-OCT scan of a patient with phakic IOL showing a vault of 410 µm*

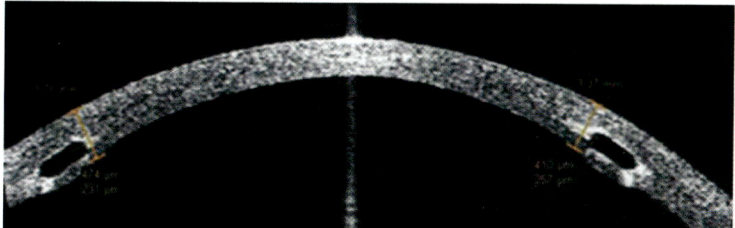

Fig. 10.19: *Horizontal AS-OCT cross-section and measurement of the intrastromal ring depth. Both rings are placed at an adequate depth*

platforms have an integrated OCT system to analyse the anterior segment and to focus the laser in a 3D manner (Fig. 10.20).[16]

5. MICROBIAL KERATITIS

OCT can also be used for corneal imaging and assessment, in conjunction with slit-lamp

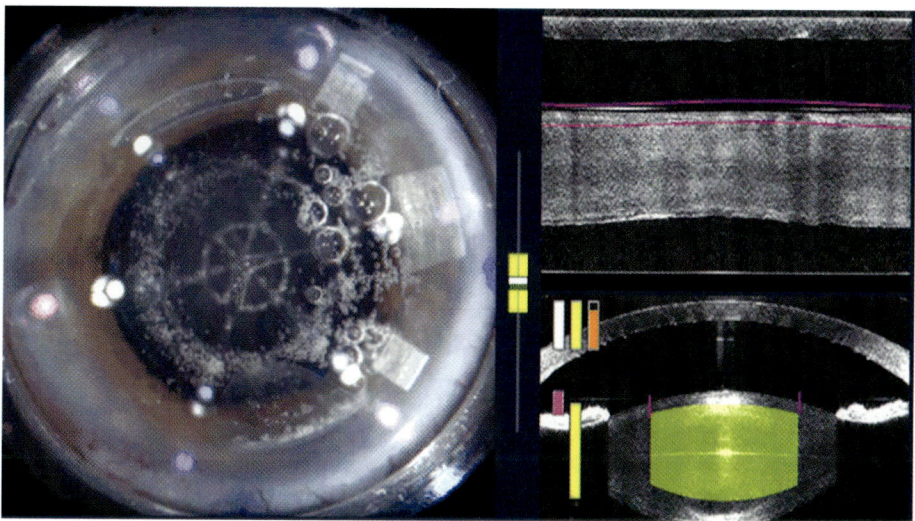

Fig. 10.20: *Integrated AS-OCT system with femtosecond laser-assisted cataract surgery which helps in 3D visualisation of the lens and posterior capsule*

biomicroscopy in cases of microbial keratitis to monitor progression of the disease. OCT can be useful in assessing the depth of corneal ulcers (Fig. 10.21). The depth of infiltrates (Fig. 10.22), areas of thinning, amount of endothelial exudates and changing therapy in cases of no response.

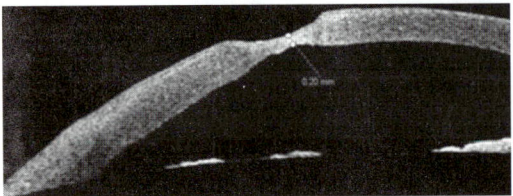

Fig. 10.21: *AS-OCT scan of a case of fungal keratitis showing the depth of ulcer associated with corneal thinning with remaining corneal thickness of only 200 μm*

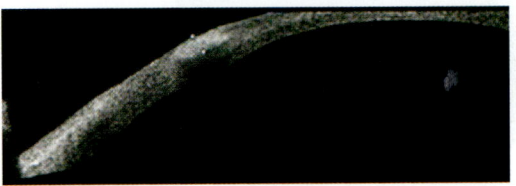

Fig. 10.22: *AS-OCT scan of a case of bacterial keratitis showing the presence of infiltrates in the epithelium and superficial stroma*

The affected area of keratitis is represented by the OCT as higher intense regions. In deciding the response of keratitis to treatment, OCT images can be followed by examining the depth and density of affected areas. When indicated, the area for corneal biopsy can be ascertained by identifying the densest areas of infiltration. Areas of impending perforation and severe thinning can also be imaged on AS-OCT. Decision on performing either lamellar keratoplasty or full-thickness penetrating keratoplasty can be made by examining the depth of infection on AS-OCT. AS-OCT allows the precise localization of microcystic edema and keratic precipitate. Infiltrate is seen as hyper-reflective areas in corneal stroma on high resolution scans. Retrocorneal pathologic features, anterior chamber inflammation, and width of endothelial plaque can be assessed by AS-OCT.

6. INTRACORNEAL FOREIGN BODY

In ocular trauma, AS-OCT may reveal unexpected lesions that are invisible or difficult to recognize on routine slit-lamp examination. It provides rapid imaging of various depths into ocular tissue and therefore provides accurate measurements of foreign body location, number and dimensions (Fig. 10.23). Different reflectivity is appreciable depending on nature of foreign body. Glass foreign body is well delineated on AS-OCT with no internal reflectivity. Wood foreign body showed moderate internal reflectivity while metal and stone foreign bodies showed high anterior reflectivity with shadowing. However, reflectivity in the anterior chamber or iris adhesion to the site of entry may suggest penetration into anterior chamber. AS-OCT provides vital detail about status of DM integrity and site of entry of foreign body. This information can be utilized to plan surgical removal. This prevents any intra- or postoperative surprises, thus providing best possible outcomes. In certain cases, corneal thinning might be suspected after removal of foreign body. AS-OCT is extremely advantageous in such situations as it gives quantitative assessment of remnant corneal thickness and hints the risk of impeding perforation. Cyanoacrylate glue and bandage contact lens can be performed in such cases if the defect is less than 2 mm in dimensions.

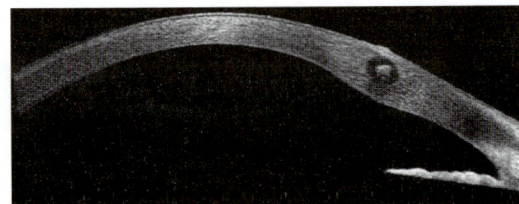

Fig. 10.23: *AS-OCT showing intracorneal foreign body*

7. EVALUATION OF CORNEA AFTER CATARACT SURGERY

AS-OCT imaging has been used to analyse the structure, integrity and configuration of the corneal incisions after cataract surgery[11] such as DMD (Fig. 10.24), posterior wound gape (Fig. 10.25) and wound retraction (Fig. 10.26). Postoperative localized Descemet detachment was found in 40–82% of the patients on postoperative day 1.[12] Stromal hydration was associated with prolonged stromal swelling, which lasted for up to 7 days.

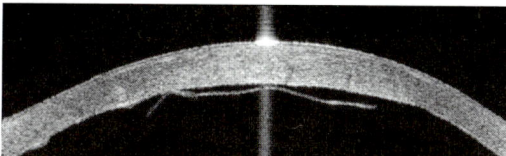

Fig. 10.24: *Descemet's membrane detachment on first postoperative day after cataract surgery associated with central corneal oedema*

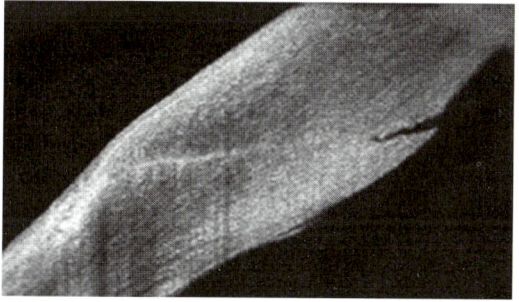

Fig. 10.25: *AS-OCT scan depicting a posterior wound gape following cataract surgery*

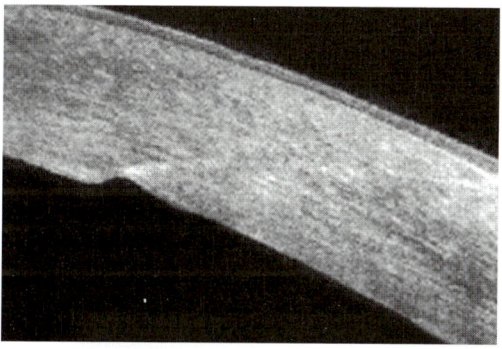

Fig. 10.26: *AS-OCT scan showing a clear corneal incision with posterior wound retraction*

AS-OCT plays an important role in finding the location and extent of DMD especially in cloudy corneas and in deciding the appropriate management of the same. In cases of large DMDs involving the visual axis, intracameral air/gas is injected and sequential AS-OCT scans help to know the resolution of the detachment.

8. ANTERIOR SEGMENT TUMOURS

Anterior iris pathology can be imaged by AS-OCT and is able to differentiate small cystic from solid lesions. It can image small non-pigmented tumours but cannot penetrate larger tumours, pigmented tumours or tumours involving the

ciliary body. Visualisation of the posterior chamber is suboptimal as the infrared light is significantly attenuated by the iris pigment epithelium.

9. ACCURATE MEASUREMENT OF OPACITIES AND RINGS

AS-OCT allows surgeons to accurately determine the depth of corneal opacities (Fig. 10.27), enabling them to choose the most appropriate treatment: Excimer laser or lamellar or penetrating keratoplasty. Insertion of shallow intrastromal corneal ring segments increases the incidence of epithelial and stromal breakdown and ring extrusion. AS-OCT can assess the depth and position of intracorneal rings to determine the risk of extrusion.

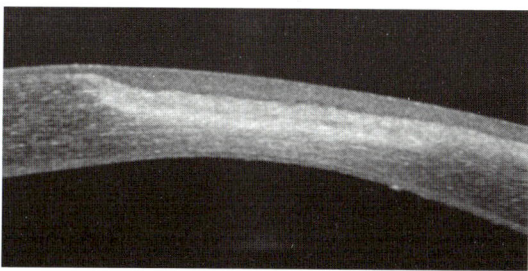

Fig. 10.27: *AS-OCT showing corneal opacity*

ADVANTAGES AND LIMITATIONS OF AS-OCT

ADVANTAGES OF AS-OCT

1. *It is a non-contact method* therefore do not cause indentation of the angle by placement of scleral cup on the eye (which is required to maintain the water bath in UBM) Also, no possibility of corneal abrasion or punctate epithelial erosions (possible with UBM).

2. *Shorter imaging time* (patient setup in UBM takes longer. Also, only one angle is imaged at a time with the UBM).

3. *Rapid image acquisition.* Eight frames can be captured per second, allowing operator to choose the best centred image.

4. *Requires less expertise to perform,* i.e. small learning curve for the operator.

   • Target may be used to induce accommodation in the eye being imaged. (This is specially useful in the evaluation of accommodative intraocular lenses.)

- More comfortable for the patient, due to non-contact technique, upright position and rapid imaging acquisition.

LIMITATIONS OF AS-OCT

AS-OCT does not completely penetrate the posterior pigment epithelium of the iris and hence cannot capture the area of the sulcus in the majority of cases. Infrared light is also absorbed by the sclera, obscuring the ciliary body. Amongst other limitations, AS-OCT cannot obtain clear images through opaque media and the iris, obstruction by the eyelids also makes imaging of the superior and inferior angles difficult.

RECENT ADVANCES IN AS-OCT IMAGING

INTRAOPERATIVE OCT

Intraoperative OCT systems have been developed which give a real-time imaging of intraoperative manoeuvres with the help of attachment to the operating microscope. This helps in planning appropriate treatment, modifying the surgical decisions and confirmation of the anatomical outcome in the operating room itself (Fig. 10.28).[17]

IOL MASTER 700

OCT systems (swept-source OCT) have also been incorporated into the IOL Master which will help in reducing refractive surprises by ensuring more accurate biometry with the help of real-time OCT imaging.

OPTICAL COHERENCE TOMOGRAPHY ANGIOGRAPHY

Optical coherence tomography angiography (OCTA) is a non-invasive modality and shows similar potential for anterior segment vasculature as for retinal diseases. The study of vasculature is important to monitor progression of disease and follow the response to treatment. The assessment of conjunctiva, tumour development, bleb formation after glaucoma surgery and corneal vascularization are potential applications of OCTA. It targets blood vessels as well as lymphatics. It detects blood flow by analysing signal decorrelation or phase deviations between ultra high speed scans.

APPLICATIONS OF OPTICAL COHERENCE TOMOGRAPHY ANGIOGRAPHY IN CORNEAL DISEASES

OCT angiography can be performed for various corneal pathologies like corneal vascularization, fungal keratitis, pterygium, postherpetic or

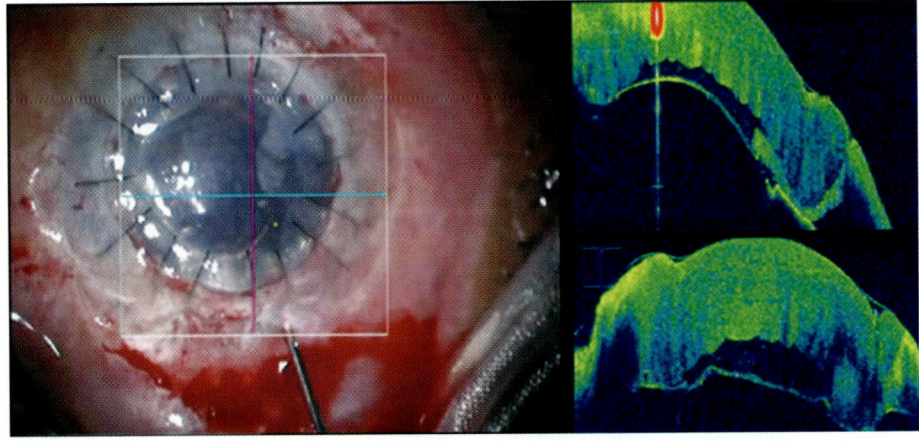

Fig. 10.28: *Anterior segment intraoperative optical coherence tomography (iOCT) showing insertion of a 30 G needle with 20% SF6 injection into the anterior chamber at the 11 o'clock position in a case of post-keratoplasty DMD*

limbal stem cell deficiency. Slight changes may be missed by slit-lamp examination, which makes OCTA a major tool for early evaluation of such pathologies. OCTA can clearly determine the extent of corneal vessels invading the corneal graft. It also shows clearly the abnormal vascular loops and the demarcation between normal and abnormal vessels. It can also be useful to assess abnormal vascularization in stromal keratitis, specially when stromal scarring causes loss of transparency. Although fluorescein and ICG angiography are useful for anterior segment vasculature, these invasive techniques are not performed in routine for evaluation of anterior segment.

CORNEAL VASCULARIZATION

Corneal vascularization is the pathological infiltration of blood vessels into cornea due to disturbance of balance between pro- and anti-angiogenic factors. It can develop due to infection, immunological process, surgery and trauma. It can cause visual impairment due to corneal oedema, lipid exudation and corneal scarring. Due to invasive and time intensive nature of corneal angiography, optical coherence tomography (OCT) angiography has considered as a non-invasive imaging modality of choice for diagnosis of corneal vascularization.

CORNEAL TRANSPLANT REJECTION

Corneal transplantation has increased risk of immune rejection in the setting of preexisting or developing corneal vascularization. Migration of vessels into corneal graft often heralds stromal rejection and can lead to rapid deterioration of a clear graft. Photographic methods to monitor the extent of creeping vessel progression over time are essential for objective assessment of risk of rejection. Early treatment of these vessels may improve rates of graft survival. Numerous pathologies can shift the balance in inflammatory signals in the clear tissue matrix of the cornea to drive growth of blood vessels.

ADVANTAGES OF OCT ANGIOGRAPHY OVER CONVENTIONAL ANGIOGRAPHY

- OCTA does not require the injection of contrast medium. Contrast dyes have rare but known risk including anaphylaxis and complications in patients with liver and renal dysfunction.
- OCTA image acquisition is also more rapid and may perform better with motion artifacts, including unsteady fixation encountered in eyes with significant pathology.
- OCTA can be repeated to capture extra information or additional regions of interest without additional contrast infusions.
- OCTA generates 3D data that can be segmented to evaluate vessel depth and to focus on features of vessels at specific corneal depths.

LIMITATIONS OF OCT ANGIOGRAPHY

- Lack of eye tracking during imaging and image distortions due to eye/patient movement during the scan.
- Limited resolution with small field of view.
- Slow or minimal blood flow vessels may not be detected, and dense opacities in the cornea may block angiographic signals, leading to false conclusions about the extent of corneal vascularization.

These limitations can be overcome by swept source OCT devices with faster scan speed and improved resolution of deeper vessels.

REFERENCES

1. Huang D, Swanson EA, Lin CP, et al. Optical coherence tomography. Science 1991; 254: 1178–81.
2. Izatt JA, Hee MR, Swanson EA, et al. Micrometer-scale resolution imaging of the anterior eye *in vivo* with optical coherence tomography. Arch Ophthalmol 1994; 112: 1584–89.
3. Maldonado MJ, Ruiz-OL, Munuera JM, et al. Optical coherence tomography evaluation of the corneal cap and stromal bed features after laser *in situ* keratomileusis for high myopia and astigmatism. Ophthalmology 2000; 107: 81–87.
4. Ramos, Jose Luiz Branco, Yan Li, and David Huang. Clinical and Research Applications of Anterior Segment Optical Coherence Tomography—a Review. Clinical and Experimental Ophthalmology 2009; 37(1): 81–89.
5. Birnbaum F, Maier P, Reinhard T. Femtosecond laser-assisted penetrating keratoplasty. Ophthalmologe. 2010; 107(2): 186–88.
6. Khurana RN, Li Y, Tang M, Lai MM, Huang D. High-speed optical coherence tomography of

corneal opacities. Ophthalmology 2007; 114: 1278–85.

7. Tarnawska D, Wylegala E. Monitoring cornea and graft morphometric dynamics after Descemet stripping and endothelial keratoplasty with anterior segment optical coherence tomography. Cornea 2010; 29: 272–77.

8. Konstantopoulos AAuthor Vitae, Kuo J, Anderson D, Hossain P. Assessment of the Use of Anterior Segment Optical Coherence Tomography in Microbial Keratitis. American Journal of ophthalmology 2008; 146(4): 534–42.

9. Qin B, Chen S, Brass R, Li Y, et al. Keratoconus diagnosis with optical coherence tomography–based pachymetric scoring system. J Cataract Refract Surg 2013; 39: 1864–71.

10. Maharana PK, Sharma N, Vajpayee RB. Acute corneal hydrops in keratoconus. Indian J Ophthalmol 2013; 61(8): 461–64.

11. Calladine D, Packard R. Clear corneal incision architecture in the immediate postoperative period evaluated using optical coherence tomography. J Cataract Refract Surg 2007; 33: 1429–35.

12. Zhou SY, Wang CX, Cai XY, Liu YZ. Anterior segment OCT-based diagnosis and management of Descemet's membrane detachment. Ophthalmologica 2012; 227: 215–22.

13. Li Y, Netto MV, Shekhar R, Krueger RR. A longitudinal study of LASIK flap and stromal thickness with high speed optical coherence tomography. Ophthalmology 2007; 114: 1124–32.

14. Baïkoff G. Anterior segment OCT and phakic intraocular lenses: a perspective. J Cataract Refract Surg 2006; 32: 1827–35.

15. Lai MM, Tang M, Andrade EMM, et al. Optical coherence tomography to assess intrastromal corneal ring segment depth in keratoconic eyes. J Cataract Refract Surg 2006; 32: 1860–65.

16. Nguyen P, Chopra V. Applications of optical coherence tomography in cataract surgery. Curr Opin Ophthalmol 2013; 24(1): 47–52.

17. Sharma N, Aron N, Kakkar P, et al. Continuous intraoperative OCT-guided management of post-deep anterior lamellar keratoplasty Descemet's membrane detachment. Saudi Journal of Ophthalmology 2016; 30: 133–36.

Section

III

Developmental Anomalies and Metabolic Disorders of Conjunctiva and Cornea

Embryology and Developmental Anomalies of Conjunctiva

EMBRYOLOGY OF CONJUNCTIVA

GENERAL CONSIDERATIONS

Eyelids are formed by reduplication of surface ectoderm above and below the cornea during 2nd month of gestation (Fig. 11.1). The folds enlarge and their margins meet and fuse with each other. The lids cut off a space called conjunctival sac.

DEVELOPMENT OF CONJUNCTIVA

Conjunctiva develops from the ectoderm lining of the lids and covering the globe (Fig. 11.1).
Conjunctival glands develop as growth of the basal cells of upper conjunctival fornix. Fewer glands develop from the lower fornix.

CONGENITAL DISORDERS OF CONJUNCTIVA

A few of the congenital disorders of conjunctiva worth mentioning include:
- Conjunctival choristoma
- Congenital pigmented lesions of conjunctiva
- Congenital epitarsus
- Conjunctival telangiectasia

CONJUNCTIVAL CHORISTOMA

Choristoma refers to benign tumour consisting of microscopically normal tissue derived from germ cell layers foreign to that body site. Conjunctival choristoma possess little growth potential and contain both dermal and epithelial elements that are not normally found in the conjunctiva.

Types of conjunctival choristomas

There are four types of conjunctival choristoma:
- Solid epibulbar dermoid
- Diffuse dermolipoma
- Complex choristomas, and
- Single-tissue choristoma

SOLID EPIBULBAR DERMOID

Demography

- *Frequency.* The estimated worldwide incidence of limbal dermoids ranges from 1 case per 10,000 population to 3 cases per 10,000 population.
- *Race.* No racial predisposition exists.
- *Sex.* Limbal dermoids occur with equal frequency in males and in females.

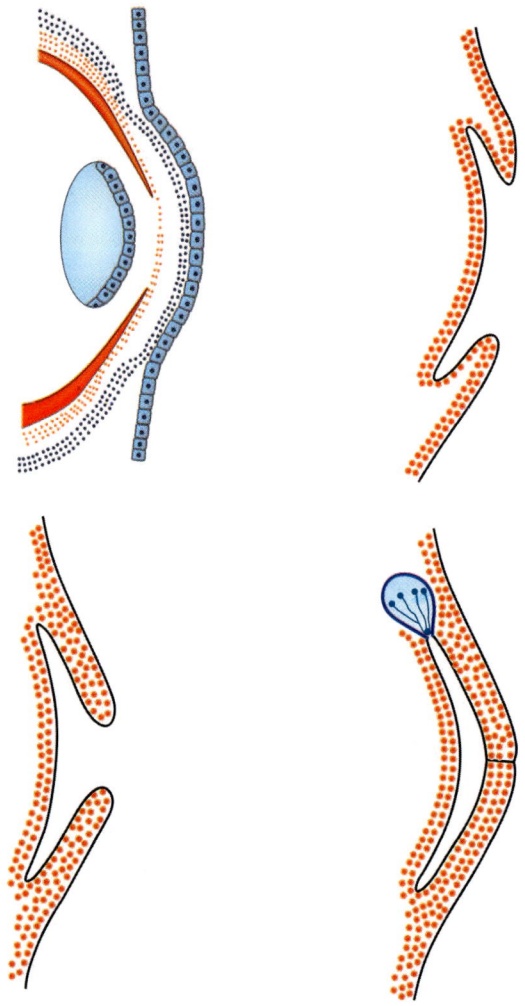

Fig. 11.1: *Development of eyelids and conjunctiva*

- *Age.* Limbal dermoids are present at birth but may not be recognized until the first or second decade of life. They may also appear to enlarge as the body matures.
- *Inheritance.* Limbal dermoids generally are not inherited, although some exceptions have been reported. Familial presentation of limbal dermoids in association with systemic disorders, such as Goldenhar syndrome, is well recognized and follows a multifactorial pattern of inheritance. Two rare forms of epibulbar dermoid (i.e. the annular limbal form, the corneal dystrophy form) presenting in multiple family members have been reported.

Pathophysiology

Several theories have been proposed to explain the development of limbal dermoids. Two important ones are:

1. *Theory of metaplastic transformation of the mesoblast.* According to this theory there occurs an early developmental error in between the rim of the optic nerve and the surface ectoderm.
2. *Theory of sequestration of the pluripotential cells* during embryonic development of the surrounding ocular structures, has also been suggested in pathophysiology.

Note. The exact pathogenesis probably varies from case to case.

Clinical features

Solid epibulbar dermoids are compact, pale yellow growths that typically occur unilaterally at the inferotemporal limbus (Fig. 11.2). Most limbal dermoids are superficial and only minimally involve the cornea and sclera. However, some tumours can penetrate deeply into the cornea, sclera, and conjunctiva.

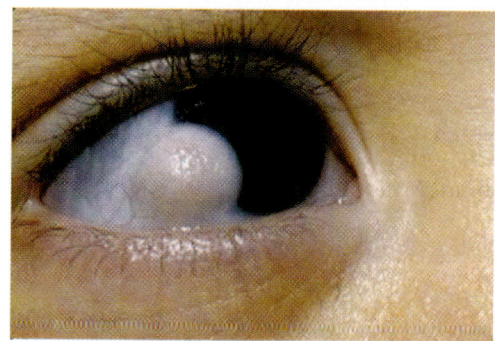

Fig. 11.2: *Limbal dermoid*

Types. Based on the location, there are three broad categories of epibulbar dermoids:

- *First type of epibulbar dermoid is the limbal dermoid* which is the most common type, in which the tumour straddles the limbus. Limbal dermoids are usually superficial lesions but rarely may involve deeper ocular structures.
- *Second type of epibulbar dermoid* involves only the superficial cornea, sparing the limbus, the Descemet membrane, and the endothelium.

- *Third type of epibulbar dermoid* involves the entire anterior segment, replacing the cornea with a dermolipoma that may involve the iris, the ciliary body, and the lens.

Associations. Limbal dermoids may be associated with Goldenhar syndrome, linear naevus sebaceous syndrome, and encephalo-craniocutaneous lipomatosis. Eyelid colobomas may also occur in association with limbal dermoids, which suggest the postulate that both anomalies may result from incomplete fusion of the lids with displacement of skin elements into the dermoid tumour.

Histological features

Histological examination reveals a thick, collagenous lesion that may contain hair, sweat glands, fat, sebaceous glands, or teeth (Fig. 11.3).

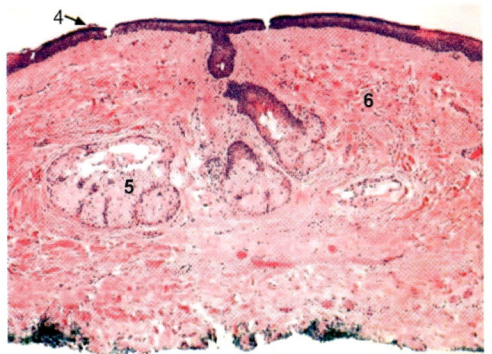

Fig. 11.3: *Histological structure of limbal dermoid*

Treatment

Treatment of limbal dermoids may consist of:

Periodic removal of irritating cilia, and *topical lubrication* to prevent foreign body sensation.

Or

Excision of the dermoid if it is causing significant cosmetic disfigurement or interfering with vision. Surgical treatment should be instituted only when the risk of subsequent scar formation or surgical complications are outweighed by the likelihood of improving the patient's vision or cosmetic appearance.

Surgical excision usually involves:
- *A superficial sclerokeratectomy*, cutting flush with the surface of the globe (shaving the lesion off the cornea and sclera) is the procedure of choice for removal of the dermoid. Excised tissue always should be sent to the pathologist for examination.
- *Exposed sclera should be covered* by relaxing the adjacent conjunctiva and sewing it into the scleral defect.
- *Lamellar keratoplasty* can be performed to reinforce the site of excision, when a deep excision is necessary.
- *Amniotic membrane graft*. Large patches of bare sclera can be treated with application of single or multilayered amniotic membrane graft tissue. The amniotic membrane can be secured to underlying sclera using sutures and/or fibrin-glue adhesive.

DIFFUSE DERMOLIPOMA

Dermolipomas are less dense than solid epibulbar dermoids and contain more adipose tissue. These are true choristomas, because fatty tissue is usually not found anterior to the orbital septum. They are typically found on the superior temporal bulbar conjunctiva. These masses can extend from the limbus anteriorly to the posterior aspect of the globe and in the orbit between the superior and lateral rectus. It appears as soft, yellowish white, movable subconjunctival mass (Fig. 11.4). It consists of fatty tissue and the surrounding dermis-like connective tissue, hence the name lipodermoid.

Treatment

Surgical excision is required only in the presence of significant cosmetic disfigurement. Usually,

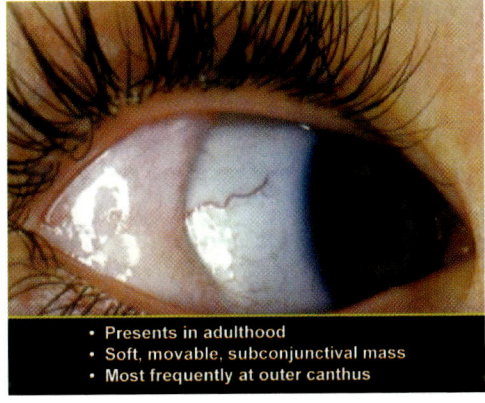

- Presents in adulthood
- Soft, movable, subconjunctival mass
- Most frequently at outer canthus

Fig. 11.4: *Lipodermoid*

surgery is restricted to partial resection of the anterior portion of the tumour. Complete removal is usually not possible. Care must be taken during surgical removal not to damage the extraocular muscles, levator muscle, or lacrimal gland.

COMPLEX CHORISTOMAS

Complex choristomas consist of variable combinations of ectopic tissues such as cartilage, adipose tissue, smooth muscle, and acinar glands.

Clinical features

Clinically, these lesions resemble dermoids and lipodermoids. When acinar elements compose the majority of the tumour, complex choristomas may assume a fleshier, vascularized appearance with raised translucent nodules. These raised nodules have been referred to as ectopic lacrimal glands. Although mild growth may occur, especially during puberty, malignant transformation is rare.

Treatment

As these tumours also tend to invade deeply into the globe, excision is usually avoided. For cosmetic reasons, partial resection of the anterior portion of the tumour may be done.

SINGLE-TISSUE CHORISTOMA

Single-tissue choristomas include choristomas of lacrimal gland, respiratory tissue, and osseous choristomas.

Epibulbar osseous choristoma is the rarest type of choristoma of the eye. These are composed of firm deposits of bone and are most commonly found in the superotemporal conjunctiva (Fig. 11.5) occasionally, the mass is firmly attached to the sclera. As with all choristomas, osseous choristomas are believed to be congenital. Due to its location underneath the eyelid, the mass is usually detected once the child becomes old enough to palpate it. Osseous choristomas are solitary nodules that resemble dermoids. However, they can be differentiated from dermoids clinically because of their location about 5–10 mm posterior to the limbus and their more discrete borders.

Treatment. Usually, excision is performed for cosmetic reasons only.

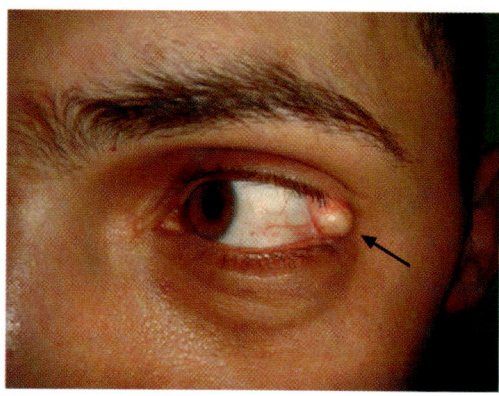

Fig. 11.5: *Epibulbar osseous choristoma*

■ CONGENITAL PIGMENTED LESIONS OF CONJUNCTIVA

Congenital melanocytic pigmented lesions of conjunctiva include:

- Conjunctival naevi
- Conjunctival epithelial melanosis
- Conjunctival subepithelial melanosis.

CONJUNCTIVAL NAEVI

Clinical features

Naevi or congenital moles are common pigmented lesions, usually presenting as grey gelatinous, brown or black, flat or slightly raised nodules on the bulbar conjunctiva, mostly near the limbus (Fig. 11.6). Melanocytic naevi are the most common tumours of the conjunctiva, accounting for 28% of all tumours. These lesions most commonly arise in the bulbar conjunctiva

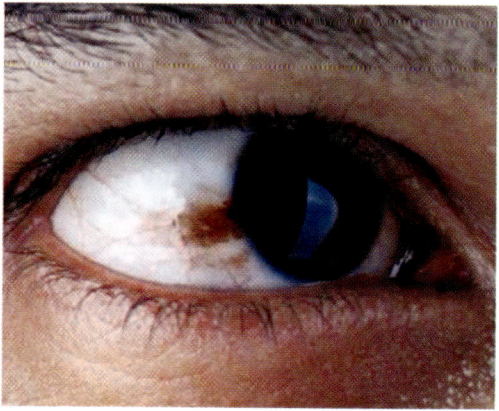

Fig. 11.6: *Conjunctival naevus*

can also occur on caruncle, or plica semilunaris. They usually appear during early childhood and may increase in size at puberty or during pregnancy.

- Naevi present clinically as circumscribed, flat to slightly raised macules or papules.
- Naevi in children often lack pigmentation, but usually acquire pigmentation after puberty. However, up to 30% of naevi remain amelanotic.
- Naevi on the bulbar conjunctiva move freely over the sclera and appear well circumscribed without extension into the cornea. A common and characteristic feature of conjunctival naevi is the presence of intralesional cysts.
- Malignant melanoma will develop in less than 1% of conjunctival naevi. Clinical features particularly suggestive of evolving melanoma include extension into the cornea, attachment to the sclera, and development of multiple "feeder vessels" seen by slit-lamp examination. There are no specific clinical signs that can accurately predict malignant transformation in a conjunctival naevus.

Histopathology

Biopsy is indicated when a pigmented naevus shows clinical characteristics of possible malignancy such as rapid growth, change in shape and/or colour, recurrence after prior biopsy, and unusual location such as the palpebral conjunctiva or the fornix. Histologically, conjunctival melanocytic naevi are classified similarly as in the skin, including junctional, compound, and subepithelial naevi.

- *Junctional naevi.* About 5% of conjunctival naevi are junctional, characterized by nested but sometimes also lentiginous proliferations of type A or type B cells confined to the epithelium. They may show occasional mitotic activity. Most junctional naevi are found in patients in the younger age groups. Therefore, they are believed to be at an early stage in the evolution of compound naevi.
- *Compound naevi* are the most common type of conjunctival naevus, comprising about 70–78% of all naevi. A very characteristic and diagnostically useful feature of conjunctival

naevi is induction of epithelial protrusions into the lamina propria and formation of intralesional epithelial cysts lined by conjunctival epithelium and goblet cells. These cysts are present in 50% of cases. It seems that cyst formation is a function of time, as they are less frequent in early lesions.

- *Subepithelial naevi* are the conjunctival counterpart of the dermal naevus and represent about 9% of all naevi. These are more prevalent in the older age groups and have predominantly type B or C nevomelanocytes in the substantia propria, without an intraepithelial component.

Treatment

Conjunctival naevi do not require treatment if clinically stable.

- *Excision or rebiopsy* is recommended in lesions that change in size or color, recur, or show other clinical features of possible malignancy, or for cosmetic indications.
- Excision should be complete, whatever may be the indication.
- Reexcising of conjunctival naevi showing focal cytologic atypia is of no clinical benefit.

CONJUNCTIVAL EPITHELIAL MELANOSIS

Conjunctival epithelial melanosis (Fig. 11.7) develops in early childhood, and then remains stationary. It is found in 90% of the blacks. The pigmented spot freely moves with the movement of conjunctiva. It has got no malignant potential and hence no treatment is required.

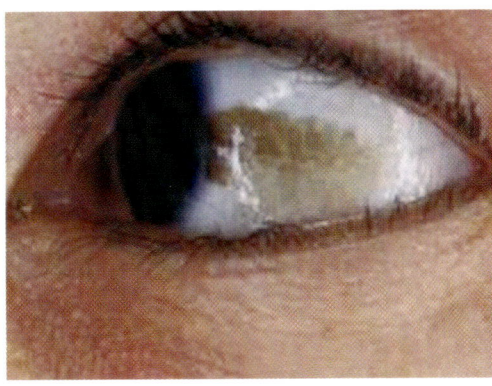

Fig. 11.7: *Conjunctival epithelial melanosis*

CONJUNCTIVAL SUBEPITHELIAL MELANOSIS

Subepithelial melanosis may occur as:

- An isolated anomaly of conjunctiva (congenital melanosis oculi, Fig. 11.8) or
- In association with the ipsilateral hyper-pigmentation of the face (oculodermal melanosis or naevus of Ota).

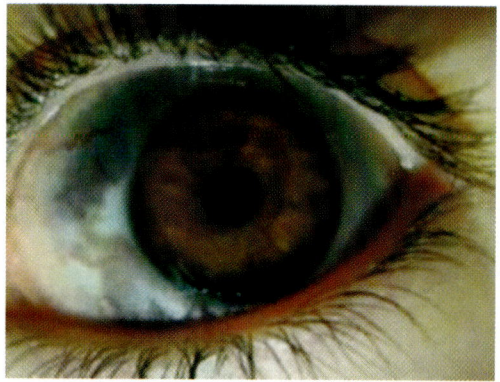

Fig. 11.8: *Congenital melanosis oculi*

NAEVUS OF OTA

Melanosis bulbi associated with ipsilateral hyperpigmentation of the face, is also known as naevus of Ota or oculomucodermal melano-cytosis. This condition was first described by Dr. Ota, a Japanese physician, in 1939, and hence the term naevus of Ota. Naevus of Ota should not be confused with Mongolian spots. Unlike Mongolian spots, naevus of Ota does not disappear with time.

Demography

- *Age.* Naevus of Ota is a skin condition that is normally present at birth, but can occur during adolescence too.
- *Sex.* Both males and females are affected, but females are affected much more than males in a 5:1 ratio.
- *Race.* All racial and ethnic groups are at risk, though naevus of Ota is more frequent among the Japanese population and other Asian races compared to Europeans, Americans, or Africans.

Etiology

- Exact cause of naevus of Ota formation is not known.

- Some researchers believe that it may be formed due to abnormal accumulation of melanocytes (cells producing melanin) in the fetal development stage.
- Even though a congenital presentation is noted, but naevus of Ota is not a hereditary condition.

Clinical features

Naevus of Ota may not present any major signs and symptoms in most cases. The general features of the skin condition include:

- *Skin pigmentation.* It is a benign skin lesion that occurs as a hyperpigmented skin patch. The skin patch may be bluish to bluish-brown in colour.
- *Head and neck region* is mostly affected, especially the face; either one side, or both sides of the face may be involved.
- *Ocular melanosis* is seen in two-thirds of the cases, the sclera of the eye is affected. The condition may be unilateral or bilateral, meaning that either one eye or both eyes may be affected.

Complications

Complications from naevus of Ota may include:

- *Cosmetic concerns* and stress may occur in some cases.
- *Glaucoma* risk is higher if along with skin lesion is present in the eye(s).
- *Malignant melanoma* is known to develop rarely from the site of the lesion, and hence, close follow-up is important and necessary.

Treatment measures for naevus of Ota include:

- *No treatment* is generally required in mild cases. A regularly observation is all that may be required, i.e. a "wait and watch" approach may be followed.
- *Laser surgery* is found to be beneficial in case of cosmetic reasons.
- *Surgical excision.* Naevus of Ota can also be excised through electrocautery surgical procedure.

Prognosis of naevus of Ota is excellent even if no treatment is provided and only periodic observation maintained, since typically it is a benign skin condition.

EPITARSUS

Epitarsus is a peculiar condition which typically occurs as an apron-like fold of conjunctiva attached to the inner surface of the upper lid but occasionally as a bridge of tissue under which a probe may be passed.

Types: Etiologically epitarsus is of two types:
1. *Primary epitarsus,* occurring purely as a congenital anomaly; and
2. *Secondary epitarsus,* following neglected cases of conjunctivitis.

Congenital epitarsus

Epitarsus occurring as a congenital anomaly is rare. The deformity is almost invariably seen in the upper lid, though its bilateral occurrence in the lower lids has also been reported.

Four clinical varieties of epitarsus depending on the extent of the deformity reported are:
- Intrafornix
- Fornix-tarsal
- Fornix-limbal, and
- Interfornix (Fig. 11.9A)

Histopathological examination following resection of the fold shows moderately dense fibrovascular connective tissue covered by stratified squamous epithelium on both the sides (Fig. 11.10).

Treatment. Simple excision gives good cosmetic and functional results (Fig. 11.9B).

CONJUNCTIVAL TELANGIECTASIA

Conjunctival telangiectasia refers to abnormal, dilated conjunctival capillary formation, which usually develop between 3 and 5 years of age.

Clinical features

Conjunctival telangiectasia appears as dot-like, corkscrew, irregular vessels near the limbus (Fig. 11.11).
- Subconjunctival haemorrhage may occur from the telangiectatic vessels.
- Patients usually have no symptoms except the asymptomatic red spots on eye.

Associations include epistaxis and gastrointestinal bleeding.

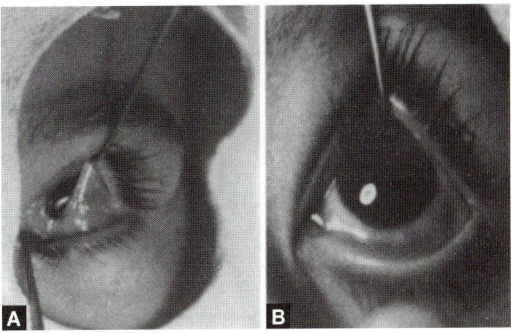

Fig. 11.9: *A, Interfornix epitarsus—the membrane extending from upper fornix to lower fornix; B, After excision of the membrane, underlying eyeball is normal*

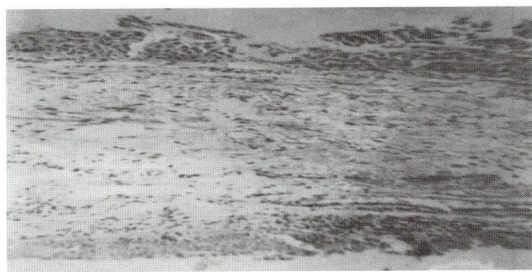

Fig. 11.10: *The mucosa on either side comprises stratified squamous epithelium. Subepithelial soft tissue contains few mononuclear cells. (Haematoxylin and eosin ×120)*

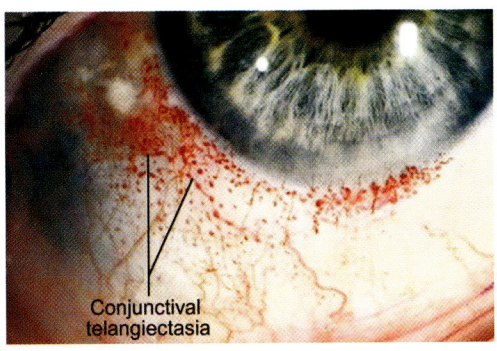

Conjunctival telangiectasia

Fig. 11.11: *Conjunctival telangiectasia appearing as dot-like, corkscrew, irregular vessels near the limbus*

Evaluation should include:
- *Complete ophthalmic history and eye examination* with attention to conjunctiva, cornea, lens, and ophthalmoscopy.
- *CT scan* may need to be considered for multisystem disorders.
- *Medical consultation* to rule out systemic disease.

Differential diagnosis

Differential diagnosis consists of an idiopathic lesion, Osler-Weber-Rendu syndrome, ataxia-telangiectasia, Fabry's disease, and Sturge-Weber syndrome.

Management. No treatment is recommended.

Prognosis. Usually benign; may bleed; depends on etiology.

◼ CONGENITAL ANOMALIES OF CARUNCLE

CONGENITAL BIFURCATED CARUNCLE

It is a rare anomaly which can be seen in the presence of normal plica semilunaris (Fig. 11.12).

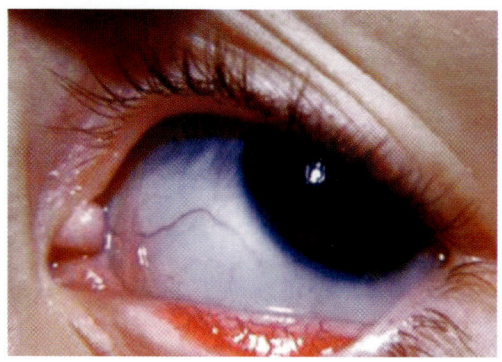

Fig. 11.12: *Congenital bifurcated caruncle*

OTHER CONGENITAL ANOMALIES OF CARUNCLE

Congenital anomalies of caruncle are in general rare. The rare case reports in the literature are on:

- *Dysplastic caruncle*, which may occur isolated or as part of Goldenhar syndrome.
- *Ectopic caruncle*
- *Congenital megacaruncle*
- *Supernumerary caruncles* are always unilateral and unassociated with other ocular abnormalities or Goldenhar syndrome.
- *Caruncular dermoid* has also been reported in the literature. Histopathology of caruncular dermoid shows a keratinizing epidermis-like surface and dense, thick collagen in place of substantia propria.

◼ BIBLIOGRAPHY

1. AB Fuhrmann S, Levine EM, Reh TA. Extra-ocular mesenchyme patterns the optic vesicle during early eye development in the embryonic chick. Development 2000; 127: 4599-4609.
2. AB Sadler TW. Langman's medical embryology (6th ed.). Williams and Wilkins. ISBN 978-0683074932. 1990.
3. Hosseini Hadi S, Beebe David C, Taber Larry A. Mechanical effects of the surface ectoderm on optic vesicle morphogenesis in the chick embryo. *Journal of Biomechanics*. 2014; 47(16): 3837-46. doi:10.1016/j.jbiomech.2014.10.018. PMC 4261019. PMID 25458577.
4. Hosseini Hadi S, Taber Larry A. How mechanical forces shape the developing eye? Progress in Biophysics and Molecular Biology. 2018; 137(16): 25-36. doi:10.1016/j.pbiomolbio.2018.01.004. PMC 6085168. PMID 29432780.
5. Keller AMV. Embryonic Development of the Eye. Retrieved 22 April 2015.
6. LifeMap Science, Inc. Embryonic and Postnatal Development of the Eye. Retrieved 22 April 2015.
7. Ort D, David H. Development of the Eye. Retrieved 22 April 2015.

12
Embryology, Developmental Anomalies and Metabolic Disorders of Cornea

Chapter Outline

EMBRYOLOGY OF CORNEA

GENERAL CONSIDERATIONS

Development of the eyeball can be considered to commence around day 22 when the embryo has eight pairs of somites and is around 2 mm in length. The eyeball and its related structures are derived from the following primordial:

- *Optic vesicle*, an outgrowth from prosencephalon (neuroectodermal structure).

- *Lens placode,* a specialised area of surface ectoderm called the surrounding surface ectoderm.
- *Mesenchyme* surrounding the optic vesicle.
- *Visceral mesoderm* of maxillary process.

Changes in neuroectoderm destined to form ocular tissue

Optic vesicle is formed from the part of neuroectoderm destined to form prosencephalon (Fig. 12.1).

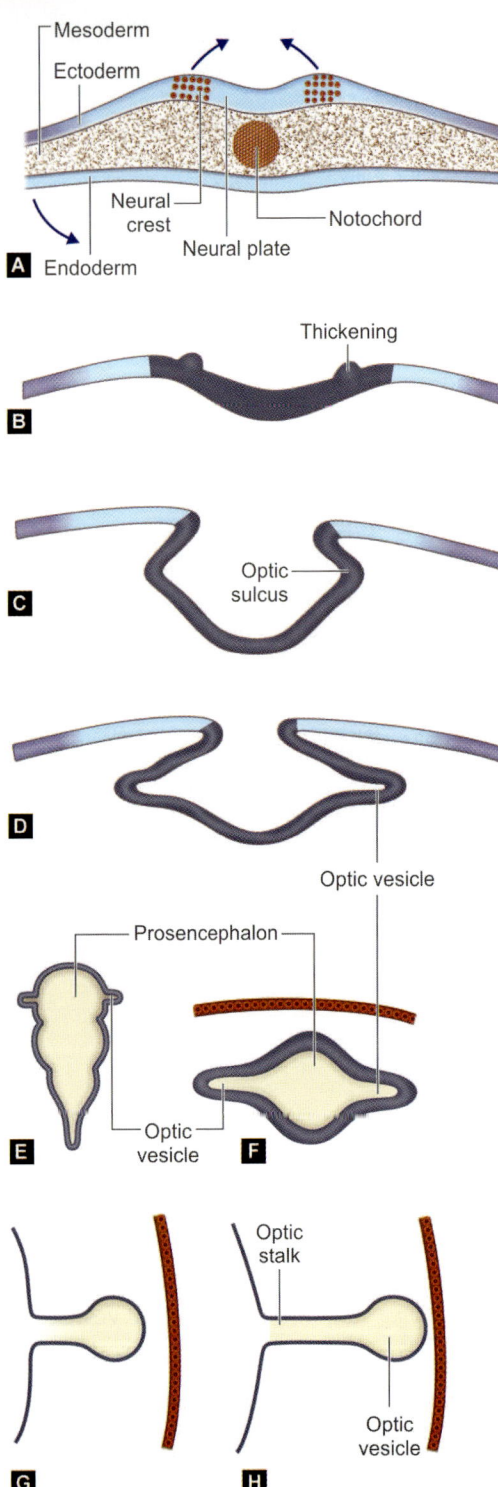

Fig. 12.1A to H: *Formation of the optic vesicle and optic stalk*

Optic cup formation: Optic vesicle is converted into the optic cup by 4 weeks of gestation (Fig. 12.2).

Changes in mesenchyme surrounding optic cup

Changes in the mesenchyme surrounding the optic cup occur and it differentiates to form (Fig. 12.3):

- *Superficial fibrous layer* (corresponding to dura of developing brain), which will ultimately form the cornea and sclera.
- *Deeper vascular layer* (corresponding to pia arachnoid), which will form stroma of uveal tissue.

Changes in surface ectoderm surrounding the developing eyeball

Reduplication of the surface ectoderm above and below the developing cornea occurs during 2nd month of gestation (Fig. 12.4). The reduplicated folds of ectoderm enlarge and their margins meet and fuse with each other. The lids cut off a space called conjunctival space (Fig. 12.4). The ectoderm covering the developing eyeball will form the epithelium of cornea and conjunctiva.

Changes in mesenchymal mass of neural crest origin

Mesenchymal mass of neural crest origin is now considered to give rise to the cornea, iris and anterior chamber angle (rather than that of mesodermal origin as thought originally). Three waves of tissue come forward, between the surface ectoderm and developing lens, from the undifferentiated mesenchymal mass of neural crest cell origin and contribute to formation of structures of anterior segment of eyeball as below (Fig. 12.5):

- *First wave* differentiates into primordial corneal endothelium by 8th week and subsequently produces Descemet's membrane as well.
- *Second wave* grows between the corneal epithelium and endothelium and produces corneal stroma.
- *Third wave* insinuates between the developing cornea and lens and gives rise to the pupillary membrane and stroma of iris.

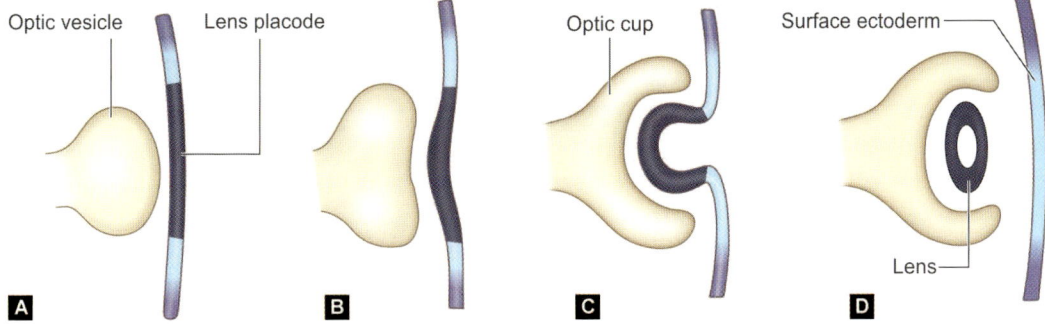

Fig. 12.2A to D: *Formation of lens vesicle and optic cup*

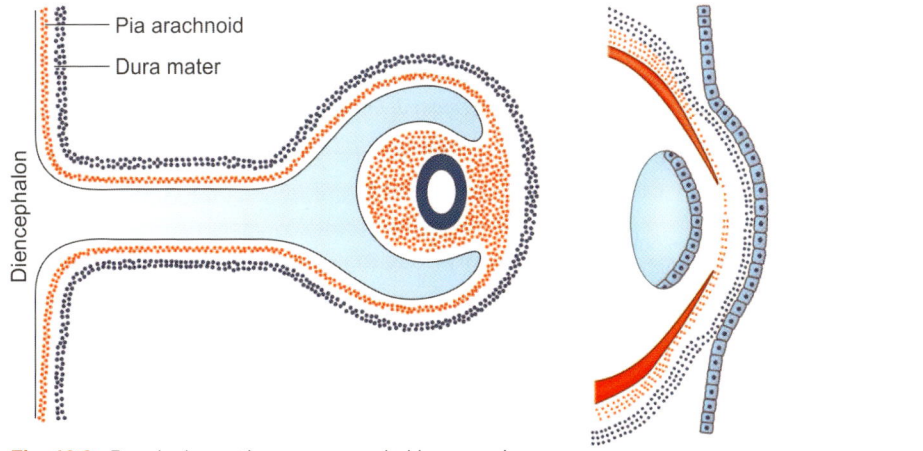

Fig. 12.3: *Developing optic cup surrounded by mesoderm*

DEVELOPMENT OF VARIOUS LAYERS OF CORNEA

Development of various layers of cornea is summarized below (Figs 12.5 to 12.7):

Epithelium is formed from the surface ectoderm. At about 40 days of gestation (embryo 17–18 mm), corneal epithelium consists of a superficial squamous cell layer and a basal cuboidal epithelial cell layer (Fig. 12.7A). By 3 months of gestation, epithelium is 3-layered (Fig. 12.7D) and by the time the eyelids open at 5–6 months of gestation, the corneal epithelium attains an almost adult appearance.

Endothelium and Descemet's membrane are formed from mesenchymal cells derived from neural crest, which are situated at the margins of the rim of the optic cup. These cells migrate into the developing eye beneath the basal lamina of the corneal epithelium and form the primordial corneal endothelium.

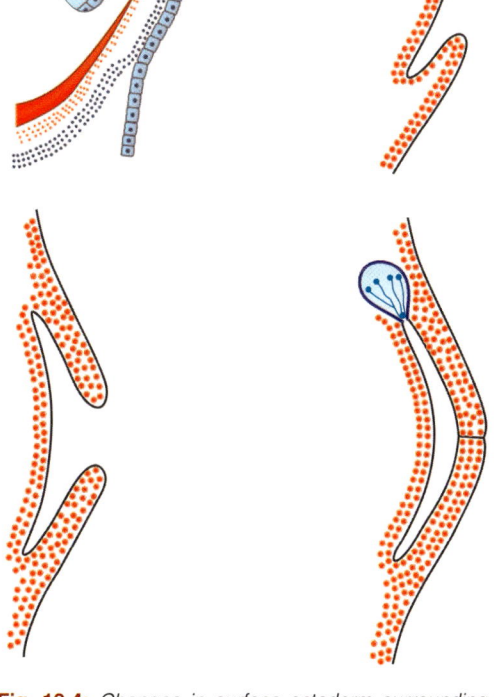

Fig. 12.4: *Changes in surface ectoderm surrounding the eyeball*

- At about 40 days of gestation (17–18 mm embryo), the corneal endothelium consists of two layers of flattened cells (Fig. 12.7A).

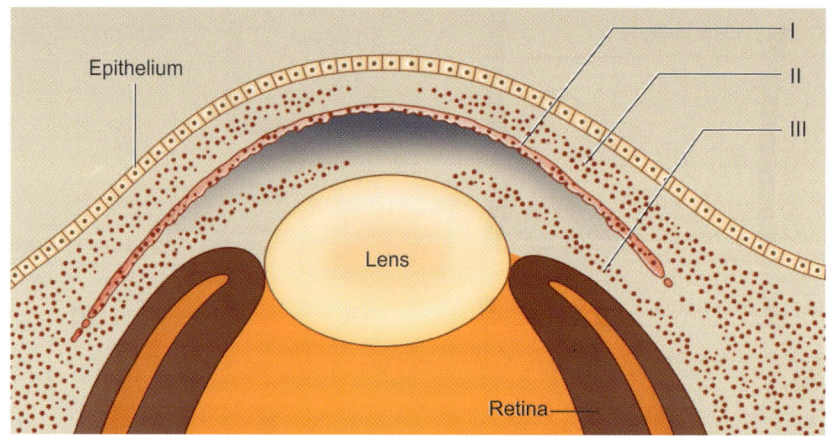

Fig. 12.5: *Three successive waves of ingrowth of neural crest cells contributing to formation of structures of anterior segment. I, First wave forms the corneal endothelium; II, Second wave forms corneal stroma; III, Third wave forms the iris and part of the pupillary membrane (from: Tripathi BJ, Tripathi RC, Wisdom J. Embryology of the anterior segment. Elds MB, Krupin T, eds. The Glaucomas. 2nd ed. St Louis: Mosby: 1996)*

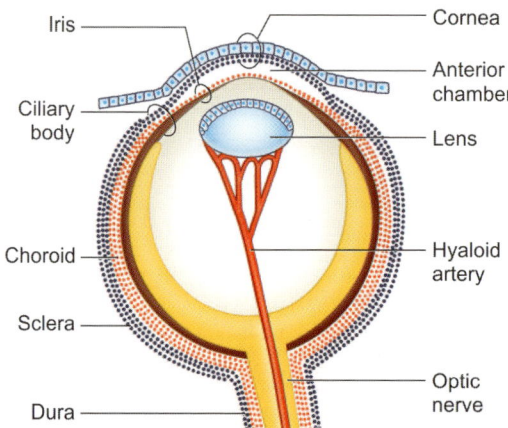

Fig. 12.6: *Derivation of various structures of the eyeball*

- By the third month (embryo 63 mm), the endothelium in the central region of cornea becomes a single layer of flattened cells that rest on their interrupted basal lamina—the future Descemet's membrane (Fig. 12.7D).
- Apices of the endothelial cells are joined by zonulae occludentes in the middle of the 4th month, which corresponds to the production of aqueous humour by the ciliary processes.
- At the 6th month of gestation, Descemet's membrane is demarcated clearly.

Stroma and Bowman's layers are derived from the mesenchymal cells that insinuate between the surface ectoderm and the developing lens.

- *Primary corneal storma* is secreted by basal layer of epithelium and consists of fine filaments, amorphous material and only a few collagen fibrils.
- *At about 22–24 mm stage* (7th–8th week), the mesenchymal cells migrate into the primary corneal stroma (between epithelium and endothelium) and contribute to the further development of corneal stroma (Fig. 12.7B).
- *The invading mesenchymal cells differentiate into stromal fibroblasts* or keratocytes that actively secrete the type I collagen fibrils and the matrix of mature (secondary) corneal stroma.
- *Bowman's layer* starts forming by condensation of most superficial acellular part of corneal stroma after 4 months of gestation and is fully developed at birth.
- *By 5 months*, corneal nerves are present. It is important to note that the fetal cornea is very hydrated compared to the adult form and is, therefore, translucent rather than transparent.

CONGENITAL DISORDERS OF CORNEA

ANOMALIES OF SIZE, SHAPE AND CURVATURE OF CORNEA

ABSENCE OF CORNEA

Absence of cornea *per se* is not reported so strictly speaking as a clinical entity the absence of cornea

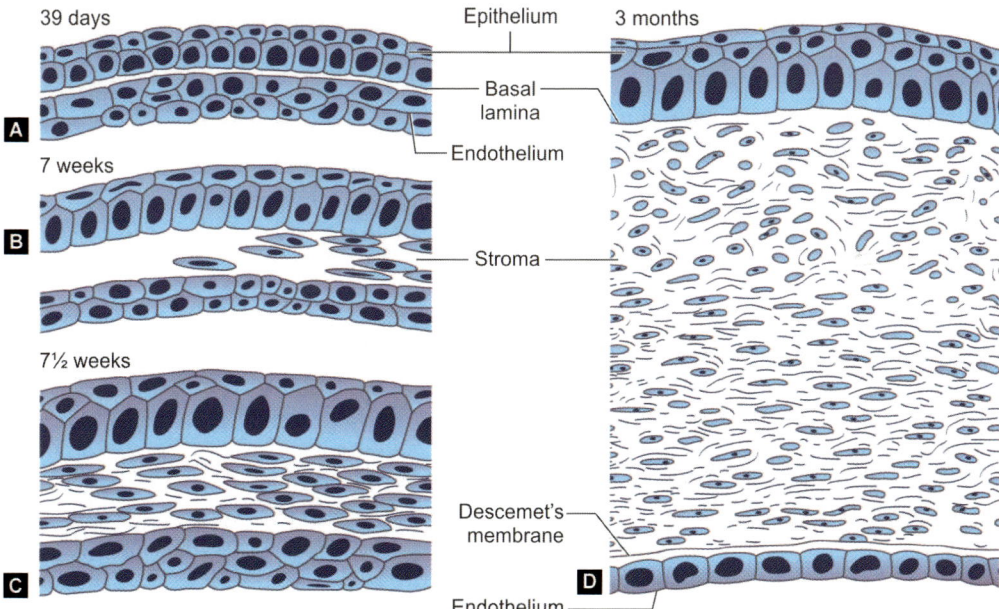

Fig. 12.7: *Development of the cornea in the central region. A, At day 39,2-layered epithelium rests on the basal lamina and is separated from the endothelium (2–3 layers) by a narrow acellular space; B, At week 7, mesenchymal cells from the peiphery migrate into the space between the epithelium; C, Mesenchymal cells (future keratocytes) are arranged in 4–5 incomplete layers by 7½ weeks; a few collagen fibrils are present among the cells; D, By 3 months, the epithelium has 2–3 layers of cells, and the stroma has about 25–30 layers of keratocytes that are arranged more regularly in the posterior half*

does not exist. However, it may be a component of the generalized developmental anomalies of the anterior segment or whole of the eyeball. Some of such anomalies are listed below:

Anophthalmos, i.e. developmentally absence of eyeball forms the condition of extreme absence of cornea and other ocular structures (Fig. 12.8).

Cryptophthalmos. True cryptophthalmos (ablepharon) is a rare anomaly in which lids fails to develop and the exposed cornea undergoes metaplasia to skin and so appears to be absent.

Pseudocryptophthalmos (total ankyloble-pharon) in which skin passes continuously from the eyebrow to the cheek hiding the underlying eyeball (Fig. 12.9).

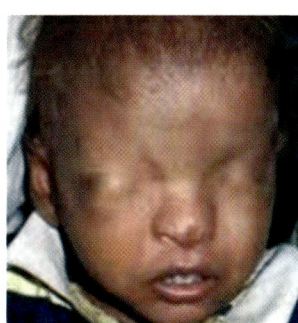

Fig. 12.9: *Pseudocryptophthalmos*

- *Main differentiating feature* of true crypto-phthalmos from pseudocryptopthalmos is absence of eyebrow and eyelashes which are present in the later.
- *Association of cryptophthalmos* with other anomalies such as syndactyly and genito-urinary anomalies forms the so-called *Faser syndrome*.

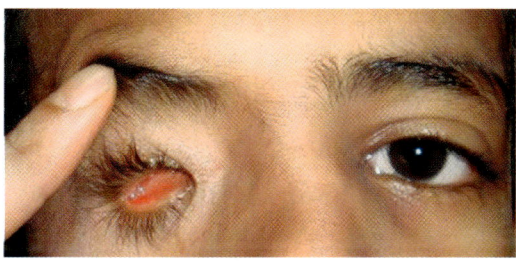

Fig. 12.8: *Congenital anophthalmos*

Corneal dermoid of extreme level also looks as if there is no cornea (*see* page 177).

Rudimentary cystic eyeball is another examples of extreme level developmental anomaly in which anterior segment is absent.

MICROCORNEA

In microcornea horizontal diameter of cornea is less than 10 mm since childhood and same is maintained in adulthood (Fig. 12.10).

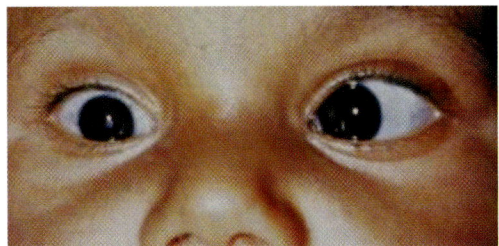

Fig. 12.10: *Microcornea*

Heredity

Most of the cases of microcornea are sporadic, although autosomal recessive and autosomal dominant pedigrees have been reported.

Clinical profile

Microcornea may occur *per se* or in association with microphthalmos, nanophthalmos and other congenital malformation of ocular structures.

Isolated microcornea

Isolated microcornea is a comparatively rare anomaly. In isolated microcornea, as the remainder of the ocular structures are normal in size, angle-closure glaucoma may occur as the lens enlarges.

Microcornea associated with other ocular and systemic anomalies

Ocular and systemic anomalies associated with microcornea are summarised in Table 12.1.

Microphthalmos

Microphthalmos refers to developmentally abnormal small eyeball. Anomalies associated with small eyeball includes coloboma of iris, retina, choroid and even optic disc.

Table 12.1: *Abnormalities associated with microcornea*

Ocular
Hyperopia (other refractive errors possible)
Cornea plana
Corneal leukoma
Mesodermal remnants in angle
Aniridia
Uveal coloboma
Corectopia
Persistent pupillary membrane
Congenital cataract
Microphakia
Open-angle glaucoma
Angle-closure glaucoma
Congenital glaucoma
Retinopathy of prematurity
Microblepharon
Small orbit

Systemic
Weill-Marchesani syndrome or similar habitus
Ehlers-Danlos syndrome
Meyer-Schwickerath and Weyers syndrome
Rieger's syndrome
Partial deletion of long arm of chromosome 18
Nance-Horan (X-linked cataract-dental) syndrome

Syndromes with microphthalmos as a component include:

- *MIDAS syndrome* refers to micropthalmos associated with dermal aplasia and sclerocornea.
- *MICRO syndrome of microcornea* congenital cataract, mental retardations, retinal dystrophy, optic atrophy, hypogenitalism and microcephaly.

Treatment

- *Correction of refractive error*, usually hyperopia resulting from the flat cornea.
- *Treatment of associated disorders* such as cataract and glaucoma.

MEGALOCORNEA

Definition

Horizontal diameter of cornea at birth is about 10 mm and the adult size of about 11.7 mm is attained by the age of 2 years. Megalocornea is labelled when the horizontal diameter of cornea is of adult size at birth or 13 mm or greater after the age of 2 years (Fig. 12.11).

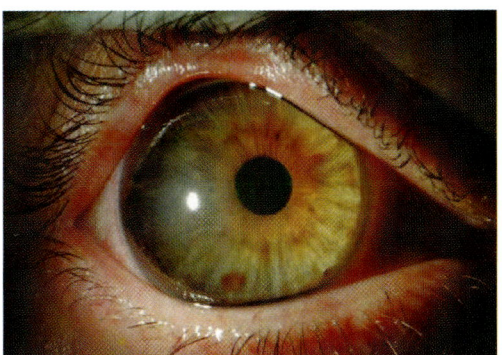

Fig. 12.11: *Congenital megalocornea*

Pathogenesis

Megalocornea is suggested to be resulting from the defective growth of optic cup, which leaves a larger space for development of the cornea.

Heredity

Two forms of megalocornea are reported:
- *X-linked recessive megalocornea* is more common and is associated with other anomalies also. The genetic locus for X-linked megalocornea appears to be in the region of Xq21–q22.6.
- *Autosomal dominant megalocornea* is less common and is not associated with other ocular anomalies.

Clinical features

Enlarged cornea may occur as an isolated anomaly (*simple megalocornea*) or in association with enlargement of the ciliary ring and lens (*anterior megalophthalmos*).

Simple megalocornea

Simple megalocornea is usually bilateral symmetric conditions in which cornea is usually clear with normal thickness and vision. The condition is not progressive.

Megalocornea associated with other ocular and systemic anomalies

- *Associated ocular anomalies*, seen in X-linked cases include iris transillumination, pigment dispersion, lens subluxation, arcus, and central crocodile shagreen.
- *Other ocular anomalies* associated with megalocornea include congenital miosis, ectopia lentis, and ectopia pupillae.
- *Ocular and systemic anomalies* associated with megalocornea are listed in Table 12.2.

Differential diagnosis

1. Buphthalmos. In this condition, IOP is raised and the eyeball is enlarged as a whole. The enlarged cornea is usually associated with central or peripheral clouding and Descemet's tears (Haab's striae).

2. Keratoglobus. In this condition, there is thinning and excessive protrusion of cornea, which seems enlarged; but its diameter is usually normal.

3. Macrophthalmos. In it the enlarged cornea is part of an overall enlarged eyeball (axial length often around 30 mm), which is not associated with glaucoma. It is an autosomal recessive condition. It is associated with juvenile cataract, and high myopia.

Treament

- *Correction of refractive error*, i.e. associated myopia.

Table 12.2: *Abnormalities associated with megalocornea*
Ocular
Myopia
Astigmatism
Arcus juvenilis
Krukenberg's spindle
Mosaic corneal dystrophy
Hypoplasia of iris stroma and pigment epithelium
Miosis (hypoplasia of iris dilator)
Prominent iris processes
Pigmentation of trabecular meshwork
Open-angle glaucoma
Congenital glaucoma (rare)
Cataract (usually posterior subcapsular)
Ectopia lentis
Systemic
Marfan's syndrome
Craniosynostosis
Lamellar ichthyosis
Mental retardation (with recessive megalocornea)

- *Juvenile cataract*, when associated may be surgically treated.

CORNEA PLANA

This is a rare anomaly in which bilaterally cornea is comparatively flat since birth. It is more often seen in association with microcornea or sclerocornea.

- *Limbus* in cornea plana is usually indistinct, whereas it is typically well defined in simple microcornea. Cornea plana usually results in hyperopia and marked astigmatic refractive error.
- *Anterior chamber* is shallow and angle closure glaucoma may be associated.
- *Ocular and systemic anomalies* associated with corneal plana are listed in Table 12.3.

Table 12.3: *Abnormalities associated with cornea plana*
Ocular
Hyperopia (other refractive errors possible)
Blue sclera
Sclerocornea
Microcornea
Arcus juvenilis
Nonspecific corneal opacities
Anterior segment dysgenesis
Absence of normal iris markings and collarette
Uveal and retinal coloboma
Aniridia
Congenital cataract
Ectopia lentis
Retinal and macular aplasia
Angle-closure glaucoma
Open-angle glaucoma
Pseudoptosis (Streiff's sign)
Systemic
Osteogenesis imperfecta
Hurler's syndrome (mucopolysaccharidosis I–H)
Maroteaux-Lamy syndrome (mucopolysaccharidosis VI) a Trisomy 13

CONGENITAL CORNEAL ECTASIA

Congenital corneal ectasia is characterized by thinning and bulging of cornea. It presumably results as a consequences of the developmental abnormalities in the migration of mesenchyme.

It is typically unilateral condition and is often associated with developmental defects of the iris.

Congenital anterior staphyloma with associated corneal ectasia is also reported in the literature. It may occur as:

- An association of Peter's anomaly, or
- A result of infectious or inflammatory corneal thinning *in utero*.

ANOMALIES OF CORNEAL STRUCTURE AND TRANSPARENCY

Some common congenital anomalies in which normal corneal structure and/or transparency is disturbed, are described briefly.

ANTERIOR EMBRYOTOXON

Anterior embryotoxon is characterized by (Fig. 12.12):

- *Congenital broad limbus superiorly*, i.e. superiorly transition between the cornea and sclera is broader.
- *Anterior segment* is otherwise normal in such cases.
- *Genetics*. Most cases are sporadic in occurrence but autosomal dominant as well as autosomal recessive cases are reported.

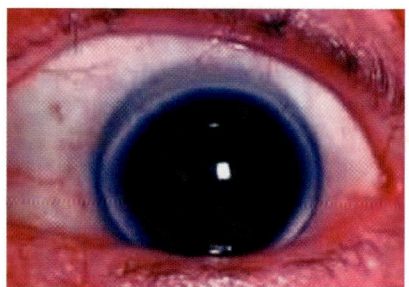

Fig. 12.12: *Anterior embryotoxon*

POSTERIOR EMBRYOTOXON

- Posterior embrytoxon refers to thickening and anterior displacement of Schwalbe's line, which is most marked temporally on slit lamp examination (Fig. 12.13).
- It is the most common congenital anomaly of the eye (seen in about 24% of population).
- It has no functional significance.

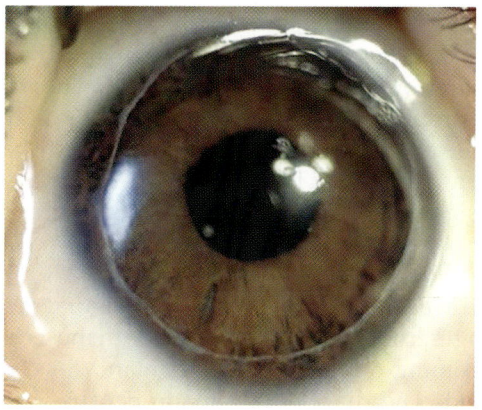

Fig. 12.13: *Posterior embryotoxon*

AXENFELD-RIEGER SYNDROME

Eponyms commonly encountered in scientific literature regarding developmental anomalies of anterior segment of eye includes:

- *Axenfeld's anomaly.* Limited to peripheral anterior segment defects.
- *Rieger's anomaly.* Peripheral abnormalities with additional changes in the iris.
- *Rieger's syndrome.* Ocular anomalies plus systemic developmental defects.

The similarity of anterior chamber angle abnormalities in Axenfeld's anomaly and Rieger's anomaly and syndrome points towards the fact that these three arbitrary categories represent a spectrum of developmental disorders. Hence, nowadays, Axenfeld-Rieger syndrome (A-R syndrome), is used for all clinical variations within this spectrum of developmental disorders.

General features

All patients with the A-R syndrome share the same general features:

- Bilateral, developmental disorder of the eyes
- Frequent family history (autosomal dominant mode of inheritance)
- No sex predilection
- Frequent systemic developmental defects
- High incidence of associated glaucoma.

Ocular features

Ocular defects in the A-R syndrome are typically bilateral. The structures most commonly involved are the peripheral cornea, anterior chamber angle, and iris.

Cornea. The characteristic abnormality is a white line on the posterior cornea near the limbus which corresponds to an anteriorly displaced Schwalbe's line. The cornea is otherwise normal in the typical case of the A-R syndrome, with the exception of occasional patients with variation in the overall size. The corneal endothelium is typically normal.

Anterior chamber angle. Gonioscopic examination reveals a prominent Schwalbe's line, although there is considerable variation among patients in the extent to which Schwalbe's line is enlarged and anteriorly displaced. Tissue strands bridge the anterior chamber angle from the peripheral iris to the prominent ridge (Fig. 12.14). These iridocorneal adhesions are typically similar in colour and texture to the adjacent iris. The strands range in size from thread-like structures to broad bands extending for a clock hour or more of the circumference. Iris abnormalities include peripheral abnormalities, mild stromal thinning (Fig. 12.15) or in some cases, marked atrophy with hole formation,

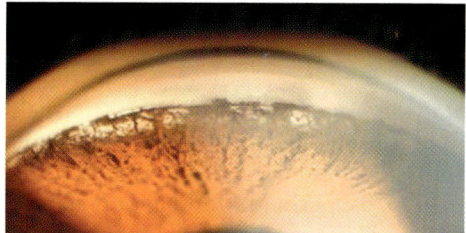

Fig. 12.14: *Gonioscopy shows dense iridocorneal strands*

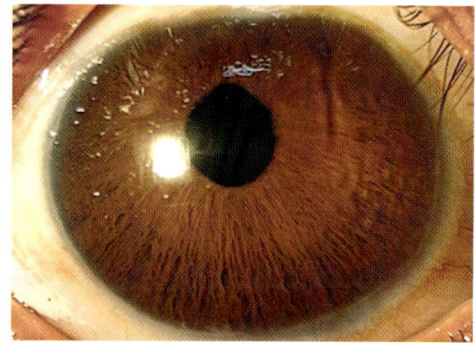

Fig. 12.15: *AR syndrome, note the posterior embryotoxon, anterior stromal iris atrophy and up-drawn pupil*

corectopia, and ectropion uveae. In cases with corectopia, the pupil is usually displaced towards a prominent peripheral tissue strand. The atrophy and hole formation occur in the quadrant away from the direction of the corectopia. The progressive changes usually consist of displacement or distortion of the pupil and occasional thinning or hole formation of the iris. In some cases, these progressive iris changes may be confused with those of iridocorneal endothelial (ICE) syndrome.

Glaucoma. Approximately half of the patients with the A-R syndrome develop glaucoma. The glaucoma may manifest during infancy, although it more commonly appears in childhood or young adulthood. The extent of the iris defects and iridocorneal strands does not correlate precisely with the presence or severity of the glaucoma.

Other ocular abnormalities include strabismus, limbal dermoids, corneal pannus, cataracts, congenital ectropion uveae, congenital pupillary-iris-lens membrane, peripheral spoke-like transillumination defects of the iris, retinal detachment, macular degeneration, chorioretinal colobomas, choroidal hypoplasia, and hypoplasia of the optic nerve heads.

Systemic features

Dental abnormalities. The dental abnormalities include a reduction in crown size (i.e. microdontia), a decreased but evenly spaced number of teeth (i.e. hypodontia), and a focal absence of teeth (i.e. oligodontia or anodontia) The teeth most commonly missing are anterior maxillary and primary and permanent central incisors.

Facial anomalies. These include maxillary hypoplasia with flattening of the midface and a receding upper lip and prominent lower lip, especially in association with dental hypoplasia. Hypertelorism, telecanthus, a broad flat nose, micrognathia, and mandibular prognathism have also been described. Other abnormalities reported in association with the A-R syndrome include redundant periumbilical skin and hypospadias, oculocutaneous albinism, heart defects, middle ear deafness, mental deficiency, and a variety of neurologic, dermatologic, and skeletal disorders.

Genetic linkage

Three chromosomal loci have been linked to A-R syndrome and related phenotypes. These loci are on chromosomes 4q25, 6p25, and 13q14. The genes at chromosomes 4q25 and 6p25 have been identified as PITX2 and FOXC1 (formerly designated FKHL7), respectively.

Diagnosis

The age at which the A-R syndrome is diagnosed ranges from birth to adulthood, with most cases becoming recognized during infancy or childhood. The diagnosis is made because of an abnormal iris or other ocular anomaly, signs of congenital glaucoma, reduced vision in older patients, or systemic anomalies.

Differential diagnosis

- *Iridocorneal endothelial syndrome.* Clinical features that distinguish the iridocorneal endothelial (ICE) syndrome from A-R syndrome include corneal endothelial abnormalities, unilaterality, absence of family history, and onset in young adulthood. The membrane in the A-R syndrome represents a primordial remnant that of the ICE syndrome results from proliferation of the abnormal corneal endothelium.
- *Posterior polymorphous dystrophy.* Differentiation can be made on the basis of the typical corneal endothelial abnormality.
- *Peters' anomaly.* The spectrum of disorders that constitutes Peters' anomaly involves the central portion of the cornea, iris, and lens.
- *Iridogoniodysgenesis.* Congenital hypoplasia of the iris.
- *Ectopia lentis et pupillae.* The corectopia in this disorder may resemble that of the A-R syndrome, but the absence of anterior chamber angle defects is a differential feature.
- *Oculodentodigital dysplasia*, and
- *Aniridia*

Management

Intraocular pressure elevation most often develops between childhood and early adulthood, but it may appear in infancy. With the exception of infantile cases, medical therapy should usually be initiated before surgical intervention is recommended. Trabeculectomy is the surgical procedure of choice for most patients with glaucoma associated with the A-R syndrome. These patients must be followed throughout their lives to detect glaucoma. In infants and in cases refractory to medication and trabeculectomy, glaucoma implant surgery and cycloablation remain options for treatment.

PETERS' ANOMALY

General features

- The condition is present at birth and is usually bilateral.
- Peters' anomaly can be caused by mutation in the PAX6 gene, the PITX2 gene, the CYP1B1 gene, or the FOXC1 gene. Most cases are sporadic, although there are reported cases of autosomal recessive inheritance.
- Peters' anomaly is considered to be a morphologic finding rather than a distinct entity because of the varied genetic and nongenetic patterns and the spectrum of ocular and systemic abnormalities.

Ocular features

The disorder has been subdivided into three groups, each of which may have more than one pathogenetic mechanism.

- *Peters' anomaly not associated with kerato-lenticular contact or cataract*
  The defect in Descemet's membrane may represent primary failure of corneal endothelial development.
- *Peters' anomaly associated with kerato-lenticular contact or cataract*
  This variation involves normal development of lens, which gets secondarily pushed forward against the cornea causing the loss of Descemet's membrane. Some cases may result from incomplete separation of the lens vesicle from surface ectoderm.
- *Peters' anomaly associated with Axenfeld-Rieger syndrome*

Corneal defects

Hallmark of Peters' anomaly is a central defect in Descemet's membrane and corneal endothelium with thinning and opacification of the corresponding area of corneal stroma.

Bowman's layer may also be absent centrally. Iris adhesions may extend to the borders of this corneal defect.

Glaucoma

Approximately one-half of the patients with Peters' anomaly develop glaucoma, which is frequently present at birth. The mechanism of the glaucoma is uncertain, because the anterior chamber angle is usually grossly normal by clinical examination.

Differential diagnosis

- Causes of central corneal opacities: Congenital glaucoma, birth trauma, the mucopolysaccharidoses, and congenital hereditary endothelial dystrophy.
- Posterior keratoconus
- Congenital corneal leukomas and staphylomas.

Management

- *Trabeculotomy or trabeculectomy* may be sufficient in milder cases where there is adequate anterior chamber depth.
- *Drainage implant device or cyclodestructive surgery* is often needed in refractory or more severely affected cases.
- *Penetrating keratoplasty* is also frequently necessary, although the results are typically poor, which probably is caused in part by the associated glaucoma and its surgical treatment.

CONGENITAL CORNEAL OPACITY

Corneal opacity, i.e. scarring of corneal stroma, is often an acquired condition but has been reported to occur congenitally in isolation and also in association with Lowe's syndrome, Axenfeld's anomaly, Rieger's syndrome and Peters' anomaly.

SCLEROCORNEA

Sclerocornea refers to sclera-like cloudy cornea, which may be peripheral or diffuse.
- Conditions are usually bilateral
- Sclerocornea is sporadic in 50% of cases and autosomal recessive or dominant in rest of the 50% of cases.

- Cornea plana and horizontal oval cornea are associations of sclerocornea.

Ocular and systemic anomalies associated with sclerocornea are listed in Table 12.4.

Table 12.4: *Abnormalities associated with sclerocornea*

Ocular

High refractive errors
Blue sclera
Cornea plana
Horizontally oval cornea
Aniridia
Anterior segment dysgenesis
Uveal and retinal coloboma
Cataract
Open-angle glaucoma
Angle-closure glaucoma
Pseudoptosis
Microphthalmos

Systemic

Anomalies of skull and facial bones
Deformities of the external ear
Deafness
Polydactyly
Cerebellar dysfunction
Testicular abnormalities
Hereditary osteo-onychodysplasia
Osteogenesis imperfecta
Others (numerous and variable)

CORNEAL DERMOID

Dermoids usually occur at inferotemporal limbus and are round, dome shaped, and pink to white to yellow in colour. Rarely the dermoids may involve large area of cornea, the entire limbus, the entire cornea, or even the interior of the eye.

Corneal dermoid is a type of choriostoma, for details *see* page 163.

Associations of epibulbar dermoids are listed in Table 12.5.

Goldenhar's syndrome

Epibulbar dermoid is common in Goldenhar syndrome which comprises *triad of*:
- Epibulbar usually limbal dermoid

Table 12.5: *Systemic malformation syndromes sometimes associated with epibulbar dermoids*

Branchial arch syndromes

Goldenhar's syndrome (oculoauriculovertebral dysplasia)
Franceschetti (or Treacher Collins) syndrome (mandibulofacial dysostosis)

Congenital neurocutaneous syndromes

Bloch-Sulzberger syndrome (incontinentia pigmenti)
Encephalocraniocutaneous lipomatosis
Linear sebaceous naevus syndrome

Chromosomal abnormalities

Cri-du-chat syndrome (deletion of short arm of chromosome 5)

- Abnormalities of ear such as auricular appendages or pretarsal fistula, and
- Anomalies of vertebral coloumns.

Other ocular and systemic anomalies which may be associated with Goldenhar syndrome are listed in Table 12.6.

Table 12.6: *Abnormalities associated with Goldenhar's syndrome*

Ocular

Coloboma of upper eyelid
Uveal coloboma
Aniridia
Miliary retinal aneurysms
Duane's retraction strabismus syndrome
Lacrimal stenosis
Microphthalmos

Systemic

Mandibular and malar hypoplasia
Hemifacial microsomia
Other facial and oral abnormalities
Cardiac abnormalities
Renal abnormalities
Gastrointestinal abnormalities
Genitourinary abnormalities
Mental retardation

DIFFERENTIAL DIAGNOSIS OF NEONATAL CLOUDY CORNEA

The acronym 'STUMPED' helps to remember the common conditions to be included in differential diagnosis of neonatal cloudy cornea. The conditions are as follows:

- Sclerocornea
- Tears in Descemet's membrane
- Ulcer
- Metabolic conditions
- Posterior corneal defect
- Endothelial dystrophy
- Dermoid

Note. Most of the causes of neonatal cloudy cornea have been described elsewhere.

METABOLIC DISORDERS INVOLVING CORNEA

INTRODUCTION

Some of the inherited metabolic diseases which may be associated with cloudy cornea and/or other ocular manifestations described briefly here can be classified as below:

Disorders of Carbohydrate Metabolism
- Mucopolysaccharidoses
- Diabetes mellitus

Disorders of Lipid Metabolism and Storage
- Hyperlipoproteinemias
- Hypolipoproteinemias
- Sphingolipidoses
- Mucolipidoses

Disorders of Protein and Amino Acid Metabolism
- Cystinosis
- Tyrosinemia
- Alkaptonuria
- Amyloidosis

Noninflammatory Disorders of Connective Tissue
- Ehlers-Danlos syndrome
- Marfan syndrome

Disorders of Nucleotide Metabolism
- Gout
- Porphyria

Disorders of Mineral Metabolism
- Wilson disease
- Hypercalcemia
- Hemochromatosis

DISORDERS OF CARBOHYDRATE METABOLISM

MUCOPOLYSACCHARIDOSES

Mucopolysaccharidoses (MPSes) refers to a group of inherited lysosomal storage diseases in which mucopolysaccharides or glycosaminoglycans and progressively accumulated in lysosomes. These are characterized by corneal clouding and other ocular and systemic manifestations.

PATHOGENESIS AND TYPES OF MPS

Pathogenesis

Inherited disorder. All the MPSes are autosomal recessive, with the exception of Hunter syndrome, which is X-linked.

Gene locus is shown in Table 12.7.

Enzyme deficiency responsible for each type of MPS is given below and summarised in Table 12.7.

Metabolite deposited in each type of MPS is shown in Table 12.7.

Types of mucopolysaccharidoses

Following MPS syndromes have been described. The enzyme deficient in each type is mentioned in parentheses:

MPS I syndrome includes three disorders:
- Hurler syndrome (MPS I-H) [α-L-iduronidase]
- Scheie syndrome (MPS I-S) [α-L-iduronidase (partial)]
- Hurler-Scheie syndrome (MPS I-H/S)

MPS II syndrome includes:
- Hunter A (MPS IIA) due to deficiency of iduronate sulfate, and
- Hunter B (MPS IIB)

MPS III syndrome includes:
- Sanfilippo A (IIIA) [heparan sulfate sulfamidase]
- Sanfilippo B [N-acetyl-α-D-glucosaminidase]
- Sanfilippo C [acetyl CoA alphaglucosaminidase]
- Sanfilippo D [N-acetylglucosamine-6-sulphatase]

MPS IV syndrome includes:
- Morquio [N-acetyl-galactosamine sulfatase]

MPS VI syndrome includes:
- Maroteaux-Lamy A (MPS VIA) (severe phenotype) [Arylsulfatase B]
- Maroteaux-Lamy B (MPS VIB) (mild phenotype) [Arylsulfatase B]

MPS VII syndrome includes:
- Sly's syndrome due to β-*glucuronidase* *deficiency*

MPS IX syndrome includes:
- Natowicz syndrome due to hyaluronidase deficiency.

CLINICAL FEATURES

Most common type is MPS III followed by MPS I and MPS II.

Ocular and systemic features of different types of MPS are listed in Tables 12.7 to 12.9. Figure 12.16 depicts clinical features of MPS I (Hurler's disease).

Ocular features include:
1. *Corneal clouding* occurs due to accumulation of incompletely degraded glycosaminoglycans (GAGs) within the keratocytes, corneal epithelium, corneal endothelium, and extracellular matrix of cornea. Corneal clouding which occurs within a few days to months of birth, slowly progresses from periphery to the centre involving the whole cornea.
2. *Retinopathy* characterized by degeneration of retinal pigment epithelium.
3. *Optic atrophy* is also a consistant feature.
4. *Glaucoma* has also been reported in some patients due to deposition of mucopolysaccharide laden macrophage in the trabecular meshwork.

Systemic features are summarised in Table 12.8.

DIAGNOSIS

Clinical diagnosis is supported by laboratory diagnosis.

Laboratory diagnosis is made by following tests.
- *Urine analysis* for presence of GAGs

- *Specific enzyme assay* from plasma or leucocyte
- *Conjunctval biopsy* is confirmatory, however, it is rarely needed.

MANAGEMENT

- *Enzyme replacement therapy* is being used in many MPS syndromes.
- *Donor stem cell bone marrow transplantation* is reported to be successful in about one-third of cases.
- *Gene transfer therapy* is under investigations.
- *Keratoplasty* may be considered for cloudy cornea, provided retina and optic nerve are not damaged.
- *Deep anterior lamellar keratoplasty* has been recommended over penetrating keratoplasty due to decreased risk of rejection. However, re-opacification may develop as early as 1 year after surgery.

◼ DIABETIC KERATOPATHY

Diabetes mellitus, the most common disorder of carbohydrates metabolism, involves almost all parts of eyeball, of course diabetic retinopathy and diabetic cataract being more conspicuous. Diabetic keratopathy is not an uncommon manifestation.

PATHOGENESIS

Various factors implicated in diabetic keratopathy are:
- *Ultrastructural abnormalities of the basement membrane complex* contribute to defective epithelial stromal adhesions.
- *Sorbital accumulation* from increased aldose reductase activity also play role in diabetic keratopathy.
- *Diabetic neuropathy*, in the form of irregularities in the basal lamina of Schwann cells and axonal degeneration, of corneal nerves also plays important role in diabetic keratopathy.

CLINICAL FEATURES

Clinical features of diabetic keratopathy include:
- *Decreased corneal sensations* are often noted in most long-standing cases of diabetes mellitus.
- *Punctate epithelial staining* and *neurotrophic corneal ulceration* have also been reported.

Table 12.7: Summary of mucopolysaccharidosis syndrome

Category	Disease	Enzyme deficiency	Accumulating substance	Gene (locus)	INH	Incidence
MPS type I-S	Scheie syndrome	α-L-iduronidase	Dematan sulfate, heparan sulfate	IDUA (4p163)	AR	Severe: 1/100,000
MPS type I-HS	Hurler syndrome	α-L-iduronidase	Dematan sulfate, heparan sulfate	IDUA (4p163)	AR	Attenuated: 1/500,000
MPS type I-H	Hurler syndrome	α-L-iduronidase	Dematan sulfate, heparan sulfate	IDUA (4p163)	AR	to 1/115,000 live birth
MPS type II	Hunter syndrome	Iduronate sulfatase	Dematan sulfate, heparan sulfate	IDS (Xq28)	XR	1/150,000 to 1/100,000 male births
MPS type IIIA	Sanfilippo syndrome A	Heparan N-sulfatase (sulfamidase)	Heparan sulfate	SGSH (17q25.3)	AR	1 in 70,000 live births
MPS type IIIB	Sanfilippo syndrome B	α-N-acetylgluco-saminidase	Heparan sulfate	NAGLU (17q21)	AR	–
MPS type IIIC	Sanfilippo syndrome C	Acetyl-CoA-α-glucosaminide	Heparan sulfate	HGSNT (8p11.1)	AR	–
MPS type IIID	Sanfilippo syndrome D	N-acetylglucosamine-6-sulfatase	Heparan sulfate	GNS (12p14)	AR	–
MPS type IVA	Morquio syndrome type A	N-acetylglucosamine-6-sulfatase	Heparan sulfate	GALNS (16q24.3)	AR	1 in 200,000 live birth
MPS type IVB	Morquio syndrome type B	β-galactosidase	Keratan sulfate	GLB1 (3p21.33)	AR	–
MPS type VI	Maroteaux-Lany syndrome	N-acetylglucosamine-4-sulfatase (Arylsulfatase B)	Keratan sulfate	ARSB (5q11–q13)	AR	1/600,000 to 1/250,000 live births
MPS type VII	Sty syndrome	β-Glucuronidase	Heparan sulfate, dematan sulfate	GUSB (7q21.11)	AR	1/250,000 live birth
MPS type IX	Natowicz syndrome	Hyaluronan	Hyaluronan	NYAL1 (3p21.3–p21.2)	AR	Unknown

Table 12.8: *Summary of ocular features of mucopolysaccharidosis*					
MPS type (eponym)	*Ocular manifestations*				
	Corneal	*Retinopathy*	*Glaucoma*	*Optic nerve*	*Other*
MPS I-S (Scheie)	+	++	+	+	
MPS I-HS (Hurler-Scheie)	++	++	++	++	
MPS I-H (Hurler)	+++	++	++	++	
MPS II (Hunter)	+	++	+	++	
MPS III (Sanfilippo)	+	+++	+	+	Bushy eyebrows, late blindness
MPS IV (Morquio)	+	++	+	+	Pseudo-exophthalmos
MPS VI (Maroteaux-Lamy)	+++	Unknown	++	++	
MPS VII (Sly)	++	Unknown	++	++	Colobomas of the iris
MPS IX (Natowicz)	Unknown	Unknown	Unknown	Unknown	

- *Poor healing and persistent epithelial defects* are common following removal of epithelium in vitreo-retinal surgery.
- *Faint vertical folds in Descemet's membrane and deep stroma* (Waite Beetham lines), a sign of early endothelial dysfunction and increased stromal hydration, may be seen.
- *Corneal endothelium in diabetics* recovers late than non-diabetics, following cataract surgery.

LABORATORY TESTS

Glycosylated haemoglobin (HbA1c), levels are associated diabetic retinopathy as well as diabetic keratopathy.

MANAGEMENT

Depending upon the severity of diabetic keratopathy, following measures may be required:
- *Lubricating* eye drops
- *Minimising epithelial debridement* in VR surgery
- *Avoiding* toxic topical eye drops
- *Therapeutic contact lens* may be needed in non-healing epithelial lesions
- *Management of associated meibomian gland dysfunction should also be done.*

GLUCOSE-6-PHOSPHATASE DEFICIENCY

Glucose-6-phosphatase deficiency is a glycogen storage diseases due to deficiency of the enzyme glucose-6-phosphatase. It is also known as *Gierke disease.*

Clinical features

General features, like other glycogen storage diseases include:

- Enlargement of the liver and kidney
- Bouts of severe hypoglycemia
- Xanthomas with prominent lipaemia are characteristic
- Seizures and vomiting are also reported.

Ocular features include:
- *Corneal lesions.* Faint brown peripheral corneal clouding
- *Retinal lesions.* Discrete yellow perimacular lesion

DISORDERS OF LIPID METABOLISM AND STORAGE

MUCOLIPIDOSES

Mucolipidoses (MLs) are autosomal recessive inherited metabolic diseases characterized by abnormal deposition of mucopolysaccharides, glycolipids and sphingolipids.

Types

Mucolipidosis of following types is known:

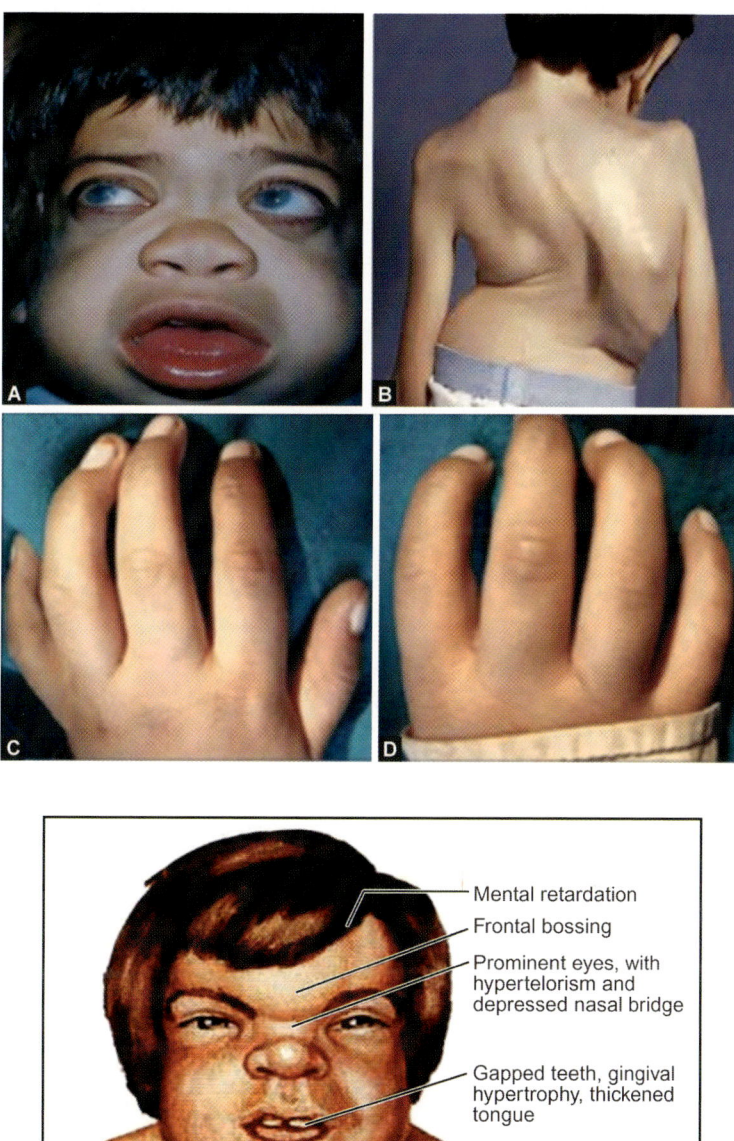

Mental retardation

Frontal bossing

Prominent eyes, with hypertelorism and depressed nasal bridge

Gapped teeth, gingival hypertrophy, thickened tongue

Fig. 12.16: *Clinical features of a patient with Hurler disease (A to D) and diagrammatic depiction of features (E)*

- *Mucolipidosis* I is also known as dysmorphic sialidosis. It is recessively inherited but the specific enzymatic defect is unknown.
- *Mucolipidosis* II , also known as inclusion cell disease, is associated with a deficiency of β-galactosidase.

- *Mucolipidosis* III, also known as pseudo-Hurler polydystrophy, is associated with an unknown enzymatic defect.
- *Mucolipidosis* IV, is also associated with an unknown enzymatic defect. It occurs more commonly in Ashkenazi Jews.

Table 12.9: *Summary of systemic features of mucopolysaccharidosis*

Manifestations	*Overview of systemic features in MPS*								
	I-S	*I-HS*	*I-H*	*II*	*III*	*IV*	*VI*	*VII*	*IX*
Mental deficiency	–	–	+	±	+	–	–	±	–
Coarse facial features	±	+	+	+	+	–	+	±	+
Middle ear disease/deafness	+	+	+	+	+	+	+	+	–
Cardiorespiratory disease	+	+	+	+	+	+	+	+	–
Visceromegaly	±	+	+	+	±	–	+	+	–
Short stature	±	+	+	+	–	+	+	+	±
Joint contractures	+	+	+	+	–	–	+	+	–
Dysostosis multiplex	±	+	+	+	±	+	+	+	–
Leukocyte inclusions	±	+	+	+	+	–	+	+	+
Mucopolysacchari-duria	+	+	+	+	+	+	+	+	–
Other				Seizures	Behavioural disturbance, hirsutism, irregular sleep		Hydrocephalus, spinal stenosis	Hydrocephalus, hydrops fetalis	Soft tissue masses, acetabular erosions

Clinical features

General features include:
- *Growth retardation* of varying degree.
- *Mental retardation* of varying degree.
- *Psychomotor retardation* of varying degree.
- *Organomegaly* especially hepatomegaly may be present in some types.

Ocular features include:
- *Corneal haze*/opacity of varying degree.
- *Cherry red spot* may be associated in some form of mucolipidosis.
- *Spoke-like cataract* may be present in some form of mucolipidosis.

Management

Laboratory confirmation
- Plasma lysosomal hydrolase levels are high.
- Conjunctival biopsy shows fibroblast inclusion bodies in mucolipidosis IV.

Treatment
- *Keratoplasty*, both penetrating and lamellar, done for corneal haze is generally a failure.
- *Allograft limbal stem cell transplantation* is being considered an option.
- *Bone marrow transplantation* is also being considered.

■ SPHINGOLIPODOSES

These include:
- Fabry's disease
- GM2 gangliosidosis II
- Metachromatic leucodystrophy (Austin's juvenile form)

FABRY'S DISEASE

Fabry's disease (sphingolipodosis) is a multisystemic disorder occurring due to the deficiency of the enzyme alpha-galactosidase.

Transmitted as an X-linked recessive trait.

Clinical features

Systemic features occur due to deposition of sphingolipids in skin, organs of genitourinary, cardiovascular, musculoskeletal and central nervous systems.
- Skin lesions are clusters of punctate, brown to maroon spots, typically involving skin of genitalia and lumbosacral areas.

- Pain in the fingers and toes is common.
- Neurological lesions include hemiplegia, aphasia, cerebellar symptoms and features of stroke.

Ocular features include:
- *Cornea verticillata* characterized by whorl-like superficial corneal opacities is a typical feature. It occurs due to the deposition of sphingolipids in the corneal epithelium.
- *Conjunctival changes* are dilated and tortuous vessels.
- *Spoke-like posterior sutural cataract* may occur. There may be associated cream-coloured anterior capsular deposits.
- *Posterior segment changes* in the form of retinal oedema, dilated and tortuous retinal veins, papilloedema and optic atrophy.
- *Periorbital oedema* may also occur.

Management

Diagnosis is confirmed by demonstrating sediments of glycolipids in urine with the help of high performance liquid chromatography.

Treatment. Fabrazyme, a drug that helps by reducing fat deposition in organs may be useful.

■ DYSLIPOPROTEINEMIAS

Metabolic disorders of lipoproteins associated with large number of lipid metabolic processes. They are characterized by accumulation of lipids in the cornea, retinal blood vessels and/or in the eyelid skin. These are summarized in Table 12.10.

LANGERHANS CELL HISTIOCYTOSIS

Langerhans cell histiocytosis, formerly known as histiocytosis X, is a group of diseases characterized by an idiopathic abnormal proliferation of histiocytes with granuloma formation. These diseases primarily affect children with an orbital involvement in 20% of cases. This group includes following three diseases:

1. Hand-Schuller-Christian disease. It is a chronic disseminated form of histiocytosis involving both soft tissues and bones in older children of either sex. It is characterized by a triad of proptosis, diabetes insipidus and bony defects in the skull.

Table 12.10: *Summary of features of dyslipoproteinemia*

Disorder	Deficiency	Gene locus	Metabolite accumulated	Mode of inheritance	Ocular manifestations	Systemic manifestations
Lecithin-cholesterol acyltransferase (LCAT) deficiency	LCAT	16q22.1	Free cholesterol	Autosomal recessive	Dense peripheral arcus, gray dots in central stroma, no visual changes	Atherosclerosis, renal insufficiency
Fish eye disease (high-density lipoprotein LCAT)	α-LCAT	16q22.1	Triglycerides, very low density lipoproteins (VLDL); low density lipoproteins (LDL)	Autosomal dominant	Progressive corneal clouding, increased corneal thickness	None
Tangier disease (an alpha-lipoproteinemia)	High density lipoprotein	9q22-q31	Triglycerides, low levels of high density lipoproteins (HDL), cholesterol and phospholipids	Autosomal recessive	Fine dot corneal clouding, severe visual loss, incomplete eyelid closure, ectropion, no arcus	Lymphadenopathy, hepatosplenomegaly, coronary artery disease
Hyperlipoproteinemia I (hyperchylomicronemia)	Lipoprotein lipase	8p22	Triglycerides, chylomicrons	Autosomal recessive	Lipaemia retinalis, palpebral eruptive xanthomata	Xanthomas
Hyperlipoproteinemia II, hyper-β-lipoproteinemia IIa, hyper-β-lipoproteinemia IIb	Low density lipoprotein LDL receptor (type IIa); defective lipid metabolism in type IIb	19p13 (type IIa); 1q21-23 (type IIb); others	Type IIa: LDL, cholesterol Type IIb: LDL, VLDL, cholesterol, triglycerides	Autosomal dominant	Both forms: corneal arcus, conjunctival xanthomata, xanthelasma	Coronary artery disease
Hyperlipoproteinemia III, dys-β-lipoproteinemia, broad β disease	Abnormality in apolipoprotein E	19q13.2	VLDL remnants, cholesterol, triglycerides	Autosomal recessive with pseudo-dominance	Arcus, xanthelasma, lipaemia retinalis	Peripheral vascular disease, diabetes mellitus
Hyperlipoproteinemia IV (hyperpre-β-lipoproteinemia)	Lipoprotein lipase; apolipoprotein A	15q11-13; 21q11; others	Triglycerides, VLDL	Autosomal dominant	Arcus, xanthelasma, lipaemia retinalis	Vascular disease, diabetes mellitus
Hyperlipoproteinemia V (hyperprelipoproteinemia and hyperchylomicronemia)	Apolipoprotein A	11q23	VLDL, chylomicrons	Uncertain	Lipaemia retinalis, no arcus	Xanthomas, hepatosplenomegaly

2. Letterer-Siwe disease. Now termed 'diffuse soft tissue histiocytosis' is a systemic form of histiocytosis characterized by widespread soft tissue and visceral involvement with or without bony changes. The disease has a slight male preponderance and often occurs in the first three years of life. Orbital involvement is comparatively rare.

3. Unifocal or multifocal eosinophilic granuloma is characterized by a solitary or multiple granulomas involving the bones. The disease occurs in elder children and frequently involves the orbital bones.

Corneal involvement, though infrequent, may be seen as peripheral, yellow white infiltrates present in all layers of cornea.

DISORDERS OF PROTEIN AND AMINO ACID METABOLISM

Common disorders of amino acid metabolism include:
- Cystinosis
- Tyrosinemia
- Alkaptonuria
- Wilson's disease, and
- Lattice dystrophy type II (Meretoja's syndrome)

CYSTINOSIS

Cystinosis, also known as Lignae-Fanconi syndrome, is a rare autosomal recessive disorder of cystine storage characterized by intracellular deposition of cystine in the reticuloendothelial cells of the bone marrow, liver, spleen, lymphatic system and kidney.

Clinical features

General features

Depending upon the age of onset and severity of symptoms cystinosis has been grouped as below:

I. Nephropathic cystinosis which is further divided into two subtypes:

a. *Infantile or classic cystinosis* is characterized by:
   - Dwarfism, and
   - Progressive dysfunction

b. *Juvenile/adolescent or intermediate cystinosis.* Dwarfism and renal dysfunction are less severe.

II. Non-nephropathic cystinosis or adult cystinosis.

Ocular features

All three types, i.e. infantile, juvenile and adult cystinosis are characterized by:

- Deposition of cystine crystals (fine and polychromatic) in the conjunctiva, cornea and other parts of the eye.
- Band keratopathy
- Photophobia
- Retinal abnormalities in the form of macular changes are seen occasionally.

TYROSINEMIA

Pathogenesis

Pathogenesis of tyrosinemia type II (tyrosinosis, Richner-Hanhart syndrome) includes:

- *Enzyme deficient:* Tyrosine transaminase
- *Mode of inheritance:* Autosomal recessive
- *Gene locus:* 16q22.1-22.3
- *Metabolite accumulated:* Tyrosine

Clinical features

Ocular features

Ocular features include:

- Red eye
- Photophobia
- Dendriform corneal epithelial changes seen as branches or snowflake opacities.

Systemic associations

Systemic manifestations associated include:

- Palmar-Plantar hyperkeratosis,
- Mental retardation, and
- Growth retardation

ALKAPTONURIA

Pathogenesis

Pathogenesis of alkaptonuria includes:
- *Inherited disorder* with autosomal recessive inheritance
- *Gene locus:* 3q21-q23

- *Enzyme deficient:* Homogentisate-1,2-dioxygenase
- *Metabolite accumulated:* Homogentisic acid

Clinical features

Ocular features

- *Conjunctiva:* Pigmented pingueculae
- *Cornea:* Oil droplet opacities in limbal corneal epithelium and Bowman's membrane
- *Sclera:* Pigmentation of sclera near insertion of horizontal rectus muscle.

Systemic associations

Joint pain and stiffness

WILSON'S DISEASE

Pathogenesis

Pathogenesis of Wilson's disease includes:
- *Inherited disorder* with autosomal recessive inheritance
- *Gene locus:* 13q14.3-q21.1
- *Enzyme deficit:* Defective excretion of copper from hepatic lysosomes
- *Metabolite accumulated:* Copper

Clinical features

Ocular features

- *Cornea:* Kayser-Fleischer ring
- *Lens:* Sunflower cataract (Fig. 12.14)

Systemic features

- *Liver:* Dysfunction
- *Kidney*: Nephrotic syndrome
- *Muscles*: Spasticity
- *CNS*: Behaviour disturbances

LATTICE DYSTROPHY TYPE II

Pathogenesis

- *Inherited disorder:* Autosomal dominant
- *Gene locus:* 9q34
- *Enzyme deficient:* Gelsolin gene defect
- *Metabolite accumulated:* Amyloid

Clinical features

Ocular features

- Lattice dystrophy of cornea

- Glaucoma
- Ptosis

Systemic features

- Progressive cranial neuropathy
- Cardiac disease

BIBLIOGRAPHY

1. Al Hazimi A, Khan A (2013). Axial lengths in children with recessive cornea plana. Ophthalmic Genet (in press).
2. Al-Rajhi A, Wagoner M (1997). Penetrating keratoplasty in congenital hereditary endothelial dystrophy. Ophthalmology; 104(6): 956–961.
3. Aldave AJ, Han J, Frausto RF. Genetics of the corneal endothelial dystrophies: an evidence-based review. Clin Genet 2013a; 84(2): 109–119.
4. Aldave A, Ann L, Frausto R, Nguyen C, Yu F, Raber I (2013b) Classification of posterior polymorphous corneal dystrophy as a corneal ectatic disorder following confirmation of associated significant corneal steepening. JAMA Ophthalmology.
5. Ali M, Buentello-Volante B, McKibbin M, Rocha-Medina J, Fernandez-Fuentes N, Koga-Nakamura W, Ashiq A, Khan K, Booth A, Wiilliams G, Raashid Y, Jafri H, Rice A, Inglehearm C, Zenteno J. Homozygous FOXE3 mutations cause non-syndromic, bilateral, total sclerocornea, aphakia, microphthalmia and optic disc coloboma. Mol Vis 2010; 16: 1162–1168.
6. Collins, ET. The development of the posterior elastic lamina of the cornea or membrane of Descemet. Roy. Ophthal. Hosp. Rep. 1897; 14, 305-11.
7. Corneal development, II. Transparency changes during rapid hydration. Amer. J. Ophthal. 46, 276–81.
8. Coulombre, AJ, Coulombre, JL. Corneal development. I. Corneal transparency/ cell.comp. Physiol. 1958fl; 51, 1–11.
9. Development of stromal collagen patterns. Amer. J. Ophthal. 1958c; 45, 291.
10. Natalie Afshari (2018-10-05). "Macular corneal dystrophy". eMedicine.
11. The role of intraocular pressure in the development of the chick eye. Arch. Ophthal. N.Y. 1958J; 59: 502–6.

Section
IV

Diseases of Conjunctiva and Ocular Surface

Conjunctivitis

DEFINITION AND CLASSIFICATION

DEFINITION

Inflammation of the conjunctiva (conjunctivitis) is classically defined as conjunctival hyperaemia associated with a discharge which may be watery, mucoid, mucopurulent or purulent.

CLASSIFICATION

Etiologically conjunctivitis can be classified as below:

A. Infective conjunctivitis

1. Bacterial conjunctivitis

- Acute bacterial conjunctivitis
- Hyperacute bacterial conjunctivitis
- Chronic bacterial conjunctivitis
- Angular bacterial conjunctivitis

Chlamydial conjunctivitis

- Trachoma
- Adult inclusion conjunctivitis
- Neonatal chlamydial conjunctivitis

2. Viral conjunctivitis

- Adenovirus conjunctivitis
  - Epidemic keratoconjunctivitis
  - Pharyngoconjunctival fever
- Enterovirus conjunctivitis
- Molluscum contagiosum conjunctivitis
- Herpes simplex conjunctivitis

3. Ophthalmia neonatorum (a separate entity)

4. Granulomatous conjunctivitis

- Parinaud oculoglandular syndrome.

B. Allergic conjunctivitis

1. Simple allergic conjunctivitis
- Hay fever conjunctivitis (rhinoconjunctivitis)
- Seasonal allergic conjunctivitis (SAC)
- Perennial allergic conjunctivitis (PAC)

2. Vernal keratoconjunctivitis (VKC)

3. Atopic keratoconjunctivitis (AKC)

4. Giant papillary conjunctivitis (GPC)

5. Phlyctenular conjunctivitis (PKC)

6. Contact dermoconjunctivitis (drop conjunctivitis).

C. Cicatricial conjunctivitis

- Ocular mucous membrane pemphigoid (OMMP),
- Stevens-Johnson syndrome (SJS),
- Toxic epidermal necrolysis (TeN), and
- Secondary cicatricial conjunctivitis.

D. Toxic conjunctivitis

- Toxic conjunctivitis secondary to molluscum contagiosum
- Chemical toxic conjunctivitis

INFECTIVE CONJUNCTIVITIS

Infective conjunctivitis, i.e. inflammation of the conjunctiva caused by micro-organisms is the commonest variety. This is in spite of the fact that the conjunctiva has been provided with *natural protective mechanisms* in the form of:

- Low temperature due to exposure to air,
- Physical protection by lids,
- Flushing action of tears,
- Antibacterial activity of lysozymes, and
- Humoral protection by the tear immunoglobulins.

BACTERIAL CONJUNCTIVITIS

There has occurred a relative decrease in the incidence of bacterial conjunctivitis in general and those caused by gonococcus and *Corynebacterium diphtheriae* in particular. However, in developing countries, it still continues to be the commonest type of conjunctivitis. It can occur as sporadic and epidemic cases. Outbreaks of bacterial conjunctivitis, epidemics are quite frequent during monsoon season.

Etiology

A. Predisposing factors for bacterial conjunctivitis, especially epidemic forms, are flies, poor hygienic conditions, hot dry climate, poor sanitation and dirty habits. These factors help the infection to establish, as the disease is highly contagious.

B. Causative organisms. It may be caused by a wide range of organisms in the following approximate order of frequency:
- *Staphylococcus aureus* is the most common cause of bacterial conjunctivitis and blepharoconjunctivitis.
- *Staphylococcus epidermidis* is an innocuous flora of lid and conjunctiva. It can also produce blepharoconjunctivitis.
- *Streptococcus pneumoniae* (*Pneumococcus*) produces acute conjunctivitis usually associated with petechial subconjunctival haemorrhages. The disease has a self-limiting course of 9–10 days.
- *Streptococcus pyogenes* (haemolyticus) is virulent and usually produces pseudomembranous conjunctivitis.
- *Haemophilus influenzae* (aegyptius, Koch-Weeks bacillus). It classically causes epidemics of mucopurulent conjunctivitis, known as 'red-eye' especially in semitropical countries.
- *Moraxella lacunata* (Morax-Axenfeld bacillus) is most common cause of angular conjunctivitis and angular blepharoconjunctivitis.
- *Pseudomonas pyocyanea* is a virulent organism, which readily invades the cornea.
- *Neisseria gonorrhoeae* typically produces acute purulent conjunctivitis in adults and ophthalmia neonatorum in newborn. It is capable of invading intact corneal epithelium.
- *Neisseria meningitidis* (*Meningococcus*) may produce mucopurulent conjunctivitis.
- *Corynebacterium diphtheriae* causes acute membranous conjunctivitis. Such infections are not known nowadays.

C. Mode of infection. Conjunctiva may get infected from three sources, viz. exogenous, local surrounding structures and endogenous, by following modes:

1. *Exogenous infections* are the commonest and may spread:
- *Directly* through close contact, as airborne infections or as waterborne infections.
- *Vector transmission* (e.g. flies)
- *Material transfer* such as infected fingers of doctors, nurses, common towels, handkerchiefs, and infected tonometers.
2. *Local spread* may occur sometimes from neighbouring structures such as infected lacrimal sac, lids, and nasopharynx. In addition to these, a change in the character of relatively innocuous organisms present in the conjunctival sac itself may cause infections.
3. *Endogenous infections* may occur very rarely through blood, e.g. gonococcal and meningococcal infections.

PATHOLOGY

Pathological changes of bacterial conjunctivitis consist of:
1. *Vascular response.* It is characterised by congestion and increased permeability of the conjunctival vessels associated with proliferation of capillaries.
2. *Cellular response.* It is in the form of exudation of polymorphonuclear cells and other inflammatory cells into the substantia propria of conjunctiva as well as in the conjunctival sac.
3. *Conjunctival tissue response.* Conjunctiva becomes oedematous. The superficial epithelial cells degenerate, become loose and even desquamate. There occurs proliferation of basal layers of conjunctival epithelium and increase in the number of mucin-secreting goblet cells.
4. *Conjunctival discharge.* It consists of tears, mucus, inflammatory cells, desquamated epithelial cells, fibrin and bacteria. If the inflammation is very severe, diapedesis of red blood cells may occur and discharge may become blood stained.

Severity of pathological changes varies depending upon the severity of inflammation and the causative organism. The changes are thus more marked in purulent conjunctivitis than mucopurulent conjunctivitis.

CLINICAL TYPES OF BACTERIAL CONJUNCTIVITIS

Depending upon the causative bacteria and the severity of infection, bacterial conjunctivitis may present in following clinical forms:
- Acute bacterial conjunctivitis,
- Hyperacute bacterial conjunctivitis,
- Chronic bacterial conjunctivitis, and
- Angular bacterial conjunctivitis.

◼ ACUTE BACTERIAL CONJUNCTIVITIS

Acute bacterial conjunctivitis is characterised by marked conjunctival hyperaemia and mucopurulent discharge from the eye. So, clinically, it is called *acute mucopurulent conjunctivitis*. It is the most common type of bacterial conjunctivitis.

Common causative bacteria are: *Staphylococcus aureus, Koch-Weeks bacillus, Streptococcus pneumoniae, Haemophilus influenzae* (Table 13.1). Mucopurulent conjunctivitis generally accompanies exanthemata such as measles and scarlet fever.

CLINICAL FEATURES

Symptoms

- *Discomfort, foreign body, grittiness, blurring and redness* of sudden onset (due to engorgement of vessels) are the usual presenting symptoms.
- *Mild to moderate pain* is often experienced by the patients.

Table 13.1: *Common pathogens causing acute, hyperacute and chronic bacterial conjunctivitis*

Acute conjunctivitis	Hyperacute conjunctivitis	Chronic conjunctivitis
• *Staphylococcus aureus*	• *Neisseria gonorrhoeae*	• *Staphylococcus aureus*
• *Streptococcus pneumoniae*	• *Neisseria meningitidis*	• *Moraxella lacunata*
• *Koch-Weeks bacillus*		• *Proteus mirabilis*
• *Haemophilus influenzae*		• *Klebsiella pneumoniae*
		• *Escherichia coli*

- *Mild photophobia*, i.e. difficulty to tolerate light.
- *Mucopurulent discharge* from the eyes.
- *Sticking together of lid margins* with discharge during sleep.
- *Slight blurring* of vision due to mucous flakes in front of cornea.
- *Coloured halos*, may be complained by some patients due to prismatic effect of mucus present on cornea.

Signs (Fig. 13.1)

- *Flakes of mucopus* seen in the fornices, canthi and lid margins is a critical sign.
- *Conjunctival congestion*, which is more marked in palpebral conjunctiva, fornices and peripheral part of bulbar conjunctiva, giving the appearance of 'fiery red eye'. The congestion is typically less marked in circumcorneal zone.
- *Chemosis*, i.e. swelling of conjunctiva.
- *Papillae* of fine type may be seen.
- *Petechial haemorrhages* are seen when the causative organism is *Streptococcus pneumoniae*.
- *Cilia are usually matted* together with yellow crusts.
- *Eyelids* may be slightly oedematous.

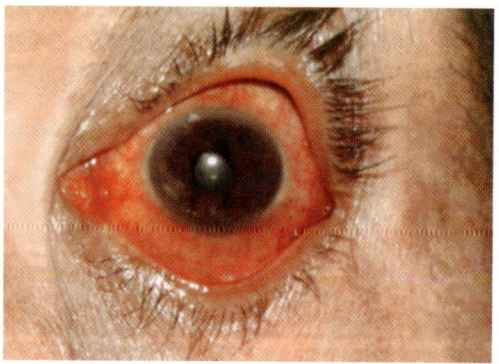

Fig. 13.1: *Signs of acute mucopurulent conjunctivitis*

Clinical course

Acute mucopurulent conjunctivitis is usually bilateral, although one eye may become affected 1–2 days before the other. The disease usually reaches its height in three to four days. If untreated, in mild cases the infection may be overcome and the condition is cured in 10–15 days; or it may pass to less intense form, the 'chronic catarrhal conjunctivitis'.

Complications

Occasionally, the disease may be complicated by superficial punctate corneal epitheliopathy, marginal corneal ulceration, superficial keratitis, blepharitis, or dacryocystitis.

DIFFERENTIAL DIAGNOSIS

1. *From other causes of acute red eye* (Table 13.2).
2. *From other types of conjunctivitis*. It is made out from the typical clinical feature of disease and is confirmed by conjunctival cytology and bacteriological examination of secretions and scrapings (Table 13.3).

TREATMENT

*1. **Topical antibiotics*** to control the infection constitute the main treatment of acute bacterial conjunctivitis. Ideally, the antibiotic should be selected after culture and sensitivity tests but in practice, it is difficult. However, in routine, most of the patients respond well to broad spectrum antibiotics. Therefore, treatment may be started with chloramphenicol (1%), or gentamicin (0.3%), or tobramycin 0.3% or framycetin 0.3% eye drops 3–4 hourly in day and ointment used at night will not only provide antibiotic cover but also help to reduce the early morning stickiness. If the patient does not respond to these antibiotics, then the quinolone antibiotic drops such as ciprofloxacin (0.3%), ofloxacin (0.3%), gatifloxacin (0.3%) or moxifloxacin (0.5%) may be used.

*2. **Irrigation of conjunctival sac*** with sterile lukewarm saline once or twice a day will help by removing the deleterious material. Frequent eyewash (as advocated earlier) is, however, contraindicated as it will wash away the lysozyme and other protective proteins present in the tears.

*3. **Dark goggles*** should be used to prevent photophobia.

*4. **No bandage*** should be applied in patients with mucopurulent conjunctivitis. Exposure to air keeps the temperature of conjunctival cul-de-sac low which inhibits the bacterial growth; while after bandaging, conjunctival sac is converted

Table 13.2: *Distinguishing features between acute conjunctitis, acute iridocyclitis and acute congestive glaucoma*

Features	Acute conjunctivitis	Acute iridocyclitis	Acute congestive glaucoma
1. Onset	Gradual	Usually gradual	Sudden
2. Pain	Mild discomfort	Moderate in eye and along the first division of trigeminal nerve	Severe in eye and the entire trigeminal area
3. Discharge	Mucopurulent	Watery	Watery
4. Coloured halos	May be present	Absent	Present
5. Vision	Good	Slightly impaired	Markedly impaired
6. Congestion	Superficial conjunctival	Deep ciliary	Deep ciliary
7. Tenderness	Absent	Marked	Marked
8. Pupil	Normal	Small and irregular	Large and vertically oval
9. Media	Clear	Hazy due to KPs, aqueous flare and pupillary exudates	Hazy due to oedematous cornea
10. Anterior chamber	Normal	May be deep	Very shallow
11. Iris	Normal	Muddy	Oedematous
12. Intraocular pressure	Normal	Usually normal	Raised
13. Constitutional symptoms	Absent	Little	Prostration and vomiting

Table 13.3: *Differentiating features of common types of conjunctivitis*

	Bacterial	Viral	Allergic	Chlamydial (TRIC)
(A) Clinical signs				
1. Congestion	Marked	Moderate	Mild to moderate	Moderate
2. Chemosis	++	±	++	±
3. Subconjunctival haemorrhages	±	±	–	–
4. Discharge	Purulent or mucopurulent	Watery	Ropy/watery	Mucopurulent
5. Papillae	±	–	++	±
6. Follicles	–	+	–	++
7. Pseudomembrane	±	±	–	–
8. Pannus	–	–	– (Except vernal)	+
9. Preauricular lymph nodes	+	++	–	±
(B) Cytological features				
1. Neutrophils	+	+ (Early)	–	+
2. Eosinophils	–	–	+	–
3. Lymphocytes	–	+	–	+
4. Plasma cells	–	–	–	+
5. Multinuclear cells	–	+	–	–
6. Inclusion bodies:				
Cytoplasmic	–	+ (Pox)	–	+
Nuclear	–	+ (Herpes)	–	–
7. Micro-organisms	+	–	–	–

into an incubator, and thus infection flares to a severe degree within 24 hours. Further, bandaging of eye will also prevent the escape of discharge.

5. No steroids should be applied, otherwise infection will flare up and bacterial corneal ulcer may develop.

6. Anti-inflammatory and analgesic drugs (e.g. ibuprofen and paracetamol) may be given orally for 2–3 days to provide symptomatic relief from mild pain especially in sensitive patients.

Preventive measures to reduce risk of transmission to the close contacts

* Frequent handwashing, and
* Avoidance of sharing towel, handkerchief and pillow with others.

◼ HYPERACUTE BACTERIAL CONJUNCTIVITIS

Hyperacute bacterial conjunctivitis also known as acute purulent conjunctivitis or *acute blennorrhoea* is characterised by a violent inflammatory response.

It occurs in two forms:
1. Adult purulent conjunctivitis
2. Ophthalmia neonatorum in newborn (*see* page 76).

◼ HYPERACUTE CONJUNCTIVITIS OF ADULTS (GONOCOCCAL CONJUNCTIVITIS)

ETIOLOGY

The disease affects adults, predominantly males.
* *Gonococcal infection* directly spreads from genitals to eye. Presently, incidence of gonococcal conjunctivitis has markedly decreased.
* *Other pathogen* causing hyperacute conjunctivitis is *Neisseria meningitidis* (Table 13.1).

CLINICAL FEATURES

Gonococcal conjunctivitis

Onset is hyperacute (12 to 24 hours).

Symptoms include:
* *Pain* which is moderate to severe.
* *Purulent discharge,* which is usually copious.
* *Swelling of eyelids,* which is usually marked.
* *Mild photophobia*, i.e. difficulty to tolerate light.

* *Sticking together of lid margins* with discharge during sleep.
* *Slight blurring* of vision due to mucous flakes in front of cornea.

Signs are as follows (Fig. 13.2)
* *Eyelids* are tense and swollen.
* *Tenderness* is marked.
* *Discharge* is thick purulent, copious trickling down the cheeks.
* *Conjunctiva shows* marked chemosis, congestion and papillae, giving bright red velvety appearance. Frequently, a pseudomembrane may be seen on the conjunctival surface (Fig. 13.3).
* *Preauricular lymph nodes* are usually enlarged and tender.

Associations. Gonococcal conjunctivitis is usually associated with urethritis and arthritis.

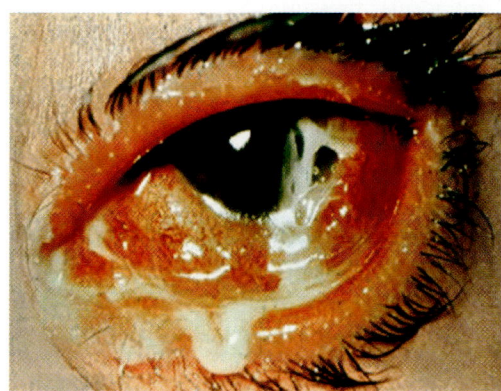

Fig. 13.2: *Hyperacute conjunctivitis*

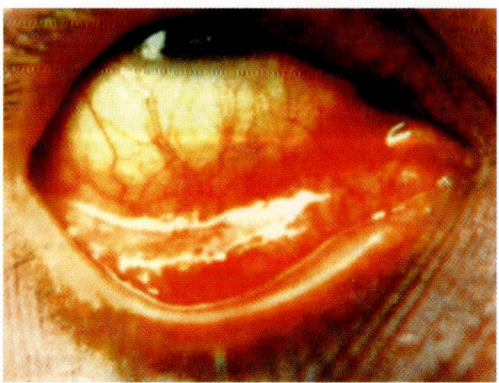

Fig. 13.3: *Pseudomembranous conjunctivitis*

COMPLICATIONS

1. *Corneal involvement* is quite frequent as the gonococcus can invade the normal cornea through an intact epithelium. It may occur in the form of diffuse haze and oedema, central necrosis, corneal ulceration or even perforation.
2. *Iridocyclitis* may also occur, but is not as common as corneal involvement.
3. *Systemic complications*, though rare, include gonorrhoea arthritis, endocarditis and septicaemia.

TREATMENT

1. Systemic therapy is far more critical than the topical therapy for the infections caused by *N. gonorrhoeae*. Any of the following regimes can be adopted:

- *Third generation cephalosporin* such as cefoxitin 1.0 g or cefotaxime 500 mg IV qid or ceftriaxone 1.0 g IM qid, all for 5 days; should be preferred treatment.
- *Quinolones* such as norfloxacin 1.2 g orally qid for 5 days, or
- *Spectinomycin* 2.0 g IM for 3 days, may be used alternatively.

All of the above regimes should then be followed by a one week course of either doxycycline 100 mg bid or erythromycin 250–500 mg orally qid.

2. Topical antibiotic therapy, presently recommended includes ofloxacin, ciprofloxacin or tobramycin eye drops or bacitracin or erythromycin eye ointment every 2 hours for the first 2–3 days and then 5 times daily for 7 days.

3. Irrigation of the eyes frequently with sterile saline is very therapeutic in washing away infected debris.

4. Other general measures are similar to acute mucopurulent conjunctivitis.

5. Topical atropine 1% eye drops should be instilled once or twice a day if cornea is involved.

Note. Sexual partner should also be treated with systemic antibiotics. Further, both the patient and the sexual partner should be referred for evaluation of other sexually transmitted diseases.

Meningococcal conjunctivitis

Hyperacute conjunctivitis caused by *Neisseria meningitidis* is comparatively milder than gonococcal conjunctivitis. It may be of two types: Primary and secondary.

Primary meningococcal conjunctivitis is extremely rare in adults and can be:

- *Invasive disease*, which is followed by systemic meningococcal disease.
- *Non-invasive disease*, i.e. isolated conjunctival infection.

Treatment of meningococcal conjunctivitis

- *Topical treatment* in similar to gonococcal conjunctivitis.
- *Systemic treatment* includes intravenous penicillin or intravenous cefotaxime or ceftriaxone (in penicillin-resistant cases).

Note. *Close contacts* of invasive meningococcal conjunctivitis should receive prophylaxis with a single dose of ciprofloxacin 500 mg or rifampin 600 mg twice daily for two days.

CHRONIC BACTERIAL CONJUNCTIVITIS

Chronic bacterial conjunctivitis also known as 'Chronic catarrhal conjunctivitis' or 'simple chronic conjunctivitis' is characterised by mild catarrhal inflammation of the conjunctiva. Chronic bacterial conjunctivitis lasts more than 3 weeks and is often associated with blepharitis.

ETIOLOGY

A. Predisposing factors

1. *Chronic exposure* to dust, smoke, and chemical irritants.
2. *Local cause of irritation* such as trichiasis, concretions, foreign body and seborrhoeic scales.
3. *Eye strain* due to refractive errors, phorias or convergence insufficiency.
4. *Abuse of alcohol*, insomnia and metabolic disorders.

B. Causative organisms (Table 13.1)

- *Staphylococcus aureus* is the commonest cause of chronic bacterial conjunctivitis. It colourizes the eyelid margin and then causes direct infection of conjunctiva or conjunctival inflammation through the exotoxins released.

- *Gram-negative rods* such as *Proteus mirabilis, Klebsiella pneumoniae, Escherichia coli, Moraxella lacunata, Serratia marcescens,* and *Branhamella catarrhalis* are other rare causes.

C. Source and mode of infection. Chronic conjunctivitis may occur:

1. *As continuation of acute mucopurulent conjunctivitis* when untreated or partially treated.
2. *As chronic infection* from associated chronic dacryocystitis, chronic rhinitis or chronic upper respiratory catarrh.
3. *As a mild exogenous infection* which results from direct contact, airborne or material transfer of infection.

CLINICAL FEATURES

Symptoms of simple chronic conjunctivitis include:

- *Burning and grittiness* in the eyes, especially in the evening.
- *Mild chronic redness* in the eyes. Feeling of heat and dryness on the lid margins.
- *Difficulty in keeping the eyes open.*
- *Mild mucoid discharge* especially in the canthi.
- *Watering,* off and on is often a complaint.
- *Feeling of sleepiness* and tiredness in the eyes.

Signs. Grossly the eyes look normal but careful examination may reveal following signs:

- *Congestion* of posterior conjunctival vessels which is mild and diffuse.
- *Mild papillary hypertrophy* of the palpebral conjunctiva.
- *Follicles,* may also occur
- *Conjunctival thickening*
- *Sticky look* of surface of the conjunctiva.
- *Lid margins* may show congestion, telangiectasis, loss of lashes and blepharitis.
- *Cornea* may develop marginal corneal ulcer.

TREATMENT

1. *Eliminate predisposing factors* when associated.
2. *Topical antibiotics* such as chloramphenicol, tobramycin or gentamicin should be instilled 3–4 times a day for about 2 weeks to eliminate the mild chronic infection.
3. *Astringent eye drops* such as zinc–boric acid drops provide symptomatic relief.

4. *Treatment of blepharitis,* which is usually associated needs to be done by good lid hygiene with warm compresses, and eyelid scrubs followed by rubbing of combination of antibiotic and corticosteroid eye ointment.
   - Systemic therapy with oral tetracycline 250 mg 4 times a day, or doxycycline 100 mg 1–2 times a day, may be needed for severe cases of blepharitis.

■ ANGULAR BACTERIAL CONJUNCTIVITIS

It is a type of chronic conjunctivitis characterised by mild grade inflammation confined to the conjunctiva and lid margins near the angles (hence the name) associated with maceration of the surrounding skin.

ETIOLOGY

1. *Predisposing factors* are same as for 'simple chronic conjunctivitis'.
2. *Causative organisms. Moraxella-Axenfeld* (MA) is the commonest causative organism. MA bacilli are placed end to end, so the disease is also called 'diplobacillary conjunctivitis'. Rarely, staphylococci may also cause angular conjunctivitis.
3. *Source of infection* is usually nasal cavity.
4. *Mode of infection.* Infection is transmitted from nasal cavity to the eyes by contaminated fingers or handkerchief.

PATHOLOGY

The causative organism, i.e. MA bacillus produces a proteolytic enzyme which acts by macerating the epithelium. This proteolytic enzyme collects at the angles by the action of tears and thus macerates the epithelium of the conjunctiva, lid margin and the skin, the surrounding angles of eye. The maceration is followed by vascular and cellular responses in the form of mild grade chronic inflammation. Skin may show eczematous changes.

CLINICAL FEATURES

Symptoms include:
- Irritation, burning sensation and feeling of discomfort in the eyes.
- History of collection of dirty-white foamy discharge at the angles.
- Redness in the angles of eyes.

Signs include (Fig. 13.4):
- *Hyperaemia of bulbar conjunctiva* near the canthi.
- *Hyperaemia of lid margins* near the angles.
- *Excoriation of the skin* around the angles.
- *Foamy mucopurulent discharge* at the angles is usually present.

Complications include blepharitis and shallow marginal catarrhal corneal ulceration.

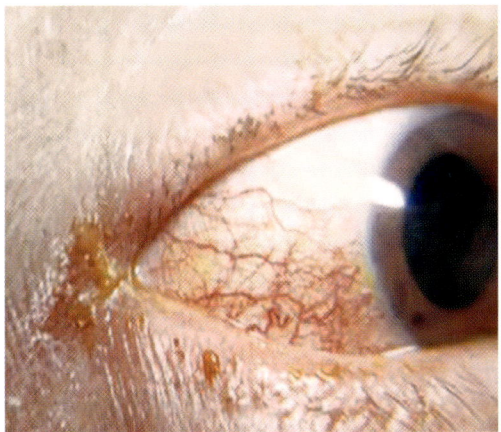

Fig. 13.4: *Signs of angular conjunctivitis*

TREATMENT

A. Prophylaxis includes treatment of associated nasal infection and good personal hygiene.

B. Curative treatment consists of:
1. *Oxytetracycline* (1%) eye ointment, 2–3 times a day for 9–14 days will eradicate the infection.
2. *Zinc lotion* instilled in daytime and zinc oxide ointment at bed time inhibits the proteolytic ferment and thus helps in reducing the maceration.

CHLAMYDIAL CONJUNCTIVITIS

Chlamydia, earlier classified as a separate organism in between bacteria and viruses, has now been classified as bacterium belonging to the family Chlamydiaceae having two genera: Chlamydia and Chlamydophilia.

Characteristics of Chlamydia

- Small, obligate intracellular, Gram-negative bacteria.
- Possess both RNA and DNA, ribosomes and cell wall similar to that of Gram-negative bacteria.
- Differ from most true bacteria is not having peptidoglycan.
- Lack the ability to produce their own ATP, therefore, use host's ATP (energy parasites).
- Multiply by binary fission.
- Inclusion bodies are basophilic in nature.
- Multiply in the cytoplasm of the host cell forming microcolonies or inclusion bodies which drape around the nucleus like a cloak or mantle (*chlamys* means mantle).
- Possess a genus-specific lipopolysaccharide-protein complex antigen.
- Exist in two morphologically distinct forms, namely elementary body (EB) and reticulate body (RB).

Life cycle of Chlamydia

Chlamydia exists in two morphological forms: The elementary body (EB) and reticulate body (RB). Life cycle of Chlamydia is shown in Fig. 13.5):

- *Elementary bodies* (EBs) are extracellular infectious particles (Fig. 13.5A). These initiate infection by attaching to the susceptible host cells (Fig. 13.5B). After attachment, the EB enters the cytoplasm of the host cells within a vesicle (Fig. 13.5C), where it increases in size and differentiates into reticulate body (RB) (Fig. 13.5D).
- *Reticulate body* (RB) is thus intracellular, metabolically active form that divides by binary fission (Fig. 13.5E). Soon there occurs condensation of DNA within the RBs, disulphide bonds are formed in the outer membrane proteins and new EBs develop within the enlarging vesicle. The developing chlamydiaceal microcolony within the vesicle is termed inclusion body which is typically perinuclear and may contain 100–500 EBs (Fig. 13.5F).
- *Release of new* EBs into the extracellular space occurs following rupture of the inclusion body (Fig. 13.5E). The liberated EBs then infect the new cells where the whole cycle is repeated (Fig. 13.5).

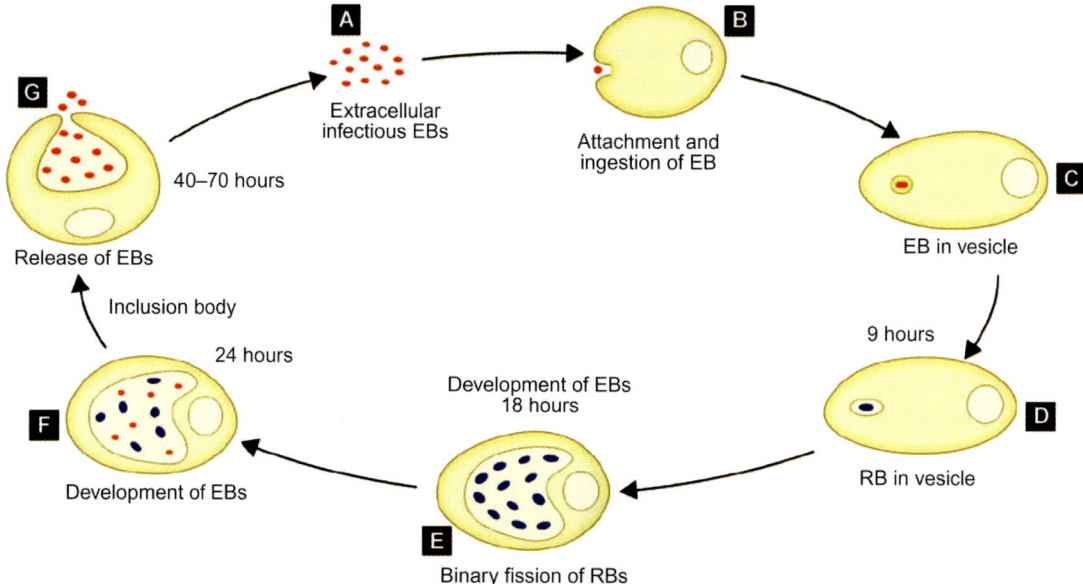

Fig. 13.5A to G: *Life cycle of Chlamydia*

Ocular infections produced by Chlamydia

Ocular infections produced by Chlamydia in human beings are summarised in Table 13.4.

■ TRACHOMA

Trachoma (previously known as *Egyptian ophthalmia*) is a chronic keratoconjunctivitis, primarily affecting the superficial epithelium of conjunctiva and cornea simultaneously. It is characterised by a mixed follicular and papillary response of conjunctival tissue, pannus formation and in late stages cicatrization giving rough appearance. The word 'trachoma' comes from the Greek word for 'rough' which describes the surface appearance of the conjunctiva in chronic trachoma. It is still one of the leading causes of preventable blindness in the world.

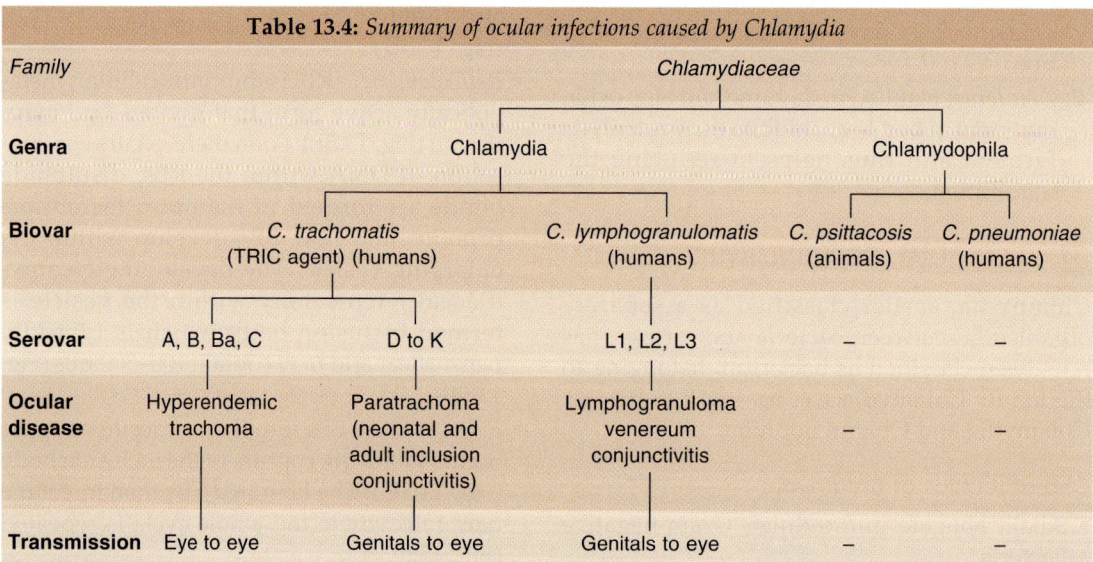

Table 13.4: *Summary of ocular infections caused by Chlamydia*					
Family			Chlamydiaceae		
Genra		Chlamydia			Chlamydophila
Biovar	C. trachomatis (TRIC agent) (humans)		C. lymphogranulomatis (humans)	C. psittacosis (animals)	C. pneumoniae (humans)
Serovar	A, B, Ba, C	D to K	L1, L2, L3	–	–
Ocular disease	Hyperendemic trachoma	Paratrachoma (neonatal and adult inclusion conjunctivitis)	Lymphogranuloma venereum conjunctivitis	–	–
Transmission	Eye to eye	Genitals to eye	Genitals to eye	–	–

ETIOLOGY

A. Causative organism. Trachoma is caused by the bacterium *Chlamydia trachomatis,* biovar TRIC. The organism is epitheliotropic and produces intracytoplasmic inclusion bodies called *HP bodies (Halberstaedter-Prowazek bodies).* Presently, 12 serovars of *Chlamydia trachomatis* biovar TRIC (A, B, Ba, C, D, E, F, G, H, I, J and K) have been identified using microimmuno-fluorescence techniques.

- *Serovars A, B, Ba and C* are associated with hyperendemic (blinding) trachoma.
- *Serovars D to K* are associated with inclusion conjunctivitis (oculogenital chlamydial disease).

B. Predisposing factors include:

- *Age.* The infection is usually contracted during infancy and early childhood. Otherwise, there is no age bar.
- *Sex.* As far as sex is concerned, there is general agreement that preponderance exists in the females both in number and in severity of disease.
- *Race.* No race is immune to trachoma, but the disease is very common in Jews and comparatively less common among Negroes.
- *Climate.* Trachoma is more common in areas with dry and dusty weather.
- *Socioeconomic status.* The disease is more common in poor classes owing to unhygienic living conditions, overcrowding, unsanitary conditions, abundant fly population, paucity of water, lack of materials like separate towels and handkerchiefs, and lack of education and understanding about spread of contagious diseases.
- *Environmental factors* like exposure to dust, smoke, irritants, sunlight, etc. increase the risk of contracting disease. Therefore, outdoor workers are more affected in comparison to office workers.

C. Source of infection. In trachoma endemic zones, the main source of infection is the conjunctival discharge of the affected person. Therefore, superimposed other bacterial infections help in transmission of the disease by increasing the conjunctival secretions.

D. Modes of infection. Infection may spread from eye to eye by any of the following modes:

1. *Direct spread* of infection may occur through contact by airborne or waterborne modes.
2. *Vector transmission* of trachoma is common through flies.
3. *Material transfer* plays an important role in the spread of trachoma. Material transfer can occur through contaminated fingers of doctors, nurses and contaminated tonometers. Other sources of material transfer of infection are use of common towel, handkerchief, bedding and *surma*-rods.

PREVALENCE

Trachoma is a worldwide disease, but it is highly prevalent in North Africa, Middle East and certain regions of South-East Asia. It is believed to affect some 500 million people in the world. There are about 150 million cases with active trachoma and about 30 million having trichiasis, needing lid surgery. Trachoma is responsible for 15–20% of the world's blindness, being second only to cataract.

CLINICAL AND PATHOLOGICAL FEATURES

Clinical features of trachoma can be described into two phases.

I. Phase of active trachoma

Phase of active trachoma usually occurs during childhood due to active chlamydial infection.

- *Incubation period* of active trachoma varies from 7 to 14 days.
- *Onset of disease* is usually insidious (subacute), however, rarely it may present in acute form.

Symptoms

Symptoms of active trachoma are determined by the absence or presence of secondary other bacterial infection (a very common situation).

- *In the absence of secondary infection*, a pure trachoma is characterized by following symptoms:
- Mild foreign body sensation
- Occasional lacrimation
- Slight stickiness of the lids
- Scanty mucoid discharge.

Note. The above symptoms are so mild that the disease is usually neglected so, the term *trachoma dubium* was suggested.

■ *In the presence of secondary other bacterial infection,* typical symptoms of acute mucopurulent conjunctivitis develop (*see* page 63).

Signs

A. Conjunctival signs

1. *Congestion* of upper tarsal and forniceal conjunctiva.

2. *Conjunctival follicles.* Follicles (Fig. 13.6) look like boiled sago-grains and are commonly seen on upper tarsal conjunctiva and fornix; but may also be present in the lower fornix, plica semilunaris and caruncle. Sometimes, follicles may be seen on the bulbar conjunctiva (pathognomonic of trachoma).

■ *Pathological structure of follicle.* Follicles are formed due to scattered aggregation of lymphocytes and other cells in the adenoid layer. Central part of each follicle is made up of mononuclear histiocytes, few lymphocytes and large multinucleated cells called *Leber cells.* The cortical part is made up of a zone of lymphocytes showing active proliferation. Blood vessels are present in the most peripheral part. In later stages, signs of necrosis are also seen. Presence of Leber cells and signs of necrosis differentiate trachoma follicles from follicles of other forms of follicular conjunctivitis.

3. *Papillary hyperplasia.* Papillae are reddish, flat topped raised areas which give red and velvety appearance to the tarsal conjunctiva (Fig. 13.7).

■ *Pathologically* each papilla consists of central core of numerous dilated blood vessels surrounded by lymphocytes and covered by hypertrophic epithelium.

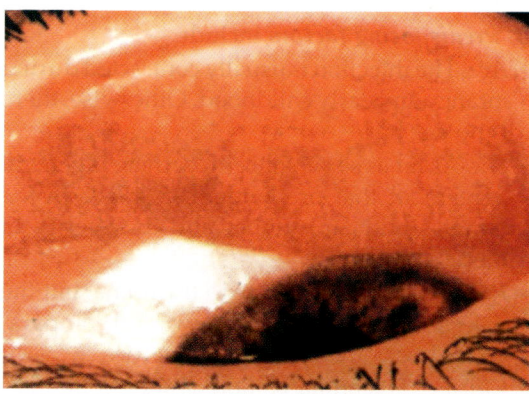

Fig. 13.7: *Trachomatous inflammation (TI) intense*

B. Corneal signs

1. *Superficial keratitis* may be present in the upper part.

2. *Herbert follicles* refer to typical follicles present in the limbal area. *Histologically* these are similar to conjunctival follicles.

3. *Progressive pannus,* i.e. infiltration of the cornea associated with vascularization is seen in upper part (Fig. 13.8). The vessels are superficial and lie between epithelium and Bowman's membrane. Later on, Bowman's membrane is also destroyed. Pannus in active trachoma is progressive in which infiltration of cornea is ahead of vascularization (Fig. 13.8A).

4. *Corneal ulcer* may sometime develop at the advancing edge of pannus. Such ulcers are usually shallow which may become chronic and indolent.

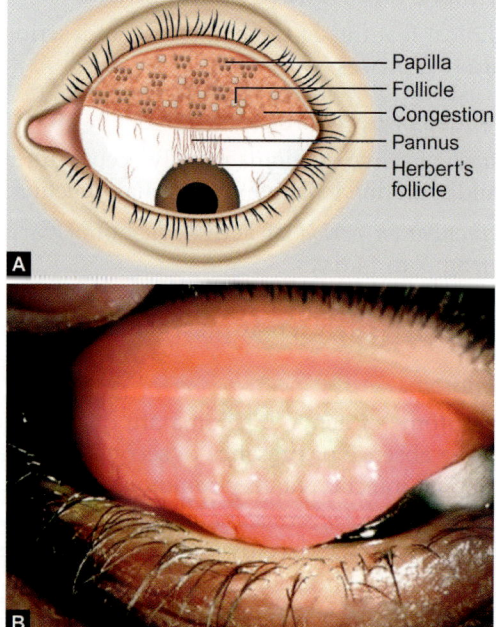

Papilla
Follicle
Congestion
Pannus
Herbert's follicle

Fig. 13.6: *Signs of active trachoma. A, Diagrammatic; B, Clinical photograph of trachomatous inflammation (TF) follicular*

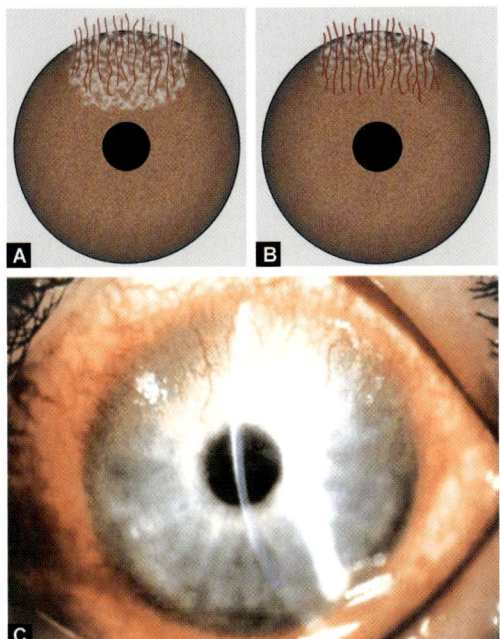

Fig. 13.8: *Trachomatous pannus. A, Progressive; B, Regressive (diagrammatic); C, Clinical photograph*

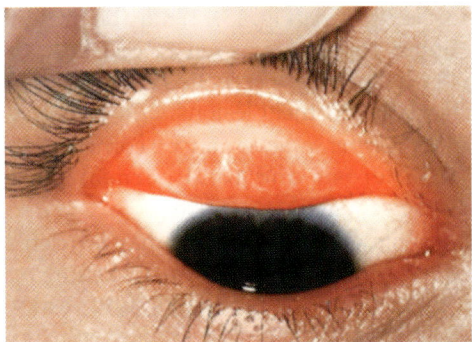

Fig. 13.9: *Trachomatous scarring (TS)*

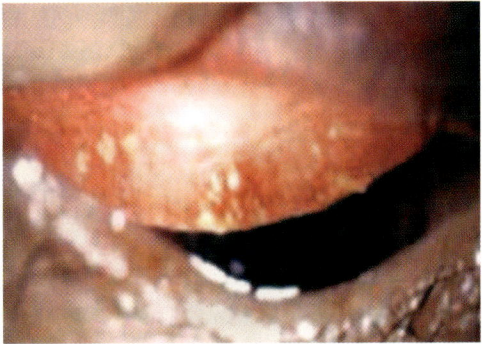

Fig. 13.10: *Concretions in upper palpebral conjunctiva*

II. *Phase of cicatricial trachoma*

Cicatricial phase of trachoma manifests in middle age. It results due to continued mild grade chronic inflammation. In fact recurrent infection elicits chronic immune response consisting of cell-mediated delayed hyper-sensitivity (type IV) reaction to the intermittent presence of chlamydial antigen, which is responsible for cicatricial phase of trachoma. The end stage of cicatricial trachoma is also referred to as sequelae of trachoma. This phase is characterized by following clinical features.

A. Conjunctival signs

i. *Conjunctival scarring* (Fig. 13.9), which may be irregular, star-shaped or linear. Linear scar present in the sulcus subtarsalis is called *Arlt's line.*

ii. *Concretions* are hard looking whitish deposits varying from pinpoint to 2 mm in size (Fig. 13.10). These are not calcareous deposits, but are formed due to accumulation of dead epithelial cells and inspissated mucus in the depressions called *glands of Henle*. Hence, the name is misnomer.

iii. *Other conjunctival sequelae* include *concretions, pseudocyst, xerosis* and *symblepharon.*

B. Corneal sign

i. *Regressive pannus* (pannus siccus) in which (Fig. 13.8B) vessels extend a short distance beyond the area of infiltration.

ii. *Herbert pits* are the oval or circular pitted scars, left after healing of Herbert follicles in the limbal area (Fig. 13.11).

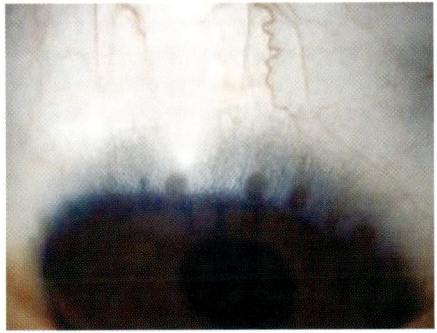

Fig. 13.11: *Trachomatous Herbert's pits*

iii. *Corneal opacity* (Fig. 13.12) may be present in the upper part. It may even extend down and involve the papillary area. It is the end result of trachomatous corneal lesions.

iv. *Other corneal sequelae* may be corneal ectasia, corneal xerosis and total corneal pannus (blinding sequelae).

C. Lid signs. *Sequelae in the lids* may be trichiasis (Fig. 13.13), entropion, tylosis (thickening of lid margin), ptosis, madarosis and ankyloblepharon.

D. Lacrimal apparatus sequelae may be chronic dacryocystitis, and chronic dacryoadenitis.

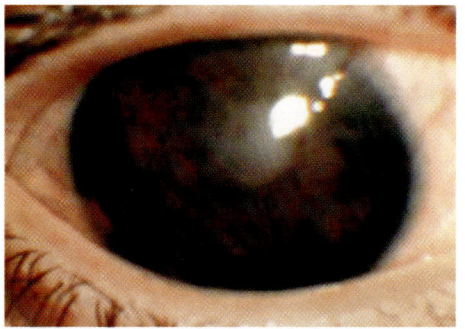

Fig. 13.12: *Trachomatous corneal opacity (CO)*

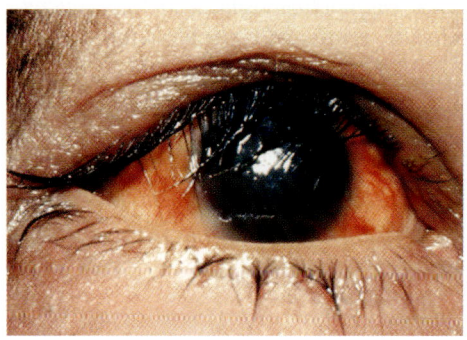

Fig. 13.13: *Trachomatous trichiasis (TT)*

GRADING OF TRACHOMA

McCallan's classification

McCallan, in 1908, divided the clinical course of the trachoma into four stages:

1. *Stage* I (incipient trachoma or stage of infiltration). It is characterized by hyperaemia of palpebral conjunctiva and immature follicles.
2. *Stage* II (established trachoma or stage of florid infiltration). It is characterized by

appearance of mature follicles, papillae and progressive corneal pannus.

3. *Stage* III (cicatrising trachoma or stage of scarring). It includes obvious scarring of palpebral conjunctiva.
4. *Stage* IV (healed trachoma or stage of sequelae). The disease is quiet and cured but sequelae due to cicatrisation, give rise to symptoms.

WHO classification

The latest simplified classification suggested by WHO in 1987 is as follows (FISTO):

1. *TF: Trachomatous inflammation-follicular*. It is the stage of active trachoma with predominantly follicular inflammation. To diagnose this stage at least five or more follicles (each 0.5 mm or more in diameter) must be present on the upper tarsal conjunctiva (*see* Fig. 13.6). Further, the deep tarsal vessels should be visible through the follicles and papillae.

2. *TI: Trachomatous inflammation intense*. This stage is diagnosed when pronounced inflammatory thickening of the upper tarsal conjunctiva obscures more than half of the normal deep tarsal vessels (*see* Fig. 13.7).

3. *TS: Trachomatous scarring*. This stage is diagnosed by the presence of scarring in the tarsal conjunctiva. These scars are easily visible as white, bands or sheets (fibrosis) in the tarsal conjunctiva (*see* Fig. 13.9).

4. *TT: Trachomatous trichiasis*. TT is labelled when at least one eyelash rubs the eyeball. Evidence of recent removal of inturned eyelashes should also be graded as trachomatous trichiasis (Fig. 13.13).

5. *CO: Corneal opacity*. This stage is labelled when easily visible corneal opacity is present over the pupil (Fig. 13.12). This sign refers to corneal scarring that is so dense that at least part of pupil margin is blurred when seen through the opacity. The definition is intended to detect corneal opacities that cause significant visual impairment (less than 6/18).

COMPLICATIONS

The only complication of trachoma is corneal ulcer which may occur due to rubbing by concretions, or trichiasis with superimposed bacterial infection.

DIAGNOSIS

A. Clinical diagnosis of trachoma is made from its typical signs. Clinical grading of each case should be done as per WHO classification into TF, TI, TS, TT or CO.

B. Laboratory diagnosis. Advanced laboratory tests are employed for research purposes only. Laboratory diagnosis of trachoma includes:

1. *Conjunctival cytology.* Giemsa-stained smears showing a predominantly polymorphonuclear reaction with presence of plasma cells and Leber cells is suggestive of trachoma.

2. *Detection of inclusion bodies* in conjunctival smear may be possible by Giemsa stain, iodine stain or immunofluorescent staining, especially in cases with active trachoma.

3. *Enzyme-linked immunosorbent assay* (ELISA) for chlamydial antigens.

4. *Polymerase chain reaction* (PCR) is also useful.

5. *Isolation of Chlamydia* is possible by yolk sac inoculation method and tissue culture technique. Standard single-passage McCoy cell culture requires at least 3 days.

6. *Serotyping of TRIC agents* is done by detecting specific antibodies using microimmunofluorescence (micro-IF) method. *Direct monoclonal fluorescent antibody microscopy* of conjunctival smear is rapid and inexpensive.

DIFFERENTIAL DIAGNOSIS

1. Active trachoma with follicular hypertrophy must be differentiated from acute adenoviral follicular conjunctivitis (epidemic keratoconjunctivitis) as follows:

- *Distribution of follicles* in trachoma is mainly on upper palpebral conjunctiva and upper fornix, while in EKC lower palpebral conjunctiva and lower fornix is predominantly involved.
- *Associated signs* such as papillae and pannus are characteristic of trachoma.
- *Laboratory diagnosis* of trachoma helps in differentiation of clinically indistinguishable cases.

2. Active trachoma with predominant papillary hypertrophy needs to be differentiated from palpebral form of spring catarrh as follows:

- *Papillae* are large in size and usually there is typical cobble-stone arrangement in spring catarrh.
- *pH of tears* is usually alkaline in spring catarrh, while in trachoma it is acidic.
- *Discharge* is ropy in spring catarrh.
- *Follicles and pannus* may also be present in trachoma.
- *Conjunctival cytology* and other laboratory tests for trachoma usually help in diagnosis in clinically indistinguishable cases.

MANAGEMENT

Management of trachoma includes curative as well as prophylactic measures.

A. Treatment of trachoma

I. Treatment of active trachoma

Stage TF and TI of WHO classification constitute active trachoma in which acute infection is present, and therefore, treatment is directed at eliminating the Chlamydia organism.

Antibiotics, thus constitute the mainstay of treatment of active trachoma. These can be given topically or systemically or in combination.

1. *Topical therapy regimes* are best for individual cases and consist of:

- *Tetracycline* (1%) or erythromycin (1%) eye ointment twice daily for 6 weeks, or
- *Sulfacetamide* (20%) eye drops three times a day along with 1% tetracycline eye ointment at bed time for 6 weeks.

2. *Systemic antibiotic therapy regimes* include:

- *Tetracycline* or *erythromycin* 250 mg orally, four times a day for 3–4 weeks, or
- *Doxycycline* 100 mg orally twice daily for 3–4 weeks, constitute the traditional standard systemic therapy.
- *Azithromycin* 20 mg/kg body weight up to maximum 1 g as single oral dose is as effective as 6 weeks of topical therapy and so is presently considered the first drug of choice. It is not used in pregnancy and children below 6 years of age.

3. *Combined topical and systemic therapy regime.* It is preferred when the ocular infection is severe (TI) or when there is associated genital infection. It includes:

- *Tetracycline* (1%) or *erythromycin* eye ointment 2 times a day for 6 weeks; and
- *Azithromycin* single oral dose (first choice) or tetracycline or erythromycin 250 mg orally 4 times a day for 2 weeks.

II. Treatment of cicatricial (inactive) trachoma

Stages TS, TI and CO of WHO classification constitute the inactive trachoma during which infection is no longer present, i.e. only trachoma sequelae are present, and therefore, treatment is directed towards these sequelae as below:

Stage TS measures include:
- *Concretions* should be removed with a hypodermic needle.
- *Conjunctival xerosis* should be treated by artificial tears (lubricating drops).

Stage TI includes trichiasis and cicatricial entropion.
- *Trichiasis,* a few misdirected cilia, should be treated with permanent lash removal measures such as electrolysis, cryolysis, and radiofrequency epilation.
- *Bilamellar tarsal resection* is the surgical procedure of choice for multiple misdirected lashes.
- *Cicatricial entropion* should be corrected surgically.

Stage CO (corneal opacification) constitutes stage of marked visual disability or blindness. After treating other trachoma sequelae, following measures must be taken:
- *Penetrating keratoplasty (PK)* is indicated for significant corneal scarring. However, the outcome is less than optimum, as these patients have extensive corneal vascularisation.
- *Keratoprosthesis (KP)* is indicated in bilateral blind cases with extensive corneal scarring and ocular surface problems.
- *Punctal occlusion and lateral tarsorrhaphy,* which takes care of the coexistent ocular surface problems, may be useful adjuncts for increasing the success of the above surgeries.

B. Prophylaxis for trachoma infection and blindness

Since immunity is very poor and short lived, so reinfections and recurrences are likely to occur. So, prophylactic measures are essential.

WHO defines blinding trachoma elimination as:
- TF prevalence, 5% in 1–9 years children, and
- TI prevalence, 1 per 1000 in total population.

SAFE strategy

The WHO's GET 2020 program (Global Elimination of Trachoma by 2020), has adopted the so-called SAFE strategy for prophylaxis against trachoma infection and prevention of blindness.

SAFE strategy includes:

S : Surgery (tertiary prevention)
A : Antibiotic use (secondary prevention)
F : Facial hygiene (primary prevention)
E : Environmental changes (primordial prevention).

1. *Environmental changes (primordial prevention).* Flies and other fomites are the common causes of spread of trachoma. So, environmental sanitation will constitute the primordial prevention for trachoma. Recommended environmental sanitation measures include:

- Provision of water latrines and good water supply to reduce flies and improve washing habits,
- Refuse dumps,
- Sprays to control flies,
- Animal pens away from human household, and
- Health education to improve personal and environmental hygiene.

2. *Facial hygiene (primary prevention).* Facial hygiene is critical measure for primary prevention of trachoma and should include:

- *Frequent face wash* with clean water to eliminate the potentially infectious ocular secretions.
- *Avoidance of common use* of towel, handkerchief, surma-rods, etc. are important facial hygienic measures to prevent spread of trachoma infections.

3. *Antibiotics for prevention against trachoma (secondary prevention).* Use of antibiotics constitutes the secondary prevention against trachoma. Current WHO recommendations for community-based mass antibiotic therapy in endemic areas are as follows:

i. *In areas with 10% or more prevalence of active trachoma (TF in children 1–9 years) recommendation are as below:*

- *Oral azithromycin* (single dose of 20 mg/kg up to 1 g), should be administered to all community members.
- *Tetracycline eye ointment* twice daily for 6 weeks is recommended for all pregnant women, children, 6 months and those allergic to macrolides.

Note. The mass antibiotic therapy should be given once in a year for continuous three years, after which reassessment of prevalence should be made. The annual treatment should be continued till the TF prevalence in 1–9 years children of that area becomes less than 5%.

ii. *In areas with prevalence between more than 5% and less than 10%,* the targeted antibiotic therapy is recommended only among family members and close contacts of the patients.

iii. *In areas with prevalence less than 5%,* treatment of the patients only is recommended.

4. *Surgery (tertiary prevention).* Surgery for trichiasis and entropion constitutes tertiary prevention for trachomatous corneal blindness. WHO recommends bilamellar tarsal rotation surgery at community level for the affected persons.

ADULT INCLUSION CONJUNCTIVITIS

It is a type of acute follicular conjunctivitis associated with mucopurulent discharge. It usually affects the sexually active young adults.

ETIOLOGY

- *Serotypes D to K of Chlamydia trachomatis* are associated with adult inclusion conjunctivitis.
- *Primary source of infection* is urethritis in males and cervicitis in females.
- *Transmission of infection* may occur to eyes either through contaminated genital-hand-eye or genital-eye contact.
- *Spread of infection may also occur* through contaminated water of swimming pools (hence the name *swimming pool conjunctivitis*).

CLINICAL FEATURES

Incubation period of the disease is 5–14 days.

Symptoms are similar to acute mucopurulent conjunctivitis and include:

- *Ocular discomfort, foreign body sensation,*
- *Mild photophobia,* and
- *Mucopurulent discharge* from the eyes.

Signs of inclusion conjunctivitis are (Fig. 13.14):

- *Conjunctival hyperaemia,* more marked in the lower palpebral conjunctiva and fornix.
- *Acute follicular hypertrophy* predominantly of lower palpebral conjunctiva and fornix.
- *Superficial keratitis* in upper half of cornea. Sometimes, superior micropannus may also occur.
- *Pre-auricular lymphadenopathy* (non-tender) is a usual finding on the ipsilateral side.

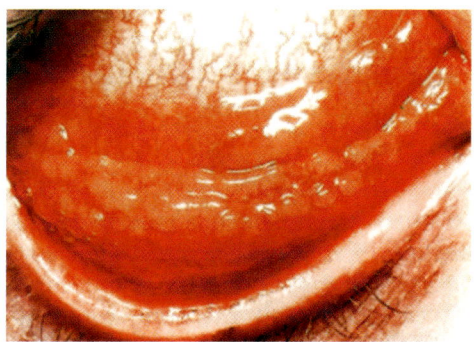

Fig. 13.14: *Signs of acute follicular conjunctivitis*

Clinical course. The disease runs a benign course and often evolves into the chronic follicular conjunctivitis.

Investigations required, their role and status is same as described above for trachoma.

Differential diagnosis must be made from other causes of acute follicular conjunctivitis.

MANAGEMENT

Treatment

1. *Topical therapy.* It consists of tetracycline (1%) eye ointment 4 times a day for 6 weeks.

2. *Systemic therapy* is very important, since the condition is often associated with an asymptomatic venereal infection. Commonly employed antibiotics are:

- *Azithromycin* 1 g as a single dose repeated after one week is currently drug of choice, a 3rd dose is required in 30% of cases.

- *Tetracycline* 250 mg four times a day for 3–4 weeks, or
- *Erythromycin* 250 mg four times a day for 3–4 weeks (only when the tetracycline is contraindicated, e.g. in pregnant and lactating females), or
- *Doxycycline* 100 mg twice a day for 3 weeks.

3. *Referral to genitourinary specialist* is mandatory. Sexual partners should be treated simultaneously. Attention should also be given to other sexually transmitted diseases, contact tracing and pregnancy testing.

Prophylaxis

- Improvement in personal hygiene.
- Regular chlorination of swimming pool water will definitely decrease the spread of disease.
- Patient's sexual partner should be examined and treated. Abstinence of sexual contact until completion of treatment.

VIRAL CONJUNCTIVITIS

Most of the viral infections tend to affect the epithelium, both of the conjunctiva and cornea; so, the typical viral lesion is a 'keratoconjunctivitis'. In some viral infections, conjunctival involvement is more prominent (e.g. pharyngoconjunctival fever), while in others cornea is more involved (e.g. herpes simplex).

Viral infections of conjunctiva include:
- Adenovirus conjunctivitis
- Herpes simplex keratoconjunctivitis
- Herpes zoster conjunctivitis
- Molluscum contagiosum conjunctivitis
- Poxvirus conjunctivitis
- Myxovirus conjunctivitis
- Paramyxovirus conjunctivitis
- Arbor virus conjunctivitis.

Clinical presentations of acute viral conjunctivitis include:
- Acute follicular conjunctivitis
- Acute haemorrhagic conjunctivitis.

ADENOVIRAL CONJUNCTIVITIS

Adenoviruses are the commonest causes of viral conjunctivitis. These are non-enveloped, double-stranded DNA viruses, which replicate within the nucleus of host cells. General reservoir of adenoviruses is only human. Fifty-one distinct human adenoviral serotypes have been described and are classified into six subgenera (A–F). More than half of all adenoviral subtypes (32) belong to subgenus D. With a few exceptions, most adenoviral conjunctivitis is caused by this genus.

Clinical types of adenoviral conjunctivitis include:
- Epidemic keratoconjunctivitis (EKC)
- Nonspecific acute follicular conjunctivitis
- Pharyngoconjunctival fever (PCF)
- Chronic relapsing adenoviral conjunctivitis.

EPIDEMIC KERATOCONJUNCTIVITIS (EKC)

It is a type of acute follicular conjunctivitis mostly associated with superficial punctate keratitis and usually occurs in epidemics, hence the name epidemic keratoconjunctivitis (EKC).

Etiology

EKC is mostly caused by adenoviruses type 8, 19 and 37 with type 8 being the classic cause. The condition is markedly contagious and spreads through contact with contaminated fingers, solutions and tonometers.

Clinical features

Incubation period after infection is about 8 days and virus is shed from the inflamed eye for 2–3 weeks.

Symptoms

Symptoms are similar to severe form of acute catarrhal conjunctivitis and include:
- *Redness* of sudden onset associated with *watering*, usually profuse, with mild mucoid discharge.
- *Ocular discomfort* and foreign body sensation.
- *Photophobia*, usually mild, becomes marked when cornea is involved.

Signs

I. *Eyelids are swollen* causing narrowing of palpebral aperture.

II. *Conjunctival signs* are:
- *Hyperaemia* is usually marked and prominent.

- *Chemosis* of conjunctiva is often present.
- *Follicles* of small to moderate size typically involving the lower fornix and palpebral conjunctiva form the characteristic feature (Fig. 13.15).
- *Papillary reaction* may also be seen in many cases.
- *Petechial subconjunctival haemorrhages* may be seen in severe adenoviral conjunctivitis (Fig. 13.16).
- *Pseudomembrane* lining the lower fornix and palpebral conjunctiva (Fig. 13.16) may be formed in about 3% patients with severe inflammation.

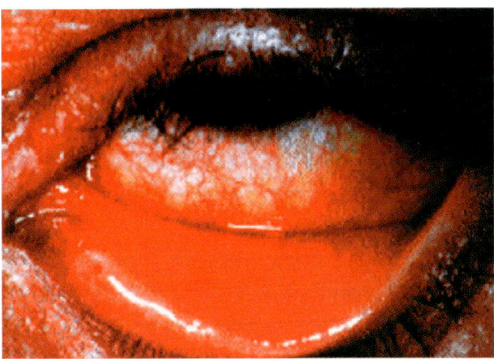

Fig. 13.15: *Acute follicular adenoviral conjunctivitis*

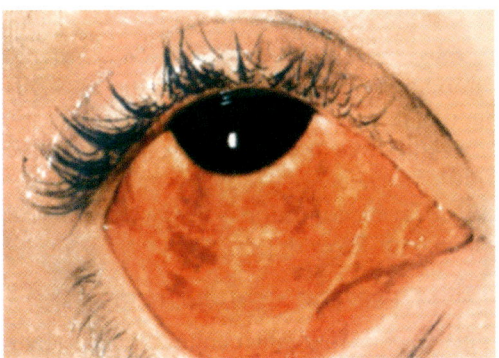

Fig. 13.16: *Pseudomembrane and petechial subconjunctival haemorrhage in acute epidemic keratoconjunctivitis (EKC)*

III. Corneal involvement occurs in about 80% of cases and is characterized by following lesions:

- *Epithelial microcystic* diffuse fine non-staining lesions are common during the early stage.

- *Superficial punctate keratitis* (SPK), a typical feature of EKC (Fig. 13.17), usually occurs after 10 days of onset of symptoms and lasts for 3 weeks even after subsidence of conjunctival inflammation.
- *Subepithelial infiltrates* may develop under the focal epithelial lesions in 20–50% of cases. These opacities may be initially disabling and may persist for months to years.

IV. Pre-auricular lymphadenopathy is associated in almost all cases of EKC.

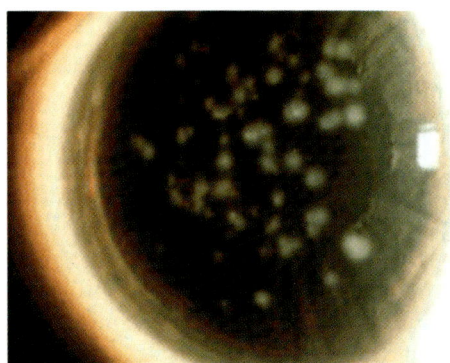

Fig. 13.17: *Superficial punctate keratitis in EKC*

Differential diagnosis

EKC needs to be differentiated from *other causes of acute follicular conjunctivitis* which include:

- *Other types of adenoviral keratoconjunctivitis* such as:
  - Nonspecific acute follicular conjunctivitis, and
  - Pharyngoconjunctival fever.
- *Acute haemorrhagic conjunctivitis*
- *Herpes simplex virus conjunctivitis*
- *Systemic viral infections* such as herpes zoster conjunctivitis, measles, mumps and chikungunya virus conjunctivitis
- *Adult inclusion conjunctivitis.*

Differentiation is made from:

- *Typical clinical features* of each entity described.
- *Investigations* are required mainly for research purposes and in some nonresolving cases, and include:
  - *Conjunctival cytology* with Giemsa stain shows predominantly mononuclear cells in adenoviral conjunctivitis and multinucleated gaint cells in herpetic conjunctivitis.

- *Polymerase chain reaction (PCR) test* is sensitive and specific for viral DNA.
- *Point-of-care immunochromatography test* takes only 10 minutes to detect adenoviral antigens in tears and have excellent sensitivity and specificity.
- *Viral cultures* are tedious and time consuming with variable sensitivity but 100% specificity.

Treatment

1. *Supportive treatment* for amelioration of symptoms is the only treatment required and includes:

- Cold compresses, and sun glasses to decrease glare.
- Decongestant and lubricant tear drops to decrease discomfort.

2. *Topical antibiotics* help to prevent superadded bacterial infections.

3. *Topical antiviral drugs* are not beneficial in adenoviral conjunctivitis. Recently promising results are reported with adenine arabinosides (Ara-A) and cidofovir.

4. *Topical steroids should not be used during active inflammation* as these may enhance viral replication and extend the period of infectivity. Weak steroids such as fluorometholone or loteprednol (0.5%) are indicated in patients with subepithelial infiltrates, and in those with membrane formation.

Prevention of spread of infection to the contacts

It is very important as the adenoviral conjunctivitis is highly contagious and patients may be infectious for up to 11 days after onset.

Transmission usually occurs
- From eye to fingers to eyes.
- *Tonometers, contact lenses* and *eye drops* are other routes of transmission.

Preventive measures include:
- Frequent handwashing,
- Relative isolation of infected individual,
- Avoiding eye rubbing and common use of towel or handkerchief sharing, and
- Disinfection of ophthalmic instruments and clinical surfaces after examination of a patient is essential.

NONSPECIFIC ACUTE FOLLICULAR CONJUNCTIVITIS

- *Most common* form of acute follicular conjunctivitis.
- *Caused by* adenovirus serotypes 1 to 11 and 19.
- *Clinical features* are of milder form of acute follicular conjunctivitis. Corneal involvement is not known.
- *Treatment and preventive measures* are similar to as described for EKC.

PHARYNGOCONJUNCTIVAL FEVER

Etiology. It is a highly infectiveness adenoviral infection commonly associated with subtypes 3, 4 and 7. *Transmitted by* three routes: Personal contact, fomites or through swimming pools or ponds.

Clinical features. Pharyngoconjunctival fever (PCF) primarily affects children and appears in epidemic form. It is characterised by an:
- Acute follicular conjunctivitis, associated with pharyngitis.
- Fever and pre-auricular lymphadenopathy.
- Corneal involvement in the form of superficial punctate keratitis is seen only in 30% of cases.

Treatment is usually supportive as described for EKC.

NEWCASTLE CONJUNCTIVITIS

Etiology. It is a rare type of acute follicular conjunctivitis caused by Newcastle virus. The infection is derived from contact with diseased owls; and thus the condition mainly affects poultry workers.

Clinically, the condition is similar to pharyngoconjunctival fever.

ACUTE HERPETIC CONJUNCTIVITIS

Acute herpetic follicular conjunctivitis is always an accompaniment of the 'primary herpetic infection', which mainly occurs in small children and in adolescents.

Etiology

The disease is commonly caused by herpes simplex virus type 1 and spreads by kissing or other close personal contacts. HSV type 2 associated with genital infections, may also involve the eyes in adults as well as children, though rarely.

Clinical features

Acute herpetic follicular conjunctivitis is usually a unilateral affection with an incubation period of 5–14 days. It may occur in two clinical forms— typical and atypical.

- In *typical form*, the follicular conjunctivitis is usually associated with other lesions of primary infection such as vesicular lesions of face and lids.
- In *atypical form*, the follicular conjunctivitis occurs without lesions of the face, eyelid and the condition then resembles epidemic kerato-conjunctivitis. The condition may evolve through phases of no-specific hyperaemia, follicular hyperplasia and pseudomembrane formation.
- *Corneal involvement*, though rare, is not uncommon in primary herpes. It may be in the form of fine or coarse epithelial keratitis or typical dendritic keratitis.
- *Preauricular lymphadenopathy* occurs almost always.

Treatment

Primary herpetic infection is usually self-limiting.
- The topical antiviral drugs control the infection effectively and prevent recurrences.
- Supportive measures are similar to EKC.

ACUTE HAEMORRHAGIC CONJUNCTIVITIS

It is an acute inflammation of conjunctiva characterised by multiple conjunctival haemo-rrhages, conjunctival hyperaemia and mild follicular hyperplasia.

Etiology

The disease is caused by picornaviruses (enterovirus type 70) which are RNA viruses of small (pico) size. The disease is very contagious and is transmitted by direct hand-to-eye contact.

Clinical features

The disease has occurred in an epidemic form in the far East, Africa and England and hence the name 'epidemic haemorrhagic conjunctivitis (EHC)' has been suggested. An epidemic of the disease was first recognized in Ghana in 1969 at the time when Apollo XI spacecraft was launched, hence the name '*Apollo conjunctivitis*'.

- *Incubation period* of EHC is very short (1–2 days).
- *Symptoms* include pain, redness, watering, mild photophobia, transient blurring of vision and lid swelling.
- *Signs* of EHC are conjunctival congestion, chemosis, multiple haemorrhages in bulbar conjunctiva, mild follicular hyperplasia, lid oedema and pre-auricular lymphadenopathy (Fig. 13.18).
- *Corneal involvement* may occur in the form of fine epithelial keratitis.

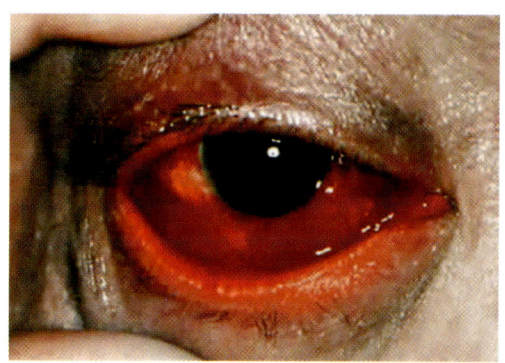

Fig. 13.18: *Acute haemorrhagic conjunctivitis*

Treatment

EHC is very infectious and poses major potential problems of cross-infection.
- *Prophylactic measures* are very important and are same as described for EKC.
- *No specific effective curative treatment* is known. However, broad-spectrum antibiotic eye drops may be used to prevent secondary bacterial infections.
- Usually the disease has a *self-limiting course of 7 days*.
- *Supportive measures* are same as EKC.

OPHTHALMIA NEONATORUM

Ophthalmia neonatorum, or neonatal conjuncti-vitis is the name given to bilateral inflammation of the conjunctiva occurring in an infant, less than 30 days old. It is a preventable disease usually occurring as a result of carelessness at the time of birth. As a matter of fact *any discharge or even watering from the eyes in the first week of life should arouse suspicion of ophthalmia neonatorum,* as tears are not formed till then.

ETIOLOGY

Source and mode of infection

Infection may occur in three ways: Before birth, during birth and after birth.

1. *Before birth* infection is very rare through infected liquor amnii in mothers with ruptured membranes.

2. *During birth.* In vaginally delivered infants, the most common mode of infection is from the infected birth canal especially when the child is born with face presentation or with forceps.

3. *After birth.* Infection may occur during first bath of newborn or from soiled clothes or fingers with infected lochia.

Causative agents

1. Chemical neonatal conjunctivitis. It is caused by (in older days silver nitrate was the common cause) or antibiotics used for prophylaxis.

2. Gonococcal infection was considered a serious disease in the past, as it used to be responsible for 50% of blindness in children. But, the decline in the incidence of gonorrhoea as well as effective methods of prophylaxis and treatment have almost eliminated it in developed countries. However, in many developing countries, it still continues to be a problem.

3. Other bacterial infections, responsible for ophthalmia neonatorum are *Staphylococcus aureus, Haemophilus* species, *Streptococcus haemolyticus,* and *Streptococcus pneumoniae.*

4. Neonatal inclusion conjunctivitis caused by serotypes D to K of *Chlamydia trachomatis* is at present the commonest cause of ophthalmia neonatorum in developed countries.

5. Herpes simplex ophthalmia neonatorum is a rare condition caused by herpes simplex II virus from the infected birth canal.

CLINICAL FEATURES

Incubation period

It varies depending on the type of the causative agent as shown below:

Causative agent	Incubation period
• Chemical	6 hours
• Gonococcal	2–5 days
• Other bacterial	5–8 days
• Neonatal inclusion conjunctivitis	5–14 days
• Herpes simplex	6–15 days

Symptoms and signs

1. *Pain* and *tenderness* in the eyeball.

2. *Conjunctival discharge.* It is purulent in gonococcal ophthalmia neonatorum (Fig. 13.19) and mucoid or mucopurulent in other bacterial cases and neonatal inclusion conjunctivitis.

3. *Lids* are usually swollen in infective cases. Eyelids and periocular vesicles may occur in HSV infection.

4. *Conjunctiva* may show hyperaemia and chemosis. There might be mild papillary response in neonatal inclusion conjunctivitis and herpes simplex ophthalmia neonatorum. Follicular response is typically absent in infants because of immaturity of lymphoid system up to 6–8 weeks of life.

5. *Corneal involvement,* though rare, may occur in the form of superficial punctate keratitis especially in herpes simplex ophthalmia neonatorum.

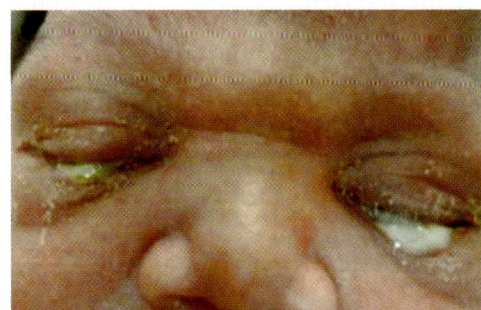

Fig. 13.19: *Gonococcal ophthalmic neonatorum*

Complications

Untreated cases, especially of gonococcal ophthalmia neonatorum, may develop corneal ulceration, which may perforate rapidly resulting in corneal opacification or staphyloma formation.

MANAGEMENT

Prophylaxis

Prophylactic treatment is always better than curative. Prophylaxis needs antenatal, natal and postnatal care.

1. *Antenatal measures* include thorough care of mother and treatment of genital infections when suspected. Surveillance of women during the third trimester of pregnancy for evidence of chlamydial, herpetic or gonococcal infection is critical in prevention of neonatal conjunctivitis.

2. *Natal measures* are of utmost importance, as mostly infection occurs during childbirth.

- Deliveries should be conducted under hygienic conditions taking all aseptic measures.
- The newborn baby's closed lids should be thoroughly cleansed and dried.

3. *Postnatal measures* include:

- *Povidone-iodine* 2.5% solution is effective against the common pathogens, and is widely used.
- *Use of either 1% tetracycline ointment* or 0.5% erythromycin ointment into the eyes of the babies immediately after birth are useful for preventing bacterial and chlamydial ophthalmia neonatorum.
- *Single injection of ceftriaxone* 50 mg/kg IM or IV (not to exceed 125 mg) should be given to infants born to mothers with untreated gonococcal infection.

Note. In the past, 1% silver nitrate solution was put in the eyes of babies immediately after birth (Crede's method). It is mentioned here just for the historical value.

Treatment

As a rule, conjunctival cytology samples and culture sensitivity swabs should be taken before starting the treatment.

1. *Chemical ophthalmia neonatorum* is a self-limiting condition, and does not require any treatment.

2. *Gonococcal ophthalmia neonatorum* needs prompt treatment to prevent complications.

- *Topical therapy* should include:
  - *Saline lavage* hourly till the discharge is eliminated.
  - *Bacitracin eye ointment* 4 times/day. Because of resistant strains topical penicillin therapy is not reliable. However, in cases with proved penicillin susceptibility, *penicillin drops* 5000 to 10000 units per millilitre should be instilled every minute for half an hour, every 5 minutes for next half an hour and then half hourly till the infection is controlled.
  - *If cornea is involved* then atropine sulphate ointment should be applied.

- *Systemic therapy.* Neonates with gonococcal ophthalmia should be treated for 7 days with one of the following regimes:
  - Ceftriaxone 75–100 mg/kg/day IV or IM, qid, or
  - Cefotaxime 100–150 mg/kg/day IV or IM, 12 hourly, or
  - Ciprofloxacin 10–20 mg/kg/day or nor-floxacin 10 mg/kg/day, or
  - If the gonococcal isolate is proved to be susceptible to penicillin, crystalline benzyl penicillin G 50,000 units to full term, normal weight babies and 20,000 units to premature or low weight babies should be given intra-muscularly twice daily for 3 days.

3. *Other bacterial ophthalmia neonatorum* should be treated for 2 weeks by broad-spectrum antibiotic drops and ointments such as neomycin-bacitracin or tobramycin.

4. *Neonatal inclusion conjunctivitis* responds well to topical tetracycline 1% or erythromycin 0.5% eye ointment qid for 3 weeks. However, systemic erythromycin 50 mg/kg/day in 3 or 4 divided days for 2 to 3 weeks should also be given since the presence of Chlamydia agents in the conjunctiva implies colonization of upper respiratory tract as well. Alternatively azithro-mycin suspension 20 mg/kg either as a single dose or once daily for 3 days should be administered. Both parents should also be treated with systemic erythromycin.

5. *Herpes simplex conjunctivitis* is usually a self-limiting disease. However, topical antiviral drugs control the infection more effectively and may prevent the recurrence. High dose intravenous acyclovir is indicated in cases suspected of systemic herpes infection.

GRANULOMATOUS CONJUNCTIVAL INFLAMMATIONS

Granulomatous inflammations of the conjunctiva are characterised by proliferative lesions which usually tend to remain localised to one eye and are mostly associated with regional lymphadenitis.

Common granulomatous conjunctival inflammations are:
- Tuberculosis of conjunctiva
- Sarcoidosis of conjunctiva
- Syphilitic conjunctivitis
- Leprotic conjunctivitis
- Conjunctivitis in tularaemia
- Ophthalmia nodosa.

PARINAUD'S OCULOGLANDULAR SYNDROME

Clinical features: It is the name given to a group of conditions characterised by:
- Unilateral granulomatous conjunctivitis (nodular elevations surrounded by follicles),
- Pre-auricular lymphadenopathy, and
- Fever.

Common causes are tularaemia, cat-scratch disease (*Bartonella henselae* infection), tuberculosis, syphilis, sporotrichosis, lymphogranuloma venereum, etc.

Note. This term (Parinaud's oculoglandular syndrome) is largely obsolete, since the infecting agents can now be usually determined.

OPHTHALMIA NODOSA (CATERPILLAR HAIR CONJUNCTIVITIS)

It is a granulomatous inflammation of the conjunctiva characterized by:
- *Formation of a nodule* on the bulbar conjunctiva in response to irritation caused by the retained *hair of caterpillar*. The disease is, therefore, common in summers.

- The condition may be often mistaken for a tubercular nodule. Histopathological examination reveals hair surrounded by giant cells and lymphocyte.

Treatment consists of excision biopsy of the nodule.

ALLERGIC CONJUNCTIVITIS

It is the inflammation of conjunctiva due to allergic or hypersensitivity reactions which may be immediate (humoral) or delayed (cellular). The conjunctiva is ten times more sensitive than the skin to allergens.

Types
1. Acute allergic conjunctivitis
    - Seasonal allergic conjunctivitis (SAC)
    - Perennial allergic conjunctivitis (PAC)
2. Vernal keratoconjunctivitis (VKC)
3. Atopic keratoconjunctivitis (AKC)
4. Giant papillary conjunctivitis (GPC)
5. Phlyctenular keratoconjunctivitis (PKC)
6. Allergic dermatoconjunctivitis (ADC)

ACUTE ALLERGIC CONJUNCTIVITIS

It is a non-specific allergic conjunctivitis characterised by itching, hyperaemia and mild papillary response. Basically, it is an acute or subacute urticarial reaction.

ETIOLOGY

Acute allergic conjunctivitis, is a type I immediate hypersensitivity reaction mediated by IgE and subsequent mast cell activation, following exposure of ocular surface to airborne allergens. Family history of atopy might be present. Acute allergic conjunctivitis is known to occur in two forms:

1. *Seasonal allergic conjunctivitis (SAC)*. SAC is a response to seasonal allergens such as tree and grass pollens. It is of very common occurrence and may be associated with hay fever (allergic rhinitis) and also known as *hay fever conjunctivitis*. It manifests as acute allergic conjunctivitis.

2. *Perennial allergic conjunctivitis (PAC)* is a response to perennial allergens such as house dust, animal dander and mite. It is not so common. The onset is subacute, the condition is chronic in nature and occurring all through the year.

PATHOLOGY

Pathological features of simple allergic conjunctivitis comprise vascular, cellular and conjunctival responses.

1. *Vascular response* is characterised by sudden and extreme vasodilation and increased permeability of conjunctival vessels leading to exudation.
2. *Cellular response* is in the form of conjunctival infiltration and exudation in the discharge of eosinophils, plasma cells and mast cells producing histamine and histamine-like substances.
3. *Conjunctival response* is in the form of boggy swelling of conjunctiva followed by increased connective tissue formation and mild papillary hyperplasia.

CLINICAL FEATURES

Clinical features are typically bilateral, i.e. both eyes are simultaneously involved.

Symptoms

- *Intense itching* and burning sensation in the eyes associated with
- *Watery, mucus, stringy discharge,* and
- *Mild photophobia.*

Signs

- *Hyperaemia and chemosis* which give a swollen juicy appearance to the conjunctiva.
- *Mild papillary reaction* may be seen on palpebral conjunctiva.
- *Oedema of lids* is often present.

DIAGNOSIS

Diagnosis is made from:
- Typical symptoms and signs,
- Normal conjunctival flora, and
- Cytological examination of conjunctival scrapings shows eosinophilic infiltration.
- Tear film shows elevated levels of IgE and histamine.

TREATMENT

1. *Avoiding known allergen triggers* is critical. Possible strategies for avoiding allergens include:
- SAC patients may benefit from staying indoor during times of high pollen counts, using room and car air conditioners, and keeping windows closed.
- *PAC patients* may benefit from covering beddings with plastic covers, removing carpets and avoiding pets.

2. *Cold compresses* may reduce swelling and may provide some additional relief.

3. *Artificial tears* like carboxymethyl cellulose provide soothing effect.

4. *Topical vasoconstrictors* like naphazoline, antizoline and tetrahydrozoline provide immediate decongestion.

5. *Mast cell stabilizers* such as sodium cromoglycate and nedocromil sodium are very effective in preventing recurrences in atopic cases.

6. *Dual action antihistamines and mast cell stabilizers* such as azelastine, olopatadine and ketotifen are very effective for exacerbations.

7. *Non-steroidal anti-inflammatory drugs (NSAIDs)* like ketorolac tromethamine and diclofenac help by decreasing the activity of cyclo-oxygenase an enzyme responsible for arachidonic acid metabolism which in turn reduce prostaglandin production.

8. *Steroid eye drops* should preferably be avoided. However, these may be prescribed for short duration in severe and non-responsive patients. These help by blocking most allergic inflammatory cascade.

9. *Systemic antihistaminic drugs* are useful in acute cases with marked itching.

VERNAL KERATOCONJUNCTIVITIS (VKC) OR SPRING CATARRH

VKC is a recurrent, bilateral, interstitial, self-limiting, allergic inflammation of the conjunctiva having a periodic seasonal incidence.

ETIOPATHOGENESIS

VKC is found in individuals with predisposed atopic background. It has been considered classically an atopic disorder, mainly type I IgE-mediated hypersensitivity reaction to pollen allergens. However, few studies have reported that pathogenesis of VKC is characterized by Th2 lymphocyte alteration and that the exaggerated IgE response to common allergens is a secondary event.

Predisposing factors

1. *Age and sex.* 4–20 years with a peace incidence between 11 and 13 years; more common in boys than girls.

2. *Season.* More common in summer; hence the name spring catarrh seems to be a misnomer. Recently, it is being labelled as *'warm weather conjunctivitis'*. Seasonal exacerbation, is common, but patients may have symptoms year-round.

3. *Climate.* More prevalent in tropics, less in temperate zones and almost non-existent in cold climate.

4. *Other atopic manifestations,* such as eczema or asthma, are associated in 40–75% patients with VKC.

5. *Family history of atopy* is found in 40–60% of patients.

PATHOLOGY

The typical lesions seen in VKC are palpebral papillae, limbal papillae and Florence-Trantas' spots.

Palpebral papillae are characterised by following histopathological changes:

- *Conjunctival epithelium* contains large number of mast cells, eosinophils and in the area of papilla formation undergoes hyperplasia and sends downward projections into the subepithelial tissue.
- *Adenoid layer* shows marked cellular infiltration by mast cells eosinophils, plasma cells, lymphocytes and histiocytes.
- *Fibrous layer* shows proliferation which later on undergoes hyaline changes.
- *Conjunctival vessels* also show proliferation, increased permeability and vasodilation.

All these pathological changes lead to formation of multiple papillae in the upper tarsal conjunctiva.

Limbal papillae, arranged as confluent lumps around the limbus, histopathologically are characterised by:

- hyperplasia of limbal epithelial cells infiltrated with lymphocytes, plasma cells, macrophages, basophils, many eosinophils and an increased number of conjunctival goblet cells.

Horner-Trantas' spots, which grossly appear as white chalk-like gelatinous nodules are composed of eosinophils and epithelial debris located at the limbus.

CLINICAL FEATURES

Symptoms

Spring catarrh is characterised by:

- *Marked burning and itching sensation* which is usually intolerable and accentuated when patient comes in a warm humid atmosphere. Itching is more marked with palpebral form of disease.
- *Other associated symptoms* include: Mild photophobia, lacrimation, stringy (ropy) discharge and heaviness of lids.

Signs

Signs of vernal keratoconjunctivitis can be described in following three clinical forms:

1. *Palpebral form.* Usually upper tarsal conjunctiva of both eyes is involved. The typical lesion is the presence of hard, flat topped, papillae arranged in a *'cobble-stone'* or *'pavement stone'*, fashion along with conjunctival hyperaemia (Fig. 13.20). Tiny twigs of vessels are found in the centres of the papillae, which

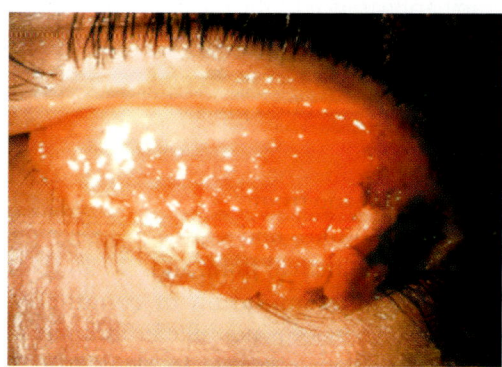

Fig. 13.20: *Palpebral form of vernal keratoconjunctivitis*

help to differentiate these from large follicles such as seen in trachoma. In severe cases, papillae may hypertrophy to produce cauliflower-like excrescences of 'giant papillae'. Conjunctival changes are associated with white ropy discharge.

2. Bulbar limbal form. It is characterised by:

- *Dusky red triangular congestion* of bulbar conjunctiva in palpebral area.
- *Limbal papillae occur as gelatinous, thickened accumulation* of tissue around the limbus as confluent rounded lumps (Fig. 13.21A). Tiny twig-like vessel arising in the centre of each lump differentiate it from limbal follicles. The gelatinous opacification around the limbus may override the cornea.
- *Presence of discrete whitish raised dots* along the limbus (Horner-Trantas' spots) (Fig. 13.21B).

3. Mixed form. It shows combined features of both palpebral and bulbar forms (Fig. 13.22).

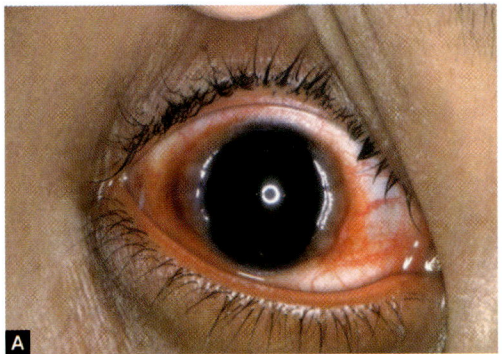

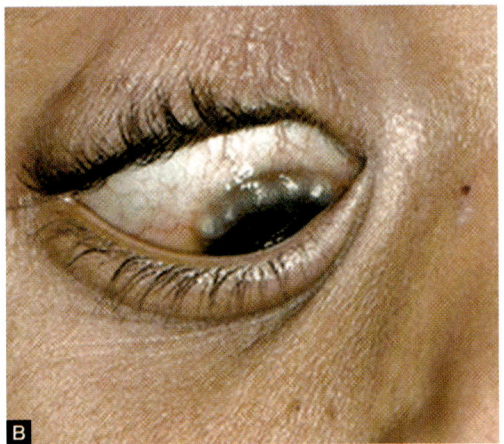

Fig. 13.21: *Bulbar form of VKC depicting. A, Gelatinous membrane around limbus; B, Trantas' spots at limbus*

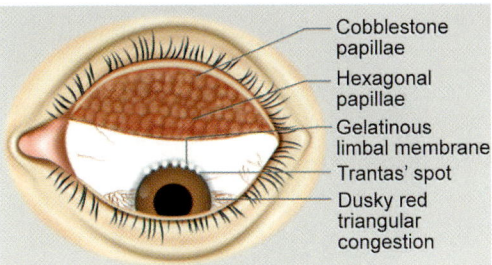

Fig. 13.22: *Artist's diagram of mixed form of vernal kerato-conjunctivitis*

Vernal keratopathy

Corneal involvement in VKC may be primary or secondary due to extension of limbal lesions. Vernal keratopathy is more frequent with palpebral form and includes following types of lesions:

1. *Punctate epithelial keratitis,* involving upper cornea, is usually associated with palpebral form of disease and is caused by:

- Direct mechanical effect of raised palpebral papillae on the corneal epithelium, and
- Toxic effect of inflammatory mediators released from the inflamed tarsal conjunctiva.

The lesions always stain with rose bengal and invariably with fluorescein dye.

2. *Frank epithelial erosions,* leaving Bowman's membrane intact, result due to coalescence of punctate epithelial lesions.

3. *Vernal corneal plaques* result due to coating of bare areas of epithelial macroerosions with a layer of mucus and calcium phosphate (Fig. 13.23A).

4. *Ulcerative vernal keratitis (shield ulceration)* presents as a shallow transverse ulcer in upper part of cornea (Fig. 13.23B). The ulceration results due to epithelial macroerosions. It is a serious problem which may be complicated by bacterial keratitis.

5. *Subepithelial scarring* occurs in the form of a grey and oval ring scar.

6. *Pseudogerontoxon* can develop in recurrent limbal disease and is characterised by a classical 'cupid's bow' outline.

7. *Keratoconus* and other corneal ectasis, seen in patients with long-standing disease are thought, at least partly, to occur because of the affect of eye rubbing.

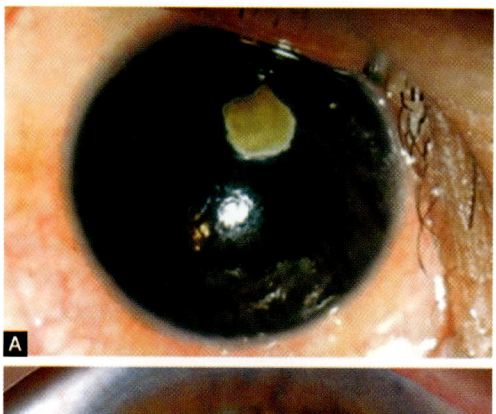

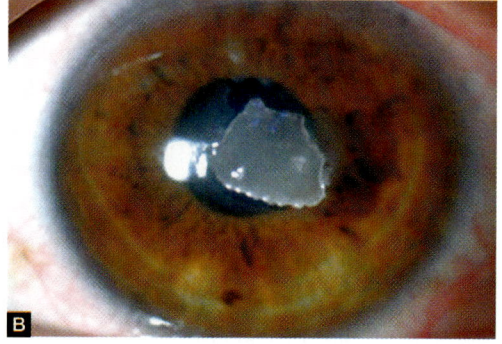

Fig. 13.23: *Vernal keratopathy. A, Vernal corneal plaque; B, Shield ulcer*

Table 13.5 *Comparison of VKC and AKC*		
	VKC	*AKC*
Age	Younger	Older
Sex	Male > female	No predilection
Duration of disease	Limited; resolves at puberty	Chronic
Time of year	Spring	Perennial
Conjunctival involvement	Upper tarsus	Lower tarsus
Cornea	Shield ulcer	Persistent epithelial defects
Corneal scar	Comon; not vision threatening	Common; vision threatening
Conjunctival vascularisation	Rare	Common

Vernal eyelid disease

In long-standing care allergic dermatitis of eyelid skin may occur and is usually mild in contrast to atopic keratoconjunctivitis.

Clinical course of disease is often self-limiting and usually burns out spontaneously after 5–10 years.

Differential diagnosis. Palpebral form of VKC needs to be differentiated from trachoma with pre-dominant papillary hypertrophy (see page 209).

Atopic keratoconjunctivitis (AKC) forms the principal differential diagnostic entity. Table 13.5 summarises the comparison and contrast between VKC and AKC.

TREATMENT

A. *Topical anti-inflammatory therapy*

Topical anti-inflammatory therapy with combined steroids, mast cell stabilisers, antihistamines, and NSAIDs forms the mainstay of treatment of VKC.

1. *Topical steroids.* These are effective in all forms of spring catarrh. However, their use should be minimised, as they frequently cause steroid-induced glaucoma. Therefore, monitoring of intraocular pressure is very important during steroid therapy. Frequent instillation (2 hourly) to start with (7 days) should be followed by maintenance therapy for 4 times a day for 2 weeks.

Commonly used steroid solutions are of fluorometholone, medrysone, betamethasone or dexamethasone. Medrysone and fluoro-metholone are safest of all these.

2. *Mast cell stabilizers* such as sodium cromo-glycate (2%) drops 5 times a day are quite effective in controlling VKC, especially atopic cases.

3. *Dual action antihistamines and mast cell stabilisers* such as azelastine, olopatadine and ketotifen are very effective for control and prevention of exacerbations.

4. *NSAIDs eye drops* such as ketorolac and diclofenac give added benefits.

5. *Topical cyclosporine* (0.5 to 1%), the immune modulator, is indicated when steroids are ineffective, inadequate, or poorly tolerated, or when given as a steroid-sparing agent in patients with severe disease.

6. *Tacrolimus* (0.03% ointment) is another immunomodulator, which can be useful in refractory cases.

B. *Topical lubricating and mucolytics*

1. *Artificial tears,* such as carboxymethyl cellulose, provide soothing effect.

2. *Acetylcysteine* (0.5%) used topically has mucolytic properties and is useful in the treatment of early plaque formation.

C. *Systemic therapy*

1. *Oral antihistaminics* may provide some relief from itching in severe cases.

2. *Oral steroids* for a short duration have been recommended for advanced, very severe, non-responsive cases.

D. *Treatment of large papillae*

Very large (giant) papillae can be tackled either by:
- *Supratarsal injection* of long acting steroid, or
- Cryo application, or
- Surgical excision is recommended for extra-ordinarily large papillae.

E. *Supportive measures* include:
- Dark goggles to prevent photophobia.
- Cold compresses and ice packs have soothing effects.
- Maintenance of air conditioned atmosphere.
- Change of place from hot to cold area is recommended for recalcitrant cases.

F. *Desensitization*

Desensitization has also been tried without much rewarding results.

G. *Treatment of vernal keratopathy*
- *Punctate epithelial keratitis* requires no extra treatment except that instillation of steroids should be increased.
- *A large vernal plaque* requires surgical excision by superficial keratectomy.
- *Severe shield ulcer* resistant to medical therapy may need surgical treatment in the form of debridement, superficial keratectomy, excimer laser therapeutic keratectomy as well as amniotic membrane transplantation to enhance re-epithelialization.

ATOPIC KERATOCONJUNCTIVITIS (AKC)

It can be thought of as an adult equivalent of vernal keratoconjunctivitis and is often associated with atopic dermatitis. Most of the patients are young atopic adults, with male predominance.

PATHOGENESIS

In AKC, both IgE and cell-mediated immune mechanisms play role, i.e. type I as well as type IV hypersensitivity reactions are responsible for the inflammatory changes of conjunctiva, cornea, lid margin and skin of eyelids. Mast cells and eosinophils are found in the conjunctival epithelium of AKC patients. Furthermore, a complex immune cell profile implicates more than the mast cells alone, but the details of those cellular interaction remain speculative.

CLINICAL FEATURES

Symptoms
- Itching, soreness, dry sensation.
- Mucoid discharge.
- Photophobia or blurred vision.

Signs

1. Eyelid signs
- *Lid margins* are chronically inflamed with rounded posterior borders.
- *Extra lid folds* (Dennie-Morgan fold) may occur due to chronic eyelid rubbing.
- *Loss of lateral eyebrows* (Hertoghe's sign) may be seen.
- *Blepharitis, meibomianitis,* and tarsal margin keratinization are also reported.
- *Trichiasis, madarosis, punctal ectropion,* ectropion and entropion may occur as sequelae of inflammation.

2. Conjunctival signs
- *Tarsal conjunctiva* has a milky appearance. There are very fine papillae, hyperaemia and scarring with shrinkage. Inferior palpebral conjunctiva is more severly involved in contrast to VKC, where superior palpebral conjunctiva is predominantly involved.
- *Bulbar conjunctiva* is chemosed and congested.
- *Limbal conjunctiva* may show gelatinous deposits and Tranta's dots as seen in VKC.
- *Subepithelial fibrosis,* fornix shortening and symblepharon are also noticed.

3. Corneal signs
- *Punctate epithelial erosions,* often more severe in the lower half of cornea, may be seen.
- *Persistent epithelial defects,* sometimes associated with focal thinning, can also occur.

- *Filamentary keratitis may also occur.*
- *Plaque formation* may occur similar to VKC.
- *Peripheral vascularization* and stromal scarring are more common than VKC.

4. Associations

- *Keratoconus* is associated in about 15% of cases.
- *Atopic cataract*, in the form of anterior or posterior subcapsular opacities, may be associated.
- *Retinal detachment*, incidence is more higher than in general public.

Clinical course. Like the atopic dermatitis eczema with which it is associated, AKC has a protracted course with exacerbations and remissions. Like vernal keratoconjunctivitis, it tends to become inactive when patient reaches the fifth decade.

Differential diagnosis of AKC needs to be made from VKC in many patients (*see* Table 13.5).

TREATMENT

- *Treatment of AKC* is exactly on the same lines as described for VKC (*see* page 222), except that the AKC is generally less responsive and requires more intensive and prolonged therapy.
- *Lid margin inflammation and facial eczema* should be treated by oral NSAIDs, oral antibiotics (doxycycline or azithromycin) and local application of steroids and antibiotic eye ointment.

◼ GIANT PAPILLARY CONJUNCTIVITIS (GPC)

GPC is the inflammation of conjunctiva with formation of very large-sized papillae greater than 1 mm in size (currently defined as papillae greater than 0.3 mm in diameter).

ETIOPATHOGENESIS

GPC, also known as mechanically-induced papillary conjunctivitis, is a localised allergic response to a physically rough or deposited surface (contact lens, prosthesis, exposed nylon sutures and scleral buckle). Exact pathogenesis of GPC is not clear, but is most frequently attributed to the combined effect of mechanical trauma and the subsequent immune response to antigens in the form of surface deposits or environmental factors. It has been postulated that the antigens from surface coating of contact lens or other materials are first processed by the membrane antigen processing cells (M cells) in the area of conjunctival-associated lymphoid tissue (CALT) before being presented to B lymphocytes, which then mediate the subsequent immune response.

CLINICAL FEATURES

Symptoms include mild irritation and itching, stringy discharge and reduced wearing time of contact lens or prosthetic shell.

Signs. Papillary hypertrophy (often ranging between 0.6 mm and 1.75 mm in diameter) of the upper tarsal conjunctiva, similar to that seen in palpebral form of VKC with hyperaemia are the main signs (Fig. 13.24). Size and pattern of papillae vary with the offending cause.

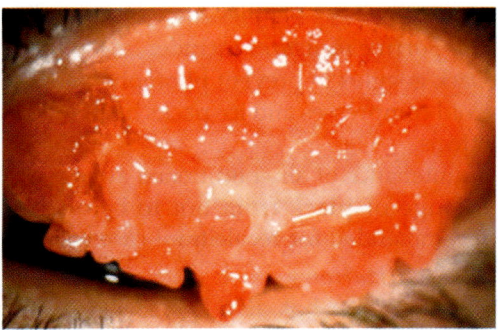

Fig. 13.24: *Giant papillary conjunctivitis (GPC)*

TREATMENT

1. *Offending cause should be removed.* After discontinuation of contact lens or artificial eye or removal of nylon sutures, the papillae resolve over a period of one month.
2. *Mast cell stabilizer* such as sodium cromoglycate and nedocromil are known to relieve the symptoms and enhance the rate of resolution.
3. *Combined antihistamines and mast cell stabilizers* like azelastine and olopatadine are very effective.
4. *Steroids* may be required in resistant cases.

◼ MICROBIALLERGIC CONJUNCTIVITIS

Microbiallergic conjunctivitis refers to type IV hypersensitivity response to the bacterial toxic protein breakdown products.

Types. Two types of microbiallergic conjunctivitis are known:

- Chronic staphylococcal allergic blepharo-conjunctivitis, and
- Phlyctenular keratoconjunctivitis.

CHRONIC STAPHYLOCOCCAL ALLERGIC BLEPHAROCONJUNCTIVITIS

This is a chronic type of blepharoconjunctivitis occurring as type IV hypersensitivity response to the staphylococcal bacterial breakdown products. It is the most common form of microbiallergic conjunctivitis. The staphylococcal bacterial breakdown products cause an allergic response in the conjunctiva as well as cornea.

Clinical features and treatment. It is similar to chronic blepharoconjunctivitis (*see* page 202). It is pertinent to note that:

- Typically such patients do not have history of atopy.
- Marginal corneal infiltrates are commonly associated with chronic blepharoconjunctivitis.

PHLYCTENULAR KERATOCONJUNCTIVITIS

Phlyctenular keratoconjunctivitis is a characteristic nodular affection (phlycten) occurring as an allergic response of the conjunctival and corneal epithelium to some *endogenous allergens* to which they have become sensitized. Phlyctenular conjunctivitis is of worldwide distribution. However, its incidence is higher in developing countries.

Etiology

It is believed to be a delayed hypersensitivity (type IV cell mediated) response to endogenous microbial proteins so-called as *microbial allergic conjunctivitis*.

I. Causative allergens

1. *Tuberculous proteins* were considered, previously, a common cause.
2. *Staphylococcus proteins* are now thought to account for most of the cases.
3. *Other allergens* may be proteins of Moraxella-Axenfeld bacillus, certain parasites (worm infestation). *Candida albicans, Coccidioides*

immitis, Chlamydia and lymphogranuloma venereum.

II. Predisposing factors

1. *Age.* Peak age group is 3–15 years.
2. *Sex.* Incidence is higher in girls than boys.
3. *Undernourishment.* Disease is more common in undernourished children.
4. *Living conditions.* Overcrowded and un-hygienic.
5. *Season.* It occurs in all climates but incidence is high in spring and summer seasons.

PATHOLOGY

1. *Stage of nodule formation.* In this stage, there occurs exudation and infiltration of leucocytes into the deeper layers of conjunctiva leading to a nodule formation. The central cells are polymorphonuclear and peripheral cells are lymphocytes. The neighbouring blood vessels dilate and their endothelium proliferates.

2. *Stage of ulceration.* Later on necrosis occurs at the apex of the nodule and an ulcer is formed. Leucocytic infiltration increases with plasma cells and mast cells.

3. *Stage of granulation.* Eventually, floor of the ulcer becomes covered by granulation tissue.

4. *Stage of healing.* Healing occurs usually with minimal scarring.

CLINICAL FEATURES

Disease is usually unilateral (in contrast to vernal keratoconjunctivitis which is bilateral).

Symptoms in simple phlyctenular conjunctivitis are few, like mild discomfort in the eye, irritation and reflex watering. However, usually there is associated mucopurulent conjunctivitis due to secondary bacterial infection.

Signs. The phlyctenular conjunctivitis can present in three forms: Simple, necrotizing and miliary.

1. *Simple phlyctenular conjunctivitis.* It is the most commonly seen variety. It is characterised by the presence of a typical pinkish white nodule surrounded by hyperaemia on the bulbar conjunctiva, usually near the limbus. Most of the times, there is solitary nodule but at times, there may be two nodules (Fig. 13.25). In a few days, the nodule ulcerates at apex which later on gets epithelised. Rest of the conjunctiva is normal.

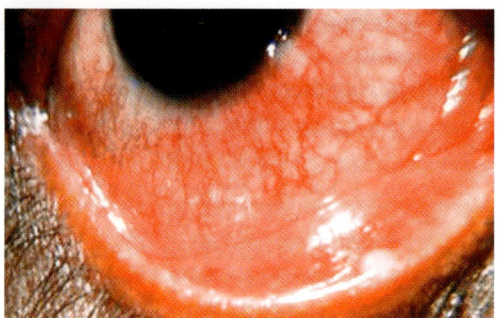

Fig. 13.25: *Phlyctenular conjunctivitis*

2. *Necrotizing phlyctenular conjunctivitis* is characterised by the presence of a very large phlycten with necrosis and ulceration leading to a severe pustular conjunctivitis.

3. *Miliary phlyctenular conjunctivitis* is characterised by the presence of multiple phlyctens which may be arranged haphazardly or in the form of a ring around the limbus and may even form a ring ulcer.

Phlyctenular keratitis. Corneal involvement may occur secondarily from extension of conjunctival phlycten; or rarely as a primary disease. It may present in two forms: The 'ulcerative phlyctenular keratitis' or 'diffuse infiltrative keratitis'.

A. Ulcerative phlyctenular keratitis may occur in the following three forms:

1. *Scrofulous ulcer* is a shallow marginal ulcer formed due to breakdown of small limbal phlycten. It differs from the catarrhal ulcer in that there is no clear space between the ulcer and the limbus and its long axis is frequently perpendicular to limbus. Such an ulcer usually clears up without leaving any opacity.

2. *Fascicular ulcer* has a prominent parallel leash of blood vessels (Fig. 13.26). This ulcer usually remains superficial but leaves behind a band-shaped superficial opacity after healing.

3. *Miliary ulcer.* In this form multiple small ulcers are scattered over a portion of or whole of the cornea.

B. Diffuse infiltrative phlyctenular keratitis may appear in the form of central infiltration of cornea with characteristic rich vascularization from the periphery, all around the limbus. It may be superficial or deep.

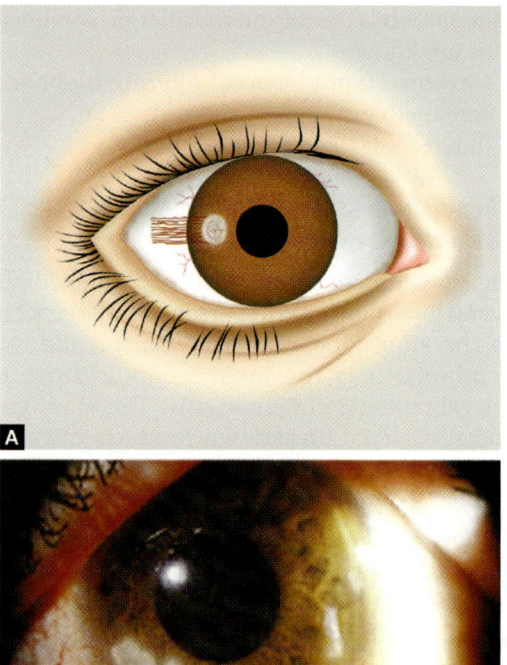

Fig. 13.26: *Fascicular corneal ulcer. A, Diagrammatic; B, Clinical photograph*

Clinical course is usually self-limiting and phlycten disappears in 8–10 days leaving no trace. However, recurrences are very common.

DIFFERENTIAL DIAGNOSIS

Phlyctenular conjunctivitis needs to be differentiated from the *episcleritis, scleritis,* and *conjunctival foreign body granuloma.*

Presence of one or more whitish raised nodules on the bulbar conjunctiva near the limbus, with hyperaemia usually of the surrounding conjunctiva, in a child living in bad hygienic conditions (most of the times) are the diagnostic features of the phlyctenular conjunctivitis.

MANAGEMENT

It includes treatment of phlyctenular conjunctivitis by local therapy, investigations and specific therapy aimed at eliminating the causative allergen and general measures to improve the health of the child.

1. Local therapy

i. *Topical steroids*, in the form of eye drops or ointment (dexamethasone or betamethasone) produce dramatic effect in phlyctenular keratoconjunctivitis.

ii. *Antibiotic drops and ointment* should be added to take care of the associated secondary infection (mucopurulent conjunctivitis).

iii. *Atropine (1%) eye ointment* should be applied once daily when cornea is involved.

2. Specific therapy

Attempts must be made to search and eradicate the following causative conditions:

i. *Tuberculous infection* should be excluded by X-rays chest, Mantoux test, TLC, DLC and ESR. In case, a tubercular focus is discovered, antitubercular treatment should be started to combat the infection.

ii. *Septic focus,* in the form of tonsillitis, adenoiditis, or caries teeth, when present should be adequately treated by systemic antibiotics and necessary surgical measures.

iii. *Parasitic infestation* should be ruled out by repeated stool examination and when discovered should be adequately treated for complete eradication.

3. General measures

General measures aimed to improve the health of child are equally important. Attempts should be made to provide high protein diet supplemented with vitamins A, C and D.

ALLERGIC DERMATOCONJUNCTIVITIS

Allergic dermatoconjunctivitis, also known as 'contact allergic blepharoconjunctivitis', is an allergic disorder, involving conjunctiva and skin of lids along with surrounding area of face, occurring as a reaction to the eye drops, eye ointment and contact lenses solution.

Etiology

It is in fact a delayed hypersensitivity (type IV) response to prolonged contact with chemicals and drugs. A few common topical ophthalmic medications known to produce contact dermatoconjunctivitis are atropine, penicillin, neomycin, soframycin, gentamicin and contact lens solutions.

Clinical features

Clinically, it is the most common form of allergic reaction seen by the ophthalmologists and contact lenses practitioners (optometes). Its features include:

1. *Cutaneous involvement* is in the form of weeping eczematous reaction, involving all areas with which medication comes in contact

2. *Conjunctival response* is in the form of hyperaemia with a generalised papillary response affecting the lower fornix and lower palpebral conjunctiva more than the upper.

3. *Cornea* may show punctate epithelial keratitis and erosions.

Diagnosis

- *Clinical features* are usually typical.
- *Conjunctival cytology* shows a lymphocytic response with masses of eosinophils.
- *Skin test* to the causative allergen is positive in most of the cases.

Treatment

1. Discontinuation of the causative medication
2. Topical steroid eye drops to relieve symptoms
3. Application of steroid ointment on the involved skin.

NON-ALLERGIC EOSINOPHILIC CONJUNCTIVITIS

The term non-allergic eosinophilic conjunctivitis (NAEC) has recently been proposed to denote a chronic non-atopic conjunctivitis predominantly occurring in women, most of whom also have associated dry eye. The condition is relatively common but under diagnosed.

Pathogenesis is similar to non-allergic eosinophilic rhinitis.

Symptoms are similar to allergic conjunctivitis and include itching, redness foreign body sensation and mild watery discharge.

Conjunctival scrapings show eosinophilia without significant IgE levels in serum and tear film.

Treatment includes:

- *Topical steroids* for 1–2 weeks
- *Topical mast cell stabilisers* and topical NSAIDs are required as maintenance therapy for 3–4 weeks.

CICATRICIAL CONJUNCTIVITIS

Cicatricial conjunctivitis may be devided into two groups: Primary (immunologic) and secondary.

Primary (immunologic) cicatricial conjunctivitis

Primary cicatricial conjunctivitis is basically immunologic conjunctivitis seen in the following conditions:

- Ocular mucous membrane pemphigoid (OMMP)
- Stenvens-Johnson syndrome (SJS)
- Toxic epidermal necrosis

Note. For details, *see* Chapter 16, page 268.

Secondary cicatricial conjunctivitis

Cicatricial conjunctivitis may occur secondary to:

- *Injuries to conjunctiva* (such as thermal, radiational or chemical burns), and
- *Infective conjunctivitis* (such as trachoma and viral pseudomembranous conjunctivitis).

TOXIC CONJUNCTIVITIS

TOXIC CONJUNCTIVITIS: SECONDARY TO MOLLUSCUM CONTAGIOSUM

It is a type of chronic follicular conjunctivitis that occurs as a response to toxic cellular debris desquamated into the conjunctival sac from the molluscum contagiosum nodules present on the lid margin (the primary lesion).

CHEMICAL TOXIC CONJUNCTIVITIS

Also known as toxic keratoconjunctivitis related to topical medication is an irritative follicular conjunctival response which occurs after prolonged administration of topical medication.

Common topical preparations associated with chronic follicular conjunctivitis are: Idoxuridine (IDU), eserine, pilocarpine, DFP, adrenaline, topical beta-adrenergic blocker dorzolamide, prostaglandin graph of glaucoma medication neomycin, preservatives including contact lens solutions and topical anaesthetise.

Other causes of toxic keratoconjunctivitis include:

- Cosmetics and skin care products,
- Hair care products, and
- Tear gas weapons and lacrimating agents.

Treatment

- Cessation of use of offending agent
- Lubricating drops and ointments provide symptomatic relief.
- Measures for persistent corneal epithelial defects depending upon the severity, include: Bandage contact lens, tarsorrhaphy and amniotic membrane transplants.

BIBLIOGRAPHY

1. American Academy of Ophthalmology. Cornea/External Disease Panel. Preferred Practice Pattern Guidelines: Conjunctivitis-Limited Revision. American Academy of Ophthalmology; San Francisco, CA: 2011 [Google Scholar]
2. Bielory BP, O'Brien TP, Bielory L. Management of seasonal allergic conjunctivitis: guide to therapy. Acta Ophthalmol 2012; 90(5): 399–407. [PubMed] [Google Scholar]
3. Chestler R J, deVenecia G. Calcific eyelid margin lesions in chronic renal failure. Am J Ophthalmol 1989; 107: 556–57. PubMed Web of Science. Google Scholar
4. Cronau H, Kankanala RR, Mauger T. Diagnosis and management of red eye in primary care. Am Fam Physician 2010; 81(2): 137–44. [PubMed] [Google Scholar]
5. Demco TA, Mc Cormick AQ, Richards JSF. Conjunctival and corneal changes in chronic renal failure. Can J Ophthalmol 1974; 9: 208–13. PubMedWeb of Science Google Scholar
6. Ehlers N, Kruse Hansen F, Hansen HE, et al. (1972) Corneo-conjunctival changes in uremia. Acta Ophthalmol 50: 83–94. Google Scholar
7. Gallenga PE, Lobefalo L, Colangelo L, et al. Topical lomefloxacin 0.3% twice daily versus tobramycin 0.3% in acute bacterial conjunctivitis: a multicenter double-blind phase III study.

Ophthalmologica 1999; 213(4): 250–57. [PubMed] [Google Scholar]

8. Huerva V, Ascaso FJ, Latre B. Tolerancia y eficacia de la tobramicina topica vs cloranfenicol en el tratamiento de las conjunctivitis bacterianas. Ciencia Pharmaceutica 1991; 1: 221–24 [Google Scholar]

9. Jackson WB, Low DE, Dattani D, Whitsitt PF, Leeder RG, MacDougall R. Treatment of acute bacterial conjunctivitis: 1% fusidic acid viscous drops vs 0.3% tobramycin drops. Can J Ophthalmol. 2002; 37(4): 228–37. Discussion 237. [PubMed] [Google Scholar]

10. Karpecki P, Depaolis M, Hunter JA, et al. Besifloxacin ophthalmic suspension 0.6% in patients with bacterial conjunctivitis: a multicenter, prospective, randomized, double-masked, vehicle-controlled, 5-day efficacy and safety study. Clin Ther 2009; 31(3): 514–26. [PubMed] [Google Scholar]

11. Leibowitz HM. Antibacterial effectiveness of ciprofloxacin 0.3% ophthalmic solution in the treatment of bacterial conjunctivitis. Am J Ophthalmol 1991; 112((4)(Suppl)): 29S–33S. [PubMed] [Google Scholar]

12. Nelson JD, Havener VR, Cameron JD. Cellulose acetate impressions of the ocular surface: dry eye states. Arch Ophthalmol 1983; 101: 1869–72.

13. Paridaens ADA, McCartney ACE, Curling OM, et al. Impression cytology of conjunctival melanosis and melanoma. Br J Ophthalmol 1992; 76: 198–201.

14. Schwab IR, Friedlaender M, McCulley J, et al. A phase III clinical trial of 0.5% levofloxacin ophthalmic solution versus 0.3% ofloxacin ophthalmic solution for the treatment of bacterial conjunctivitis. Ophthalmology. 2003; 110(3): 457–65. [PubMed] [Google Scholar]

15. Tseng SCG. Staging of conjunctival squamous metaplasia by impression cytology. Ophthalmology 1985; 92: 728–33.

16. Vannucchi MT, Vannucchi H, Humphreys M(1992) Serum levels of vitamin A and retinol binding protein in chronic renal failure patients treated by continous ambulatorial peritoneal dialysis. Int J Vitam Nutr Res 62: 107-112.

17. Zhang M, Hu Y, Chen F. Clinical investigation of 0.3% levofloxacin eyedrops on the treatment of cases with acute bacterial conjunctivitis and bacterial keratitis [in Chinese] Yan Ke Xue Bao. 2000; 16(2): 146-148. [PubMed] [Google Scholar]

Tear Film and Dry Eye Disease

TEAR FILM

The value of tear fluid in preserving a clear cornea has been understood since ages. The fact that the blinking action of lids was essential for spreading the tears and maintaining a moist surface on anterior portion of globe was obvious even in olden age. That is why in the ancient times, as a crueler form of punishment eyelids used to be excised, invariably leading to blindness due to desiccation and opacification of cornea. Hence, the knowledge of the precorneal liquid is of long-standing and so is the knowledge that the cornea will dry up, if the blinking is prevented.

The presence of precorneal layer of liquid was first demonstrated by Fischer in 1928,[1] by using light reflected from the corneal surface on a photographic plate (reflectography). Further studies showed it to be an important part of cornea and Rollet[2] even described it as the most superficial, sixth layer of cornea.

FUNCTIONS, STRUCTURE, PROPERTIES AND COMPOSITION OF TEAR FILM

FUNCTIONS OF TEAR FILM

1. The most important function of the tear film is *to form an almost perfectly smooth optical*

surface on the cornea by filling in and smoothening out small surface irregularities in the corneal epithelium.

2. *It serves to keep the surface of cornea and conjunctiva moist.* It is unlikely that the sensitive epithelial cells could survive, if the surfaces were dry.

3. *It serves as a lubricant for the preocular surface and lids*, thereby decreasing the frictional forces that are generated during the constant blinking movements of the eyelids and rotational movements of the eyeball.

4. *It transfers oxygen* from the ambient air to the cornea.

5. *It prevents infection* due to the presence of antibacterial substances such as lysozyme, betalysin, lactoferrin, immunoglobulins and other proteins.

6. *It washes away debris* and noxious irritants.

7. *It provides a pathway for white blood cells* in case of injury.

STRUCTURE OF TEAR FILM

Wolff (1946) was the first to describe in detail the structure of tear film. He gave a clinical description of the fluid in the conjunctival sac with special reference to the lid margin. He coined the term "precorneal film" and assumed that it consisted of three layers, viz. an outer oily layer, an intermediate aqueous layer and an inner mucoid layer (Fig. 14.1A). This description still holds good in understanding tear film and its various abnormalities.[3] Another model with six layers has also been proposed by Tiffany,[3a] which included the original three layers proposed by Wolff, along with air–lipid, lipid–aqueous and aqueous–mucin interfaces.

Further, it has also been suggested that there are dissolved mucins in the aqueous layer which decrease in concentration towards the lipid layer.[3b] The most current concept is that the tear film is a bilayer structure consisting of an aqueous–mucinous phase, with a overlying superficial lipid phase (Figs 14.1B and C). However, for understanding, the description given below is as per classical concept.

Lipid layer

Outermost superficial oily layer of tear film derived from the secretions of Meibomian, Zeiss and Moll glands covers the entire free surface of the tear fluid.

Marginal tear strip. Wolff[3] found that this layer on the lid margins forms a strip which extends to the posterior margin of the openings of the meibomian glands and limits the anterior end of the tear fluid reservoirs. He called it marginal tear strips.

Physical integrity of lipid layer. Thickness of lipid layer is about 0.1–0.2 mm and depends on the palpebral fissure width, i.e. it increases when the lids are partially closed.

Brauninger *et al*[4] demonstrated the existence and physical integrity of oily layer by simple physical method of bombarding the tear film with microdroplets of oil and water, and then observing their behaviour upon striking the surface. The water particles rolled off the tear film surface, while the oily particles were immediately absorbed into the anterior surface of the tear film, indicating that the anterior surface of the tear film is an oily layer.

Chemically, this layer consists of lipids having low polarity, such as wax and cholesterol esters. These lipids are fluid at body temperature despite their considerable cholesterol contents and high average molecular weight. Lipid layer is formed from polar and neutral lipids. The polar lipids face the aqueous component of the tear film and non-polar lipids face the air. There are a number of different types of lipid secreted. High polarity lipids such as triglycerides, free fatty acids and phospholipids are present in negligible amounts.

Control of lipid secretion is neuroendocrinal:
- *Androgen sex hormones* regulate lipid synthesis and secretion.
- *Neurotransmitters* from the nerves surrounding the acini can alter lipid synthesis or alveolar cell rupture.

Functions of lipid layer include:
- *Oily layer of tear film prevents the overflow of tears and retards their evaporation.* The latter fact accrues from the observation that cauterization of the orifices of meibomian glands increases the evaporation by more than 10 times and results in absence of oily layer.
- *It prevents migration of skin lipids* onto the ocular surface.

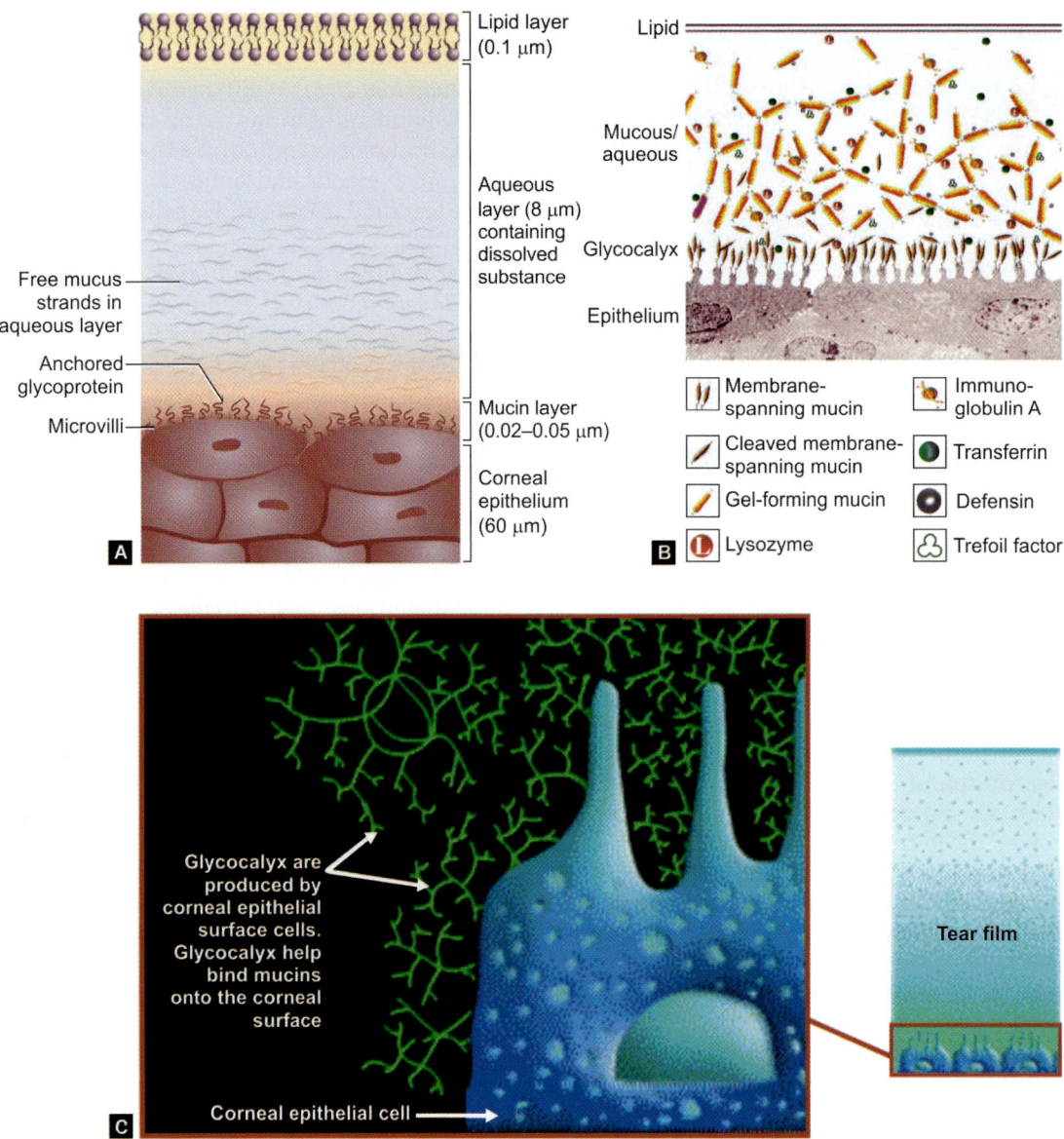

Fig. 14.1A to C: *Structure of tear film*

- *It provides a clear ocular medium* and smooth surface for refraction of light.
- *Acts as a barrier for preventing contamination of tear film.*
- *It acts as a surfactant layer* which makes an effective bridge between the non-polar lipid phase and aqueous–mucinous phase.
- *It acts as a lubricant* to facilitate smooth movement of eyelids during blinking.

Aqueous layer

Middle aqueous layer of tear film is secreted by the lacrimal gland and the accessory glands of Krause and Wolfring as depicted in Fig. 14.2. Main bulk of thickness of tear film is constituted by this layer. Aqueous layer comprises 60% of the tear film. Thickness of aqueous layer of pre-corneal tear film is uniform over the cornea and is about 7 μm. The film covering the cornea is

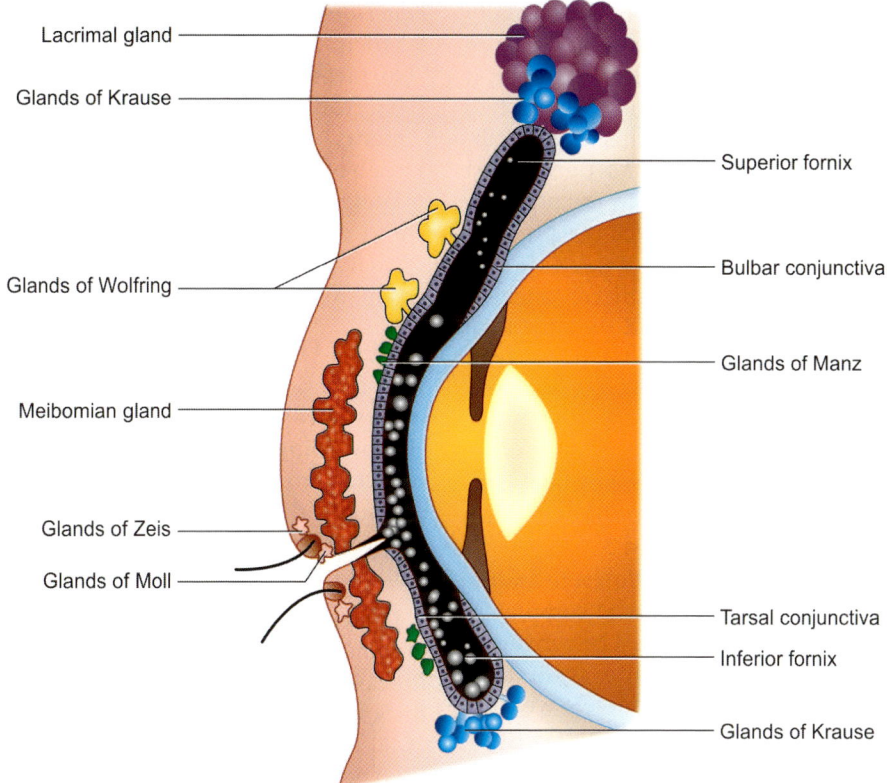

Fig. 14.2: *Parts of conjunctiva and conjunctiva glands*

considerably thinner than over the conjunctiva. Recently, it has also been suggested that there are dissolved mucins in the aqueous layer which decrease in concentration towards the lipid layer and form the so-called aqueous–mucinous phase.[3b, 3c]

Composition. This layer is an aqueous solution of low viscosity, containing ions of inorganic salts, glucose, urea and various biopolymers such as enzymes, proteins and glycoproteins. Lysozyme, lactoferrin, tear specific prealbumin and secretory immunoglobulin A are the main constituents of protein fraction. Because some bicarbonate ions as well as proteins are present, the tear fluid has some buffering capacity. It has been observed that only the macromolecular solutes of the tears have surface activity. The electrolyte concentration of aqueous layer varies with flow rate. At low flow rates, the fluid is hypertonic, whereas at high flow rates it becomes isotonic.

Surface tension of normal aqueous tears varies between 40 and 42 dyn/cm. All the surface active substances in the aqueous tear that determine its surface tension are macromolecular and believed to be mucous glycoproteins.

Functions. It serves to provide atmospheric oxygen to the epithelium, washes away debris and noxious irritants and contains antibacterial substances like lysozyme and betalysin. Thus, the aqueous layer has antibacterial, antiadhesive and lubricant properties.

Mucus layer

Deepest stratum of the precorneal tear film is the mucus coat. Being in a highly hydrated, semisolid state, the mucus layer is not strictly a part of fluid film. It plays a vital role in the stability of the tear film. That is why Holly and Lemp[5] found it reasonable to consider it as the third layer of tear film. They also observed that in healthy eyes the mucus layer is rather thin (only 0.02–0.04 μm), so its morphology usually resembles the microvillous, ridged appearance of superficial epithelial cell walls. However, it has been suggested that tear mucins are of two types, i.e. aqueous soluble mucins and membrane adherent mucins, and as per recent concepts the mucins dissolved in the aqueous forms the so-called aqueous–mucinous phase of tear film.[3b, 3c]

Mucin layer is mainly secreted by conjunctival goblet cells, crypts of Henle and the glands of Manz. But mucus has also been identified both histochemically and biochemically in the secretions of the main lacrimal gland. Mucus layer is made from the epithelial cell *glycocalyx* and a layer of tear mucins (*glycoprotein*). MUC5AC is the main tear mucin which is produced along with the trefoil protein TFF1 and 3.

Clear corneal epithelium is a relatively hydrophobic surface. In order for tears to completely cover the cornea, the surface must be converted from its natural hydrophobic state to a hydrophilic state that allows complete wetting. Mucin converts the hydrophobic corneal surface to a hydrophilic surface by adhering to the glycocalyx on the corneal microvilli.

- *Glycocalyx* are long chain molecules that help hold mucin to the corneal surface. Formed by corneal cells, glycocalyx migrate out from the surface of the corneal microvilli to form a hydrophilic network that holds mucin on the ocular surface (Fig. 14.1C).
- Holding mucin to the ocular surface creates a water attraction, as well as protection against bacterial pathogens. Mucin (a glycoprotein) produced by goblet cells, mixed and spread by action of lids, gets adsorbed on the cell membrane of epithelial cells and anchored by their microvilli forming a new hydrophilic surface on which aqueous and lipid layers spread spontaneously. It thus plays a vital role in the stability of preocular tear film, as the latter depends upon the constant supply of mucin to maintain proper hydration of ocular surface tissues.

Thickness. Electron micrographs of epithelial sections stained with Mowry's colloidal iron stain revealed that mucous layer has a thickness ranging from 200 to 500 Å (0.02 to 0.04 μm).[6]

Functions of mucus are as below:
- Mucin lubricates the ocular and palpebral surfaces, so that minimal energy is lost as friction during blinking and eye movements.
- It also provides a slippery coating over the foreign bodies, thereby protecting the cornea and conjunctiva against abrasive effects of such particles as they move about with blinking.

PHYSICAL PROPERTIES OF TEAR FILM

Tear fluid is clear, salty, slightly alkaline and watery. It varies somewhat in its appearance and composition, depending on whether it is collected from the ducts of gland or from the conjunctival sac. Some of the important physical characteristics of the tear film are described in Table 14.1:

1. *Thickness of tear film.* The average thickness of tear film varies from 7 to 8 μm. The film is thickest after a blink, measuring about 9 μm. The thickness then decreases in a linear manner until at 30 seconds it has decreased to its minimal thickness of 4 μm. However, recent confocal microscopy has shown that tear film is about 40 μm thick.

2. *Volume of tear film.* The average volume of tear film has been reported to be 7 μl with a range from 4 to 13 μl (one to two drops) during basal conditions. The volume is highest in youth and then begins to decline in a linear manner until it reaches a value of 10% the youthful value by the age of 70 years. This constant slow decrease in tear film volume is accompanied by signs and symptoms of dryness.

Table 14.1: *Physical properties of tear film*	
1. Thickness	7–8 μm
2. Volume	4–13 μl
3. Rate of tear secretion	1.2 μl/min
4. Turnover rate	18% per min
5. Refractive index	1.357
6. pH	7.3–7.7
7. Osmotic pressure	0.90–0.95% NaCl soln
8. Temperature	35°C at the limbus; 30°C at the centre
9. O_2 tension (PO_2)	40–160 mm Hg

3. Rate of tear secretion. In the non-stimulated subjects, the average rate of tear secretion is 1.2 µl per min, with a total 24-hour secreting volume of about 10 cu ml.

4. Turnover rate. The tear turnover rate is 18% per minute. This high turnover rate with low volume of conjunctival sac (20 ml) is responsible for poor retention of instilled medication.

5. Refractive index. Refractive index of tear film is about 1.357.

6. pH of tears. The pH of tears is nearly 7.4 and approximates that of blood plasma. Although, wide variations have been found in normal individuals (between 5.2 and 8.35), the usual range is from 7.3 to 7.7.[8] Reflex tears are somewhat more consistent with pH values ranging between 7.5 and 8. Tear pH is the lowest on awakening due to acid byproducts associated with relatively anaerobic conditions in prolonged lid closure and increases due to loss of carbon dioxide as eyes are open. Tear pH is maintained at constant level during waking hours by the normal buffering mechanism. When solutions having a pH lower than 6.6 and above 7.8 are instilled into the conjunctival sac, subjective discomfort occurs. Corneal injuries tend to produce an alkaline reaction in the tears.

Age, sex, time of examination, the presence of pterygium or pinguecula seem to have a little effect on pH of tears. Inflammatory conditions of conjunctiva and cornea tend to produce a shift towards a more acid tear film.

7. Osmotic pressure. The osmotic pressure of the tear film in normal eyes is equivalent to 0.90 to 0.95% sodium chloride solution.[9] The optical integrity of the cornea is significantly influenced by the tonicity of tears. Variation in osmotic pressure between 0.6% and 1.3% sodium chloride equivalent is well tolerated by the eye, but beyond these limits discomfort is experienced. Total osmotic pressure is proportional to the dissolved crystalloids. The osmotic pressure of tears is slightly below that of the blood. There is no difference in osmotic pressure between tears and the aqueous humour. Osmotic pressure is significantly changed with reflex stimulation of tears. Corneal oedema often seen in early stages of contact lens adaptation occurs due to relative hypotonicity of tears resulting from a reflex stimulation.

8. Temperature of tear film. Under basal conditions with a normal blink rate, temperature of the tear film and anterior cornea with eyelids open ranges from 35°C at the limbus to a low of 30°C at the centre of cornea.[10] It varies with extremely cold or hot environment, under windy conditions, and with the eyelids tightly closed or held open for prolonged period of time.

9. Oxygen tension (PO_2). In the normal tear film under basal conditions, PO_2 varies from 40 to 160 mm Hg. Under a tightly fitting contact lens it may drop to a value as low as 20 mm Hg. With a well fitted contact lens a more normal PO_2 is retained during blinking as the tidal flow of tears changes beneath the lens.[11]

CHEMICAL COMPOSITION OF TEARS

Regarding composition of tear film, there seems a general agreement that it mainly consists of water with a certain content of salts and low molecular weight substances. The continuous evaporation of water from the tears makes defining a "tear composition" very difficult. A second confusing factor is the sensitivity of the tear-producing processes to stimulation while the tears are being collected for analysis. Table 14.2 depicts the chemical composition of tears. The data includes consensus values from different studies. The constituent of the tears is as follows.

Water

The aqueous phase of tear film is a dilute watery solution of salts and dissolved organic materials. The water forms the largest part of tear liquid; 98.2% with 1.8% dissolved solids.

Proteins

The total tear protein content strongly depends on the method of collection of tears. Small unstimulated tears show levels of about 2 gm% while stimulated tears show much lower values in the range of 0.3 to 0.7 gm% reflecting the level of lacrimal gland fluid. As in practice, reflex tearing is difficult to avoid; a mixture of stimulated and unstimulated tears can be obtained giving normal values in the range from 0.6 to 2.0 gm%. A number of protein components have been isolated from human tears. The major fractions include, specific tear protein (STP) or

Table 14.2: *Chemical composition of human tears and plasma*

	Tears	Plasma
Water	98.2 g%	94 gm/100 ml
Solids, total	1.8%	6 gm/100 ml
Na^+	142 mEq/L	137–142 mEq/L
K^+	15–29 mEq/L	5 mEq/L
Cl^-	120–135 mEq/L	102 mEq/L
HCO_3^-	26 mEq/L	24.3 mEq/L
Ca^{++}	2.29 mg/100 ml	
Total proteins	0.6–2 gm/100 ml	6.78 gm/100 ml
Amino acids	8 mg/100 ml	
Urea	0.04 mg/100 ml	20–40 mg/100 ml
Glucose	3–10 mg/100 ml	80–90 mg/100 ml

prealbumin, albumin, immunoglobulin, metal carrying protein, lysozyme and other enzymes. These proteins can be divided into two groups as follows:[12]

Group A. The components of this group are similar to serum proteins. They are in a low concentration representing less than 15% of all tear proteins. Immunoglobulin G, albumin, transferrin, alpha-1 antitrypsin, alpha-1 antichymotrypsin and beta-2-microglobulins are always present. Others which occur sporadically are ceruloplasmin, haptoglobulins and zinc alpha-2-glucoproteins.

Group B. These are specific proteins, synthesized by tear glands, also known as "rapid migrating proteins". They are also present in other external secretions. Electrophoretically, they correspond to three main peaks. Protein migrating to cathode is lysozyme and the one migrating to anode is lactoferrin and third peak of immunoglobulin A.

Albumin

The albumin represents 58.2% of total protein in basic tears and 20.2% of total protein in reflex tears (Table 14.3).

Tear specific protein (prealbumin)

It is an acidic protein constituting most of the albumin content of tears. Albumin identical with serum albumin forms only a minor component of continuous tears but rises markedly in reflex tearing. While the total albumin content decreases in reflex tearing as compared with that present in continuous tears (Table 14.3), the

Table 14.3: *Proteins found in human tears*

Protein	Normal undisturbed state (%)	Reflex tears (%)
Albumin	58.2	20.2
Globulin	23.9	56.9
Lysozyme	17.9	22.9

From Iwata S (1973): Chemical composition of aqueous phase. In Holly and Kemp (eds): The preocular tear film and dry eye syndrome. International ophthalmic clinics. Boston, Little Brown.

amount of serum albumin increases relative to specific tear albumin. The exact function of albumin in the tears is not known; perhaps aids the oily meibomian secretion in stabilizing the thin tear film.

Immunoglobulins

Approximate levels of tear immunoglobulin *vis-à vis* plasma immunoglobulin are given in Table 14.4. IgA is the most prominent tear immunoglobulin as compared to IgA in the serum. Tear IgA is a secretory immunoglobulin produced locally by plasma cells located in adenoid layer of the conjunctiva. It differs from the circulating IgA in having an additional secretory piece. While the circulating immunoglobulins function in blocking systemic infection, locally produced antibody provides a more effective defence against externally invasive viral or bacterial antigens. Tear IgM and IgE are also produced locally in the conjunctiva. In general, tear immunoglobulins are found in higher concentration in reflex tears than in continuous tears.

Table 14.4: *Levels of tear and serum immunoglobulins*		
Class	Tear	Plasma
IgA	14–24 mg/100 ml	170–200 mg/100 ml
IgG	17 mg/100 ml	1000 mg/100 ml
IgM	<1 mg/100 ml	125 mg/100 ml
IgD	<1 mg/100 ml	3 mg/100 ml
IgE	250 mg/ml	2000 mg/100 ml

Lysozyme

Lysozyme also termed muramidase is a proteolytic enzyme, first discovered by Fleming in 1922.[13] Tear lysozyme concentration is highest amongst all the body fluids, forming nearly 20% of the tear proteins. In fact, lysozyme is one of the most important protein contents of the human tear film.

Lysozyme, probably produced by the acinar cells of the lacrimal gland, is a strongly basic protein of molecular weight 14000–25000 with an isoelectric point 10.5 to 11. It has a net positive charge at physiological pH so that it migrates to the cathode, in contrast with the other proteins which have a net negative charge.

Lysozyme acts as a protective agent against bacterial infections. It causes lysis by hydrolysis of the polymer N-glucosamine-N-acetyl muramic acid present in the bacterial cell wall. In addition to its bactericidal activity it has also been reported to facilitate secretory IgA-mediated bacteriolysis in the presence of complement and to promote contact inhibition of cells. Perhaps, it also helps in determining the role of lysis in an IgM antibody complement system.

The total antibacterial activity of human tears is some 200 times greater than that could be ascribed to lysozyme; depicting thereby an important role of non-lysozomal fraction. It has been reported that the non-lysozomal fraction is active against many gram-negative organisms while lysozyme is active only against certain gram-positive organisms.

Other enzymes

Glycolytic enzymes and the enzymes of tricyclic citric acid cycle can be detected in high levels, only in tear samples collected in paper strips or in small volumes of unstimulated tears. The source of these enzymes is conjunctiva, where they are secreted in small amounts. *Lactate dehydrogenase* (LDH) is the enzyme in highest concentration in tears. Electrophoretically, it can be separated into its fine isoenzymes. Tear LDH originates from the corneal epithelium. In patients suffering from various corneal diseases, the distribution of the LDH isoenzymes in tears can differ from those found in healthy individuals.[14] *Betalysin* is an antibacterial agent presents in higher concentration in tears than in human serum, but its activity is found to be poor as compared to lysozyme.[15]

Various workers have demonstrated the presence of amylase and peroxidase in normal tears and collagenases in tears from patients of corneal ulceration due to infection, chemical burns, trauma or desiccation.

Mucopolysaccharides

Mucopolysaccharides are found in tear fluid as indicated by electrophoretic and histochemical studies. The surface of corneal epithelium can also be stained with Alcian blue or with Mowry's modification of the colloidal iron reaction, both methods indicating the presence of mucopolysaccharides.

Glycoproteins

Glycoproteins are found in the mucoid layer as well as in the tear fluid, since they are highly soluble in water. Iwata and Kabasawa[16] fractionated three types of glycoproteins by gel filtration from tear mucoid clots collected from the conjunctival surface of rabbit eye.

Amino acids

Some 17-amino acids have been isolated from human tears. Whether all or part of the amino acid component of tears is due to secretion, filtration, local synthesis or local degradation of proteins and polypeptides is unknown. Also not much is known about the role of amino acids in conjunctival and corneal diseases.

Amino acids are present in small amount (8 mg per 100 ml) in the tears.

Lipids

Lipids are present in small amount in tears as they are contained only in very thin superficial oily layer of the tear film. Tiffany (1978) found out all possible lipids in meibomian gland secretions, namely hydrocarbon, wax esters, cholesterol ester, triglycerides and less amounts of—diglycerides, monoglycerides, free fatty acids, free cholesterol and phospholipids. The profile of free fatty acids and the proportion of lipid classes varies considerably between individuals, and may be a factor that predisposes to the development of chronic blepharitis. The composition of lipid after release is altered by the action of lipolytic lid margin bacteria and is invariably different from that of the lipid originally produced by the meibomian glands.

Metabolites

- *Glucose* is present in minimum amounts, about 3 to 10 mg/ml, in tear fluid collected in capillary tubes during stimulation in normoglycemic persons. This concentration is one-tenth of the concentration in the blood. Tokyda[17] found a corresponding rise in tear glucose with elevation of plasma glucose above 100 mg% while other workers found no significant elevation in the tear glucose level in diabetics with blood glucose levels of more than 20 mmol/L.
- *Lactate* levels of 1–5 mmol/L in tears are far higher than the normal blood levels of 0.5–0.8 mmol/L.
- *Pyruvate* level is about the same as is normal for blood.
- *Urea* concentration in tear fluid is about 0.04 mg per 100 ml.

Electrolytes

Sodium and potassium are the main positively charged electrolytes while chlorides and bicarbonates are main negatively charged electrolytes in tears. An equal concentration of Na^+ in tears and plasma suggests its passive diffusion in tears. In fact, the primary secretion from the acinar region of lacrimal gland is essentially an ultrafiltrate of plasma, it is later modified by ductal secretion of potassium chloride. A much higher concentration of K^+ (3.5 times) than the corresponding plasma concentration explains this active secretion of K^+ in the tears. Ca^{++} is independent of the tear production and is lower than the free fraction in plasma.

TEAR FILM DYNAMICS

The main role of the lacrimal system is to establish and maintain a continuous tear film over the preocular surface. The primary role of tear film is to establish a refractive surface of high quality for the cornea and to ensure the well-being of the cornea and conjunctival epithelium.

Tear film accomplishes its functions by the highly specialized and well-organized dynamic activities which starting from the secretion to the elimination of tears in a chronological order include the following:

- Secretion of tears
- Formation of preocular tear film
- Retention and redistribution of tear film
- Displacement phenomenon
- Evaporation of tear film
- Stability drying and rupture of tear film
- Dynamic events during blinking
- Elimination of tears

SECRETION OF TEARS

Tears are continuously secreted throughout the day by accessory (basal secretion) and main (reflex secretion) lacrimal glands. This concept of 'basal tear secretion' is presently thought to be redundant one; as even minimal tear production in the undisturbed eye is thought to be secondary to light or temperature stimulation or both. (Proprioceptors in the lids may also play a part.)

- *Reflex secretion* occurs in response to sensations from the cornea and conjunctiva, probably produced by evaporation and break-up of tear film.
- *Hyperlacrimation* occurs due to irritative sensations from the cornea and conjunctiva.
- *Afferent pathway of this secretion* is formed by fifth nerve and efferent by parasympathetic (secretomotor) supply of lacrimal gland.

Normal rate of tear production is about 1.2 μl/min, the tear volume in the eye at any time is about 7 μl and the turnover rate is about 5 to 7 min.[19] Abnormal lacrimation brought about by ocular surface irritation or emotion can increase the production rate several hundred folds. *Most (82%) of the full term newborn babies secrete tear within 24 hours* and 95% of all full term infants have normal tear secretory rate within the first week of life.[20] However, it is of interest to note that abnormal tearing starts only after an infant is 4 months old. A newborn baby produces no excess tear fluid even when crying loudly. The absence of excess tearing in very young infants may be connected with the low innervation of the cornea. A newborn can tolerate large particles on the cornea without being uncomfortable.

It is generally accepted that the main lacrimal gland secretes water and electrolytes only during reflex tearing and that its contribution to the normal tear film is negligible. However, occasional reports indicate that, following excision of the main gland, a dry eye syndrome may follow. Conversely blocking the lacrimal puncta or excision of the lacrimal sac, i.e. dacryocystectomy results in an appropriate decrease in lacrimal secretion on the ipsilateral side, so that tears do not overflow the lid margin. The exact mechanism of these fluids and electrolyte secretory changes is unknown.

Continuous preocular tear film is formed by the secretions of the main lacrimal gland, accessory lacrimal gland, meibomian gland and mucous glands of the conjunctiva, which flows over the ocular surface.

FORMATION OF PREOCULAR TEAR FILM

Wettability of a surface is characterised by the tendency of liquids to spread on it. A drop of liquid placed on a solid surface will either spread completely or form a certain boundary line beyond which it will not spread. At this boundary, a positive angle (contact angle, theta) is formed between the liquid and solid surfaces. A solid surface, on which a liquid forms such a positive contact angle is said to be only partially wetted (non-wetted) by the liquid. In contrast, liquids that wet (spread on) a solid surface completely show a contact angle of zero.[21]

With respect to water, surfaces on which water forms the angle θ greater than 90° are said to be hydrophobic; those with angle q between zero and 90° are relatively hydrophobic; and those with zero angle q are hydrophilic.[22]

Corneal epithelium is a relatively hydrophobic surface. Experiments conducted by Lemp and Holly[22] have indicated that principal constituent of tears, responsible for the wetting of corneal surface, is conjunctival mucus which spreads on to the cornea by the action of lids and converts its surface to a hydrophilic one.

Doane in 1980 studied the interaction of eyelids and tears in corneal wetting and held the blinking process responsible for distributing tear fluid over the ocular surface or wiping away the excess fluid.[23]

Sequence of events in the formation of a continuous precorneal tear film can be summarized as follows:

- *Lids surfacing cornea* with a thin layer of mucus.
- *On this new surface, the aqueous component* of tears now spreads spontaneously.
- *Then the superficial lipid layer spreads over the aqueous film,* probably contributing to its stability and retarding evaporation between blinks.

Tear film thus formed has three distinctive phases layered one above the other. The mucin adsorbed onto the corneal epithelium, together with any excess mucin not yet dissolved and coating the adsorbed mucin layer, forms the bottom layer. The outermost layer is superficial lipid layer.

RETENTION AND REDISTRIBUTION OF TEAR FILM

The tear film is retained at a uniform thickness over the corneal surface against a gravitational force, since it is normally positioned almost vertically. The absence of downward flow of the precorneal tear film was suggested by Wolff in 1954.[24] Further, studies indicated that the outermost layer of corneal epithelium, along with mucopolysaccharides play an important role in retaining the fluid layer on the corneal surface.[25]

The fluid in the precorneal tear film is stagnant, unless it is mixed by blinking and eye movements with the tear fluid in the marginal strip. Redistribution occurs in the form of bringing of new tear fluid by way of marginal strip where there is constant flow of tears.

DISPLACEMENT PHENOMENON

If with a finger the lower eyelid is carefully displaced upwards over the eyeball, the particles in the film are seen to move up the cornea as an integral whole all particles on the surface including those lying far away from the margin of the eyelid, moving upward.

Based on this phenomenon, it has been concluded that surface of cornea is covered by a film possessing a certain stability, compressibility and elasticity and that it is more or less unaffected by gravity. It has been postulated that the displacement phenomenon is possible due to thin monomolecular layer on the surface of cornea that is displaced in the aforesaid manner and not the whole of the precorneal film.[26]

EVAPORATION OF TEAR FILM

It has been shown that almost all lipid films including those of wax esters and cholesterol esters retard the evaporation of water. With proper type of measurement technique, specific resistance to evaporation due to lipid layer can be determined. Using such an approach, evaporation retarding effect has been demonstrated both *in vivo* and *in vitro*.[27]

Such a retarding effect of superficial lipid layer is important, especially under conditions of low humidity and turbulent air flow near the cornea such as exists in a windy and arid climate.[28]

Evaporation from the tear film is estimated to be about 10% of the production rate. That makes the evaporation 0.12 µl/min since the tear production rate is 1.2 µl/min. There is a little effect of air motion on the evaporation rate because most of the resistance to evaporation is the oily layer on the tear film.

STABILITY DRYING AND RUPTURE OF TEAR FILM

The tears can function properly only if the tear film covers the entire preocular surface and is re-established quickly and completely after a blink. In the normal human eye, the precorneal tear film has a short-lived stability. When blinking is prevented, after a brief time interval of 15–40 seconds, the tear film ruptures and dry spots appear on various parts of cornea.[29] The drying of the corneal surface cannot be a result of evaporation of water alone, because at least ten minutes would be required to eliminate the whole tear film by drying only according to evaporation rates observed *in vivo* with the oily

layer in place.[27] It is interesting to note that among the lower animals, the tear film can remain complete for as long as 600 seconds between blinks. Following mechanisms have been put forward to explain the break-up of tear film in humans.

Mechanism of tear film break up

Holly (1973) has described a mechanism of tear film rupture (Fig. 14.3). The steps involved in the break-up of tear film as per Holly (also known as Holly and Lemp's mechanisms) are as follows:

- First of all the tear film thins uniformly by evaporation (Fig. 14.3A).
- When the tear film is thinned out to some critical thickness, a significant number of lipid molecules begin to be attracted by the mucin layer and migrate down to this layer. This migration process is enhanced, if there is any spontaneous local thinning (Fig. 14.3B).
- When the mucin layer on the epithelium is sufficiently contaminated by lipid migrating down from the top surface of the tear film, the mucin becomes hydrophobic and the tear film ruptures (Fig. 14.3C).

Of course, the blinking can supposedly repair the rupture by removing the lipid contaminant from the mucin layer and restoring a thick aqueous layer.

Thus, the dry spot formation is essentially localised non-wetting, and not localised drying caused by discontinuities in the superficial lipid layer. As regards the location of these dry spots, it has been noticed that these occur twice more in temporal quadrant as compared to nasal one. The suggested reason for these differences is that nasal areas are more protected against air currents and have comparatively higher temperature.[26]

DYNAMIC EVENTS DURING BLINKING

Holly (1980) has given a brief account of events during blinking.[30] A complex series of events take place (Fig. 14.4). As the upper lid moves downwards, the superficial layer is compressed. As it thickens, it begins to exhibit interference colours. The whole lipid layer together with the

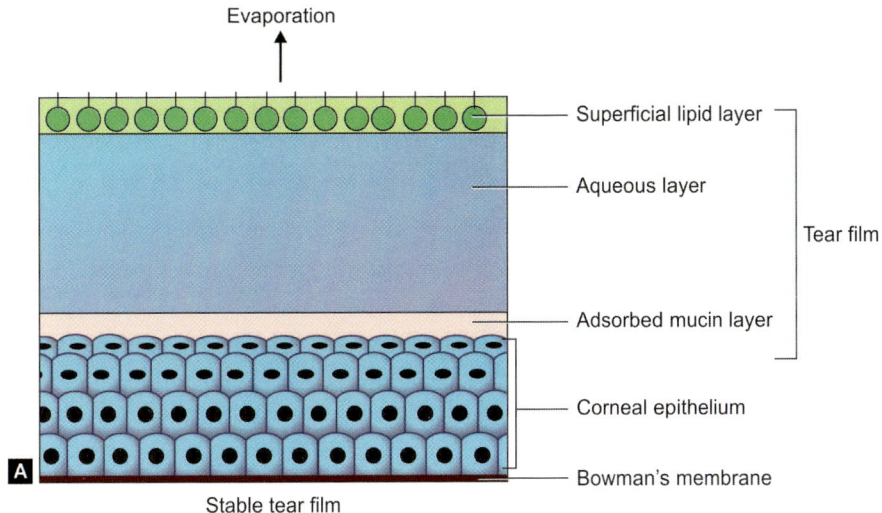

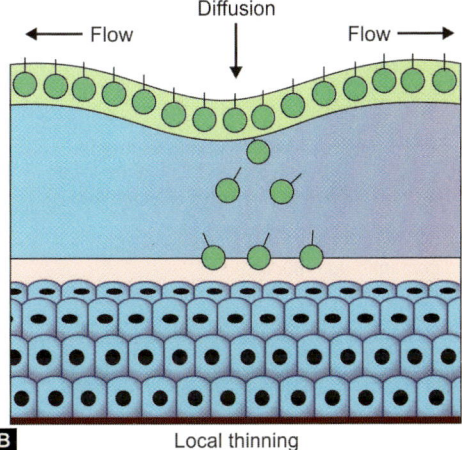

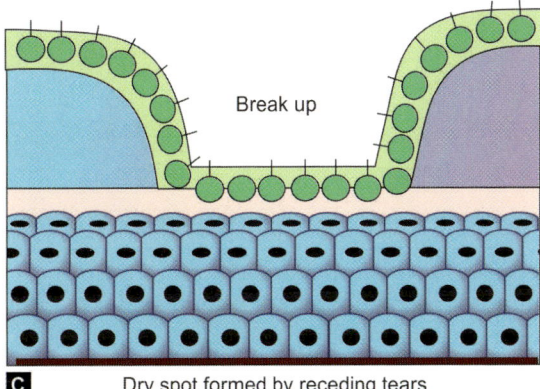

Fig. 14.3A to C: *Mechanism of rupture of tears*

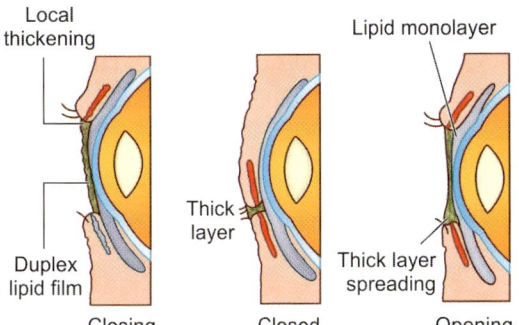

Fig. 14.4: *Dynamic events during blinking*

associated biopolymers is compressed between the lid edges. Lipid epiphora almost never occurs as the compressed lipid layer between

closed eyelids has a thickness only of the order of 0.1 μm.

This lipid contaminated mucus according to Norn[31] is rolled up in a thread-like shape and dragged into lower fornix (Fig. 14.5).

When the eye opens, at first the lipid spreads in the form of a monolayer against the upper eyelid. In this spreading process, the limiting factor is the motion of eyelid. The spreading of the excess lipid follows and in about 1 sec. multimolecular layer of lipid is formed. The spreading lipid drags some aqueous tears with it, thereby thickening the tear film. The magnitude of this effect is controlled by the size and shape of tear meniscus adjacent to lid edges. As

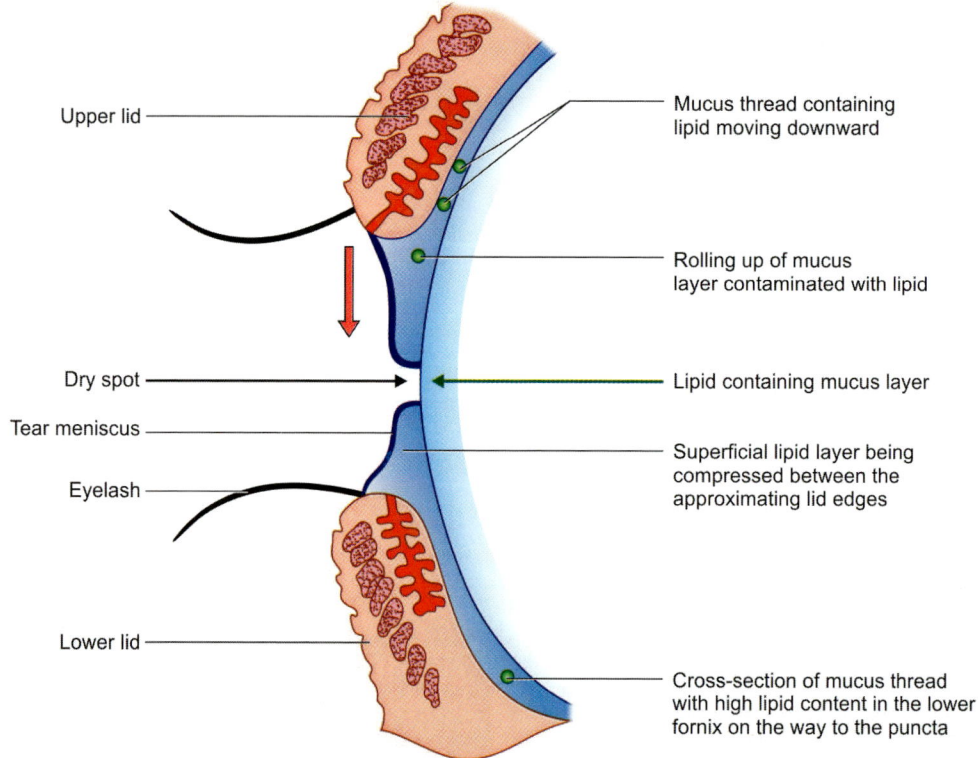

Upper lid

Mucus thread containing lipid moving downward

Rolling up of mucus layer contaminated with lipid

Dry spot

Lipid containing mucus layer

Tear meniscus

Eyelash

Superficial lipid layer being compressed between the approximating lid edges

Lower lid

Cross-section of mucus thread with high lipid content in the lower fornix on the way to the puncta

Fig. 14.5: *Mechanism of removal of lipid contaminated mucus*

soon as there are insufficient tears to form a saturated meniscus, a local thinning adjacent to the meniscus, takes place which effectively prevents further fluid flow from the meniscus to the tear film.[32]

ELIMINATION OF TEARS

Drainage of lacrimal fluid from lacus lacrimalis into the nasolacrimal duct

The lacrimal fluid flows over the precocular surface and reaches the marginal tear strip running along the ciliary margin of each eyelid and collects as lacus lacrimalis in the inner canthus. 25% of tears are lost by evaporation. From the lacus lacrimalis and along the marginal tear strip, the lacrimal fluid is then drained by the lacrimal passages into the nasal cavity (Fig. 14.6). Capillary action plays an important role in conducting the tears into the punctum and vertical limb of canaliculus. Flow along the lacrimal passages is brought about by an *active lacrimal pump mechanism* constituted by fibres of

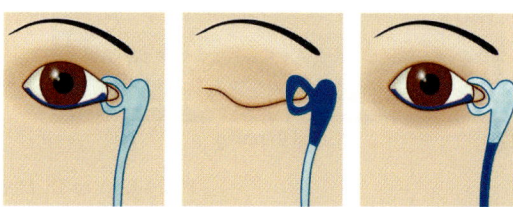

Fig. 14.6: *Elimination of tears by lacrimal pump mechanism*

the preseptal portion of the orbicularis which arise from the lacrimal fascia and posterior lacrimal crest (Horner's muscle). This lacrimal pump operates with the blinking movements of the eyelids as follows:[33]

A. *On eyelid closing movement,* following three events occur concomitantly (Fig. 14.7A):

1. *Contraction of pretarsal fibres* of the orbicularis compresses the ampulla and shortens the canaliculi. This movement propels the tear fluid present in the ampulla and horizontal part of the canaliculi toward the lacrimal sac.

2. *Contraction of preseptal fibres of orbicularis pulls* the lacrimal fascia and lateral wall of the

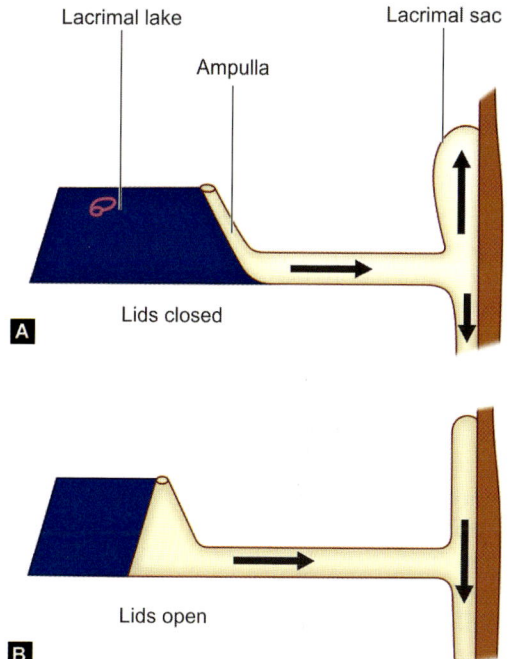

Fig. 14.7: *Lacrimal pump mechanism. A, When lids close; B, When lids open (see text for explanation)*

lacrimal sac laterally, thereby opening the normally closed lacrimal sac. This produces a relative negative pressure and draws the tears from the canaliculi into lacrimal sac.

3. *Along with the increased tension on the lacrimal fascia* (which opens the lacrimal sac), the inferior portion closes more tightly, thereby preventing aspiration of air from the nose.

B. When the eyelids open, tone in the orbicularis muscle is decreased and following events occur concomitantly (Fig. 14.7B):

1. *Relaxation of pretarsal fibres* of the orbicular allows the canaliculi to expand and reopen. The expansion of the canaliculi and ampullae draws in the lacrimal fluid through the puncti from the lacrimal lake.

2. *Relaxation of the portion of the preseptal fibres* (Horner's muscle) allows the lacrimal sac to collapse. The collapse of the lacrimal sac expels the fluid therein downwards into the now open nasolacrimal duct. Therefore, in atony of the sac tears is not drained rough the lacrimal passages, in spite of anatomical patency, resulting in epiphora.

Drainage of lacrimal fluid from nasolacrimal duct (NLD) into the nasal cavity

Once the lacrimal fluid enters the upper end of the NLD, the influence of eyelid movements on its further downward flow ends.

Factors which influence the flow of tears along the NLD are as follows:

- *Gravity* helps in downward flow.
- *Air current movement within the nose:* The opening of NLD in the nasal cavity is so placed that air currents passing either inward or outward, induce a negative pressure within the NLD and thus draw the fluid down the potential lumen of the duct into the nose.
- *Hasner's valve* present at the lower end of NLD remains open as long as the pressure within the nose is less than the NLD and thus allows the tears to flow from the NLD into the nose. However, when the intranasal pressure increases (as on blowing the nose), the Hasner's valve closes, thereby preventing the reflux upward.

From the nose, the tears pass posteriorly with the nasal mucus secretions.

DRY EYE DISEASE

DEFINITION, CLASSIFICATION AND CAUSES

DEFINITION

TFOS International Dry Eye Workshop (DEWS) II, new definition of dry eye disease (DED) is as follows: "Dry eye is a multifactorial disease of the ocular surface characterised by a loss of homeostasis of the tear film, and accompanied by ocular symptoms, in which tear film instability and hyperosmolarity, ocular surface inflammation and damage, and neurosensory abnormalities play etiological roles".

CLASSIFICATION AND CAUSES OF DED

According to International Dry Eye Workshop report (DEWS report 2007), the causes of dry eye can be classified as below.

I. AQUEOUS DEFICIENCY DRY EYE

Aqueous deficiency dry eye (ADDE) also known as keratoconjunctivitis sicca (KCS). Its causes include:

a. *Sjögren's syndrome* (primary keratoconjunctivitis sicca).

b. *Non-Sjögren's keratoconjunctivitis sicca.* Causes can be grouped as below:

1. *Primary age-related hyposecretion* is the most common cause.

2. *Lacrimal gland deficiencies* as seen in congenital alacrima, infiltrations of lacrimal gland, e.g. in sarcoidosis, tumours, post-radiation fibrosis of lacrimal gland and surgical removal.

3. *Lacrimal gland duct obstruction* as seen in old trachoma, chemical burns, cicatricial pemphigoid and Stevens-Johnson syndrome.

4. *Reflex hyposecretion* (neurogenic causes) as seen in familial dysautonomia (Riley-Day syndrome), Parkinson disease, reflex sensory block, reflex motor blade, 7th cranial nerve damage, reduced corneal sensations after refractive surgery and corneal lens wear.

II. EVAPORATIVE DRY EYE

It is caused by the conditions which decrease tear film stability and thus increase evaporation.

Causes can be grouped as:

1. *Meibomian gland dysfunction* as seen in chronic posterior blepharitis, rosacea, and congenital absence of meibomian glands.

2. *Lagophthalmos* as seen in facial nerve palsy, severe proptosis, symblepharon and eyelid scarring.

3. *Defective blinking* such as low blink rate as seen in prolonged computer users and other causes.

4. *Vitamin A deficiency and other factors* affecting ocular surface, e.g. topical drugs, preservatives, contact lens wear, ocular surface allergic disease and scarring disorders.

PATHOGENESIS

Dry eye disease (DED) is a chronic inflammatory condition that can be initiated by numerous extrinsic or intrinsic factors that promote an unstable and hyperosmolar tear film.

Core mechanism of DED is evaporation-induced tear hyperosmolarity, which is the hallmark of the disease, as concluded by the TFOS DEWS II pathophysiology subcommittee. It damages the ocular surface both directly as well as by initiating inflammation. The broad outlines of cycle of events, described as the *vicious circle of DED* is shown in Fig. 14.8 and details are shown in Fig. 14.9.

Two forms of DED are recognized. Aqueous deficiency dry eye (ADDE) and evaporative dry eye (EDE).

- *In ADDE,* tear hyperosmolarity results when lacrimal secretion is reduced, in conditions of normal evaporation from the eye.

- *In EDE,* tear hyperosmolarity is caused by excessive evaporation from the exposed tear film in the presence of a normally functioning lacrimal gland.

Since tear osmolarity is a function of tear evaporation in either ADDE or EDE, tear hyperosmolarity arises due to evaporation from the ocular surface and, in that sense, all forms of DED are evaporative. In other words, EDE is more accurately considered a hyper-evaporative state. EDE is associated with meibomian gland dysfunction (MGD) (*see* page 288 for pathogenesis of MGD).

Tear hyperosmolarity activates stress signalling pathways in the ocular surface epithelium as well as resident immune cells and triggers production of innate inflammatory molecules that initiate a vicious self-perpetuating cycle (Figs 14.8 and 14.9) that may lead to further decline in tear function and worsen the symptoms. The numerous extrinsic factors (e.g. desiccating environment, exposure) and intrinsic (e.g. ageing, autoimmunity, drying medications) factors that can contribute to this inflammatory cycle demonstrate why it is often difficult to ascribe a single cause for most cases of dry eye disease and the importance of addressing all modifiable risk factors.

Hyperosmolar stress has a direct pro-inflammatory effect on the ocular surface epithelium. It has been shown to activate mitogen-activated protein kinases (MAPKs), stimulate secretion of pro-inflammatory cytokines (e.g. IL-1β, TNF-α, and IL-6), chemokines and matrix metalloproteinases such as MMP-3 and MMP-9 and induce apoptosis. The interaction of these inflammatory mediators is complex and they have been shown to upregulate each other; thus

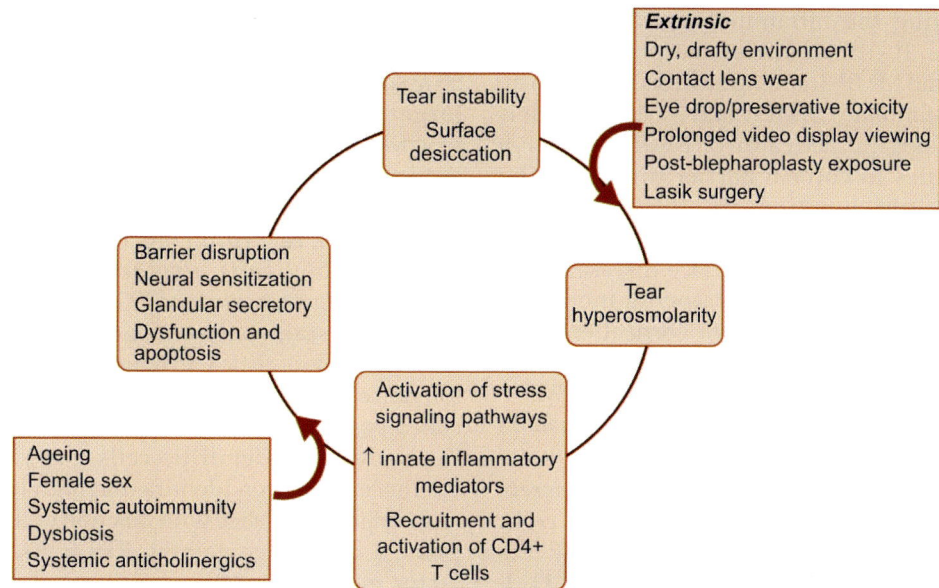

Fig. 14.8: *Broad outlines of vicious cycle of events involved in pathogenesis of dry eye*

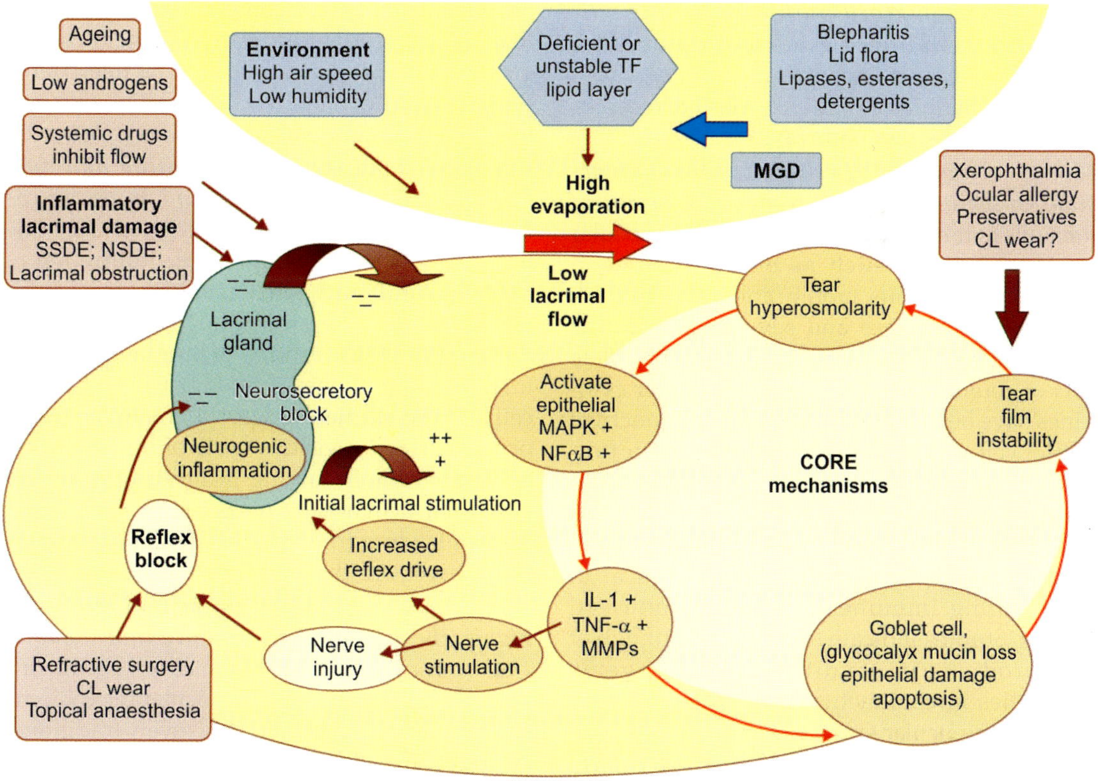

Fig. 14.9: *Detailed outlines of vicious cycle of events involved in pathogenesis of dry eye*

amplifying the inflammatory cascade. For example, IL-1β stimulates the production of TNF-α and MMP-3, among other factors. In turn, TNF-α stimulates MMP-9 and MMP-3 which is a physiological activator of MMP-9. MMP-9 contributes to corneal barrier disruption by lysing tight junctions in the superficial epithelium. Increased tear MMP-9 has also been detected in other ocular surface diseases, such as atopic and vernal keratoconjunctivitis, corneal ulceration, recurrent corneal erosions and ocular burns that also have corneal barrier disruption. *Detection of elevated tear MMP-9 provides a rationale for use of anti-inflammatory/ protease therapies in these conditions.*

Ocular surface epithelial cells also secrete chemokines that attract inflammatory cells. Increased levels of chemokines CCL20 (MIP-3α), CXCL9 (MIG), CXCL10 (IP-10) and CXCL11 (I-TAC) and their receptors were noted in ocular surface cells and/or tears of dry eye patients.

Another effect of desiccation is upregulation of innate inflammatory pathways in the epithelium, including the nucleotide-binding domain, leucine-rich-containing family, pyrin domain-containing 3 (NLRP3), toll-like receptor and oxidative stress pathways.

Metaplasia and goblet cell loss in the conjunctival epithelium is a well-recognized feature of aqueous tear deficiency. The most severe ocular surface disease, such as Stevens-Johnson syndrome, mucous membrane pemphigoid, graft-*vs*-host disease and severe alkali burns involving the conjunctiva often have complete loss of conjunctival goblet cells. T helper cytokines have been found to modulate conjunctival goblet cell differentiation. In addition to producing tear-stabilizing mucins, goblet cells also produce immunoregulatory factors, such as TGF-β and retinoic acid. Crosstalk between goblet cells and dendritic cells is critical to maintaining immune tolerance in mucosal tissues. Studies indicate a critical role of goblet cell products in conditioning tolerogenic properties in conjunctival dendritic cells and maintaining ocular surface immune tolerance.

Evidence indicates that the initial innate immune response to dryness is followed by an adaptive CD4+ T cell autoimmune response in mice exposed to desiccating stress and in patients with Sjögren syndrome (SS) and non-SS associated aqueous tear deficiency. While the target autoantigen(s) in this autoimmune reaction have not been identified, members of the kallikrein family have been implicated as putative antigens in some studies.

In addition to producing tear-stabilizing mucins, goblet cells also produce immunoregulatory factors, such as TGF-β and retinoic acid. Crosstalk between goblet cells and dendritic cells is critical to maintaining immune tolerance in mucosal tissues. Goblet cell associated passages that deliver surface antigens to the underlying dendritic cells and promote tolerance have been identified in both intestine and conjunctiva. Mice with deletion of the SAM pointed domain containing ETS transcription factor gene (Spdef knockout) are devoid of goblet cells, develop conjunctival inflammation and lose immune tolerance to topically applied antigens, as has been found in other mouse dry eye models that are accompanied by goblet cell loss. These studies indicate a critical role of goblet cell products in conditioning tolerogenic properties in conjunctival dendritic cells and maintaining ocular surface immune tolerance.

Lacrimal gland (LG) inflammation and dysfunction develop with age and in the autoimmune disease Sjögren syndrome (SS). The hallmarks of SS are lymphocytic infiltration of the lacrimal and salivary glands, serum autoantibodies, keratoconjunctivitis sicca and dry mouth. Mouse models of SS and aging have identified a pathogenic role for CD4+ T and B cells. These studies suggest that similar to the ocular surface, a vicious cycle of inflammation and apoptosis involving infiltrating cells and glandular acinar cells perpetuates LG inflammation leading to glandular dysfunction in SS and age-related dry eye.

There is evidence demonstrating that the microbiome, the microbial community that inhabits the human body, has immunoregulatory functions. The presence of an ocular microbiome has long been suspected; however, traditional swab cultures of the conjunctiva are often negative. Studies using 16S genomic sequencing have demonstrated an ocular surface microbiome that may have the lowest biomass of any tissue in the mice that had an antibiotic-induced depletion of the microbiome with a cocktail of five oral antibiotics prior to experimental desiccating stress developed significantly worse dry eye than control mice that did not receive antibiotics.

CLINICAL FEATURES

Symptoms suggestive of dry eye include irritation, foreign body (sandy) sensation, feeling of dryness, itching, nonspecific ocular discomfort and chronically sore eyes not responding to a veriety of drops instilled earlier.

Signs of dry eye are as below:

- *Tear film signs.* It may show presence of stingy mucous and particulate matter. Marginal tear strip is reduced or absent (normal height is 1 mm).
- *Conjunctival sign.* It becomes lustureless, mildly congested, conjunctival xerosis and keratinization may occur. Rose bengal or lissamine green staining may be positive (details given in tear film tests).
- *Corneal sign.* It may show punctate epithelial erosions, filaments and mucus plaques. Cornea may loose lusture. Vital stains, fluorescein, rose bengal or lissamine green may delineate the above lesions.
- *Signs of causative disease* such as posterior blepharitis, conjunctival scarring diseases (trachoma, Stevens-Johnson syndrome, chemical burns, ocular pemphigoid) and lagophthalmos may be depicted.

Sjögren syndrome (SjS, SS) is a *long-term auto-immune disease* that affects the body's moisture-producing *glands*. Primary symptoms are a *dry mouth* and *dry eyes*. Other symptoms can include *dry skin*, vaginal dryness, a *chronic cough, numb-ness* in the arms and legs, *feeling tired, muscle and joint pains*, and *thyroid problems*. Those affected are at an increased risk (5%) of *lymphoma*.

- While the exact cause is unclear, it is believed to involve a combination of *genetics* and an *environmental trigger* such as exposure to a *virus* or *bacteria*. It can occur independently of other health problems (primary Sjögren syndrome) or as a result of another *connective tissue disorder* (secondary Sjögren syndrome).

The *inflammation* that results progressively damages the glands. Diagnosis is by biopsy of moisture-producing glands and *blood tests* looking for specific *antibodies*. On *biopsy* there are typically *lymphocytes* within the glands

- Treatment is directed at the person's *symptoms*. For dry eyes *artificial tears*, medications to reduce inflammation, *punctal plugs*, or surgery to shut the *tear ducts*, may be tried. For a dry mouth, *chewing gum* (preferably *sugar free*), sipping water, or a *saliva substitute* may be used. In those with joint or muscle pain, *ibuprofen* may be used. Medications that can cause dryness, such as *antihistamines*, may also be stopped.

TESTS FOR TEAR FILM ADEQUACY

A number of tests of tear function have been developed to aid in the diagnosis of dry eye conditions.

SCHIRMER TEST

It is the test for tear quantity. Schirmer[38] investi-gated the extent of wetting of a 5 × 35 mm blotting paper strip after folding 5 mm from one end and placing it in the lower fornix, at the junction of outer one-third and inner two-thirds for 5 minutes (Fig. 14.10). He found that normal secretion varied from 0.50 to 0.67 ml of tears per day and more than 15 mm of wetting in 5 minutes, measured from the folded end, was normal. Later, Whatman filter paper number 41 was standardised for this test. This test became

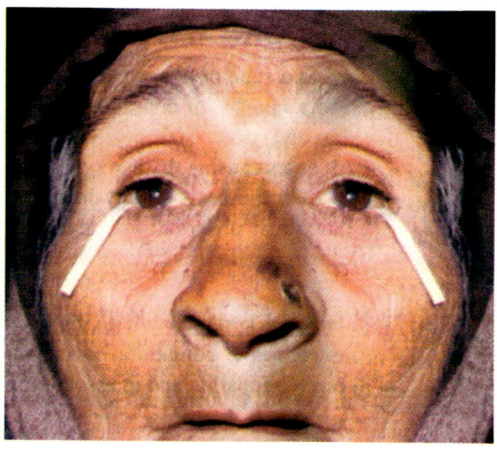

Fig. 14.10: *Technique of Schirmer I test*

popular as *Schirmer I* (or simply Schirmer) *test* and gives the value for both basic and reflex secretions of tears. It involves an open eye technique as closure of eyes during the test is believed to give false positive results.

A basal secretion test has been described in which the conjunctiva is anaesthetised before performing the test in a similar manner as above.[39] The difference between Schirmer I test and this test is a measure of basal secretion of tears. No statistical data supports this test as it is believed that conjunctiva is not fully anaesthetised to block reflex secretion.

Schirmer II test. To know the reflex secretion of tears, Schirmer II test was described. It is performed in the same way, after rubbing the unanaesthetised nasal mucosa with a dry cotton and noting the wetting after 2 minutes. But, since reflex secretion is not of major clinical sequence, this test is seldom used and Schirmer testing without anaesthesia or stimulation usually gives most useful and reproducible clinical information.

Schirmer III test. Schirmer extended his observations to know the reflex secretion and described a Schirmer III test, which required the patient to look directly in the sun. It has no diagnostic value and is potentially dangerous.

The Schirmer values were found to be age dependent, decreasing beyond age 60. One-third of persons above the age of 40 years were observed to have a wetting of 15 mm or less, the cut-off line suggested by Schirmer. Young women were reported to have more active lacrimation than young men while older women produced lesser amount of tears than older men.

Different cut-off values have been suggested for Schirmer test. Beetham, later on supported by Jones, suggested that wetting of less than 10 mm/5 minutes would indicate a diminished lacrimal secretion, whereas in another study, the safest cut-off value was reported to be 5 mm/ 5 minutes.

Modifications of Schirmer test have been described in an attempt to make it more appropriate and reproducible. Jones multiplied the distance of wetting of a standard strip placed for one minute by a factor of three and found it to correlate with a 5-minute reading.

A modified Schirmer test, in which the standard strip intended to be placed for 5 minutes was moved to a different place if there was no wetting after first 2 minutes, has been reported to obviate false positive results.[44]

Thread test is claimed to measure tear component more efficiently than the filter paper.[45]

Kinetic tear flow test has also been devised in which capillary tear flow in a Schirmer strip is prevented from evaporating by plastic cuff around the filter paper.[46]

TEAR FILM BREAK-UP TIME

Break-up time (BUT) has been defined as the interval between a complete blink and the appearance of the first randomly distributed dry spot on the cornea.[47] It is noted after instilling a drop of fluorescein and examining in the cobalt-blue light of a slit-lamp.

In the literature, there has been a wide fluctuation in the normal duration of BUT as studies by various workers. No significant relation between age, sex or corneal sensation and BUT has been observed.[47] In other studies, however, females and older people were reported to have a shorter BUT. Similarly, no correlation of palpebral fissure width, intra-ocular pressure, humidity or temperature with BUT has been observed.[48] A significant decrease in BUT on holding the lids apart has, however, been reported.

A BUT of 10 seconds has been recommended as a cut-off point for normal individuals by both Western[47] and Indian[49] authors. Values less than this are reported to indicate an abnormal, unstable tear film suggestive of mucin deficiency.[34] One study showed, a definite correlation between goblet cell population and BUT.[50]

BUT was found to be decreased significantly after use of benzalkonium chloride[51] and topical beta-blockers. Exposure to cigarette smoke also resulted in substantial (30–40%) fall in BUT.[52]

VITAL STAINING

Normally, the corneal surface is regular, smooth and shiny, and the tear film covering the epithelium is not directly seen. The histological principle of making transparent structures visible by admixing dyes has been applied to ocular tissues as well. The literature on vital staining of the eye is comprehensive and dates back to the end of last century. It became more popular with the introduction of slit-lamp biomicroscopy.[53]

Many dyes, like fluorescein, rose bengal, lissamine green, Alcian blue, scarlet red, etc., have been used for vital staining of the cornea and conjunctiva.

Fluorescein staining

It was synthesized by Baeyer in 1871. Chemically, fluorescein is resorcinolphthalein with molecular weight 376.27 and formula $C_{20}H_oNa_2$. Sodium salt of fluorescein is an orange red hygroscopic powder producing an intense green fluorescent colour in alkaline (pH above 5.0) solution. It was used in nineteenth century to delineate abrasions or minute ulcerations.

The intact corneal epithelium because of its high lipid content resists penetration of water soluble fluorescein and is not stained by it. Any break in the epithelial barrier permits rapid flourescein penetration and staining of areas denuded of epithelium. Due to slight acidic reaction of normal tear film, staining appears yellow or orange; the more alkaline aqueous humour colours fluorescein brilliant green in denuded areas. Fluorescein staining of the eye is transient and disappears within 30 minutes. Fluorescein staining is considered a sensitive test for detection of KCS and a positive staining was found in 96% cases of Sjögren's syndrome in a clinical study.[35]

Rose bengal staining

It is a dark red powder soluble in water. It is employed as 1% aqueous solution which is very irritating especially in tear deficient eyes. Unlike fluorescein, rose bengal selectively stains the mucus, debris and devitalised cells of corneal and conjunctival epithelium as readily visible red colour.

Bijsterveld[54] found the dye to be very useful in diagnosis of KCS. He suggested a grading system of rose bengal staining in such patients.

The palpebral aperture was divided into three areas, nasal and temporal conjunctiva and the cornea. A score of 0 for absent, 1 for just present, 2 for moderate staining, and 3 for gross staining was suggested in each of these areas; a total score was used for interpretation and a score of 3.5 out of 9 was considered abnormal.

The staining patterns have also been classified as A, B and C according to severity of KCS.[35] 'C' pattern represents mild or early cases with fine punctate stains in the interpalpebral area 'B' the moderate cases with extensive staining of entire exposed area; and in 'A' pattern there is confluent rose bengal staining on the exposed bulbar conjunctiva and blotchy and confluent on the cornea.

The staining pattern has been quantified by a point system. The number of stained dots on cornea, medial and lateral bulbar conjunctiva were estimated on a slit-lamp and were given points from 1 to 5 for <30, <100, < 000, <10,000 and >10,000 stained dots, respectively. Points more than 6 (out of a total of 15) were considered pathological.[55]

Lissamine green staining

It is a dark green, water-soluble substance used for colouring articles of food. It is an acidic, synthetically produced organic dye with a molecular weight of 576.6.

Norn[56] first employed this dye for vital staining of the cornea and conjunctiva. He investigated 171 eyes and 99 specimens of mucus threads, epithelial scrapings, and conjunctival fluid using 1% lissamine green solution, subjected to biomicroscopy. He concluded that lissamine green has vital staining properties almost identical with those of rose bengal and it stains degenerated and dead cells and mucus. It was further noted that lissamine green is far less irritating as compared to rose bengal.

OTHER TEAR FILM TESTS

Marginal tear strip characteristics

Marginal tear strip or tear meniscus is a continuous, full and slightly concave meniscus formed by tears between the eyelid margin and the inferior bulbar conjunctiva where the lid touches the globe. A height of 0.5 mm of tear strip on slit-lamp examination considered normal. A scanty, discontinuous or absent tear meniscus is an important sign of dry eye and suggests tear deficiency.[35]

pH (hydrogen ion concentration)

Normal pH is necessary for buffering action of tears. A wide difference in normal values tear pH is reported in the literature. In the early literature, the value reported was about 7.4 while the more modern it is about 7.0. The results depend upon the method of its determination, viz. vital staining, glass electrode, indicator paper or microcombination glass pH probe technique and sources of error, most common being due to CO_2 evaporation.

Abelson et al[57] suggested that tear pH measured by pH indicator paper, if adjusted by a correction factor of +0.70 pH units, would yield an equivalent pH as measured by an electrode. Indicator paper, however, was not found to be reliable for measuring tear pH.

Tear pH is known to change in many ocular conditions. A little has been reported in the literature about tear pH studies in dry eye syndrome. Recently, KCS patients were found to exhibit slight alkaline shift which, however, was statistically insignificant.[58]

Tear lysozyme levels

It is a bacteriolytic enzyme produced by tubuloacinar epithelial cells of main and accessory lacrimal glands. It presents 20% of protein contents of tear.[35]

It can be determined qualitatively and quantitatively. Tear lysozyme levels are decreased in early stages of dry eye and is thus an important test for early diagnosis of dry eye.[35]

Tear lactoferrin levels

Recently, the role of tear lactoferrin in the diagnosis of dry eye has been identified. Lactoferrin levels were observed to correlate closely to tear lysozyme assay. It may form a useful clinical tool in diagnosing dry eye syndrome, either singly or in combination with other tests.[59]

Tear evaporation

Rolando and Refojo[60] devised a tear evaporimeter and measured tear film evaporation in normal and dry eye patients. They reported a significant increased rate of evaporation in certain conditions like KCS, Stevens-Johnson syndrome, ocular pemphigoid and meibomitis. The instrument, though complex for routine diagnosis, serves as a non-invasive diagnostic and research tool.

Tear film osmolarity

Osmolarity of tear film has been reported to be isotonic (3.02 + 6.3 mOsm/L) in normal subjects and hypertonic (330 to 340 mOsm/L) in KCS. Though unsuitable for routine use, it is believed to be a very specific diagnostic test for KCS.[35]

Conjunctival biopsy and scrapings

Conjunctival biopsy and scrapings have been advocated to detect the histological changes in dry eye. After staining the material, goblet cell densities and their morphology, and keratinisation of epithelial cells, which is very specific in dry eye, can be seen microscopically.[35]

Conjunctival impression cytology

Recently, a non-invasive technique of impression cytology, where conjunctival impressions are taken to examine cellular structure, has been used for the diagnosis of dry eye. Ocular surface cells are obtained by using cellulose acetate filter material to make an impression.[35]

Squamous metaplasia involves three major steps, namely loss of goblet cells, increase in cellular stratification and keratinization. On the basis of cellular changes occurring in course of squamous metaplasia, the findings on conjunctival impression cytology have been graded according to the severity of dry eye state from 0 to 5 as follows:[61]

Stage 0: Normal cellular structure.

Stage 1: Early loss of goblet cells without keratinization.

Stage 2: Total loss of goblet cells with slight enlargement of epithelial cells.

Stage 3: Early and mild keratinization.

Stage 4: Moderate keratinization.

Stage 5: Advanced keratinization.

Fluorophotometry

Fluorescein dilution test or fluorophotometry is used to estimate tear flow, tear film thickness and various subvolumes of the total volume by measuring the dilution of an initial concentration of fluorescein in tear. The test is limited because of unavailability of fluorophotometer attachment with a slit-lamp routinely.[35]

OCULAR SURFACE ANALYSIS

Ocular surface analysers are now commercially available on sophisticated gadgets for comprehensive analysis of ocular surface.

Ocular surface disease index (OSDI) is determined with the help of a symptoms questionnaire.

▇ STEPS IN DIAGNOSIS OF DRY EYE DISEASE

Step 1: *DED confirmation with 'Positive symptom score* using:
1. Dry eye questionare 5 (DEQ 5), and/or
2. Ocular surface disease index (OSDI).

Step 2: *DED confirmation with 'Positive homeostasis markers* using:
1. Reduced non-invasive break-up time
2. Elevated or a large interocular disparity in tear osmolarity
3. Ocular surface staining

Step 3: *DED subtype (ADDE or EDE) classi-fication tests*
1. Tear volume measurement
2. Meibography
3. Lipid interferometry

▇ GRADING OF DRY EYE SEVERITY

Various criteria have been proposed to grade severity of dry eye. Recently accepted system based on severity of signs and tear film tests recommended by Dry Eye Workshop (DEWS) Report (2007) grades the severity of dry eye into 4 levels:
• Level 1 (mild dry eye),
• Level 2 (moderate dry eye),
• Level 3 (severe dry eye), and
• Level 4 (very severe dry eye).

DEWS system of grading of severity of dry eye is summarized in Table 14.5.

▇ TREATMENT OF DRY EYE DISEASE

Treatment of dry eye disease can be described as *step-ladder treatment* based on the severity level of dry eye.

STEP I: FOR LEVEL 1 (MILD) DRY EYE DISEASE

1. Patient education and supportive measures
• About dry eye disease, its management, and prognosis.
• Regarding lifestyle changes especially the importance of blinding while reading, watching television or using a computer screen.
• Potential dietary modification. Environmental review and modification.

2. Managing the potential affecting topical and systemic drugs being used by the patients. Tables 14.6 and 14.7 show the topical and systemic drugs associated with dry eye. These drugs showed be eliminated or changed with those having lesser side effects.

3. Supplementation with tear substitutes. Artificial tears remain the mainstay in the treatment of dry eye. These are available as drops, ointments and slow-release inserts. Mostly available artificial tear drops contain either cellulose derivatives (e.g. 0.25 to 0.7% methylcellulose and 0.3% hypromellose) or polyvinyl alcohol (1.4%).

4. Treatment of the causative disease of dry eye when discovered is very useful, e.g.:
• *Systemic tetracycline*, lid hygiene and warm compressor in patients with chronic posterior blepharitis (meibomitis).
• *Vitamin A supplement* for the deficiency.
• Treat the cause of lagophthalmos, entropion, ectropion, etc. when present.

STEP II: FOR LEVEL 2 (MODERATE SEVERITY) DRY EYE DISEASE

In patients with level 2 dry eye or when step I measures are inadequate following measures are recommended:
1. *Preservative-free artificial tear* to minimize preservative-induced toxicity.
2. *Anti-inflammatory drugs* to control the ocular surface inflammation should be added. These include:
   • *Topical cyclosporine* (0.05%, 0.1%) is reported to be very effective drug for dry eye

Table 14.5: *Dry eye severity grading scheme*

Symptoms, signs and tear film test	Dry eye severity level			
	1	*2*	*3*	*4**
Discomfort, severity	Mild and/or episodic; occurs under environmental stress	Moderate episodic or chronic, stress or no stress	Severe frequent or constant without stress	Severe and/or disabling and constant
Visual symptoms	None or episodic mild fatigue	Annoying and/or activity-limiting	Annoying, chronic and/or constant, limiting activity	Constant and/or possibly disabling
Conjunctival injection	None to mild	None to mild	+/−	+/++
Conjunctival staining	None to mild	Variable	Moderate to marked	Marked
Conjunctival staining	None to mild punctate erosions	Variable (severity/location)	Marked central	Severe
Corneal/tear signs	None to mild	Mild debris, ↓meniscus	Filamentary keratitis, mucus clumping, ↓ tear debris	Filamentary keratitis, mucus clumping, ↓ tear debris, ulceration
Lid/meibomian	MGD variably present	MGD variably present	Frequent	Trichiasis, keratinization, symblepharon
TFBUT (sec)	Variable	≤10	≤5	Immediate
Schirmer score (mm/5 min)	Variable	≤10	≤5	≤2

* Must have signs and symptoms. TBUT: Fluorescein tear break-up time. MGD: Meibomian gland disease.

Reprinted from Behrens A, Doyle JJ, Stem L, et al. Dysfunctional tear syndrome. A Delphi approach to treatment recommendations. Cornea 2006; 25: 90–7.

Table 14.6: *Topical ocular drugs that may cause or aggravate dry eye*[13]

Class	Examples
Agents used to treat glaucoma	
• Beta-blocking agents	Betaxolol, carteolol, levobunolol, metipranolol, timolol
• Adrenergic agonist drugs	Apraclonidine, brimonidine
• Carbonic anhydrase inhibitors	Brinzolamide, dorzolamide
• Cholinergic agents	Pilocarpine
• Prostaglandins	Bimatoprost, latanoprost, travoprost, dipivefrine, unoprostone
Agents used to treat allergies	Emedastine, olopatadine
Antiviral agents	Aciclovir, idoxuridine, trifluridine
Decongestants	Naphazoline, tetryzoline
Miotics	Dapiprazole
Mydriatics and cycloplegics	Cyclopentolate, tropicamide, hydroxyamfetamine
Preservatives	Benzalkonium chloride
Topical local anaesthetics	Cocaine, proxymetacaine, tetracaine
Topical ocular NSAIDs	Bromfenac, diclofenac, ketorolac, nepafenac

Table 14.7: *Systemic drugs probably causing or aggravating dry eyes*[13]

Class	Examples
Antihypertensive agents (beta-agonists)	Acebutolol
Antihypertensive agents (alpha-agonists)	Atenolol
Antiarrhythmic agents (beta-blockers)	Carvedilol, labetalol, metoprolol, nadolol, pindolol, clonidine, prazosin, oxprenolol, propranolol
Antipsychotic agents	Chlorpromazine, fluphenazine, lithium carbonate, perphenazine, prochlorperazine, promethazine, quetiapine, thiethylperazine, thioridazine, brompheniramine, carbinoxamine, chlorphenamine (chlorpheniramine), clemastine, cyproheptadine, dexchlorpheniramine
Bronchodilators	Diphenhydramine
Antispasmodics/antimuscarinic	Doxylamine
Antiarrhythmic agents	Ipratropium, atropine, homatropine, tolterodine, hyoscine (scopolamine), hyoscine methobromide (methscopolamine), disopyramide
Antineoplastic agents	Busulfan, cyclophosphamide, interferon (alpha, beta, gamma or PEG), vinblastine, cetuximab, erlotinib, gefitinib
Antihistamines	Cetirizine, desloratadine, fexofenadine, loratadine, olopatadine, tripelennamine
Antidepressants	Citalopram, fluoxetine, fluvoxamine, paroxetine, sertraline
Antileprosy agents	Clofazimine
Antirheumatic agents/analgesics	Aspirin, ibuprofen
Sedatives and hypnotics	Primidone
Drugs secreted in tears	Aspirin, chloroquine, clofazimine, docetaxel, ethyl alcohol, hydroxychloroquine, ibuprofen, isotretinoin
Antiandrogens	Tamsulosin, terazosin, doxazosin, alfuzosin
Neurotoxins	Botulinum A or B toxin
Antimalarial agents	Chloroquine, hydroxychloroquine
Retinoids	Isotretinoin
Antiviral	Aciclovir
Thiazides	Bendroflumethiazide, chlorothiazide, chlortalidone, hydrochlorothiazide, hydroflumethiazide, indapamide, methyclothiazide, metolazone, polythiazide, trichlormethiazide
Cannabinoids	Dronabinol, hashish, marijuana
Chelating agents	Methoxsalen
Strong analgesics	Morphine, opium/opioids
Antipsychotic agents	Pimozide

- *Topical steroids* used for limited duration are effective
- *Oral omega fatty acids* were also reported useful. However, recently the DREAM study has concluded that omega fatty acids play not much role in the treatment of dry eye diseases.

3. *Secretogogues* such as pilocarpine, cevimeline, and rebamipide.

4. *Tear conservation* by use of:
   - *Punctal occlusion* with temporary measures
   - *Moist chamber* spectacles and spectacle with side shields.

5. *Measure for MGD,* associated dry eye, includes:
   - *Oral macrolide* or tetracycline antibiotic
   - *Topical antibiotics* or antibiotic–steroid combination eye ointment to be rubbed at lid margin.
   - *Physical heating* and expression of the meibomian glands (including device-assisted therapies such as lipi-flow.
   - *In-office intense pulsed* light therapy for MGD.

   Note: For detailed management of MGD, *see* Chapter 18, page 296.

6. *Demodex,* when present, should be treated with tea tree oil.

STEP III: FOR LEVEL 3 (SEVERE) DRY EYE DISEASE

Following additional measures over those described in step II include:

1. *Serum eye drops,* autologous or allogenic
2. *Oral secretogogues*
3. *Therapeutic contact lens options* are:
   - Soft bandage lenses,
   - Rigid scleral lenses.

STEP IV: FOR LEVEL 4 (VERY SEVERE) DRY EYE DISEASE

The additional measures include:

1. *Topical steroids* for longer duration
2. *Systemic anti-inflammatory agents*
3. *Surgical measures*
   - *Permanent punctal occlusion,* surgically, for preserving the tear
   - *Tarsorrhaphy* is useful for ocular surface recovery
   - *Mucous membrane or amniotic membrane transplantation* for corneal complications
   - *Salivary gland* autotransplantation may be required in very severe cases.

REFERENCES

1. Fischer FP. Arch Augenheilk 98: Erganzungsheft 1–84, 1928. Cited by Ehlers N Acta Ophthalmol. 1965; (Suppl 81): 12.
2. Rollet J. La couch de liquide pre corneenne. Arch. Ophthal. Paris, 53: 5–24, 1936. Cited by Ehlers, N: Acta ophthalmol, 1965; (Suppl 81): 12.
3. Wolff E. Macocutaneous junction of lid margin and the distribution of the tear fluid. Trans. Opthal Soc UK 1946; 66: 291–308.
3a. Tiffany J. Tear film stability and contact lens wear. J Br Contact Lens Assoc 1988; 11: 35–38.
3b. Dilly PN. Structure and function of the tear film. Adv Exp Med Biol 1994; 350: 239–47.
3c. Ptlugfelder SC, Liu Z, monroy D, Li DQ, Carvajal ME, Price-Schiavi SA, Idris N, Solomon A, Perez A, Carraway KL. Detection of sialomucin complex (MUC4) in human ocular surface epithelium and tear fluid. Invest Ophthalmol Vis Sci 2000; 41: 1316–26.
4. Brauninger GE, Shah DO and kaufman HE. Direct physical demonstration of oil layer on tear film surface. Am J Ophthalmol 1972; 73: 132–134.
5. Holly FJ, Lemp MA. Tear Physiology and dry eyes. Surv. Ophthalmol 1977; 22: 69–87.
6. Holly FJ and Lemp MA. Surface chemistry of the tear film: Implications for dry eye syndromes, contact lenses and ophthalmic polymers. Cont Lens Soc Am J 1971; 5: 12.
7. Mishima S. Some physiological aspects of the precorneal tear film. Arch. Ophthalmol 1965; 73: 213–41.
8. Altaman PL. Blood and other body fluids. Federation of American Society for experimental Biology, Washington, DD 1961; 488.
9. Mastman GL, Blades EJ, Henderson JW. The total osmotic pressure of tears in normal and various pathological conditions, Arch Ophthalmol 1961; 65: 509–13.
10. Mizukawa T, et al. Physiology of tears. Acta Soc Ophthalmol Jap 1971; 75: 1953–73.
11. Hill RM, Schoessler JP. Tear pumps: Reservoir oxygen measurement *in situ.* J Am Optom 1969; 40: 1103–05.
12. Liotet S, Warnet VM, Arrata M. Functional exploration of lacrimal gland by tear electrophoresis. Ophthalmologica, Basel 1982; 184: 87.
13. Fleming A. On a remarkable bacteriolytic element found in tissues and secretion, Proc. R. Soc. Lond. (Biol.) 1922; 93: 306.
14. Kahan IL, Ottovay E. The significance of tear lactate dehydrogenase in health and external eye diseases. Albrecht von Graefes Arch. Ophthalmol 1975; 194: 267.
15. Ford LC, Delange RJ, Petty RW. Identification of a non-lysozomal bacteriocidal factors (betalysin) in human tear and aqueous humour. Am J Ophthalmol 1976; 81: 30.

16. Iwata S, Kabasawa I. Fraction-action and chemical properties of tear mucoids. Exp. Eye Res 1971; 12: 360–67.

17. Tokyda H. Glucose detection in tears in diabetes. Jpn. J. Clin. Ophthalmol 1969; 23: 517.

18. Van-Haeringen NJ, Glassius E. Collection method dependent upon concentration of some metabolites in human tear fluid, with special reference to glucose in hyperglycaemic conditions. Albrecht von Grafes Arch. Ophthalmol 1977; 202: 1.

19. Doane MG, Gleason WJ. Tear layer mechanisms. In Bennett ES, Weissman BA (eds). Clinical contact lens practice, Philadelphia, JB Lippincott 1991; pp 1–17.

20. Patrick RK. Lacrimal secretion in full-term and premature babies. Trans Ophthalmol Soc UK 1974; 94: 283. (cited in Am J Ophthalmol 1975; 79: 713.

21. Adamson AW. Physical chemistry of the surfaces. 2nd ed. New York. Interscience Publishers 1967; p. 363.

22. Lemp MA, Holly FJ. Recent advances in ocular surface chemistry Am J Optom 1970; 47: 669–72.

23. Doane MG. Interaction of eyelids and tears in corneal wetting and the dynamics of normal human eyeblink. Am J Ophthalmol 1980; 89: 507–16.

24. Wolff E. Anatomy of eye and orbit. New York, Blakiston Co. 1954; ed. 4: 207–09.

25. Mishima S. Some physiological film. Acta Ophthalmol 1965 (Suppl. 81).

26. Ehlers N. The precorneal film. Acta Ophthalmol 1965 (Suppl. 81).

27. Iwata S, Lemp MA, Holly FJ, Dohlman CH. Evaporation rate of water from the precorneal tear film and cornea in rabbit. Invest Ophthalmol 1969; 8: 613–19.

28. Holly FJ. Formation and stability of the tear film I Int. Ophthalmol. Clinic 1973a; 13: 73–96.

29. Norn MS. Desiccation of precorneal tear film I corneal wetting time. Arch Ophthalmol 1969a; 47: 865–80.

30. Holly FJ. Tear film physiology. Am J Optom and Physiol. Optics 1980; 57: 252–57.

31. Norn MS. Mucous flow in the conjunctiva. Rate of migration of the mucous thread in the inferior conjunctival fornic towards the inner canthus. Acta Ophthalmol 1969b; 47: 129–46.

32. Holly FJ. Surface chemical evaluation of artificial tears and their ingredients. I. Interfacil, activity at equilibrium. Contact intraocul. Lens, Med J 1978; 4: 14–31.

33. Jones LT. The cure of epiphora due to canalicular disorders, trauma ad surgical failures on the lacrimal passages. Trans. Am. Acad. Ophthalmol. Otolaryngol 1962; 66: 506.

34. Holly FJ, Lemp MA. Tear Physiology and dry eyes. Surv Ophthalmol Clin 1977; 22(2): 69–87.

35. Whitcher JP. Clinical diagnosis of the dry eys. In: Smolin G, Friedlaender MH, eds. The dry eye. Int Ophthalmol Clin 1987; 27(1): 7–24.

36. Moudgil SS, Singh M, Parmar IPS, Khurana AK. Tear film flow and stability in herpes simplex keratitis and chronic blepharitis. Acta Ophthalmol (Copenhagen) 1986; 64: 509–11.

37. Gaule VJ. Effect of trigeminal nerve on the cornea. Z Physiologie 1891–92; 5: 409–15.

38. Schirmer O. Studien Zur physiologie and pathologieder Tranenadsondeung und Tranenabfuhr. Arch Ophthalmol 1903; 56: 197.

39. Jones LT. The lacrimal secretory system and its treatment. Am J Ophthalmol 1966; 62: 47–60.

40. Doughman DJ. Clinical tests film. In: Holly FJ, Lemp MA, eds. The preocular tear film and dry eye syndromes. Int Ophthalmol Clin 1973; 13 (1): 199–217.

41. deRoeth A. On the hypofunction of the lacrimal gland. Am J Ophthalmol Soc 1941; 24: 20–23.

42. Beetham WP. Filamentary keratitis. Trans Am Ophthalmol Soc 1935; 33: 413–17.

43. Jones LT, Marquis MM, Vincent NJ. Lacrimal function. Am J Ophthalmol 1972; 73: 658–59.

44. Mackie LA, Seat DV. The questionably dry eye. Br J Ophthalmol 1981; 65: 2–9.

45. Kurihashi K, Yanogihara N, Honda Ya. A modified Schirmer test. The fine-thread method for measuring lacrimation. J Paediatr Ophthalmol 1977; 14: 309–08.

46. Holly FJ, Lambers DW, Esquival ED. Kinetics of capillary tear flow in the Schirmer strip. Curr Eye Res 1983; 2: 57–59.

47. Lemp Ma, Hamil JR. Factors affecting tear film breakfilm time in normal eyes. Arch Ophthalmol 1973; 89: 103–05.

48. Norn MS. Cytology of the conjunctival fluid. Acta Ophthalmol Suppl 1960; 59.

49. Moudgil SS, Khurana AK, Singh M, et al. Tear film flow and stability in normal Indian subjects. Ind J Ophthalmol 1989; 37(4): 182–83.

50. Lemp MA. Dohlman CH, Kuwabara T, et al. Dry eye secondary to mucous deficiency. Trans Am Acad Ophthalmol Otolaryngol 1971; 75: 1223–27.

51. Wilson WS, DuncanAJ, Jay JL. Effect of benzalkonium chloride on the stability of precorneal

tear film in rabbit and man. Br J Ophthalmol 1975; 59: 667–69.

52. Basu PK, Pimm PE, Shephard RJ. Cigarette smoke and tear film—the effect of cigarette smoke on human tear film. Can J Ophthalmol 1978; 13: 22–26.

53. Ehlers N. The precorneal film. Acta Ophthalmol Suppl 1965: 81.

54. Van Bijsterveld OP. Diagnostic tests in the sicca syndrome. Arch Ophthalmol 1969; 82: 10–14.

55. Norn MS. Treatment of keratoconjunctivitis sicca with liquid paraffin or polyvinyl alcohol in double-blind trials. Acta Ophthalmol 1977; 55: 945–50.

56. Norn MS. Lissamine green. Vital staining of cornea and conjunctiva. Acta Ophthalmol (KBh) 1973; 51: 483–91.

57. Abelson MB, Sadun AA, Udel IJ, et al. Alkaline tear pH in ocular rosacea. Am J Ophthalmol 1980; 90: 866–69.

58. Norn MS. Tear fluid pH in normals, contact lens wearers, and pathological cases. Acta Ophthalmol 1988; 66: 485–89.

59. Goren MB, Goren SB. Diagnostic tests in patients with symptoms of keratoconjunctivitis sicca. Am J Ophthalmol 1988; 106: 570–74.

60. Rolando M, Refojo MF. Tear evaporimeter for measuring water evaporation rate from the tear film under controlled conditions in humans. Exp Eye Res 1983; 36: 25–33.

61. Tseng S. Staging of conjunctival squamous metaplasia by impression cytology. Ophthalmology 1985; 92: 728–33.

Chapter

15

Effects of Contact Lens, Environment and Topical Medication on Ocular Surface

Chapter Outline

EFFECTS OF CONTACT LENSES ON THE OCULAR SURFACE
- Contact lens-induced corneal thinning
- Contact lens-associated red eye
- Contact lens-induced conjunctivitis
- Contact lens-induced dry eyes
- Contact lens-induced corneal inflammatory events

EFFECTS OF ENVIRONMENTAL POLLUTION ON THE OCULAR SURFACE

- Mechanism

TOXIC EFFECTS OF TOPICAL MEDICATIONS ON THE OCULAR SURFACE

Drug Formulation Toxicity Effects

Toxicity of Preservatives
- Types of preservatives
- Effects of commonly used preservatives
- Modulation of toxicity of preservatives
- Characterstics of an ideal topical formulation

EFFECTS OF CONTACT LENSES ON THE OCULAR SURFACE

The physiological effects of soft contact lens wear on the cornea were first studied and published by Göteborg in 1985. The wearing of contact lens on an eye results in a significantly thinner corneal epithelium, low rate of oxygen uptake, great number of corneal epithelial microcysts, thin corneal stroma, significant oedema during the day and a greater degree of corneal endothelial polymegethism (variation in the size of endothelial cells of the cornea as a result of disturbed metabolism) than the fellow eye. Great amount of limbal hyperaemia has been noticed in long-term wearers of hydrogel lenses as compared to the non-lens wearers with an encroachment of limbal vessels into the cornea. The epithelial and stromal changes reverse after one month of cessation of contact lens wear. All these effects are discussed in detail below.

1. CONTACT LENS-INDUCED CORNEAL THINNING

Mechanism: The cornea, conjunctiva and the tear film are main components of ocular surface that interact with a contact lens. Soft contact lenses have diameters 2 to 3 mm larger than the cornea so that their periphery directly interacts with the limbus and the surrounding bulbar conjunctiva. Factors responsible for corneal thinning are:

i. *Hypoxia:* The physiological changes induced on the cornea by chronic lens wear are due to long-standing hypoxia. Corneal epithelium and stroma are dependant on oxygen supply from the pre-corneal tear film. When the eyes are closed during sleep, the supply of oxygen to the corneal surface from the atmosphere is blocked and the ocular environment is in a state of hypoxia, resulting in a subclinical inflammation. Also, during sleep, the upper palpebral conjunctiva is in constant physical contact with the lens surface; as the tear film is reduced in the absence of blink mechanism (that normally

257

replenishes the tear film over the cornea), lens wetting is decreased and the rapid eye movements further produce frictional affects on the corneal epithelium.

The most reliable clinical indicators of chronic hypoxic stress are epithelial microcysts noticed in extended contact lens wearers. Microcysts form in the basal layer of corneal epithelium by hypoxia-induced cell apoptosis and move to the surface during cell turnover. They appear as small (10 to 50 μm diameter) translucent, irregular dots distributed as a ring in the mid-periphery of cornea, when seen under high magnification on the slit-lamp microscopy and marginal retroillumination. With daily wear lenses, less hypoxic damage occurs and less than 10 microcysts may be visible; more than 50 microcysts indicate a severe and chronic hypoxic stress.

Lens-induced hypoxia is also a major risk factor for infection by *Pseudomonas aeruginosa* as it can bind to the exfoliated surface epithelial cells in all soft contact lens wearers as compared to those wearing rigid gas permeable lenses; irrespective of the lens wearing schedule, significantly greater binding of Pseudomonas occurs with hydrogel lenses as compared to silicone lens.

ii. *Effects on the limbal stem cells:* The limbal stem cells are located at the basal level of limbal conjunctival and corneal epithelium. They produce daughter basal epithelial cells which have a great proliferative potential. They differentiate vertically upwards (from basal cells towards the surface epithelial cells) and migrate horizontally to replace the old surface epithelial cells that have undergone apoptosis-mediated cell death and exfoliation into the pre-corneal tear film. This cell cycle continues to replace the desiccated or damaged corneal epithelium and repairs superficial damage.

Soft contact lenses that cover the limbus result in hypoxic as well as mechanical trauma to the stem cells by the lens edge. Loss or injury of even 10% of these cells, makes the cornea vulnerable to deficient epithelialisation, resulting in recurrent erosions, chronic keratitis, and corneal vascularization. Various studies have confirmed that contact lens wear significantly slows the turnover of corneal epithelium by suppressing epithelial cell proliferation, migration and by decreasing the rate of exfoliation. The reduced epithelial thickness may result from a reduced demand for new surface cells, which signals to suppress the proliferation of basal cells. As a result, insufficient proliferation and movement of epithelial cells to the corneal surface results in corneal thinning.

Highly oxygen transmissible silicone hydro-gel lenses have a less pronounced affect on epithelial proliferation than hydrogel lenses (lower oxygen transmissibility) or rigid gas permeable lenses (equivalent oxygen transmissibility), and they show greater evidence of adaptive recovery during long-term extended wear.

2. CONTACT LENS ASSOCIATED RED EYE (CLARE)

The limbal region has a superficial blood supply from the episcleral arterial circle situated 1–5 mm the limbus and formed by branches of the anterior ciliary arteries. At a deeper level, it also receives communicating branches from the long posterior ciliary arteries situated deep within the eye. From the episcleral circle, two types of vessels emerge: One group passes anteriorly, among the palisades of Vogt, subdivides and recombines extensively to form the limbal arcade. The second group comprises recurrent vessels, which contribute partially to the limbal arcade but mainly travel posteriorly to supply the anterior 3–6 mm of the conjunctiva. Capillary vessels are mainly confined to the upper stromal levels of the conjunctiva, whereas larger vessels and nerves penetrate the lower stratum.

The cornea itself is avascular and relies on the limbal arcade to provide the blood-borne defence mechanism. To promote vascular growth into the cornea, the stimulus has to be strong, of the right character and long duration, so as to disturb the dynamic equilibrium of pro- and anti-angiogenic factors that maintains the normal avascular state of the cornea. Such a stimulus upregulates messenger molecule like vascular endothelial growth factor (VEGF), which is normally held at a low level through-out the cornea. The various stimuli that can initiate the neovascularization of cornea are:

i. *Mechanical abrasion* of the corneal surface: It can result from debris trapped under the lens or ill fitting/defective lenses. Also, specific components of the lens care solutions adsorb to the lens surface, and desorb after lenses are inserted in the eye.

ii. *Any corneal injury (hypoxic, traumatic), initiates an inflammatory response;* the initial line of defence is provided by the polymorphonuclear leukocytes which invade the area and try to kill and localise the offending agent. Then they are replaced by monocytes which change to macrophages to clear up the debris. These macrophages release VEGF and fibroblast growth factor (FGF) at the site of corneal injury.

As the concentration of angiogenic factors substantially increases, the local blood flow increases (hyperaemia, Fig. 15.1), promotes the chemotaxis of monocytes and macrophages, and initiates mitosis of vascular endothelial cells. Because the surrounding cornea is quite dense, the VEGF upregulates enzymes like matrix metalloproteinase 2 (MMP-2), a collagenase that digests the collagen matrix of the cornea. If the original stimulus persists, the growth of new vessels into the cornea continues at a rate of about 0.5 mm per day, and the blood cell movement starts within 72 hours after the event. Once the stimulus ceases, the persistence of neovessels depends upon whether they have been covered over by the pericytes. Pericytes are similar to smooth muscle cells; they are recruited to neovessels rapidly once they are formed. Around 80% of vessels get surrounded by the pericytes within 2 weeks of the initial injury, and once this has happened, vessel regression is

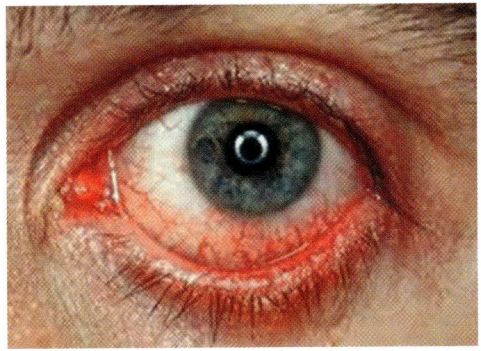

Fig. 15.1: *Contact lens-induced red eye*

unlikely. Hence, stimuli causing vascularisation must be removed or cleared within 2 weeks of onset for the corneal vessels to regress and prevent them from becoming permanent.

When the entire cornea as well as the limbal vascular arcade is covered with the soft lenses, the whole cornea gets hypoxic and the rate of corneal vascularization is much higher than when the peripheral cornea is exposed to the atmosphere by the rigid gas permeable lens.

3. CONTACT LENS-INDUCED CONJUNCTIVITIS (CLIC)

The basal epithelium of palpebral conjunctiva consists of a greater concentration of goblet cells, which move to the surface and discharge mucins into the tear film as well as covering the glycocalyx layer of the corneal epithelium, thus making it hydrophilic. The conjunctival stroma is highly immunosensitive due to the presence of large number of mast cells and memory cells.

Mechanism

Contact lens-induced conjunctivitis affects the upper palpebral conjunctiva. It may result from:

i. *Direct mechanical injury* due to constant rubbing of conjunctiva by the lens edge, resulting in the release of cytokines by the damaged cells and the resultant inflammation.

ii. *Allergic response to the lens material or deposits* (debris, desquamated epithelial cells, and microorganisms) accumulated on the under surface of lens. The allergic response is a type 1 hypersensitivity reaction mediated by degranulation of mast cells and release of histamine, producing symptoms of foreign body sensation, watering, itchiness, mucoid discharge. The upper and lower palpebral conjunctiva becomes congested (Fig. 15.2), oedematous and raised papillae are noted overlying the tarsal conjunctiva; the papillae (Fig. 15.3) are swollen conjunctival epithelium with a central core containing a blood vessel surrounded by lymphocytes and plasma cells. The symptoms improve after discontinuing the use of contact lens.

iii. *Delayed type IV hypersensitivity reaction:* The papillae and memory cells may persist in the stroma and predispose a person to recurrent

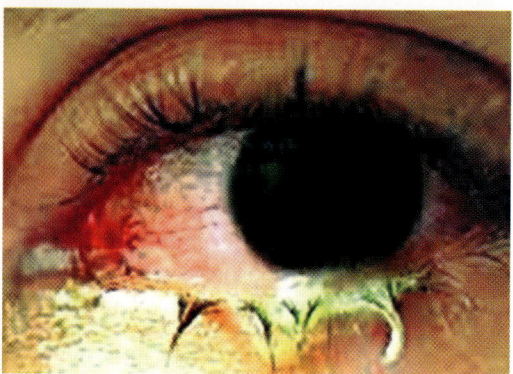

Fig. 15.2: *Contact lens-induced conjunctivitis*

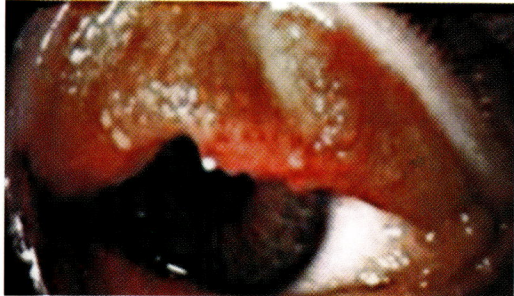

Fig. 15.3: *Papillae upper tarsus*

CLIC whenever the lens wear is resumed. The memory cells trigger a delayed type IV hypersensitivity reaction mediated by T-lymphocytes; this results in cytokine-induced inflammation, a further release of inflammatory mediators and an accelerated immune response after successive exposure to lens antigens.

4. CONTACT LENS-INDUCED DRY EYES (CLIDE)

Contact lens wear affects the structure, physiology and stability of the tear film by causing:

i. *Compartmentalisation of the tear film into pre-corneal and pre-lens components.* Normal pre-corneal tear film is 3 microns thick while a contact lens is 30 microns thick. It splits the tear film into two, resulting in an enhanced evaporation, and thinning.

ii. *Accumulation of debris,* inflammatory cells, metabolic by-products and microorganisms under the lens surface which promote the ocular surface inflammation and reduced tear production.

iii. *Affecting the structure of tear film:* Contact lens results in hypoxia as well as degradation of the lipid layer of tear film, with a lower level of stable non-polar lipids and an increase in polar lipids. This results in increased evaporation of the pre-lens tear film, its hyperosmolarity, thinning of the whole tear film and a reduced tear film break-up time; this affect is exaggerated in hot climate, by lenses of large diameter and by prolonged wearing of lenses.

iv. *Altered defence mechanisms of tear film* such as phagocytosis and microbial killing with prolonged retention time of microorganisms on the ocular surface. This is due to reduced secretion of IgA, increase in fibronectins and cytokines, reduced recruitment of polymorphs. This affect is exaggerated by overnight lens wear as the tear film stagnates and intensifies the subclinical inflammation.

v. *Damage to the conjunctival goblet cells* with resultant loss of mucins destabilises the tear film by making the corneal surface hydrophobic. The loss of soluble mucins in the tear film further interferes with the natural defence mechanisms and promotes surface inflammation.

Tear film instability results in contact lens dehydration which increases corneal hypoxia, increased formation of lens deposits, corneal staining, and patient symptoms of watering and an irritable red eye. All these affects are worsened by overnight lens wear.

5. CONTACT LENS-INDUCED CORNEAL INFLAMMATORY EVENTS

There is a range of adverse effects due to contact lens wear, as discussed above, the most harmful being 'corneal inflammatory events' (CIEs). They can range in severity from small infiltrates (Fig.15.4: Asymptomatic aggregation of small clusters of white blood cells in the peripheral cornea) to a sight-threatening microbial keratitis (Fig. 15.5). CIEs can result from either direct microbial infection or the release of their toxins only.

Normally the ocular surface has a strong defence mechanism against microbial infection and most contact lens wearers do not develop such a problem. The key elements in the defence process are blinking, lacrimation and the drainage system which are able to remove microorganisms rapidly from the ocular surface,

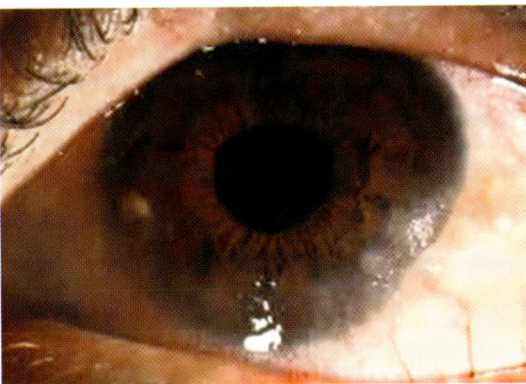

Fig. 15.4: *Peripheral corneal infiltrates*

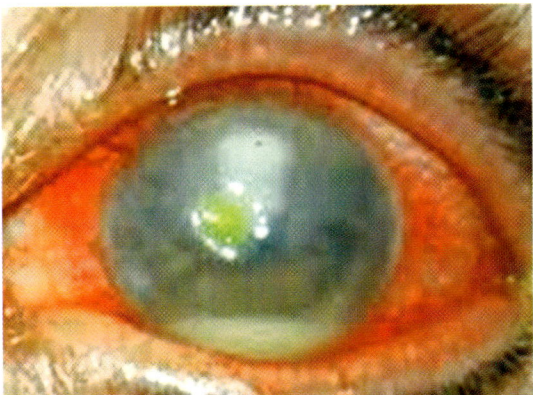

Fig. 15.5: *Hypopyon ulcer*

preventing their adherence and invasion of the cornea.

However, this system is rendered less potent when bacteria adhere to the under surface of contact lens, which acts as a vehicle for transferring them to the corneal surface. They get trapped between the lens and the cornea for a long period of time and have a chance to invade the cornea.

Bacteria can also be introduced to the eye via unclean hands of the contact lens wearer or from the unsterilised contact lens storage case in which the lenses have been stored. A greater number of microorganisms can reach the ocular surface and the eye's ability to clear a conta-minated tear film is compromised by the presence of the contact lens itself.

Key factors associated with CIEs

• Inadequate hand washing

• Non-prescribed overnight wear
• Excessive duration of overnight wear
• Excessive lens replacement interval
• Inadequate/poor case cleaning, demonstrated by almost all contact lens wearers
• Failure to use the correct disinfecting solution
• Failure to rub and rinse lenses and 'topping off' solution.
• Inadequate hand washing.

METHODS TO IMPROVE THE SAFETY PROFILE OF CONTACT LENSES

I. Contact lens care systems

Their primary purpose is to minimise the number of microorganisms which may reach the eye when a contact lens is applied, thereby enhancing patient's comfort and maintaining good vision.

It has been noted in various studies that the three common behaviours of hand washing, case cleaning and lens rinsing:
• are associated with CIEs,
• are performed poorly by most contact lens wearers, and
• they can be improved with repeated instruction.

II. Important instructions to the contact lens wearers

1. Always wash hands before handling contact lenses to reduce the chance of contaminating the lens.
2. Clean and disinfect lenses properly accord-ing to the labelling instructions. Rub and rinse contact lenses with sterile saline.
3. The contact lens solutions should not be used beyond the expiration or discard date. Do not "top-off" the solutions in the lens case; all of the left over contact lens solution should be discarded after each use. Never reuse any lens solution.
4. Contact lenses should never be exposed to any water: Tap, distilled, bottled, lake or ocean water because of the strong risk of Acanthamoeba keratitis.
5. Remove contact lenses before swimming as bacteria can adhere to contact lens and cause infection.

6. Clean and rinse the lens case with disinfecting solution (never tap water), each time the lenses are removed. A biofilm (persistent microbial coating) may form in the storage case with ongoing use. Immediately tissue dry the lens case and leave to air dry face down on a clean tissue.

7. The lens storage case should never be kept in a bathroom to avoid the aerosol effect from toilet flushing as it mobilises microorganisms through the room. It should be kept dry during the day. At night, when contact lens has to be placed in the case, it should be half filled with the lens solution.

8. Replace the contact lens storage case every 3 months.

9. Do not transfer contact lens solutions into smaller size travel-containers as this can effect the sterility of the solution.

10. Remove the lenses immediately if the eyes become red, irritated.

11. Do not put your lenses in your mouth to wet them as saliva is not a sterile solution.

EFFECTS OF ENVIRONMENTAL POLLUTION ON THE OCULAR SURFACE

Climate change and pollution have a strong impact on human health. Sources of pollution are variable in different areas. It ranges from toxic gases (CO_2, NO_2, O_3 and SO_2) and particulate matter discharged as exhaust fumes from automobiles; smoke from burning coal, fossil fuels, burning of crop-stubs and garden waste; environmental dust; pollen from trees; air-conditioning in offices, cigarette smoke. These toxic fumes and particles come into contact with the ocular surface and produce disease by causing an oxidative stress, ocular toxicity and inflammation. As the level of pollution increases, not only the respiratory and cardiovascular ailments become more prevalent, but eye-related complaints like ocular irritation, redness, watering, grittiness, and blurring of vision become common.

When people are chronically exposed to environmental pollutants, homeostatic mechanisms occur in the whole body to adapt to such changes and the affected people are not always symptomatic. However, a person who has pre-existing chronic allergies or an atopic tendency, the mucosal lining of eyes, respiratory tracts are in a state of heightened immune sensitivity. When such a person is exposed to further environmental antigenic stimulation, an exaggerated allergic reaction occurs, and continues for a long time so the quality of life is significantly impaired.

Mechanism

Environmental pollutants affect the ocular surface by the following mechanisms:

1. *Exposure to air pollutants* results in a selective binding of toxic particles to the ocular surface membrane receptors, leading to activation of pro-inflammatory signalling pathways.

2. *Desiccating environment* (hot, dry air, low humidity), seen particularly in air-conditioned offices, results in an increased tear film evaporation, its thinning and an increase in its osmolarity. This causes ocular surface inflammation.

3. *Reduced blinking* while working for long hours on computer screens, reading results in a decline in the tear film turnover and its clearance.

4. *Combined exposure to indoor and outdoor factors* reduce the conjunctival goblet cell density, the tear film break up time (TFBUT), and promote corneal epithelial damage. This compromises the barrier function of corneal epithelium resulting in ocular surface inflammation.

5. *Exposure to antigens* in a sensitised individual results in mast cell degranulation and triggering of type 1 hypersensitive reaction as seen in acute allergic conjunctivitis, seasonal allergic conjunctivitis and vernal conjunctivitis.

It is important to identify environmental agents either as the primary factors causing dry eyes and allergic conjunctivitis or secondarily worsening pre-existing chronic allergies. Steps should be taken as a part of therapy to eliminate the possible factors like ambient humidity, airflow, purity of air in a room and temperature to tolerable levels.

TOXIC EFFECTS OF TOPICAL MEDICATIONS ON THE OCULAR SURFACE

Topical medications are used for the ocular surface and anterior segment disorders because of the high exposure and an easy penetration of drugs into the ocular surface. Also, it is an easy, non-invasive and effective method of drug administration. Bioavailability of a drug into the aqueous is dependant upon factors like its hydrophilic or lipophilic nature, its ionisation/unionisation, molecular weight and drug concentration in the formulation. Upon instillation into an eye, the drug is distributed via two routes: Transconjunctival and transcorneal.

Absorption into the cornea and anterior chamber is along a concentration gradient of the drug, which in turn, depends upon its concentration in the tear film, blinking (drugs are drained from ocular surface by blinking), loss of integrity of corneal epithelium (promotes entry of hydrophilic drugs into the eye). The concentration of a drug entering the vitreous and reaching the retina or choroid is very low so there is a low bioavailability at the posterior segment of the eye. If a drug is injected into the sub-tenon space, then by diffusion through the posterior sclera, it does reach the posterior retina and choroid.

Short-term use of topical medications is highly effective usually with a little ocular toxicity. However, their chronic use not only increases the likelihood of toxicity from the drug formulation itself but also from the preservatives. The mechanisms involved are an acute allergy, toxicity, or inflammation. The inflammatory reactions are mediated by the release of pro-inflammatory cytokines, apoptosis, oxidative stress, and direct interactions with the lipid components of the tear film and cell membranes.

Drug formulation toxicity effects

The drug concentration is highest on the ocular surface after topical application therefore, the side-effects noted are also common, and include:

1. *Conjunctival hyperaemia:* It may be transient/temporary if the drug has a vaso-dilator affect. However, if the drug causes cytotoxicity, the resultant tissue inflammation and conjunctival congestion, papillae and follicles may be apparent as long as the drug is being used.

2. *Dryness of the ocular surface:* Many drugs reduce aqueous production from the lacrimal glands resulting in a dry eye.

3. *Raised intraocular pressure:* This may occur either by dilation of pupil in patients with narrow angles or by producing changes in the trabecular meshwork (steroids).

4. *Heterochromia:* Prostaglandin analogues increase melanin synthesis and produce hyperpigmentation of the iris, which is permanent.

5. *Corneal deposits:* Amiodarone causing cornea verticillata (Fig. 15.6).

6. *Lens opacities:* The drugs entering the anterior chamber alters the metabolism of lenticular cells, denature lens proteins and produce lens opacities.

7. *Affect of local anaesthetic drugs:* The cornea is richly supplied by nerve endings from the long and short ciliary nerves (branches of nasociliary nerve). Topical anaesthetics block nerve conduction by reducing sodium permeability, thus preventing the generation and conduction of nerve impulses. This prevents the brain from detecting painful stimuli.

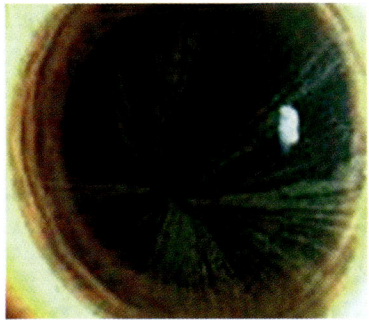

Fig. 15.6: *Cornea verticillata*

At the same time, they are directly toxic to the corneal epithelium, stroma and the endothelium. The cell injury releases antigens and incites an inflammatory response resulting in the formation of corneal infiltrates, a ring-shaped infiltrate and oedema. The preservatives in anaesthetics further add to the toxicity. Frequent use results in toxicity to the limbal stem cells and result in persistent epithelial defects, corneal ulceration, thinning and even perforation.

Toxicity of preservatives

Besides the direct toxic effects of medications in the eyedrops, the preservatives added to enhance the shelf-life have their own inherent toxicity. Preservative-free topical medication can develop contamination either through the ambient air or touching the bottle-dropper/ nozzle with fingers, eyelids or eyelashes during the instillation of eyedrops. In one study, the contamination rate of containers was found to be 8.4%. The most common microbial agents identified were Pseudomonas and *Staphylococcus aureus* (coagulase negative).

Types of preservatives

Over time, many preservatives have been developed. Common types of preservatives are listed in Table 15.1. Because of their anti-microbial activity against bacteria and fungi, they are added to the ophthalmic preparations to prevent their contamination, thereby increasing their shelf-life. They have anti-microbial properties by causing the rupture of outer membrane of microorganisms, by lowering the surface tension, and inhibiting the DNA synthesis at 37°C.

Effects of commonly used preservatives

Table 15.2 summarises the mode of action of common preservatives and their toxic effects are given below.

Benzalkonium chloride (BAK) is the most frequently used preservative. It is a quaternary ammonium compound that is weakly allergenic but highly toxic.

- *It acts as a cationic surfactant* that breaks up or dissolves the tight junctions between the corneal surface epithelial cells (zona occludens) as well as in the conjunctival epithelium, thereby increasing the space between the epithelial cells and results in enhanced transcorneal/transconjunctival penetration of the medicinal substances.
- *It also causes conjunctival squamous metaplasia and apoptosis, loss of goblet cells,* the solubilisation of lipophilic protective layer (loss of epithelial microvillar brush, the glycocalyx and mucin), resulting in an instability or breakdown of the tear film.
- *Its detergent affect disrupts the lipid layer of the tear film* resulting in an enhanced evaporation of the aqueous component with resultant corneal dryness. For this reason, it is not used in combination with topical anaesthetic agents.
- *It stimulates conjunctival fibroblasts* that may result in subconjunctival fibrosis, and the potential risk of failure for further glaucoma surgery.

BAK toxicity is direct as well as indirect

- *Direct toxicity affect* is dose and time-dependant; it depends upon the amount administrated daily, the duration of treatment and its concentration in the administered solution. It is manifested as a subclinical inflammatory response in which the patient

Table 15.1: *Types of preservatives*		
Chemical class	*Compound*	*Commercial name*
Quaternary ammoniums	Benzalkonium chloride (BAK)	BAK
	Cetrimide	Cetrimide
	Polyquaternium-1	Polyquad®
Mercury derivatives	Thiomersal	
Oxidative complexes (soft preservatives)	Sodium perborate (NaBO$_3$)	GenAqua®-Novartis
	SOC (stabilized oxychloro complex)	Purite-Allergan Ocupure-AMO
	SCP (stabilized chlorite peroxide)	Oxyd-Tubilux
Amidines	Chlorobutanol	
Alcohols	Phenylethanol	
Parabens	Methylparaben	

Table 15.2: *Mode of action of common preservatives*

Compound	Mode of action
Sodium perborate	In presence of water, the perborate is transformed in ion borate and hydrogen peroxide (H_2O_2), which is an oxidative compound
	Claim: "It turns into pure water and oxygen upon contact with your eye"
Stabilized oxychloro complex	Chlorite acts by producing a high degree of oxidation of glutathione, thus reducing the cell's defenses against oxidative stress
	Claim: "Dissipates into water and sodium chloride—components of natural tears when exposed to ambient light"
Stabilized chlorite complex	Chlorite acts by producing a high degree of oxidation of glutathione, thus reducing the cell's defenses against oxidative stress.
	The H_2O_2 is eliminated in water and oxygen by enzymes of the tissues
Benzalkonium chloride	A cationic surfactant, dissolves interepithelial tight junctions, loss of goblet cells, tearful instability

develops discomfort after instillation of eyedrops, a foreign body or a burning sensation, ocular dryness, lacrimation, itchy eyes. The signs of ocular surface damage are conjunctival injection, follicles on the lower conjunctival fornix, superficial punctate keratitis, anterior blepharitis, meibomitis and eyelid eczema (Fig. 15.7).

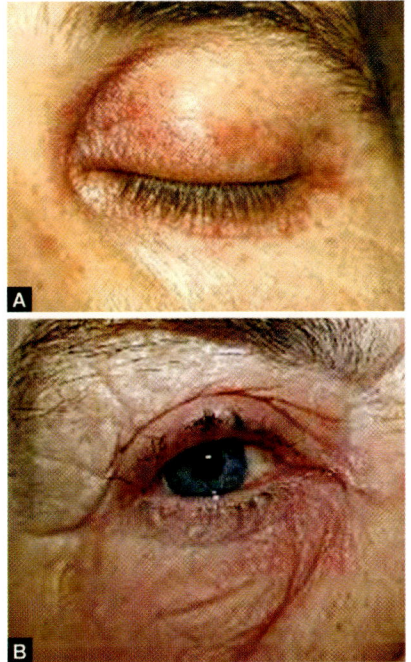

Fig. 15.7A and B: *Drug-incluced eyelid enzyme*

• *Indirect cytotoxicity* is mediated as a delayed type IV hypersensitive reaction, manifested as eczema and blepharitis. The allergen is formed by the binding of a hapten (with a high molecular weight of 1000 daltons) contained in the eye drop, with a protein molecule of the subject. Therefore, to prevent this reaction, all constituents of an eye drop should have a molecular weight less than 1000 daltons.

Care should especially be taken in patients who are prescribed high doses for prolonged time-period, those suffering from a pre-existing or concomitant ocular surface disease, and those who are already experiencing side effects related to other topical medications. In these instances, it would be advisable to use benzalkonium-free or preservative-free solutions whenever possible.

Chlorobutanol, sodium perborate, and stabilized oxychloro complex (SOC) have been studied and all preservatives cause harmful affects on the ocular surface. Compared with other preservatives, SOC caused the least amount of damage to rabbit corneal epithelial cells. BAK has demonstrated cytotoxic effects in cell culture, as well as in animal and human studies. Physicians should consider treatment with new-generation preparations containing low-risk preservatives such as SOC, especially in patients receiving multiple ophthalmic medications.

In order of decreasing toxicity, they are: Thiomersal > BAK > chlorobutanol > methylparaben > sodium perborate ≈ EDTA ≈ PBS.

Polyquad is a preservative derived from benzalkonium chloride. It is also a quaternary ammonium compound and is highly effective in preventing microbial growth, especially of fungus. It is not absorbed into hydrogel lenses because of its high molecular weight therefore, it is used in the storage solutions for contact lenses. Currently, it is increasingly used as a preservative in ophthalmic solutions particularly in the treatment of glaucoma. Bacterial cells attract Polyquad, but human corneal epithelial cells tend to reject the compound. Though it seems to be better tolerated by patients, and toxic or allergic reactions are rare, but it reduces the number of conjunctival goblet cells and affects the production of aqueous in the tear film.

Modulation of toxicity of preservatives

- The preservatives used in ophthalmic preparations are well tolerated when they are in normal concentrations and small doses are used for a short period.
- Ocular tolerance can be modified by the concentration of preservatives, combination of preservatives, their chemical purity, frequency of instillation, the duration of treatment, the condition of the cornea, wearing contact lenses and using polymers in formulating ophthalmic preparations.
- Recently developed oxidising and ionising preservatives are less toxic than detergent preservatives (BAK).
- Newer agents and newer technology multidose bottles have been developed to minimise drug toxicity, while enhancing drug delivery.

Characteristics of an ideal topical formulation

- It should be free of preservatives and phosphates.
- Should mimic the behaviour of the tear film.
- The pH should be near neutral or slightly alkaline.
- Should protect the ocular surface against osmolar challenge (addresses the hyperosmolarity of a dry eye).
- Should have an efficient drug delivery to the site intended.

BIBLIOGRAPHY

1. Albietz JM, Bruce AS. The conjunctival epithelium in dry eye subtypes effect of preserved and non-preserved topical treatments. Curr Eye Res 2001; 22: 8-18 [PubMed].
2. Baudoin C. Detrimental effect of preservatives in eye drops: Implications for the treatment of glaucoma. Acta Ophthalmol 2008; 86(7): 16–26.
3. Efron N, Morgan PB. Rethinking contact lens associated keratitis. Clinical and Experimental Optometry 2006; 89: 280–98.
4. Fleiszig SMJ, Evans DJ. Pathogenesis of contact lens-associated microbial keratitis. Optometry and Vision Science 2010; 87: 225–32.
5. Furrer P, Mayer J, Gurny R. Ocular tolerance of preservatives and alternatives. Eur. J. Pharm. Biopharm 2002; 53(3): 363–80.
6. Harris MG. Survival of contaminating bacteria in over the counter artificial tears. Jam. Optom. Assoc 1996; 67(11): 676–80 [PubMed].
7. Kallings L, Rigertz O, Silverstolpe I. Microbial contamination of medical preparations. Acta Pharm. Sue 1966; 3: 199–213.
8. Krishnan S. Secondary pseudomonas infection of fungal keratitis following use of contaminated natamycin eye drops: a case series. Eye (Lond). 2009; 23(2): 477–79 [PubMed].
9. Labbe A, Pauly A, Liang H, Brignole-Baudouin F, Martin C, Warnet JM, Baudouin C. Comparison of toxicological profiles of benzalkonium chloride and polyquaternium-1: An experimental study. J Ocul Pharmacol Ther 2006; 22: 267–78 [PubMed].
10. Raham MQ. Microbial contamination of preservative free eye drops in multiple application containers. Br. J. Ophthalmol 2006; 90(2): 139–41 [PMC free article] [PubMed].
11. Rosenthal R, Henry C, Stone R, Stone R, Schlech B. Anatomy of a regimen: consideration of multipurpose solutions during non-compliant use. Cont. Lens Anterior Eye 2003; 26: 17–26. [PubMed].
12. Wu P, Stapleton F, Willcox MDP. The Causes of and Cures for Contact Lens-induced Peripheral Ulcer. Eye and Contact Lens: Science and Clinical Practice S63-S66 (2003). do:10.1097/00140068-200301001-00018

Immunological Disorders of Ocular Surface

INTRODUCTION

The eye is a common target of inflammatory responses induced by local and systemic immunologic hypersensitivity reactions. Inflammatory ocular conditions resulting from immune responses are highly prominent because of the eye's considerable vascularization and the sensitivity of the vessels in the conjunctiva, which are embedded in a transparent medium. The eye and its surrounding tissues are also involved in a variety of other immunologically mediated disorders (Table 16.1).

Table 16.1: *Immunologic involvement of the eye*	
Ocular structures	*Lesions*
Lids	Blepharitis, contact dermatitis
Conjunctiva	Allergic conjunctivitis, atopic conjunctivitis, vernal conjunctivitis, GPC pemphigus/pemphigoid, Stevens-Johnson syndrome
Sclera	Episcleritis, scleritis
Cornea	Corneal allograft rejection, amyloid deposition
Iris	Iritis, cyclitis, pars planitis
Vitreous	Vitreitis
Retina	Retinitis
Choroid	Choroiditis
Optic nerve	Optic neuritis, vasculitis (e.g. temporal arteritis)
Extraocular muscles	Myasthenia gravis, orbital pseudotumour vasculitis

When such reactions occur, they are not infrequently seen first by the clinical allergist/immunologist, who then is in a position to correlate ocular and systemic findings and to coordinate therapy so as to treat underlying disease (if present) rather than only local eye symptoms.

While all the above conditions have been discussed in detail in respective chapters, few are being discussed here.

COMMON IMMUNOLOGICAL DISORDERS OF OCULAR SURFACE

PEMPHIGUS

Ocular pemphigus has been established as a clinical entity since 1858, when White Cooper, in the first volume of the Royal London Ophthalmic Hospital Reports, described a case. The term "pemphigus" comes from the Greek word *pemphis*, meaning blisters. It is certain that prior to this date the disease occurred, but was confused with the various conjunctival degenerations known at that time, notably as conjunctival xerosis. Subsequent to this date the exact pathological differentiation of the condition occasioned dispute amongst dermatologists and ophthalmologists, a controversy which was engendered by the rarity of the disease, until von Graefe, in 1879, identified pemphigus with what had hitherto been called "essential shrinking of the conjunctiva". Various authors (Pergens and others) have testified to the rarity of the condition; the average for eye cases is about 1 case per 20,000 and for skin cases 1 per 300 (Pusey).

ETIOPATHOGENESIS

Etiology is still uncertain for both pemphigus and ocular pemphigus but the isolation of a virus from pemphigus vulgaris has been claimed, current reports however suggest an autoimmune aetiology.

Autoimmune bullous diseases are associated with autoimmunity against structural components that maintain cell-cell and cell-matrix adhesion in the skin and mucous membranes. They include those where the skin blisters at the basement membrane zone and those where the skin blisters within the epidermis.

Clinical subtypes

The variants of pemphigus are determined according to the level of intraepidermal split formation.
- Pemphigus vulgaris (most common)
- Pemphigus foliaceus
- Pemphigus erythematosus
- Drug-induced pemphigus
- Paraneoplastic pemphigus

Pathophysiology

Pemphigus vulgaris (PV) is caused by auto-antibodies against desmoglein 3 (Dsg 3), a glycoprotein that localizes to the core of desmosomes. These autoantibodies cause acantholysis in the deeper suprabasal epidermis which is where Dsg 3 is mainly located. Dsg 3 is also located throughout the oral and other mucous membranes including the conjunctiva where blisters also occur in PV. ELISA tests for autoantibodies against desmoglein 1 (Dsg 1) and Dsg 3 are recently available that differentiate pemphigus vulgaris (anti-Dsg 3 IgG detected) from pemphigus foliaceus (only anti-Dsg 1 IgG detected), and the clinical subtypes of PV, i.e. mucosal dominant (anti-Dsg 3 IgG detected) and mucocutaneous (anti-Dsg 3 IgG and anti-Dsg 1 IgG detected).

In general, binding of autoantibodies results in loss of cell cohesion due to compromised function of specific cell-cell contact structures, the desmosomes. Autoantibody-induced interference with Dsg interaction and subsequently altered intracellular signaling seem to be required for full loss of cell cohesion and blister formation.

CLINICAL FEATURES

Pemphigus vulgaris is a rare, acute or chronic, usually fatal disease, characterized by a generalised eruption of bullae, containing, serous, haemorrhagic or purulent material on a previously normal skin (Fig. 16.1). Mucous membrane complications may occur simultaneously with the skin eruption in the mouth and throat (Fig. 16.2) which often interfere with mastication

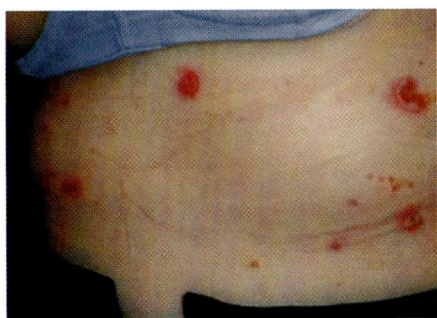

Fig. 16.1: *Ulcerated skin lesions*

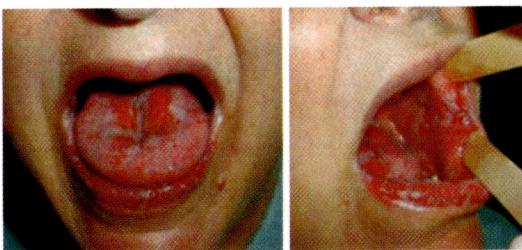

Fig. 16.2: *Ulcerated lesions on the buccal mucosa, the lip and the back of the tongue*

and swallowing and in late state the mucous membrane of the eyes (Fig. 16.3) may be involved. Death usually ensues in a matter of weeks from sepsis or bronchopneumonia.

Ocular manifestations

The conjunctiva is nearly always involved and the lesions in both acute and chronic types are similar. Non-cicatricial conjunctivitis is the most frequent, and ulcerated lesions on the eyelid and ocular mucosa are uncommon. Occlusion of the tear duct, subepithelial fibrosis, formation of the symblepharon and perforation of the cornea are also described in the literature.

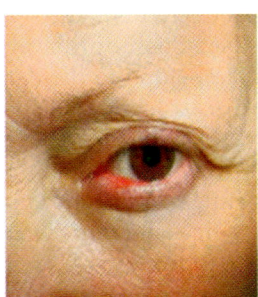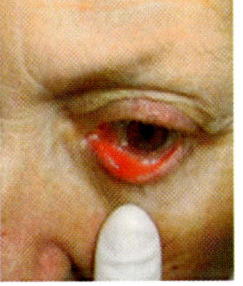

Fig. 16.3: *Vesicular lesion on the mucosa of the eyelid*

Acute ocular pemphigus consists of bullae which rupture rapidly leaving ulcerated base. The bullae are transient. It is often difficult to find a case with an intact bullae. In acute cases death supervenes before cicatricial changes can develop.

Chronic ocular pemphigus (benign mucous membrane pemphigoid) may occur either with or without associated mucous membrane lesions of the nose, and throat and in the absence of skin changes. When there are no mouth changes the diagnosis is difficult but it can be made on the basis of bullous lesions on the conjunctiva with progressive cicatrization which is most marked in the lower fornix over a period of month. The low grade conjunctival eosinophilia of pemphigus is usual in differentiating it from erythema multiforme bullosum.

Prognosis is poor in acute case and death results in a matter of weeks (in some cases steriod gives temporary effect). Chronic cases are characterised by long remissions and exacerbation until death finally ensues. Death may not occur however until vision has been greatly diminished or lost through cicatrization of the conjunctiva and cornea. Loss of tear function due to cicatrization in the upper fornix results in keratinization of the corneal epithelium and contributes to loss of vision.

DIAGNOSIS

Diagnosis of PV is made by a characteristic clinical presentation, histological suprabasilar intraepithelial acantholysis, IgG autoantibodies on the cell surface by direct immunofluorescence testing of a biopsied lesion and the presence of circulating antiepithelial autoantibodies.

Differential Diagnosis

PV is a differential diagnosis of several pathologies of autoimmune and vesicle-bullous origin, such as
- Benign mucosal pemphigoid,
- Systemic lupus erythematosus,
- Epidermolysis bullosa,
- Erosive lichen planus,
- Erythema multiforme, and
- Herpes simplex and zoster.

TREATMENT

The treatment should have a multidisciplinary approach, involving a dermatologist, ophthalmologist and immunologist.

Systemic treatment

The recommended therapeutic regimen for PV and being a systemic autoimmune disease should first be treated with *systemic corticosteroid therapy*, and this procedure may be associated or in combination with *other immunosuppressants* such as azathioprine and other alternatives include cyclosporine, cyclophosphamide, prostaglandin, chlorambucil, levamisole and immunoglobulins. The expected outcome of the isolated or combined use of these drugs is the reduction of the production of autoantibodies. These therapies should be prescribed by a physician experienced in immunosuppressive therapy.

Currently, low-power laser therapy combined with immunosuppressants becomes an effective and recommended alternative therapeutic option, providing improvements in the health and quality of life of patients.

Ocular treatment

Adequate eye care is required in particular in infection prevention, scar development and corneal perforation. Surgical treatment of trichiasis, poor eyelid position and perforation of the cornea are performed in the more severe cases of pemphigus vulgaris.

OCULAR MUCOUS MEMBRANE PEMPHIGOID

Mucous membrane pemphigoid (ocular mucous membrane pemphigoid/cicatricial pemphigoid/ocular cicatricial pemphigoid/benign mucous membrane pemphigoid) is an autoimmune disease in which binding of anticonjunctival basement membrane antibodies results in conjunctival inflammation. It is unrelated to bullous pemphigoid.

Ocular cicatricial pemphigoid (OCP) or ocular mucous membrane pemphigoid (OMMP) is considered a subtype of mucous membrane pemphigoid (abbreviated MMP), and thus these terms are sometimes used interchangeably.

OCP is a type of autoimmune conjunctivitis that leads to cicatrization (i.e. scarring) of the conjunctiva. If OCP is left untreated, it can lead to blindness.

ETIOLOGY

The exact pathogenesis of OMMP remains to be elucidated but the existing evidence supports a Type II hypersensitivity response caused by an autoantibody to a cell surface antigen in the basement membrane of the conjunctival epithelium and other similar squamous epithelia.

Studies of HLA (human leukocyte antigen) typing have found an increased susceptibility to the disease in patients with HLA-DR4. The **HLA-DQB1*0301** allele in particular shows a strong association with OCP and other forms of pemphigoid disease. HLA-DQB1*0301 is thought to bind to the beta-4 subunit of the alpha-6 beta-4 integrin (the suspected autoantigen in OCP).

PATHOPHYSIOLOGY

Although the exact mechanism remains to be elucidated, the existing evidence supports the production of an autoantibody in susceptible individuals to the beta-4 subunit of the alpha-6 beta-4 integrin of hemidesmosomes in the lamina lucida of the conjunctival basement membrane.

Binding of the autoantibody to the autoantigen activates complement, resulting in the cytotoxic destruction of the conjunctival membrane. Disruption of the conjunctival basement membrane subsequently leads to bullae formation.

The associated cellular inflammatory infiltrate of the epithelium and substantia propria manifests as chronic conjunctivitis that is the hallmark of this disease. Eosinophils and neutrophils mediate inflammation in the early and acute phases of the disease, similar to what is observed in the skin. Chronic disease has largely lymphocytic infiltration. Fibroblast activation leads to subepithelial fibrosis, which in early disease appears as fine white striae most easily seen in the inferior fornix. A scar in the upper palpebral conjunctiva may also be seen. Over time, the fibrotic striae contract, leading to conjunctival shrinkage, symblepharon formation, and forniceal shortening. In severe cases of conjunctival fibrosis, entropion, trichiasis and symblepharon may develop, leading to associated keratopathy and corneal vascularization, scarring, ulceration, and epidermalization.

The clinical course and severity is variable. Recurrent inflammation causes loss of goblet cells and obstruction of lacrimal gland ductules, leading to aqueous and mucous tear deficiency. The resulting xerosis is severe, and along with progressive subepithelial fibrosis and destruction of limbal stem cells leads to limbal stem cell deficiency and ocular keratinization.

Several pro-inflammatory cytokines are found to be elevated in the conjunctival tissues of patients with OCP. Levels of interleukin 1 (IL-1), tumour necrosis factor α (TNF-α), migration inhibition factor, and macrophage colony-stimulating factor, and IL-13 have been found to be elevated. IL-13 has been found to have a pro-fibrotic and pro-inflammatory effect on conjunctival fibroblasts, and may be implicated in the progressive conjunctival fibrosis that can occur despite clinical quiescence.

Additionally, testing of the tears of patients with OCP found elevated levels of IL-8, matrix metalloproteinase 8 (MMP-8), MMP-9, and myeloperoxidase (MPO), which are thought to result from neutrophilic infiltrate in patients with OCP.

CLINICAL FEATURES

In patients with MMP, oral involvement is most common (in 90% of cases), followed by ocular involvement (in 61% of cases). Ocular involvement of MMP is considered high risk and carries a poorer prognosis (despite treatment) than when oral mucosa and/or skin alone are affected. Up to one-third of patients with oral disease progress to ocular involvement.

Additional sites of involvement include the oropharynx, nasopharynx, esophagus, larynx, genitalia, and anus. The skin is involved in approximately 15% of cases. Dysphagia may be a presenting symptom.

Ocular features

Foster's classification system has 4 stages as well and is based on specific clinical signs:

Stage I: Early stage

May include nonspecific symptoms and minimal findings which lead to under-recognition of the disease. Commonly presents as chronic conjunctivitis, tear dysfunction, and subepithelial fibrosis. Subepithelial fibrosis manifests as fine gray-white striae in the inferior fornix. Signs and symptoms are usually bilateral, and may be asymmetric.

Stage II: Shortening of the fornices

A normal inferior forniceal depth is approximately 11 mm. A reduced inferior forniceal depth is abnormal and should prompt further investigations.

Stage III: Symblepharon formation

Can be detected by pulling the lower eyelid down while the patient looks up and vice versa (Fig. 16.4).

Stage IV: Ankyloblepharon

Represents end-stage disease, with surface keratinization, and extensive adhesions between the eyelid and the globe, resulting in restricted motility (Figs 16.5 and 16.6).

Patients with OCP vary significantly in disease severity and rate of progression, but untreated disease often progresses in up to 75% of patients. Additionally, the subepithelial fibrosis in OCP can progress even despite clinical quiescence. A study conducted in the UK found that 42% of patients had disease progression in the absence of clinical inflammation.

Histological analysis of these patients has found significant inflammatory cellular infiltrate despite the white and quiet appearance of the conjunctiva clinically, and this has been termed

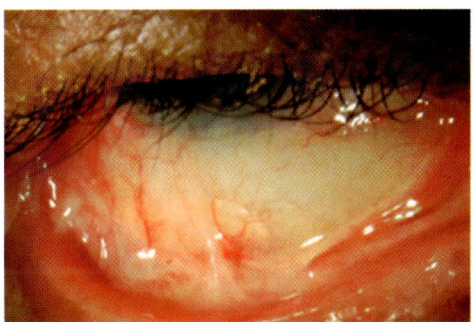

Fig. 16.4: *Symblepharon formation in the inferior fornix of a patient with OCP*

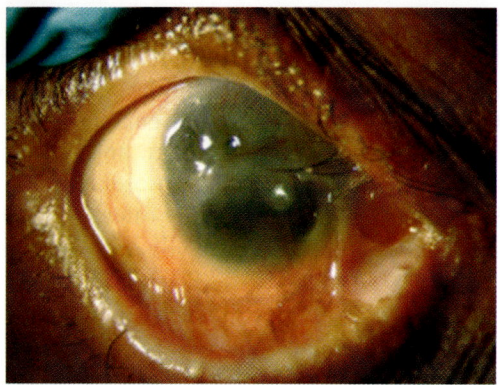

Fig. 16.5: *Patient with advanced, end-stage disease. Note the extensive surface keratinization and symblepharon*

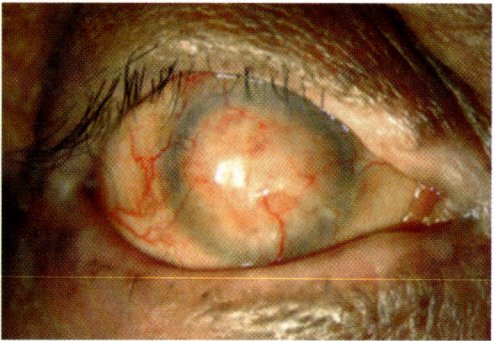

Fig. 16.6: *Complete keratinization of the ocular surface in a patient with end-stage OCP*

"white inflammation". This is particularly important as 30% of patients with advanced conjunctival fibrosis become blind and represent a clinical challenge to treatment of disease.

Differences between pemphigus and pemphigoid are summarised in Table 16.2.

DIAGNOSIS

Diagnosis is based on clinical signs and positive direct immunofluorescence testing of the conjunctiva.

Conjunctival biopsy of an actively involved area is needed and the conjunctival tissue must be submitted unfixed for analysis. If involvement is diffuse, biopsy of the inferior conjunctival fornix is recommended. Judicious biopsy is advisable as OCP is an obliterating disease of the conjunctiva and only the minimal amount of tissue necessary should be removed. Alternatively, biopsy of an active oral mucosa lesion can be diagnostic as well.

Immunofluorescence reveals linear staining of the epithelial basement membrane zone. The sensitivity of immunofluorescence may be as low as 50%, especially for long-standing/severe cicatrization because of the loss of immuno-reactants and the destruction of basement membrane in long-standing disease.

Serological testing is not routinely used in diagnosis.

Sequential photographs are useful to monitor clinical progression.

Differential diagnosis

Differential diagnosis of OCP is broad as it encompasses the differential for cicatricial conjunctivitis. The differential includes:
- Infectious etiologies such as trachoma,
- Inflammatory etiologies such as rosacea,
- Autoimmune etiologies such as linear IgA disease, graft-versus-host disease (GVHD), and Stevens Johnson syndrome (SJS), and

Table 16.2: *Differences between pemphigus vulgaris and bullous pemphigoid*		
Characteristics	*Pemphigus vulgaris*	*Bullous pemphigoid*
Age	Middle-aged people	Elderly people
Clinical features	Monomorphic	Polymorphic
Blisters	Rupture easily, flaccid	Tense, firm
Content of blisters	Fluid-filled	Often haemorrhagic
Oral lesions	Common	Rare
Nikolsky's sign	Positive	Negative
Tzanck smear	Acantholysis	No acantholysis
Direct immunofluorescence	Intraepidermal deposits	Deposits at the epidermal basement membrane
Zone	Target antigen	Desmoglein 1 and 3 BPAG2 (type 17 collagen)

- Allergic etiologies such as atopy, conjunctival trauma, chemical burns, medicamentosa, radiation, and neoplasia.

TREATMENT

Without treatment, the disease progresses in up to 75% of patients. While systemic treatment stops progression of cicatrization in most patients, it fails in approximately 10% of them.

1. *Topical treatment* comprises:
   - Tear substitutes, to be used frequently.
   - Antibiotics for secondary infection.
   - Steroids may help in reducing inflammation (caution for corneal melting).

2. *Systemic immunosuppression:* Systemic therapy is necessary in OCP as ocular involvement comprises a high risk subset of MMP and is insufficiently treated with topical therapy alone. Systemic treatment is best managed by a physician trained in the management of anti-inflammatory and immunomodulatory treatment given the significant risk of systemic complications necessitating frequent blood test monitoring. Several drugs are effective in treating OCP and a stepwise approach of escalation of therapy when there is insufficient response, is recommended:

   - Mild disease—use dapsone (1 mg/kg).
   - Moderate disease—use antimetabolite such as methotrexate or azathioprine.
   - Severe disease—use intravenous methyl-prednisolone with or without cyclophosphamide for 4 days, followed by oral prednisolone.

3. *Surgical intervention* required in late stage (depending upon the condition) may be:
   - Punctal occlusion for dry eye.
   - Silicon hydrogel contact lens use.
   - Correction of trichiasis and entropion.
   - Ocular surface reconstruction for advanced scarring.
   - Corneal transplantation.
   - Keratoprosthesis in extensive corneal and ocular surface scarring.

Note. Seemingly trivial surgical intervention and conjunctival trauma can lead to serious exacerbation of disease. Surgical intervention, such as treatment of trichiasis, entropion and cataract should be deferred if possible until control of active disease is achieved. In some situations this may not be possible and a multi-disciplinary approach is best.

Inferior eyelid retractor plication for trichiasis avoids surgery on the conjunctiva and has been shown to be safe and effective when undertaken in the setting of clinically quiescent OCP. Cryotherapy for the treatment of trichiasis has also been shown to be safe and moderately effective when undertaken in the setting of clinically quiescent OCP.

STEVENS-JOHNSON SYNDROME AND TOXIC EPIDERMAL NECROLYSIS

Stevens-Johnson syndrome and toxic epidermal necrolysis (SJS/TEN) are on a spectrum of a rare immune-mediated mucocutaneous disease usually associated with severe ocular complications.

SJS/TEN is a severe immune-mediated disease which can lead to blindness. Seemingly mild disease in the acute or subacute stage can lead to end-stage blindness if left unaddressed. Attentive examination and management in the acute stage provides the best opportunity to prevent or mitigate chronic disease. There are changes in the ocular surface at every stage of the disease, which if left unaddressed, can become irreversible, and a lost opportunity to improve the visual function and quality of life of these patients.

SUBDIVISIONS OF STEVENS-JOHNSON SYNDROME AND TOXIC EPIDERMAL NECROLYSIS

- Stevens-Johnson syndrome (SJS)
- SJS/TEN overlap
- Toxic epidermal necrolysis (TEN)

Stevens-Johnson syndrome (SJS) and toxic epidermal necrolysis (TEN) represent opposite ends of a spectrum of disease that results from an adverse reaction, most often to certain medications. SJS is the less severe end, but still represents a serious condition and potential medical emergency. TEN is a severe, life-threatening disorder. These disorders are differentiated by the degree of skin detachment.

SJS affects less than 10% of the body surface area; TEN affects more than 30% of the body surface area. The term SJS/TEN overlap syndrome is used to describe cases in which 10–30% of the body surface area is detached.

The reaction may start with a persistent fever and nonspecific, flu-like symptoms followed by appearance of erythematous macules (red spots) that may cover a large part of the body, and painful blistering of the skin and mucous membranes. The eyes are often involved.

ETIOPATHOGENESIS

The exact pathogenesis of SJS/TEN is unknown but appears to involve cell-mediated keratinocyte apoptosis via the Fas signaling cascade and granulysin release. The syndrome can result from exposure to certain medications, infections, or malignancy, though almost a quarter of cases have no known trigger.

Numerous drugs have been reported to cause SJS and TEN and the following have shown an increased risk in larger studies (Table 16.3):
- Antibacterial sulfonamides
- Non-steroidal anti-inflammatory drugs of the oxicam type
- Certain anti-seizure drugs (antiepileptics)
- Allopurinol
- Nevirapine.

Table 16.3: *Most common causes of SJS/TEN[2]*

Pharmacologic	Infectious
• Allopurinol	• Bacterial
• Anticonvulsants	– Mycoplasma pneumoniae
– Carbamazepine	– Group A β-hemolytic streptococcus
– Phenytoin	• Viral
Lamotrigine	– Cytomegalovirus
• Barbiturates	– Herpes simplex virus
• Sulfonamides	– HIV
• NSAIDs	

However, approximately one quarter (25%) of cases are not caused by drugs, but potentially by infections or have to be considered as idiopathic (of unknown cause).

CLINICAL FEATURES

Systemic features

Most cases involve the development of general, nonspecific symptoms including a persistent

fever, burning or stinging eyes, body aches, and discomfort or difficulty swallowing.

Additional nonspecific symptoms include headaches, chills, joint paint, and a general feeling of poor health (malaise).

A pus-producing (purulent) cough that also brings up mucous, phlegm and saliva (sputum) may also occur. Such symptoms may precede the development of skin involvement by a few days.

Skin lesions include often the development of a superficial reddening of the skin (erythema) or reddish spots on the skins (macules) that rapidly spread and come together (coalesce) to form a rash. In some cases, these lesions may resemble a target or bull's eye, so-called "target" lesions. A rash often first develops on the upper chest, face, and the palms and soles. The rash may remain limited to these areas or it may spread, within a few hours or days, to cover a significant portion of the body. The rash may be itchy (pruritic) or painful. Blisters appear on the confluent eruption leading to detachment of the skin and leaving erosions.

Ocular features

Ocular involvement begins with oedema, erythema and crusting of the eyelids.

Palpebral conjunctiva becomes hyperaemic and distinct vesicles or bullae may occur (Fig. 16.7).
- In many instances, a concomitant conjunctivitis appears that is characterised by watery discharge with mucoid strands.
- Secondary infection, most commonly with *Staphylococcus species*, may develop.
- In severe cases, a membranous or pseudo membranous conjunctivitis may result from coalescence of fibrin and necrotic cellular debris (Fig. 16.8).
- *Symblepharon formation* (Fig. 16.9) may occur with severe pseudomembranous conjunctivitis.
- Primary corneal involvement and iritis are rare ocular manifestations of disease.

Late ocular complications occur in approximately 20% of patients, and include:

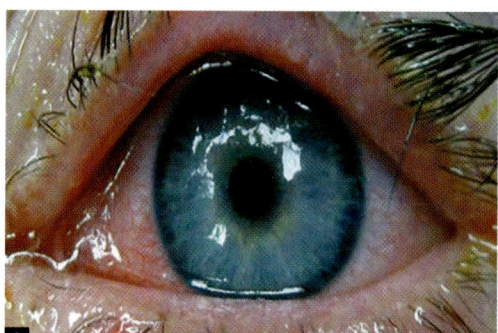

Fig. 16.7: *External photograph of the left eye showing a corneal epithelial defect and diffuse conjunctival injection*

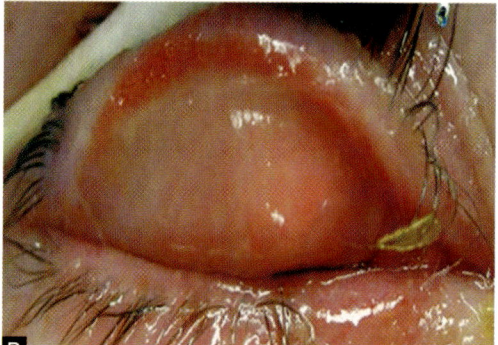

Fig. 16.8: *Eversion of the right upper eyelid shows a conjunctival membrane*

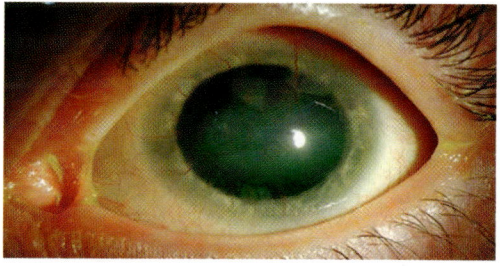

Fig. 16.9: *Slit-lamp photograph showing the long-term consequences of SJS/TEN, which can include limbal stem cell deficiency and symblepharon*

- *Structural anomalies of lid* position (ectropion and entropion), trichiasis and symblepharon.
- *Dry eye syndrome* may also result from deficiencies in the tear film—either in the aqueous layer, from scarring of lacrimal duct orifice, or more commonly, in the mucin layer, from destruction of the conjunctival goblet cells.

DIFFERENTIAL DIAGNOSIS

- Erythema multiforme
- Cicatricial pemphigoid
- Paraneoplastic pemphigus
- Epidermolysis bullosa acquisita
- Graft-versus-host disease
- Atopic keratoconjunctivitis
- Infectious conjunctivitis—adenovirus, trachoma, *C. diphtheriae*.

TREATMENT

Systemic treatment in acute phase includes: Removal (e.g. causative drugs) or treatment (e.g. of causative infection) of the inciting factor:

- Intravenous immunoglobulin,
- Role of systemic steroids is controversial,
- Maintenance of hydration, and
- Debridement and replacement of sloughing skin.

Ocular treatment during acute phase includes:

- *Topical tear drops* and prevention of exposure,
- *Topical antibiotics* and steroid eye drops, and
- *Pseudomembrane peel* and symblepharon lysis with glass rod or moistened cotton swab should be done daily.
- *Amniotic membrane transplantation:* It may be used as either a temporary bandage or permanent graft. Not every case of SJS/TEN is suitable for AMT. This technique is generally reserved for patients with moderate or severe conjunctival involvement, as these are the patients at greatest risk of visual loss from ocular surface scarring. Patients with minimal epithelial sloughing may instead be treated medically.

Ocular treatment during chronic SJS/TEN includes:

- *Patients with cicatrizing diseases, including SJS/TEN, are poor candidates for traditional penetrating keratoplasty (PKP) due to the development of lid abnormalities and severe surface dryness.*
- *End-stage corneal blindness that is unresponsive to the above measures may necessitate a keratoprosthesis.* Keratoprostheses can restore vision almost immediately after surgery but not

indefinitely, and postoperative complications are higher in these patients than in those who receive keratoprostheses for other indications.

- *Keratoprosthesis and limbal allografting:* Rarely match the success of early surgical treatment, but these methods can provide some visual recovery despite limbal stem cell loss and corneal conjunctivalization.

- *Keratolimbal allografting (KLAL)* is a technique that transplants cadaveric keratolimbal tissue to correct limbal stem cell deficiency.

BIBLIOGRAPHY

1. Chang YS, Huang FC, Tseng SH, et al. Erythema multiforme, Stevens-Johnson syndrome, and toxic epidermal necrolysis: acute ocular manifestations, causes, and management. Cornea 2007; 26: 123–29.

2. Hazin R, Ibrahimi OA, Hazin MI, et al. Stevens-Johnson syndrome: pathogenesis, diagnosis, and management. Annals of Medicine 2008; 40: 129–38.

3. Hoang-Xuan T, Robin H, Demers PE, et al. Pure ocular cicatricial pemphigoid. A distinct immunopathologic subset of cicatricial pemphigoid. Ophthalmology 1999; 106: 355.

4. Koulu L, Kusumi A, Steinberg MS, Klaus-Kovtun V, Stanley JR. Human autoantibodies against a desmosomal core protein in pemphigus foliaceus. J Exp Med 1984; 160: 1509–18.

5. Neumann R, Tauber J, Foster CS. Remission and recurrence after withdrawal of therapy for ocular cicatricial pemphigoid. Ophthalmology 1991; 98: 858.

6. Solomon A, Ellies P, Anderson D, et al. Long-term outcome of keratolimbal allograft with or without penetrating keratoplasty for total limbal stem cell deficiency. Ophthalmology 2002; 109: 1159–66.

7. Sotozono C, Ueta M, Koizumi N, et al. Diagnosis and treatment of Stevens-Johnson syndrome and toxic epidermal necrolysis with ocular complications. Ophthalmology 2009; 116: 685–90.

8. Thorne JE, Woreta FA, Jabs DA, Anhalt GJ. Treatment of ocular mucous membrane pemphigoid with immunosuppressive drug therapy. Ophthalmology 2008; 115: 2146.

Chemical Burns of Ocular Surface

ETIOPATHOGENESIS

Chemical injuries form a large chunk of 'Ophthalmic emergencies'. Ranging from just a mild discomfort and minimal tissue damage; to severe, irreversible tissue damage; the manifestations could be varied. Depending upon access of the patient to prompt and adequate management, the prognosis could change from 'good' to 'grim'.

SOURCE OF COMMON CHEMICAL AGENTS

Source of common chemical agents implicated in chemical injuries of eyes are summarised in Table 17.1.

General comments about chemical agents causing ocular injuries are:

- *Alkali injuries* are more common, compared to acid injuries, because of their more frequent household use.
- *Ammonia*, that is found in fertilisers, refrigerants and cleaning solutions, is the most common cause of chemical eye injuries.
- *Other chemicals*, besides ammonia, such as hydroxides of sodium, potassium and

Table 17.1: *Source of chemical agents implicated in eye injuries*

Chemical agent	Source
Calcium hydroxide	Cement, mortar, white-wash
Potassium hydroxide	Caustic potash
Magnesium hydroxide	Sparklers
Ammonia	Fertilizers, refrigerants
Sulphuric acid	Battery, industrial cleaner
Acetic acid	Vinegar, glacial acetic acid
Sulphurous acid	Bleach, refrigerants, food preservative
Hydrofluoric acid	Glass polishing, gasoline alkylation, silicone production
Hydrochloric acid	Chemical laboratories

magnesium are also important etiological agents.
- *Most common acid* implicated in ocular trauma is sulphuric acid, which is commonly used in invertor batteries, car batteries, fertilisers,

manufacturing of dyes, explosives and refining petroleum.

- *Other acids* such as nitric acid, chromic acid and hydrofluoric acid also contribute to ocular trauma.

MODES OF CHEMICAL INJURIES

Chemical injuries usually occur due to external contact with chemicals under following circumstances:

- *Domestic accidents*, with ammonia, solvents, detergents and cosmetics.
- *Agricultural accidents*, due to fertilisers, insecticides, toxins of vegetable and animal origin.
- *Chemical laboratory accidents*, with acids and alkalies.
- *Deliberate chemical attacks*, especially with acids to disfigure the face.
- *Chemical warfare injuries*.
- *Self-inflicted chemical injuries* are seen in malingerers and psychopaths.

PATHOGENESIS

Pathogenesis of alkali burns

Alkalis cause damage to the cornea and ocular surface by causing pH change, proteolysis and collagen synthesis defects.

Rise in pH leads to saponification of fatty acids of cell membranes, leading to cell destruction thus allowing the alkalis to enter the anterior chamber. This in turn leads to damage to all anterior segment structures.

Proteolysis. The damaged tissue and inflammatory cells secrete proteolytic enzymes, the response which leads to further tissue damage.

Collagen synthesis defect. Alkalis also damage ciliary body to reduce aqueous ascorbate levels that is necessary for conversion of proline and lysine to hydroxyproline and hydroxylysine, respectively, which is an important step of collagen synthesis.

Pathogenesis of acid burns

Acids damage the ocular surface by lowering the pH thereby precipitating tissue proteins, thus creating a barrier to further ocular penetration. Due to this, acid injuries are less severe than alkali injuries.

GRADING (CLASSIFICATION) OF CHEMICAL BURNS

Depending upon the severity of damage caused to the limbus and cornea, the extent of chemical burns may be graded as in Roper-Hall classification (Table 17.2) and Dua's classification (Table 17.3).

CLINICAL COURSE OF CHEMICAL BURNS

The clinical course following an acute chemical injury can be divided in three stages (Fig. 17.1).

1. ACUTE STAGE (IMMEDIATE TO ONE WEEK)

This stage is characterized by (Fig. 17.1):

- *Conjunctiva* shows marked oedema, congestion, widespread necrosis and a copious purulent discharge.
- *Limbal ischaemia* (Fig. 17.2) may or may not be present depending upon the grade of chemical burn (Tables 17.2 and 17.3).
- *Cornea* develops widespread sloughing of the epithelium, oedema and opalescence of the stroma.
- *Iris* becomes violently inflamed and in severe cases both iris and ciliary body are replaced by granulation tissue.
- *Rise in intraocular pressure* due to compression of globe because of shortening of collagen fibrils and impedance of aqueous humor outflow.

2. EARLY REPARATIVE STAGE (ONE TO THREE WEEKS)

During this period there is clearing off of necrotic tissue and regeneration of the denuded

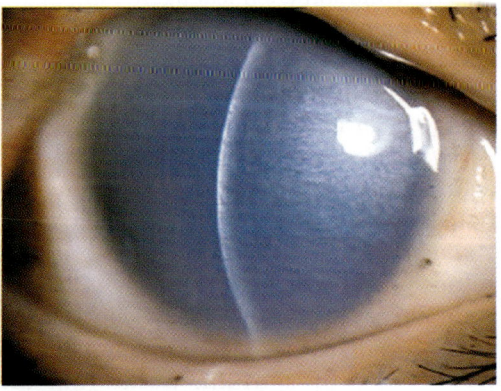

Fig. 17.1: *Limbal ischaemia in a case of chemical burn*

Table 17.2: *Roper-Hall classification (1965)*

Grade	Prognosis	Cornea	Conjunctiva/limbus
I	Good	Corneal epithelial damage	No limbal ischaemia
II	Good	Corneal haze, iris details visible	<1/3 limbal ischaemia
III	Guarded	Total epithelial loss, stromal haze, iris details obscured	1/3-1/2 limbal ischaemia
IV	Poor	Cornea opaque, iris and pupil obscured	>1/2 limbal ischaemia

Table 17.3: *Dua classification of ocular surface burns (2001)*

Grade	Prognosis	Clinical findings	Conjunctival involvement	Analogue scale
I	Very good	0 clock hours limbal involvement	0%	0/0%
II	Good	≤3 clock hours limbal involvement	≤30%	0.1–3/1–29.9%
III	Good	>3–6 clock hours limbal involvement	>30–50%	3.1–6/31–50%
IV	Good to guarded	>6–9 clock hours limbal involvement	>50–75%	6.1–9/51–75%
V	Guarded to poor	>9–< 12 clock hours limbal involvement	>75–< 100%	9.1–11.9/75.1–99.9%
VI	Very poor	Total (12 clock hours) limbal involvement	100%	12/100%

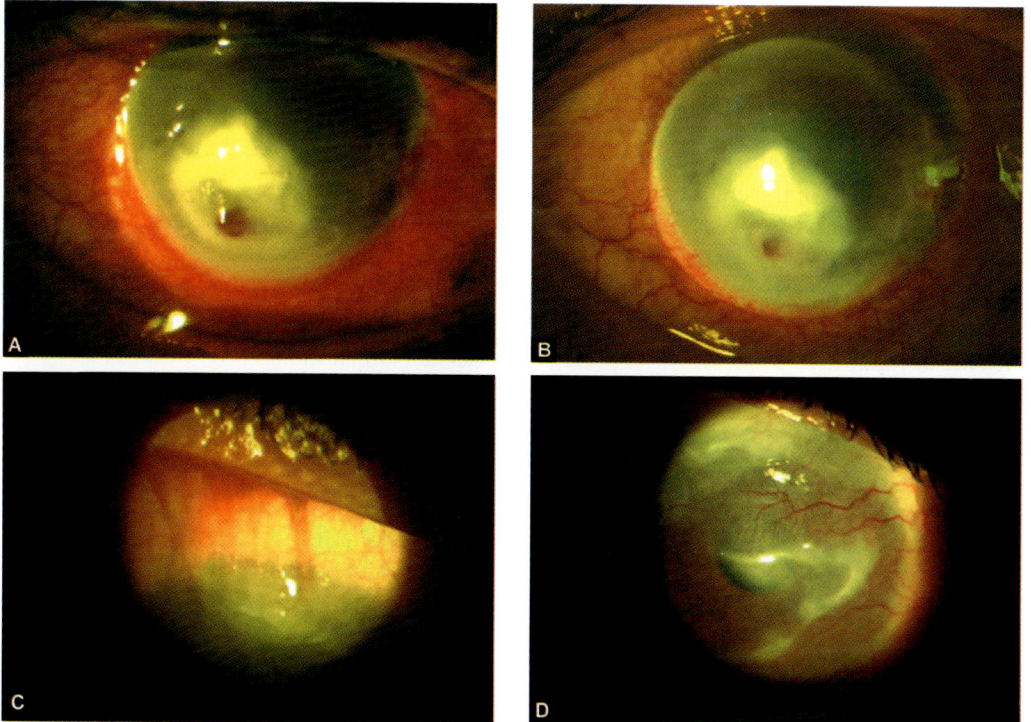

Fig. 17.2: *A, Acute phase; B, Sequelae developed 3 months after mild chemical injury with a liquid cleansing agent; C, Symblepharon formation due to lime injury; and D, Result after symblepharon release and amniotic membrane grafting*

area. *Clinical findings* depending on the grade of burns are as below:

- *Grade I/II burns.* Epithelium regeneration brings along clearing of stromal haze and synthesis of stromal collagen.
- *Grade III/IV burns.* Epithelium regeneration is difficult. Stroma remains hazy and stromal ulceration takes place due to action of digestive enzymes such as collagenases, matrix metalloproteinases (MMP), and other proteases released due to inflammation.

3. LATE REPARATIVE STAGE AND SEQUELAE (≥ THREE WEEKS)

- *Grade I/II burns.* In such cases complete healing may occur without much sequelae.
- *Grade III/IV burns.* Sequelae occur in such cases and include corneal scarring, xerosis, symblepharon (Figs 17.2C and 17.3), ankyloblepharon, secondary glaucoma, uveitis, complicated cataract, lagophthalmos, cicatricial entropion or ectropion, trichiasis and dry eye disease.

■ MANAGEMENT

GENERAL PRINCIPLES AND GOALS OF TREATMENT

General principles and goals of management in a case of chemical burns are:

- Thorough removal of the chemical agent and necrotic debris from the eyes.
- Restoration of intact ocular surface.
- Control of acute inflammation.
- Prevention of superadded infection.
- Support of reparative process.
- Prevention and management of sequelae.

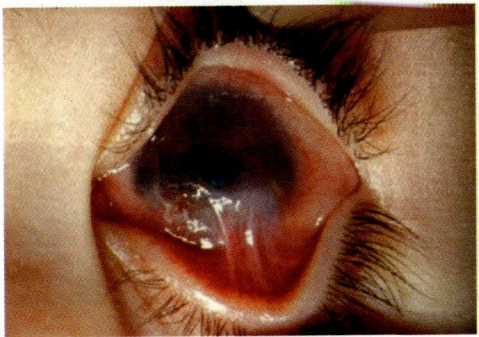

Fig. 17.3: *Post-chemical burn symblepharon*

MANAGEMENT PROTOCOL

A. Immediate treatment

Aim of immediate treatment is to minimise tissue damage due to the chemical agent. *Emergency kit*, should preferably, be maintained by the treating ophthalmologists for management of acute burns (Table 17.4).

Treatment protocol includes:

1. *Irrigation of the cul-de-sac.* Immediate copious irrigation of the eye must be initiated without wasting time on history and examination.

- *Irrigating solution* includes normal saline, Ringer's lactate, balanced salt solution, tap water, borate buffer solution or diphoterine (high buffer capacity amphoteric hypertonic polyvalent compound depending upon the availability).
- *Use of acidic solution* to neutralise alkali is dangerous and NOT recommended.
- *Duration of irrigation* may vary with the severity of injury:
  - 15–20 min in Grade 1 and 2 burns
  - 30–35 min in Grade 3 and 4 burns
  - 45–50 min in Grade 5 and 6 burns.
- *pH of conjunctival cul-de-sac should be measured* after completion of irrigation, and further irrigation should be done till pH approaches normal level.

Table 17.4: *Emergency kit for the management of acute chemical injuries*

Constituents of the kit	Purpose
Bottles of Ringer's lactate/normal saline and IV drip sets	Copious irrigation
Litmus paper strips	See the change in pH
Topical anaesthetic	Anaesthetize the eye to facilitate ocular examination
Swab stick	Clean the ocular surface
Desmarres retractor	Retract the eyelids to allow thorough ocular examination
26 gauge needle	Remove embedded chemical particles
Fluorescein strips	Extent of epithelial defects
Topical medication	Promote healing

2. *Examination with everted lids* should always be done after thorough irrigation. The fornices along with the ocular surface should be examined after topical anaesthesia, by double eversion of eyelids or with Desmarres retractor. Often this is very difficult in the inflamed eye, but it is a very important step. Efforts should be made to note for presence of any particulate matter.

3. *Mechanical removal of contaminant.* If any particles are left behind, particularly in the case of lime, these should be removed carefully with a swab stick.

4. *Removal of contaminated and necrotic tissue.* Necrosed conjunctiva should be excised. Contaminated and necrosed corneal epithelium should be removed with a cotton swab stick.

B. Early reparative stage management

During this stage, intent of the treatment is to control inflammation-mediated damage, promote healing and prevent symblepharon formation.

I. **Controlling inflammation mediated damage.** This approach incorporates use of drugs such as anti-inflammatory drugs, enzyme inhibitors, and cycloplegics.

a. *Topical anti-inflammatory drugs*
- *Topical steroids* used in the initial seven to ten days after injury to reduce inflammatory cells infiltrating the corneal stroma. Steroids should be rapidly tapered after this period if the epithelium is not intact, as it slows the repair process.
- *Topical nonsteroidal anti-inflammatory drugs (NSAIDs)* should be used cautiously due to their known ocular surface toxicity. Corneal melting is known to occur due to some NSAIDs.

b. *Enzyme inhibitory drugs* which help in controlling inflammation include:
- *Tetracycline eye ointment*, to be used two to three times a day.
- *Systemic tetracycline.* Doxycycline (100 mg BD) helps by inhibiting gene expression of neutrophil collagenase and epithelial gelatinase.

- *Collagenase inhibitors.* These include 10% sodium citrate drops made in artificial tears, cysteine, acetylcysteine, EDTA and penicillamine.

c. *Cycloplegics*, e.g. atropine, may improve the comfort.

II. **Promoting healing.** This can be achieved by use of:

a. *Medications promoting healing* include:
- *Tear substitutes.* Most important medication, because adequate lubrication and prevention of symblepharon formation is one of the prime concerns. Preservative-free artificial tears help in stabilising tear film thereby hastening epithelial regeneration.
- *Autologous serum eye drops* (20–40%) contain growth factors.
- *Ascorbate.* Oral ascorbate 500 mg QID or topical 10% solution in artificial tears administered hourly promotes epithelial healing by replenishing ascorbic acid to fibroblasts of cornea.
- *Epidermal growth factor.* May be of help as it promotes epithelial migration.
- *Retinoic acid.* Promotes goblet cell recovery and tear film stabilisation.
- *Fibronectin.* It is still in experimental phase.

b. *Mechanical methods which help in healing,* depending upon the prevailing situation, include:
- *Debridement.* Excision of necrotic tissues hastens the re-epithelialisation as necrotic tissue acts as a source of inflammatory mediators.
- *Bandage contact lens.* Prevents the ocular surface from windshield-wiper effect prouced by movement of the eyelids.
- *Conjunctival/tenon advancement (tenoplasty).* It involves excision of the necrotic conjunctiva and cornea, followed by the advancement of Tenon's over the cornea.
- *Tissue adhesives* such as cyanoacrylate glue may be used along with a bandage contact lens, in the presence of a small corneal perforation.
- *Tectonic penetrating keratoplasty or patch graft* may be required.

- *Amniotic membrane transplantation*. May be of use in grade II–III chemical burns as amniotic membrane facilitates epithelialisation and prevents symblepharon formation, vascularisation and scarring.

III. **Prevention of symblepharon formation** can be done by using a glass shell or sweeping a glass rod in the fornices twice daily.

C. Treatment of sequelae

1. *Ocular surface rehabilitation* measures needed include symblepharon lysis, fornix formation, entropion surgery, and ectropion surgery. Keratoplasty, which provides corneal tissue for tectonic support, may be needed, in some cases.

2. *Limbal stem cell deficiency* can be treated by limbal stem cell transplantation using either conjunctival limbal autografts, or graft from living related or cadaveric donors or cultured limbal epithelium. This is especially useful in high grade chemical injuries with extensive perilimbal ischaemia.

3. *Secondary glaucoma* should be treated by topical 0.5% timolol, instilled twice a day along with oral acetazolamide 250 mg 3–4 times a day.

4. *Pseudopterygium*, when formed, should be excised together with conjunctival autograft (if adequate host conjunctiva) or amniotic membrane facilitated by antimitotic drugs (e.g. mitomycin C).

5. *Visual rehabilitation in the presence of corneal opacity* is done with:

- *Penetrating keratoplasty* may be performed after acute inflammatory stage has subsided
- *Keratoprosthesis* remains a surgical option in severely damaged eyes where keratoplasty is not possible.

BIBLIOGRAPHY

1. Ballen PH. Treatment of chemical burns of the eye. Eye, Ear, Nose, Throat Mon. 1964; 43: 57–61.
2. Clare G, et al. Amniotic membrane transplantation for acute ocular burns. Cochrane database of systematic reviews, 2012.
3. Colby K. Chemical injuries of the Cornea. Focal Points in American Academy of Ophthalmology. 2010; 28(1): 1–14.
4. Davis AR, Ali QK, Aclimandos WA, Hunter PA. Topical steroid use in the treatment of ocular alkali burns. Br J Ophthalmol. 1997; 81: 732–4.
5. Dohlman CH, Schneider HA, Doane MG. Prosthokeratoplasty. Am J Ophthalmol. 1974; 77: 694–70.
6. Dua HS, King AJ, Joseph A. A new classification of ocular surface burns. Br J Ophthalmol. 2001; 85: 1379–83.
7. Fish R, RS Davidson. Management of ocular thermal and chemical injuries, including amniotic membrane therapy. Current opinion in ophthalmology, 2010; 21(4): 317–21.
8. Holekamp TL. Ocular injuries from automobile batteries. Trans Sect Ophthalmol Am Acad Ophthalmol Otolaryngol. 1977; 83: 805–10.
9. Kuckelkorn R, Makropoulos W, Kottek A, Reim M. Retrospective study of severe alkali burns of the eyes. Klin Monbl Augenheilkd. 1993; 203: 397–402.
10. Paterson CA, Pfister RR. Intraocular pressure changes after alkali burns. Arch Ophthalmol. 1974; 91: 211–8.
11. Pfister RR. Chemical injuries of the eye. Ophthalmology. 1983; 90: 1246–53.
12. Roper-Hall MJ. Thermal and chemical burns. Trans Ophthalmol Soc U K. 1965; 85: 631–53.
13. Wagoner MD. Chemical Injuries of the eye: current concepts in pathophysiology and therapy. Survey of ophthalmology, 1997; 41(4): 275–313.

Blepharitis and Meibomian Gland Dysfunction

BLEPHARITIS

DEFINITION AND CLASSIFICATION

The term 'blepharitis', means inflammation of the eyelid margin. Blepharitis is divided into an anterior and a posterior variety.

Anterior blepharitis refers to inflammation of the lid margin anterior to the grey line, i.e. of the skin, eyelashes, and lash follicles.

Posterior blepharitis means the inflammation of structures posterior to the grey line; that includes the meibomian duct orifices, meibomian glands, tarsal plate, and the blepharoconjunctival junction.

Mixed variety of blepharitis may be seen frequently as the inflammatory process spreads from one structure to the next.

ANTERIOR BLEPHARITIS

Blepharitis is a subacute or chronic inflammation of the lid margins. It is an extremely common disease which can be divided into following clinical types:
- Bacterial blepharitis,
- Seborrhoeic or squamous blepharitis,
- Mixed staphylococcal with seborrhoeic blepharitis,
- Posterior blepharitis or meibomitis, and
- Parasitic blepharitis.

Bacterial Blepharitis

Bacterial blepharitis, also known as chronic anterior blepharitis, or staphylococcal blepharitis or ulcerative blepharitis, is a chronic infection of the anterior part of the lid margin. It is a common cause of ocular discomfort and irritation. The disorder usually starts in child-hood and may continue throughout life.

Etiology

Causative organisms, most commonly involved, are coagulase positive Staphylococci. Rarely, Streptococci, *Propionibacterium acnes,* and Mora-xella may be involved.

Predisposing factors, usually none, may rarely include chronic conjunctivitis and dacryo-cystitis.

Clinical features

Symptoms include chronic irritation, itching, mild lacrimation, gluing of cilia, and mild photophobia. The symptoms are character-istically worse in the morning. Remissions and exacerbations in symptoms are quite common.

Signs (Fig. 18.1) are as below:

- *Yellow crusts* are seen at the root of cilia which glue them together.
- *Small ulcers,* which bleed easily, are seen on removing the crusts.
- *Red, thickened lid margins* are seen with dilated blood vessels (rosettes).
- *Mild papillary conjunctivitis* and conjunctival hyperaemia are common associations.

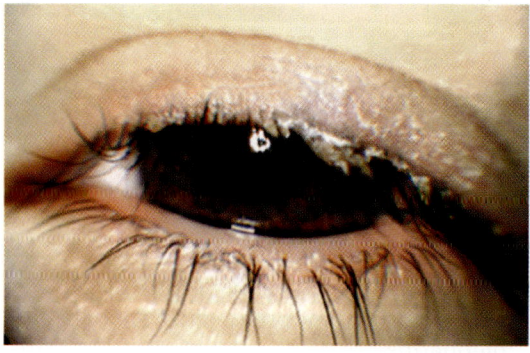

Fig. 18.1: *Bacterial blepharitis*

Complications and sequelae of long-standing bacterial blepharitis include:

- *Lash abnormalities* such as madarosis (spar-seness or absence of cilia), trichiasis (mis-directed cilia), and poliosis (graying of lashes).
- *Tylosis,* i.e. thickening and scarring of lid margin.

- *Eversion of punctum* leading to epiphora.
- *Eczema of skin and ectropion* may develop due to prolonged watering.
- *Recurrent styes* (external hordeola) are a common complication.
- *Marginal keratitis,* and occasionally phlycte-nulosis may develop.
- *Tear film instability,* and dry eye may result.
- *Secondary inflammatory and mechanical changes in the conjunctiva and cornea* are common because of intimate relationship between the lid margins and ocular surface.

Treatment

Bacterial blepharitis should be treated promptly, as below, to avoid complications and sequelae:

1. Lid hygiene is essential at least twice daily and should include:

- *Warm compresses* for 5–10 minutes to soften the crusts,
- *Crust removal and lid margin cleaning* with the help of cotton buds dipped in the dilute baby shampoo or solution of 3% sodium bicarbo-nate.
- *Avoid rubbing of the eyes* or fingering of the lids.

2. Antibiotics should be used as below:

- *Eye ointment* should be applied at the lid mar-gin, immediately after removal of the crusts.
- *Antibiotic eye drops* should be used 3–4 times a day.
- *Oral antibiotics* such as erythromycin or doxycycline may be useful in unresponsive patients and those complicated by external hordeola and abscess of lash follicle.

3. Topical steroids (low potency) such as fluoro-metholone may be required in patients with papillary conjunctivitis, marginal keratitis and phlyctenulosis.

4. Ocular lubricants, i.e. artificial tear drops, are required for associated tear film instability and dry eye.

Seborrhoeic or squamous blepharitis

Seborrhoeic blepharitis is primarily anterior blepharitis with some spillover posteriorly. It is of common occurrence.

Etiology. It is usually associated with sebor-rhoea of scalp (dandruff). Some constitutional and metabolic factors play a part in its etiology. In it, glands of Zeis secrete abnormal excessive neutral lipids which are split by *Corynebacterium acne* into irritating free fatty acids.

Symptoms. Patients usually complain of deposition of whitish material (soft scales) at the lid margin associated with mild discomfort, irritation, occasional watering and a history of falling of eyelashes.

Signs include:

- *Accumulation of white dandruff-like scales* is seen on the lid margin, among the lashes (Fig. 18.2). On removing these scales underlying surface is found to be hyperaemic and greasy (no ulcers).
- *The lashes fall out easily* but are usually replaced quickly without distortion.
- *Lid margin* is thickened and the sharp posterior border tends to be rounded leading to epiphora, in long-standing cases.
- *Signs of bacterial blepharitis,* as described above, may be superadded in patients with mixed seborrhoeic and bacterial blepharitis.

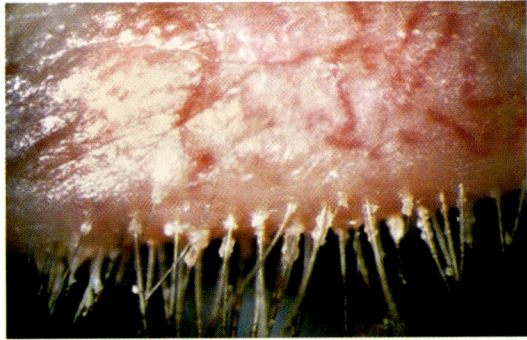

Fig. 18.2: *Seborrhoeic blepharitis*

Complications are similar to bacterial blepharitis with comparatively lesser frequency (*see* page 284).

Treatment includes:

- *General measures* include improvement of health and balanced diet.
- Associated *seborrhoea of the scalp* should be adequately treated.
- *Local measures* include removal of scales from the lid margin with the help of lukewarm solution of 3% soda bicarb or baby shampoo

and frequent application of combined antibiotic and steroid eye ointment at the lid margin.

- *Antibiotics*, as described above in bacterial blepharitis, may be required in patients with mixed seborrhoeic and bacterial blepharitis.

POSTERIOR BLEPHARITIS (MEIBOMITIS)

Meibomitis, i.e. inflammation of meibomian glands occurs in chronic and acute forms.

1. Chronic meibomitis

Chronic meibomitis is a commonly occurring meibomian gland dysfunction, seen more commonly in middle-aged persons, especially those with acne rosacea and/or seborrhoeic dermatitis. Bacterial lipases are being blamed to play main role in the pathogenesis of chronic meibomitis.

Clinical features

Symptoms include chronic irritation, burning, itching, grittiness, mild lacrimation with remissions and exacerbations intermittently. Symptoms are characteristically worse in the morning.

Signs include (Fig. 18.3):

- *White frothy (foam-like) secretions* are frequently seen on the eyelid margins and canthi (meibomian seborrhoea).
- *Opening of meibomian glands* become prominent with thick secretions which can be expressed out by pressure on the lids giving toothpaste appearance. Meibomian gland orifices may also show capping with oil globules, pouting, recession, or plugging.
- *Vertical yellowish streaks shining* through conjunctiva can be seen on eversion of the lids.

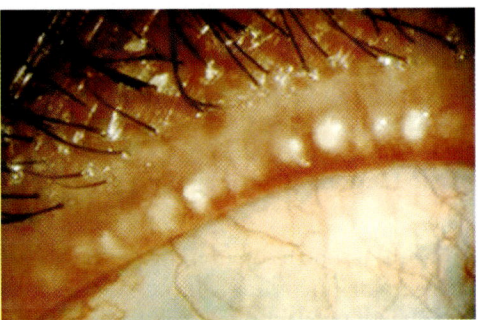

Fig. 18.3: *Chronic meibomitis*

These represent the meibomian ducts filled with thick secretion.

- *Hyperaemia and telangiectasia* of posterior lid margin around the orifices of meibomian glands can be seen frequently.
- *Oily and foamy tear film* with accumulation of froth on the lid margins or inner canthus.
- *Secondary changes* in the form of papillary conjunctivitis, and inferior corneal punctate epithelial erosions may be seen.

2. Acute meibomitis

Acute meibomitis occurs due to staphylococcal infection. It is characterised by painful swelling around the involved gland. Pressure on it results in expression of pus bead followed by sero-sanguineous discharge.

Treatment of meibomitis

1. **Lid hygiene** is essential at least once a day and should include:
- *Warm compresses* for several minutes.
- *Expression* of accumulated secretions by repeated vertical massage of lids in the form of milking.

2. **Topical antibiotics** in the form of eye oint-ment should be rubbed at the lid margin immediately after massage.
- Eye drops may be used 3–4 times a day.

3. **Systemic tetracyclines,** e.g. doxycycline 100 mg b.d. for 1 week and then o.d. for 6–12 weeks, remain the mainstay of treatment of posterior blepharitis because of their ability to block staphylococcal lipase production. Erythromycin may be used where tetracyclines are con-traindicated.

4. **Ocular lubricants,** i.e. artificial tear drops are required for associated tear film instability and dry eye disease.

5. **Topical steroids** (weak) such as fluorometho-lone may be required in patients with papillary conjunctivitis.

Parasitic blepharitis (lash infestation)

Etiology

Blepharitis associated with infestation of lashes by lice is not uncommon in persons living in poor hygienic conditions. The lice infestations include the following:

- *Phthiriasis palpebrarum* refers to the infestation by *phthirus pubis* (crab louse). It is most commonly seen in adults in whom it is usually acquired as a sexually transmitted infection.
- *Pediculosis* refers to the infestation by *pediculus humanus corporis* or *capitis* (head louse). If heavily infested the lice may spread to involve lashes.
- *Demodex blepharitis* is caused by two distinct species: Demodex folliculorum which causes anterior blepharitis and demodex brevis which causes posterior blepharitis.

Clinical features

Infestation of lashes with lice causes chronic blepharitis and chronic follicular conjunctivitis.

Symptoms include chronic irritation, itching, burning, and mild lacrimation.

Signs are as below (Fig. 18.4):
- *Lid margins* are red and inflamed.
- *Lice* anchoring the lashes with their claws may be seen on slit-lamp examination.
- *Nits (eggs)* may be seen as opalescent pearls adherent to the base of cilia.
- *Conjunctival congestion* and follicles may be seen in long-standing cases.

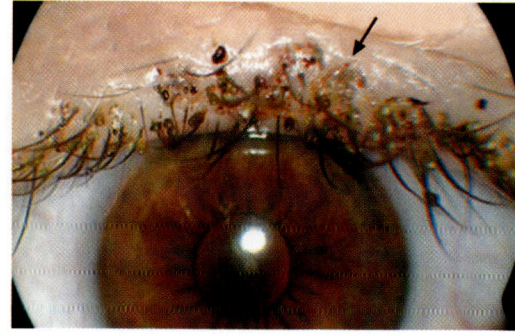

Fig. 18.4: *Phthiriasis palpebrarum*

Treatment

- *Mechanical removal* of the lices and nits with forceps.
- *Application of antibiotic ointment* and yellow mercuric oxide 1% to the lid margins and lashes.
- *Delousing* of the patient, family members, clothing and bedding is important to prevent recurrences.

MEIBOMIAN GLAND DYSFUNCTION

ANATOMY AND PHYSIOLOGY OF MEIBOMIAN GLANDS

The meibomian glands were first described in detail by Heinrich Meibom in 1666. These are modified sebaceous glands with a tubuloacinar structure. Each gland consists of clusters of 10–15 secretory acini, arranged circularly around a long central duct and connected to it by short ductules. There are 30–40 glands in the upper tarsal plate and 25 in the lower; the glands in the upper tarsus are 5.5 mm long while the lower ones are 2 mm long.

Innervation. Meibomian glands are densely innervated by the sympathetic and para-sympathetic nerve fibres via the V nerve which also supplies the lacrimal and accessory lacrimal glands, thereby ensuring an optimal composition of the tear film.

Hormonal control. Meibomian glands are also under a strong hormonal control mediated by androgens, oestrogens, progestins, retinoic acid, growth factors and neurotransmitters.

Secretion of meibomian glands is called meibum which is made up of mostly non-polar lipids (>90%: primarily wax and, sterol esters and tri-acylglycerols), while less than 10% are polar lipids [(O-acyl)-ω-hydroxy fatty acids (OAHFA)], and a small amount of proteins and electrolytes. The tear film lipid layer is a multi-layered structure formed of a thin, mono-molecular layer of polar lipids present at the aqueous–lipid interface and act as a surfactant. This is essential in the uniform spreading and stability of the tear film. It is covered over by a thick layer of non-polar lipids, which form the outermost eye–air interface that resists the evaporation of the aqueous component of the tear film.

Mode of secretion of meibum is holocrine, which means that the secretion is produced in the cyto-plasm of an acinar cell; the cell membrane ruptures, releases its secretions into the gland's lumen while the cell itself is destroyed in the process. The secretion from multiple acini are poured via tiny ductules into the central duct that opens at the grey line of the lid margin. The terminal part of the central duct and the terminal acini close to the lid margin are encircled by a thin strip of orbicularis muscle fibres (Riolan's muscle). During a blink, the pre-tarsal orbicularis muscle produces uniform compression of the tarsal plate and of the enclosed meibomian glands, and promotes the flow of secretion towards the duct opening by a milking action. Meibum is squirted out of the duct openings by the contraction of Riolan muscle at the end of a blink.

Meibum is in a liquid/fluid state at the body temperature; this allows it to coat the lid margins, thus making their movement smooth over the ocular surface, and to be delivered to the tear meniscus. From there, it is picked up by the upper lid margin (as it comes down during a blink up picks up the tear meniscus) and is spread uniformly over the aqueous layer of the tear film. This prevents the excess evaporation and thinning in-between the blinks, thus making the tear film stable.

If a person fails to blink for a long time, e.g. staring at a computer screen, or during sleep, meibum accumulates within the ducts and is delivered in increased amounts when the person blinks on waking up in the morning. This excess amount of oil in the precorneal tear film makes the vision misty and blurred in the morning, and explains the diurnal variation in meibum secretion.

Functions of a healthy meibomian secretion (in particular the lipids) are:

- To provide a smooth optical surface at the air–lipid interface for the cornea.
- To reduce excess evaporation of the tear film in-between blinks.
- To enhance the stability of the pre-corneal tear film.
- To enhance a uniform spreading of tear film over the cornea.
- To prevent spillover of tears from the lid margin.
- To prevent contamination of tear film by the sebum.
- To seal the apposing lid margins during sleep.

DEFINITION AND CLASSIFICATION

DEFINITION

The term meibomian gland dysfunction (MGD) was first described by Korb and Henriquez in the early 1980s, previously, there was no firmly established definition in the literature. MGD is generally considered by the clinicians as a *posterior blepharitis*. In 2011, the International Workshop on MGD conducted by the Tear Film and Ocular Surface Society (TFOS) defined it as *"A chronic, diffuse abnormality of the meibomian glands, characterised by the terminal duct obstruction and/or qualitative/quantitative changes in the glandular secretion. It may result in an alteration of the tear film, symptoms of ocular irritation, clinically apparent inflammation, and ocular surface disease"*. It is a very common condition, with a prevalence of more than 60% in Asian populations; while in Caucasians, it spans from 3.5 to 19.9%. It is *considered as the leading cause of dry eye disease throughout the world.*

Dry eye disease had been classically considered an aqueous deficiency problem, but after the report by TFOS, there has been a paradigm shift towards "not producing enough lipids to retain the tears that are being produced". This has led to a huge impact on the treatment proto-

cols which are now targeting MGD as the primary underlying cause, rather than being focused on a symptomatic treatment of dry eyes. It has now been accepted worldwide that dry eye occurs when the ocular surface system cannot adequately protect itself from the desiccating stress due to the lack of healthy meibomian gland secretion.

CLASSIFICATION OF MGD
Etiological types of MGD
I. Primary MGD

In primary MGD only meibomian glands are affected. With age, there is an increase in meibomian gland dropout, particularly after the age of 50 years, which correlates with the appearance of primary MGD. A fall in bioavailable androgens may contribute to these events.

II. Secondary MGD

Secondary MGD is associated with either some other ocular pathology or systemic pathology (Fig. 18.5).

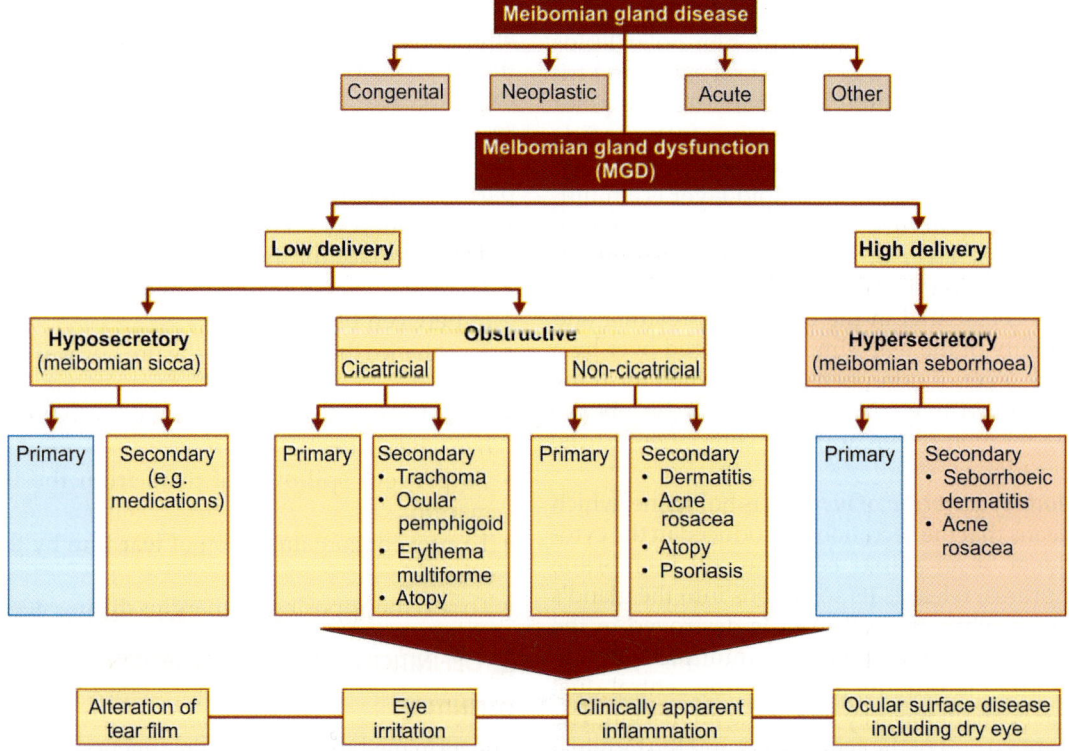

Fig. 18.5: *The new classification system proposed by the International Workshop on MGD*

Classification of MGD proposed by the International Workshop on MGD

A new classification system proposed by the International Workshop on MGD is shown in Fig. 18.5.

PATHOPHYSIOLOGY OF MGD

MGD is a highly complex disease that is caused by a variety of hormonal, microbial, metabolic and environmental factors. Pathophysiology of various types of MGD is summarised below (Fig. 18.5).

A. LOW DELIVERY MGD

Low delivery MGD may be hyposecretory or obstructive. It may be primary or secondary.

I. Hyposecretory MGD

Secondary hyposecretory MGD (meibomian sicca) occurs in seborrhoeic dermatitis, acne rosacea, and as a side effect of certain medications (hormone replacement therapy, anti-histamines, antidepressants, isotretinoin for acne).

II. Obstructive MGD

Obstructive MGD may be cicatricial or non-cicatricial.

Non-cicatricial MGD

A key event in non-cicatricial MGD is hyper-keratinisation of the terminal ducts. Due to *hyperkeratinisation* of the terminal ducts and lid margin; the desquamated cells clump together to form plaques which block the duct openings. Obstruction may be exacerbated by changes in oil composition that increase meibum viscosity. Obstruction of duct opening results in stasis of meibum within the duct; the back pressure produces a cystic dilation of the glands and finally pressure/disuse atrophy of acini and gland dropout. The loss of acini further results in meibum hyposecretion.

In addition, stasis of meibum inside the ducts promotes the growth of commensal bacteria; the bacterial lipases cause degradation of lipids in the meibum and release of toxic mediators. All these factors aggravate the primary hyperkera-tinisation and compositional disturbance of meibum, consequently, the MGD becomes a progressive and a chronic inflammatory disease. The degree to which inflammatory changes are found around affected glands varies in different reports, but signs of inflammation are common at the lid margin. Chronic obstruction leads to degeneration of the secretory gland tissue, and even if the primary obstruction is later resolved by therapeutic approaches, the damage is permanent.

Primary non-cicatricial MGD. Hyperkeratini-sation is commonly due to hormonal imbalance as a part of the ageing process. With age, there is an increase in meibomian gland dropout, particularly after the age of 50 years, which correlates with the appearance of primary MGD. A fall in bioavailable androgens may contribute to these events.

Secondary non-cicatricial MGD is seen in the following conditions:

- *Skin disorders*, such as acne rosacea, atopic dermatitis, seborrhoeic dermatitis, and psoriasis.
- *Topical medications* which can promote MGD are:
  - Antiglaucoma drugs such as pilocarpine, timolol, carbonic anhydrase inhibitor
  - Retinoic acid
- Blink abnormality
- Prolonged contact lens wear
- Antiandrogen medications
- Decreased expression of androgen receptors as a result of anti-androgen therapy.

Polychlorinated biphenyls are also reported to cause MGD.

Cicatricial MGD

In cicatricial MGD, submucosal conjunctival scarring drags the meibomian orifices, terminal ducts and mucocutaneous junction posteriorly, across the posterior lid border and onto the tarsal plate, where the narrowed and displaced ducts can no longer deliver meibum effectively to the tear film lipid layer. Low meibum delivery and changes in oil composition can lead to tear film instability, increased tear evaporation and ultimately to EDE. Cicatricial MGD can also be primary or secondary.

Causes of secondary cicatricial MGD include:
- Trachoma,
- Chronic ocular surface inflammation,
- Chemical injuries,
- Stevens-Johnson syndrome,
- Erythema multiforme, and
- Ocular pemphigoid.

B. HIGH DELIVERY MGD

Hypersecretory MGD (meibomian seborrhoea)

Hypersecretion of meibum occurs in meibomitis (meibomian gland inflammation); excessive amount of meibum with an altered chemical composition is produced that is toxic to the ocular surface.

Primary hypersecretory MGD occurs due to abnormalities of meibum-secreting cells seen as a result of ageing.

Secondary hypersecretory MGD occurs due to *Staphylococcus aureus* or *Demodex folliculorum* infection, environmental factors (hot, dry climate) and nutritional disorders such as generalised malnutrition, a diet low in omega-3 fatty acids, protein deficiency, vitamin A deficiency. All these conditions have been associated with the production of a poor quality meibum.

RISK FACTORS FOR MGD

1. Ageing and hormonal imbalance. This is the most common cause of MGD. Oestrogen and androgen and receptors are present within the meibomian glands. Meibocytes contain enzymes which are necessary for the intracrine synthesis and metabolism of sex steroids. Androgens stimulate meibum secretion, promote the synthesis of proteins and lipids, suppress inflammation within the glands and prevent keratinisation of ductules, while oestrogens have all the opposite effects.

With increasing age, there is a decline in the total androgen pool in both genders, but the effects of androgen deficiency are more pronounced in post-menopausal women. In autoimmune diseases, like rheumatoid arthritis, Sjögren's syndrome and systemic lupus erythematosus, total androgen production in the body is reduced. The aged meibomian glands exhibit decreased meibocyte differentiation, cell renewal, gland size, and an increased inflammatory cell infiltration. These changes lead to gland atrophy and a hyposecretory state.

Similar changes in meibomian glands occur in individuals on anti-androgen therapy for benign prostatic hypertrophy or prostate cancer.

2. Gender. More common in women particularly with oily skin conditions, post-menopausal state and hormonal imbalance due to polycystic ovaries.

The key ingredient of many anti-ageing cosmetics for use around the eye is retinoid acid. It suppresses the action of androgens on meibomian glands, leading to their atrophy.

3. Environment. Hot and dry environment with a low humidity results in an alteration of meibocyte structure and function; there is an increase in basal acinar cell proliferation, a high meibum protein/lipid ratio that increases the viscosity of meibum, with a negative impact on the tear film stability. Increased production of meibum causes ductal dilation as well as depletion in the number of functioning meibocytes (as it is a holocrine secretion), with subsequent gland atrophy and hyposecretion. Exhaustion of the basal cells leads to the loss of acinar meibocytes and meibomian gland dropout.

4. Topical medications. Anti-glaucoma medications, like beta blockers, prostaglandin analogs, carbonic anhydrase inhibitors, are associated with changes in meibomian gland morphology, including decreased acinar area and cell density. Chemical formulations, which contain adrenaline or phenylephrine, promote keratinisation of the lid margin and blocking of meibomian ducts. Retinoic acid reduces meibum production and alters its quality.

Topical medications contain preservatives to enhance their shelf life. The most commonly used preservative is benzalkonium chloride, which is most toxic to the ocular surface.

5. Dietary factors. Malnutrition (explained above) alters the quality of meibum. The use of oral fatty acids improves the quality and expressibility of meibum, especially the omega-3 fatty acids which alter the polar lipid profile and a decrease in the saturated fatty acid content of meibum. This helps in reducing ocular surface inflammation (by reduced production of pro-inflammatory mediators—prostaglandins, thromboxane and leukotriens). Foods rich in omega-3 fatty acids include flaxseed oil, fish oil, and olive oil. Taking 2 capsules of fish oil provide a daily dose of eicosapentaenoic acid 2 gm and decosahexanoic acid 1 gm.

6. Microbial infection. Cholesterol esters present in meibum stimulate the proliferation of commensal organisms, in particular *Staphylococcus aureus*, on the eyelid margin. Bacterial lipases, in turn, breakdown the neutral fats and esters of meibum, releasing glycerides and free fatty acids into the tear film, destroy the mucin layer and make the cornea hydrophobic. This causes the tear film to become unstable. The free fatty acids also stimulate hyperkeratinisation of the lid margins, with keratin plugs adding to the blockage of meibomian ducts.

7. Infestation with the Demodex mite. It is a microscopic ectoparasite of the human skin and constitutes a part of the normal flora. It produces disease when its cell population increases, and is associated with MGD in about 46.8% of such patients. It is of two distinct varieties: *Demodex folliculorum* that infests the eyelash follicles, and *Demodex brevis* that burrows deep into sebaceous and meibomian glands. It causes a direct mechanical damage to the epithelial cells of eyelash follicles (by feeding on them), and by laying eggs at the base of eyelashes, causing follicular distension and misdirected lashes. *D. brevis* mechanically blocks the orifice of meibomian glands and results in a granuloma formation in the infected gland (chlazion). Therefore, it should be considered in the differential diagnosis of a chronic ocular surface disease not responding to the usual therapy.

Diagnosis can be made by random epilation of non-adjacent eyelashes placed on a glass slide, mounted to a coverslip with the addition of a droplet of oil, sodium fluorescein, peanut oil, or 75% alcohol which helps release embedded *Demodex* in the hair follicles.

8. Contact lens wear. Contact lens wear can result in the following harmful effects on the ocular surface:

  i. *Thinning of tear film:* The thickness of a pre-corneal tear film is 3 m (approximately),

while the average central thickness of a contact lens is 30 m. When the contact lens is worn, it splits the tear film both above and below the lens, the altered thickness results in an excessive evaporation and further thinning of the tear film.

  ii. *Contact lenses cause a direct mechanical trauma to the lid margin:* By constant rubbing, it desquamates the surface epithelium, pluggs the meibomian duct orifices, resulting in the gland atrophy.

  iii. *It causes a chronic ocular surface inflammation* which further affects the gland morphology and function, secretion of an altered meibum that adds to the ocular surface inflammation. All these changes are positively correlated with the duration of contact lens wear.

9. Congenital anomalies of meibomian glands. The number of meibomian glands can be decreased or they may be totally absent at birth, as seen in Turner syndrome, ectodermal dysplasia and cleft-lip and palate (ECC syndrome), and in anhidronic ectodermal dysplastic syndrome. Stub-like rudiments may be visible as yellow streaks on the tarsal conjunctival surface or the glands may be totally absent.

Primary distichiasis (aberrant row of eyelashes) may be present at birth in which meibomian glands are replaced by an extra row of eyelashes at the grey line. This results in meibum deficiency and ocular surface trauma due to the misdirected eyelashes. Secondary distichiasis can also occur as a result of meta-plastic reaction caused by repeated rubbing of eyelids (in VKC or chronic allergic conjunctivitis or due to the autosomal dominant lympho-edema).

CLINICAL PRESENTATION OF MGD

MGD is asymptomatic and may remain undiagnosed in its early stages. It only becomes symptomatic when it has worsened enough to cause the tear film instability or eyelid inflammation. Its symptoms and signs vary, and include changes due to (Table 18.1):

- Altered morphology of the lid margin, altered meibum secretion, bacterial overgrowth and gland dropout,
- Tear film instability, and
- Ocular surface inflammation.

Table 18.1: *Summary of MGD clinical features*

Symptoms	Clinical signs
A. Due to tear film instability	
• Visual fluctuation	• Reduce visual acuity
• Blurred vision	• Meibomian gland obstruction
• Visual 'fatigue' and 'trouble focusing'	• Meibomian gland inspissated secretions
• Monocular diplopia	• Rapid tear film break-up time
• Epiphora	• Punctate epithelial erosions
• Foreign body sensation	
• All worse under evaporative conditions	
B. Due to ocular surface inflammation	
• Itching (especially if atopic)	• Conjunctival injection
• Burning	• Conjunctival chemosis
• Photophobia	• Conjunctivochalasis
• Tend to be worse upon awakening	• Fornix foreshortening
	• Symblepharon
	• Inferior punctate epithelial erosions
	• Sterile keratitis (marginal)
C. Due to bacterial overgrowth	
• Morning discharge	• Eyelid seborrhoea, crusting, and loss of lashes
• History of recurrent conjunctivitis	• Conjunctival discharge
• History of recurrent hordeolum	• Papillary conjunctivitis
	• Microbial keratitis

SYMPTOMS

I. Symptoms due to tear film instability include:

- *Fluctuation in vision* that occurs during the tasks associated with decreased blinking, such as reading, driving, staring at a computer screen or watching television is the most common symptom of MGD.
- *Blurred vision.* The thinning of pre-corneal tear film and reduced central corneal thickness, reduce the overall refractive power of the eye, this results in blurring of vision, reduced focusing ability, and sometimes even diplopia.
- *Epiphora.* Despite the presence of a dry eye, a foreign body sensation a paradoxical reflex watering may occur (as the lacrimal gland function is normal and dry spots on cornea stimulate the reflex), particularly when patient is exposed to low environmental humidity and blowing air (in air-conditioned rooms, under a fan).

II. Symptoms related to chronic lid margin inflammation include chronic lid discomfort, pain, redness and irritation.

III. Symptoms related to ocular surface inflammation are burning, itching, frequent blinking and photophobia that gradually worsen to produce severe blepharospasm.

- *Symptoms of ocular irritation* tend to be worse in the morning due to a prolonged exposure of the ocular surface to toxic meibum and hyperosmolar tears (due to poor clearance of the tear film) during sleep.
- *Symptoms get worsened after the insertion of punctal plugs* due to reduced clearance of toxic tears.
- *Most troublesome symptom is a chronic burning sensation* in the eyes which is presumably attributable to the presence of inflammatory mediators or an increased tear osmolarity of the pre-corneal tear film.
- *Itching of eyelids* is more commonly present in atopic patients.

SIGNS (MORPHOLOGICAL CHANGES) IN MGD

Morphological changes in MGD should be assessed, systematically, on a slit-lamp examination and documented. These include:

1. *Lid margin changes.* These include thickening, hyperaemia, discharge, crusts, loss of eyelashes, distichiasis, telangiectasia, keratinisation, foaminess or frothing at the canthal angles and along the lid margin. The presence of scales along eyelash follicles should be noted (keeping in mind seborrhoeic dermatitis and Demodex infestation).

2. *Meibomian duct orifice changes.* These include changes in the orifice position with respect to the mucocutaneous junction, plugging with thick meibum (Fig. 18.3), and notching (indicating lost/atrophic glands).

3. *Meibum quality* is assessed by applying pressure on the eyelid margin with your finger or a cotton-tipped applicator, and noting the ease with which meibum is expressed and its texture.

4. *Ocular surface signs.* Ocular surface inflammation is manifested as conjunctival injection, chemosis, oedema, inferior limbal punctate epithelial erosions, peripheral/marginal keratitis, perilimbal neovascularisation, symblepharon formation, keratinisation of conjunctiva and cornea.

■ DIAGNOSTIC TESTS

Clinical diagnosis of MGD is evident from typical clinical features. Diagnostic tests are required for objectively evaluation of various parameters for instituting and monitory of treatment and also for research purposes.

Routine tests, should preferably be performed in the following sequence to minimise the extent to which one test may influence the other:
- Symptom questionnaire
- Measurement of blink rate, blink interval and blink dynamics
- Measurement of lower tear meniscus height
- Measurement of tear osmolarity
- Tear film break-up time (TBUT) and ocular protection index (OPI)
- Ocular surface fluorescein staining pattern
- Schirmer's test or alternative (phenol red thread test)
- Meibomian gland expressibility (MGE)

Specialised tests, particularly required for research purposes include:

- Interferometry—LipiView
- *In vivo* confocal microscopy (IVCM)
- Meibography

ROUTINE TESTS

1. Ocular surface disease index (OSDI)

Ocular surface disease index (OSDI) is determined with the help of a symptoms questionnaire. This questionnaire is a quick assessment of the symptoms of ocular irritation and how they are affecting the visual functions (photophobia, ocular/eyelid pain, blurring of vision, problems with reading/driving/watching TV) and quality of life of patients. The OSDI assesses the quality of life measures in such patients.

It is a 12-item questionnaire with 3 sub-scales: Ocular symptoms, vision-related function, and environmental triggers. Patients rate their responses on a 0–4 scale with 0 indicating 'none of the time' and 4 indicating 'all the time.' A final score is calculated, ranging from 0 to 100 with scores of 0–12 representing normal, 13–22 representing a mild dry eye disease, 23–32 representing a moderate dry eye disease, and greater than 33 representing a severe dry eye disease.

2. Measurement of blink rate, blink interval and blink dynamics

Normal blink rate is 15–20 times/minute and once every 3–4 seconds in most people. During reading or staring at a computer/cellphone screen, the blink rate reduces to 4.5 per minute, and the blink interval increases to 13.5 seconds. The examiner evaluates, by inspection on a slit-lamp, whether the upper lid closes onto the lower lid with a blink, notes the frequency of partial and complete blinks, the area of ocular surface (cornea and conjunctiva) that remains exposed with each complete blink. If the blink rate reduces and the *blinks are incomplete,* meibum will build up at the lid margin and inside the meibomian ducts, and meibomian glands will be used less over time. This could lead to meibomian gland atrophy, if unidentified.

3. Measurement of lower tear meniscus height

Measure lower tear meniscus height and its clarity. Normal lower tear meniscus is 1.00–

2.00 mm. It can simply be measured by narrowing the vertical beam of a slit-lamp or by meniscometry (measurement of tear meniscus height, radius and cross-sectional area). A rotatable projection system with a target comprising black and white stripes is projected onto the lower central tear film meniscus. Images are recorded and then transferred to a computer for calculation of the radius of curvature.

4. Measurement of tear osmolarity

This measures the concentration of solutes/salts in the tear film. As the aqueous component of the tear film evaporates, the concentration of solutes (mainly salts) increases. This test has become a critical part of dry eye management. It requires only a microlitre sample of tears (≤ 0.2 µl) which is collected by a micro-pen from the lateral canthal tear meniscus. It is placed in an instrument, called the osmometer, which gives the reading in a minute. The disadvantages are the need for an expensive equipment and its constant maintenance.

The osmolarity of both eyes is measured simultaneously; a difference of 8 mOsm/L or more between the two eyes is considered abnormal.

The osmolarity score of 300 mOsm/L or greater in the higher scoring eye is considered abnormal. From 300–320 mOsm/L, is graded as mild; from 320 to 340 mOsm/L, is graded as moderate; and greater than 340 mOsm/L, is graded as a severe dry eye disease.

5. Tear film break-up time (TFBUT)

It is assessed by applying a fluorescein strip to the conjunctiva and using a slit-lamp with cobalt blue illumination. Time is noted between the last blink and the appearance of a black island in the normal green fluorescence of the tear film, or the first dry spot on the cornea. The test is performed prior to the instillation of anaesthetic eye drops (as they are toxic to the corneal epithelium and produce dry spots). Normal TFBUT is 15–45 seconds. If it is >5 seconds, the patient is usually asymptomatic, but when it becomes less than 2 seconds, the patients are almost invariably symptomatic.

6. Ocular surface staining by fluorescein

It stains the corneal stroma under the desquamated epithelium but does not stain a dry spot (it becomes hydrophobic after losing its mucin coating), and appears as a blue spot in the uniform green fluorescence of the tear film. Fluorescein pools in the areas of epithelial erosions/thinning. The area of ocular surface stained should be noted as an interpalpebral staining is due to excess evaporation of aqueous while an inferior limbal staining is due to a toxic meibum production.

Early or mild cases of dry eye disease can be detected more easily with rose bengal or lissamine staining than with fluorescein as they stain dead/devitalised epithelial cells, healthy cells that have lost their mucin coating and the conjunctiva more intensely than the cornea.

7. Schirmer's test

It is of two types: Schirmer I and Schirmer II test. *Schirmer I test can be performed without the anaesthesia* in which it measures the basal tear secretion (which is from the accessory lacrimal glands) as well as the reflex secretion from the main lacrimal gland whose secretory activity is stimulated by the irritating nature of the filter paper. Less than 10 mm of wetting after 5 minutes is diagnostic of ATD. The test is relatively specific, but it is poorly sensitive.

Schirmer I test performed *after topical anaesthesia* measures only the basal lacrimal secretion. *It is highly specific and sensitive for a dry eye disease due to aqueous deficiency.* After instilling a topical anaesthetic, a thin strip of filter paper (5 × 35 mm) is placed in the inferior cul de-sac in the lateral canthus. The excess tears should be wiped off prior to measuring the basal aqueous production. This distinguishes a dry eye due to less aqueous production from the one due to excess aqueous evaporation (due to MGD).

8. Meibomian gland expressibility score

Meibomian gland expressibility (MGE) is a clinical score that helps in assessing the severity of disease at initial presentation, and its improvement with treatment. The number of glands that can be expressed with mild pressure are counted (either with a cotton-tipped swab or a commercially available device). Five glands in the nasal, middle, and lateral thirds of the lower eyelid (total 15 glands) are expressed and scored at each visit. A score of 15 indicates almost all glands are expressible throughout the lower eyelid. A score of zero indicates a complete blockage of ducts and total absence of meibum. Patients with MGE score 0–5 are always symptomatic, while those with a score of 7 or more are usually asymptomatic. The quality of secretion expressed is also noted whether it is clear, opaque, vivid or cheesy.

Grading of MGD

Grade 0 MGD: Normal, clear meibum seen squirting out of the duct orifices with each blink, and can be easily expressed by lightly touching the lid margin.

Grade 1 MGD: Meibum looking opaque, viscous and needs pressure on the lid margin to be expressed. Patient is asymptomatic at this stage and has no corneal staining. MGE score is more than 7.

Grade 2 MGD: Meibum becomes very thick, cheese-like and expressed with difficulty; frothing may be noted at the lid margins (indicating lipid breakdown by bacterial lipases). Patient may be asymptomatic or may have slight discomfort of lid margins, mild conjunctival hyperaemia, mild corneal staining detected by fluorescein at the inferior limbus and an MGE score of 7.

Grade 3 MGD: Most of the ducts are plugged with thick meibum that cannot be expressed by pressure. MGE score is 3–7. Excessive frothing at the canthal angles or along the lid margins. Patient is moderately symptomatic with irritable lid margins, injected, watery eyes with inferior corneal and conjunctival staining.

Grade 4 MGD: Meibomian gland dropout is detected by the presence of notching at the grey line and by transillumination with a pen-light through everted eyelids or by infrared photography. MGE score is 0–3. At this stage, patient presents with severe dry eye symptoms and corneal staining.

SPECIALISED TESTS

1. Meibography

Meibography documents morphology and meibomian gland count in upper and lower lids by infrared camera (LipiView, Fig. 18.6), confocal microscopy, spectral-domain optical coherence tomography. Normal meibomian glands are long, vertical, extending from the lid margin to the end of tarsal plate. They become dilated and tortuous in early/mild disease. In disease of intermediate duration/moderate severity, the gland dropout increases with loss of identifiable gland architecture. In prolonged/severe disease, all glands are markedly shortened or absent.

2. Interferometry

Interferometry is required to analyse the lipid layer of tear film. Following techniques have been recommended over the period:

- *Gearscope* (Keeler Ltd, Windsor, UK) was the first device used for this purpose. It projects a cylindrical white fluorescent light on the tear film lipid layer (TFLL) and the interference images generated are used to evaluate the tear film.
- *DR-1 Camera* (Kowa, Nagoya, Japan) has also been derised to capture the tear film lipid layer and grade the severity of disease according to the *Yokoi dry eye grading system.*
- *LipiView interferometer* (Tear Science, Inc., Morrisville, NC, USA) is the most recent device, which uses white-light interferometry to form a pattern termed *interferogram*. This technique is used for:
  - *Lipid layer thickness measurement,* which is decreased in MGD.
  - *Dynamic lipid layer interference pattern (DLIP) test.* It measures the interference pattern of lipid layer on the control layer of tear film in between the blinks and provides a quantitative analysis of tear film lipid layer (TFLL).

3. *In vivo* confocal laser microscopy

In vivo confocal laser microscopy (IVCM) allows direct visualisation of the meibomian glands. It provides information about acinar density and diameter, secretion reflectivity and peri-

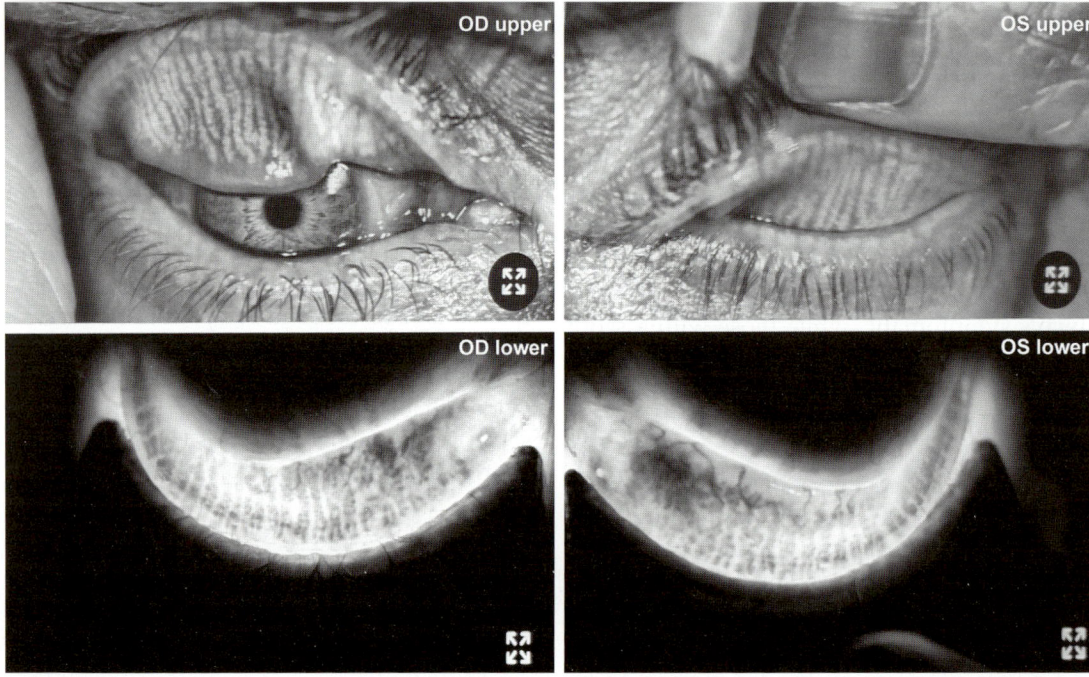

Fig. 18.6: *Infrared camera (LipiView) meibography depicting normal meibomian glands in upper eyelids and some gland dropouts in lower eyelids*

glandular inflammation in patients with MGD. It can also be used to image the resident Demodex mites in the meibomian gland orifices.

MANAGEMENT OF MGD

PRINCIPLES OF MGD MANAGEMENT

MGD is an extremely common clinical entity and is the leading cause of an evaporative dry eye. It should be specifically looked for, and treated in its early stages even in an asymptomatic patient; if untreated, it progresses to meibomian gland atrophy and drop out which is an irreversible stage. The goal of therapy is to improve the flow and the quality of meibum so as to restore the stability of the tear film. Since the therapy has to be continued for 2–3 months, patient education is mandatory to ensure compliance.

A. *Restore tear film stability*
1. *Relieve meibomian gland obstruction*
   - Hot compresses (>108.5°F)
   - Expression
   – Digital massage (patient)
   – Manual (eye care provider)
   – LipiFlow Thermal Pulsation System or equivalent
2. *Improve meibomian gland oils*
   - Fish oil supplementation
   - Systemic tetracycline or macrolide antibiotics
3. *Prevent desiccation*
   - Environmental manipulation
   - Blink exercises
   - Control atopy
   - Lipid layer supplementation
   - Aqueous layer supplementation
   - Correct eyelid and orbicularis muscle abnormalities

B. *Control ocular surface inflammation*
   - Topical steroids
   - Topical cyclosporine

C. *Reduce bacterial overgrowth*
   - Eyelid hygiene
   - Topical/systemic antibiotics

MANAGEMENT MEASURES

1. *Patient education.* As MGD is a chronic disease, in order to ensure compliance to the therapy, this is the most important part of treatment. Patients need to be educated regarding the nature of their disease, its prolonged therapy, the beneficial effects of diet containing omega-3 fatty acids (flaxseed oil, fish oil, and olive oil), how to combat environmental dryness/low humidity (by humidifiers in an air-conditioned rooms) and the drying effects of topical or systemic medications.

2. *Lid hygiene.* Lids should be scrubbed gently with a diluted baby shampoo, applied on cotton-tipped applicator, and rinsed with lukewarm water. This removes the toxic, foamy meibum and reduces the microbial load.

3. *Warm compresses* or application of heat is the mainstay of therapy. Normal meibum is liquid at body temperature, but denatured meibum becomes thick and hard. It blocks the duct openings as well as their entire lumen. Heat therapy helps in liquifying the thick meibum, but to be effective, the glands have to be consistently heated to at least 45°C (113°F). This can be done with application of warm wet towel or cotton pads, soaked in hot (not boiling) water; with the eyes closed, the hot towel is held onto the eyelids for 2 minutes. It is made wet again with hot water and the process repeated five times, so that total heat application is for 10 minutes. This needs to be done daily for at least a month. Heat masks are available commercially, or devices (LipiFlow, Thermal Pulsation System, MiBo Thermaflow) that can be applied to the lid margin and the emitted heat helps liquefy the meibum and massages it upwards towards the duct openings, from where it can easily be expressed.

4. *Gentle lid massage.* After the application of heat, upper eyelid should be massaged downwards with the fingers, while the lower lid massaged upwards to establish meibum flow out of the glands.

5. *Blinking exercises.* They help improve meibum flow and spread of the tear film over the ocular surface by contraction of pre-tarsal orbicularis and Riolan muscle. Patients should be advised to do 10 good blinks at a time; the eyes should be fully closed for 2 seconds, squeezed for another 2 seconds. This should be done for every hour of digital device use.

6. *Topical lubricants.* To relieve the symptoms, reduce tear film evaporation, stabilise lipids in the tear film and prevent aqueous evaporation; preservative-free preparations should be preferred.

7. *Topical or systemic antibiotics* to control infections: Low-dose oral doxycycline (50–100 mg/day for 6 weeks) helps to reduce inflammation in the eyelid tissue, it is anti-angiogenic and reduces lid swelling and hyperaemia, and helps in restoring healthy meibum secretion.

Topical tetracycline, erythromycin or azithromycin eye ointments have similar but more enhanced effects.

Topical cyclosporin eye drops and tacrolimus ointment are specific immunomodulators that affect primarily T lymphocytes. They are found to be highly effective in reducing inflammation of the meibomian glands and reduce their plugging and dysfunction.

8. *Treating Demodex mite infestation.* The aim of therapy is to reduce the number of Demodex mites; total eradication is not required as it is a part of the normal flora of the skin. This can be achieved by a combination of lid scrubs (scrubbing the eyelids twice daily with a baby shampoo diluted with water to yield a 50% dilution and applying an antibiotic ointment at night until resolution of symptoms) and removal of the eyelash collarettes with the use of a cotton-tipped applicator and lid foam. Demodex mites are resistant to a wide range of antiseptic agents including 10% povidone-iodine, 75% alcohol and erythromycin. The most effective and commonly used treatment is tea tree oil. Chemically, it is Terpinen-4-ol—a terpene that has an antimicrobial, antifungal, and antiseptic properties. Many commercially available products contain tea tree oil like shampoos, soaps, ointment, skin creams. Hypochlorous acid and mercury oxide 1% ointment are also effective. Patients should be instructed to avoid

oil-based facial cleansers and greasy makeup as they can provide further 'food' for the mites. They should discard the previously used make-up, use hot water to wash clothes, and a hot dryer to dry them.

9. *Intraductal probing.* This can clear the obstruction of ducts and allows the meibum to flow, thereby reducing the intraductal pressure (IDP), inflammation, lid congestion and improvement of symptoms.

10. *Intense pulsed light (IPL) therapy.* This also liquifies the meibum and improves its drainage by delivering a combination of heat and gentle pressure to the eyelids. It is an in-office therapy and requires 1–2 sessions.

Staged treatment algorithm

The International Workshop on MGD recommended a Staged Treatment Algorithm, depending upon the grade of MGD:

Grade 1
  i. Patient education regarding MGD, diet, environment.
 ii. Lid hygiene
iii. Warm compresses

Grade 2
  i. Advise patient to improve humidity and increase dietary intake of omega-3 fatty acids, or dietary supplements containing conjugated linoleic acid (vegetables, fruits, nuts, grains and seeds; linseed oil) or docosahexaenoic acid (DHA) 1000 mg daily.
 ii. Warm compresses followed by firm lid massage
iii. Blinking exercises
 iv. Topical lubricants
  v. Topical tetracycline/azithromycin eye ointment massaged to lid margin.
 vi. Oral tetracycline, 50–100 mg or azithromycin, 250 mg daily for a month.

Grade 3: All in Grade 2 plus:
  i. Add anti-inflammatory therapy for dry eyes (topical cyclosporin, tacrolimus)
 ii. Ductal probing.

Grade 4: All of Grade 3 therapy.

BIBLIOGRAPHY

1. Alan Tomlinson, Santosh Khanal, Kanna Ramaesh, Charles Diaper, Angus McFadyen. Tear film osmolarity: Determination of a referent for dry eye diagnosis. Investigative Ophthalmology & Visual Science 2006; 47: 4309–15.
2. Baudouin C, Messmer EM, Aragona P, et al. Revisiting the vicious circle of dry eye disease: a focus on the pathophysiology of meibomian gland dysfunction. Br J Ophthalmol 2016; 100: 300–06.
3. Cheng AM, Sheha H, Tseng SC. Recent advances on ocular Demodex infestation. Curr Opin Ophthalmol 2015; 26(4): 295–300 [PubMed].
4. Craig J, Tomlinson A. Importance of the lipid layer in human tear film stability and evaporation. Optom Vis Sci 1997; 74:8–13 [PubMed].
5. Dell SJ. Intense pulsed light for evaporative dry eye disease. Clin Ophthalmol 2017; 11: 1167–73.
6. Foulks GN, Bron AJ. Meibomian gland dysfunction: a clinical scheme for description, diagnosis, classification, and grading. Ocul Surf 2003; 1: 107–26.
7. Irfan S. Is Benign Essential Blepharospasm a 'Benign' and or an 'Essential' Condition? Major Review Paper. The American Journal of Cosmetic Surgery. 2018; 35(2): 83–91. DOI10.1177/0488/6817740185 journals.sagepub.com/home/acs
8. Jones L, Downie LE, Korb D, et al. TFOS DEWS II management and therapy report. Ocul Surf 2017; 15(3): 575–628.
9. Knop E, Knop N, Miller T, Sullivan DA. The International Workshop of meibomian gland dysfunction: report of the subcommittee on anatomy, physiology, and pathophysiology of the meibomian gland. Invest Ophthalmol Vis Sci 2011; 52(4): 1938–78.
10. Korb DR, Henriquez AS. Meibomian gland dysfunction and contact lens intolerance. J Am Optom Assoc 1980; 51: 243–51.
11. McCulley JP, Dougherty JM, Deneau DG. Classification of chronic blepharitis. Ophthalmology 1982; 89: 1173–80 [PubMed].
12. Na Li, Xin-Guo Deng, Mei-Feng He. Comparison of the Schirmer I test with and without topical anaesthesia for diagnosing dry eye. Int J Ophthalmol 2012; 5(4): 478–81.
13. Nelson JD, Shimazaki J, Benitez-del-Castillo JM, et al. The International Workshop on meibomian gland dysfunction: report of the

definition and classification subcommittee. Invest Ophthalmol Vis Sci 2011; 52: 1930–37.

14. Özcura F, Aydin S, Helvaci MR. Ocular surface disease index for the diagnosis of dry eye syndrome. Ocular immunology and inflammation 2007; 15(5): 389–93.

15. Schaumberg DA, Nichols JJ, Papas EB, et al. The International Workshop on meibomian gland dysfunction: report of the subcommittee on the epidemiology of, and associated risk factors for, MGD. Invest Ophthalmol Vis Sci.

2011; 52: 1994–2005. [PMC free article] [PubMed].

16. Schaumberg DA, Nichols JJ, Papas EB, Tong L, Uchino M, Nichols KK. The International Workshop on meibomian gland dysfunction: report of the subcommittee on the epidemiology of, associated risk factors for, MGD. Invest Ophthalmol Vis Sci 2011; 52(4): 1994–2005.

17. Truong S, Cole N, Stapleton F, Golebiowski B. Sex hormones and the dry eye. Clin Exp Optom 2014; 97(4): 324–36.

Xerophthalmia

■ GENERAL CONSIDERATIONS

DEFINITION

"Xerophthalmia" (Greek word for dry eyes) refers to an array of ocular manifestations caused due to vitamin A deficiency. As there is depletion of vitamin A stores in the body, manifestations occur with increasing severity in the form of night blindness, conjunctival xerosis, Bitot's spot, corneal xerosis, and corneal ulceration/keratomalacia. All of them usually respond rapidly to vitamin A therapy, the milder ones often clearing without sequelae while corneal scarring and opacification occurs when there is loss of deep corneal tissue from ulceration.

PREVALENCE

Xerophthalmia although can occur in any age group, it is especially prevalent in preschool-age children, adolescents and pregnant women owing to their greater vitamin A requirements for growth. Children are also at higher risk of intestinal infestations and infections, which may impair the absorption of vitamin A thereby causing deficiency. In India, prevalence of subclinical vitamin "A" deficiency (VAD) ranges from 31 to 57% among preschool children and a further 1 to 2% of children suffer from clinical VAD.

■ ETIOPATHOGENESIS

- Xerophthalmia is primarily caused by depletion of vitamin A in the body, it is especially prevalent in infants suffering from protein energy malnutrition (PEM).
- In addition, it is seen in association with certain systemic diseases such as Sjögren's syndrome, SLE, rheumatoid arthritis, scleroderma, sarcoidosis, amyloidosis and hypothyroidism.
- Certain medications such as antihistamines, nasal decongestants, tranquillizers and anti-

depressants are associated with milder forms of xerophthalmia.

VITAMIN A AND ITS METABOLISM

Vitamin A, or retinol, is a fat-soluble vitamin required for gene expression, epithelial cell differentiation, normal growth, photopic vision and immunity. It is found in liver (particularly fish liver), egg yolk and dairy products. Carotenoids and potential provitamin A precursors that can be converted to retinol in the wall of the gut, are present in green leafy vegetables, red palm oil and yellow fruits. The relative biological values of these various substances were formerly expressed in international units (IU) of vitamin A activity, 1 IU being equivalent to 0. 3 µg of retinol, 0.55 µg of retinyl palmitate, 0.6 µg of 13-carotene, and 1.2 µg of other provitamin A carotenoids. 90% of ingested retinol is absorbed in the small intestine and transported, in association with chylomicrons, to the liver, where it is stored as retinyl palmitate. When needed, it is released into the bloodstream as retinol in combination with retinol-binding protein (RBP), a specific carrier protein elaborated by the liver. In the serum RBP—retinol complex combines with transthyretin, a large protein also synthesized in the liver. The retinol is then removed from the serum and utilized by target cells, such as retinal photoreceptors and epithelial linings throughout the body. Specific receptors exist on the cell surface and nucleus for the vitamin A complex or its active metabolites, particularly retinoic acid. Liver stores form an important buffer against variations in the intake of vitamin A and provitamin A carotenoids. When intake surpasses requirements, the excess is stored in the liver. If intake is less than this amount, liver stores are drained to maintain serum retinol at a normal level (well above 0.7 µmol/litre or 200 µg/litre). If intake remains low for prolonged periods there is depletion of liver stores followed by decrease in serum retinol levels resulting in impaired cellular function, abnormal differen-tiation (e.g. xerophthalmia) and other physio-logical consequences and clinical manifestations of deficiency (e.g. anaemia, impaired resistance to infection).

CLINICAL MANIFESTATIONS AND CLASSIFICATION

The first symptom of vitamin A deficiency is characterised by impaired adaptation to the dark, which can begin when serum retinol concentrations fall below 1.0 µmol/L, but occurs more often when they fall below 0.7 µmol/L. Xerophthalmia occurs when serum retinol concentrations fall below 0.35 µmol/L.[1,2] Night blindness generally responds rapidly to vitamin A therapy, within 1–2 days,[3–5] and prompt treatment of xerophthalmia generally results in the full preservation of eyesight up to the stage of corneal xerosis.[6]

WHO CLASSIFICATION

Xerophthalmia manifestations have been classified by WHO (1982) into various categories as per Table 19.1.

XN: Night blindness

Retinol is essential for the elaboration of rhodopsin (visual purple) by the rods, the sensory receptors of the retina responsible for vision under low levels of illumination. Vitamin A deficiency can interfere with rhodopsin production, impair rod function, and result in night blindness. Night blindness is generally the earliest manifestation of vitamin A deficiency. When mild, it may become apparent only after a photic stress, such as flying a kite on a sunny day. It takes some time for the eyes to adjust from brightly lit areas to dim ones. It is also associated with decrease in contrast vision.

Table 19.1: WHO classification of xerophthalmia signs[7]

Classification	Ocular signs
XN	Night blindness
X1A	Conjunctival xerosis
X1B	Bitot's spots
X2	Corneal xerosis
X3A	Corneal ulceration/keratomalacia involving one-third or less of cornea
X3B	Corneal ulceration/keratomalacia involving one-half or more of cornea
XS	Corneal scar
XF	Xerophthalmic fundus

Night blindness responds rapidly, usually within 24–48 hours, to vitamin A therapy. In some instances term 'chicken eyes' has been used to describe night blindness as chicken lack rods and hence are night blind.[4]

X1A, X1B: Conjunctival xerosis and Bitot's spot

Vitamin A deficiency causes alterations in epithelial architecture termed "keratinizing metaplasia". The columnar epithelium of the conjunctiva is transformed to the stratified squamous type, with a resultant loss of goblet cells, formation of a granular cell layer and keratinization of the surface. The distended squamous cells have large, open nuclei with prominent nucleoli. Clinically, this causes marked dryness of the conjunctiva which appears roughened with fine droplets or bubbles on the surface. These changes may not be seen in the presence of tears but as the tears drain off the affected area will emerge like "sandbanks at receding tide" which is best detected with an oblique illumination. Conjunctival xerosis first appears in the temporal quadrant, as an oval or triangular patch adjacent to the limbus in the interpalpebral fissure, usually in both eyes. In some individuals keratin and saprophytic bacilli accumulate on the xerotic surface, giving it a foamy or cheesy appearance. Such lesions are known as Bitot's spots. The overlying material can be easily wiped off and the amount can vary from day to day. With increase in deficiency of vitamin A, similar, though less prominent lesions are seen in the nasal quadrant.

Generalized conjunctival xerosis, involving the interior and/or superior quadrants, suggests advanced vitamin A deficiency. The entire conjunctiva appears dry, roughened, and corrugated, sometimes skin like. There may be prominent conjunctival thickening and folds (Fig. 19.1). This is an advanced lesion, almost always accompanied by gross corneal involvement. Isolated, usually temporal, patches of conjunctival xerosis or Bitot's spot are sometimes encountered in the absence of active vitamin A deficiency. The affected individuals are usually of school-age or older and may have a history of previous bouts of night blindness or xerophthalmia. In most instances, these patches represent persistent areas of squamous

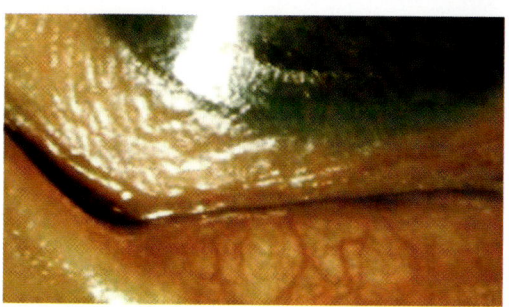

Fig. 19.1: *Conjunctival xerosis (X1A)*

metaplasia-induced during a prior episode of vitamin A deficiency. The only certain means of distinguishing active from inactive lesions is to observe their response to vitamin A therapy. Active conjunctival xerosis and Bitot's spot begin to resolve within 2–5 days. Most will disappear within 2 weeks, though a significant proportion of temporal lesions may persist for months in shrunken form.

X2: Corneal xerosis

Corneal changes begin early in vitamin A deficiency, long before they can be seen with the naked eye. Many children with night blindness (without clinically evident conjunctival xerosis) have superficial punctate lesions over inferior nasal aspects of cornea that stain brightly with fiuorescein. With more severe disease the punctate lesions become more numerous and spread upwards over the central cornea, and the corneal stroma becomes edematous (Fig. 19.2). Clinically, the cornea develops classical xerosis, a hazy, lustreless, dry appearance, first apparent near the inferior limbus. Thick, keratinized

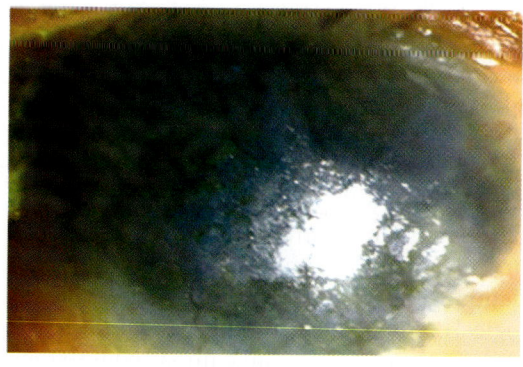

Fig. 19.2: *Corneal xerosis (X2)*

plaques resembling Bitot's spot may form, on the corneal surface. These are often dense in the interpalpebral zone. With treatment, these corneal plaques peel off, sometimes leaving a superficial erosion which quickly heals. Corneal xerosis responds within 2–5 days to vitamin A therapy, the cornea regaining its normal appearance in 1–2 weeks.

X3A, X3B: Corneal ulceration/keratomalacia

Ulceration/keratomalacia indicates permanent destruction of part or all of the corneal stroma, resulting in permanent structural alteration. Ulcers are classically round to oval "punched-out" defects, as if a trephine or cork-borer had been applied to the eye (Fig. 19.3). The surrounding cornea is generally xerotic but otherwise clear, and typically lacks the grey, infiltrated appearance of ulcers of bacterial origin. There may be more than one ulcer. Small ulcers are almost invariably confined to the periphery of the cornea, especially its inferior and nasal aspects. The ulceration may be shallow, but is commonly deep. Perforations become plugged with iris, thereby preserving the anterior chamber. Histologically, the sharply demarcated area of stromal necrosis is covered by keratinized epithelium.

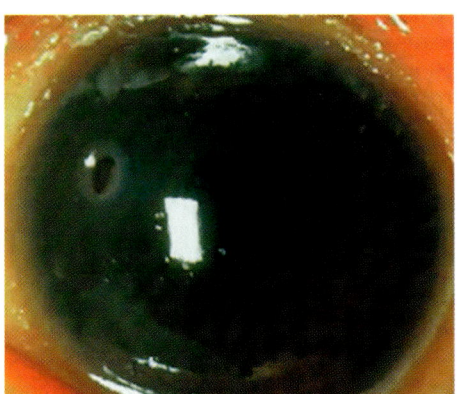

Fig. 19.3: *Corneal ulceration (X3A)*

With therapy, superficial ulcers often heal with surprisingly little scarring; deeper ulcers, especially perforations, form dense peripheral adherent leukomas. Localized keratomalacia is a rapidly progressive condition affecting the full thickness of the cornea. It first appears as an opaque, grey to yellow mound or outpouching of the corneal surface. In more advanced disease the necrotic stroma sloughs, leaving a large ulcer or descemetocele. As with smaller ulcers, these are usually peripheral and heal as dense, white, adherent leukomas. Ulceration/keratomalacia involving less than one-third of the corneal surface (X3A) generally spares the central pupillary zone; prompt therapy ordinarily preserves useful vision. More widespread involvement (Fig. 19.4) (X3B), especially generalized liquefactive necrosis, usually results in perforation, extrusion of intraocular contents, and loss of the globe. Prompt therapy may still save the other eye and the child's life. It is not always possible to distinguish cases of ulceration/necrosis due to vitamin A deficiency from those due to bacterial or fungal infections. The most obvious reason is that vitamin A-related lesions can become secondarily infected. In addition, however, once ulceration/keratomalacia occurs, the conjunctiva usually becomes inflamed, and for reasons that are not well understood, inflammation commonly masks or reverses conjunctival xerosis. Examination of the other, unulcerated eye, may then reveal the true nature of the problem although not always. When vitamin A status deteriorates precipitously, as occurs with measles, severe gastroenteritis, or kwashiorkor in children previously in borderline vitamin A balance-corneal necrosis can precede the appearance of night blindness or conjunctival xerosis. In such instances it is safest to assume that both vitamin A deficiency and infection are present and the child should be treated accordingly.

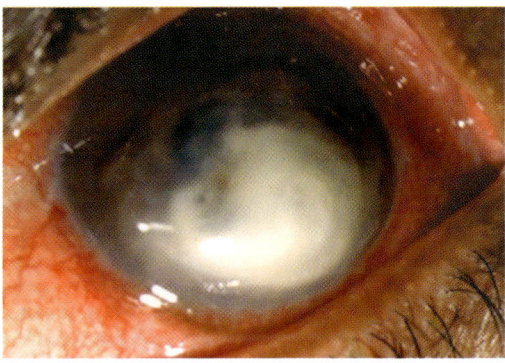

Fig. 19.4: *Corneal ulceration (X3B)*

Children suffering from forms of the disease destructive to the cornea are usually younger (often less than 1 year of age), more severely malnourished, and more deficient in vitamin A. History of a recent precipitating event (pneumonia, measles, gastroenteritis, tuberculosis, etc.) is common, and the mortality is often quite high (20–50%).

XS: Scars

Healed sequelae of prior corneal disease related to vitamin A deficiency include opacities or scars of varying density (nebula, macula, leukoma) (Fig. 19.5), weakening and outpouching of the remaining corneal layers (staphyloma, and descemetocele) and, where loss of intraocular contents had occurred, phthisis bulbi, a scarred shrunken globe. Such end-stage lesions are not specific for xerophthalmia and may arise from numerous other conditions, notably trauma and infection.

XF: Xerophthalmic fundus

It is characterized by small white retinal lesions which may be accompanied by constriction of the visual fields and will largely disappear within 2–4 months of vitamin A therapy.

■ DIAGNOSIS

Clinical diagnosis of xerophthalmia is based on clinical manifestations.

Laboratory investigations are rarely required but may be useful in few instances when there is doubt.

Serum retinol study is an expensive but direct measure to assess vitamin A deficiency. A value

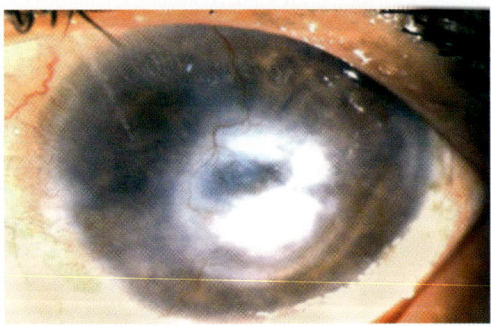

Fig. 19.5: *Corneal scar (XS)*

of <1.0 mg/dl indicates gross deficiency and >2.0 mg/dl indicates adequate vitamin A in the body. A value of <0.7 mg/L in children younger than 12 years is considered low.

Total retinol binding protein (RBP) is a less costly and easier to perform immunologic assay. Although it is a more stable compound than retinol, its measure is less accurate as it is affected by serum protein concentration and also zinc deficiency interferes with production of RBP.

■ TREATMENT AND PREVENTION

TREATMENT

1. **Vitamin a therapy:** Xerophthalmia is a medical emergency, requiring prompt administration of massive amounts of vitamin A. Oral administration is just as effective as parenteral administration.

i. *All patients above the age of 1 year (except woman of reproductive age should be* administered 110 mg oil- or water-miscible retinol palmitate or 66 mg retinol acetate (200,000 IU vitamin A) by mouth immediately upon diagnosis and repeat the dose of the following days.

• *An additional dose* should be given 1–2 weeks later to boost liver reserves.

• Because children with severe protein-energy deficiency handle a massive dose poorly, they should receive an additional dose, every 2 weeks, until protein status improves.

• *For children unable to swallow, or suffering from repeated vomiting or profuse diarrhoea,* an intramuscular injection of 55 mg *water-miscible* retinol palmitate (l00,000 IU) should be substituted for the first oral dose. Oil-miscible preparations should never be given by injection because they are poorly absorbed from the injection site.

ii. *For children less than 12 months* of age the doses should be reduced by half.

iii. *Women of reproductive age* (pregnant or otherwise). Special attention is required while providing vitamin A supplementation to women of reproductive age because of the potential teratogenic effects of very high dose retinol if given early in pregnancy. Women of reproductive age with night blindness or Bitot's spots should be treated with a daily oral dose of 5,000–10,000 IU of vitamin A for at least 4 weeks. Such a daily dose should never exceed 10,000 IU, although a weekly dose not exceeding 25,000 IU may be substituted. All women of reproductive age, whether or not pregnant, who exhibit severe signs of xerophthalmia (i.e. acute corneal lesions) should be treated with three-dose treatment.

2. **Treatment of underlying conditions:** Malnutrition to be corrected by including plenty of milk, butter, dark green leafy vegetables, carrots, orange, cod-liver oil in the diet.

3. **Local ocular therapy:** Topical lubrication and antibiotics to be used as adjunctive measures.

Note: Vitamin A supplementation in excess can result in toxicity which is characterised by dermatitis with xanthosis cutis, hepatosplenomegaly, bone pain and increased risk of fracture and pseudotumor cerebri.

PREVENTION

I. **Prolongation of breast-feeding and early food supplementation (preferably by 6 months of age)** with tasty, easily digested provitamin A-rich fruits (e.g. mango and papaya) or appropriately prepared dark-green leafy vegetables are likely to have a significant impact. Dark-green leafy vegetables are often the least expensive and most widely and consistently available source of vitamin A activity. The same amount of vitamin A is obtained from 68 g of spinach as from 63 g of liver, 227 g of hens' eggs, 1.7 litres of whole cow's milk, or 6 kg of beef or mutton. The recommended dietary allowance (RDA) for children, adults and lactating women is 400 µg, 900 µg and 1200 µg respectively. *This is the best long term approach.*

II. **Food fortification with vitamin A** serves as *medium term approach* for preventing vitamin A deficiency, where people cannot afford vitamin A-rich foodstuffs. Foodstuffs commonly used by poor and middle class population which can be fortified are:
- Vanaspati ghee or oil used to cook food.

III. **Prophylactic vitamin A supplementation** periodically serves as *short-term approach* for preventing vitamin A deficiency, especially in poor economic strata/population. This approach is mostly in vogue in Asian and African countries.

WHO recommended universal distribution of schedule of prophylactic vitamin A supplementation is as follows (Table 19.2):

1. *Newborn:* 27.5 mg retinol palmitate at birth (50,000 IU)
2. *Infant 6–12 month and older children who weigh less than 8 kg:* 100,000 IU orally every 4–6 months
3. *Children over 2 years and under 6 years of age:* 200,000 IU orally every 4–6 months.
4. *Women of childbearing age:* 165 mg retinol palmitate in 1 month (300,000 IU) of giving birth.
5. *Pregnant and lactating women:* 2.75 mg retinol palmitate every day (5000 IU) or 11 mg retinol palmitate once every week (20,000 IU).

Table 19.2 summarises prophylaxis schedule of vitamin A to prevent debilitating effects of xerophthalmia.

Table 19.2: *Vitamin A prophylaxis schedule*	
Newborn	27.5 mg retinol palmitate at birth (50,000 IU)
Children <12 months	55 mg retinol palmitate once every 4–6 (100,000 IU) months
Children >12 months	110 mg retinol palmitate once every 4–6 (200,000 IU) months
Women of childbearing age	165 mg retinol palmitate within 1 month (300,000 IU) of giving birth
Pregnant and lactating women	2.75 mg retinol palmitate every day (5000 IU) or 11 mg retinol palmitate once every week (20,000 IU)

REFERENCES

1. Natadisastra G, Wittpenn JR, West KP Jr, Muhilal, Sommer A. Impression cytology for detection of vitamin A deficiency. Arch Ophthalmol 1987; 105: 1224–8.
2. Sommer A. Nutritional blindness: xerophthalmia and keratomalacia. New York: Oxford University Press; 1982.

3. Spence JC. A clinical study of nutritional xerophthalmia and night blindness. Arch Dis Child 1931; 6: 17–26.

4. Sommer A. Vitamin A deficiency and its consequences. A field guide to detection and control, 3rd ed. Geneva: World Health Organization; 1995 (http://whqlibdoc.who.int/publications/1995/92415447783_eng.pdf).

5. WHO/UNICEF/IVACG Task Force. Vitamin A supplements. A guide to their use in the treatment and prevention of vitamin A deficiency and xerophthalmia, 2nd ed. Geneva: World Health Organization; 1997 (http://whqlibdoc.who.int/publications/1997/9241545062.pdf).

6. McLaren DS, Kraemer K, editors. Manual on vitamin A deficiency disorders (VADD), third edition. Basel: Sight and Life Press; 2012.

7. Control of vitamin A deficiency and xerophthalmia. Report of a joint WHO/UNICEF/USAID/Helen Keller International/IVACG meeting. Geneva: World Health Organization; 1982 (WHO Technical Report Series, No. 672) (http://whqlibdoc.who.int/trs/WHO_TRS_672.pdf).

Chapter

20

Pterygium and Conjunctival Degenerations

PINGUECULA

Pinguecula is an extremely common degenerative condition of the conjunctiva. It is characterised by formation of a yellowish white patch on the bulbar conjunctiva near the limbus. This condition is termed pinguecula, because of its resemblance to fat, which means pinguis.

Etiology of pinguecula is not known exactly. It has been considered as *an age-change*, occurring more commonly in persons chronically exposed to strong sunlight, dust and wind. Its predominant nasal location has been presumed to be due to reflection of light by the nose to the nasal conjunctiva. It has been suggested that the effect of ultraviolet light may be mediated by mutations in the p53 gene. Earlier it was considered a precursor of pterygium. However, currently it is suggested that pinguecula does not progress to pterygium and that the two are distinct disorders.

Pathology

There is an elastotic degeneration of collagen fibres of the substantia propria of conjunctiva, coupled with deposition of basophilic elastotic fibres and granular deposits in the substance of conjunctiva. Cornea is never involved.

Clinical features

Pinguecula is a bilateral, usually stationary condition, presenting as yellowish white triangular patch near the limbus (Fig. 20.1). Apex of the triangle is away from the cornea. It affects the nasal side more commonly than the temporal side. When conjunctiva is congested, it stands out as an avascular prominence.

Complications

Complications of pinguecula include its inflammation, intraepithelial abscess formation and rarely calcification and doubtful conversion into pterygium.

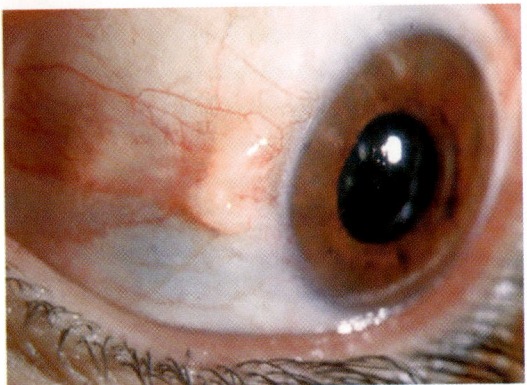

Fig. 20.1: *Pinguecula*

Differential diagnosis

Pinguecula is usually differentiated from:
• Diagnosis is obvious due to its typical appearance
• However, it needs to be differentiated from *conjunctival intraepithelial neoplasia*
• Gaucher's disease type I.

Treatment

In routine no treatment is required for pinguecula. However, when cosmetically unaccepted and if so desired, it may be excised. When inflamed it is treated with topical steroids.

PTERYGIUM

Pterygium (L. Pterygion = a wing) is a wing-shaped fold of conjunctiva encroaching upon the cornea from either side within the interpalpebral fissure. Recent evidence suggest that pterygium is a proliferative lesion rather than a degenerative condition characterised by proliferation of fibrovascular tissues, inflammatory infiltration, fibrosis, angiogenesis and breakdown of extracellular matrix.

ETIOLOGY

Etiology of pterygium is not definitely known. But the disease is more common in people living in hot climates. Therefore, the most accepted view is that it is a response to prolonged effect of environmental factors such as exposure to sun (ultraviolet rays), dry heat, high wind and abundance of dust.

Ultraviolet-induced damage to limbal stem cells and activation of matrix metalloproteinase is considered the basic mechanism for causation of pterygium.

Hereditary factors have been implicated for prediction. Molecular genetic alterations reported include loss of heterozygosity (LOH), and point mutations of proto-oncogeners.

Ocular surface markers, such as overexpresion of defensins, phospholipases D3 and upregulation of growth factors, have also been implicated in pathogenesis of pterygium.

PATHOLOGY

Pathologically pterygium is a degenerative and hyperplastic condition of conjunctiva. The subconjunctival tissue undergoes elastotic degeneration and proliferates as vascularised granulation tissue under the epithelium, which ultimately encroaches the cornea. The corneal epithelium, Bowman's layer and superficial stroma are often destroyed.

• *Abnormal elastic fibres* form the significant part of pterygium tissue. These are called elastotic fibres, as they do not degrade with elastase.
• *Fibroblasts* are also seen in abundance in the vicinity of elastodysplasia, indicating probably an actinic-induced damage.

CLINICAL FEATURES

Demography
• *Age*: Usually seen in old age.
• *Sex*: More common in males doing outdoor work than females.
  More common nasal occurrence has been postulated to be due to reflection of ultraviolet rays from the nose in this region.
• *Laterality*: It may be unilateral or bilateral. Usually present on the nasal side but may also occur on the temporal side.
• *Region*: Occur more frequently and most severely in hot and dry climatic region, i.e. in tropical areas near the equator and to a lesser and milder degrees in cooler climates.
• *Profession:* Outdoor workers are exposed to sunlight, especially those working in the setting of highly reflective surfaces are more prone Both blue and ultraviolet rays/radiation have been implicated to cause it.

Symptoms

- *Cosmetic intolerance* may be the only issue in otherwise asymptomatic condition in early stages.
- *Foreign body* sensation, irritation and mild watering may be experienced by many patients.
- *Defective vision* occurs when it encroaches the pupillary area or due to corneal astigmatism induced by fibrosis in the regressive stage.
- *Diplopia* may occur occasionally due to limitation of ocular movements.

Signs

Pterygium presents as a triangular fold of conjunctiva encroaching on the cornea in the area of palpebral aperture usually on the nasal side (Fig. 20.2) but may also occur on the temporal side. Very rarely, both nasal and temporal sides are involved (*primary double pterygium*).

Parts of a fully-developed pterygium are as follows (Fig. 20.2):

- *Head:* Apical part present on the cornea, as elevated whitish mass.
- *Neck:* Constricted part present in the limbal area.
- *Body:* Scleral part, extending between limbus and the canthus.
- *Cap:* Semilunar whitish infiltrate present just in front of the head.

Types. Depending upon the progression it may be progressive or regressive pterygium.

- *Progressive pterygium* is thick, fleshy and vascular with a few whitish infiltrates in the cornea, in front of the head of the pterygium

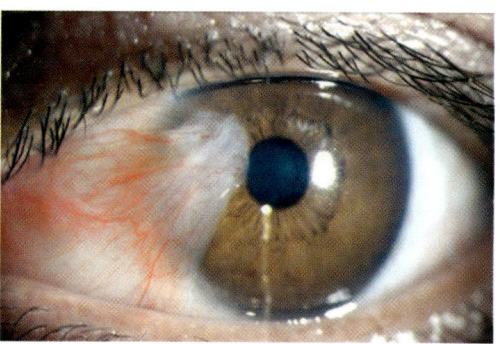

Fig. 20.2: *Pterygium*

known as *Fuch's spots* or *islets of Vogt* also called cap of pterygium.

- *Regressive pterygium* is thin, atrophic, attenuated with very little vascularity. There is no cap, but deposition of iron (*Stocker's line*) may be seen sometimes, just anterior to the head of pterygium. Ultimately, it becomes membranous but never disappears.
- *Corneal astigmatism* is an important sign of pterygium and varies depending upon its extent and severity, usually with-the-rule astigmatism is induced. However, obliquely against-the-rule and irregular astigmatism may also occur.
- *Anterior segment optical coherence tomography (ASOCT)* examination reveals pterygium as a wedge-shaped mass of tissue separating the corneal epithelium from the Bowman's membrane. The Bowman's membrane is often seen as wavy, interspersed and destroyed. ASOCT also reveals stellate mass of sub-epithelial pterygium tissue beyond the clinically seen margin.

COMPLICATIONS

- *Cystic degeneration and infection* are of infrequent occurrence.
- *Neoplastic change* to epithelioma, fibrosarcoma or malignant melanoma, may occur rarely.

DIFFERENTIAL DIAGNOSIS

Pterygium must be differentiated from pseudo-pterygium. Pseudopterygium is a fold of bulbar conjunctiva attached to the cornea. It is formed due to adhesions of chemosed bulbar conjunctiva to the marginal corneal ulcer. It usually occurs following chemical burns of the eye. Differences between pterygium and pseudo-pterygium are given in Table 20.1.

TREATMENT

Surgical excision is the only satisfactory treatment.

Indications of pterygium surgery are:

- *Cosmetic disfigurement* is the common indication
- *Visual impairment* due to significant regular or irregular astigmatism.

Table 20.1: *Differences between pterygium and pseudopterygium*

		Pterygium	Pseudopterygium
1.	Etiology	Degenerative process	Inflammatory process
2.	Age	Usually occurs in elder persons	Can occur at any age
3.	Sex	More common in male	Equally common
4.	Site	Always situated in the palpebral aperture	Can occur at any site
5.	Stages	Either progressive, regressive or stationary	Always stationary
6.	Probe test	Probe cannot be passed underneath	A probe can be passed under the neck

- *Continued progression* threatening to encroach onto the pupillary area (once the pterygium has encroached pupillary area, wait till it crosses on the other side).
- *Diplopia* due to interference in ocular movements.
- *Atypical appearance* such as possible dysplasia.

Recurrence of the pterygium after surgical excision is the main problem (30–50%). Therefore, primary goal of treatment is to excise the pterygium and prevent recurrence. Following measures are recommended to reduce recurrences:

- *Surgical excision with free conjunctival limbal autograft* (CLAU) taken from the same eye or other eye is presently the preferred technique.
- *Surgical excision with amniotic membrane graft and mitomycin C* (MMC) (0.02%) application may be required in recurrent pterygium or when dealing with a very large pterygium.
- *Surgical excision with lamellar keratectomy and lamellar keratoplasty* may be required in deeply infiltrating recurrent recalcitrant pterygia.
- *Old methods to prevent recurrence* (not preferred now) included transplantation of pterygium in the lower fornix (McRaynold's operation) and postoperative use of beta irradiations.

Surgical technique of pterygium excision

1. *After topical anaesthesia,* eye is cleansed, draped and exposed using universal eye speculum.
2. *Head of the pterygium is lifted* and dissected off the cornea very meticulously (Fig. 20.3A).
3. *Main mass of pterygium is then separated* from the sclera underneath and the conjunctiva superficially.

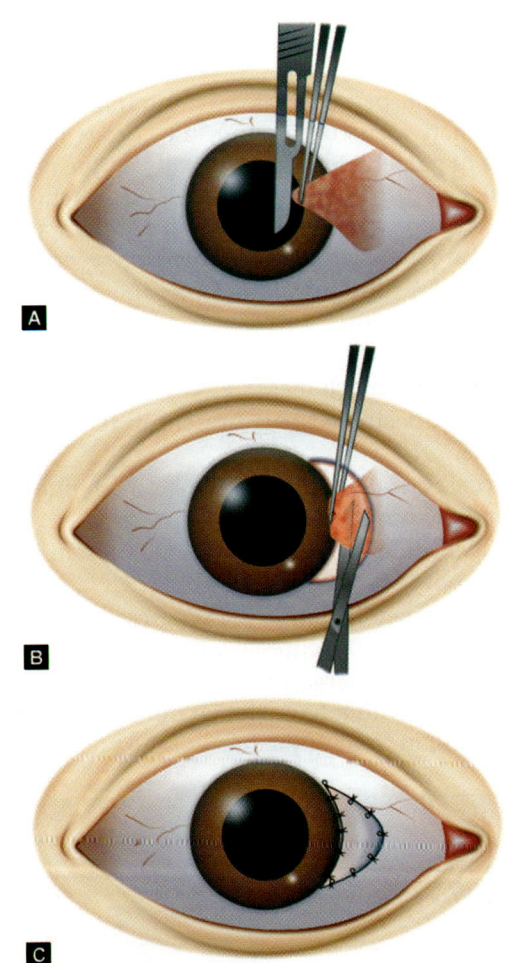

Fig. 20.3: *Surgical technique of pterygium excision. A, Dissection of head from the cornea; B, Excision of pterygium tissue under the conjunctiva; C, Conjunctival limbal autograft after excising the pterygium*

4. *Pterygium tissue is then excised* taking care not to damage the underlying medial rectus muscle (Fig. 20.3B).

5. *Haemostasis* is achieved and the episcleral tissue exposed is cauterised thoroughly.
6. *Conjunctival limbal autograft (CLAU)* transplantation to cover the defect after pterygium excision (Fig. 20.3C). It is the latest and most effective technique in the management of pterygium. Use of fibrin glue to stick the autograft in place reduces operating time as well as discomfort associated with the sutures.

Note: For further details, *see* Chapter 35.

CONCRETIONS

Etiology. Concretions are formed due to accumulation of inspissated mucus and dead epithelial cell debris into the conjunctival depressions called *loops of Henle*. They are commonly seen in elderly people in a degenerative condition and also in patients with scarring stage of trachoma. The name concretion is a misnomer, as they are not calcareous deposits.

Clinical features
• *Locations.* Concretions are seen on palpebral conjunctiva, more commonly on upper than the lower. They may also be seen in lower fornix.
• *Appearance.* These are yellowish white, hard looking, raised areas, varying in size from pin point to pin head (Fig. 20.4).
• *Symptoms.* Being hard, they may produce foreign body sensations and lacrimation by rubbing the corneal surface. Occasionally, they may even cause corneal abrasions.

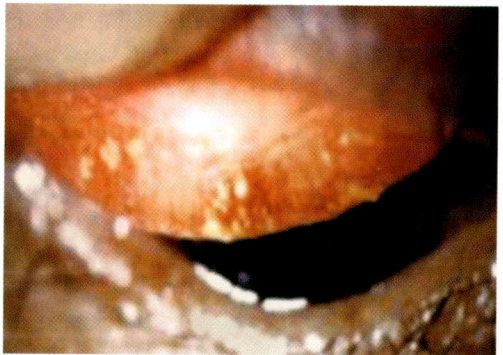

Fig. 20.4: *Concretions in upper palpebral conjunctiva*

Treatment. It consists of their removal with the help of a hypodermic needle under topical anaesthesia.

AMYLOID DEGENERATION OF CONJUNCTIVA

Etiology
Conjunctival amyloid, though rare, is reported to occur in two forms:
• *Primary conjunctival amyloid* is associated with deposition of light-chain immunoglobulin by the monoclonal B cells and plasma cells.
• *Secondary conjunctival amyloid* may occur secondary to systemic diseases or secondary to chronic conjunctival inflammations.

CLINICAL FEATURES
• Deposition of yellowish, well-demarcated, irregular amyloid material in the conjunctiva with superior fornix and tarsal conjunctiva being more commonly involved areas.
• Subconjunctival haemorrhages, recurrent may be associated with amyloid deposition in blood vessels.
• Amyloid involving stain of eyelid may be associated in patients with conjunctival amyloid secondary to systemic diseases.

TREATMENT
• *Lubricating drops* are sufficient for mild symptoms.
• *Excision biopsy* can be performed in patients with marked irritation due to raised lesions. Surgical excision may not cause full regression of the deposited amyloid.
• *Radiotherapy* may be tried in recurrent cases to present progression.

BIBLIOGRAPHY

1. Clearfield E, Muthappan V, Wang X, Kuo IC (2016). "Cojunctival autograft for pterygium". Cochrane Database Syst Rev. 2: CD011349. doi:10.1002/14651858.CD011349.pub2. PMC 5032146. PMID 26867004.
2. Gulani, A; Dastur, YK (January – March 1995). "Simultaneous pterygium and cataract surgery". Journal of Postgraduate Medicine. 41 (1): 8–11.

PMID 10740692.Archived from the original on 8 February 2012. Retrieved 30 November 2012.

3. Mackenzie F.D., Hirst L.W., Battistutta D., Green A. (1992). Risk Analysis in the Development of Pterygia". Ophthalmology. 99 (7): 1056–1061. doi:10.1016/s0161-6420(92)31850-0.

4. Martins, TG; Costa, AL; Alves, MR; Chammas, R; Schor, P (2016). "Mitomycin C in pterygium treatment". International journal of ophthalmology. 9 (3): 465–8. doi:10.18240/ijo.2016.03.25. PMC 4844053. PMID 27158622.

5. Ophthalmology. 1997 Jun;104(6):974-85. Comparison of conjunctival autografts, amniotic membrane grafts, and primary closure for pterygium excision. Prabhasawat P1, Barton K, Burkett G, Tseng S

6. Perkins ES (1985) The association between pinguecula, sunlight, and cataract. Ophthalmic Res 17:325–330

7. Pham TQ, Wang JT, Rochtchina E, Mitchell P (2005) Pterygium/pinguecula and the five-year incidence of age related maculopathy. Am J Ophthalmol 139:536–537

8. Kisling, David (2010-06-26). "Eye Growth & Bumps Often Pinguecula". Retrieved 2018-02-21.

Symptomatic Conditions of Conjunctiva

COMMON SYMPTOMATIC CONDITIONS OF CONJUNCTIVA

INTRODUCTION

Conjunctival lesions are frequently seen in the eye clinic, because the conjunctiva is readily seen and patients notice some change in their ocular appearance. This discussion does not attempt to classify lesions, but only highlights some of the more common lesions that are seen.

Always obtain a full medical and ocular history. In the consulting room the conjunctiva can be examined with a bright light and magnifying glass. Examine what you can see and evert the upper lid to look at the tarsal conjunctiva. Always test the visual acuity, look at the cornea and feel for pre-auricular and submandibular lymph nodes.

Common symptomatic conditions

Common symptomatic conditions of conjunctiva include:
• Hyperaemia of conjunctiva
• Chemosis of conjunctiva
• Ecchymosis of conjunctiva
• Xerosis of conjunctiva
• Discolouration of conjunctiva
• Conjunctival lacerations
• Conjunctival foreign body
• Conjunctival bleb

SIMPLE HYPERAEMIA OF CONJUNCTIVA

Simple hyperaemia of conjunctiva means congestion of the conjunctival vessels due to acute exposure to some minor irritants without being associated with any of the established eye disease. The pattern of hyperaemia often appears with the greatest redness at the fornices and fades moving toward the limbus.

Etiology

It may be acute and transient, or recurrent and chronic.

1. Acute transient hyperaemia. It results due to temporary irritation caused by: (i) *Direct irritants* such as a foreign body, misdirected cilia, concretions, dust, chemical fumes, smoke, stormy wind, bright light, extreme cold, extreme heat and simple rubbing of eyes with hands. (ii) *Reflex hyperaemia* due to eye strain, from inflammations of nasal cavity, lacrimal passages and lids. (iii) *Hyperaemia associated with systemic febrile conditions.* (iv) *Nonspecific inflammation* of conjunctiva.

2. *Recurrent or chronic hyperaemia.* It often occurs due to chronic exposure to irritant as in chronic smokers, chronic alcoholics, people residing in dusty, ill-ventilated rooms, workers exposed to prolonged heat, in patients suffering from rosacea and insomnia or otherwise having less sleep.

Clinical features

- Feeling of discomfort, heaviness, grittiness, tiredness and tightness in the eyes are common complaints of patients with conjunctival hyperaemia.
- Mild lacrimation and minimal mucoid discharge, may occur.
- On cursory examination, the conjunctiva often looks normal. However, eversion of the lids may reveal mild to moderate congestion being more marked in fornices (Fig. 21.1).

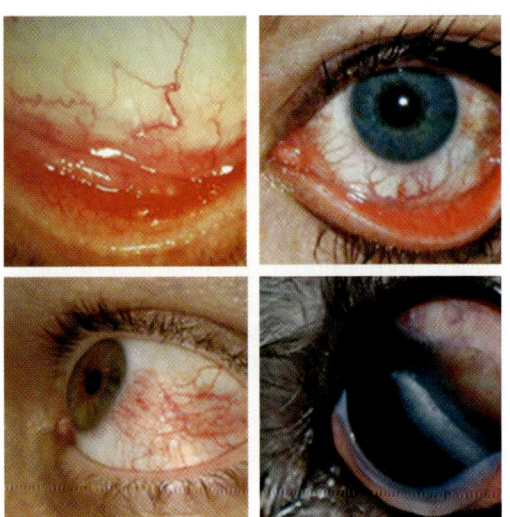

Fig. 21.1: *Hyperaemia of conjunctiva*

Treatment

- *Removal of the cause of hyperaemia,* e.g. in acute transient hyperaemia the removal of irritants (e.g. misdirected cilia) gives prompt relief.
- *Symptomatic relief* may be achieved by use of topical decongestants (e.g. 1:10000 adrenaline drops) or naphazoline drops.

■ CHEMOSIS OF CONJUNCTIVA

Chemosis or oedema of the conjunctiva is of frequent occurrence owing to laxity of the tissue.

The conjunctiva also serves as a defense against potential microbes from entering the eye that may potentially cause harm. When the defenses of the conjunctiva are active, it can become swollen, increasing the production of fluid leakage from abnormally permeable capillaries. This leads to the commonly seen presentation of chemosis, watery eyes (Fig. 21.2).

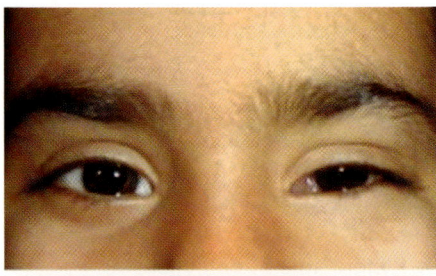

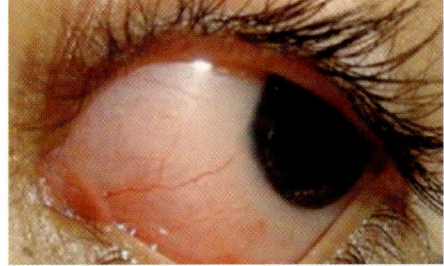

Fig. 21.2: *Chemosis of conjunctiva*

CAUSES

There are a variety of causes of chemosis, with the most usual one being allergies, viral and bacterial infections, and constant rubbing of the eyes themselves. Any factor that can lead to eye irritation can lead to the development of chemosis.

Common causes of chemosis

- ***Allergies:*** Seasonal changes, pet dander, pollen, and virtually anything else you may be allergic to has a high chance of making your eyes water and become itchy.
- ***Infections:*** Commonly caused by bacterial or viral infections leading to a condition called conjunctivitis. While these types of infection can be contagious, leading the eyes to become red, itchy, and watery, the specific symptom of chemosis cannot be transmitted alone. Some other conditions like corneal ulcers, fulminating iridocyclitis, endophthalmitis, panophthalmitis,

styes, acute meibomitis, orbital cellulitis, acute dacryoadenitis, acute dacryocystitis, tendonitis and so on may also lead to chemosis.

• *Eye surgeries:* Performing any type of surgery to the eye or eyelid frequently leads to the development of chemosis. Fortunately, these symptoms usually only last a couple of days with appropriate treatment using eye drops, cold compresses, or temporary eye patching.

• *Hyperthyroidism:* A disorder of the thyroid gland leading to the overproduction of thyroid hormone. This condition can lead to several types of eye problems such as bulging of the eyes, eye puffiness, and retraction of the eyelids.

• *Excessive rubbing:* Constantly touching, rubbing, or scratching the eyes is a common cause of chemosis. Rubbing the eyes is never recommended as this will induce more irritation and possibly even cause eye damage.

• *Systemic causes:* These include severe anaemia and hypoproteinaemia, congestive heart failure, nephrotic syndrome, urticaria, and angioneurotic oedema.

• *Local obstruction to flow of blood and/or lymph:* It may occur in patients with orbital tumours, cysts, endocrine exophthalmos, orbital pseudotumours, cavernous sinus thrombosis, caroticocavernous fistula, blockage of orbital lymphatics following orbital surgery, acute congestive glaucoma, etc.

Less common causes of chemosis

• Orbital cellulitis
• Acute glaucoma
• Obstruction of the superior vena cava
• Cluster headaches
• Urticaria
• Rhabdomyosarcoma of the orbit
• Parasitic infections
• Systemic lupus erythematosus
• Angioedema
• Dacryocystitis
• Carotid cavernous fistula

SYMPTOMS OF CHEMOSIS

Symptoms of chemosis often include:
• Watery eyes
• Excessive tearing
• Eye itchiness
• Double or blurred vision
• Chemosis sufferers may also have trouble closing the affected eye completely due to the swelling.

It is recommended to seek medical attention if one begins to experience eye pain of any kind in combination with watery eyes as it may signal a more severe underlying eye condition.

TREATMENT AND PREVENTION OF CHEMOSIS

Treatment methodologies generally depend on the underlying cause of particular case of chemosis. The following are examples of various treatments

• *Lubricating eye drops:* Help combat dryness and irritation of the eye and is commonly prescribed in case of mild swelling.

• *Cold compress:* Can provide immediate relief to reduce the intensity of chemosis, but only for mild cases.

• *Patching:* Commonly done for patients who have difficulty closing the eye. Patching helps to prevent the eye from becoming excessively irritated and drying out.

• *Corticosteroids:* Commonly given in the form of eyedrops to aid in reducing the eye's inflammatory response and subsequently reduce eye swelling.

• *Anti-inflammatory medication:* Can be topical or oral medication to aid in the reduction of inflammation and pain.

• *Anti-histamines:* A common treatment for allergic reactions to suppress the release of histamine, a substance produced by the body when exposed to allergens.

• *Adrenaline or epinephrine:* Standard emergency treatment for life-threatening anaphylactic reactions. An absolute must in cases where the patient is having difficulty breathing or swallowing.

• *Antibiotics:* May be prescribed for bacterial infections that result in chemosis or post-surgical to reduce the risk of a secondary infection. This may come in the form of medicated eye drops or ointments. Unfortunately, antibiotics are not effective against viruses.

• *Conjunctivoplasty:* A minor surgery that involves performing a small incision into the conjunctiva and the removal of the excess membrane. This may be required in cases of prolonged swelling.

By avoiding potential allergic triggers, one can help reduce the occurrence of chemosis. It is also recommended to maintain a high level of personal hygiene, to limit the sharing of personal items that may come into contact with the eyes, such as towels or cosmetic products. However, it is important to keep in mind that chemosis may not be preventable in some cases.

ECCHYMOSIS OF CONJUNCTIVA

Ecchymosis or subconjunctival haemorrhage is a benign condition and is of very common occurrence. It is characterised by painless acute redness due to bleeding underneath conjunctiva in the absence of discharge or inflammation. It may vary in extent from small petechial haemorrhage to an extensive one spreading under the whole of the bulbar conjunctiva and thus making the white sclera of the eye invisible (Fig. 21.3). The condition though draws the attention of the patients immediately as an emergency but is most of the time trivial.

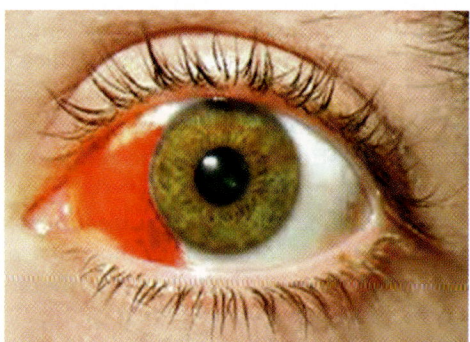

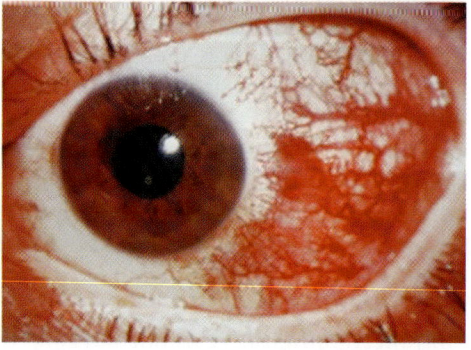

Fig. 21.3: *Subconjunctival haemorrhage*

Whereas a bruise typically appears black or blue underneath the skin, a subconjunctival bleeding initially appears bright-red underneath the transparent conjunctiva. Later, the haemorrhage may spread and become green or yellow, like a bruise. Usually this disappears within 2 weeks.

The vision is usually unaffected by the haemorrhage. An extensive subconjunctival haemorrhage may track into the eyelids.

Recurrent or persistent subconjunctival haemorrhage needs to be investigated for systemic hypertension, ocular or systemic malignancies, bleeding disorders and any side effects of drugs.

Etiology

Subconjunctival haemorrhage may be associated with the following conditions:

1. *Trauma.* It is the most common cause of subconjunctival haemorrhage. It may be in the form of (i) local trauma to the conjunctiva including that due to surgery and subconjunctival injections, (ii) retrobulbar haemorrhage which almost immediately spreads below the bulbar conjunctiva. Mostly, it results from a retrobulbar injection and from trauma involving various walls of the orbit.

2. *Inflammations of the conjunctiva.* Petechial subconjunctival haemorrhages are usually associated with acute haemorrhagic conjunctivitis caused by picornaviruses, pneumococcal conjunctivitis and leptospirosis, icterohaemorrhagica conjunctivitis.

3. *Sudden venous congestion of head.* The subconjunctival haemorrhages may occur owing to rupture of conjunctival capillaries due to sudden rise in pressure. Common conditions are whooping cough, epileptic fits, strangulation or compression of jugular veins and violent compression of thorax and abdomen as seen in crush injuries.

4. *Spontaneous rupture of fragile capillaries* may occur in vascular diseases such as arteriosclerosis, hypertension and diabetes mellitus.

5. *Local vascular anomalies* like telangiectasia, varicosities, aneurysm or angiomatous tumour.

6. *Blood dyscrasias* like anaemias, leukaemias and dysproteinaemias.

7. Bleeding disorders like purpura, haemophilia and scurvy.

8. Acute febrile systemic infections such as malaria, typhoid, diphtheria, meningococcal septicaemia, measles and scarlet fever.

9. Vicarious bleeding associated with menstruation is an extremely rare cause of subconjunctival haemorrhage.

Clinical features

Symptoms. Subconjunctival haemorrhage per se is symptomless. Except for red discolouration noted by patients as a serious symptom. However, there may be symptoms of associated causative disease.

Signs. On examination, subconjunctival haemorrhage looks as a flat sheet of homogeneous bright red colour with well-defined limits (Fig. 21.3).

Natural course. In traumatic subconjunctival haemorrhage, posterior limit is visible when it is due to local trauma to eyeball, and not visible when it is due to head injury or injury to the orbit. Most of the time it is absorbed completely within 7 to 21 days. During absorption, colour changes are noted from bright red to orange and then yellow. In severe cases, some pigmentation may be left behind after absorption.

Treatment

- *Treat the cause* when discovered.
- *Cold compresses* to check the bleeding in the initial stage and hot compresses may help in absorption of blood in late stages.
- *Placebo therapy* with astringent and lubricant eye drops.
- *Psychotherapy and assurance* to the patient is most important part of treatment.

◼ XEROSIS OF CONJUNCTIVA

Xerosis of the conjunctiva is a symptomatic condition in which conjunctiva becomes dry and lustreless (Fig. 21.4). Normal conjunctiva is kept moist by its own secretions, mucin from goblet cells and aqueous solution from accessory lacrimal glands. Therefore, even if the main lacrimal gland is removed, xerosis does not occur.

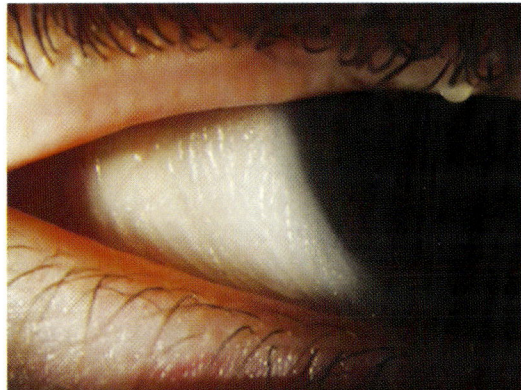
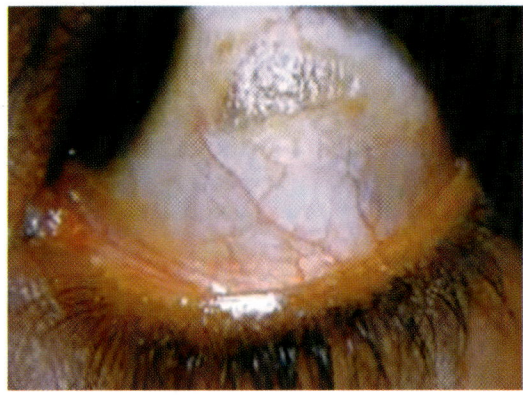

Fig. 21.4: *Xerosis of conjunctiva*

Etiology

Depending upon the aetiology, conjunctival xerosis can be divided into two groups, parenchymatous and epithelial xerosis.

1. Parenchymatous xerosis. It occurs following cicatricial disorganization of the conjunctiva due to local causes which can be in the form of:

- *Destructive interstitial conjunctivitis* as seen in trachoma, diphtheric membranous conjunctivitis, Stevens-Johnson syndrome, pemphigus or pemphigoid conjunctivitis, thermal, chemical or radiational burns of conjunctiva.
- *Exposure of conjunctiva to air* as seen in marked degree of proptosis, facial palsy, ectropion, lack of blinking (as in coma), and lagophthalmos due to symblepharon.

2. Epithelial xerosis. It occurs due to *hypovitaminosis A*. Epithelial xerosis may be seen in association with night blindness or as a part and parcel of the xerophthalmia (the term which is applied to all ocular manifestations of vitamin

A deficiency) which range from night blindness to keratomalacia (*see* page 301).

Clinical features

Parenchymatous xerosis is characterised by marked dryness, thickening, scarring and even keratinization associated with features and complication of the causative disease.

Epithelial xerosis typically occurs in children and is characterised by varying degree of conjunctival dryness, thickening, wrinkling and pigmentation.

Treatment

Treatment of conjunctival xerosis consists of:
- *Treatment of the cause,* and their complications
- *Symptomatic local treatment* with artificial tear preparations (0.7% methylcellulose or 0.3% hypromellose or polyvinyl alcohol), which should be instilled frequently.

■ DISCOLOURATION OF CONJUNCTIVA

Normal conjunctiva is a thin transparent structure. In the bulbar region, underlying sclera and a fine network of episcleral and conjunctival vessels can be easily visualised. In the palpebral region and fornices, it looks pinkish because of underlying fibrovascular tissue.

Causes

Conjunctiva may show discolouration in various local and systemic diseases given below:

1. ***Red discolouration***. A bright red homogeneous discolouration suggests subconjunctival haemorrhage (*see* Fig. 21.3).

2. ***Yellow discolouration***. It may occur due to: (i) Bile pigments in jaundice, (ii) blood pigments in malaria and yellow fever, (iii) conjunctival fat in elder and Negro patients.

3. ***Greyish discolouration***. It may occur due to application of kajal (surma or soot) and mascara in females.

4. ***Brownish grey discolouration***. It is typically seen in argyrosis, following prolonged application of silver nitrate for treatment of chronic conjunctival inflammations. The discolouration is most marked in lower fornix.

5. ***Blue discolouration***. It is usually due to ink tattoo from pens or effects of manganese dust.

Blue discolouration may also be due to pseudopigmentation as occurs in patients with blue sclera and scleromalacia perforans.

6. ***Brown pigmentation***. Its common causes can be grouped as under:

a. *Non-melanocytic pigmentation*
   i. *Endogenous pigmentation*. It is seen in patients with Addison's disease and ochronosis.
   ii. *Exogenous pigmentation*. It may follow long-term use of adrenaline for glaucoma. Argyrosis may also present as dark brown pigmentation.

b. *Melanocytic pigmentation*
   i. *Conjunctival epithelial melanosis* (Fig. 21.5). It develops in early childhood, and then remains stationary. It is found in 90% of the blacks. The pigmented spot freely moves with the movement of conjunctiva. It has got no malignant potential and hence no treatment is required.

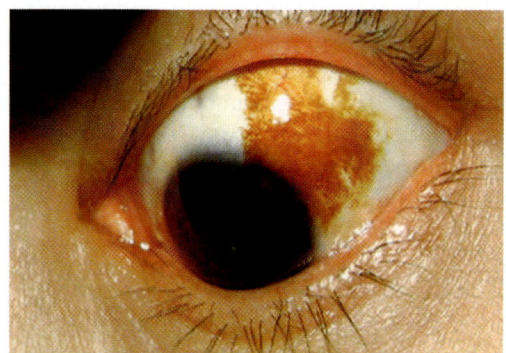

Fig. 21.5: *Conjunctival epithelial melanosis*

   ii. *Subepithelial melanosis*. It may occur as an isolated anomaly of conjunctiva (congenital melanosis oculi, Fig. 21.6) or in association with the ipsilateral hyperpigmentation of the face (oculodermal melanosis or naevus of Ota).
   iii. *Pigmented tumours*. These can be benign naevi, precancerous melanosis or malignant melanoma (refer to melanocytic tumours of conjunctiva).

■ CONJUNCTIVAL LACERATIONS

Due to its exposed position, thinness, and mobility, the conjunctiva is susceptible to lacerations,

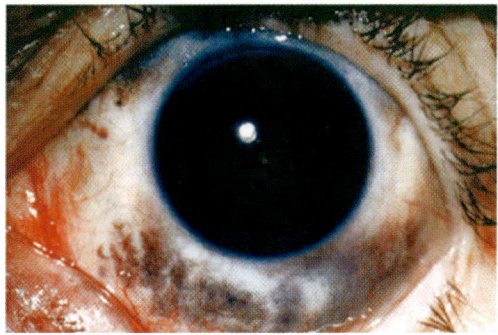

Fig. 21.6: *Congenital melanosis oculi*

which are usually associated with sub-conjunctival haemorrhage.

Etiology

Conjunctival lacerations most commonly occur as a result of penetrating wounds (such as from bending over a spiked-leaf palm tree or from a branch that snaps back onto the eye).

Clinical features

The patient experiences a foreign body sensation. Usually this will be rather mild. Examination will reveal circumscribed conjunctival reddening or subconjunctival haemorrhage in the injured area (Fig. 21.7). Chemosis may also be present. Occasionally only application of fluorescein dye to the injury will reveal the size of the conjunctival gap.

In such cases, it is important to rule out underlying scleral perforation. The fundus should be examined for any retinal tear or intraocular foreign body. An ultrasound may be done for the posterior segment evaluation.

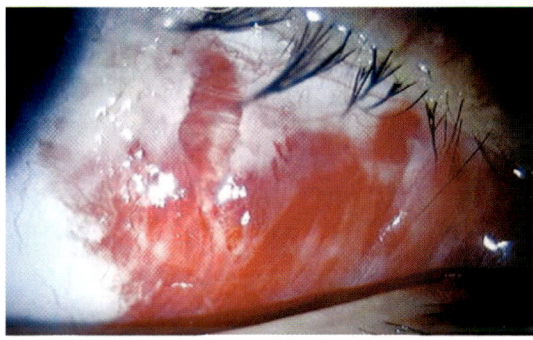

Fig. 21.7: *Conjunctival laceration with subconjunctival haemorrhage*

Seidel test should be done to rule out open globe injury and CT scan to rule out intraocular foreign body.

Treatment

Such cases are managed with observation and topical antibiotics in mild cases and in large lacerations, surgical repair may be needed using 8–0 vicryl suture.

■ CONJUNCTIVAL FOREIGN BODY

Foreign bodies can lodge in the inferior cul-de-sac or can be located on the conjunctival surface under the upper eyelid (Fig. 21.8). The most common foreign bodies in the conjunctiva include the following:
• Dust
• Dirt
• Contact lenses
• Sand
• Cosmetics

Clinical features

Symptoms include ocular irritation, pain, foreign body sensation, tearing or red eye.

Examination

It is imperative to evert the upper eyelid to examine the superior tarsal plate and eyelid margin in all patients with a history that suggests a foreign body. If several foreign bodies are suspected or particulate matter is present, double eversion of the eyelid with a Desmarres retractor or a bent paperclip is advised to allow the examiner to effectively search the entire arc of the superior cul-de-sac. Foreign bodies on the conjunctival surface are best recognized with slit-lamp examination.

Following eversion of the upper eyelid, copious irrigation should be used to cleanse the fornix. This procedure should then be repeated using a Desmarres retractor for the upper and lower eyelids. Glass particles, cactus spines, and insect hairs are often difficult to see, but a careful search of the cul-de-sac with high magnification aids in identification and removal. With slit-lamp magnification, the clinician can gently use a moistened cotton-tipped applicator to remove superficial foreign material. Occasionally, saline

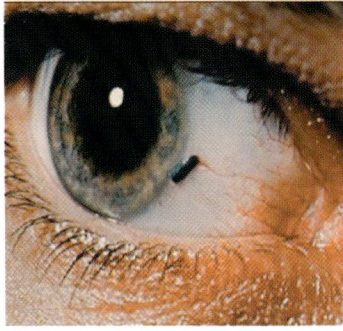 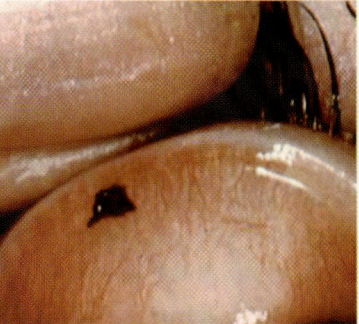 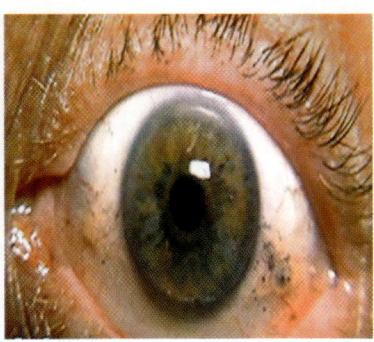

Fig. 21.8: *Conjunctival foreign bodies*

lavage of the cornea or cul-de-sac washes out debris that is not embedded in tissue.

When a patient complains of foreign body sensation, topical fluorescein should be instilled to check for the fine, linear, vertical corneal abrasions that are characteristic of retained foreign bodies on the eyelid margin or superior tarsal plate. Foreign matter embedded in tissue is removed with a sterile, disposable hypodermic needle. Glass or particulate matter may be removed with a fine-tipped jeweler's forceps or blunt spatula. If a foreign body is suspected but not seen, the cul-de-sac should be irrigated and wiped with a moistened cotton-tipped applicator.

Treatment

- Careful examination of the entire eye is mandatory to rule out intraocular foreign bodies including a thorough slit lamp and dilated retinal examination.
- B scan ultrasonography, X ray film or CT scanning is sometimes indicated to rule out intraocular foreign body.
- MRI is contraindicated, since intraocular foreign body may be metallic.
- Multiple small fragments or debris can be removed with saline irrigation.
- Localized/embedded foreign body can be removed under topical anaesthesia at the slit lamp using cotton-tipped applicator or forceps.
- Short course of topical antibiotic after foreign body removal may be given to prevent secondary infection.

CONJUNCTIVAL BLEB

A conjunctival bleb is formed when there is a direct connection of the aqueous in the anterior chamber to the subconjunctival space (Fig. 21.9). This bleb can be formed deliberately, e.g. in glaucoma surgery or after corneoscleral laceration repair. Ask the patient about any ocular trauma or surgery. It is extremely important never to try to puncture or deflate these cysts as it may lead to hypotonia of the eye or even endophthalmitis.

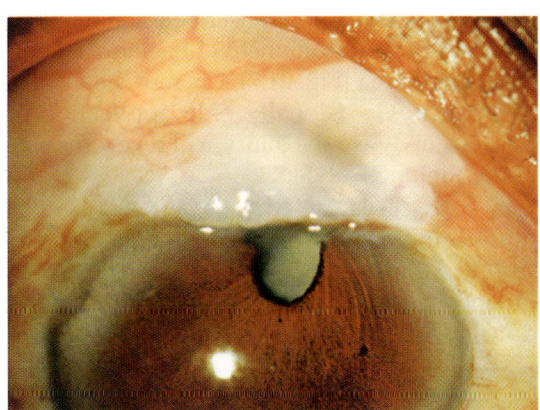

Fig. 21.9: *Conjunctival bleb after trauma*

BIBLIOGRAPHY

1. Basic and Clinical Science Course, American Academy of Ophthalmology, Section 8. External Disease and Cornea, 2009–2010. San Francisco, CA: American Academy of Ophthalmolgy, 2010.
2. Cronau H, Kankanala RR, Mauger T. Diagnosis and management of red eye in primary care. Am Fam Physician 2010; 81(2): 137–44.

3. Ehlers J, Shah C. The Wills Eye Manual. Office and Emergency Room Diagnosis and Treatment of Eye Disease. 5th ed. Philadelphia: Lippincott, Williams and Wilkins, 2008.

4. Kanski JJ, Bowling B. Clinical Ophthalmology. A Systematic Approach. 7th ed. Philadelphia: Elsevier, 2007.

5. Mahmood AR, Narang AT. Diagnosis and management of the acute red eye. Emerg Med Clin North Am 2008; 26(1): 35–55.

6. O'Brien TP, Jeng BH, McDonald M, Raizman MB. Acute conjunctivitis: truth and misconceptions. Curr Med Res Opin 2009; 25(8): 1953–61.

7. Rietveld RP, van Weert HC, ter Riet G, Bindels PJ. Diagnostic impact of signs and symptoms in acute infectious conjunctivitis: systematic literature research. BMJ 2003; 327(7418): 789.

8. Yannof J, Duker JS, editors. Ophthalmology. 2nd ed, Mosby; Spain: 2004. Disorders of the conjunctiva and limbus 2004; 397–412.

Cysts and Tumours of Conjunctiva

CYSTS OF CONJUNCTIVA

Conjunctival cysts are mostly thin walled and slowly progressive. They are fluid-filled sacs, but can sometimes look more like a solid mass. These lesions are most common during first three decades of life. They are usually symptomless but can cause cosmetic disfigurement, reduced motility, foreign body sensation, dry eye due to unstable tear film and proptosis when they increase in size.

CLASSIFICATION

- Congenital cystic lesions
  - Congenital corneoscleral cysts
  - Cystic epibulbar dermoid
- Epithelial implantation cysts
- Epithelial cysts due to downgrowth of epithelium

- Lymphatic cysts
  - Lymphangiectasia
  - Lymphangioma
- Retention cysts
- Aqueous cysts
- Parasitic cysts
  - Hydatid cyst
  - Cysticercus
  - Filarial cyst
- Pigmented epithelial cysts: Prolonged topical use of cocaine/epinephrine.

CONGENITAL CYSTIC LESIONS

These are of rare occurrence and include congenital corneoscleral cyst and cystic form of epibulbar dermoid.

Conjunctival dermoids (Fig. 22.1) are usually noticed in adulthood, are located nasally or

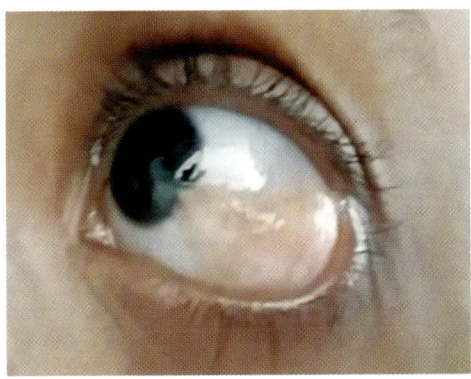

Fig. 22.1: *Conjunctival dermoid*

superonasally, lack an associated osseous defect and are lined by a non-keratinizing epithelium with goblet cells. The cut surface of the cyst contains cheesy material and hair shafts, sweat and sebaceous glands. The lumen contains granular keratin material.

EPITHELIAL CYSTS

Epithelial implantation cysts

Implantation cysts are benign cysts filled with clear serous fluid containing shed cells or gelatinous mucous material. Cyst wall consists of several layers of non-keratinised lining epithelium and connective tissue. The implantation cysts are the commonest cystic lesions of conjunctiva, 80% of the entire cystic lesions of

conjunctiva being implantation cysts. These can be primary and secondary.

Primary implantation cyst

Pathogenesis of primary implantation cyst is due to excessive invagination of the caruncular epithelium or the fornix during embryonic development.

Age of presentation of these cysts range from birth to 70 years.

Typically located. These are in the superonasal part of the orbit and less commonly temporally (Fig. 22.2).

Typical clinical features. These consist of painless cystic masses of small to moderate size having thin walls and low pressure which generally do not induce significant mechanical alterations, however they can rarely erode adjacent bony structures and cause visual symptoms.

Secondary implantation cysts

Secondary implantation cysts are more common, they occur either naturally or under inflammatory conditions of the conjunctiva. In most cases these developed by detachment of a portion of conjunctival epithelium by surgery or trauma and even subtenon anaesthesia. Following implantation into the conjunctival epithelium, conjunctiva is especially vulnerable

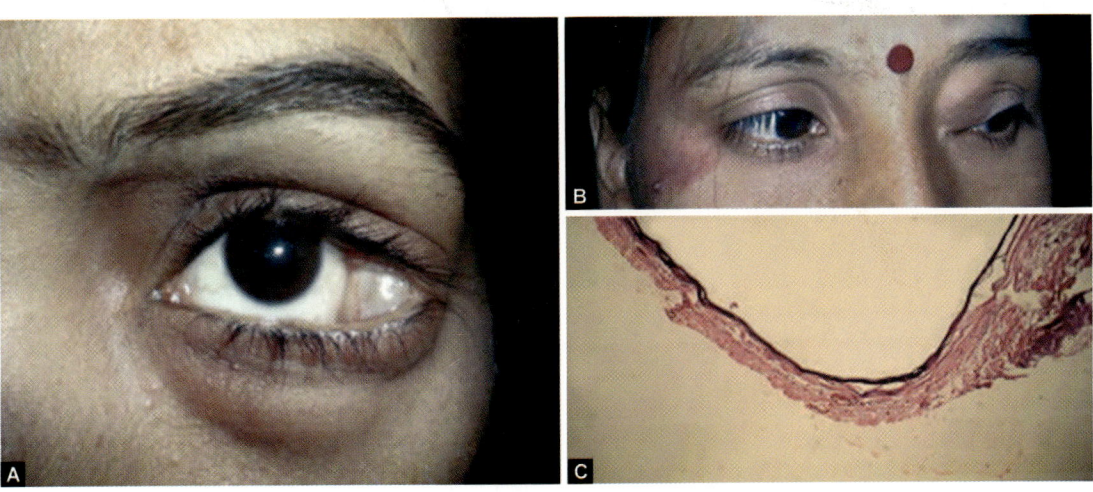

Fig. 22.2: *Primary conjunctival cyst. A, On temporal side; B, On nasal side; and C, Histopathology—cyst lined with single layer of stratified squamous epithelium containing amorphous material*

to injuries because of its presence on our outer eye. Any type of blow to the eye or vigrous rubbing can cause a conjunctival cyst to develop. Epithelial inclusion cysts occupy the major bulk.

In normal conjunctiva a mild degree of trauma may not lead to embedding of conjunctival epithelium into the deeper tissues. However, once there is conjunctival inflammation, the epithelium becomes loose and the deeper tissues get oedematous and even with mildest trauma the epithelial cells may get exfoliated and buried into the deeper tissues where mild fibrosis, shallowing of fornices and adhesions may progress slowly. Proliferation of these cells results in the formation of cysts. Hence, simultaneous occurrence of inflammation and trauma may contribute to its genesis.

Implantation cysts following small incision cataract surgery have also been reported (Fig. 22.3). This complication occurs due to implan-

tation of conjunctival tissue during construction of tunnel or dragging of conjunctiva during IOL implantation. Chief differential diagnosis is the filtering bleb. This can be prevented by careful reflection of the conjunctiva during surgery. Inclusion cysts have also been reported in conditions of chronic inflammation like VKC.

Epithelial cysts due to downgrowth of epithelium

These are rarely seen in chronic inflammatory or degenerative conditions, e.g. cystic change in pterygium.

In such cases cyst may commonly be located at the head of the pterygium or embedded in the body (Fig. 22.4). There is no adherence of the cyst to the underlying structures. These cases are managed by excision of the cyst along with the reverse peeling of pterygium. Histopathology shows pterygium with stratified squamous epithelium lining with cystic changes, mild chronic inflammatory reaction can be seen around the cyst.

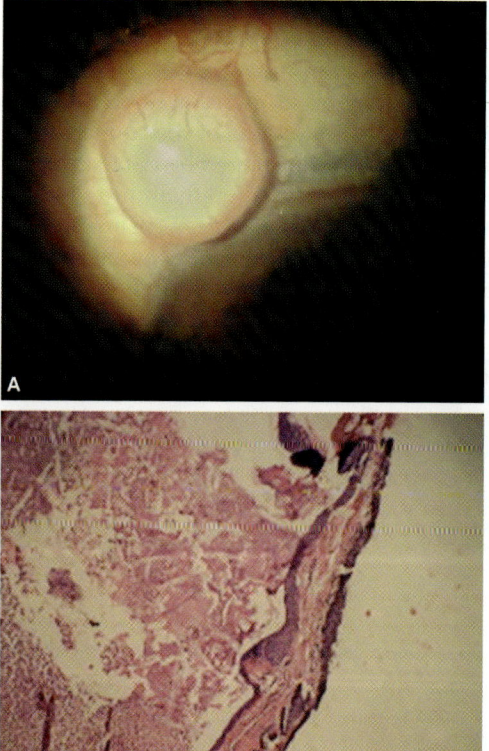

Fig. 22.3: Post-SICS cyst. A, Clinical photograph; B, HPE: Cyst lined by stratified squamous epithelium filled with amorphous material inside

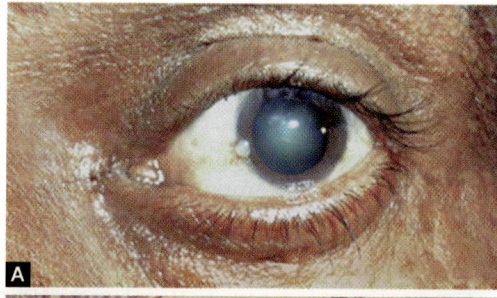

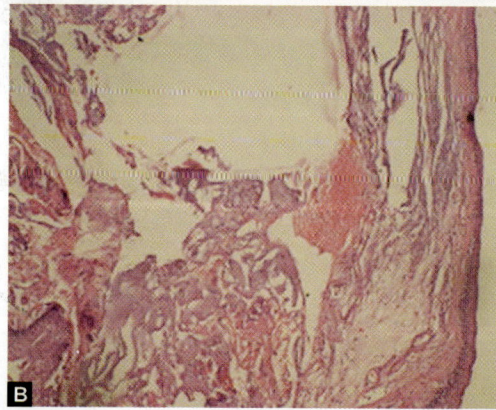

Fig. 22.4: Cystic change in pterygium. A, Clinical photograph with cyst; B, HPE: Pterygium with stratified squamous epithelium with cystic changes and mild chronic inflammatory reaction around the cyst

LYMPHATIC CYSTS

These are common and present under the bulbar conjunctiva and upper fornix (Fig. 22.5). Usually occur due to dilatation of lymph spaces in the bulbar conjunctiva. They are transparent, multilocular and filled with clear fluid. Rarely the cyst can be pedunculated. Histopathological examination shows dilated lymphatic spaces lined with endothelium. The dilated lymphatics which cannot be emptied are considered to develop into lymphatic cysts.

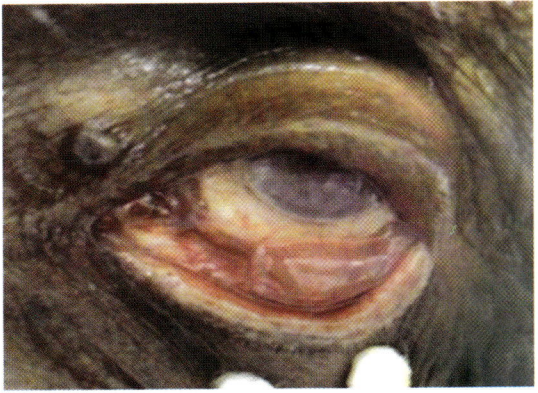

Fig. 22.5: *Lymphatic cyst*

Lymphangiectasis is characterized by a row of small cysts. They can present either as cystic lesions of the conjunctiva which mimic allergic chemosis or as beaded dilatation of lymphatic vessels with a string of pearl appearance. Treatment modalities for conjunctival lymphangiectasia are surgical resection, marsupialization and obliteration of abnormal lymphatics by liquid nitrogen cryotherapy. Rarely, lymphangioma may occur as a single multilocular cyst.

RETENTION CYSTS

These occur occasionally due to blockage of ducts of accessory lacrimal glands of Krause in chronic inflammatory conditions, viz. trachoma and pemphigus. Retention cysts are more common in upper fornix.

AQUEOUS CYST

It may be due to healing by cystoid cicatrix formation, following surgical or non-surgical perforating limbal wounds.

PARASITIC CYSTS

Parasitic cysts such as subconjunctival cysticercosis, hydatid cyst and filarial cyst are not infrequent in developing countries.

Conjunctival cysticercosis

Parasitic conjunctival cysts due to cysticercus appear to be most common. The size of the parasitic cysts may vary and their shape may be circular or oval. These look whitish with a chalky white spot in the cavity representing the scolex of the parasite (Fig. 22.6A). Histopathological examination of these cysts showed the body canal of cysticercus cellulosae lined by the epithelium (Fig. 22.6C). The left eye seems to be involved more with a predisposition to nasal side. This may be explained on the basis of anatomical reasons, i.e. the course of ophthalmic artery.

At times, the cyst may prolapse from the subconjunctival tissue. No obvious cause for the spontaneous expulsions could be elicited. However, mechanical stretching due to the presence of the cyst and weak conjunctiva (due to associated inflammation) could possibly explain the spontaneous expulsion.

Hydatid cyst

Hydatid cysts mostly occur in young people between 10 and 30 years. They most frequently present as exophthalmos, chemosis, lid oedema, visual impairment and restriction of extraocular movement. Sudden exacerbation of pain, increase in proptosis, and local inflammatory reaction in eye is an important diagnostic clue to the hydatid cyst. Definitive treatment is surgical excision.

PIGMENTED EPITHELIAL CYST

It may be formed sometimes following prolonged topical use of cocaine or epinephrine. Histopathological examination reveals the presence of aggregates of melanocytes under epithelium with a tendency to form adenomatous arrangement.

■ TREATMENT OF CONJUNCTIVAL CYSTS

Conjunctival cysts do not always require treatment, especially if they are small and are not

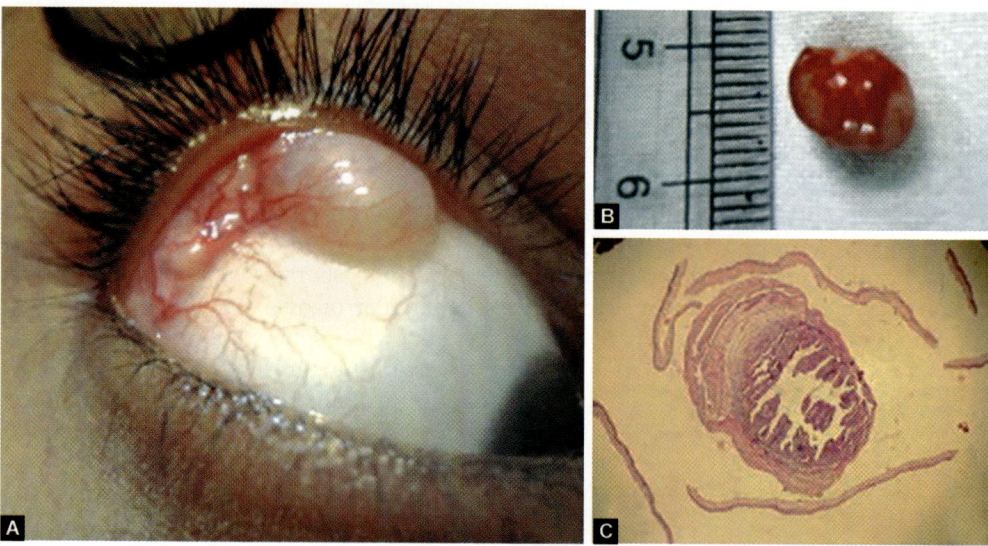

Fig. 22.6: *Conjunctival cysticercosis cyst: A, Clinical photograph; B, Excised cysticercosis cyst; C, HPE: Cyst with embedded parasite, with chronic inflammatory cell infiltrate with lymphocytes, eosinophils and giant cells in the cyst wall*

causing any symptoms. In some cases, they go away on their own over time.

Conservative treatment in the form of lubricating eye drops may help with any dryness or discomfort. Steroid eye drops can also help to reduce inflammation and prevent the cyst from getting bigger. This is especially helpful if the cyst is due to an allergic reaction to something.

Surgical excision is required in cases of large and symptomatic conjunctival cysts. As the cysts are thin walled, rupture is common during excision. Recurrence is the main postoperative concern. B scan USG and MRI of cyst can be done whenever required to see the posterior extent. Careful and intact removal of conjunctival cyst is important to prevent recurrence. Minor modifications in surgical technique according to the size, site and nature of cyst help in intact removal and prevent recurrence. The excised cyst should always be subjected to histopathological examination.

OCULAR SURFACE TUMOURS

Ocular surface tumours are rare but potentially deadly diseases of the conjunctiva and/or cornea. These tumours are grouped into two major categories of congenital and acquired lesions. The acquired lesions are further subdivided based on origin of the mass into surface epithelial, mucoepidermoid, melanocytic, vascular, fibrous, neural, histiocytic, myxoid, myogenic, lipomatous, lymphoid, leukaemic, metastatic and secondary tumours. It is important for ophthalmologists to recognise the characteristics of ocular surface tumours and to have an understanding of their management. Some common ocular surface tumours are described in this chapter.

Classification of ocular surface tumours

Primary tumours

Epithelial tumours
- Nonmelanocytic
- Melanocytic

Stromal tumours
- Vascular
- Fibrous
- Neural
- Histiocytic
- Myogenic
- Lipomatous
- Lymphoproliferative
- Choristoma

Caruncular tumours

Metastasis and secondary tumours

PRIMARY TUMOURS

EPITHELIAL TUMOURS

CONJUNCTIVAL NONMELANOCYTIC EPITHELIAL TUMOURS

CLASSIFICATION

A simplified classification of conjunctival nonmelanocytic tumours is given in Table 22.1.

CONJUNCTIVAL BENIGN NONMELANOCYTIC EPITHELIAL TUMOURS

1. Conjunctival papilloma

Etiology

Conjunctival papillomas occur in both children and adults with variable presentation.

In children, it results from infection of the conjunctival epithelium with human papillomavirus (HPV) 6, 11 or 16.

In adults, clinically, it may resemble squamous cell carcinoma (SCC). It may be associated with HPV infection and immunocompromised status.

Prevalence

Prevalence of conjunctival papillomas ranges from 4 to 12%.

Types of conjunctival papilloma

Conjunctival papillomas are categorized based on appearance, location, patient's age, propensity to recur after excision, and histopathology into:

- Squamous cell papilloma (infectious papilloma),
- Limbal papilloma, and
- Inverted papilloma.

They demonstrate an exophytic growth pattern. Interestingly, inverted papillomas exhibit exophytic and endophytic growth patterns.

Conjunctival papilloma also can be classified based on gross clinical appearance, as either pedunculated or sessile.

- *Pedunculated type* is synonymous with infectious conjunctival papilloma and squamous cell papilloma.
- *Sessile papilloma.* The limbal conjunctival papilloma often is referred to as noninfectious conjunctival papilloma because it is believed that limbal papillomas arise from UV radiation exposure. Because of its gross appearance, limbal papillomas are typed as sessile.

Clinical features

Squamous cell papilloma (infectious papilloma)

- This lesion is benign and self-limiting.
- It is seen commonly in children and young adults.
- Most lesions are asymptomatic without associated conjunctivitis or folliculitis.

Table 22.1: *A simplified classification of conjunctival nonmelanocytic tumour*		
	Child	*Adult*
Benign	• Conjunctival papilloma • Conjunctival hereditary benign intraepithelial dyskeratosis	• Conjunctival papilloma • Papilloma of caruncle • Conjunctival pseudoepitheliomatous hyperplasia • Keratoacanthoma • Conjunctival hereditary benign intraepithelial dyskeratosis • Conjunctival dacryoadenoma • Epithelial inclusion cyst
Premalignant	• Conjunctival intraepithelial neoplasia	• Conjunctival keratotic plaque • Actinic keratosis • Conjunctival intraepithelial neoplasia
Malignant	• Conjunctival invasive squamous cell carcinoma	• Conjunctival invasive squamous cell carcinoma • Mucoepidermoid carcinoma • Spindle cells carcinoma

- Anatomically, it is commonly located in the inferior fornix, but it also may arise in the limbus, caruncle, and palpebral regions.
- The lesion may be bilateral and multiple. It becomes confluent in extreme cases to form massive papillomatosis.
- Grossly, squamous cell papilloma appears as a greyish red, fleshy, soft, pedunculated mass with an irregular surface (cauliflower-like) (Fig. 22.7A).

Limbal papilloma

Characteristic features of limbal papilloma are (Fig. 22.7B):
- This lesion is typically benign.
- It is seen commonly in older adults.
- Anatomically, the lesion commonly occurs at the limbus or the bulbar conjunctiva.
- These lesions may spread centrally toward the cornea or laterally toward the conjunctiva.
- Visual acuity may be affected if the lesion grows centrally.
- These lesions almost always are unilateral and single.
- It has a lighter pink colour than the childhood variety.
- They tend to have variable proliferation potential with a tendency to slowly enlarge in size.

Inverted conjunctival papilloma

- This lesion (Fig. 22.7C) is slow growing and is seen commonly in the nose, paranasal sinuses, or both. The lacrimal sac and the conjunctiva are uncommon sites.

- The papilloma may invaginate inward into the underlying conjunctiva and substantia propria to present as a mixed inverted exophytic papilloma.
- Rarely, it appears as solid or cystic solitary nodule at the limbus, plica semilunaris, and tarsal conjunctiva.
- The lesion is unilateral and unifocal and does not recur after surgical excision.

Histopathology

Squamous cell papillomas (e.g. infectious papilloma, viral conjunctival papilloma) are composed of multiple branching fronds emanating from a narrow pedunculated base. Individual fronds are surrounded by connective tissue, each having a central vascularized core. Acute and chronic inflammatory cells are found within these fronds. The epithelium is acanthotic, nonkeratinized stratified squamous epithelium without atypia. Numerous goblet cells are seen along with acute inflammatory cells. Koilocytosis is exhibited. The basement membrane is intact (Fig. 22.8).

Squamous papilloma is reported to have low malignant potential. Occasionally, as a variant, it can assume an inverted growth pattern, which has a greater tendency towards malignant transformation into transitional cell carcinoma, SCC, or mucoepidermoid carcinoma.

Limbal papillomas are sessile lesions arising from a broad base with a gelatinous appearance. Corkscrew vascular loops and feeder vessels are seen. The epithelium is acanthotic, displaying

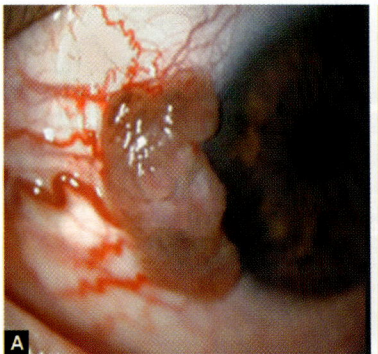 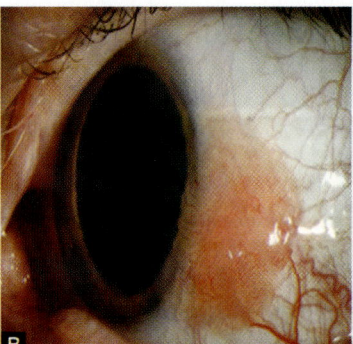 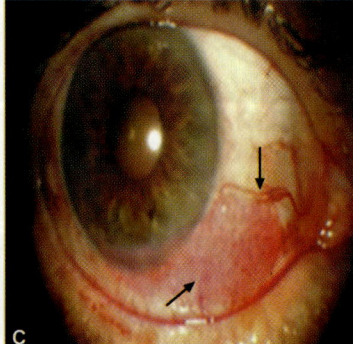

Fig. 22.7: *Conjunctival papilloma. A, Squamous papilloma; B, Limbal papilloma; C, Inverted papilloma*

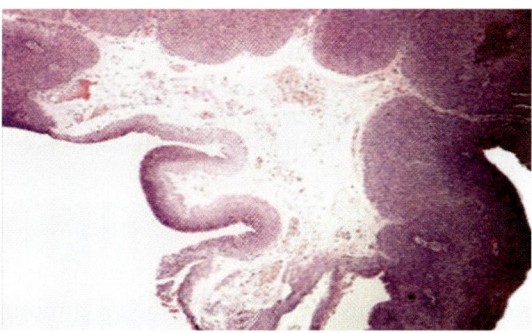

Fig. 22.8: *Microphotograph of squamous papilloma. The lesion shows numerous vascularized papillary fronds lined by acanthotic epithelium*

varying degrees of pleomorphism and dysplasia. The epithelium surface may be keratinized with foci of parakeratosis within the papillary folds. The basement membrane is intact.

Inverted papillomas exhibit exophytic and endophytic growth patterns. Those arising from the conjunctiva tend to be less aggressive in malignant transformation, than those present in nose and paranasal sinuses. The lesions are composed of lobules of epithelial cells extending down into the stroma. The lesion may be elevated or umbilicated. Epithelial cells do not demonstrate atypia, and dysplastic changes are uncommon for conjunctival inverted papillomas. The cytoplasm is vacuolated in some cells. They may resemble squamous papilloma or pyogenic granuloma. Numerous goblet cells are intermixed with the epithelium. Cystic lesions may be seen secondary to the confluence of goblet cells. The lesion may contain melanin granules and/or melanocytes.

Differential diagnosis

- Ichthyosis
- Sebaceous gland carcinoma
- Conjunctival squamous cell carcinoma

Treatment

Observation and patient reassurance are indicated for squamous cell papillomas. These lesions may regress spontaneously over time. Seeding may follow excision, resulting in multiple new lesions.

Surgical excision by the "no-touch technique" followed by cryotherapy is the treatment of choice. For limbal papillomas, excision is indicated to rule out neoplastic changes.

Other reported treatment modalities include:
- Laser
- Dinitrochlorobenzene immunotherapy
- Interferon alpha 2b (IFN-α-2b)
- Topical mitomycin C (MMC) drops
- Recent reports show significant role of oral cimetidine in treating recalcitrant and recurrent conjunctival papillomatosis. It enhances the immune system by inhibiting certain T-cell functions.

2. Papilloma of caruncle

Santos-Gómez Leal et al reported in their series that this lesion has a prevalence of 25.66% of the tumours of the caruncle, with a mean age of 27 years (3–65 years old). It was more common in women 1.2:1. The characteristics are the same of the papilloma of conjunctiva in adults, with the same treatment.

3. Conjunctival pseudoepitheliomatous hyperplasia

Etiology

Pseudoepitheliomatous hyperplasia (PEH) is a benign reactive inflammatory proliferation of the epithelial cells, which simulates carcinoma clinically and histopathologically. It occurs as a conjunctival lesion secondary to irritation by concurrent or preexisting stromal inflammation such as pterygium, pinguecula, allergic conjunctivitis, and foreign body. It can be a result of various conditions such as infections, inflammation, trauma, and malignancy and is also referred to as pseudocarcinomatous hyperplasia.

Clinical features

It appears as an elevated leukoplakic pink lesion in the limbal area. Usually, PEH appears as a well-demarcated plaque or nodule with scaling and crusting. Papules or nodules may range from <1 cm to several centimetres in size. The colour of the lesion may be as that of the mucosa or pigmented as in case of melanoma (Fig. 22.9A).

Histopathology

Histopathologically, it is characterised by massive acanthosis, hyperkeratosis, and parakeratosis of the conjunctival epithelium (Fig. 22.9B).

Differential diagnosis

The differential diagnosis of PEH is SCC, keratoacanthoma, granular cell tumour, necrotizing sialometaplasia, malignant melanoma, and verrucous carcinoma. The presence of a nodular lesion with feeder vessels and intrinsic vascularity should raise a suspicion of invasive SCC and hence, the word "diagnostic dilemma" is one of the most appropriate words for this lesion.

Treatment

- *Complete excision and additional cryotherapy* would constitute optimal management, as difficulty prevails in clinically and histologically differentiating the lesion from low-grade SCC.
- *Use of photodynamic therapy and microdebrider shaver* in its treatment has also been reported.

4. Keratoacanthoma

Etiology

Keratoacanthoma, a benign epithelial tumour that grows rapidly and shows spontaneous regression, has a characteristic central crater filled with keratin. Keratoacanthomas arise most commonly in sun-exposed skin and only rarely in mucosa. The few reported cases of conjunctival keratoacanthoma have occurred mostly in whites. It is a variant of conjunctival pseudoepitheliomatous hyperplasia. Though it is a benign lesion, some believe that it may represent an abortive malignancy that rarely progresses to SCC.

Clinical features

Appearance of keratoacanthoma is that of a nodule with rounded edges and a central keratin filled crater in its mature form approximately 1–2 cm in diameter in size.

Presenting symptoms include a sudden onset of conjunctival injection or irritation or a rapidly enlarging mass.

Onset as well as the progression is rapid (Fig. 22.10A).

Histopathology

It shows a central crater containing a keratotic plug surrounded by acanthotic conjunctival epithelium that includes horn pearls. The tumour cells have abundant, glassy, eosinophilic cytoplasm and small nuclei. In the deeper regions, tumour cells show cellular atypia and infiltrative growth associated with an inflammatory reaction (Fig. 22.10B).

Differential diagnosis

The main differential diagnosis of keratoacanthoma is squamous cell carcinoma which develops more slowly than keratoacanthoma, is less well demarcated, and is not usually characterised by the central keratin filled crater.

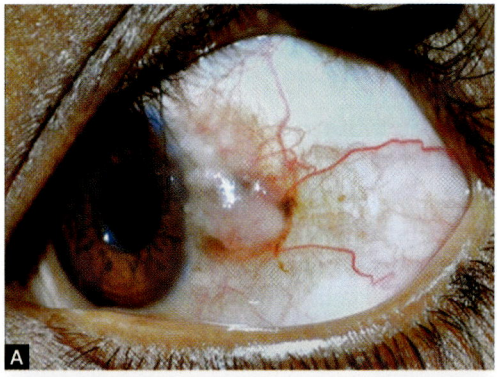

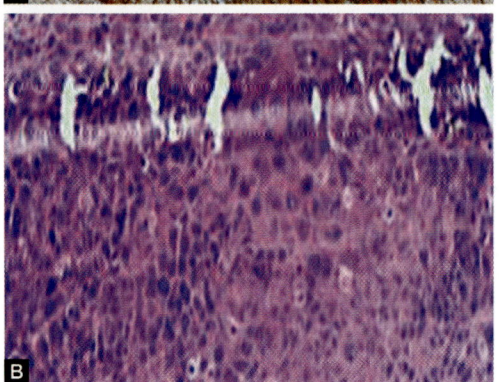

Fig. 22.9: A, *Pseudoepitheliomatous hyperplasia. Elevated leukoplakic pink lesion in the temporal limbal area with apparent feeder vessels and pigmentation. Resembles a nodular OSSN; B, HPE shows hyperplasia, acanthosis, elongation of rete ridges*

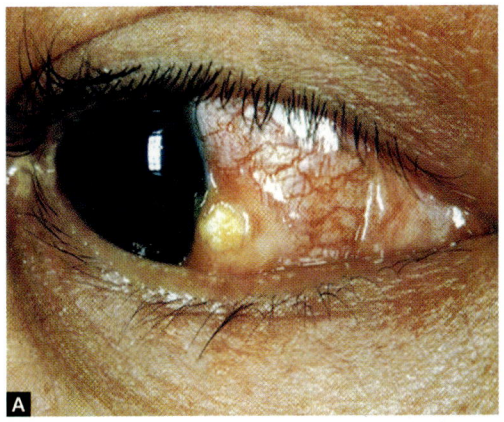

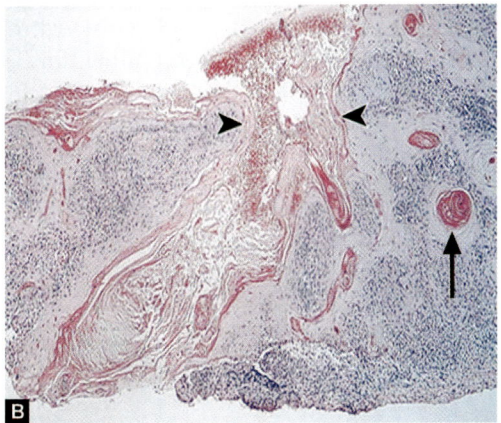

Fig. 22.10: *Keratoacanthoma of conjunctiva: A, White, dome-shaped mass with a central crater filled with white material; B, HPE showing a central crater containing a keratotic plug (arrowheads), surrounded by acanthotic conjunctival epithelium including horn pearls (arrow)*

Although it remains controversial whether squamous cell carcinoma can arise from keratoacanthoma, it is more likely that such tumours are well differentiated squamous cell carcinoma mimicking closely the histological features of keratoacanthoma. Such cases underline the importance of close follow-up of all patients with diagnosed conjunctival keratoacanthoma.

Treatment

Complete excision of the tumour and cryotherapy is the treatment of choice.

5. Dacryoadenoma

Etiology

Dacryoadenoma is a rare condition affecting children and young adults. It is not known if it is congenital or acquired. It originates from the surface epithelium by the downward invagination of tubular formations that undergo secondary and tertiary ramifications and develop glandular lobules similar to those seen in normal lacrimal glands but with abundant goblet cells.

Clinical features

It appears as a translucent and fleshy pink lesion in the bulbar, forniceal or palpebral conjunctiva (Fig. 22.11A).

Histopathology

The surface epithelium overlying the mass is not normal conjunctival squamous epithelium, but it is a modification in the form of a superficial layer of columnar to cuboidal cells surmounting several nuclei similar to the cells lining the subepithelial lumen-forming units. Scattered myoepithelial cells were associated with the acinar-type epithelium of the tumour, and there were goblet cells intermixed. Neither light nor electron microscopy disclosed the presence of true ducts (Fig. 22.11B).

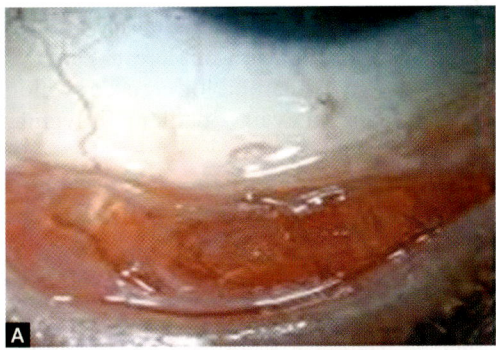

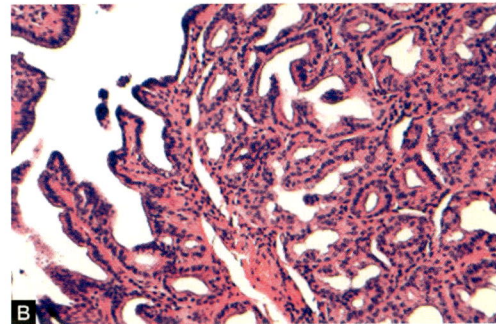

Fig. 22.11: *A, Conjunctival dacryoadenoma; B, HPE showing acinar type of epithelium*

Differential diagnosis

Differential diagnosis includes lymphoma and other pink- or salmon-coloured masses in the conjunctiva.

Treatment

Because of the benign nature of this disease, it can be followed with careful monitoring and photography. However, because of the rarity of this condition and the concern for other more serious problems, an excisional biopsy can help to differentiate this from other possible diseases.

6. Hereditary benign intraepithelial dyskeratosis

Etiology

This is a rare autosomal dominant condition of the conjunctiva and other mucous membranes. It is specifically seen among the inbred Caucasians, African-Americans, and Native Americans known as Haliwa Indians but, is also seen in the population of other descent. Due to the classic sign of marked, bilateral conjunctival hyperaemia, this disease is sometimes referred to as the **"red eye"** disease.

Clinical features

Hereditary benign intraepithelial dyskeratosis (HBID) has a distinct clinical picture. Diagnosis can be made by slit lamp biomicroscopy alone. Affected patients may have ocular involvement, oral involvement, or both.

Oral manifestations of the disease include white, spongy plaques of the buccal mucosa, tongue, or lips.

Ocular manifestations of the disease are characterised by:

- *Bilateral, conjunctival injection* with whitish-grey, elevated, gelatinous corneal plaques located in the perilimbal area, most often nasally or temporally.
- *Corneal plaques* may become visually significant with extension into the central visual axis, disruption of the normal ocular surface, or induction of astigmatism.
- *Corneal neovascularization* can occur around areas of plaque formation. Most commonly, neovascularization develops superficially, but involvement of the mid to deep stroma has been reported (Fig. 22.12A).

Although originally thought to be congenital, HBID is not present at birth. Symptoms begin in early childhood and follow a waxing and waning pattern throughout life. Few reports have suggested that plaques spontaneously shed, however, there has never been photographic documentation of this phenomenon. Excision of plaques leads to recurrence and further exacerbation in most cases.

Histopathology

In addition to clinical diagnosis, HBID can also be diagnosed histopathologically. Ocular and oral plaques are distinctively characterised by acanthosis, dyskeratosis, and parakeratosis within the stratified squamous epithelium. The hallmark dyskeratotic cells in hereditary benign intraepithelial dyskeratosis have a dense cytoplasm and pyknotic nuclei. Beneath the epithelium in the stroma lies a chronic, mild to moderate lymphocytic inflammatory response. The adjacent stratified squamous epithelium of the conjunctiva can be normal or acanthotic (Fig. 22.12B).

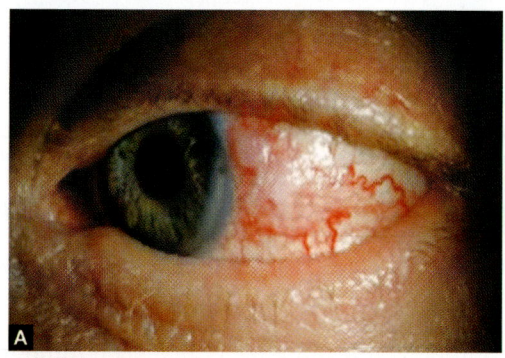

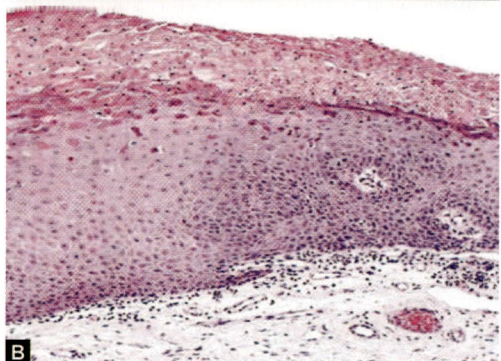

Fig. 22.12: *A, Hereditary benign intraepithelial dyskeratosis; B, Acanthosis and underlying chronic lymphocytic infiltrate in HBID*

Treatment

Treatment of HBID has proven to be very difficult and there is no cure to date.

- *Medical management* with ATTs, topical corticosteroids, and systemic immunosuppression only minimally improves the symptoms.
- *Topical management* alone has not shown to reduce plaque size in the majority of cases.

Smaller symptomatic lesions are treated conservatively with lubricants and topical steroids while *larger lesions* require *local resection* with ocular surface reconstruction. It carries no risk of malignancy, but recurrence is common. Hence, complete excision with clear margins is warranted.

7. Epithelial inclusion cyst

The epithelial inclusion cyst could be spontaneous or occur after inflammation, surgery or trauma. It has round form lined by conjunctival epithelium with clear fluid inside. If the fluid has epithelial cells, they can go to the bottom of the cyst and form a pseudohypopyon. If they are asymptomatic they can be observed, but if it is too large it can be excised completely with primary closure of the conjunctiva.

This entity has been covered in detail in this chapter (cysts of conjunctiva, page 322).

CONJUNCTIVAL PREMALIGNANT NONMELANOCYTIC EPITHELIAL NEOPLASMS

1. Conjunctival keratotic plaque and actinic keratosis

The conjunctival keratotic plaque and actinic keratosis are two lesions that cannot be clinically differentiated from each other. Shields et al in their clinical series of 1663 conjunctival tumours had four conjunctival keratotic plaques and four actinic keratoses, each representing less than 1% of the entire conjunctival tumour.

Clinical features

The two lesions develop on the limbal or the bulbar conjunctiva in the interpalpebral region. They are a flat and white plaque that appear gradually. They are a lot similar to the conjunctival intraepithelial neoplasia (CIN).

Keratotic plaque denotes local hyperplasia and cornification of the conjunctival and the corneal epithelium. It is a rare pathologic lesion when affecting the eye. Many other names have been used in the literature for these lesions, such as tyloma (Gallenga), cornification of the conjunctiva (Best), keratosis (Mohr and Schein) and conjunctival callosities (Saemisch).

Actinic keratosis is seen commonly as a focal leukoplakic lesion occurring at the interpalpebral area presenting as flat, white plaque sometimes with a frothy covering. Actinic keratosis progresses very gradually and shows no tendency towards aggressive growth. Clinically, it may often be indistinguishable from conjunctival intraepithelial neoplasia (CIN). Rose bengal staining of the surface of the lesion tips the clinical suspicion in favour of CIN (Fig. 22.13).

Histopathology

The histopathology of the keratotic plaque shows acanthosis of the epithelium and keratinization of the conjunctival epithelium and parakeratosis.

The actinic keratosis also called senile keratosis shows a similar histopathologic aspect with prominent keratosis and usually appears over a chronic inflammation like a pingueculum or pterygium.

Treatment

- *Document and observe:* Some ophthalmologists prefer to document the lesion and follow it, particularly in elderly patients, because the prognosis is excellent.

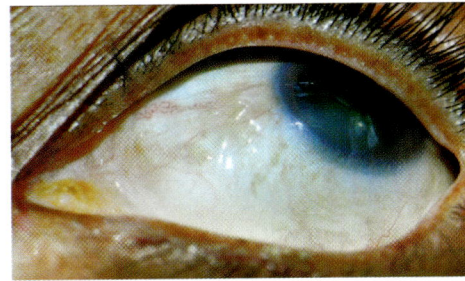

Fig. 22.13: *Actinic keratosis, a focal leukoplakic lesion seen in the interpalpebral area. It can easily be misdiagnosed as pinguecula*

- *Excision and supplementary cryotherapy:* Because of the clinical similarity with CIN, the finding of leukoplakia in the conjunctiva is a relative indication of excision and cryotherapy.

2. Conjunctival intraepithelial neoplasia

The conjunctival intraepithelial neoplasia is a squamous neoplasia confined to the conjunctival epithelium that sometimes transgresses the basement membrane but strictly do not have the potential to metastasize, unlike the invasive squamous carcinoma. Some authors are talking about an entire spectrum of epithelial neoplasia called "ocular surface squamous neoplasia", that includes dysplasia, CIN and invasive squamous cell carcinoma.

Etiology

CIN is more common in elderly and immuno-suppressed patients with considerable sunlight exposure, but children can develop it.

The human papillomavirus (HPV) and sunlight are considered the main predisposing factors for the conjunctival intraepithelial neoplasia. But nevertheless, in some CIN there is not to be found the HPV with the polymerase chain reaction.

Shields et al found in their series that the CIN corresponded to 39% of all premalignant and malignant lesions and to 4% of all the conjunctival lesions.

Clinical features

Conjunctival intraepithelial neoplasia could be a fleshy, sessile or minimally elevated lesion that frequently appears perilimbal in the inter-palpebral zone or less commonly begins in the inferior fornix or palpebral conjunctiva.

CIN can extend into the adjacent corneal epithelium. It appears like a grey superficial opacity that can be avascular or it can have fine vascularization (Fig. 22.14).

Histopathology

The histopathology of mild CIN shows a partial replacement of the surface epithelium by abnormal epithelial cells that do not have a normal maturation. In severe CIN, the histo-pathology is characterised by a total replacement

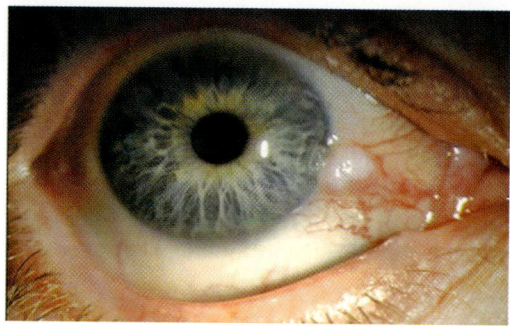

Fig. 22.14: *Conjunctival intraepithelial neoplasia. Moderate dysplasia: Limbal leukoplakic appearing lesion with feeder vessels*

of epithelium by abnormal epithelial cells with no maturation.

Treatment

- *Excision with adequate margins* is the recommended approach. Incomplete removal increases the recurrences.
- *Growth removal with alcohol corneal epithe-liectomy,* partial lamellar sclerokerato-conjunctivectomy and double freeze thaw cryotherapy: This is for more localised lesions.
- *Low dose irradiation* with strontium-90
- *Chemotherapy with topical mitomycin C* for recurrent or persistent cases. Also interferon alpha 2b and 5-fluorouracil are used.
- *Cidofovir.*

CONJUNCTIVAL MALIGNANT NONMELANOCYTIC EPITHELIAL NEOPLASMS

1. Conjunctival invasive squamous cell carcinoma

Etiology

Conjunctival invasive squamous cell carcinoma is when CIN breaks the basement membrane of the conjunctival epithelium and invades the stroma and the underlying tissues.

Conjunctival invasive squamous cell carcinoma. It tends to occur in patients with xeroderma pigmentosum and atopic eczema. It is associated to the dysfunction of T lymphocytes and the HPV type 16.

Incidence of the conjunctival invasive squamous cell carcinoma varies from 0.02 to 3.5 per 100,000, it is less frequent than the CIN, with a frequency of 60% of all conjunctival malignant epithelial tumours and 7% of all the conjunctival neoplasms. It is more common in men (75%) and elderly patients (75% >60 years old).

Clinical features

It occurs frequently in the interpalpebral region of Caucasian elderly or immunosuppressed patients. Most commonly it begins at the limbus (75%). The lesion can be a sessile, gelatinous, circumscribed or papillomatous mass with leukoplakia. Some lesions are diffuse, flat and poorly delineated that can be confused with a chronic conjunctivitis, scleritis or pagetoid invasion of sebaceous carcinoma.

The lesion is invasive to the local structures (orbit, cornea and the globe), but with a low range of metastasis (1–2%). If the invasion causes glaucoma, and the intraocular pressure is uncontrollable, that may necessitate an enucleation.

Diagnosis

Conjunctival invasive squamous cell carcinoma cannot be differentiated clinically from CIN.

- *Excisional biopsy:* If the lesion is localised and small.
- *Impression cytology:* If the lesion is diffuse.
- *Ultrasound biomicroscopy:* To determine the limbal invasion.

Histopathology

The histopathology of conjunctival invasive squamous cell shows well-differentiated neoplasm with abnormal epithelial cells that have mitotic activity and keratinic production. Some lesions can be poorly differentiated with pleomorphic cells, giant cells and a lot of mitotic figures with acanthosis and dyskeratosis.

Treatment

- *Excision with adequate margins and double freeze thaw cryotherapy:* This is the first approach. Incomplete removal increases the recurrences. If the lesion is large, adjuvant amniotic membrane grafting can be used.
- *Growth removal with alcohol corneal epitheliectomy,* partial lamellar sclerokeratoconjunctivectomy and double freeze thaw cryotherapy.

- *Chemotherapy with topical mitomycin C* for recurrent or persistent cases. Also interferon alpha 2b and 5-fluorouracil are used.
- Cidofovir
- Enucleation
- Eyelid-sparing exenteration

Note: As conjunctival invasive squamous cell carcinoma or OSSN is an extremely important topic, it has been described in detail in Chapter 23.

2. Mucoepidermoid carcinoma

Mucoepidermoid carcinoma is an aggressive variation of the conjunctival invasive squamous cell carcinoma, that is less than 5% of this lesion.

Clinical features

Mucoepidermoid carcinoma is more frequent in elderly men (>70 years old). It can be in the bulbar conjunctiva but can also be presented in the caruncle and then it can invade the orbit and paranasal sinuses. It can have a yellow, globular and cystic appearance. This neoplasm tends to invade the globe or the orbit. In the intraocular space, the mucoepidermoid carcinoma can produce a mucinous cyst in the suprauveal space. The mucin production is more frequent in the intraocular space than in the bulbar conjunctiva.

Histopathology

The histopathology of mucoepidermoid carcinoma shows an epidermoid component, mucin and goblet cells with signet cells. The pseudoadenomatous hyperplasia also have goblet cells and mucin that is why this is a differential diagnosis of the mucoepidermoid carcinoma. Other differential diagnosis is a primary mucoepidermoid carcinoma of the paranasal sinuses.

3. Spindle cell carcinoma

The spindle cell carcinoma is a more aggressive type of conjunctival invasive squamous cell carcinoma that is very rare with only 20 cases reported in the literature. It has a worst prognosis because of the tendency for intraocular invasion and metastasis to the the lung and bone.

Histopathology

The histopathology of spindle cell carcinoma shows pleomorphic spindle cells that look like fibroblasts. This can be misdiagnosed as fibrosarcoma, therefore the diagnosis must be confirmed with immunohistochemistry and electron microscopy.

MELANOCYTIC EPITHELIAL TUMOURS

CLASSIFICATION

Benign
- Conjunctival melanocytic naevi
- Congenital ocular melanosis
- Racial melanosis
- Primary acquired melanosis

Premalignant

Primary acquired melanosis

Malignant

Conjunctival melanoma

BENIGN MELANOCYTIC EPITHELIAL TUMOURS

Conjunctival melanocytic naevus

Etiology

Melanocytic tumours of the conjunctiva have a wide spectrum. Conjunctival naevus usually becomes apparent in the first to the second decade of life as a group of small nests of pigmented epithelial cells in the basal layer of the epithelium. As the cells migrate into the underlying stroma in the second to third decade, the naevus progresses to become the compound naevus. Further migration occurs, and cells reside in the stroma as subepithelial naevus during the third and fourth decades. Naevus is more commonly seen in Caucasians (89%) than Africans (6%) and Asians (5%). Although most conjunctival naevi are pigmented (84%), some may be amelanotic or partially pigmented (16%).

Clinical features

Conjunctival naevi are mostly located near the limbus in the interpalpebral area (72%) (Fig. 22.15A). Other locations are the caruncle, semilunar folds, fornix, tarsus, and cornea. Characteristic clear cysts strongly support the diagnosis. They may also clinically demonstrate feeder vessels (64%) and intrinsic vascularity (77%). It can vary in size, colour, and location.

Conjunctival naevus can increase in size in growing young children, during puberty, pregnancy, and sun exposure.

Malignant transformation was estimated to be <1%. Sudden increase in size, alteration in colour, and increased thickness with prominent feeder vessels indicates malignant transformation.

Histopathology

Histopathologically, a conjunctival naevus is composed of nests of benign melanocytes in the stroma near the basal layers of the epithelium (Fig. 22.15B). Positive immunostaining for HMB-45 and Ki-67 are useful adjuncts in differentiating benign melanocytic lesion from suspected malignant entities.

Differential diagnosis

Irregular and diffuse growth pattern poses a diagnostic confusion with primary acquired melanosis (PAM), melanoma, lymphoma, and pigmented OSSN.

Treatment

Periodic (annual) observation with slit lamp measurements and serial photographs is the management of choice. If excision is performed for cosmesis or suspected growth, it is preferable not to leave any residual lesion.

Indications for excision of conjunctival naevus
- Distinct onset in middle age or later life
- Location in the fornix or palpebral conjunctiva
- Lesions more than 10 mm in diameter
- Exuberant feeder blood vessels
- Exuberant intrinsic vascularity and haemorrhage
- Lesions with no cysts
- Lesions with dark uniform pigmentation
- Corneal epithelial invasion >3 clock hours and 3 mm from limbus
- Episcleral fixity
- Cosmetic concern

Congenital ocular melanosis

Ocular melanocytosis is a congenital pigmentary condition of the periocular skin, sclera, orbit, meninges, and soft palate. It appears as irregular patches of scleral and episcleral pigmentation

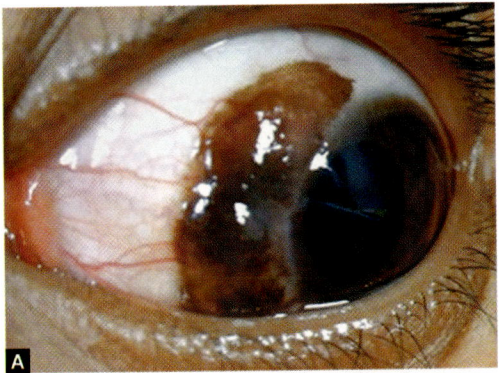

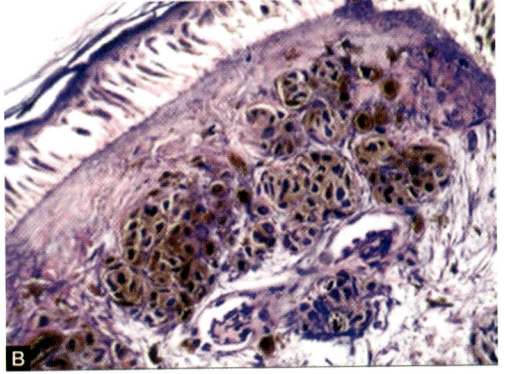

Fig. 22.15: *A, Conjunctival naevus with intralesional cysts and feeder vessels; B, microphotograph of a subepithelial naevus showing clumps of melanocytes with no cellular atypia (OM ×40)*

varying in colour from brown to grey. Typically, there is no conjunctival pigment. It can involve the underlying uveal tract. Since it has an episcleral involvement, it does not move with manipulation of the conjunctiva. This condition imparts a 1 in 400 risk for the development of uveal melanoma.

The scleral pigmentation of congenital ocular melanocytosis has typical features and location (Fig. 22.16). It must be differentiated from other diffuse epibulbar pigmentary conditions like primary acquired melanosis and complexion related pigmentation. Unlike these other conditions it is attached to the sclera and does not move with manipulation of conjunctiva.

If associated with the dermal component, it is known as oculodermal melanocytosis or naevus of Ota. It is mandatory that all patients with oculodermal melanocytosis undergo fundus

examination to exclude uveal melanocytosis or melanoma. Associated hairline pigmentation predisposes them for meningeal melanoma and palate pigmentation to esophageal melanoma, therefore, these signs should be elicited with appropriate referrals when needed.

Racial melanosis or complexion-related conjunctival pigmentation

Etiology

The most common benign conjunctival lesions are due to racial (secondary) melanosis. Racial melanosis is present in 92.5% of African Americans, 35.7% of Asians, 28% of Hispanics, and 4.9% of Caucasians. This benign entity is the result of epithelial melanocytes producing excessive melanin which is transferred into surrounding keratinocytes. Typically racial melanosis is bilateral, asymmetric, occurs in the interpalpebral fissures, and does not contain cysts.

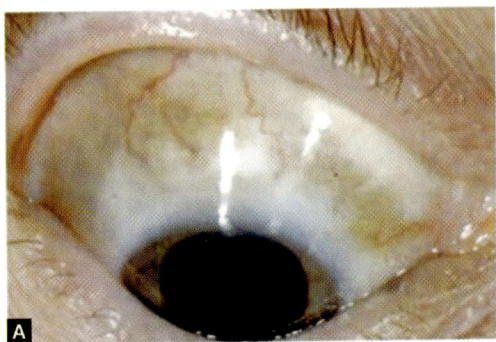

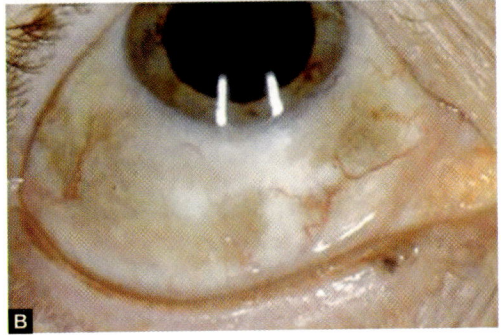

Fig. 22.16: *A, Scleral melanocytosis showing diffuse patchy brown pigment in superior aspect of the right eye; B, Same patient shown in Fig. 22.16A demonstrating pigment in the inferior aspect of the right eye*

Clinical features

Complexion-related conjunctival pigmentation is a relatively common bilateral, flat, diffuse conjunctival pigmentation (Fig. 22.17). It is more concentrated in the limbus, often for 360°, with variable pigmentation at the perilimbal bulbar conjunctiva and cornea. Uncommonly, it may also involve the fornix and rarely the palpebral conjunctiva. Periodic observation is recommended.

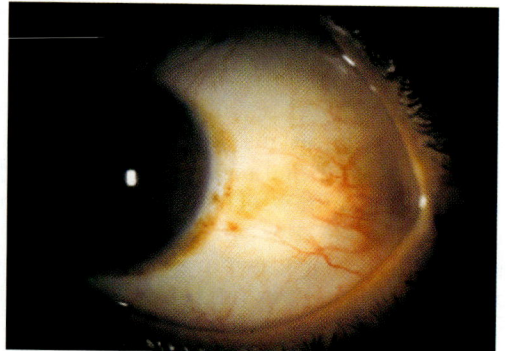

Fig. 22.17: *Physiologic (racial) melanosis. Flat conjunctival pigmentation present bilaterally starting at the limbus and most prominent in the interpalpebral zone is likely to be racial melanosis in a darkly pigmented patient*

PREMALIGNANT MELANOCYTIC EPITHELIAL TUMOURS

Primary acquired melanosis

Reese noted the tendency of a certain type of acquired conjunctival pigmentation to evolve into melanoma and named it precancerous melanosis. Zimmerman replaced the term with benign acquired melanosis, which was further modified by WHO as Primary Acquired Melanosis (PAM) in 1980.

Primary acquired melanosis (PAM) can either be regarded as benign (PAM without atypia) or represent a precancerous lesion (PAM with atypia).

Etiology

Sunlight exposure may play a role in the development of PAM. It has also been seen in patients with neurofibromatosis raising suspicion that it may have a developmental relationship to the neural crest.

Clinical features

Primary acquired melanosis usually manifests in the middle age as unilateral, superficial, solitary, patchy, diffuse or multifocal pigmentation of the bulbar, forniceal and palpebral conjunctiva, and cornea (Figs 22.18 and 22.19). Occasionally, PAM can be amelanotic. In PAM without atypia, there occurs melanin pigmentation of the basal epithelium with or without hyperplasia of cytological benign melanocytes. This may progress to cytological atypical melanocytes to form PAM with atypia, where there is an increased risk of developing melanoma.

Malignant transformation. Clinically, larger the extent of PAM, greater the risk of malignant transformation. The PAM risk factors are summarised in Table 22.2.

Indications for biopsy of PAM
- Lesion diameter >5 mm
- Documented progression
- Thickening of involved conjunctiva
- Distant nodule arising within the lesion
- Nutrient vessels
- Involvement of the cornea

Table 22.2: *Primary acquired melanosis (PAM) risk factors*

Higher risk	Lower risk
>3 clock hours involvement of conjunctiva	Small, circumscribed without extensive involvement of conjunctiva
Extension onto cornea	Confinement to the conjunctiva
Nodular	Flat
Multifocal	One lesion
Highly vascular	Minimal vasculature
History of skin or conjunctival melanoma	No history of skin or conjunctival melanoma
Older age	Young age

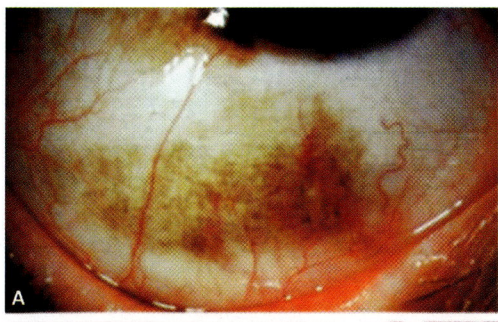

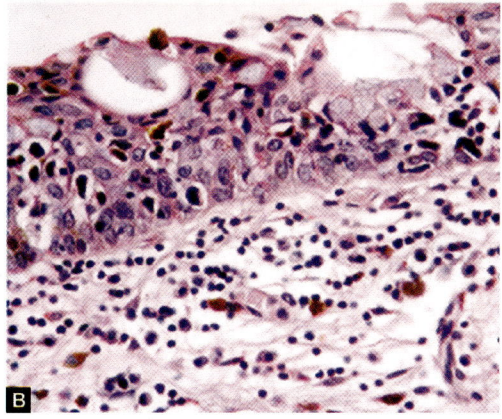

Fig. 22.18: *Primary acquired melanosis: A, Diffuse pigmentation of bulbar conjunctiva in an elderly male; B, HPE of PAM with cellular atypia*

- Involvement of the palpebral conjunctiva
- Personal history of cutaneous/uveal melanoma
- Dysplastic naevus syndrome in patient or close relative.

A simple biopsy can determine whether a pigmented conjunctival tumour is a naevus, primary acquired melanosis, or conjunctival melanoma. As seen below, primary acquired melanosis typically affects one eye, in middle-aged, fair-skinned people.

Histopathology

A PAM without atypia is best characterised by minimal melanocytic hyperplasia along the basal epithelial layer of the conjunctiva. PAM with atypia shows usually isolated or confluent nests of atypical melanocytes. Pagetoid spread can also be observed. The melanocytes exhibit varying signs of atypia as large abnormal cells, prominent nucleoli, a high nuclear-cytoplasmic ratio, and mitotic figures.

It can be differentiated histologically by the degree of atypia of melanocytes. Without atypia, PAM is a benign melanocytic proliferation. With atypia, PAM may progress to malignant melanoma. Progression to melanoma occurred in 0% of PAM without atypia, 0% of PAM with mild atypia, and 13% of PAM with severe atypia. Multivariable analysis revealed that the most significant factor for both PAM recurrence and progression to melanoma was extent of PAM in clock hours.

Differential diagnosis

- *Racial melanosis*—almost always bilateral.
- *Conjunctival naevus*—does not extend into cornea or fornices, may have very little pigmentation, and can have cysts.
- *Secondary acquired melanosis*, e.g. foreign body, ciliary body melanoma, blood filled cysts.
- *Oculodermal melanocytosis* (naevus of Ota)—mostly in Blacks and Asians, unilateral, blue/grey colour, and does not move with the conjunctival epithelium.
- *Malignant melanoma*—growth and biopsy makes the diagnosis.
- *Congenital melanocytosis*—present at birth.
- *Conjunctival foreign body*
- *Exogenous pigmentation* (e.g. mascara)

Treatment

Management strategies are:

- *Observation* for PAM without atypia
- *Cryotherapy* for PAM with atypia <3 clock hours
- *Excision with excision edge cryotherapy* for PAM >3 clock hours
- *Topical MMC* for diffuse PAM with atypia.

MALIGNANT MELANOCYTIC EPITHELIAL TUMOURS

Conjunctival melanoma

Etiology

Conjunctival melanomas (CM) comprise approximately 2% of all ocular surface malignancies and 0.25% of all melanomas. Non-Hispanic Caucasians are most commonly affected, with an incidence of 0.2–0.8 per million.

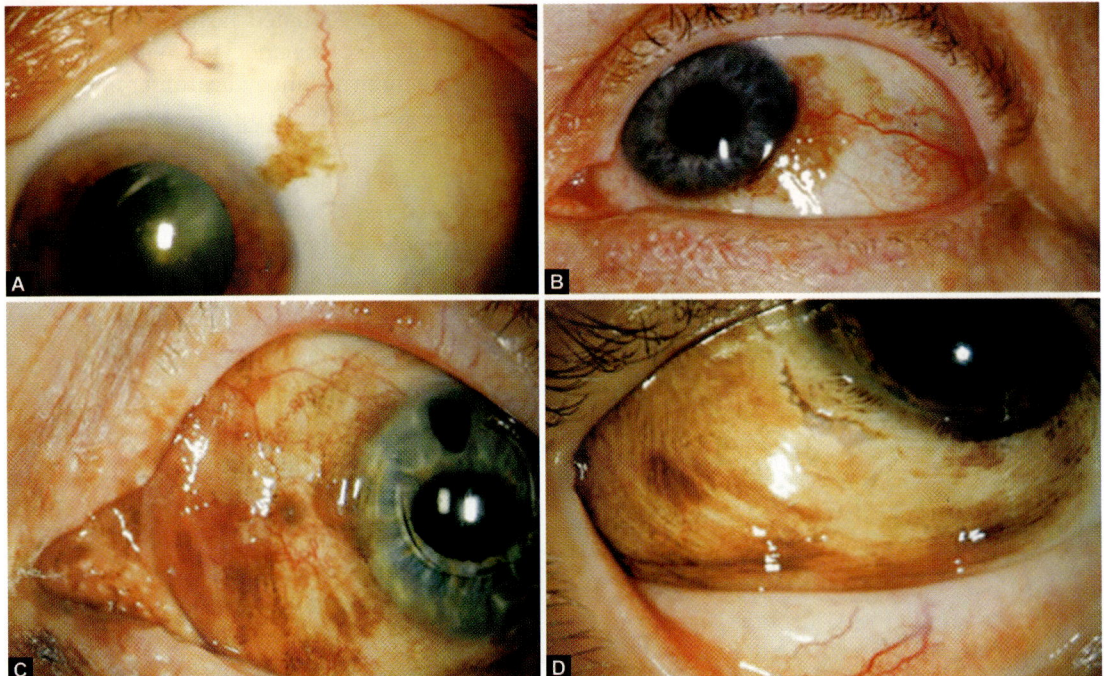

Fig. 22.19: *Primary acquired melanosis (PAM) with varying extent of involvement. A, PAM involving less than 1 clock hour of bulbar conjunctiva; B, PAM involving 4 clock hours of conjunctiva with slight corneal extension; C, PAM involving more than 6 clock hours of bulbar conjunctiva with extension into the cornea; D, PAM involving entire bulbar conjunctiva (12 clock hours)*

Conjunctival melanoma is most common in light-skinned individuals. Non-Whites are rarely affected.

Age and sex. Studies have failed to show consistent predilection for sex. It usually presents in the middle-aged or elderly. The median age of presentation is approximately 60 years.

Risk factors have been difficult to ascertain due to the low incidence of disease. However, studies have reported risk for those with fair skin and hair, a family history, certain genetic syndromes (familial melanoma syndromes, xeroderma pigmentosum), and significant ultraviolet (UV) light exposure. Sunlight exposure is also suggested as a cause, but that fails to explain the occurrence of melanoma in the fornices and palpebral conjunctiva.

The surveillance, epidemiology, and end results (SEER) study reported an increased incidence of conjunctival melanoma in White males. The mechanism is hypothesized to be secondary to increased UV light exposure. There is also a strong association between primary acquired melanosis (PAM) and conjunctival naevi with CM. In particular, PAM with severe atypia transforms into CM in 13% of cases, with greater risk associated with more extensive circumferential spread of PAM. PAM without atypia or with mild atypia does not demonstrate a predisposition for progression to melanoma. Conjunctival melanomas arise from three sources: PAM (75%), *de novo* (20%), and naevus (5%); with PAM being most common and naevus being least common. Other risk factors are dysplastic naevus syndrome, neurofibromatosis, and xeroderma pigmentosum.

Conjunctival melanoma may rarely develop secondary to continuous touch from an eyelid margin melanoma (implantation melanoma).

Clinical features

Conjunctival melanoma appears (Fig. 22.20A) as a pigmented fleshy mass located in the bulbar, forniceal or palpebral conjunctiva. As a variant, it may appear as diffuse or multifocal with ill-defined margins particularly if arising from PAM. It occasionally originates in the forniceal and palpebral conjunctivae. It may extend to cover the cornea or even arise as a primary corneal tumour. Melanoma can be sparsely pigmented or amelanotic. It is typically amelanotic, fleshy, and vascular when it recurs after prior excision.

Classification. Conjunctival melanoma is classified according to the AJCC-TNM classification (Table 22.3).

Table 22.3: *AJCC–TNM classification of conjunctival melanoma*			
Stage	*Clinical*	*Stage*	*Pathological*
Primary tumour (T)			
Tx	Primary tumour cannot be assessed	Tx	Primary tumour cannot be assessed
T0	No evidence of primary tumour	T0	No evidence of primary tumour
T (is)	Malignant melanoma confined to conjunctival epithelium	T (is)	Malignant melanoma confined to conjunctival epithelium
T1	Malignant melanoma of the bulbar conjunctiva	pT1	Malignant melanoma of the bulbar conjunctiva
T1a	<1 quadrant	pT1a	<0.5 mm thick with invasion of substantia propria
T1b	>1 but <2 quadrant		
T1c	>2 but <3 quadrant	pT1b	>0.5–1.5 mm thick, with invasion of substantia propria
T1d	>3 quadrant		
		pT1c	>1.5 mm thick, with invasion of substantia propria
T2	Malignant melanoma of palpebral conjunctiva, forniceal conjunctiva, and/or caruncle	pT2	Malignant melanoma of palpebral conjunctiva, forniceal conjunctiva, and/or caruncle
T2a	<1 quadrant	pT2a	≤0.5 mm thick, with invasion of substantia propria
T2b	>1 quadrant but not involving caruncle	pT2b	>0.5–1.5 mm thick, with invasion of substantia propria
T2c	<1 quadrant and involving caruncle	pT2c	>1.5 mm thick, with invasion of substantia propria
T2d	>1 quadrant and involving caruncle		
T3	Malignant melanoma with local invasion	pT3	Malignant melanoma invading the eye, eyelid, nasolacrimal system, sinuses or orbit
T3a	Globe		
T3b	Eyelid		
T3c	Orbit		
T3d	Paranasal sinus		
T4	Malignant melanoma with local invasion	pT4	Malignant melanoma with intracranial extension
Regional lymph node (N)			
Nx	Regional lymph node cannot be assessed		
N0a	No regional lymph node metastasis, biopsy done		
N0b	No regional lymph node metastasis, no biopsy done		
N1	Regional lymph node metastasis		
Distant metastasis (M)			
M0	No distant metastasis		
M1	Distant metastasis		

Source: Edge SB, Byrd DR. Complon CC, et al. (Eds). Carcinoma of the conjunctiva. In: AJCC Cancer Staging Manual. 7th ed., New York. Springer, 2010. ***AJCC: American Joint Committee on Cancer. TNM: Tumour, node and metastasis***

Regional metastasis involves preauricular and submandibular lymph nodes. Sentinel lymphangiography makes it possible to accurately remove lymph nodes and is indicated in tumours more than 2 mm in thickness. Distant metastasis occurs in the brain, liver, skin, and bone.

Histopathology

Histopathologically (Fig. 22.20B), conjunctival melanoma is composed of variably pigmented malignant melanocytes. The cells may range from relatively low grade spindle cells to more anaplastic epithelioid cells. It initially affects the basal area of the epithelium but readily invades the stroma where it has access to conjunctival lymphatic channels.

Immunophenotype studies have shown that these cells are positive for S-100 protein, tyrosinase, melan-A, HMB-45, HMB-50, and microphthalmia conscription factor at high

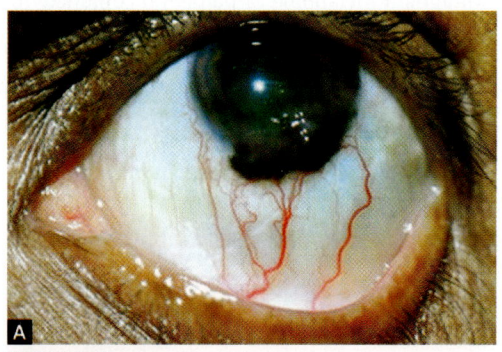
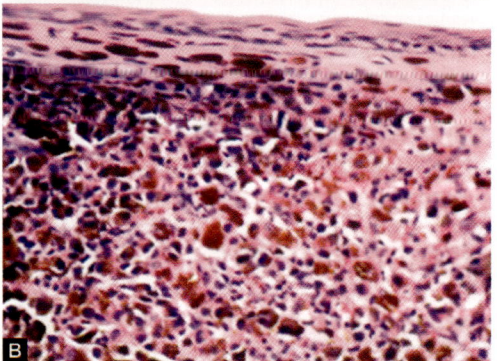

Fig. 22.20: *Conjunctival melanoma. A, Elevated, nodular, pigmented mass at the inferior limbus with extension into the peripheral cornea. Feeder vessels and intrinsic vessels present; B, HPE of CM showing variably pigmented melanocytes with mitotic activity*

levels, suggesting that these are good diagnostic markers for these tumours.

Differential diagnosis

Differential diagnoses are the same as for PAM (*see* page 339).

Treatment

Treatment of conjunctival melanoma is based on certain established principles:
- *Complete excision* in the episcleral plane with 4 mm clinically clear margins.
- *Alcohol keratoepitheliectomy* of the corneal epithelial component.
- *Partial lamellar sclerokeratectomy* if sclera and corneal stroma are involved.
- *Double freeze-thaw cryotherapy* to the excision edge, excision base cryotherapy if sclera is involved and the extent of involvement is <3 clock hours.
- *Postoperative adjuvant plaque brachytherapy* if excision base is clinically detected to have been involved >3 clock hours and if the excision base is positive for tumour cells on histopathology. Since conjunctival melanoma is not radiosensitive, brachytherapy is not used as a sole treatment.
- *Extended enucleation with en bloc excision* if the tumour has deep corneal or scleral invasion or intraocular extension.
- *Eyelid sparing exenteration* if the tumour extends into the orbit. Proton beam radiotherapy may be used as an alternative and/or adjunct to exenteration.
- *Systemic chemotherapy* is administered with combination of IFN and interleukin-2 in disseminated melanoma.

Prognosis

- *Local recurrence* after therapy is as high as 50–70% at 10 years.
- *Overall mortality* rate is 25% in 10 years and more than 30% in 15 years.
- *Critical thickness* that may serve as a prognostic factor, according to various studies implies a value between 0.8 mm and 4 mm.
- *Conjunctival melanoma.* AJCC-TNM staging predicts the prognosis and outcome.
- *Prognostic risk factors* are summarised in Table 22.4.

Table 22.4: *Prognostic indicators for conjunctival melanoma*

Higher risk	Lower risk
Tarsus, caruncle, forniceal involvement	Localised
Deeper extension into tissue	Limbal or bulbar
Thickness >1.8 mm	Thin
Lymphadenopathy	
Lid margin involvement	

STROMAL TUMOURS OF THE OCULAR SURFACE

VASCULAR STROMAL TUMOURS

1. Pyogenic granuloma

Etiology

Pyogenic granuloma is a misnomer; it is neither pyogenic nor a granuloma, but exuberant granulation tissue. It is a fibrovascular response to a tissue insult such as surgical or nonsurgical trauma or inflammation.

Clinical features

Pyogenic granuloma (Fig. 22.21) has rapid onset and progression and presents as fleshy, elevated, red, richly vascular mass. It can be round to ovoid, typically pedunculated, rarely broad-based, and even mushroom shaped. It may be seen in any part of the conjunctiva, limbus, and the cornea.

Histopathologically, it is composed of granulation tissue with lymphocytes, plasma cells, scattered neutrophils, and numerous small caliber vessels.

Treatment

- *Topical steroids,* when diagnosed early, are effective
- *Excision at the base followed by cauterization or cryotherapy* to the excision base is the treatment of choice for larger, unsightly, symptomatic or bleeding pyogenic granuloma.
- *Care of the inciting factor,* if found to minimize the risk of recurrence is important along with excision. It is usual to find a suture knot or a foreign body at the base if the cause is prior surgery or trauma.

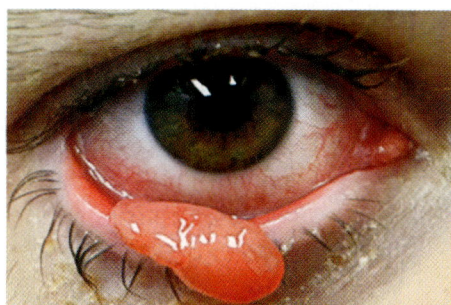

Fig. 22.21: *Pyogenic granuloma of conjunctiva*

- Low dose plaque brachytherapy can be employed for exuberant recurrence.

2. Capillary haemangioma

Etiology

Capillary haemangioma is common in the eyelids but is less common in the orbit and uncommon in the conjunctiva. It is present in 1–4% of all births and is more common in premature infants and often following chorionic villus sampling. The periocular lesion appears within the first few weeks after birth and usually has superficial or deep components. Primary conjunctival capillary haemangiomas are rarely reported. Seen as diffuse red elevated lesion, it may present as a small conjunctival component of a predominant eyelid lesion in a neonate. It may uncommonly develop as an acquired lesion in adults.

Clinical features

Capillary haemangioma (Fig. 22.22A) is usually a cutaneous, subcutaneous, or deep orbital lesion and commonly presents a few weeks after birth. The usual clinical course of infantile cutaneous or subcutaneous haemangiomas includes an initial engorgement (age 6–12 months) followed by regression (age 1–7 years). It usually regresses spontaneously and hence is kept under close observation. Spontaneous regression is often complete by 4–5 years of age.

Histopathology

Histologically, it is composed of lobules of proliferating endothelial cells separated by thin fibrous septa (Fig. 22.22B).

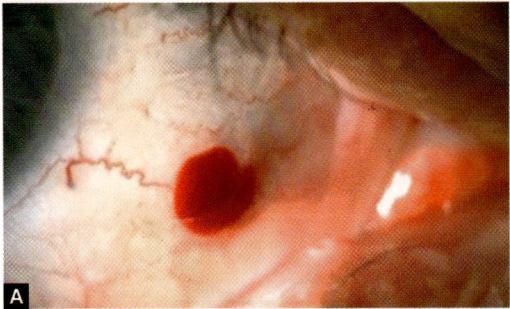

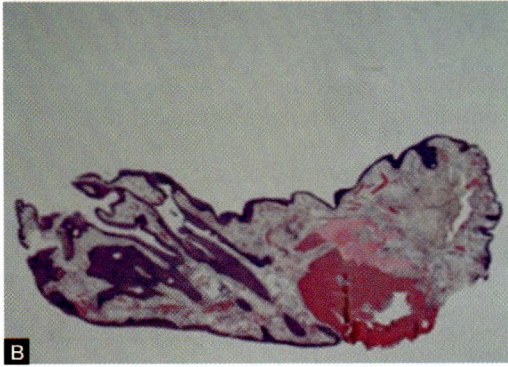

Fig. 22.22: *A, Conjunctival capillary haemangioma; B, HPE showing thin walled vascular channels filled with blood*

Differential diagnosis

The differential diagnosis for capillary haemangioma includes rhabdomyosarcoma, lymphangioma, chloroma, neuroblastoma, orbital cysts, and cellulitis.

Treatment

Management generally is observation until spontaneous regression. Active intervention is performed only if the lesion is very extensive and causes amblyopia, mechanical ptosis, exposure keratopathy, or optic neuropathy. Intervention is also considered if the lesion is unsightly, ulcerates and bleeds and relentlessly progresses.

Typical primary intervention is intralesional steroid injection. Triamcinolone is used in the maximum dose of 6 mg/kg body weight. In general, one injection results in significant involution of the lesion. Injection may be repeated at 6–8 weeks interval if there is a suboptimal response. Dermatologists favour using high-dose oral steroids over 4–6 weeks.

Systemic propranolol 2 mg/kg body weight is being tried as an alternative therapy with encouraging results. If the tumour does not respond to these measures or if there is an indication for an emergent management (as in ulcerated and bleeding lesions), controlled surgical excision or debulking may help.

3. Cavernous haemangioma

Etiology

Cavernous haemangioma is a common orbital tumour, but relatively uncommon in the conjunctiva. It arises often from the conjunctival vessels and rarely from the scleral, muscular or orbital vessels. It appears as red blue lesion in the deep conjunctival stroma.

Clinical features

Conjunctival cavernous haemangioma appears at any age as a red or blue lesion, usually in the stroma. It can be solitary or it can occur in association with other cavernous haemangiomas such as Sturge-Weber syndrome, or diffuse neonatal haemangiomatosis. The literature is not entirely clear as to whether such lesions are a pure cavernous haemangioma or a combination of types.

It consists of multiplicity of venous channels of varying calibre, shows no tendency to involution and may become larger and troublesome by bleeding sometimes giving rise to bloody tears after remaining stationary for years.

Histopathology

Histology shows dilated congested veins separated by connective tissue with smooth muscles in the walls of the blood vessels (Fig. 22.23B).

Treatment

The tumour is radiosensitive but can be treated well by surgical excision.

4. Conjunctival varix

Etiology

Varix refers to venous malformation of the conjunctiva that may range from an isolated single channel to dilated complex venous channels. Often, it is the anterior extension of an orbital varix.

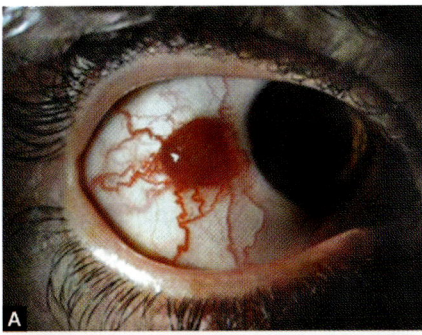

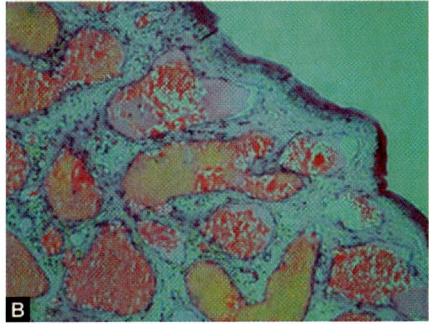

Fig. 22.23: *A, A smooth, oval, dark red, lobular surface mass in the temporal side of bulbar conjunctiva with engorged episcleral and conjunctival vessels around the lesion; B, Histopathologic examination showed multiple, endothelium-lined cavernous spaces surrounded by fibromyxoid tissue (haematoxylin and eosin, magnification × 100)*

Clinical features

Conjunctival varix (Fig. 22.24) usually is an anterior extension of an orbital varix. It may be directly visible as large, distinct blood vessels or it may be deeper and have a diffuse faint blue

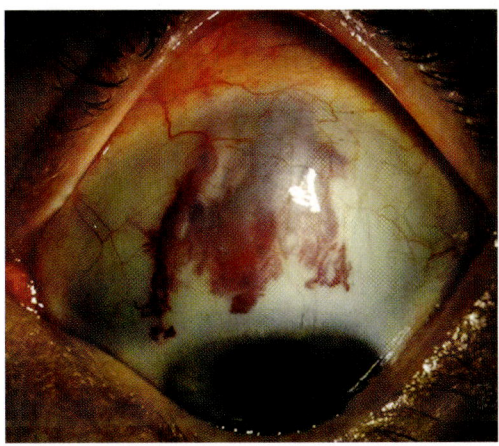

Fig. 22.24: *Conjunctival varix*

black colour. It is generally movable and not fixed to sclera.

Histopathology

Histopathologically, varix is composed of venous channels, ranging from one dilated vessel to more complex channels. Thrombosis and hyalinization are frequent.

Differential diagnosis

Lymphangioma and cavernous haemangioma as their features can overlap.

Treatment

Management is generally conservative by observation and symptomatic treatment. They can be excised for cosmetic reasons, but one should be aware that they may have orbital extensions.

5. Racemose haemangioma

Racemose haemangioma involves loops of dilated arteries and veins communicating directly without the interface of a capillary bed. The lesion is clinically seen as loops of dilated vessels in the conjunctival stroma with no evidence of a stimulus for such vascularization or planned direction. It may be associated with Wyburn-Mason syndrome. It is generally observed unless symptomatic or a cosmetic blemish.

6. Haemangiopericytoma
Etiology

Haemangiopericytoma is known to be derived from the vascular pericytes but is recently considered to be a vascular entity of the solitary fibrous tumour. It is a very rare conjunctival tumour.

Clinical features

Haemangiopericytoma (Fig. 22.25) presents as an elevated or pedunculated reddish pink mass, that has no distinct clinical features. It shows slow progressive growth and often is continuous with a more posterior orbital component.

Histopathology

It is a tumour composed of an abnormal proliferation of pericytes that surround blood

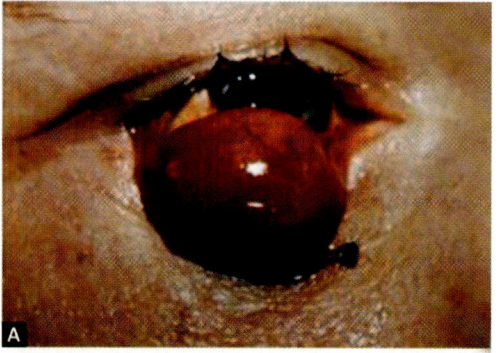

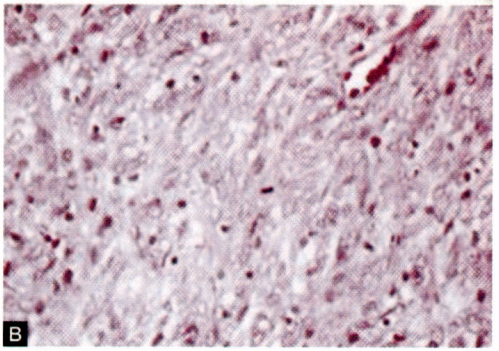

Fig. 22.25: *A, Haemangiopericytoma arising from the inferior fornix in a 40-year-old woman (Courtesy by Hans Frossnikiaus, MD); B, Histopathology of lesion in Fig. 22.25A showing solid tumour composed of spindle-shaped cells and blood vessels (haematoxylin and eosin × 63)*

vessels. With routine light microscopy, a characteristic feature is the 'staghorn' branching of blood vessels in the tumour (Fig. 22.25B).

Treatment

The diagnosis is rarely made clinically. A wide surgical resection with tumour-free margins is advocated.

7. Kaposi sarcoma

Etiology

Kaposi sarcoma was a rare tumour before the AIDS era. It is a malignant tumour seen more frequently in immunocompromised individuals, specifically with HIV, caused by the human herpesvirus 8. Sometimes the conjunctival Kaposi sarcoma is the first sign of immunocompromised status.

Clinical features

Kaposi's sarcoma (Fig. 22.26) clinically appears as single or multifocal vascular red conjunctival lesion, which may become confluent and resemble haemorrhagic conjunctivitis. May also appear as a bright red fleshy to violaceous nodular mass, commonly seen in the fornix.

Differential diagnosis

The differential diagnosis includes granuloma pyogenicum, cavernous haemangioma, foreign body granuloma, malignant melanoma, metastatic tumour, and chronic subconjunctival haemorrhage.

Treatment

- It is moderately responsive to IFN-α-2b and chemotherapy and markedly responsive to low dose radiotherapy (800–2000 cGy).
- The current thinking is in favour of the immediate institution of highly active antiretroviral therapy. The tumour is known to involute with improved immune status.

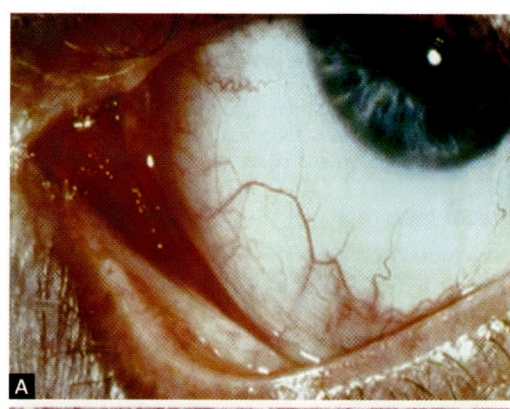

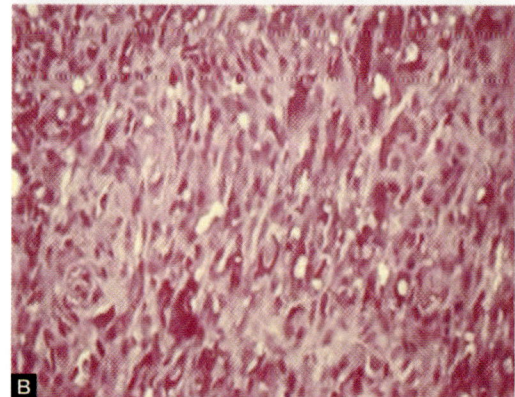

Fig. 22.26: *A, Kaposi sarcoma affecting medial aspect of conjunctiva into the fornix; B, HPE reveals myriads of vascular channels*

• Surgical excision: In extensive, large tumours, loosely connected with healthy tissue.

8. Lymphangiectasia

Etiology

When lymphatic channels in the conjunctiva are dilated and prominent, the condition is called lymphangiectasia. There exists a communication with conjunctival veins, and hence these dilated channels may often be filled with blood, termed haemorrhagic lymphangiectasia. It can occur spontaneously or after trauma or inflammation.

Clinical features

Lymphangiectasia can lead to irritation and redness from desiccation of the overlying conjunctival epithelium, epiphora, if the lacrimal puncta become functionally occluded by over-hanging conjunctiva, blurred vision, and pain.

Surrounding conjunctiva appears edematous and is occasionally associated with sub-conjunctival haemorrhage (Fig. 22.27). It is inter-mittent with a resolution between episodes.

Treatment

No treatment is required unless it is a cosmetic blemish. Liquid nitrogen cryotherapy is effective in treating conjunctival lymphangiectasia probably by collapsing the lymph vessel walls onto each other with a cryogenic burn and also by scarring down the conjunctiva to the underlying globe.

9. Lymphangioma

Etiology

Lymphangioma is a benign tumour of the lymphatic vessels that usually manifests in the first decade of life. It can occur as an isolated conjunctival lesion, but often represents a superficial component of an orbital lymph-angioma.

Clinical features

Conjunctival lymphangiomas (Fig. 22.28A) generally appear as a visible mass without affecting vision, or the globe. These are multi-oculated lesions with dilated cystic spaces. Those that contain blood are called chocolate cysts.

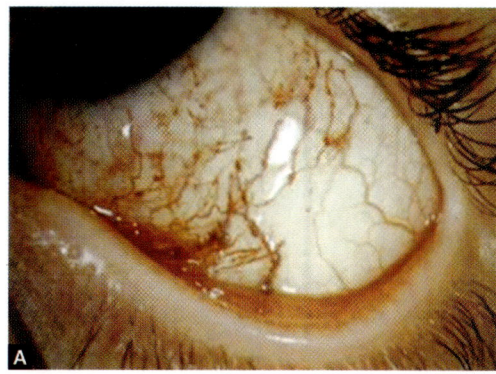
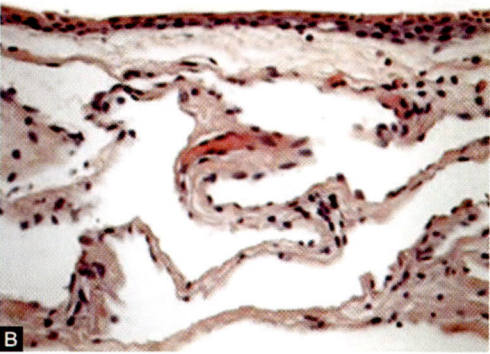

Fig. 22.27: *A, Conjunctival haemorrhagic lymphangiectasia in a 10-year-old boy; B, Histopathology of conjunctival lymphangiectasia, showing bloodless ectatic vascular channels lined by thin endothelial cells*

Histopathology

It histopathologically (Fig. 22.28B) appears as nonencapsulated, irregular mass composed of numerous cyst-like channels that contain clear fluid, blood, or a combination of the two. The ectatic channels are lined by somewhat atten-uated endothelial cells. These channels are separated by loose connective tissue that contains aggregates of small lymphocytes, sometimes forming lymph follicle.

Treatment

• Surgical debulking
• CO_2 laser-assisted debulking
• β-irradiation using strontium-90 applicator
• Brachytherapy is used with partial success.

FIBROUS TUMOURS

Fibrous tumours manifest generally as slowly progressive acquired white stromal tumours in adults. These could be a well-circumscribed

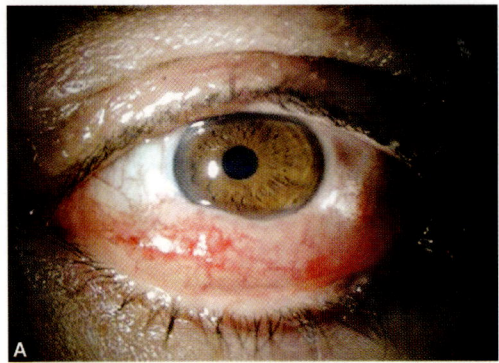

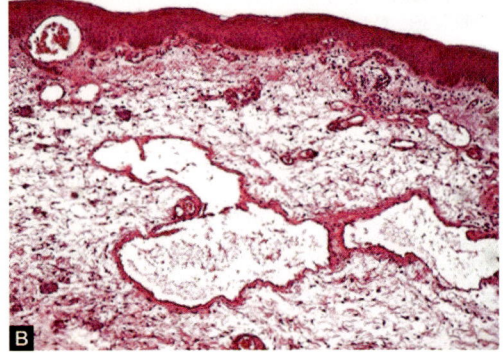

Fig. 22.28: *A, Conjunctival lymphangioma; B, Histology showing a lymphatic proliferation and ectasia with a network of empty bloodless channels lined by flattened endothelium with the presence of some blood vessels and inflammatory infiltrate*

lesion or multi-nodular. Common fibrous tumours affecting the ocular surface are fibrous histiocytoma and nodular fasciitis.

1. Fibrous histiocytoma

Etiology

Fibrous histiocytomas (FHs) are soft tissue tumours usually found on the extremities, but can occur in any part of the body, including orbital tissues. They are classified as:
• Benign fibrous histiocytoma
• Malignant fibrous histiocytoma

Case reports have described the occurrence of conjunctival FHs after trauma and radiation and in the immunosuppressed.

Clinical features

Benign fibrous histiocytomas have been reported in the orbit, eyelid, and episclera, corneoscleral limbus. Conjunctival FHs usually present as painless masses and can develop at any age, but most commonly between the ages of 20 and 40 years. Their gross appearance is of a circumscribed yellow or white mass, and they may have focal areas of haemorrhage, which can make them appear brown or black in colour. Symptoms and signs depend on the site, but may include decreased vision, pain, restricted eye movements, diplopia, and disc swelling.

In contrast, malignant **fibrous histiocytomas** of the corneoscleral limbus characteristically appear in later life, between the ages of 50 and 70 years, with an equal distribution of males to females. They are highly aggressive tumours, and have been reported to have a local recurrence rate of 100% if a limited excision is performed. Recurrence can occur within a few months of excision.

Histopathology

The histopathological appearance of a **benign fibrous histiocytoma** includes a mixture of fibroblastic and histiocytic cells that are often arranged in a cartwheel or storiform pattern, and accompanied by varying numbers of inflammatory cells, including foam cells and siderophages. No atypical nuclei or mitotic figures are present. Although some authors regard these tumours as reactive proliferations of fibroblasts, others do not accept this view because the lesions tend not to regress spontaneously. Recurrence is rare.

Malignant fibrous histiocytomas have a broad range of histological appearances; storiform-pleomorphic, myxoid, giant cell, and inflammatory. The storiform-pleomorphic type is the most common. The cells are predominantly plump pleomorphic spindle-shaped with occasional large, ovoid histiocyte-like cells. Modest amounts of inflammatory cells, such as lymphocytes and plasma cells may be present (Fig. 22.29C).

Differential diagnosis

Clearly, the diagnosis of FH is challenging. Other neoplasms (sarcomas, melanoma, sarcomatous carcinoma, and neural tumours) and reactive lesions (nodular fasciitis) must be excluded. In addition to routine histopatho-

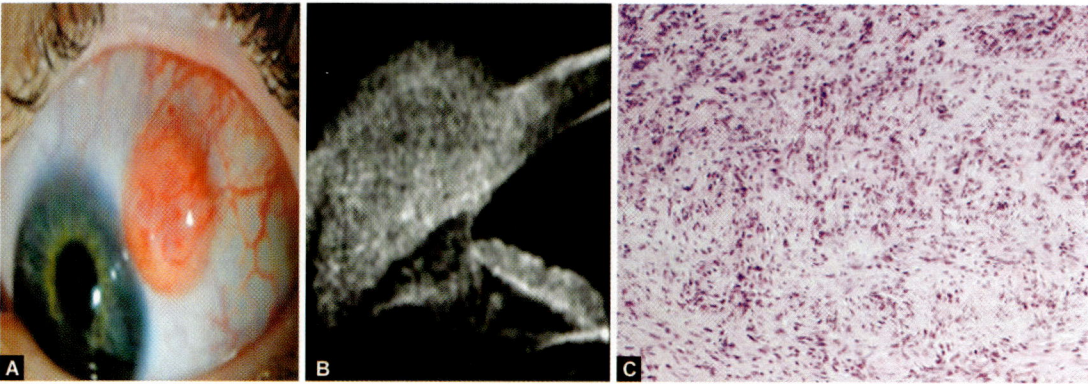

Fig. 22.29: *A, Elevated, vascularized, and fleshy-pink lesion of the left superotemporal conjunctiva extending into the peripheral cornea; B, Ultrasound biomicroscopy discloses a dome-shaped lesion with peripheral corneal and scleral involvement with reduced echogenicity; C, Microscopic high power showing spindle cells with focal storiform arrangement and lymphocytic infiltrate*

logical evaluation, immunohistochemical analysis is extremely helpful in differentiating an FH from above mentioned lesions. Fibrous histiocytoma typically displays strong immuno-reactivity for vimentin; focal immunoreactivity for factor XIIIA, smooth muscle actin, and CD68; and occasional mild immunoreactivity for CD34 and lacks immunoreactivity for cytokeratins, the neural and melanocytic marker S-100, and the melanocytic marker HMB-45.

Treatment

For those limbal fibrous histiocytomas with a benign histopathological appearance, the management should be local surgical excision. The most appropriate management of FH at any site, particularly the conjunctiva, is complete surgical excision with tumour-free margins. The lesion should be managed by resecting it with a 4 to 5 mm wide margin, planar base clearance, excision edge cryotherapy, excision base cryo-therapy for planar invasion, and appropriate ocular surface reconstruction. A pathologist should be consulted before and after surgery to ensure that appropriate measures are taken to care for the specimen. In the event of positive margins, adjuvant treatment such as brachy-therapy is recommended. In order to exclude disease recurrence, patients require close, lifelong follow-up.

Malignant fibrous histiocytomas need to be managed cautiously, preferably by wide local excision and cryotherapy at the earliest opportunity. If necessary, enucleation should be considered to fully excise a limbal malignant fibrous histiocytoma.

2. Nodular fasciitis (pseudosarcomatous fasciitis)

Etiology

Nodular fasciitis is a benign nodular reactive proliferation of fibroblasts and vascular tissue usually arising within the fascia. It occurs in a variety of anatomical locations in both adult and pediatric populations, without gender pre-dilection. In the eye, it usually manifests in the orbit, eyelid, or episclera and rarely conjunctiva. Although trauma has been suggested as a possible cause, there is no clear etiology.

Clinical features

Nodular fasciitis (Fig. 22.30) presents in the varied age group ranging from 3 to 81 years as a solitary white episcleral enlarging nodule at the limbus or over the sclera anterior to the insertion of one of the rectus muscles. The nodule may grow quickly and show signs of inflammation. Grossly, the lesions tend to be between 0.5 and 1.5 cm in diameter and tend to be round or oval. The specimen is not encapsu-lated. While benign, the tumour can be mistaken for malignancy. Proper identification is essential in helping direct appropriate treatment.

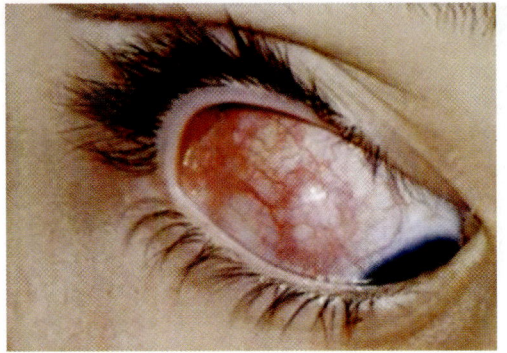

Fig. 22.30: *Nodular fasciitis in epibulbar tissues supero-temporally in an 11-year-old boy*

Histopathology

A histopathologic specimen is required for definitive diagnosis. The specimens tend to be sparsely cellular, with scant infiltration of lymphocytes and mononuclear cells. Gross samples are mostly made of spindle fibroblasts (non-atypical), myxoid ground substance, and vasculature. Mitotic figures may be identified, and it is important not to confuse this with a sarcoma.

Differential diagnosis

Nodular fasciitis may mimic episcleritis which is a benign recurring condition that often presents as hyperaemia, oedema, and infiltration, which are all limited to the episcleral tissue.

General considerations in the differentiation of nodular fasciitis and episcleritis are as follows: (1) Episcleritis tends to be a more lymphocytic reaction, whereas nodular fasciitis tends to be more of a fibrocytic reaction, (2) presence of a myxoid background points more towards nodular fasciitis, and (3) clinical history is important in making a diagnosis, i.e. the presence of systemic inflammatory illness increases the likelihood of nodular episcleritis.

Treatment

Differentiating between nodular fasciitis and episcleritis is important because the treatments differ.

For nodular fasciitis, conservative steroid treatment may be attempted first to shrink the growth. Ultimately, the standard of care treatment for nodular fasciitis is surgical excision.

In contrast, episcleritis is often managed conservatively. As it is not typically sight-threatening and is often self-limited, symptomatic relief is the goal of therapy. For example, topical lubricants and oral NSAIDs can alleviate the discomfort.

NEURAL TUMOURS

1. Simple neuroma and neurofibroma

Simple neuromas are soft mucosal neural tumours that appear in the conjunctiva and other mucous membrane in patients with multiple endocrine neoplasia. All such patients have prominent corneal nerves in 100% of cases.

Neurofibroma is a peripheral nerve sheath tumour that can occur in the conjunctiva as a solitary mass or as a diffuse or plexiform variety associated with von Recklinghausen's neurofibromatosis 1 (NF-1). Conjunctival neurofibromas can be divided into solitary, diffuse and plexiform types. The solitary type is not usually associated with NF-1, the diffuse type is sometimes associated with NF-1, and the plexiform type is generally considered to be almost pathognomic of NF-1.

Clinical features

Clinically, simple neuroma appears as pink-yellow and grows over time. There is significant association with medullary carcinoma of the thyroid and so ophthalmologists should be familiar with these conjunctival lesions.

Solitary conjunctival neurofibroma appears as a yellow-grey sessile or dome-shaped mass located in the conjunctival stroma. The sessile variant can have poorly defined margins. The plexiform variant is an ill-defined, firm, irregular mass that has been likened to a bag of worms. The conjunctival plexiform neurofibroma is often in continuity with the same lesion of eyelid and orbit (Fig. 22.31).

Histopathology

Histopathologically, diffuse and plexiform neurofibromas are composed of bundles of enlarged nerves with proliferation of Schwann cells and endoneural fibroblasts in a mucoid matrix. A distinct perineural sheath defines the individual tumour cores. The localised

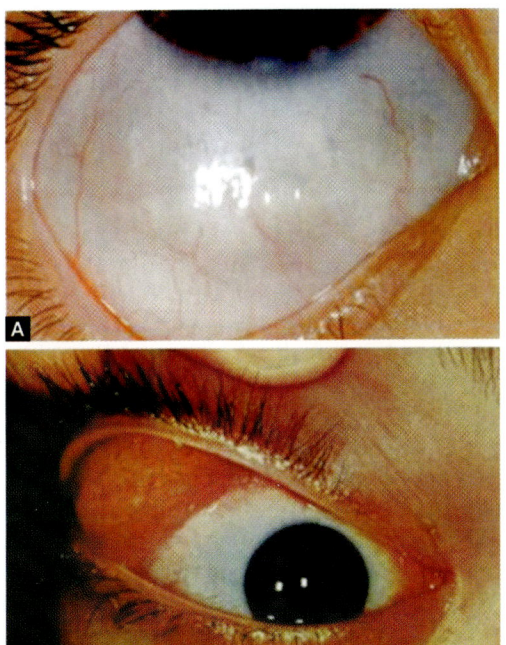

Fig. 22.31: *A, Very subtle diffuse neurofibroma of the inferior bulbar conjunctiva in a young girl with NF-1; B, Involvement of superior aspect of conjunctiva with plexiform neurofibroma in a 4-year-old girl with NF-1 (Courtesy: Frederick Blodi, MD)*

neurofibroma lacks a perineural sheath and is encapsulated. It can sometimes be difficult to differentiate from other spindle cell tumours and special stains for axons may help make the diagnosis in such cases.

Treatment

These benign neural tumours are generally asymptomatic and usually require no treatment. Occasionally, solitary tumours appear as slowly enlarging elevated stromal masses that can be managed by complete surgical resection. The plexiform type can be extremely difficult to remove intact and debulking procedures are often necessary. This can result in extensive scarring. The systemic prognosis is good, malignant transformation is extremely rare.

2. Schwannoma

Etiology

Schwannoma is the proper name for tumours developing from the Schwann cells of the neural

sheath in preference to the older terms, neurilemmoma and neurinoma, since the latter designate tumours containing connective tissue elements (i.e. neurofibromata).

Schwannomas are slow-growing, encapsulated, peripheral nerve sheath tumours that may be found in isolation or in association with von Recklinghausen neurofibromatosis. It has been proposed that these conjunctival schwannomas might arise from either the nasociliary nerves supplying the conjunctiva or the subconjunctivally lying autonomic nerve fibres. Overall, schwannomas typically appear in the third to fifth decades of life and demonstrate no sex predilection.

Clinical features

Conjunctival schwannomas have an indolent clinical course. They usually present as a slow-growing painless nodule on the conjunctiva/epibulbar surface (Fig. 22.32A). Since the bulbar conjunctiva is the most common site of this tumour, "epibulbar schwannoma" is probably the most apt description. In the conjunctiva, they present as a light pink-yellow, elevated mass that generally lies in the stroma of the bulbar conjunctiva or episcleral tissues. It is a slow-growing lesion that may have mildly dilated conjunctival or episcleral nutrient vessels.

Histopathology

Schwannomas are composed of a pure proliferation of Schwann cells. Two distinct, intermingling histologic patterns are seen (Fig. 22.32B): An Antoni A pattern of sheets of palisading spindle cells with spindle-shaped nuclei forming Verocay bodies, and an Antoni B pattern of haphazardly arranged elongated cells in a myxoid stroma. Light-microscopic features of schwannoma are usually characteristic, but immunohistochemistry may be required in some cases.

Differential diagnosis

Schwannoma is not frequently included in the differential diagnosis of nonpigmented conjunctival masses, which consists of pingueculum, naevus, foreign body, neurofibroma, leiomyoma, fibrous histiocytoma, dermoid,

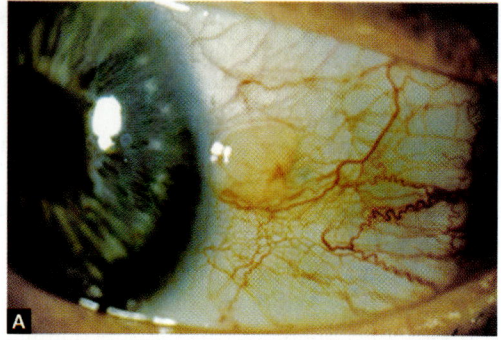

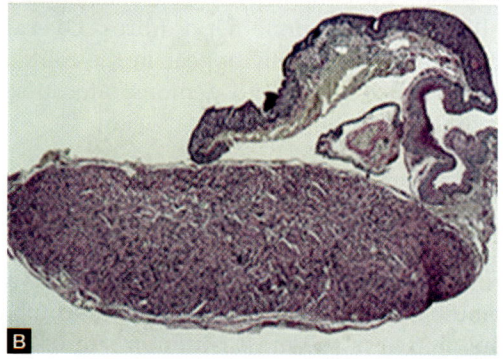

Fig. 22.32: *A, An elevated, well-circumscribed, mobile, yellow, perilimbal conjunctival lesion at the 3 o'clock position; B, HPE showing spindle cell morphologic characteristics which are suggestive of Antoni A and B patterns*

squamous and sebaceous cell carcinomas, and amelanotic malignant melanoma.

Treatment

The treatment of epibulbar schwannomas is complete excision. While excising, one must be careful to excise it in-toto and prevent damage to the underlying sclera. Additional double freeze cryotherapy to the base, namely the underlying scleral bed if the mass is found to be adherent to underlying sclera peroperatively. However, it is unlikely that cryotherapy has any role in preventing recurrence, given the benign pathology of the tumour. Furthermore, no malignant transformation is noted. Epibulbar or conjunctival schwannoma can be best described as a common tumour at an uncommon site.

3. Granular cell tumour

Etiology

Granular cell tumour (GCT), also known as myoblastoma, is extremely rare. It is an uncommon neoplasm for which the pathogenesis is uncertain and disputed. Originally thought of having a striated muscle origin, recent suggestions are that it is of neural derivative, Schwann cell origin.

Clinical features

It is seen as a pink elevated smooth mass of the conjunctival stroma. It is clinically indistinguishable from most other well circumscribed, nonpigmented conjunctival neoplasms (Fig. 22.33A).

Histopathology

Microscopically, GCT consists of (Fig. 22.33B) cords and lobules of round, benign cells with a pronounced granular cytoplasm. Pseudoepitheliomatous hyperplasia of the overlying conjunctival epithelium is a recognized feature of this tumour. Based on electromicroscopic studies, it has been suggested that the cells may be modified Schwann cells, although the precise histogenesis of the tumour is still disputed. A malignant variant of this tumour may be indistinguishable from alveolar soft part sarcoma. Granular cell tumour is rarely diagnosed clinically.

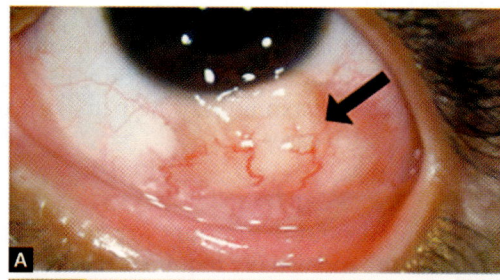

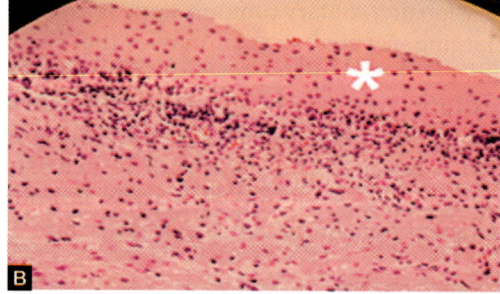

Fig. 22.33: *A clinical aspect. A, Yellowish mass in the temporal area from the bulbar conjunctiva (arrow); B, Microphotography. At lower magnification, tumour cells can be identified under a normal conjunctival epithelium (asterisk)*

Treatment

Treatment is by complete excision.

HISTIOCYTIC TUMOURS

1. Xanthoma

Etiology

Xanthomas are nodular masses of lipid-laden histiocytes which may contain scattered Touton giant cells and are usually a manifestation of a group of diseases which are collectively referred to as the xanthomatoses. They occur in the systemic lipoidoses, in patients with increased serum lipids, and in apparently normal individuals.

Clinical features

Xanthoma presents as a yellow subepithelial mass on the epibulbar surface (Fig. 22.34A). These lesions may be solitary or may be seen as multiple plaques or papules with a characteristic distribution. In xanthoma disseminatum, multiple limbal lesions are found in both the eyes.

Histopathology

Microscopic examination revealed dense infiltration of the corneal stroma by macrophages containing foamy cytoplasm. A few lymphocytes were scattered in each field. The pathological diagnosis was "xanthoma" (Fig. 22.34B).

Treatment

Treatment is by complete excision.

2. Juvenile xanthogranuloma

Etiology

Juvenile xanthogranuloma (JXG) is an idiopathic cutaneous eruption of childhood characterised by solitary or multiple, yellow red, transient papules. In ocular region it is best known for causing an iris mass that can produce a spontaneous hyphaema. It can also affect the eyelid, conjunctiva and orbital tisssues. There are isolated case reports of juvenile xanthogranuloma of the conjunctiva in children.

Clinical features

Conjunctival involvement usually occurs as a solitary lesion unassociated with the skin

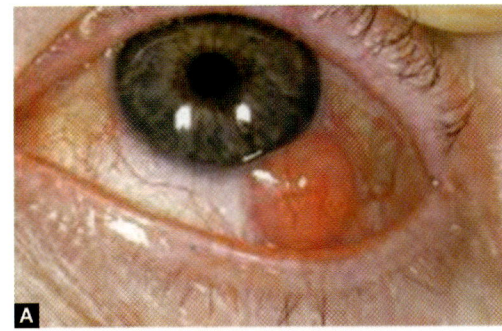

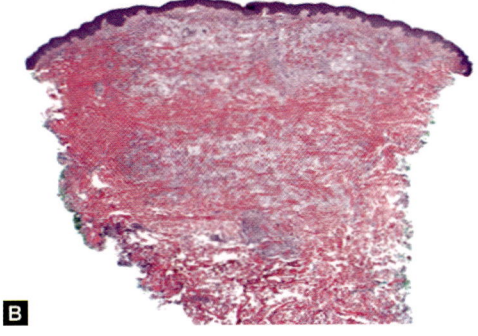

Fig. 22.34: *A, Conjunctival xanthoma; B, HPE: Dermal foamy histiocytes with admixed neutrophils and extravascular lipid*

eruption. It appears as a yellow elevated lesion, usually near the corneoscleral limbus in any quadrant. Although cutaneous and iris JXG classically appear in infancy or childhood, JXG on the conjunctiva often appears as a solitary mass and often has its onset in adulthood. This adult-onset xanthogranuloma seems to be identical clinically and histopathologically to the infantile or juvenile form (Fig. 22.35A).

Histopathology

Histopathologically, JXG is a mass composed of lipid histiocytes, chronic inflammatory cells and Touton giant cells, which typically have a ring of lipid around a focus of granulomatous inflammation. Fine blood vessels ramify through the lesion (Fig. 22.35B).

Differential diagnosis

The differential diagnosis of a yellowish conjunctival mass, with or without limbal involvement, includes epibulbar dermoid, dermolipoma, and, less frequently, phlyctenular keratoconjunctivitis, neurofibroma, fibrous histiocytoma, pterygium, pyogenic granuloma,

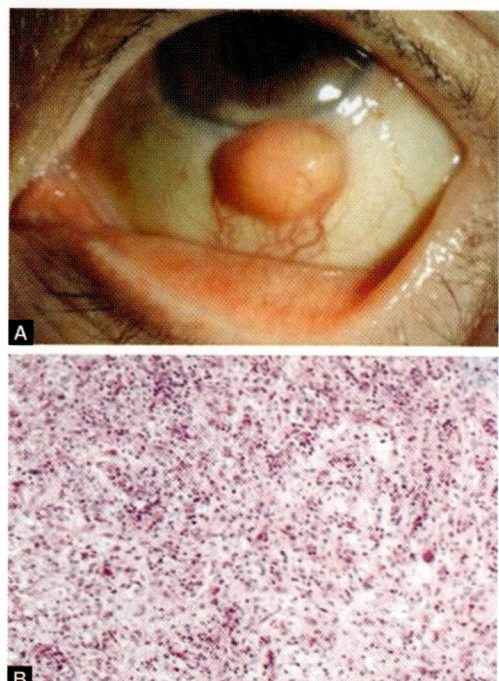

Fig. 22.35: *A, Yellow-orange subconjunctival mass with feeding vessels at the limbus. The overlying conjunctiva was intact; B, HPE showing a mixed inflammatory lesion composed of dense infiltrates of epithelioid histiocytes with foamy cytoplasm, lymphocytes, plasma cells, and multinucleate giant cells*

and foreign body granuloma, as well as other primary and secondary inflammatory lesions such as JXG and Langerhans cell histiocytosis.

Treatment

Most conjunctival JXG lesions have been excised because the diagnosis was uncertain clinically. However, if the diagnosis is suspected clinically, a period of observation is justified, the lesion is said to resolve without treatment. Topical or oral corticosteroids can be employed for cases that do not resolve. Recurrence after complete excision is rare.

3. Reticulohistiocytoma

Etiology

Reticulohistiocytoma (RH) is a rare benign histiocytic lesion that is often a part of a systemic disorder known as multicentric reticulohistiocytosis.

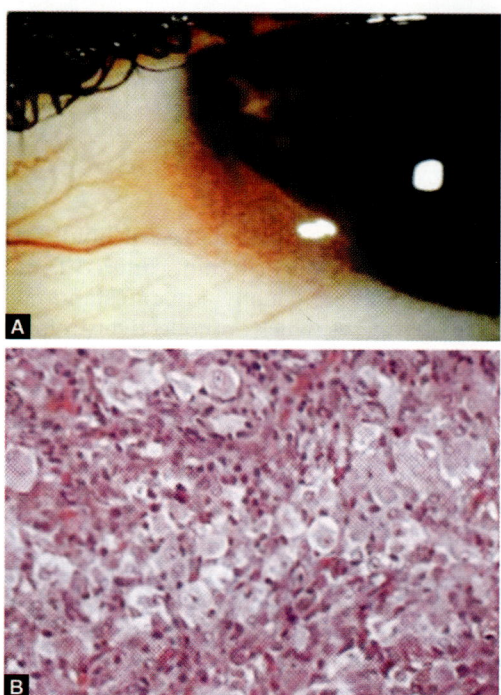

Fig. 22.36: *A, Localised reticulohistiocytosis at the limbus; B, HPE showing large histiocytes with granular cytoplasm*

Clinical features

Although multiple lesions can occur on the eyelid in association with multicentric histiocytosis, cases reported in the conjunctiva have been in adults and appeared as localised masses at the corneoscleral limbus without systemic evidence of multicentric reticulohistiocytosis (Fig. 22.36A).

Histopathology

RH is composed of large mononuclear or multinucleated cells with fine granular 'ground glass' cytoplasm and large nuclei with prominent nucleoli (Fig. 22.36B). It differs from juvenile xanthogranuloma in that it occurs in adults and lacks Touton giant cells histopathologically.

Treatment

RH should be included in the differential diagnosis of epibulbar benign histiocytic lesions. Management is complete surgical resection. The role of corticosteroids is unknown.

MYXOID TUMOURS

1. Conjunctival myxoma

Etiology

Conjunctival myxoma is a benign neoplasm presumably derived from primitive mesenchyme. It is a condition of adulthood with no predisposition for gender.

Clinical features

Myxoid tumours are rare benign stromal tumours, manifesting as slowly growing, asymptomatic freely movable unilateral, soft, pink white lesions usually seen in the temporal bulbar conjunctiva (Fig. 22.37A). Unlike naevus and lymphangioma which may appear similar, myxoma characteristically does not have cysts. However, the clear lesion can sometimes resemble a conjunctival cyst.

Carney complex

Conjunctival and eyelid myxoma can occur in association with an autosomal dominant condition called Carney complex, characterised by myxomas, spotty pigmentation of skin and mucous membranes, endocrine overactivity, and schwannomas. Most conjunctival myxomas have been solitary, without systemic evidence of Carney complex. However, any myxoma of the eyelid or conjunctiva should prompt evaluation for cardiac myxoma, a life-threatening condition. Eyelid and conjunctival myxomas can become apparent long before cardiac myxoma is recognised.

Histopathology

Histologically, they are hypocellular and are composed of stellate and spindle-shaped cells interspersed in the loose stroma. Cytoplasmic vacuoles are often present. Scattered mast cells may be present (Fig. 22.37B). Special stains and electron microscopy may help to differentiate myxoma from similar lesions like myxoid liposarcoma, spindle cell lipoma, myxoid neurofibroma, and rhabdomyosarcoma.

Treatment

Management is generally surgical resection, most excised lesions do not recur. If the

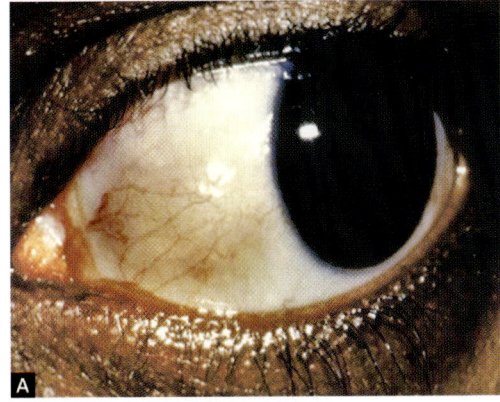

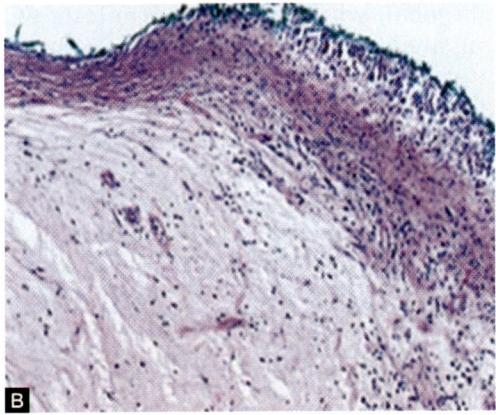

Fig. 22.37: *A, Conjunctival myxoma. Anterior segment of the left eye showing a well-circumscribed, yellow-pink, translucent mass with a solid basal part and a cystic apical part on the nasal bulbar conjunctiva; B, HPE showing relatively paucicellular nature of lesion and abundant mucoid material*

diagnosis is suspected and the lesion is small and asymptomatic, observation only may be appropriate.

MYOGENIC TUMOURS

1. Rhabdomyosarcoma

Etiology

Malignant tumours of the conjunctiva in children are rare, accounting for only 3% of conjunctival tumours. Rhabdomyosarcoma (RMS), while more commonly a primary orbital tumour, can present as a primary conjunctival lesion. The occurrence of rhabdomyosarcoma in the conjunctiva alone is rare, it generally has an orbital component. Most commonly the embryonal type manifests with a conjunctival component. Botryoid rhabdomyosarcoma may be seen in the conjunctival fornices.

Clinical features

Rhabdomyosarcoma presents as a pink, rapidly growing vascular conjunctival mass (Fig. 22.38A). It may appear as a pedunculated soft tissue mass but occasionally swelling and erythema precede the visible tumour.

Histopathology

The most common ophthalmic RMS subtype is embryonal, which typically manifests with elongated spindle or strap-like cells and scattered rhabdomyoblasts with eosinophilic cytoplasm. Although cross striations are a characteristic feature, they are absent in many cases. The botryoid variant of embryonal RMS is named for its grape-like appearance and is usually found in the mucous membrane of the urogenital tract or conjunctiva (Fig. 22.38B).

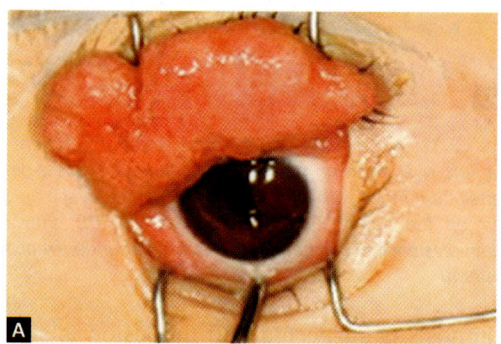
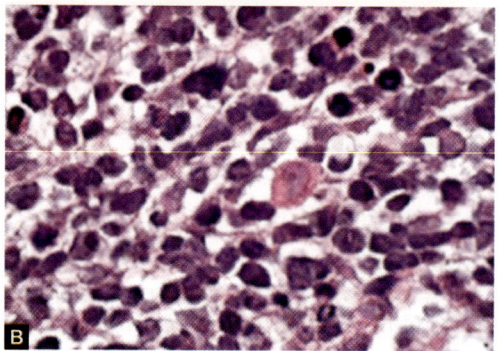

Fig. 22.38: *A, Conjunctival rhabdomyosarcoma. Eversion of the left upper eyelid revealing a large multilobulated forniceal mass; B, HPE: The conjunctival substantia propria contained scattered strap cells and rhabdomyoblasts*

Differential diagnosis

The clinical differential diagnosis includes progressive rapidly developing masses and inflammatory conditions of childhood, such as neuroblastoma, chloroma, lymphangioma, infantile haemangioma, cellulitis, and non-specific inflammatory diseases.

Treatment

Complete surgical excision with protocol-based adjuvant chemotherapy and radiotherapy is the treatment of choice for rhabdomyosarcoma localised to the conjunctiva. The prognosis for ophthalmic RMS has drastically improved during the past 40 years to a >90% survival rate based on a combination of surgery, radiotherapy, and chemotherapy.

LIPOMATOUS TUMOURS

1. Lipoma and liposarcoma

Etiology

Although lipomas, benign tumours of mature adipose tissue cells represent by far, the most common mesenchymal neoplasms, conjunctival lipomas are a very rare occurrence. Most lipomas reported at this anatomic location have been of the pleomorphic lipoma types or dermolipoma. It may exist as a hereditary condition and as a congenital anomaly.

Clinical features

It appears as a localised, circumscribed, elevated, freely mobile, non-pigmented, yellowish growth in the bulbar conjunctiva. The mass is easily compressible and does not significantly increase in size on pressing the eyeball (Fig. 22.39A).

Histopathology

Lipoma shows loose myxoid connective tissue with pleomorphic lipocytes, often with a spindle cell configuration. Floret giant cells and nuclear pyknosis, and characteristic bubbly nuclear vacuolations are also seen (Fig. 22.39B). There is an absence of mitotic activity. Liposarcoma is clinically similar to lipoma but on histopathology neoplastic stellate lipid cells and signet ring cells have been observed.

Differential diagnosis

The differential diagnoses include dermoid cyst, vasoformative and melanocytic lesions and both benign and malignant forms of epithelial and mesenchymal conjunctival tumours such as neurofibroma, dermatofibroma and a narrow range of carcinomata.

Treatment

It can be managed by surgical resection. Recurrence after complete surgical resection is unlikely.

2. Dermoid

Etiology

Conjunctival dermoid cysts are believed to result from embryonic sequestration of conjunctiva. Uncommon and small, conjunctival dermoid cysts are found anteriorly in the orbit, sometimes in the fornices or eyelids. These cysts typically involve soft tissue and do not erode bone.

Clinical features

Epibulbar dermoid is a well-circumscribed yellow white solid lesion involving the corneoscleral limbus. It most commonly occurs at the inferotemporal limbus and has fine white hairs that are best seen with slit lamp biomicroscopy (Fig. 22.40). It is not uncommon to see them associated with Goldenhar syndrome. Rarely, it can extend to the central cornea or be located in the other quadrants. In addition to becoming a cosmetic blemish, can cause severe astigmatism and amblyopia in some cases.

Histopathology

Histopathologically, epibulbar dermoid is a simple choristomatous malformation that consists of dense fibrous tissue lined by conjunctival epithelium with deeper dermal elements including hair follicles and sebaceous glands.

Treatment

Observation alone is preferred if the dermoid is small and does not cause visual symptoms. Larger demoids can be excised by lamellar keratosclerectomy with amniotic membrane grafting if the defect is superficial or closure using lamellar or full thickness corneal or sclerocorneal graft if the defect is deep or full thickness. While the cosmetic appearance does improve with surgery, the astigmatic error and visual acuity may not change significantly unless the child is treated early. It may have oncocytic differentiation.

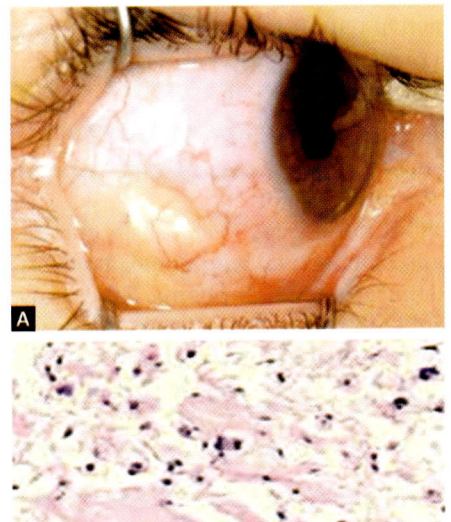

Fig. 22.39: *A, Conjunctival lipoma; B, HPE showing lobules of mature adipocytes with a delicate fibrovascular connective tissue stroma, a characteristic morphology of lipoma*

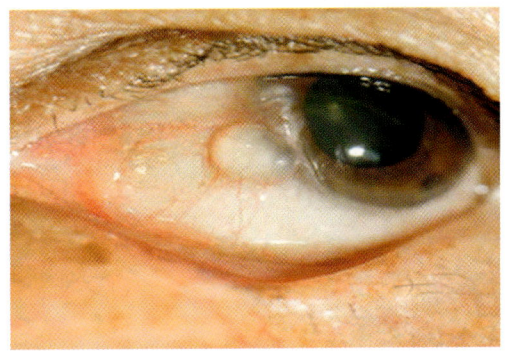

Fig. 22.40: *Conjunctival dermoid*

3. Dermolipoma

Etiology

Dermolipoma is an uncommon benign tumour. It constitutes 4.2% of all conjunctival lesions. Although dermolipoma is congenital and present at birth, it typically remains asymptomatic for years and may not be detected until adulthood.

Clinical features

The lesion presents as a pale yellow, soft, fluctuant, mass protruding from the orbit through the conjunctival fornix superotemporally (Fig. 22.41A). Unlike herniated orbital fat, dermolipoma may show the fine white hair on its surface.

Histopathology

Histopathologically, it is lined by conjunctival epithelium on its surface, and subepithelial tissue has variable quantities of collagenous

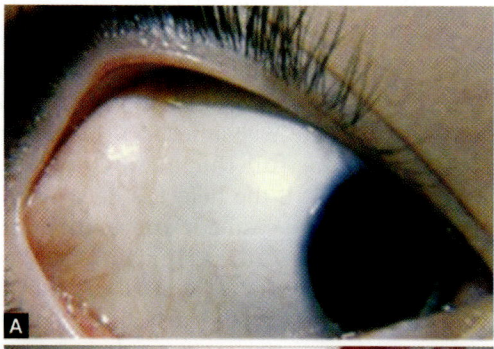

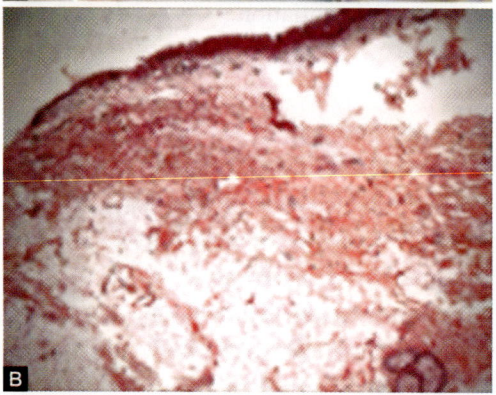

Fig. 22.41: *A, Dermolipoma; B, Conjunctival epithelium underneath which are mild mononuclear inflammatory cells and dense collagen beneath which are abundant adipose tissue containing few sebaceous glands and eccrine duct*

connective tissue and adipose elements (Fig. 22.41B). Pilosebaceous units and lacrimal gland tissue may occasionally be present.

Differential diagnosis

The appearance of dermolipoma closely resembles orbital fat prolapse and limbal dermoid and therefore, it is necessary to take this into account in diagnosis.

Treatment

No treatment is required unless for cosmetic considerations or in symptomatic patients with exuberant hair growth over the lesion. Visible portion of the dermolipoma may be debulked, and the ocular surface reconstructed with amniotic membrane graft.

LYMPHOPROLIFERATIVE TUMOURS

There are three major types of conjunctival lymphoproliferative lesions, varying from benign to malignant and present as a spectrum, but may appear identical clinically:

- Reactive lymphoid hyperplasia
- Atypical lymphoid hyperplasia
- Conjunctival lymphoma.

There is increasing emphasis that many conjunctival lymphomas may be low-grade B cell lymphomas of the mucosa-associated lymphoid tissue type (MALT). In one-third of patients, conjunctival lymphoma manifests with coexisting systemic lymphoma. Patients usually present with a conjunctival mass. They may also present with nonspecific irritation, ptosis, epiphora, blurred vision, proptosis, and diplopia.

Clinical features

Conjunctival lymphoproliferative lesions appear as diffuse, slightly elevated pink mass, resembling smoked salmon, seen mostly in the bulbar conjunctiva and fornix (Figs 22.42A and 22.43A). Some appear in the caruncle and plica, but very rarely in the palpebral conjunctiva. In the unilateral cases, chance of systemic lymphoma is 17%, and if bilateral cases, the chance is 47%. Systemic lymphoma occurs in 15% of patients at 5 years and 28% in 10 years.

Histopathology

Histopathologically, conjunctival lymphoproliferative tumours are composed of solid sheets of lymphocytes, with overlap between benign reactive lymphoid hyperplasia, atypical lymphoid hyperplasia, and malignant lymphoma. Benign reactive lymphoid hyperplasia is generally polymorphic, with well-differentiated lymphocytes and plasma cells, while lymphoma tends to be more monomorphic and poorly differentiated (Figs 22.42B and 22.43B). Most are non-Hodgkin's B cell lymphomas, whereas Hodgkin's and T cell lymphomas affect the conjunctiva rarely. Immunohistochemistry may be helpful in determining the cell types.

Prognostic factors for developing systemic lymphoma are forniceal or mid-bulbar location, multifocality, and bilaterality. There are several treatment options.

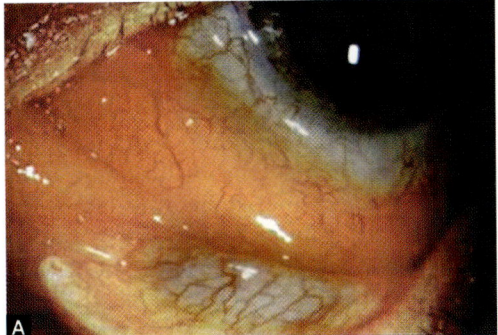
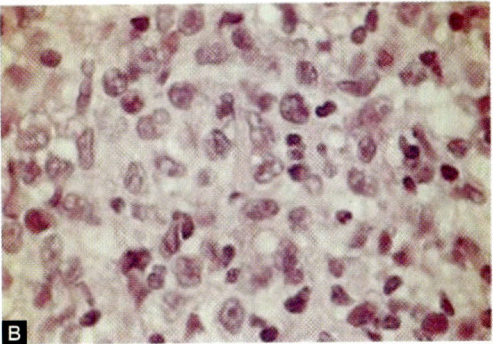

Fig. 22.43: *A, Diffuse lymphoma affecting wide area of inferior conjunctiva in a 62-year-old woman; B, Histopathology of malignant lymphoma showing more anaplastic lymphoid cells (hematoxylin and eosin × 200)*

Treatment

- Excision biopsy
- Cryotherapy
- Low-dose external beam radiotherapy
- Local injection of IFN-α
- Brachytherapy
- Chemotherapy if associated with systemic involvement.

CHORISTOMA

Etiology

Choristoma is derived from a Greek word *choristos* meaning "separated" and is defined as the presence of normal tissue in an abnormal location. It differs from hamartoma which is an excessive proliferation of normal tissue at the normal site and from teratoma which is a neoplasm comprising tissues from all three germ layers. Choristoma makes up about 3% of all conjunctival and corneal tumours. It is considered a simple choristoma when composed of

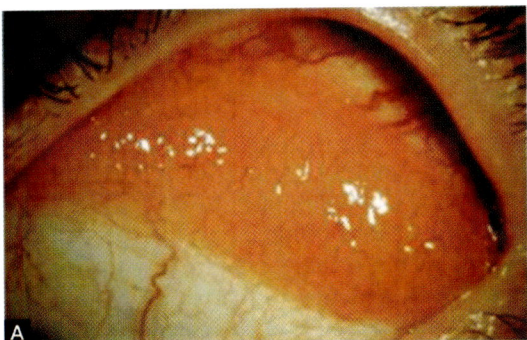
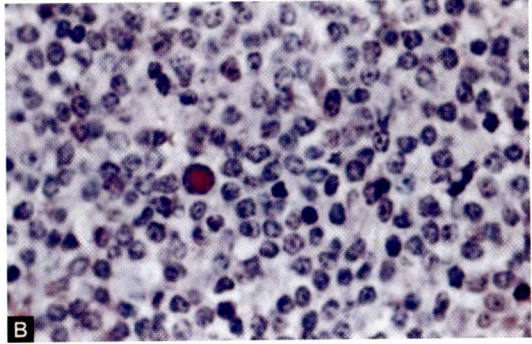

Fig. 22.42: *A, Conjunctival benign reactive lymphoid hyperplasia presenting as a diffuse elevated mass in the superior bulbar conjunctiva in a 38-year-old man; B, Histopathology of reactive lymphoid hyperplasia showing well-differentiated uniform lymphocytes. Near the centre of the field, not the cell with the large intranuclear inclusion body; referred to as a Dutcher body (hematoxyline and eosin × 200)*

one type of tissue and a complex choristoma when a combination of displaced tissue is involved.

Although choristomas can be seen in any age, these are common in children and are the most common epibulbar and orbital tumours among them. A variety of choristomatous lesions have been reported previously such as dermoid, dermolipoma, osseous choristoma, and lacrimal choristoma in different components of eye.

Clinical features

Ocular choristomas are most frequently epibulbar and located in the superotemporal quadrant near the superior and lateral rectus muscles (Fig. 22.44A). Epibulbar choristomas can be associated with eyelid and uveal coloboma, Goldenhar syndrome or organoid naevus syndrome.

Histopathology

Epipalpebral location is rare. Ocular choristomas contain a variable proportion of epithelium, dermal adnexa such as pilosebaceous or eccrine glands, adipose tissue, fibrous tissue, cartilage, bone, smooth muscle, and neural tissue (Fig. 22.44B).

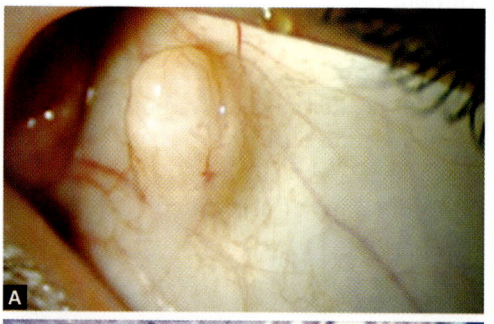

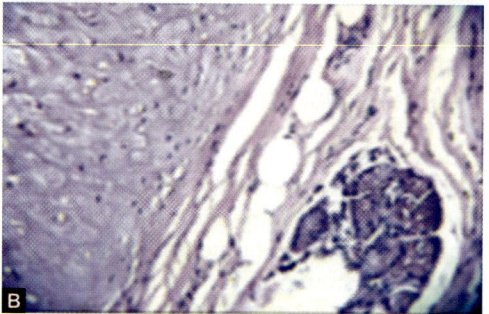

Fig. 22.44: A, Epibulbar choristoma; B, HPE showing mature cartilage and well-differentiated acinar structure

However, complex choristoma is a very rare entity which contains a variety of tissues derived from more than one germ cell layer.

Differential diagnosis

The differential diagnosis of a pediatric conjunctival mass includes the following entities: Limbal dermoid, myxoma, scleral melanocytosis, melanoma, Kaposi's sarcoma, sebaceous carcinoma, extraocular retinoblastoma extension, and intraorbital foreign body, among others.

Treatment

Treatment of complex choristoma depends on the size, location, and mechanical effect of the lesion. In general, wide excision of the lesion with closure is the treatment of choice. Sometimes, keratoplasty (when cornea is involved) and repair with amniotic membrane may be necessary.

■ CARUNCULAR TUMOURS AND CYSTS

Etiology

The caruncle lies at the inner canthus nasal to plica semilunaris, a unique anatomic structure containing elements of both conjunctiva and skin. The lesions occurring in the caruncle are similar to those that occur in mucous membranes and cutaneous structures. By histopathological analysis, 95% of the caruncular lesions are benign with the majority being either papilloma and melanocytic naevus, and 5% are malignant. Other lesions of caruncle include pyogenic granuloma, inclusion cysts, sebaceous hyperplasia, sebaceous adenoma, and oncocytoma.

Clinical features

Clinically, a caruncular tumour presents as an enlargement of the caruncle as a distinct mass arising from or displacing the caruncle. The clinical appearance varies with the type of tumour.

Papilloma generally appears as a frond-like mass with fine vascular tufts visible clinically in the central core of each frond.

Caruncular naevus usually appearing at about puberty is variably pigmented and may show slight change in size or colour with time. It generally contains clear cysts best seen with slit lamp biomicroscopy (Fig. 22.45A). Caruncular melanoma appears as a variably pigmented, usually noncystic solid mass.

Oncocytoma is a benign tumour that is believed to originate from transformed glandular epithelial cells particularly in the lacrimal gland, salivary glands and other organs. When it occurs in the caruncle, it appears as an asymptomatic slowly growing reddish blue solid or cystic mass.

Histopathology

It most often occurs in older individuals. It is composed of benign epithelial cells with abundant eosinophilic granular cytoplasm (Fig. 22.45B). Electron microscopy shows large number of abnormal mitochondria.

Several sebaceous gland tumours and cysts can arise from the caruncle. Sebaceous gland hyperplasia and sebaceous adenoma may resemble each other clinically appearing as a smooth or multinodular yellow mass. Sebaceous gland carcinoma may also arise from sebaceous gland of caruncle. It can be aggressive and can metastasize.

Other lesions that can occasionally arise in the caruncle include metastatic carcinoid neoplasms, cavernous haemangioma, Kaposi sarcoma, lymphoma, adenosquamous carcinoma, dacryops and dermoid tumour.

Treatment

Management of a caruncular tumour is complete surgical excision when possible. We generally perform a circular incision through the conjunctiva and hook the medial rectus to prevent severing it. The tumour is then removed intact using a minimal manipulation or "no touch" method. We generally use supplemental cryotherapy. Squamous papilloma requires special precautions because like that in the caruncle disruption of the lesion can lead to shedding of viral particles into the surrounding tissue. Pedunculated papilloma is sometimes managed by clamping the base of mass with a haemostat and cutting beneath the haemostat removing the tumour intact. Another alternative is to freeze

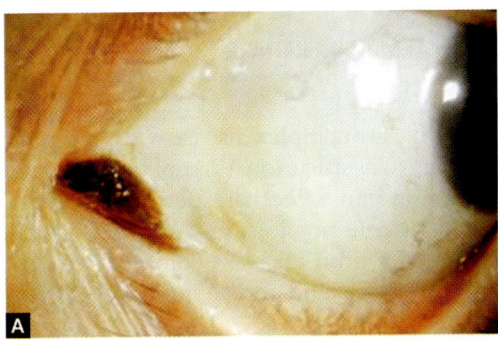

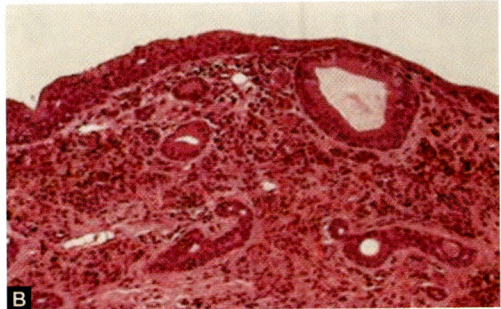

Fig. 22.45: *A, Cystic caruncular naevus in a 47-year-old woman; B, Histopathology of lesion shown in Fig. 22.45A depicting cystic structures and naevus cells in stroma of the caruncle (hematoxylin and eosin × 100)*

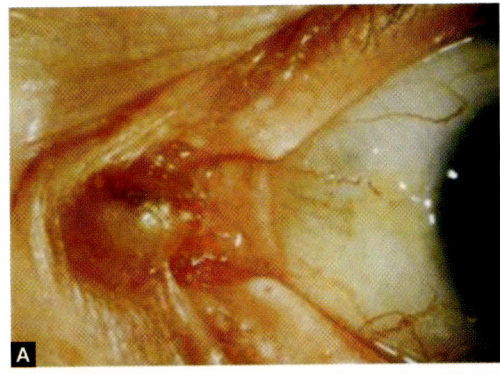

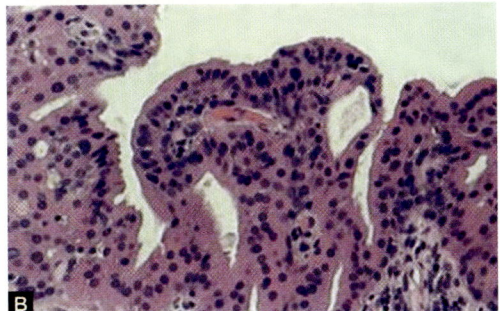

Fig. 22.46: *A, Caruncular oncocytoma in a 75-year-old man; B, Histopathology of lesion in Fig. 22.46A showing lining of cystic area with epitheilal cells with granular cytoplasm (hematoxylin and eosin × 75)*

the lesion using the cryoprobe and cutting the base. Malignant tumour-like melanoma and sebaceous carcinoma may require wider excision and heavy cryotherapy because they have a greater capacity to invade into the deeper tissue. We often use punctual plugs in cases of primary acquired melanosis and melanoma to prevent seeding of tumour cells into the lacrimal drainage system.

METASTATIC AND SECONDARY TUMOURS

METASTATIC TUMOURS

Etiology

Most metastatic cancers to the ocular region involve the uveal tract and orbit. Eyelid and conjunctival metastasis are less common and individual cases are often reported. Conjunctival metastasis can occur from breast carcinoma, cutaneous melanoma, or other primary tumours. Most patients have a history of a primary malignancy but sometimes the conjunctival metastasis is the initial manifestation of a systemic cancer.

Clinical features

Clinically conjunctival metastasis appears as a rapidly growing sessile or nodular mass that has a yellow or fleshy colour. They may also appear as one or more fleshy pink vascularized conjunctival stromal tumours. The lesion can be diffuse or multifocal. Melanoma metastatic to the conjunctiva is usually pigmented but can be nonpigmented.

Histopathology

Histopathologically, conjunctival metastasis varies with the primary tumour and degree of differentiation of the metastatic focus. Some lesions like melanoma, breast cancer or renal cell carcinoma have characteristic features. Poorly differentiated tumours may require immuno-histochemistry to assist in confirming the primary site of involvement.

Treatment

In addition to the management of the primary neoplasm, the conjunctival metastasis may require specific management. A small lesion may be removed by local excision. Larger lesions may require an incisional biopsy to confirm the diagnosis. Needle biopsy can be performed but it generally yields less tissue thus making the diagnosis more difficult. If the patient is receiving specific chemotherapy for the primary lesion a conjunctival metastasis can be observed for a period of time to assess the response to chemotherapy. If conjunctival metastasis does not respond to chemotherapy it can be treated with irradiation. Plaque brachytherapy is another option in selected cases.

LEUKAEMIC INFILTRATE

Etiology

Leukaemia is a complex disease with continually changing classification. Virtually all types of leukaemia can affect the ocular structures, specially acute myeloid leukaemia. It usually involves the orbit and less commonly extends to involve the eyelid and conjunctiva. Conjunc-

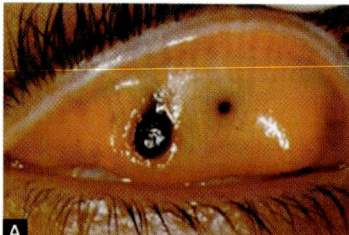 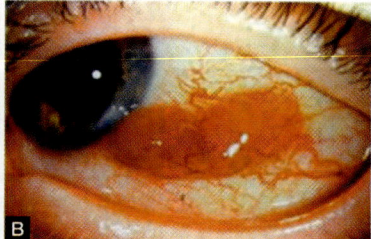 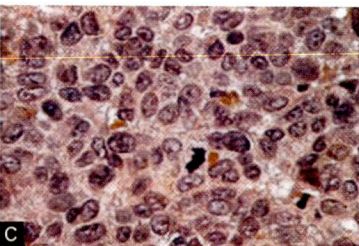

Fig. 22.47: *A, Everted left upper eyelid showing multiple foci of metastatic melanoma on the tarsal conjunctiva; B, Tan-coloured mass in bulbar conjunctiva of a 48-year-old woman with a history of cutaneous melanoma. She had no known metastasis at time of ocular presentation, but was subsequently found to have widespread metastases; C, Higher magnification of lesion in Fig. 22.47B showing the epithelioid melanoma cells. Note the mitotic figures (hematoxylin and eosin)*

tival involvement in patients with leukaemia usually takes the form of subconjunctival heamorrhage rather than direct infiltration of tissues with leukaemic cells. Conjunctival involvement can take place at any age depending on the type of leukaemia. It is often an early sign of relapse of previously treated disease.

Clinical features

In most instances, leukaemic infiltration of the conjunctiva has a similar appearance to lymphoma. It may be unilateral or bilateral with focal or diffuse lesions in the bulbar or palpebral conjunctiva. It has a spectrum of presentation, ranging from subconjunctival haemorrhage to direct infiltration of the tissue with leukaemic cells but often manifests as a firm, nontender, pink smooth mass associated with haemorrhage. It has the tendency to appear in the perilimbal tissue near the cornea.

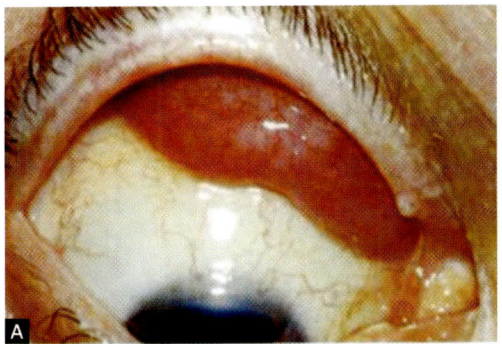

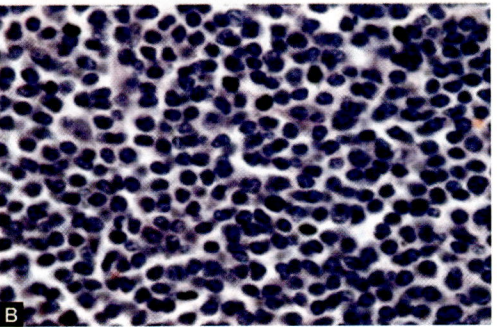

Fig. 22.48: *A, Infiltration of the superior conjunctival tissues with chronic lymphocytic leukaemia in an 87-year-old man; B, Histopathology of lesion in Fig. 22.48A, showing sheets of mononuclear cells with round to oval uniform nuclei (haematoxylin and eosin × 200)*

Histopathology

It is characterised by an infiltration of conjunctival stroma by leukaemic cells. The characteristics of the cell vary with the type of leukaemia. Special stains and immunohistochemistry may assist in characterising the nature of leukaemia.

Treatment

The management involves treatment of the systemic disease first. For cases that do not respond to such treatment, low dose radiotherapy can be very effective.

■ SECONDARY TUMOURS

Etiology

Some neoplasm can reach the conjunctiva and episcleral tissue by direct spread from an adjacent structure, such as the eyelid, orbit or sinuses. We can call such contiguous spread a "secondary conjunctival tumour" rather than a true metastasis.

The conjunctiva can be secondarily involved by tumours of adjacent structures, particularly by direct extension from the tumour of the eyelid. Intraocular and orbital tumours may also extend into the conjunctiva. Most important is the sebaceous gland carcinoma of the eyelid which can exhibit pagetoid invasion and direct invasion into the conjunctival epithelium. Uveal melanoma can extend extrasclerally into the subconjunctival tissues. Rhabdomyosarcoma of the orbit in children occasionally presents first with its conjunctival component.

■ BIBLIOGRAPHY

1. Bajaj MS, Pushker N, Kashyap S, Balasubramanya R, Chandra M, Ghose S. Conjunctival malignant melanoma. Orbit 2003; 22: 47–53.
2. Chaudhry IA, Al-Jishi Z, Shamsi FA, Riley F. Juvenile xanthogranuloma of the corneoscleral limbus: Case report and review of the literature. Surv Ophthalmol 2004; 49: 608–14.
3. Cohen VM, Tsimpida M, Hungerford JL, Jan H, Cerio R, Moir G. Prospective study of sentinel lymph node biopsy for conjunctival melanoma. Br J Ophthalmol 2013; 97: 1525–29.

4. Coupland SE, Heimann H, Kellner U, Bornfeld N, Foerster MH, Lee WR. Keratoacanthoma of the bulbar conjunctiva. Br J Ophthalmol 1998; 82: 586.

5. Folberg R. Melanocytic lesions of the conjunctiva. In: Spencer WH (Ed). Ophthalmic Pathology. An Atlas and Textbook. 4th ed. Philadelphia: WB Saunders. 1996; 125–47.

6. Jakobiec FA, Bhat P, Colby KA. Immunohistochemical studies of conjunctival naevi and melanomas. Arch Ophthalmol 2010; 128: 174–83.

7. Kaeser PF, Uffer S, Zografos L, Hamédani M. Tumours of the caruncle: A clinicopathologic correlation. Am J Ophthalmol 2006; 142: 448–55.

8. Kurumety UR, Lustbader JM. Kaposi's sarcoma of the bulbar conjunctiva as an initial clinical manifestation of acquired immunodeficiency syndrome. Arch Ophthalmol 1995; 113: 978.

9. Reddy S, Sundararama Sarma C, Ramana Rao VV, Banerjea S. Tumour and cysts of conjunctiva—A study of 175 cases. Indian Journal of Ophthalmology 1983; 31: 5: 658–660.

10. Santosh G Honavar, Fairooz P Manjandavida. Tumours of the ocular surface: A review Indian Journal of Ophthalmology 2015; 63(3): 187–203.

11. Shields CL, Demirci H, Karatza E, Shields JA. Clinical survey of 1643 melanocytic and non-melanocytic conjunctival tumours. Ophthalmology 2004; 111: 1747–54.

12. Shields CL, Shields JA. Tumours of the conjunctiva and cornea. Surv Ophthalmol 2004; 49: 3–24.

13. Shields JA, Shields CL. Eyelid, conjunctival and orbital tumours. An Atlas and Textbook. 2nd ed. Philadelphia, PA: Lippincott, Williams and Wilkins. 2008; 250–445.

14. Vassallo P, Forte R, Di Mezza A, Magli A. Treatment of infantile capillary haemangioma of the eyelid with systemic propranolol. Am J Ophthalmol 2013; 155: 165–70.

Ocular Surface
Squamous Neoplasia (OSSN)

GENERAL CONSIDERATIONS

INTRODUCTION

Ocular surface squamous neoplasia (OSSN) refers to a broad spectrum of dysplastic changes involving the epithelia of the conjunctiva, cornea, and limbus.

Histological subtypes that comprise OSSN are squamous dysplasia, conjunctival/corneal intraepithelial neoplasia, and squamous cell carcinoma (SCC). They represent the most common primary tumours of the eye among adults.[1] Also, OSSN is the most common non-pigmented malignant disease of the surface of the eye, comprising 7% of all conjunctival tumours. Although uncommon, they can cause ocular and at times systemic morbidity, hence their significance. The first case was described in 1860 by von Graefe,[1] subsequently it has been extensively studied and reported, as a result, a range of management options are now available depending on the stage of the disease.

Earlier various terms like epithelial plaque, intraepithelial epithelioma, Bowen's disease, Bowenoid epithelioma, and precancerous epithelioma were used for non-invasive forms of squamous neoplasms. Pizzarello and Jakobiec[2] classified conjunctival intraepithelial neoplasms as mild, moderate and severe dysplasia based on the extent of involvement on histopathology. Lesions that involved the basal one-third of the conjunctiva were classified as mild, those involving the inner two-thirds were classified as moderate, and lesions that were full thickness were termed severe dysplasia. Waring et al[3] extended the term to include the cornea, and Erie et al[4] further extended it to include invasive neoplasia.

The term ocular surface squamous neoplasia (OSSN) was given by Lee and Hirst[5] and it has been classified into three grades: (i) Benign dysplasia, (ii) preinvasive OSSN; and (iii) invasive OSSN. Papilloma, pseudotheliomatous hyperplasia and benign hereditary intraepithelial dyskeratosis represent benign dysplastic changes. Conjunctival/corneal carcinoma *in situ* comprise preinvasive OSSN. Invasive OSSN consists of squamous carcinoma and mucoepidermoid carcinoma.

INCIDENCE

The overall estimated prevalence of OSSN is 1.9 per 100,000 per year.[6,7] Its incidence is between 0.02 to 3.5 per 100,000; it is relatively common in Australia and African/tropical countries.[8,9] In the last few decades, an increase in the incidence of OSSN has been observed in these countries, and reported to be associated with sun exposure, human immunodeficiency virus (HIV), and human papillomavirus (HPV) infection.[10] It is predominantly seen in males, although reported to be predominant in females in sub-Saharan Africa. This may be related to Africa having the highest prevalence of both HIV and HPV, which may increase the risk of OSSN in women and gender differences in mortality of HIV infected adults.[9]

Ocular surface squamous neoplasia is mostly unilateral and is seen in middle-aged and older patients. Rarely, it is bilateral in immunosuppressed patients. The average age of occurrence has been noted to be 60 years, ranging from 20 to 88 years.[11] Patients of xeroderma pigmentosum and human immunodeficiency virus (HIV) develop OSSN at a younger age. Young patients of HIV are more prone to develop aggressive OSSN.

ETIOPATHOGENESIS

OSSN is associated with certain risk factors which include sunlight exposure, human papillomavirus infection, history of actinic skin lesions (xeroderma pigmentosum), increased p53 expression, HIV seropositivity, chemical exposure (trifluridine, beryllium, arsenicals, petroleum products), heavy cigarette smoking, light pigmentation of the hair and eyes, ocular pigmentation, ocular surface injury, vitamin A deficiency, mechanical trauma (e.g. ocular

prosthesis) and contact lens users. Other conditions in which OSSN has been reported are ocular cicatricial pemphigoid, non-Hodgkin's lymphoma, epidermodysplasia verruciformis and hepatitis C virus infection.[12–16] Chronic inflammation associated with atopic keratoconjunctivitis may be a risk factor for the development of bilateral, diffuse, invasive, and recurrent OSSN.[17] OSSN has also been reported in association with Papillon Lefèvre syndrome.[93,94]

1. **Ultraviolet B light** (UV B). Higher incidence of OSSN seen in residents of lower latitudes near to the equator, in males (predominant outdoor activity), in fair skinned individuals and in individuals with actinic skin lesions (xeroderma pigmentosum), strongly suggest sunlight exposure as a major etiological factor. UV B causes pyrimidine dimer formation and damage to nucleotide excision repair which is responsible for the repair of DNA. In addition, it has also been seen to cause p53 mutation which is reported in OSSN.[18] Xeroderma pigmentosum (XP) is an autosomal recessive disorder with defective DNA repair mechanism which predisposes to OSSN with aggressive clinical presentation at a younger age. OSSN has been reported as early as 3 years of age in a patient of XP.[19] Scholz et al identified telomerase reverse transcriptase (TERT) gene promoter mutations in 44% of 48 samples of conjunctival OSSN. They found that the TERT mutational profile supported ultraviolet light induction as the major source of the malignancy. However, there was no relationship with tumour recurrence comparing those with versus without TERT mutation.[48]

2. **Human papillomavirus.** HPV genotypes 6 and 11 have been demonstrated in a large number of papillomas as well as dysplastic and malignant lesions of the cornea and conjunctiva. Deoxyribonucleic acid (DNA) and messenger ribonucleic acid (mRNA) of HPV 16 and 18 have been shown in conjunctival intraepithelial neoplasia (CIN) cases proving a causal relationship. Further, it has been demonstrated that the protein coded by the E6 region of HPV 16 and 18 forms a complex with the protein coded by the p53 tumor suppressor gene in the host.[20]

3. **Human immunodeficiency virus.** In the HIV-positive population, there is a 12-fold increase in risk of OSSN.[21] Few studies have shown OSSN in young may be a marker for HIV infection.[21,22] OSSN in HIV-positive patients is more aggressive with larger and thicker tumours, higher incidence of deep invasion, and poorer prognosis, requiring enucleation or exenteration, than in the more common demographic of older, fair-skinned patients.[23]

4. **Stem cell theory.** OSSN may represent the abnormal maturation of corneal and conjunctival epithelium as a result of a combination of damaging factors to the limbal transition zone such as UV B irradiation and HPV.

5. Role of **ATP-binding cassette subfamily B member 5** (ABCB5). ABCB5 is a new member of the ATP-binding cassette super-family and has been identified as an important factor in regulating progenitor cell fusion, multidrug sensitivity and cellular melanogenesis. The expression of ABCB5 is upregulated in OSSN and that elevated expression of ABCB5 may be involved in the pathogenesis of OSSN.[24]

CLINICAL FEATURES

OSSN typically presents as a growth on the ocular surface and gives rise to symptoms like foreign body sensation, redness or irritation and rarely, diminution of vision due to high astigmatism or involvement of visual axis. OSSN lesions are usually located within the interpalpebral fissure at the limbus in the nasal quadrant, which receives the highest intensity of sunlight[9] (Fig. 23.1A). They are slightly elevated lesions, pearly grey in appearance, with or without well-defined borders. The tumor appears as fleshy or nodular, sessile minimally elevated lesion with surface keratin, feeder vessels (sentinel vessels), and secondary inflammation[5,25–27] (Figs 23.2A and 23.3A).

Rose bengal staining is helpful in the diagnosis and delineation of the tumor extent. Sometimes, these lesions have pigmentation (Fig. 23.3A) when it becomes difficult to distinguish it from melanoma. The tumor may extend for a variable distance into the adjacent corneal epithelium and appear as a subtle wavy, advancing, grey,

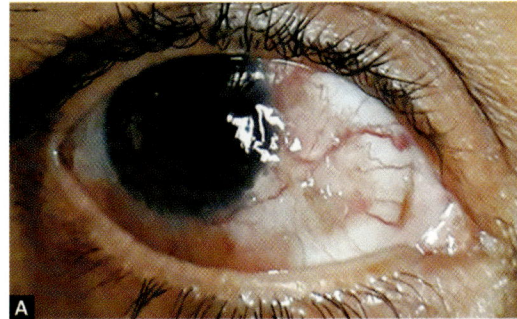
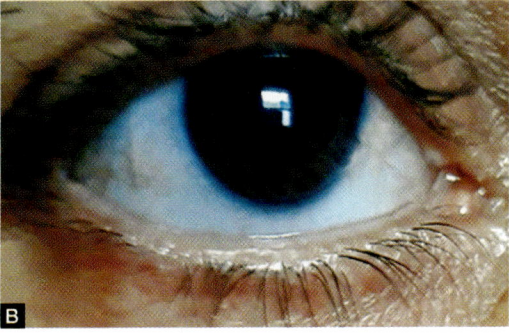

Fig. 23.1: *A, Clinical picture showing diffuse gelatinous ocular surface squamous neoplasia right eye; B, Complete resolution post-treatment with topical interferon at 3 months*

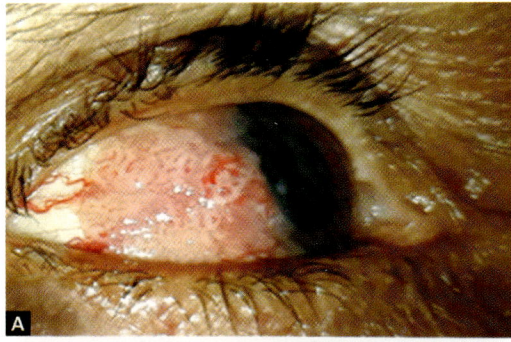
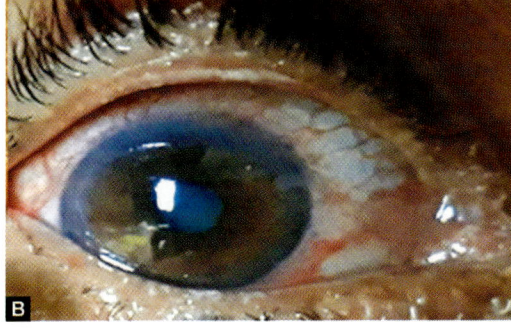

Fig. 23.2: *A, OSSN post-treatment failure with MMC drops; B, Treated with interferon eye drops*

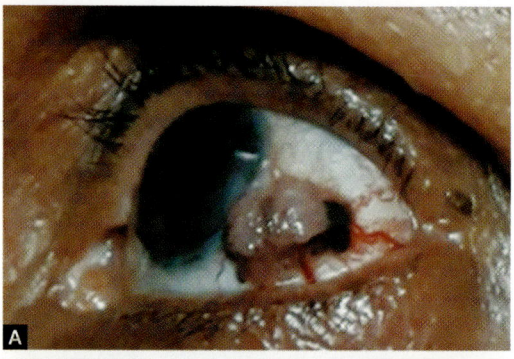

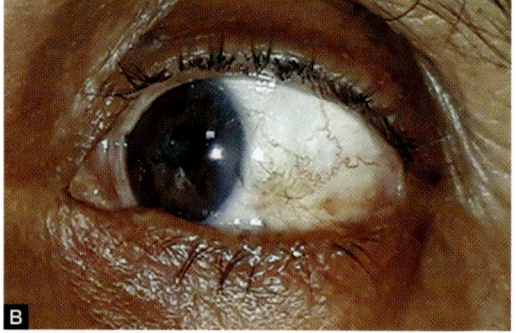

Fig. 23.3: *A, Pigmented OSSN; B, Treated with perilesional injection of interferon alpha 2b*

superficial opacity that may be relatively avascular or may have fine blood vessels. The presence of feeder vessels and intrinsic vascularity favours SCC. Although greater thickness is believed to be a sign of malignant transformation, there are thick tumors that remain within the epithelium. It is also important to examine the tarsal conjunctiva after everting the eyelid of patients with OSSN to detect contiguous or multifocal involvement of the tarsal conjunctiva.

MORPHOLOGICAL CLASSIFICATION

Conjunctival lesions

1. **Gelatinous:** Circumscribed gelatinous lesions are the most common OSSN lesions. The nodular lesion causes suspicion of invasive SCC. The nodular type is rapidly growing with a high incidence of metastasis to adjacent lymph nodes. The diffuse type is the least common and in the early stages presents as persistent redness of the conjunctiva, is slow growing and mimics chronic conjunctivitis.[28]

2. **Leukoplakic:** These are usually preinvasive. Leukoplakia is usually absent or minimal in CIN; extensive leukoplakia raises the suspicion of malignancy.

3. **Papilliform:** These are typically exophytic, strawberry like, with a stippled red appearance corresponding to its fibrovascular core. They are clinically benign.

Corneal lesions

Corneal OSSN lesions are preinvasive, with a mottled ground glass sheet appearance which is opalescent. They have sharply defined fimbriated borders, the convex leading edge spreads in an arc away from the limbus and often white dots are present over the grey epithelium. They are usually avascular. These lesions are typically indolent, slow growing and prone to recurrence.

Advanced cases can infiltrate the cornea and sclera to have the intraocular extension.[29] Noduloulcerative lesions are associated with high risk of intraocular invasion. Rarely, the tumor may extend into the orbit causing proptosis. The tumor can metastasize to the regional lymph nodes and rarely distant metastasis may occur. Aggressive variants include spindle cell squamous carcinoma, mucoepidermoid carcinoma, and adenoid SCC.[5,25,26,30,31] According to the American Joint Committee on Cancer (AJCC)—tumor, node, and metastasis (TNM) classification, SCC is classified depending on the size, tumor location, and extent of involvement (Table 23.1).

OSSN can mimic various conditions, it could present or be misdiagnosed as pannus, corneal ulcer,[32] pinguecula, pterygium,[33] pyogenic granuloma, keratoacanthoma, pseudoepitheliomatous hyperplasia, actinic keratosis, sclerokeratitis,[34] blepharoconjunctivitis,[28] nodular scleritis,[35] hereditary benign intraepithelial dyskeratosis, vitamin A deficiency, naevi, malignant melanoma and PUK.[36]

DIAGNOSTIC TESTS

IMPRESSION AND EXFOLIATIVE CYTOLOGY

Impression cytology (IC): In this superficial epithelial cells are collected by applying

Table 23.1: *AJCC 8th edition classification of conjunctival carcinoma (OSNN)*

Definition of primary tumor (T)

TX Primary tumor cannot be assessed

T0 No evidence of primary tumor

Tis Carcinoma *in situ*

T1 Tumor (≤5 mm in greatest dimension) invades through the conjunctival basement membrane without invasion of adjacent structures

T2 Tumor (>5 mm in greatest dimension) invades through the conjunctival basement membrane without invasion of adjacent structures

T3 Tumor invades adjacent structures* excluding the orbit

T4 Tumor invades the orbit with or without further extension

   T4a Tumor invades orbital soft tissues, without bone invasion

   T4b Tumor invades bone

   T4c Tumor invades adjacent paranasal sinuses

   T4d Tumor invades brain

Definition of regional lymph nodes (N)

NX Regional lymph nodes cannot be assessed

N0 Regional lymph node metastasis absent

N1 Regional lymph node metastasis present

Definition of distant metastasis (M)

M0 Distant metastasis absent

M1 Distant metastasis present

Definition of histopathologic grade (G)

GX Grade cannot be assessed

G1 Well differentiated

G2 Moderately differentiated

G3 Poorly differentiated

G4 Undifferentiated

*Adjacent structures include cornea, forniceal conjunctiva, palpebral conjunctiva, tarsal conjunctiva, lacrimal punctum and canaliculi, plica, caruncle, anterior or posterior eyelid lamellae, eyelid margin, and/or intraocular compartments. (Data adapted from AJCC Cancer Staging Manual. 8th ed. Switzerland: Springer. 2017; 787793).

collecting devices [either cellulose acetate filter paper (CAP) or Biopore membrane device (Millipore Corp, Bedford, MA)] such that the cells adhere to the surface and are removed from the eye to be fixed, stained, and then mounted on a slide for analysis.[37] It has the advantage of maintained cell-to-cell relationship as compared

to exfoliative cytology.[38] However, these specimens require immediate processing. Using CAP for specimen collection, an 80% correlation was found between impression cytology, diagnosis and histopathology specimens obtained from incisional biopsy. Biopore membrane has better cell adherence and can be stored for subsequent analysis making it the procedure of choice.[39] Nolan et al found that 55% of intraepithelial OSSN cases diagnosed by IC had keratinized dysplastic cells often accompanied by hyperkeratosis, 35% had large syncytial-like groups, and 10% had non-keratinized dysplastic cells as a predominant feature.[38] However, it is not possible to differentiate intraepithelial lesions from invasive squamous cell carcinoma given the superficial sampling of cells.[38]

Exfoliative cytology (EC): This technique uses a cytobrush which is particularly suited as malignant cells have poor cell to cell adherence and tend to desquamate when located on the mucosal surface. After instillation of anaesthetic eye drops, samples for cytology are collected with the help of a specific brush with plastic bristles and a blepharostat. The material is then smeared onto a slide and fixed with 90% alcohol spray, and subsequently sent for analysis by the cytopathologist after staining with the Papanicolaou method.[40]

Both IC and EC may also be used to monitor regression of lesion and response of the lesion to chemotherapeutic modulators. There are pitfalls using these modalities as the only diagnostic tool. Keratinizing malignancies offer the highest chance of false negatives because of paucity of cells in the specimen and should be kept in mind in such cases. Cytological features that reliably differentiate carcinoma *in situ* (CIS) from invasive carcinoma are yet to be identified. Several patients may have histological CIN or partial thickness epithelial atypia adjacent to the invasive disease, which would not necessarily yield sheets of atypical cells if sampled by impression cytology. Endophytic lesions and orbital invasion cannot be identified with impression cytology, limiting its use as a diagnostic aid.

DYE STAINING

It is another diagnostic test that is inexpensive and helpful in identifying OSSN. Diagnostic dyes like lissamine green and rose bengal are used to stain and delineate the extent of OSSN lesions but since these dyes are nonspecific and stain many other ocular surface conditions, it is not possible to diagnose OSSN with the use of these dyes alone. Other vital dyes that have been studied in the diagnosis of OSSN include toluidine blue (ToB) and methylene blue. ToB and methylene blue are acidophilic dyes that stain abnormal tissue dark royal blue. They have an affinity for nucleic acids, and given the increased nuclear material from high rates of mitoses and poor cell-to-cell adhesion in malignancy, these tissues stain more frequently than benign tissues.[22] Several studies have shown that ToB and methylene blue staining have a high sensitivity but low to moderate specificity in diagnosing OSSN compared to histopathology.[41–43]

HISTOPATHOLOGY

The gold standard for confirming diagnosis of OSSN is excisional biopsy for histopathology. The specimens may be obtained from excision biopsies in small lesions which can be removed in toto or incisional biopsies in cases of large infiltrating lesions. Papillomas demonstrate papillary fibrovascular fronds covered by acanthotic epithelium. This epithelium may show varying degrees of dysplasia, however, the cells have normal polarity and the basal layers are often unremarkable. Preinvasive OSSN are classified as mild, moderate or severe depending on the degree of involvement of the dysplastic epithelium. In mild (CIN grade I), dysplasia is confined to lower third of the epithelium. In moderate (CIN grade II), dysplasia extends into the middle third and full thickness dysplasia is termed severe (CIN grade III).

In conjunctival and corneal intraepithelial neoplasia (CCIN), epithelial cells are thickened, dysplastic, and irregular with increased cell proliferation. These changes affect less than the full thickness of the epithelium. When the abnormal cellular proliferation involves only partial thickness of the epithelium it is classified as mild CIN, a condition also called mild or moderate dysplasia. When it affects full thickness epithelium it is called severe CIN, a condition also called severe dysplasia. In these cases, there may be an intact surface layer of cells. Where there are no longer normal surface cells, that is the entire epithelium is involved but tumor cells have not yet invaded the substantia propria, the lesion is categorized as carcinoma *in situ*. Invasive squamous cell carcinoma is defined as when the lesion has affected the epithelial basement membrane and substantia propria.[44,45] CIN accounts for 39% of all premalignant and malignant lesions of the conjunctiva and for 4% of all conjunctival lesions.[46] Unlike CIN, incidence of invasive SCC is of much lesser frequency, varying from 0.02 to 3.5/100,000 population.[47] About 75% occur in men, 75% are diagnosed in older patients and over 75% occur at the limbus.[26–46] It can locally invade the sclera, uvea, eyelids, and orbit and has the ability to metastasize to distant sites thus potentially becoming life-threatening.[49]

In low-grade dysplasia cells show enlarged nuclei, hyperchromasia and irregular contour of the nuclear membrane with increased nuclear/cytoplasmic ratio. In high-grade dysplasia, there is pleomorphism of the nucleus with dyskeratotic cells.[5,50] The presence of syncytial sheath, nucleoli and infiltration of inflammatory cells is suggestive of invasive SCC.[51] Invasive OSSN show nests of infiltrating cells that have penetrated the epithelial basement membrane and spread into the conjunctival stroma. These cells can either be well differentiated and easily recognized as squamous, or poorly differentiated and difficult to distinguish. The latter are more uncommon and more aggressive. Two types of cells may be seen interspersed with squamous cells in these tumours: Spindle cells and mucoepidermoid cells.[52]

Electron microscopy: In cases of OSSN electron microscopy reveals excessive mitochondria, tonofilaments and endoplasmic reticulum; decreased desmosomes, alteration/absence of basement membrane and deposition of fibrillogranular material between the basement membrane and Bowman's layer.

ULTRASOUND BIOMICROSCOPY (UBM)

UBM provides cross-sectional visualization of the anterior segment in an intact globe at microscopic resolution.[53] In the 50 MHz mode, images to a depth of 5 to 6 mm at a resolution of 25 microns can be produced.[54] Studies on the use of UBM in diagnosing OSSN have shown that UBM is most useful in assessing intraocular tumor extension.[55,56] On UBM, the tumor surface is found to be hyperechoic while the tumor stroma is generally hypoechoic. Features suggestive of ocular tumor extension are blunting of the anterior chamber angle and uveal thickening, which correlated with histopathology findings. In patients with orbital extension, it has been reported that the relatively hypoechoic tumor can be differentiated from the more hyperechoic orbital tissues using UBM while 50 MHz images had better resolution, 20 MHz ultrasonography provided a deeper and wider field of view.[55]

ANTERIOR SEGMENT OPTICAL COHERENCE TOMOGRAPHY (ASOCT)

ASOCT provides noncontact, non-invasive, and high axial resolution cross-sectional imaging of various anterior segment conditions. The technology has undergone refinements, with transition from time-domain to spectral-domain OCT providing a better axial resolution and increasing scanning speed, leading to improved diagnostic imaging. A novel custom-built, ultra high-resolution, spectral-domain anterior segment OCT (UHR-OCT) has been developed with an axial resolution of approximately 2 μm for evaluation of corneal pathologic features.[57] UHR-OCT in ocular surface squamous neoplasia reveals epithelial thickening and increased reflectivity of the epithelium, and an abrupt demarcation from normal to abnormal tissue. Typically, there is sharp disparity in reflectivity of normal and diseased epithelium, allowing for exact localisation of the tumor margins.[58]

Using UHR-OCT, Kieval et al showed that an epithelial thickness value greater than 140 μm provided 94% sensitivity and 100% specificity for differentiating CCIN from pterygia.[59] In contrast, using HR-OCT with a resolution of 5–7 μm, Nanji et al demonstrated that an epithelial thickness cuts at greater than 120 μm provided 100% sensitivity and specificity for differentiating OSSN from pterygia.[60] Normal epithelium overlying subepithelial lesion effectively rules out OSSN.[61] UHR-OCT can also be used to diagnose pigmented CCIN, as demonstrated in the study by Shousha et al where UHR-OCT demonstrated thickened and hyperreflective epithelium in a pigmented conjunctival lesion that had been referred for conjunctival melanoma. Histopathology confirmed the diagnosis of pigmented CCIN.[61] UHR-OCT scan also be used to monitor disease resolution and detect residual subclinical disease. For lesions treated successfully with topical agents, post-treatment UHR-OCT showed normalisation of epithelial architecture at the site of the treated lesions. However, in lesions resistant to medical treatment, UHR-OCT will show persistently thickened epithelium with retained abrupt transition between normal and diseased epithelium.[62,63] UHR-OCT is also useful to rule out OSSN in the setting of complex ocular pathology and in clinically indeterminate lesions.[42] It has been used to show foci of OSSN in pterygia, Salzmann's nodular degeneration, HSV keratopathy, and atypical peripheral corneal infiltrates when the clinical diagnosis was unclear.[63]

CONFOCAL MICROSCOPY

In vivo confocal microscopy (IVCM) is a simple, safe, and relatively non-invasive diagnostic tool that can provide with the initial clinical diagnosis of OSSN, estimation of recurrence, management of treatment, and evaluation of response to topical chemotherapeutic agents in patients with conjunctival and corneal squamous lesions. When compared with a subsequent biopsy, cytological evaluation with *in vivo* confocal microscopy was capable to distinguish different stages of OSSN in all the cases.[51,64,65] The new generations of confocal scanning laser microscopes have an axial resolution of approximately 4 μm; however, the only disadvantage compared to UHR-OCT is that they provide a transverse view without reference to neighbouring corneal layers. The accuracy of diagnosis with cytological *in vivo* confocal microscopy could be improved by the implementation of automated image analysis which has been widely used in the interpretation of conjunctival and corneal exfoliative cytological analysis, and the acquired characteristics of cells were similar to those obtained from biopsies of OSSN.[66] In addition, *in vivo* confocal microscopy sampling from various ocular surface regions can offer a real-time monitoring of the extent and condition of tumor, and guide further managements.

In conjunctival and corneal intraepithelial neoplasia, IVCM shows regular conjunctival epithelium interspersed with complexes of enlarged, irregular cells with bright hyper-reflective and polymorphic nuclei.[67–69] Bright prominent nucleoli producing a starry night sky pattern has also been reported in these lesions.[70] Further, the authors have reported absence of sub-basal corneal nerves in areas of CCIN. Larger case series also demonstrated correlation between IVCM and histopathology findings.[51,70,71] Parrozzani et al in their series of 10 cases of OSSN reported that IVCM demonstrated dysplastic cells in each case and morphologic agreement with *ex vivo* scraping cytology and histology in 100% of cases.[51] A larger study conducted by Nguena et al showed a statistically significant difference between the normal controls and cases (benign and OSSN combined) but there was no difference between the benign and OSSN cases.[72] Therefore, there are limitations to the use of IVCM, it cannot reliably differentiate benign from OSSN lesions because of an overlap in IVCM features in the various ocular lesions, it provides only *en face* images in contrast to cross-sectional images obtained in tissue histology.[70] Also as it provides images at a cellular level, IVCM cannot provide a comprehensive scan of the entire ocular surface. Despite the limitations, IVCM can reliably predict the grade of dysplasia that is based on cellular morphology, nuclear atypia, and nuclear to cytoplasmic ratio, it can differentiate between invasive and *in situ* tumors, helpful in initial evaluation of subtypes of OSSN and could also be valuable in the setting of suspected recurrent tumours and in the follow-up evaluation of patients on topical chemotherapeutic agents.[73]

TREATMENT

SURGICAL TREATMENT

Surgery has been the treatment of choice as tissue diagnosis is considered essential before initiation of adjunctive therapy. Excision or incisional biopsy is an important initial step in the management as it is not possible to exclude invasive disease clinically or with impression cytology. Excision allows an immediate histopathological diagnosis, debulking, and excludes invasive carcinoma. The only disadvantage of primary excision alone is the high recurrence rate which ranges from 15 to 52%. Enucleation, and rarely exenteration may be required in cases of intraocular or intraorbital spread. In all cases a no-touch technique is used, and direct manipulation of the tumour is avoided to prevent tumour seeding.

'No-touch' surgical technique tumor resection is done under peribulbar anaesthesia. Phenylephrine 2.5% drops are used to induce vasoconstriction, thus reducing perioperative bleeding and allowing better visualisation of the corneal advancement of the tumor. A wide surgical excision with a margin of 3–4 mm on conjunctival side is done to maximize the chances of complete removal. Rose bengal/lissamine green staining is helpful to delineate the margins of the lesion. A 'no-touch' technique avoiding direct manipulation of the lesion, by holding the tissue at the healthy conjunctival borders is employed to prevent tumour seeding into new area. If the tumor is adherent to the sclera, a partial thickness sclerectomy is performed with crescent knife. The use of absolute alcohol on the corneal side of the lesion to facilitate epithelial removal as one sheet, i.e. alcohol epitheliectomy, is recommended. Once the lesion is removed *en bloc*, the specimen is marked in the proper orientation with sutures and then transferred to a piece of pencil-marked paper or the excised conjunctival specimen is placed on an absorbent paper and air-dried to prevent loss of orientation, and sent for histopathology in formalin.

Conjunctival defect so created can be closed primarily if less than three clock hours in diameter. Larger defects require either transpositonal conjunctival flaps, free conjunctival flaps from the other eye, or amniotic membrane grafts. Fibrin sealant tissue adhesive can be used to shorten the surgical time, mitigate inflammation postoperatively and improve patient discomfort.[74] Frozen section can be used to assess the adequacy of excision, and is accurate in delineating horizontal tumor spread. Bunns modification of Moh's technique of tumor margin surveillance may also be used. In this the free conjunctival edges are excised by 2 mm if residual tumor is evident even after excision of a 2 mm surgical margin.[75]

CRYOTHERAPY

Intraoperative cryotherapy is commonly used as an adjunctive therapy during excision of the lesion as it is known to decrease the recurrence rate by destruction of any residual tumour tissue beyond the horizontal or deep surgical margin of the wound. It lowers the temperature and also causes ischemic necrosis , thereby destroying the tumor cells. It has the advantage of reaching both tumor cell islands and deeply infiltrated cells, thus obviating the need for radical surgery. A nitrous oxide cryoprobe tip (2.5 or 5 mm) is used to form an ice ball extending 2 mm for conjunctiva, 1 mm for episcleral tissue and 0.5 mm for the cornea. A slow duration freeze with a slow thaw, repeated two times (freeze-thaw-refreeze) is recommended. It is important to include the limbal region during cryotherapy, and not apply the cryoprobe for more than three seconds. Both extensive surgical excision and cryotherapy can cause limbal stem cell insufficiency.

RADIOTHERAPY

Radiation as an adjuvant treatment after surgery has been used for OSSN. The various forms which have been described are external radiotherapy with protons,[76,77] electrons,[78] brachytherapy using strontium-90 (beta irradiation), orthovoltage external radiation, and stereotactic radiotherapy. For incompletely excised tumors Sr-90 brachytherapy with a concave 18 mm plaque size is an effective sole adjuvant treatment.[79] It can be given as 1 week schedule of 10 Gy daily for 5 days or a single fraction of 30 Gy as single dose treatment to facilitate compliance.

External radiotherapy using electrons is an effective treatment option for invasive orbital OSSN. It helps to preserve the eye and vision while providing good disease control and cosmesis. Electrons are the special particulate type of radiation which deliver high dose of ionizing radiation to the tumor. Electrons have the inherent capacity of treating the surface with no exit dose avoiding the collateral damage. Proton radiation delivers more three-dimensional conformal dose than electrons, especially sparing lens and posterior eye structures. Long-term studies involving larger number of patients are required to look into the efficacy and side effect profile in detail. Electron radiotherapy is inexpensive and more widely available, as compared to stereotactic radiotherapy or protons.

CHEMOTHERAPY

Topical chemotherapy is inexpensive, simple and reduces the risk of limbal stem cell deficiency, and obviates the need for clear tumor margins by treating the entire ocular surface, including the potentially dysplastic cells.[80] However, the drawback is the limited drug penetration in larger tumours, and a possibly deleterious effect on the ocular surface and nasopharyngeal epithelium on prolonged use.

1. **Mitomycin C:** It is an antimetabolite made from *Streptomyces caespitosus* and converted into an alkylating agent in tissues. It preferentially inhibits DNA synthesis in the G1 and S phases. As the hypoxia required for the intracellular reduction of MMC is greater in tumour tissue, it exhibits a certain degree of selectivity. MMC appears to produce cell death in OSSN by apoptosis and necrosis.[81] It is used in the concentration of 0.02–0.04% four times a day with one week on and one week off in alternating cycles for a maximum of 8 weeks. The one week on, one week off regimen prevents damage to more slowly dividing epithelial cells and limbal stem cells, allowing them to repair their DNA. Allowing time for complete epithelial healing before application of MMC is important in avoiding the more serious complications such as corneal epitheliopathy, scleral ulceration, uveitis, cataract, and glau-

coma. MMC related changes may persist in ocular surface epithelium for at least 8 months following MMC therapy. The other side effects include contact dermatitis, limbal stem cell deficiency and punctal stenosis.

2. **5-Fluorouracil** (5-FU): It is an antimetabolite that acts specifically during the S phase of the cell cycle. It is converted to 5-F DUMP, which inhibits thymydilate kinase thus preventing DNA and RNA synthesis. In contrast to MMC which acts on cells in all phases of the cell cycle, 5-FU inhibits cells that are in the S phase of the cell cycle, whereas dormant cells, such as part of the normal corneal and conjunctival cell population, can proliferate once treatment is completed. It is used as 1% in aqueous solution, four times a day over 4 weeks. Both MMC and 5-FU are currently being used four times daily for 1–2 weeks in a pulsed fashion, the treatment being repeated after every 1–2 weeks. This one week on and one week off drug regimen has the added advantage of good efficacy and better tolerance. Other regimens reported for topical 5-FU are 30 days on and 30 days off cycles, 2–6 courses of 2–4 days, with 30–45 days without any treatment. For nodular/thick lesions with limited superficial diffusion, surgical removal plus adjuvant topical chemotherapy remains the best option.[82–84]

IMMUNOTHERAPY

Recently immunotherapy has become a very popular modality of treatment in view of fewer side effects, better tolerability as compared to chemotherapeutic agents and high efficacy. It is being increasingly used as first line mono-therapy for OSSN lesions.

Interferon alpha 2b (IFN-α2b): It is a naturally occurring glycoprotein which binds to cell surface receptors affecting intracellular events resulting in antitumor and antiviral properties. Its efficacy in treatment of OSSN may be explained by the oncogenic link between HPV and OSSN. Topical drops and subconjunctival injections of IFN-α2b have been used as off-label therapy to treat OSSN. It has been used for extensive, multifocal or diffuse, residual, recalcitrant, recurrent lesions and for those that

involve the visual axis where surgery is not the treatment of choice. Topical IFN-α2b is used as 1 million international unit/ml (IU/ml) four times a day until resolution, and a month thereafter. The main drawback of topical interferon is its requirement of storage in refrigeration. Perilesional injections (3 million IU/ml) are being increasingly given to shorten the duration for complete resolution. Median time for resolution has been reported as 54 days (range 28–188 days), with a mean follow-up ranging from 2.9 to 18 months.[95] Experience from our centre shows a median time to complete resolution of 8 weeks with eye drops (n = 17) and 6 weeks in eyes with injections (n = 9).[96] There seems to be no significant difference between 1 million IU/ml and 3 million IU/ml for perilesional injections.[95] Medical therapy with interferons has the advantage of treating microscopic disease that may be present throughout the entire ocular surface. Peri-lesional injections have been associated with flu-like symptoms which lasted for 2 to 3 days, however, no adverse effects have been reported with topical interferons.

Pegylated interferon alpha 2b: Pegylation of therapeutic proteins is a well-established method for delaying clearance and reducing immunogenicity.[85] Pegylated interferon alpha 2b (PEGIFN-α2b), polyethylene glycol (PEG) intron, Schering-Plough, Kenilworth, NJ) is a derivative of recombinant interferon alpha 2b and was developed to reduce the clearance of traditional recombinant interferon alpha 2b. Attachment of a single straight-chain poly-ethylene glycol (PEG; molecular weight of 12,000 Da) moiety to interferon alpha 2b significantly decreases renal clearance, increasing plasma half-life tenfold compared to non-pegylated interferon without altering the volume of distribution or spectrum of activity.[86,87] This has potential advantage of significantly decreasing the dosing of the pegylated interferon. It was found in a small pilot study that PEGIFN-α2b was effective in treating OSSN with complete clinical resolution of the lesion in all patients.[88] A mean of 3 injections were needed for tumor resolution in a case series using PEGIFN-α2b.

In comparison, a previous case series using sub-conjunctival and topical recombinant interferon for the treatment of CIN reported that a mean of 5 injections were needed for tumor resolution.[89] Pegylated interferon costs approximately 3 times as much as recombinant interferon.

Other agents

Topical bevacizumab: It is effective as a neoadjuvant therapy combined with surgical excision for the treatment of OSSN. It may be used before surgery to decrease the size of the excision. In a case series of six eyes with OSSN, topical 5 mg/ml bevacizumab in the dosage of 4 times daily for a period of 8 weeks was reported to be effective as a primary and sole therapy in two cases and as neoadjuvant therapy in four cases that required surgical excision at the end of the topical treatment period.[90]

Topical cidofovir: It may provide an additional option for managing treatment-unresponsive lesions owing to potential HPV presence. Topical cidofovir use has been reported as 2.5 mg/ml drops 3 times each day for 6 weeks.[91]

RECURRENCE

Recurrence rates of OSSN ranges from 15 to 52%, average reported being 30%. Recurrences are higher in case of inadequate excision margins, and occur usually within two years of surgery. These typically exhibit a more aggressive behaviour because of the tissue disruption associated with the primary excision theoretically enhancing the ability of the tumor cells to enter the eye. The main predictors for recurrence include age, histological grade of the lesion, adequacy of margins at initial excision, corneal location, larger size (>2 mm), and a high proliferation index. Immunostaining with antibody to Ki-67, a nuclear antigen expressed in proliferating cells, allows evaluation of the growth fraction of normal and neoplastic cells yielding the proliferation index.[52]

RECOMMENDED THERAPEUTIC STRATEGY AND CURRENT THERAPEUTIC PRACTICE

According to recommendations made by Viani GA et al, incision biopsy may be done to rule out invasive lesions before starting on topical therapy in tumors of more than one quadrant size.[92] However, incision biopsy may not be representative of the whole tumour and increases the risk of tumour progression and spread. Therefore, most centres avoid incision biopsy except in cases of OSSN requiring enucleation or exenteration. Most of the studies on topical treatment have used only clinical criteria for diagnosis and assessment of tumour grade with use of UBM to rule out invasion. With 70–80% tumours responding to immune or chemotherapy, most oncologists use them as primary treatment in non-invasive cases.

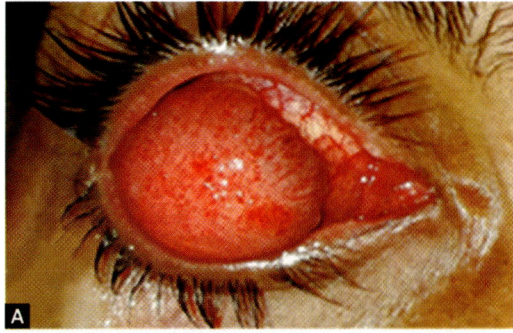

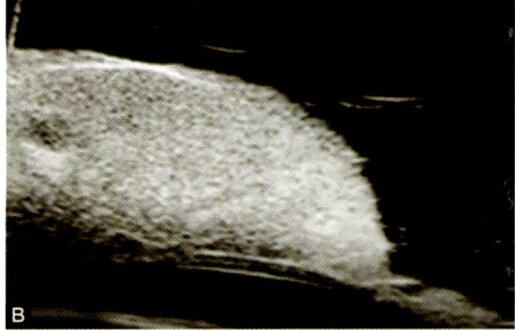

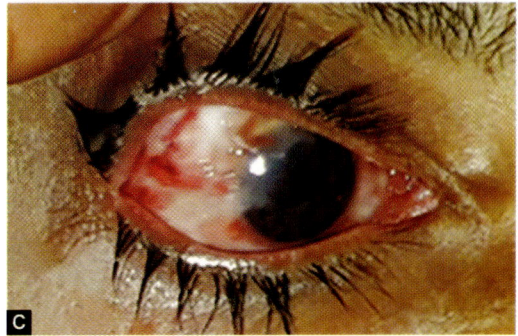

Fig. 23.4: *A and B, Invasive OSSN; C, Treated with wide local excision*

Table 23.2: *Drug classification, mechanism of action, administration and adverse effects*

Drug	Mechanism of action	Administration	Adverse effects
MMC Alkylating agent	Generates free radicals under aerobic conditions ↓ Inhibition of DNA and protein synthesis. Inhibition of cell migration and production of extracellular matrix	Topical 0.02–0.04% 0.04% (0.4 mg/ml) 4 times a day 4 days a week 4 weeks Treatment-free interval of 2 weeks	Conjunctival hyperaemia Blepharospasm Corneal punctate erosion Punctal stenosis Limbal stem cell deficiency
5-FU Pyrimidine analog	Inhibits thymidylate synthetase ↓ Inhibits production and incorporation of thymidine into DNA Inhibits RNA synthesis	Topical 1% 5-FU. 1% is used 3–4 times a day continuously for 3–4 weeks or 3–4 times daily for 4–7 days with 30–45 days off and cycles repeated	Eyelid erythema Conjunctival hyperaemia Corneal punctate erosion
IFN-α2b Type 1 IFN	Immune-mediated suppression of IL-10, stimulates IL-2 and IFN-γ mRNA Anti-proliferative Anti-viral	Topical 1 million IU/ml four times daily or intralesional 3 million IU/ml	Superficial punctate keratopathy Follicular conjunctivitis Systemic flu-like syndrome Fever/myalgia

(Data adapted from Viani GA, Fendi LI. Adjuvant treatment or primary topical monotherapy for ocular surface squamous neoplasia: a systematic review. Arq Bras Oftalmol. 2017 Mar-Apr; 80(2): 131–136)

Excision biopsy may be planned for invasive tumors, AJCC grade T1 tumors and cases with partial resolution to topical therapy. Due to absence of significant side effects, immunotherapy is emerging as primary management for immunotreatment or immunoreduction for most cases with no invasion on imaging (UBM).

CONCLUSION

Squamous lesions of the cornea and conjunctiva are uncommon but demand appropriate attention due to the potential for visual loss and systemic morbidity and mortality. Newer modalities of diagnosis allow non-invasive evaluation which correlates well with histopathological tissue diagnosis. With the advent of interferons which have minimal side effects and comparable efficacy, more conservative approach is being followed for treatment of non-invasive lesions.

REFERENCES

1. Duke-Elder S, Leigh AG. Diseases of the outer eye. In: Duke-Elder S, ed. Systems of Ophthalmology, Vol 7, Part 2. St Louis: CV Mosby, 1985: 1154–1159.

2. Pizzarello LD, Jakobiec FA. Bowen's disease of the conjunctiva: a misomer. In: Jakobiec FA, ed. Ocular Adnexal Tumors, Birmingham, AL: Aescula-pius, 1978: 553–571.

3. Waring GO III, Roth AM, Ekins MB. Clinical and pathological description of 17 cases of corneal in-traepithelial neoplasia. Am J Opthalmol 1984; 97: 547–59.

4. Erie JC, Campbell RJ, Leisgang J. Conjunctival and corneal intraepithelial and invasive neoplasia. Opthalmology 1986; 93: 176–83.

5. Lee GA, Hirst LW. Ocular surface squamous neoplasia. Surv Ophthalmol 1995; 39: 429–50.

6. Verma V, Shen D, Sieving PC, et al. The role of infectious agents in the etiology of ocular adnexal neoplasia. Surv Ophthalmol 2008; 53: 312–31.

7. Weinstein JE, Karp CL. Ocular surface neoplasias and human immunodeficiency virus infection. Curr Opin Infect Dis 2013; 26: 58–65.

8. Yang J, Foster CS. Squamous cell carcinoma of the conjunctiva. Int Ophthalmol Clin 1997; 37(4): 73–85.

9. Gichuhi S, Sagoo MS, Weiss HA, Burton MJ. Epidemiology of ocular surface squamous neoplasia in Africa. Trop Med Int Health. 2013; 18(12): 1424–43.

10. Scott IU, Karp CL, Nuovo GJ. Human papillomavirus 16 and 18 expression in conjunctival intraepithelial neoplasia. Ophthalmology. 2002; 109(3): 542–7.

11. Lee GA, Hirst LW: Incidence of ocular surface epithelial dysplasia in metropolitan Brisbane. A 10 year survey. Arch Ophthalmol 1992; 110: 525–7.

12. Choi CJ, Jakobiec FA, Zakka FR, Foster CS, Chodosh J, Freitag SK. Conjunctival Squamous Cell Neoplasia Associated With Ocular Cicatricial Pemphigoid. Ophthal Plast Reconstr Surg. 2017 May 15.

13. Sivalingam V, Shields CL, Shields JA, et al. Squamous cell carcinoma of the conjunctiva associated with benign mucous membrane pemphigoid. Ann Ophthalmol 1990; 22: 106–9.

14. Joshi RS. Ocular surface squamous neoplasia inpatient with non-Hodgkin's lymphoma. Indian J Ophthalmol 2017; 65(1): 71–72.

15. Arora T, Sharma S, Sharma N, Titiyal JS. Bilateral recurrent ocular surface squamous cell cancer associated with epidermodysplasia verruciformis. BMJ Case Rep 2015 Jan 30.

16. Choi CJ, Jakobiec FA, Zakka FR, Sanchez AV, Lee NG. Ocular Surface Squamous Neoplasia in a Patient With Hepatitis C. JAMA Ophthalmol. 2017; 135(10): 1121–3.

17. Shah A, Espana EM, Singh AD. Ocular Surface Squamous Neoplasia Associated with Atopic Keratoconjunctivitis. Ocul Oncol Pathol 2017; 3(1): 22–27.

18. Mahomed A, Chetty R Human immunodeficiency virus infection, Bci-2, p53 protein, and Ki-67 analysis in OSSN. Arch Ophthalmol. 2002; 120: 554–8.

19. Jacyk WK. Xeroderma pigmentosum in black South Africans Int J Dermatol 1999; 38: 511–4.

20. Sen S, Sharma A, Panda A. Immunohistochemical localization of human papillomavirus in conjunctival neoplasias: a retrospective study. Indian J Ophthalmol 2007; 55(5): 361–3.

21. Weinstein JE, Karp CL. Ocular surface neoplasia and human immunodeficiency virus infection. Curr Opin Infect Dis 2013; 26: 58–65.

22. Kaliki S, Kamal S, Fatima S. Ocular surface squamous neoplasia as the initial presenting sign of human immunodeficiency virus infection in 60 Asian Indian patients. Int Ophthalmol. 2017; 37(5): 1221–8.

23. Kamal S, Kaliki S, Mishra DK, et al. Ocular surface squamous neoplasia in 200 patients: a case-control study of immunosuppression resulting from human immunodeficiency virus versus immunocompetency. Ophthalmology 2015; 122: 1688–94.

24. Jongkhajornpong P, Nakamura T, Sotozono C, Nagata M, Inatomi T, Kinoshita S.Elevated expression of ABCB5 in ocular surface squamous neoplasia. Sci Rep 2016; 6: 20541.

25. Shields CL, Shields JA. Tumors of the conjunctiva and cornea. Surv Ophthalmol 2004; 49: 3–24.

26. Shields JA, Shields CL. An Atlas and Textbook. 2nd ed. Philadelphia, PA: Lippincott Williams and Wilkins; 2008. Eyelid, Conjunctival and Orbital Tumors; pp. 250–445.

27. Farah S, Baum TD, Conton MR. Tumors of cornea and conjunctiva. In: Albert DM, Jakobiec FA, editors. Principles and Practice of Ophthalmology. 2nd ed. Philadelphia: WB Saunders; 2000; 1002–19.

28. Akpek EK, Polcharoen W, Chan R, Foster CS. Ocular surface neoplasia masquerading as chronic blepharoconjunctivitis. Cornea. 1999; 18: 282–8.

29. Nicholson DH, Herschler J. Intraocular extension of squamous cell carcinoma of the conjunctiva. Arch Ophthalmol 1977; 95: 843–6.

30. Searl SS, Krigstein HJ, Albert DM, Grove AS Jr. Invasive squamous cell carcinoma with intraocular mucoepidermoid features. Conjunctival carcinoma with intraocular invasion and diphasic morphology. Arch Ophthalmol. 1982; 100: 109–11.

31. Johnson TE, Tabbara KF, Weatherhead RG, Kersten RC, Rice C, Nasr AM. Secondary squamous cell carcinoma of the orbit. Arch Ophthalmol 1997; 115: 75–8.

32. Sridhar MS, Honavar SG, Vemuganti G, et al.Conjunctival intraepithelial neoplasia presenting as corneal ulcer. Am J Ophthalmol 2000; 129: 92–94.

33. Mirza E, Gumus K, Evercklioglu C, et al. Invasive squamous cell carcinoma of the conjunctiva first misdiagnosed as a pterygium: A clinicopathologic report. Eye Contact Lens 2008; 34: 188–190.

34. Mahmood MA, Al-Rajhi A, Riley F, et al. Sclerokeratitis: An unusual presentation of squamous cell carcinoma of the conjunctiva. Ophthalmology 2001; 108: 553–8.

35. Sharma M, Sundar D, Vanathi M, Meel R, Kashyap S, Chawla R, Tandon R.Invasive Ocular Surface Squamous Neoplasia Masquerading as Nodular Scleritis. Ophthal Plast Reconstr Surg. 2017; 33(2): 45–47.

36. Ganger A, Devi S, Gupta N, Vanathi M, Tandon R. Ocular surface squamous neoplasia masquerading as peripheral ulcerative keratitis. Trop Doct 2017; 47(3): 233–6.

37. Barros Jde N, Almeida SR, Lowen MS, Cunha MC, Gomes JÁ. Impression cytology in the evaluation of ocular surface tumors: review article. Arq Bras Oftalmol 2015; 78(2): 126–32.

38. Nolan GR, Hirst LW, Bancroft BJ The cyto-morphology of ocular surface squamous neoplasia by using impression cytology. Cancer 2001; 25; 93(1): 60–5.

39. Tole DM, McKelvie PA, Daniell M. Reliability of impression cytology for the diagnosis of ocular surface squamous neoplasia employing the Biopore membrane. Br J Ophthalmol 2001; 85(9): 1115–9.

40. Kayat KV, Correa Dantas PE, Felberg S, Galvão MA, Saieg MA. Exfoliative Cytology in the Diagnosis of Ocular Surface Squamous Neoplasms. Cornea 2017; 36(1): 127–30.

41. IL Romero, JDN Barros, MC Martins, PL Ballalai. The use of 1% toluidine blue eye drops in the diagnosis of ocular surface squamous neoplasia. Cornea 2013; 32(1): 36–9.

42. J Stefen, J Rice, K Lecuona, H Carrara. Identification of ocular surface squamous neoplasia by *in vivo* staining with methylene blue. British Journal of Ophthalmology 2014; 98(1): 13–5.

43. S Gichuhi, E Macharia, J Kabiru. Toluidine blue 0.05% vital staining for the diagnosis of ocular surface squamous neoplasia in Kenya, "JAMA Ophthalmology 2015; 133(11): 1314–21.

44. JC Erie, RJ Campbell, TJ Liesegang. Conjunctival and corneal intraepithelial and invasive neoplasia. Ophthalmology 1986; 93(2): 176–83.

45. R Hamam, P Bhat, CS Foster. Conjunctival/corneal intraepithelial neoplasia. Int Ophthalmol Clin 2009 Winter; 49(1): 63–70.

46. Shields CL, Demirci H, Karatza E, Shields JA. Clinical survey of 1643 melanocytic and nonmelanocytic conjunctival tumors. Ophthalmology 2004; 111: 1747–54.

47. Tunc M, Char DH, Crawford B, Miller T. Intraepithelial and invasive squamous cell carcinoma of the conjunctiva: Analysis of 60 cases. Br J Ophthalmol 1999; 83: 98–103.

48. Scholz SL, Thomasen H, Reis H, et al. Frequent TERT promoter mutations in ocular surface squamous neoplasia. Invest Ophthalmol Vis Sci 2015; 56: 5854–61.

49. YA Yousef, PT Finger. Squamous carcinoma and dysplasia of the conjunctiva and cornea: an analysis of 101 cases. Ophthalmology 2012; 119(2): 233–40.

50. Tananuvat N, Lertprasertsuk N, Mahanupap P, Noppanakeepong P. Role of impression cytology in diagnosis of ocular surface neoplasia. Cornea 2008; 27: 269–74.

51. Parrozzani R, Lazzarini D, Dario A, et al. *In vivo* confocal microscopy of ocular surface squamous neoplasia. Eye 2011; 25: 455–60.

52. McKelvie PA, Daniell M, McNab A, Loughnan M, Santamaria JD. Squamous cell carcinoma of the conjunctiva: a series of 26 cases. Br J Ophthalmol 2002; 86(2): 168–73.

53. CJ Pavlin, MD Sherar, FS Foster. Subsurface ultra-sound microscopic imaging of the intact eye. Ophthalmology 1990; 97(2): 244–50.

54. C Bianciotto, CL Shields, JM Guzman. Assessment of anterior segment tumors with ultra-sound biomicroscopy versus anterior segment optical coherence tomography in 200 cases. Ophthalmology 2011; 118(7): 1297–302.

55. PT Finger, HV Tran, RE Turbin. High-frequency ultrasonographic evaluation of conjunctival intraepithelial neoplasia and squamous cell carcinoma. Arch Ophthalmol 2003; 121(2): 168–72.

56. DH Char, G Kundert, R Bove, JB Crawford. 20 MHz high-frequency ultrasound assessment of scleral and intraocular conjunctival squamous cell carcinoma. Br J Ophthalmol 2002; 86(6): 632–5.

57. Shousha MA, Perez VL, Wang J, et al. Use of ultra high-resolution optical coherence tomography to detect *in vivo* characteristics of Descemet's membrane in Fuchs' dystrophy. Ophthalmology 2010; 117: 1220–7.

58. Lejla M. Vajzovic, MD, Carol L. Karp, MD, Payman Haft, MD. Ultra high-resolution anterior segment optical coherence tomography in the evaluation of anterior corneal dystrophies and degenerations. Ophthalmology 2011; 118: 1291–6.

59. Kieval JZ, Karp CL, Shousha MA. Ultra high-resolution optical coherence tomography for diferentiation of ocular surface squamous neoplasia and pterygia. Ophthalmology 2012; 119(3): 481–6.

60. Nanji AA, Sayyad FE, Galor A, Dubovy S, Karp CL. High resolution optical coherence tomography as an adjunctive tool in the diagnosis of corneal and conjunctival pathology. Ocul Surf 2015; 13(3): 226–35.

61. Shousha MA, Karp CL, Canto AP. Diagnosis of ocular surface lesions using ultra high-resolution optical coherence tomography. Ophthalmology 2013; 120(5): 883–91.

62. Shousha MA, Karp CL, Perez VL. Diagnosis and management of conjunctival and corneal intraepithelial neoplasia using ultra high-resolution optical coherence tomography. Ophthalmology 2011; 118(8): 1531–7.

63. Homas BJ, Galor A, Nanji AA. Ultra high-resolution anterior segment optical coherence tomography in the diagnosis and management of ocular surface squamous neoplasia. Ocular Surface 2014; 12(1): 46–58.

64. Y Xu, Z Zhou, Y Xu, M Wang, F Liu, H Qu, J Hong. The clinical value of in vivo confocal microscopy for diagnosis of ocular surface squamous neoplasia. Eye 2012; 26: 781–7.

65. McKelvie PA, Daniell M. Impression cytology following mitomycin-C therapy for ocular surface squamous metaplasia. Br J Ophthalmol 2001; 85: 1115–9.

66. Hassani RT, Brasnu E, Amar N, Gheck L, Labbe A, Sterkers M. et al. Contribution of in vivo confocal microscopy to diagnosis of invasive ocular surface squamous neoplasia: a case report. J Fr Ophtalmol 2010; 33(3): 163–8.

67. Malandrini A, Martone G, Traversi C, Caporossi A. In vivo confocal microscopy in a patient with recurrent conjunctival intraepithelial neoplasia. Acta Ophthalmologica 2008; 86(6): 690–1.

68. Wakuta M, Chikama TI, Takahashi N, Nishida T. A case of bilateral corneal epithelial dysplasia characterized by laser confocal biomicroscopy and cytokeratin immunofluorescence. Cornea 2008; 27(1): 107–10.

69. Falke K, Zhivov A, Zimpfer A, Stachs O, Guthof RF. Diagnosis of conjunctival neoplastic lesions by confocal in vivo microscopy. Klin Monbl Augenheilkd 2012; 229(7): 724–7.

70. Alomar TS, Nubile M, Lowe J, Dua HS. Corneal intraepithelial neoplasia: in vivo confocal microscopic study with histopathologic correlation. Am J Ophthalmol 2011; 151(2): 238–47.

71. Y Xu, Z Zhou, Y Xu. The clinical value of in vivo confocal microscopy for diagnosis of ocular surface squamous neoplasia. Eye (Lond) 2012; 26(6): 781–7.

72. Nguena MB, VanDen Tweel JG, Makupa W. Diagnosing ocular surface squamous neoplasia in east Africa: case-control study of clinical and in vivo confocal microscopy assessment. Ophthalmology 2014; 121(2): 484–91.

73. Nanji AA, Sayyad FE, Galor A, Dubovy S, Karp CL. High-resolution optical coherence tomography as an adjunctive tool in the diagnosis of corneal and conjunctival pathology. Ocul Surf 2015; 13(3): 226–35.

74. Queiroz de Paiva AR, Abreu de Azevedo Fraga L, Torres VL. Surgical Reconstruction of Ocular Surface Tumors Using Fibrin Sealant Tissue Adhesive. Ocul Oncol Pathol 2016; 2(4): 207–11.

75. Buuns DR Tse. DT, Folberg R. Microscopically controlled excision of conjunctival squamous cell carcinoma. Am J Ophthalmol 1994; 117: 97–102.

76. El-Assal KS, Salvi SM, Rundle PA, Mudhar HS, Rennie IG. Treatment of invasive ocular surface squamous neoplasia with proton beam therapy. Eye (Lond) 2013; 27: 1223–4.

77. Ramonas KM, Conway RM, Daftari IK, Crawford JB, O'Brien JM. Successful treatment of intraocularly invasive conjunctival squamous cell carcinoma with proton beam therapy. Arch Ophthalmol 2006; 124: 126–8.

78. Murthy R, Gupta H, Krishnatry R, Laskar S. Electron beam radiotherapy for the management of recurrent extensive ocular surface squamous neoplasia with orbital extension. Indian J Ophthalmol. 2015; 63(8): 672–4.

79. Lecuona K, Stannard C, Hart G, Rice J, Cook C, Wetter J, Duffield M. The treatment of carcinoma in situ and squamous cell carcinoma of the conjunctiva with fractionated strontium-90 radiation in a population with a high prevalence of HIV. Br J Ophthalmol 2015; 99(9): 1158–61.

80. Chen C, Louis D, Dodd T, Muecke J Mitomycin-C as an adjunct in the treatment of localized ocular surface squamous neoplasia. Br J Ophthalmol 2004; 88(1): 17–8.

81. Sepulveda R, Pe'er J, Midena E, Seregard S, Dua H, Singh AD. Topical chemotherapy for ocular surface squamous neoplasia: current status. Current Status. Br J Ophthalmol 2010; 95(5): 532–5.

82. Galor A, Karp CL, Oellers P, et al. Predictors of ocular surface squamous neoplasia recurrence after excisional surgery. Ophthalmology 2012; 119: 1974–81.

83. Pe' er J. Ocular surface squamous neoplasia: evidence for topical chemotherapy. Int Ophthalmol Clin 2015; 55: 9–21.

84. Parrozzani R, Frizziero L, Trainiti S, Testi I, Miglionico G, Pilotto E, Blandamura S,

Fassina A, Midena E. Topical 1% 5-fluorouracil as a sole treatment of corneoconjunctival ocular surface squamous neoplasia: long-term study. Br J Ophthalmol 2017; 101(8): 1094–99.

85. Mehvar R. Modulation of the pharmacokinetics and pharmacodynamics of proteins by polyethylene glycol conjugation. J Pharm Pharm Sci 2000; 3(1): 125–36.

86. Glue P, Fang JW, Rouzier-Panis R, et al. Pegylated interferon alpha-2b: pharmaco-kinetics, pharmacodynamics, safety, and preliminary efficacy data. Hepatitis C Intervention Therapy Group. Clin Pharmacol Ther 2000; 68(5): 556–67.

87. Wang YS, Youngster S, Grace M, Bausch J, Bordens R, Wyss DF. Structural and biological characterization of pegylated recombinant interferon alpha-2b and its therapeutic implications. Adv Drug Deliv Rev 2002; 54(4): 547–70.

88. Karp CL, Galor A, Lee Y, Yoo SH. Pegylated Interferon Alpha-2b for Treatment of Ocular Surface Squamous Neoplasia: A Pilot Study. Ocular Immunology & Inflammation 2010; 18(4): 254–60.

89. Vann RR, Karp CL. Perilesional and topical interferon alfa-2b for conjunctival and corneal neoplasia. Ophthalmology 1999; 106(1): 91–7.

90. Asena L, Dursun Altýnörs D. Topical Bevacizumab for the Treatment of Ocular Surface Squamous Neoplasia. J Ocul Pharmacol Ther 2015; 31(8): 487–90.

91. Ip MH, Coroneo MT. Treatment of Previously Refractory Ocular Surface Squamous Neoplasia with Topical Cidofovir. JAMA Ophthalmol 2017; 135(5): 500–2.

92. Viani GA, Fendi LI. Adjuvant treatment or primary topical monotherapy for ocular surface squamous neoplasia: a systematic review. Arq Bras Oftalmol 2017; 80(2): 131–36.

93. Murthy R, Honavar SG, Vemuganti GK, Burman S, Naik M, Parathasaradhi A. Ocular surface squamous neoplasia in Papillon-Lefevre syndrome. Am J Ophthalmol 2005; 139(1): 207–9.

94. Kaliki S, Singh S, Gowrishankar S, Reddy VAP. Ocular Surface Squamous Neoplasia in Papillon-Lefèvre Syndrome: Outcome at Long-term Follow-up of 12 Years. Cornea 2017; 36(6): 743–46.

95. Galor A, Karp CL, Chhabra S, Barnes S, Alfonso EC. Topical Interferon Alpha-2b Eye drops for Ocular Surface Squamous Neoplasia. Br J Ophthalmol 2010; 94(5): 551–4.

96. Meel R, Dhiman R, Vanathi M, Pushker N, Tandon R, Devi S. Clinicodemographic profile and treatment outcome in patients of ocular surface squamous neoplasia. Indian J Ophthalmol 2017; 65(10): 936–41.

Section
V

Inflammatory Diseases of Cornea

Keratitis: Classification and Pathogenesis

DEFINITION

KERATITIS

Inflammation of cornea (keratitis) is characterised by corneal oedema, cellular infiltration and ciliary congestion.

CORNEAL ULCER

Corneal ulcer may be defined as discontinuation in normal epithelial surface of cornea associated with necrosis of the surrounding corneal tissue. Pathologically, it is characterised by oedema and cellular infiltration. Common types of corneal ulcers are described below.

CLASSIFICATION OF KERATITIS

It is difficult to classify and assign a group to each and every case of keratitis; as overlapping or concurrent findings tend to obscure the picture. However, the following simplified topographical and etiological classifications provide a workable knowledge.

TOPOGRAPHICAL (MORPHOLOGICAL) CLASSIFICATION

A. Ulcerative keratitis (corneal ulcer)

Corneal ulcer can be further classified variously:

1. *Depending on location*
   - Central corneal ulcer
   - Peripheral corneal ulcer
2. *Depending on purulence*
   - Purulent corneal ulcer or suppurative corneal ulcer (most bacterial and fungal corneal ulcers are suppurative).
   - Non-purulent corneal ulcers (most of viral, chlamydial and allergic corneal ulcers are non-suppurative).
3. *Depending upon association of hypopyon*
   - Simple corneal ulcer (without hypopyon)
   - Hypopyon corneal ulcer
4. *Depending upon depth of ulcer*
   - Superficial corneal ulcer
   - Deep corneal ulcer
   - Corneal ulcer with impending perforation
   - Perforated corneal ulcer

5. *Depending upon slough formation*
   - Non-sloughing corneal ulcer
   - Sloughing corneal ulcer

B. Non-ulcerative keratitis

1. *Superficial keratitis*
   - Diffuse superficial keratitis
   - Superficial punctate keratitis (SPK)
2. *Deep keratitis*
   a. Non-suppurative
      - Interstitial keratitis
      - Disciform keratitis
      - Keratitis profunda
      - Sclerosing keratitis
   b. Suppurative deep keratitis
      - Central corneal abscess
      - Posterior corneal abscess.

ETIOLOGICAL CLASSIFICATION

1. *Infective/microbial keratitis*
   - Bacterial keratitis
   - Viral keratitis
   - Fungal keratitis
   - Chlamydial keratitis
   - Protozoal keratitis
   - Spirochaetal keratitis
2. *Allergic keratitis*
   - Phlyctenular keratitis
   - Vernal keratitis
   - Atopic keratitis
3. *Trophic keratitis*
   - Exposure keratitis
   - Neurotrophic keratopathy
   - Keratomalacia
   - Atheromatous ulcer
4. *Keratitis associated with diseases of skin and mucous membrane.*
5. *Keratitis associated with systemic collagen vascular disorders.*
6. *Traumatic keratitis* which may be due to mechanical trauma, chemical trauma, thermal burns, radiations.
7. *Idiopathic keratitis,* e.g.
   - Mooren's corneal ulcer
   - Superior limbic keratoconjunctivitis
   - Superficial punctate keratitis of Thygeson.

PATHOGENESIS OF KERATITIS

Steps in pathogenesis of corneal ulceration are described below (Fig. 24.1):

Break in epithelial continuity
↓
Bacteria adheres, enters and proliferates in stroma
↓
Inflammatory response (PMN)
↓
Abscess
(appears as grayish white infiltrate in stroma)

Fig. 24.1: *Steps in development of infective keratitis*

CORNEAL EPITHELIAL DAMAGE

Corneal epithelial damage is a pre-requisite for most of the infecting organisms to produce corneal ulceration. It may occur in following conditions:
- *Epithelial damage* due to hypoxia and trauma in contact lens wears.
- *Corneal abrasion* due to small foreign body, misdirected cilia, concretions and trivial trauma.
- *Refractive corneal surgery* especially LASIK.
- *Epithelial drying as in xerosis* and exposure keratitis.
- *Necrosis of epithelium* as in keratomalacia.
- *Desquamation of epithelial cells* as a result of corneal oedema as in bullous keratopathy.
- *Epithelial damage* due to trophic changes as in neuroparalytic keratitis.

INVASION BY OFFENDING AGENT

Source and mode of invasion by various offending microorganisms such as bacteria, viruses, fungi, chlamydia, protozoa, spirochaete and others are described in respective chapters.

DEVELOPMENT AND COURSE OF KERATITIS

1. ***Once the damaged corneal epithelium is invaded by the offending agents***, the process of development of keratitis starts (Fig. 24.1). The sequence of pathological changes which occur

during development of corneal ulcer can be described under four stages:

- Stage of progressive infiltration
- Stage of active ulceration
- Stage of regression
- Stage of cicatrisation.

2. *Terminal course of corneal ulcer depends upon* the virulence of infecting agent, host defence mechanism and the treatment received.

3. *Depending upon the prevalent circumstances the course of corneal ulcer* may take one of the three forms:

- Ulcer may become localised and heal
- Penetrate deep leading to corneal perforation
- Spread fast to involve the whole cornea as sloughing corneal ulcer.

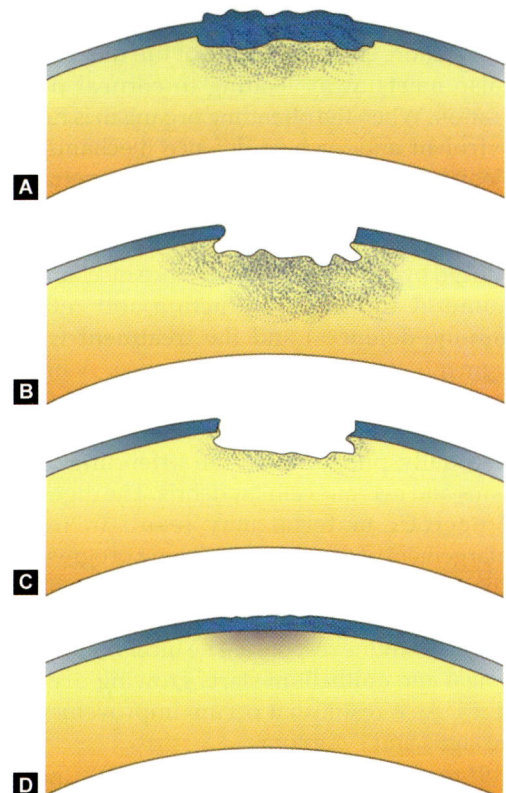

A

B

C

D

Fig. 24.2: *Pathology of corneal ulcer. A, Stage of progressive infiltration; B, Stage of active ulceration; C, Stage of regression; D, Stage of cicatrisation*

PATHOLOGY OF KERATITIS

The salient pathological features of corneal ulcer in general are described here. The specific pathological features of different etiological types of corneal ulcer are described in respective chapters.

A. PATHOLOGY OF LOCALISED CORNEAL ULCER

1. *Stage of progressive infiltration* (Fig. 24.2A). It is characterised by adherens and entry of organisms followed with the infiltration of polymorphonuclear and/or lymphocytes into the epithelium from the peripheral circulation supplemented by similar cells from the underlying stroma if this tissue is also affected. Subsequently, lytic enzymes and toxins are released by lucocytes and bacteria causing necrosis of the involved tissue extent of which will depend upon the virulence of offending agent and the strength of host defence mechanism.

2. *Stage of active ulceration* (Fig. 24.2B). Active ulceration results from necrosis and sloughing of the epithelium, Bowman's membrane and the involved stroma. The walls of the active ulcer project owing to swelling of the lamellae by the imbibition of fluid and the packing of masses of leucocytes between them. This zone of infiltration may extend to a considerable distance both around and beneath the ulcer. At this stage, sides

and floor of the ulcer may show grey infiltration and sloughing.

During this stage of active ulceration, there occurs

- *Hyperaemia* of circumcorneal network of vessels which results into accumulation of purulent exudates on the cornea.
- *Vascular congestion of the iris and ciliary* body and some degree of iritis due to absorption of toxins from the ulcer. Exudation into the anterior chamber from the vessels of iris and ciliary body may lead to formation of hypopyon.
- *Ulceration may further progress* by lateral extension resulting in diffuse superficial ulceration or it may progress by deeper penetration of the infection. Descemet's membrane (DM) in resistant to digestion by proteolytic enzymes

to some extent leading to descemetocele formation. Over the course of full disease DM also meets away leading to corneal perforation. When the offending organism is highly virulent and/or host defence mechanism is jeopardised there occurs deeper penetration during stage of active ulceration.

3. *Stage of regression* (Fig. 24.2C). Regression is induced by the natural host defence mechanisms (humoral antibody production and cellular immune defences) and the treatment which augments the normal host response. A line of demarcation develops around the ulcer, which consists of leucocytes that neutralise and eventually phagocytose the offending organisms and necrotic cellular debris. The digestion of necrotic material may result in initial enlargement of the ulcer mimicking progression. This process may be accompanied by superficial vascularization that increases the humoral and cellular immune response. The ulcer now begins to heal and epithelium starts growing over the edges. As a result that occurs improvement in the signs and symptoms.

4. *Stage of cicatrisation* (Fig. 24.2D). In this stage, healing continues by progressive epithelisation which forms a permanent covering. Beneath the epithelium, Bowman's membrane does not regenerate, fibrous tissue is laid down partly by the corneal fibroblasts and partly by the endothelial cells of the new vessels. New vessels usually regress leave a residue but of sometimes vessels. The stroma thus thickens and fills in under the epithelium, pushing the epithelial surface anteriorly.

The degree of scarring from healing varies. If the ulcer is very superficial and involves epithelium only, it heals without leaving any opacity behind. When ulcer involves Bowman's membrane and few superficial stromal lamellae, the resultant scar is called a 'nebula'. Macula and leucoma result after healing of ulcers involving up to one-third and more than that of corneal stroma, respectively.

B. PATHOLOGY OF PERFORATED CORNEAL ULCER

Perforation of corneal ulcer occurs when the ulcerative process deepens and reaches up to

Descemet's membrane. This membrane is tough and bulges out as descemetocele (Fig. 24.3). At this stage, any exertion on the part of patient, such as coughing, sneezing, straining for stool, etc., will perforate the corneal ulcer. Immediately after perforation, the aqueous escapes, intraocular pressure falls and the iris-lens diaphragm moves forward.

The effects of perforation depend upon the position and size of perforation. When the perforation is small and opposite to iris tissue, it is usually plugged and healing by cicatrisation proceeds rapidly (Fig. 24.4). Adherent leucoma is the commonest end result after such a catastrophe.

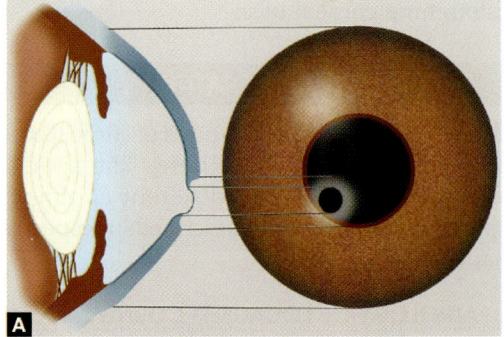
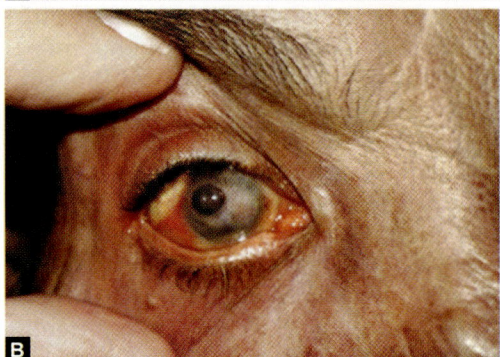

Fig. 24.3: *Descemetocele. A, Diagrammatic depiction; B, Clinical photograph*

C. PATHOLOGY OF SLOUGHING CORNEAL ULCER AND FORMATION OF ANTERIOR STAPHYLOMA

When the infecting agent is highly virulent and/or body resistance is very low, the whole cornea sloughs with the exception of a narrow rim at the margin and total prolapse of iris occurs. The iris becomes inflamed and exudates block the

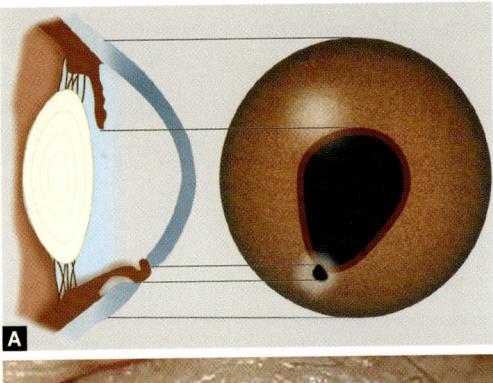

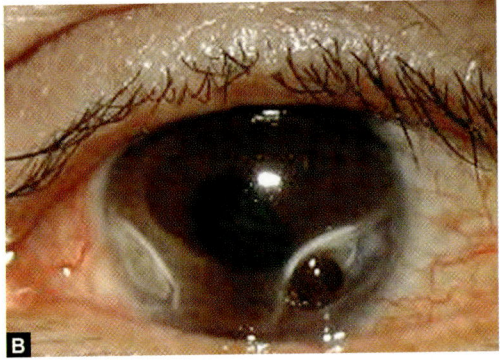

Fig. 24.4: *Perforated corneal ulcer with prolapse of iris. A, Diagrammatic depiction; B, Clinical photograph*

pupil and cover the iris surface; thus a false cornea is formed. Ultimately, these exudates organise and form a thin fibrous layer over which the conjunctival or corneal epithelium rapidly grows and thus a pseudocornea is formed. Since, the pseudocornea is thin and cannot withstand the intraocular pressure, so it usually bulges forward along with the plastered iris tissue. This ectatic cicatrix is called anterior staphyloma which, depending upon its extent, may be either partial or total. The bands of scar tissue on the staphyloma vary in breadth and thickness, producing a lobulated surface often blackened with iris tissue which resembles a bunch of black grapes (hence the name staphyloma).

BIBLIOGRAPHY

1. Bacon AS, Frazer DG, Dart JK, Matheson M, Ficker LA, Wright P. A review of 72 consecutive cases of Acanthamoeba keratitis, 1984-1992. Eye 1993;7:719-25.
2. Chan C, Li Q, Brezin A, Whitcup S, Egwuagu C, Ottesen E, Nussenblatt R. Immunopathology of ocular onchocerciasis. Th-2 helper T cells in the conjunctiva. Ocular Immunol Inflammation. 1993;1:71–77.
3. Kenyon KR, Ghinelli E, Chaves HV. Morphology and pathologic response in corneal and conjunctival disease. In: Foster CS, Azar DT, Dohlman CH (Eds): Smolin and Thoft's Cornea. Lippincott Williams and Wilkins NY; 4th edition, 2005;4:103-40.
4. Kenyon KR. Inflammatory mechanisms in corneal ulceration. Trans Am Ophthalmol Soc 1985;83:610-63.
5. Nordlund M, Pepose JS. Corneal Response to Infection. In: Krachmer JH, Mannis MJ, Holland EJ (Eds): Cornea, 2nd Edition Elseivier Co. NY. 2005;7:95-114.
6. Sharma S, Silverberg M, Mehta P, Gopinathan U, Agrawal V, Naduvilath TJ. Early diagnosis of mycotic keratitis: Predictive value of potassium hydroxide preparation. Indian J Ophthalmol 1998;46:31-5

Infective Keratitis

BACTERIAL KERATITIS

Being the most anterior part of eyeball, the cornea is exposed to atmosphere and hence prone to get infected easily. At the same time, cornea is protected from day-to-day minor infections by the normal defence mechanisms present in tears in the form of lysozyme, betalysin and other protective proteins. Therefore, infective corneal ulcer may develop when:

- Either the local ocular defence mechanism is jeopardised, or
- There is some local ocular predisposing disease, or
- Host's immunity is compromised, or
- The causative organism is very virulent.

ETIOLOGY

Main factors in the production of purulent corneal ulcer are:

- Damage to corneal epithelium
- Infection of the eroded area.

Corneal epithelial damage

Corneal epithelial damage is a pre-requisite for most of the infecting organisms to produce corneal ulceration. It may occur in the following conditions:

- *Epithelial damage* due to hypoxia and trauma in contact lens wears.
- *Corneal abrasion* due to small foreign body, misdirected cilia, concretions and trivial trauma.
- *Refractive corneal surgery* especially LASIK.
- *Epithelial drying* as in xerosis and exposure keratitis.
- *Necrosis of epithelium* as in keratomalacia.
- *Desquamation of epithelial cells* as a result of corneal oedema as in bullous keratopathy.
- *Epithelial damage due to trophic changes* as in neuroparalytic keratitis.

System risk facts which play role in establishment of infection

- Malnutritions
- Immunosuppression
- Diabetes mellitus

Invasion by organisms

Pathogens which can invade the intact corneal epithelium and produce ulceration are:

- *Neisseria gonorrhoeae*
- *Corynebacterium diphtheriae*
- *Neisseria meningitidis*
- *Haemophilus aegyptius*
- *Listeria* species.

Source of infection

Most of the times bacterial corneal infection arises from exogenous source like conjunctival sac, lacrimal sac (dacryocystitis), infected foreign bodies, infected vegetative material and waterborne or airborne infections.

Causative organisms. Bacteria reported to be associated with keratitis can be classified as below:

- *Gram-positive cocci: Staphylococcus aureus, Staphylococcus epidermidis* and *Streptococcus pneumoniae.*

- *Gram-negative cocci: Neisseria gonorrhoeae, Neisseria meningitidis.*
- *Gram-positive bacilli: Corynebacterium diphtheriae, C. xerosis, Bacillus cereus, Propionibacterium acne, Listeria* and *Clostridium.*
- *Gram-negative bacilli: Pseudomonas aeruginosa,* Enterobacteriaceae (*Klebsiella, Proteus, E. coli, Serratia*), *Moraxella lacunata* (diplobacillus), *Haemophilus influenzae* (coccobacillus).
- *Gram-positive filamentous bacteria: Actinomyces, Nocardia.*
- *Mycobacteria:* Non-tuberculous mycobacteria and *M. tuberculosis.*

Common bacteria associated with corneal ulceration include staphylococci, *Pseudomonas, Streptococcus pneumoniae,* Enterobacteriaceae and *Neisseria.*

- *Most common cause* in general is *Staphylococcus*
- Most common cause in contact lens wearers is *Pseudomonas.*

Other organisms associated with contact lens keratitis are *Staphylococcus* and *Serratia marcescens.*

Organisms causing severe and rapidly progressive ulcers

- *Staph. aureus*
- *Strepto. pneumoniae*
- Beta-haemolytic streptococci
- *Pseudomonas aeruginosa*

Organisms causing less severe and slowly progressive ulcers

- Coagulase negative *Staph. aureus*
- *Strepto. viridans*
- *Actinomyces*
- *Nocardia*
- *Moraxella*
- *Serratia marcescens*

CLINICAL FEATURES

In bacterial infections, the outcome depends upon the virulence of organism, its toxins and enzymes, and the response of host tissue.

Broadly bacterial corneal ulcers may manifest as:
- Purulent corneal ulcer without hypopyon, or
- Hypopyon corneal ulcer.

In general, following symptoms and signs may be present.

Symptoms

1. *Pain* and *foreign body sensation* occurs due to mechanical effects of lids and chemical effects of toxins on the exposed nerve endings. Pain is moderate to severe.
2. *Watering and discharge.* Watering from the eye occurs due to reflex hyperlacrimation. Mild to serve discharge is noted depending upon the causative organism.
3. *Photophobia*, i.e. intolerance to light results from stimulation of nerve endings.
4. *Blurred vision* results from corneal haze.
5. *Redness of eyes* occurs due to congestion of circumcorneal conjunctival vessels.

Signs

1. **Swelling of lid** of varying degree is present with reactive ptosis.
2. **Blepharospasm** may be moderate to severe.
3. **Conjunctiva** is chemosed and shows conjunctival hyperaemia and ciliary congestion.
4. **Tear film** may show debris and mucopurulent discharge associated with purulent corneal ulcerations.
5. **Corneal ulcer** normally starts as an epithelial defect associated with greyish-white circumscribed infiltrate (seen in early stage). Soon the epithelial defect and infiltrate enlarges and stromal oedema develops. A well-established bacterial corneal ulcer is characterised by (Fig. 25.1):

- *Yellowish-white area* of ulcer which may be oval or irregular in shape.
- *Margins* of the ulcer are swollen and over hanging.
- *Floor of the ulcer* is covered by necrotic material.
- *Stromal oedema* is present surrounding the ulcer area.

Characteristic features produced by some of the common causative bacteria are as follows:

- *Staphylococcus aureus* and *Streptococcus pneumoniae* usually produce an oval, yellowish-white densely opaque ulcer which is surrounded by relatively clear cornea (Fig. 25.1A).
- *Pseudomonas* species usually produce an irregular sharp ulcer with thick greenish mucopurulent exudate, diffuse liquefactive necrosis and semiopaque (ground glass)

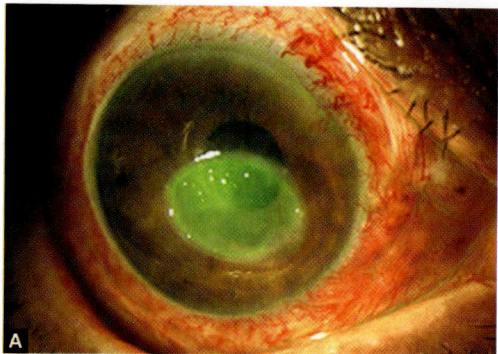
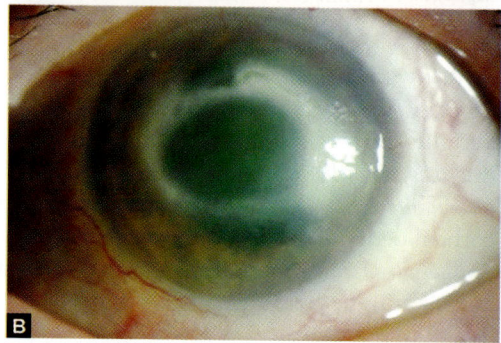

Fig. 25.1: *Bacterial corneal ulcer. A, Oval ulcer; B, Ring-shaped ulcer*

surrounding cornea. Such ulcers are usually associated with hypopyon, spread very rapidly and may even perforate within 48 to 72 hours.

- *Enterobacteriaceae* (*E. coli, Proteus* species, and *Klebsiella* species) usually produce a shallow ulcer with greyish-white pleomorphic suppuration and diffuse stromal opalescence. The endotoxins produced by these gram-negative bacilli may produce ring-shaped corneal infiltrate (Fig. 25.1B).
- *Streptococcus pneumonia keratitis* is usually seen after corneal trauma, dacryocystitis, and filtering bleb infection. It is characterstically acute, purulent and rapidly progressive with a deep stromal abscess.
- *Nocardia* causes indolent ulcer with raised superficial, pin-head infiltrates in a wreath-like configuration, brushfire border, cracked windshield appearance and satellite lesions.
- *Infectious crystalline keratopathy* is characterised by minimal stromal inflammation and fine needle-like extensions into stroma resembling a snowflake.

- *Risk factors* include corticosteroid use, anaesthetic abuse, prior surgeries (PK), BCL wear.
- *Causative organisms* are alpha haemolytic streptococci, *Strepto. pneumoniae, Staph. epidermidis*, Pseudomonas.

Clinical stages of corneal ulcer are:

Progressive stage occurring due to diffusion of toxins and enzymes and resultant tissue destruction is characterised by active ulceration (Fig. 25.2A to D).

Regressive stage: Characterised by improvement in signs and symptoms. Infiltrates decrease in size, ulcer becomes demarcated, AC reaction resolves, bacterial multiplication is controlled. Epithelium begins to heal over ulcer, pain improves, necrotic areas may slough off, mimicking progression.

Healing stage: Signs and symptoms continue to decrease and visual acuity starts to improve. Epithelium grows from all sides to cover the defect. Necrotic tissue is replaced by scar tissue. Bowman membrane does not regenerate and is therefore replaced by fibrous tissue, which may become less dense later. Vessels grow towards ulcer (Fig. 25.3), they usually regress completely but sometimes leave a residue of ghost vessels.

6. **Anterior chamber** shows reaction in the form of cells and flare. It may or may not show pus formation (hypopyon). In bacterial corneal ulcers, the hypopyon remains sterile so long as the Descemet's membrane is intact.

7. **Iris** may be slightly muddy in colour.

8. **Pupil** may be small due to associated toxin-induced iritis.

9. **Intraocular pressure** may sometimes be raised (inflammatory glaucoma).

HYPOPYON CORNEAL ULCER

Etiopathogenesis

Causative organisms. It is customary to reserve the term 'hypopyon corneal ulcer' for the characteristic ulcer caused by Pneumococcus and the term 'corneal ulcer with hypopyon' for the ulcers associated with hypopyon due to

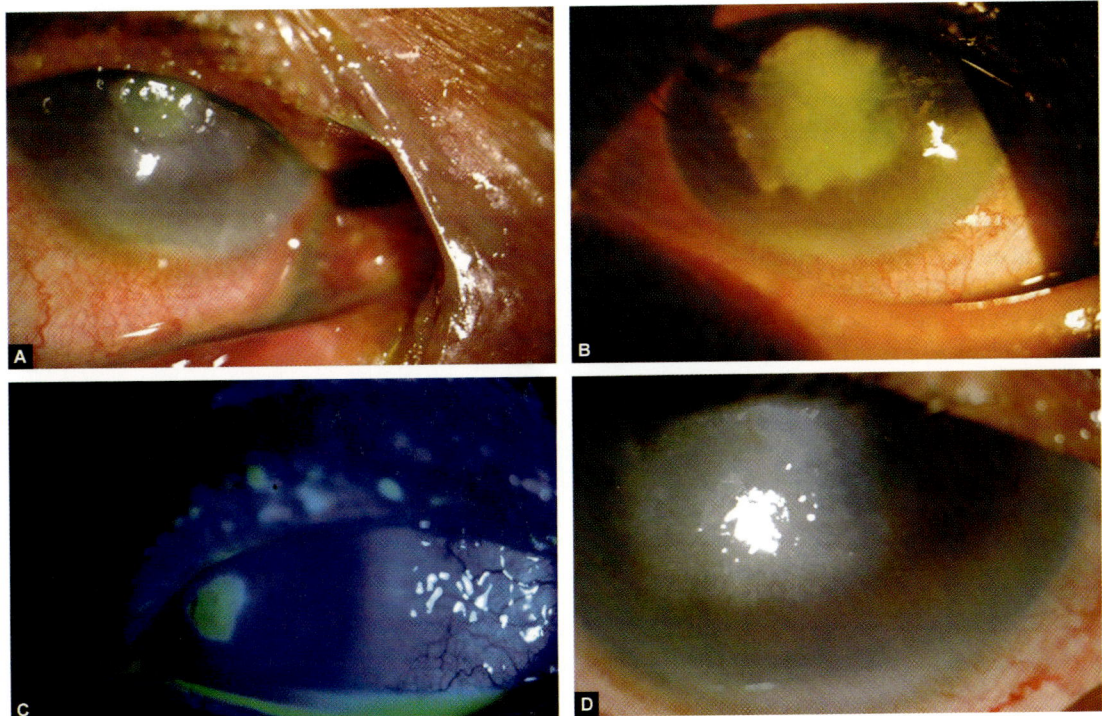

Fig. 25.2: *Progressive corneal ulceration. A, Central ulcer with hypopyon; B, Central progressive corneal ulcer; C, Fluorescein staining in corneal ulcer; D, The infiltrate may extend at deeper layers without corresponding epithelial defect*

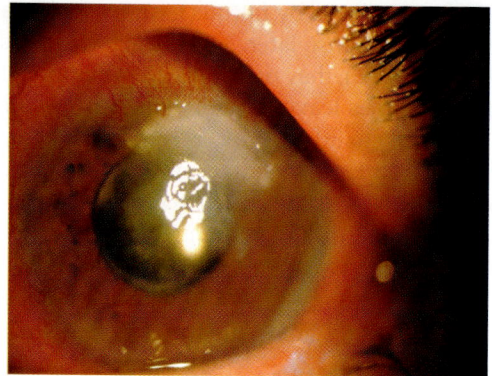

Fig. 25.3: *Healing corneal ulcer with early vascularization*

other organisms such as staphylococci, streptococci, gonococci, Moraxella and *Pseudomonas pyocyanea*. The characteristic hypopyon corneal ulcer caused by Pneumococcus is called *ulcus serpens*.

Source of infection for pneumococcal infection is usually the chronic dacryocystitis. Purulent keratitis with hypopyon is almost always exogenous, due to pyogenic organisms.

Factors predisposing to development of hypopyon. Two main factors which predispose to development of hypopyon in a patient with corneal ulcer are the virulence of the infecting organism and the resistance of the tissues. Hence, hypopyon ulcers are much more common in old debilitated or alcoholic subjects.

Mechanism of development of hypopyon. Corneal ulcer is often associated with some iritis owing to diffusion of bacterial toxins. When the iritis is severe the outpouring of leucocytes from the vessels is so great that these cells gravitate to the bottom of the anterior chamber to form a hypopyon. Thus, it is important to note that the hypopyon is sterile since the outpouring of polymorphonuclear cells is due to the toxins and not due to actual invasion by bacteria. Once the ulcerative process is controlled, the hypopyon is absorbed.

Clinical features

Symptoms are same as described above for bacterial corneal ulcer. However, it is important to note that during initial stage of ulcus serpens, there is remarkably little pain. As a result, the treatment is often unduly delayed.

Signs. In general, the signs are same as described above for the bacterial ulcer.

Characteristic features of ulcus serpens are:
- *Ulcus serpens* is a greyish-white or yellowish disc-shaped ulcer occurring near the centre of cornea (Fig. 25.4).
- *Ulcer has a tendency to creep* over the cornea in a serpiginous fashion. One edge of the ulcer, along which the ulcer spreads, shows more infiltration. The other side of the ulcer may be undergoing simultaneous cicatrisation and the edges may be covered with fresh epithelium.
- *Violent iridocyclitis* is commonly associated with a definite hypopyon.
- *Hypopyon increases in size very rapidly* and often results in secondary glaucoma.
- *Ulcer spreads rapidly* and has a great tendency for early perforation.

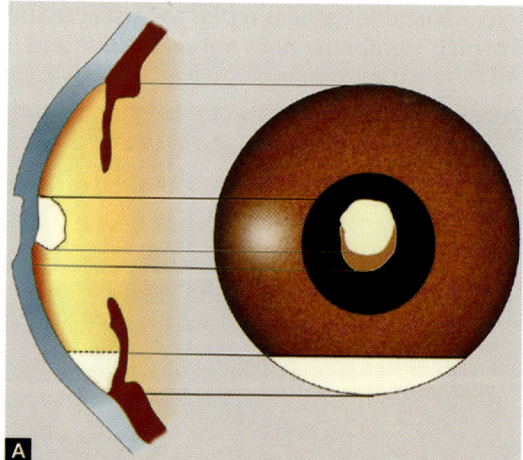

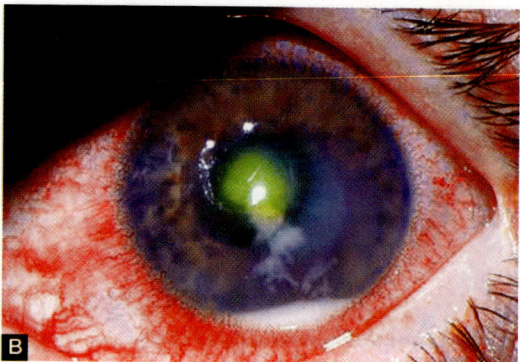

Fig. 25.4: *Hypopyon corneal ulcer. A, Diagrammatic depiction; B, Clinical photograph*

Management

Management of hypopyon corneal ulcer is same as for other bacterial corneal ulcer.

Special points which need to be considered are:

- *Secondary glaucoma* should be anticipated and treated with 0.5% timolol maleate, BID eye drops and oral acetazolamide.
- *Source of infection*, i.e. chronic dacryocystitis if detected, should be treated by dacryo-cystectomy.

COMPLICATIONS OF CORNEAL ULCER

1. *Toxic iridocyclitis.* It is usually associated with cases of purulent corneal ulcer due to absorption of toxins in the anterior chamber.

2. *Secondary glaucoma.* It occurs due to fibrinous exudates blocking the angle of anterior chamber (inflammatory glaucoma).

3. *Descemetocele.* Some ulcers caused by virulent organisms extend rapidly up to Descemet's membrane, which gives a great resistance, but due to the effect of intraocular pressure, it herniates as a transparent vesicle called the descemetocele or keratocele (Fig. 25.3). This is a sign of impending perforation and is usually associated with severe pain.

4. *Perforation of corneal ulcer.* Sudden strain due to cough, sneeze or spasm of orbicularis muscle may convert impending perforation into actual perforation (Fig. 24.4). Following perforation, immediately pain is decreased and the patient feels some hot fluid (aqueous) coming out of eyes.

Sequelae of corneal perforation include:

- *Prolapse of iris.* It occurs immediately following perforation in a bid to plug it.
- *Subluxation or anterior dislocation of lens* may occur due to sudden stretching and rupture of zonules.
- *Anterior capsular cataract.* It is formed when the lens comes in contact with the ulcer following a perforation in the pupillary area.
- *Corneal fistula.* It is formed when the perforation in the pupillary area is not plugged by iris and is lined by epithelium which gives way repeatedly. There occurs continuous leak of aqueous through the fistula.

- Purulent uveitis, endophthalmitis or even panophthalmitis may develop due to spread of intraocular infection.
- Intraocular haemorrhage in the form of either vitreous haemorrhage or expulsive choroidal haemorrhage may occur in some patients due to sudden lowering of intraocular pressure.

5. *Corneal scarring.* It is the usual end result of healed corneal ulcer. Corneal scarring leads to permanent visual impairment ranging from slight blurring to total blindness. Depending upon the clinical course of ulcer, corneal scar noted may be nebula, macula, leucoma, ectatic cicatrix or kerectasia, adherent leucoma or anterior staphyloma (for details *see* page 541).

MANAGEMENT OF A CASE OF CORNEAL ULCER

Since corneal ulcer is sight threatening ophthalmic emergency, it needs urgent treatment by identification and eradication of causative bacteria. Preferably such patients should be hospitalized. The management includes:

- Clinical evaluation
- Laboratory investigations
- Treatment.

A. Clinical evaluation

Each case with corneal ulcer should be subjected to:

1. *Thorough history taking* to elicit mode of onset.

2. *General physical examination*, specially for built, nourishment, anaemia and any immuno-compromising disease.

3. *Ocular examination* should include:

- *Diffuse light examination* for gross lesions of lids, conjunctiva and cornea including testing for sensations.
- *Regurgitation test* and syringing to rule out lacrimal sac infection.
- *Biomicroscopic examination* after staining of corneal ulcer with 2% freshly prepared aqueous solution of fluorescein dye or preferably sterilised fluorescein impregnated filter paper strip. Ulcer area stains as brilliant green, which looks opaque green when seen with blue filter. Note site, size, shape, depth, margin, floor and vascularization of corneal

ulcer. On biomicroscopy also note presence of keratic precipitates at the back of cornea, depth and contents of anterior chamber, colour and pattern of iris and condition of crystalline lens.

B. Laboratory investigations

1. *Routine laboratory investigations* such as haemoglobin, TLC, DLC, ESR, blood sugar, complete urine and stool examination should be carried out in each case.

2. *Microbiological investigations.* These studies are essential to identify causative organism, confirm the diagnosis and guide the treatment to be instituted. Material for such investigations is obtained by corneal scraping and corneal biopsy (which indicated).

Corneal scraping

Corneal scraping is done at the base and margins of the corneal ulcer (under local anaesthesia, using 2% Xylocaine or preferably paracaine) with the help of a modified Kimura spatula or by simply using the number 15 blade or bent tip of a 20 gauge hypodermic needle. The material obtained is used for the following investigations:

- *Gram and Giemsa stained* smears for possible identification of infecting organisms (bacteria, fungi, inclusion bodies and Acanthamoeba).
- *10% KOH wet preparation* for identification of fungal hyphae.
- *Calcofluor white (CFW) stain* preparation is viewed under fluorescence microscope for fungal filaments, the walls of which appear bright apple green.
- *Acridine orange stain* for Acanthamoeba and fungi.
- *Culture on blood agar*–chocolate agar medium for aerobic and facultative anaerobic organisms.
- *Culture on Sabouraud's dextrose agar* medium for fungi.
- *AFB stain* for mycobacteria and nocardia (when indicated)
- *PCR/immunodiagnostic techniques* may be used in non-responding ulcers when smear or cultues are negative.

Corneal biopsy

Indications include:
- Lack of response to treatment
- Negative culture on more than one occasion from the corneal scraping.
- Location of infiltrate in the mid or deep stroma with overlying uninvolved tissue.

Procedure. Corneal biopsy is performed under topical anaesthesia using a small trephine or blade. A small piece of stromal tissue, large enough to allow bisection is excised meticulously. One half of the biopsied tissue is sent for culture and microbiological studies and other half for histopathology. In case of a deep corneal abscess with overlying clear cornea, the biopsy can be taken from below a lamellar flap (Fig. 25.5A).

Alternative to biopsy is to pass a silk suture through the infiltrate and to culture the suture (Fig. 25.5B).

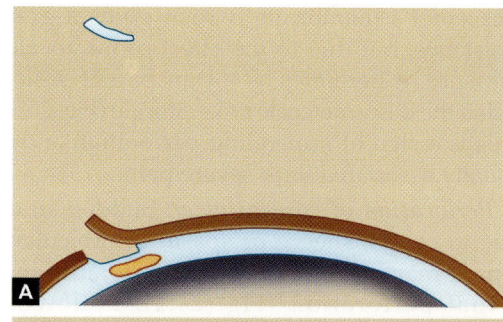
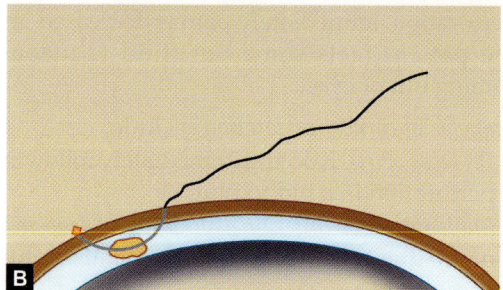

Fig. 25.5: *Corneal biopsy. A, From under the flap in patients with deep infiltrate; B, Using silk suture*

C. Treatment

Aim of treatment is to timely eliminate the organisms, reduce inflammation, prevent further structural damage and promote corneal healing and re-epithelization.

I. Treatment of uncomplicated corneal ulcer

Treatment of corneal ulcer can be discussed under three headings:

- Definitive treatment of the cause.
- Adjunctive/concurrent therapy.
- Physical and general measures.

1. Definitive treatment

a. *Topical antibiotics* form the mainstay of treatment. Initial treatment should be intensive so that the corneal tissue is rapidly saturated with a high antibiotic concentration. A high concentration (usually exceeding the minimum inhibitory concentration (MIC) by a number of log units) can be achieved within a few hours, so that 48 hours of sustained high concentration is usually enough to eliminate most bacterial infections.

Initial therapy (before results of culture and sensitivity are available) should be with combination therapy to cover both gram-negative and gram-positive organisms. To begin with any of the following two drugs may be instilled:

- Fortified cefazoline 5%, i.e. 50 mg/ml freshly prepared by adding sterile water to 500 mg powder to make 10 ml solution.
- Fortified tobramycin 1.3%, i.e. 13.6 mg/ml prepared by adding 2 ml of tobramycin injection (40 mg/ml in 5 ml bottle of commercially available 0.3% tobramycin drops).

Or

- Freshly prepared fortified vancomycin 5%, i.e. 50 mg/ml (prepared by adding sterile water to 500 mg vancomycin powder to form 10 ml solution) and one of commercially available fluoroquinolones eye drops (0.3% ciprofloxacin, or 0.3% ofloxacin or 0.3% gatifloxacin or 0.5% moxifloxacin).

Frequency of instillation. The chosen two drugs should be instilled alternately as below:

- Every 5 minutes for 30 minutes
- Every 15 minutes for 2 hours
- 1 hourly round the clock for first 48 hours
- 2 hourly during day and 4 hourly at night till healing is begins
- 4–6 hourly to allow for healing of the epithelial defect till healing occurs
- Once the favourable response is obtained, the fortified drops can be substituted by the commercially available eye drops.

Subsequent therapy. There is no need to change initial antibiotics, if the response is good. However, if the response is poor, immediately change the antibiotics as per culture and sensitivity report (Table 25.1).

Table 25.1: *Choice of antibiotics with doses for common organism in patients with bacterial corneal ulcer*

Organism	Antibiotics	Doses (topical) mg/ml	Doses (subconjunctival)
Multiple organisms or no organism	Cefazolin	50	100 mg in 0.5 ml
	Gentamicin/tobramycin	9–14	20 mg in 0.5 ml
	Fluoroquinolones	3	
Gram-positive cocci	Cefazoline	50	100 mg in 0.5 ml
	Vancomycin	15–50	25 mg in 0.5 ml
Gram-negative	Tobramycin/gentamicin	9–14	20 mg in 0.5 ml
	Ceftazidime	50	100 mg in 0.5 ml
	Fluoroquinolones	3 mg/ml	
Non-tuberculous mycobacteria	Amikacin	20–40 mg/ml	20 mg in 0.5 ml
	Clarithromycin		
Nocardia	Amikacin	20–40 mg/ml	20 mg in 0.5 ml
	Trimethoprim	16 mg/ml	
	Sulfamethoxazole	80 mg/ml	
Multidrug-resistant (MDR) bacteria	Imipenem/cilastin	1 mg/ml	
	Colistin	19 mg/ml	
	Linezolid	2 mg/ml	

b. *Systemic antibiotics* are usually not required. However, a cephalosporin and an amino-glycoside or oral ciprofloxacin (750 mg twice daily) may be given in fulminating cases with perforation or when sclera is also involved or care of systemic infections such as gonorrhoea.

2. Adjunctive/concurrent therapy

a. *Cycloplegic drugs.* Preferably 1% atropine eye drops (ointment in small children) should be used:

- To reduce pain from ciliary spasm
- To prevent the formation of posterior synechiae from secondary iridocyclitis.
- Atropine also increases the blood supply to anterior uvea by relieving pressure on the anterior ciliary arteries and so brings more antibodies in the aqueous humour.
- It also reduces exudation by decreasing hyperaemia and vascular permeability.

Other cycloplegic drug which can be used in 2% homatropine eye drops.

b. *Oral doxycycline*, 100 mg per day, is used as metalloproteinase inibitor, when the ulcer is large and there is corneal thinning.

c. *Systemic analgesics* and anti-inflammatory drugs such as paracetamol and ibuprofen relieve the pain and decrease oedema.

d. Vitamins (A, B-complex and C) help in early healing of ulcer.

- *Oral doxycycline:* When the ulcer is large and there is corneal thinning oral doxicycline as a metalloproteinase inhibitor.
- *Corticosteroid treatment:* Topical steroids are contraindicated in infective corneal ulcer. However, in later stages, corticosteroids may be required to settle the resultant inflam-mation and may be necessary to promote healing of the epithelial defect.

3. Physical and general measures

- *Hot fomentation.* Local application of heat (preferably dry) gives comfort, reduces pain and causes vasodilatation.
- *Dark goggles* may be used to prevent photo-phobia.
- *Rest,* good diet and fresh air may have a soothing effect.

II. Treatment of non-healing corneal ulcer

If the ulcer progresses despite the above therapy the following additional measures should be taken:

1. *Removal of any known cause of non-healing ulcer.* A thorough search for any already missed cause not allowing healing should be made and when found, such factors should be eliminated. Common causes of non-healing ulcers are as under:

- *Local causes:* Associated raised intraocular pressure, concretions, misdirected cilia, impacted foreign body, dacryocystitis, inade-quate therapy, wrong diagnosis, lagophtha-lmos and excessive vascularization of ulcer.
- *Systemic causes:* Diabetes mellitus, severe anaemia, malnutrition, chronic debilitating diseases and patients on systemic steroids.

2. *Mechanical debridement of ulcer* to remove necrosed material by scraping floor of the ulcer with a spatula under local anaesthesia may hasten the healing.

3. *Cauterisation of the ulcer* may also be consi-dered in non-responding cases. Cauterisation may be performed with pure carbolic acid or 10–20% trichloroacetic acid.

4. *Bandage soft contact lens* may also help in healing.

5. *Peritomy,* i.e. severing of perilimbal conjunc-tival vessels may be performed when excessive corneal vascularisation is hindering healing.

III. Treatment of impending perforation

When ulcer progresses and perforation seems imminent, the following additional measures may help to prevent perforation and its complications:

1. *No strain.* The patient should be advised to avoid sneezing, coughing and straining during stool, etc. He should be advised strict bed rest.

2. *Pressure bandage* should be applied to give some external support.

3. *Lowering of intraocular pressure* by simul-taneous use of acetazolamide 250 mg QID orally, intravenous mannitol (20%) drip stat, oral glycerol twice a day, 0.5% timolol eye drops twice a day, and even paracentesis with slow evacuation of aqueous from the anterior chamber may be performed if required.

4. *Tissue adhesive glue* such as cyanoacrylate is helpful in preventing perforation.

5. *Bandage soft contact lens* may also be used.

6. *Conjunctival flap.* The cornea may be covered completely or partly by a conjunctival flap to give support to the weak tissue.

7. *Amniotic membrane transplantation* may also be considered as an option.

8. Therapeutic penetrating keratoplasty (tectonic graft) (Fig. 25.6) may be undertaken in suitable cases, when available.

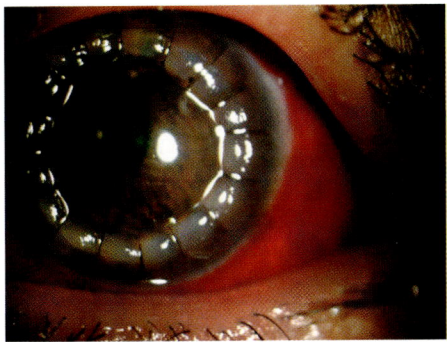

Fig. 25.6: *A large non-responsive corneal ulcer treated with therapeutic keratoplasty*

Indications include:
- Large size of ulcer
- Central location with uncontrolled progression
- Limbal involvement
- Impending scleritis

IV. Treatment of perforated corneal ulcer

Best is to prevent perforation. However, if perforation has occurred, immediate measures should be taken to restore the integrity of perforated cornea. Depending upon the size of perforation and availability, measures like use of tissue adhesive glues, covering with conjunctival flap, use of bandage soft contact lens or therapeutic keratoplasty should be undertaken. Best option is an *urgent tectonic keratoplasty.* A localised *patch graft* can be performed when perforation is small (<2 mm).

MARGINAL CATARRHAL ULCER

These superficial ulcers situated near the limbus are frequently seen especially in old people.

Etiology

Marginal catarrhal ulcer is thought to be caused by a hypersensitivity reaction to staphylococcal toxins. It occurs in association with chronic staphylococcal blepharoconjunctivitis. Moraxella and Haemophilus are also known to cause such ulcers.

Clinical features

- *Patient usually presents with* mild ocular irritation, pain, photophobia and watering.
- *Ulcer is shallow*, slightly infiltrated and often multiple, usually associated with staphylococcal conjunctivitis (Fig. 25.7).
- *Vascularization* occurs soon and is followed by resolution.
- *Recurrences* are very common.

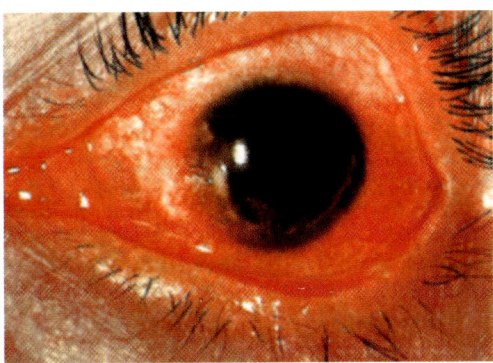

Fig. 25.7: *Marginal corneal ulcer in a patient with acute conjunctivitis*

Treatment

- A short course of topical corticosteroid drops along with adequate antibiotic therapy often heals the condition.
- Adequate treatment of associated blepharitis and chronic conjunctivitis is important to prevent recurrences.

MYCOTIC KERATITIS

The incidence of suppurative corneal ulcers caused by fungi has increased in the recent years due to injudicious use of antibiotics and steroids. Fungal keratitis is more common in tropical and developing countries as compared to temperate and developed countries.

EPIDEMIOLOGY

Fungi may be a part of normal ocular flora and can be isolated from conjunctival sac of healthy individuals. The incidence of fungal keratitis has increased over the past 30 years and varies from 22 to 50% in developing world. This increased occurrence of fungal keratitis is a result of the frequent use of topical corticosteroids in younger age group specially in cases of vernal keratoconjunctivitis and improvement in microbiological diagnostic techniques. They remain a leading cause of microbial keratitis in low income countries where major population belong to rural areas. In north India, most common cause is Aspergillus while in south India Fusarium is the most common organism isolated.

ETIOLOGY

Fungi

Fungi are eukaryotic organisms with membrane bound nucleus consisting of chromosomes of DNA that reproduce by forming spores. They can be either unicellular or formed of filamentous bodies called mycelia. They are found ubiquitously in dead decaying organic matter and can be saprophytic as well as pathogenic in nature.

Morphologically the fungi can be classified as below (Table 25.2).

i. Filamentous fungi

- *Filamentous septate fungi,* e.g. Aspergillus, Fusarium, Alternaria, Cephalosporium, Curvularia and Penicillium are septate multicellular fungi. Filamentous septate fungi, which can be pigmented (*dematiaceous*) and non-pigmented (*non-dematiaceous*).
- A feathery or powdery growth on the surface of culture media is produced by septate filamentary fungi, which are the most common cause of fungal keratitis. *Aspergillus* species is the most common isolate in fungal keratitis worldwide. Large series of fungal keratitis from India report that *Aspergillus* species is the most common isolate (27–64%), followed by *Fusarium* (6–32%) and *Penicillium* (2–29%) species. *Dematiaceous fungi* are characterised by the development of a brown, olive

Table 25.2: *Morphological classification of fungi*

Yeast
Candida species
  albicans, parapsilosis, krusei, tropicalis
Cryptococcus species
Filamentous septated
 Non-pigmented hyphae
  Fusarium species
   solani, oxysporum
  Aspergillus species
   fumigatus, flavus, niger
  Acremonium
Filamentous non-septated
  Mucor species
  Rhizopus species
  Pythium species
 Pigmented hyphae
  Alternaria species
  Curvularia species
  Cladosporum species
Dimorphic fungi
 Histoplasma
 Coccidioides
 Blastomyces

or black colour in the cell walls of their vegetative cells, conidia or both which results in pigment colonies on culture. Clinically small proportion of cases showed brown to black macroscopic pigmentation (24%). Pigmentation of fungal filaments related to melanin metabolism, linked to altered metabolic state associated with low virulence and less severe inflammation. Commonest dematiaceous fungi isolated are Curvularia (44%), Phialophora (16%) and Alternaria (12%).

- *Filamentous non-septate fungi* include Mucor and Rhizopus.

ii. Yeasts

Yeasts, e.g. Candida and Cryptococcus are unicellular fungi that reproduce by budding. Yeast produces characteristic creamy, opaque, pasty colonies on the surface of culture media. Candida is the most representative pathogen in this group, primarily affecting those corneas already compromised by topical steroids, surface pathology, or both.

iii. Dimorphic fungi

Dimorphic fungi such as Histoplasma, Coccidioides and Blastomyces demonstrate both yeast phase that occurs in the tissues and a mycelia phase that appears in culture media and on saprophytic surfaces.

Predisposing risk factors

Factors which predispose to mycotic keratitis are (Table 25.3):

- *Injury by vegetative material* such as crop leaf, branch of a tree, straw, thorn, wooden stick or decaying vegetable matter. Common sufferers are field workers especially during harvesting season.
- *Injury by animal tail* is another mode of infection.
- *Immunosuppressing* systemic (HIV diabetic) or local such as patients suffering from dry eye, herpetic keratitis, bullous keratopathy or postoperative cases of keratoplasty. Predisposes to secondary fungal ulcers.
- *Role of antibiotics and steroids.* Antibiotics disturb the symbiosis between bacteria and fungi; and the steroids make the fungi facultative pathogens which are otherwise symbiotic saprophytes. Therefore, excessive use of these drugs predisposes the patients to fungal infections.

Table 25.3: *Presenting risk factor for fungal keratitis*

Ocular	Systemic
Trauma	Immunosuppressive disorders
Vegetative foreign bodies	HIV
Contact lens use	Uncontrolled diabetes mellitus
Use of topical steroids	Hospitalised patients
Corneal surgery	Leprosy patients
Chronic keratitis	

CLINICAL FEATURES

Symptoms are similar to the central bacterial corneal ulcer (*see* page 390), but in general, they are less marked than the equal-sized bacterial ulcer and the overall course is slow and torpid. Thus, unlike bacterial keratitis, mycotic keratitis does not present acutely and patients may complain of non-specific symptoms of foreign body sensation and slowly progressive pain for several days.

Signs are more prominent than symptoms. A typical fungal corneal ulcer has following salient features (Fig. 25.8).

- *Corneal ulcer* in filamentous keratitis is greyish-white, dry-looking with elevated rolled out margins; while in candidal keratitis, it occurs as a yellow-white densely suppurative infiltrate (Fig. 25.8A).
- *Pigmented ulcer* (brownish) may be caused by some species of fungi, e.g. dermatiaceous fungi (Fig. 25.9).
- Delicate *feathery finger-like extensions* are present into the surrounding stroma under the intact epithelium.
- *Sterile immune ring* (yellow-white line of demarcation) may be present where fungal antigen and host antibodies meet.

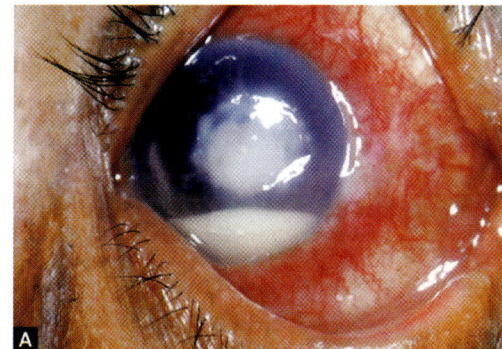

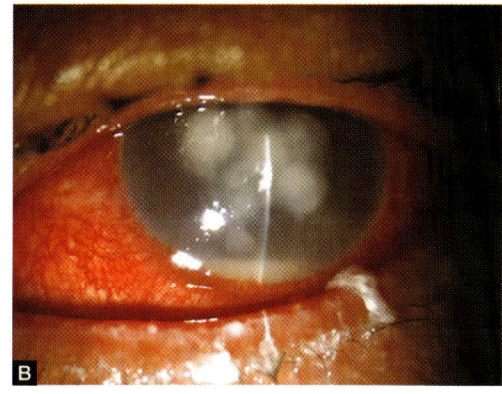

Fig. 25.8: *Fungal corneal ulcer: A, Showing thick hypopyon; B, Showing satellite lesions and hypopyon*

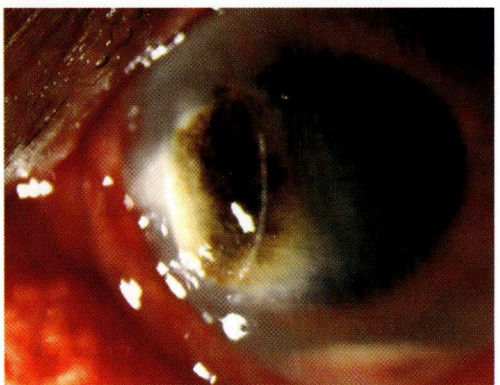

Fig. 25.9: *Mycotic keratitis caused by dermatiaceous fungi showing elevated margins with brown-black pigmentation*

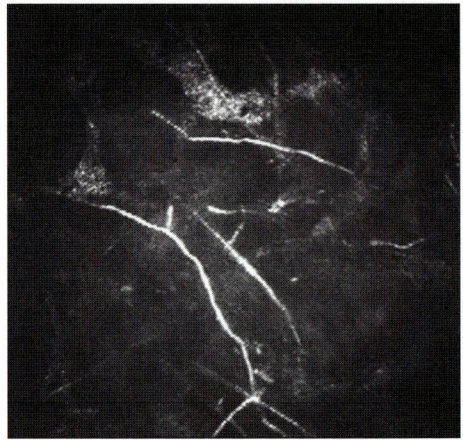

Fig. 25.10: *Confocal microscopy image showing branching fungal hyphae in the corneal stroma*

- *Multiple, small satellite lesions* may be present around the ulcer (Fig. 25.8B).
- *Hypopyon*, usually a big one, is present even if the ulcer is very small. Unlike bacterial ulcer, the hypopyon is not sterile as the fungi can penetrate into the anterior chamber without perforation.
- *Endothelial plaque*, composed of fibrin and leucocytes, may be located under the stromal lesion. It may be present in the absence of hypopyon.
- *Perforation*, in mycotic ulcer, is rare but can occur.
- Corneal vascularization is conspicuously absent in pure mycotic ulcer.

INVESTIGATIONS AND DIAGNOSIS

I. Clinical diagnosis

Clinical diagnosis is made from:
- Typical clinical manifestations associated with history of injury by vegetative material are highly suspicious of a mycotic corneal ulcer.
- Chronic ulcer worsening in spite of most efficient treatment should arouse suspicion of mycotic involvement.

II. *In vivo* scanning slit confocal microscopy

Confocal microscopic examination of cornea is reported to identify actual fungi. It is a newer investigation that works on principle of pinhole apertures to create optical sections of cornea (Fig. 25.10). Non-invasive in nature, it can identify deeply placed fungal hyphae not readily

obtained in scraping specimens and can be used wherever available. However, it is costly and artefacts may be confused with yeast cells and fungal hyphae.

III. Laboratory investigations

Laboratory investigations are required to identify the causative fungi.

Corneal scrapings should be performed under topical anaesthesia from the base and leading edge of the ulcer. Thus, the most important step in the initial management of suspected fungal keratitis is to obtain corneal material for direct smears and inoculation of media. Corneal scraping also forms a therapeutic method of ulcer debridement and better penetration of topical antifungal agents alongside obtaining material for diagnostic evaluation.

The primary isolation cultures for fungus are Sabouraud and blood agar at room temperature. Chocolate agar and thioglycolate broth can also be used to grow these organisms in laboratory. Initial growth occurs in 72 hours but may take up to 2 weeks for slow-growing fungi. Antifungal susceptibility testing may also be performed for identification of resistance to antifungal agents. The following tests should be performed from the scraped material:
- *Examination of wet KOH mount preparation* may reveal filamentous fungi as branched, septate hyphae (*Aspergillus fumigatus* or Fusarium) or nonfilamentous yeast like fungi (Candida).

- *Gram's and Giemsa stained films* may reveal fungal hyphae and inflammatory cells.
- *Culture on Sabouraud's agar medium* should also be performed for fungi.
- *Polymerase chain reaction* (PCR) has emerged as a sensitive and specific test for diagnosis of fungal keratitis. Advantage of PCR is that it is rapid and only a small sample is needed for diagnosis. Major limitation is that it is costly and not readily available at all centres. Also it can lead to overdiagnosis from fungal contamination of obtained corneal specimen. DNA-based sequence methods can be used for rapid species identification of an organism.

Note. Material for microbiological investigations may also be collected from:

Anterior chamber paracentesis may be carried out in cases with intraocular extension.

Corneal biopsy is indicated in cases with deep stromal abscess or in cases where repeated cultures from scrapings are negative. Superficial keratitis or punch biopsy may be performed.

TREATMENT

A. Definitive treatment

Definitive treatment includes antifungal drugs:

Antifungal drugs

Antifungal agents are mainstay of treatment and are classified into the groups below (Table 25.4).

I. Polyenes

Polyenes include natamycin, nystatin, and amphotericin B. Polyenes disrupt the cell by binding to fungal cell wall ergosterol and are effective against both filamentous and yeast forms.

Amphotericin B although penetrates ocular tissue poorly, it is the drug of choice for treatment of fungal keratitis caused by Candida. In addition, it has efficacy against many filamentous fungi. It is available as 50 mg powder which is reconstituted in 10 ml of sterile water. 3 ml of this reconstituted solution is then made into 10 ml by adding 7 ml sterile water to make it into concentration of 0.15% and dispensed in a dark brown bottle. Drops are clear yellow in colour, if they turn milky then it should be discarded. Usually, the prepared solution can be used for a week. Natamycin has a broad-spectrum of activity against filamentous organisms.

Natamycin is the only commercially available topical ophthalmic antifungal preparation. It is effective against filamentous fungi, particularly for infections caused by Fusarium. However, because of poor ocular penetration, it has primarily been useful in cases with superficial corneal infection. Also it can form chalky white infiltrates on the epithelial interfering with monitoring of underlying infection (Fig. 25.11).

II. Azoles

Azoles (imidazoles and triazoles) include ketoconazole, miconazole, fluconazole, itraconazole and clotrimazole. Azoles inhibit ergosterol synthesis at low concentrations, and, at higher concentrations, they appear to cause direct damage to cell walls.

Table 25.4: *Antifungal agents*		
Polyenes: Bind to fungal cell membranes, altering membrane permeability		
Amphotericin B	First line therapy for *Candida* species	
	Good to moderate activity against *Aspergillus, Fusarium* species	0.05–.30%
Natamycin	Good activity against most Fusarium	2.5–5%
Azoles: Inhibitor of ergosterol biosynthesis of the fungal cell wall		
Clotrimazole	Effective against Fusarium, Aspergillus	1% topical/cream
Econazole	Effective against Fusarium, Aspergillus, and *Candida* species	0.02–2%
Fluconazole	Effective against yeast	0.5–1%
Ketoconazole	Effective against Candida, Aspergillus	1–2%
Itraconazole		
Voriconazole	Effective against Aspergillus, Fusarium, Candida	1%

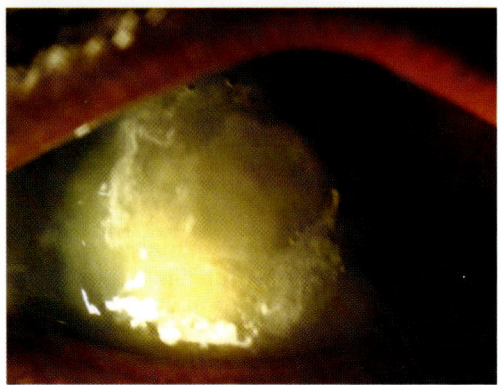

Fig. 25.11: *Natamycin deposits seen in a case of fungal keratitis*

Voriconazole is a newer synthetic azole having good efficacy against filamentous fungi. Recent reports have shown that it may not be effective against Fusarium but shows good activity against Aspergillus. It is commercially available as 30 mg powder and can be reconstituted with 3 ml of sterile water to form 1% solution. It can be used in the same concentration as intrastromal or intracameral injection in deep stromal/endothelial infections. Intravitreal injections are also used in fungal endophthalmitis.

Oral fluconazole and ketoconazole are absorbed systemically with good levels in the anterior chamber and the cornea; therefore, an oral antifungal should be considered for patients with deep stromal infection, scleral involvement or endophthalmitis. Antifungal therapy usually is maintained for 12 weeks, and patients are monitored closely. The adult dose of ketoconazole is 200–400 mg/d, which can be increased to 800 mg/d. However, because of the secondary effects, increasing the dose should be decided carefully. Gynaecomastia, oligospermia, and decreased libido have been reported in 5–15% of patients who have been taking 400 mg/d for a long period.

The potential role of topical itraconazole in treatment of fungal keratitis is still unclear. However, it may be a helpful adjunctive agent in fungal keratitis.

Posaconazole is a new triazole proved to be effective against Fusarium keratitis resistant to other azoles without significant toxicity.

III. Pyrimidines

Fluorinated pyrimidines, such as flucytosine, are other antifungal agents. Flucytosine is converted into a thymidine analog that blocks fungal thymidine synthesis. It usually is administered in combination with an azole or amphotericin B; it is synergistic with these medications. Otherwise, if flucytosine is the only drug used in therapy for Candida infections, emergence of resistance rapidly develops. Therefore, flucytosine should never be used alone.

IV. Echinocandins

These act by inhibiting synthesis of 1,3-β-d-glucan synthesis leading to cell lysis from increased cell wall permeability. Topical micafungin 0.2% can be tried in refractory mycotic keratitis cases.

Mode of administration of antifungal drugs

1. **Topical antifungal eye drops** should be used for a long period (6 to 8 weeks). These include:
   - *For filamentous fungi* (Aspergillus and Fusarium). Natamycin (5%) eye drops (drug of choice), or amphotericin B (0.1 to 0.3%), or fluconazole (0.2%), or miconazole (10 mg/ml) or voriconazole (10%) eye drops to be instilled initially one hourly around the clock, then taper slowly over 6 to 8 weeks.
   - *For yeasts* (Candida) amphotericin B (drug of choice), or nystatin (3.5%) eye ointment, five times a day is effective.

Topical agents are administered every 30 minutes for the first 24 hours, every hour for the second 24 hours, and then continued every 2 hourly according to the clinical response. Response to medical management is assessed everyday waiting for 3–7 days for resolution of signs and symptoms.

2. **Intracameral and intracorneal/intrastromal administration** of voriconazole may be considered in cases with intraocular extension or anterior chamber involvement (Fig. 25.12A and B).

3. **Systemic antifungal drugs** may be required for severe cases of deeper fungal keratitis. Tablet fluconazole or ketoconazole or voriconazole may be given for 2–3 weeks.

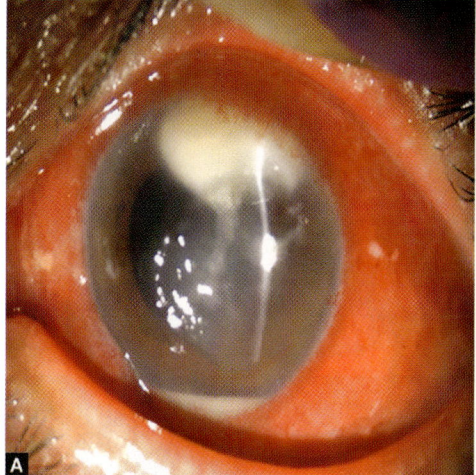

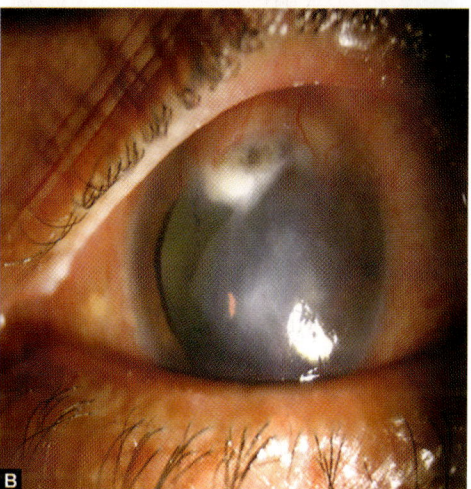

Fig. 25.12: *A case of fungal abscess near limbus responding to intrastromal voriconazole injection. A, Before injection; B, After injection*

Indications for starting systemic antifungal therapy include large ulcer >6 mm, deep ulcer >2/3 stromal involvement, scleral involvement, endophthalmitis, post-keratoplasty and patients with diabetes mellitus or immunocompromised status. Systemic side-effects of these drugs include nausea, diarrhoea, vomiting and dyspepsia. Hepatotoxicity resulting from these drugs warrants serious attention and patients should be monitored two weekly with liver function tests. Oral voriconazole appears to have a favourable side-effect profile among all azoles and is the first drug of choice. However, cost and availability are its major limitations.

Note. Topical steroids enhance fungal replication and corneal invasion and are thus contraindicated during early therapy of fungal corneal ulcer. Topical steroids are a strict contraindication and systemic steroids should be used cautiously in patients with active fungal keratitis.

B. Adjunctive/concurrent therapy

Non-specific treatment and general measures are similar to that of bacterial corneal ulcer (*see* page 396).

C. Therapeutic penetrating keratoplasty

Therapeutic penetrating keratoplasty (Fig. 25.13) may be required for non-responsive cases.

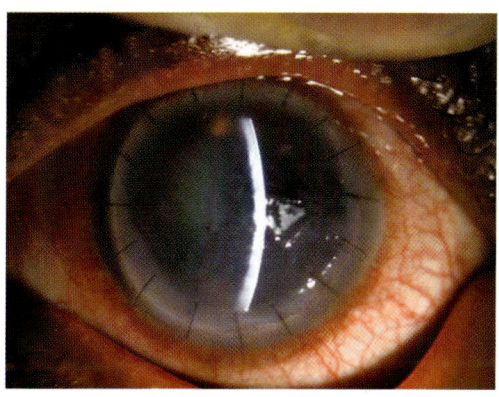

Fig. 25.13: *Edematous graft, well-formed anterior chamber and cataractous lens post-penetrating keratoplasty for patient in Fig. 25.10*

Approximately 15–30 patients require surgical treatment in the form penetrating or deep anterior lamellar keratoplasty. Recurrences are also quite common often therapeutic keratoplasty.

Note. Antifungal drugs should be continued at least 2–3 weeks postoperatively and weak steroids such as fluorometholone should be started after 2 weeks only when there are no signs of infection.

MICROSPORIDIAL KERATITIS

ETIOLOGY

Causative organism, Microsporidia, the ubiquitous obligate intracellular organism, previously classified as parasite (protozoa), have recently been re-classified as fungi. Following species are associated with ocular infection:

- *Encephalitozoon* species causes superficial keratoconjunctivitis.
- *Nosema, Vitaformia and Trachiplestophora* species are known to cause deep stromal keratitis.

Predisposing risk factors include:

- *Immunosuppression* is the main predisposed risk factor, specially the HIV infection. Local immunosuppression with typical case of corticosteroids also predisposes to the microsporidial infection. Although previously considered to occur only HIV cases, the infection is being observed in immunocompetent persons.
- *Trauma*, associated with exposure to water or mud, acts as another predisposing factor.
- *Contact lense wear* is also reported as risk factor.

CLINICAL FEATURES

Microsporidial keratitis, presenting with pain, photophobia, blurred vision and foreign body sensation, is known to occur in two distinct clinical forms:

I. *Superficial keratoconjunctivitis*, usually caused by *Encephalitozoon* species, typically occurs in immunocompromised individuals and is characterised by:

- Bilateral chronic diffuse punctate epithelial keratitis (Fig. 25.14)
- Conjunctivitis of mild form

II. *Deep stromal keratitis*, caused by *Nosema, Vitaformia*, and *Trachiplestophora* species, is usually seen in immunocompetent individuals. It is characterised by:

- Unilateral deep stromal infiltrate
- Corneal vascularization may or may not be associated
- Uveitis may also be associated.

Systemic features. In severely immunocompromised patient with HIV, the Microsporidia may involve nearly every organ system, most common being enteritis, and often being sinusitis, hepatitis, peritonitis, bronchiolitis, encephalitis, skeletal and cutaneous involvement.

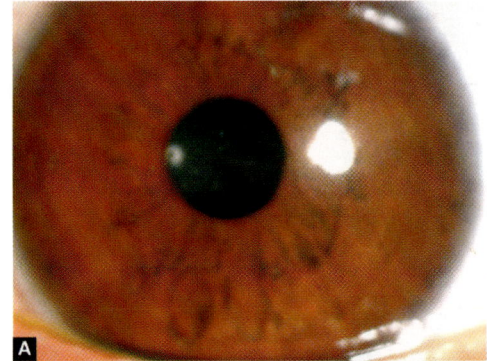
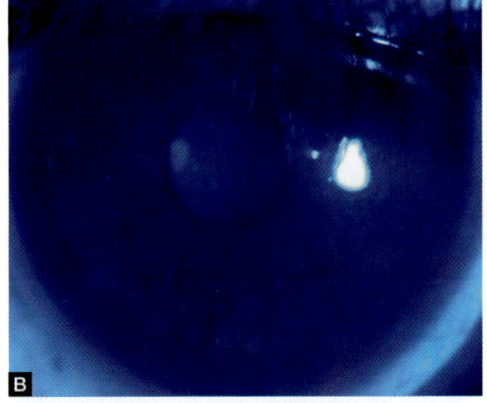

Fig. 25.14A and B: *Microsporidial keratitis*

DIAGNOSIS

1. *High level of clinical suspicion*, is required, specially in immunocompromised persons.
2. *Confocal microscopy* may reveal intraepithelial Microsporidia.
3. *Conjunctival and corneal scrapings* may show Microsporidia (Fig. 25.15) when studied with KOH, calcofluor white, Gram's and modified Ziehl-Neelsen stains.
4. *Culture* for Microsporidia is very difficult.
5. *PCR* assays have been developed, but have rare availability.
6. *Electron microscopy performed on body fluids* is considered the gold standard for diagnosis of microsporidial infection.

TREATMENT

A. *Definitive treatment* includes:

- *Topical fumagillin*, 10 mg/ml suspension used one hourly for 24 hours and then tapered, is the treatment of choice.

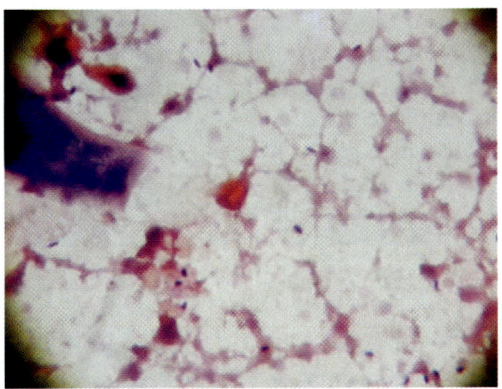

Fig. 25.15: *Microsporidia demonstrated from corneal scrapings*

- *Other topical preparations* used include propamidine, chlorhexidine, polyhexamethylene biguanide (PHMB), voriconazole and fluoroquinolone.
- *Oral albendazole,* 40 mg once a day for 2 weeks, repeated for 2 weeks often a gap of 2 weeks, is specially useful in patients with microsporidial stromal keratitis.

B. *Adjunctive/concurrent therapy.* Non-specific treatment and general measures are similar to that of bacterial corneal ulcer (*see* page 396).

C. *Highly active antiretroviral therapy (HAART)* is required in immunocompromised HIV patients.

D. *Therapeutic keratoplasty* may be indicated in non-responsive patient (Fig. 25.13). Recurrences are common, but can be reduced by cryotherapy to the residual tissue.

VIRAL KERATITIS

Incidence of viral corneal ulcers has become much greater especially because of the role of antibiotics in eliminating the pathogenic bacterial flora. Most of the viruses tend to affect the epithelium of both the conjunctiva and cornea, hence the typical viral lesions constitute the viral keratoconjunctivitis.

Viruses are acellular small (10–400 nm in diameter) infectious units which may affect the any part of the eye and cause severe ocular morbidity. Many of the viruses cause transient epithelial keratitis which heals without any sequelae, whereas viruses like herpes and adenovirus can lead to permanent corneal damage and visual loss.

Viruses causing ocular infections in humans are classified as follows.

DNA viruses
- Herpes—HSV (1 and 2), HVZ, CMV, EBV, human HSV 6–8
- Adeno
- Papova
- Poxviruses

RNA viruses
- Picorna: Enterovirus 70, coxsackie A24
- Orthomyxo: Influenza (A, B, C)
- Paramyxo: Measles, mumps, Newcastle
- Toga: Rubella, arbovirus group.

HERPES SIMPLEX KERATITIS

Ocular infections with herpes simplex virus (HSV) are extremely common and constitute herpetic keratoconjunctivitis and iritis.

ETIOLOGY

Herpes simplex virus (HSV). It is a large double-stranded DNA virus. It is the only natural host in man. According to different clinical and immunological properties, HSV is of two types:
- *HSV type I* (oral) typically causes infection above the waist.
- *HSV type II* (genital) typically causes infection below the waist (herpes genitalis) has also been reported to cause ocular lesions. It is the leading cause of herpetic infections in neonates.

Note. The severity and frequency of ocular disease may be influenced by different strains. Both HSV I and HSV II have an affinity for the sensory ganglion cells, and therefore, are called *neurotrophic viruses.*

Mode of infection is as below:
- *HSV I infection.* It is acquired by kissing or coming in close contact with a patient suffering from herpes labialis.
- *HSV II infection.* It is transmitted to eyes of neonates through infected genitalia of the mother.

Pathogenesis. The only natural reservoir of HSV in man. Children with primary disease, adults with recurrent disease and asymptomatic carriers acting as source of infections. Disease is rare below 6 months of age as there is high incidence of herpetic neutralising antibodies due to passive maternal transfer. Virus can be transferred by droplet infections, direct oral contact (HSV I). Figure 25.16 depicts the viral activity after inoculation by herpes simplex virus.

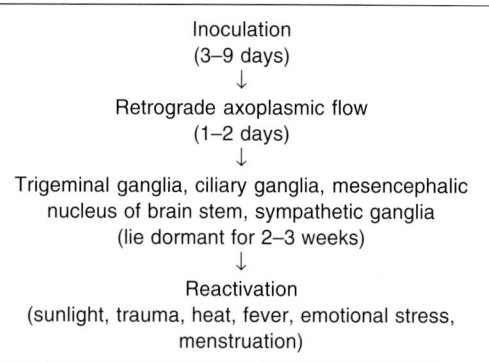

Inoculation
(3–9 days)
↓
Retrograde axoplasmic flow
(1–2 days)
↓
Trigeminal ganglia, ciliary ganglia, mesencephalic nucleus of brain stem, sympathetic ganglia
(lie dormant for 2–3 weeks)
↓
Reactivation
(sunlight, trauma, heat, fever, emotional stress, menstruation)

Fig. 25.16: *Herpes simplex virus activity after inoculation*

It has been postulated the HSV does not lie dormant but actively produces a viral RNA latency associated transcript (LAT), while the junctional region of the viral genome is retained in the host cell, the former being responsible for maintenance of latency.

Reactivation results in production of large amount of this antisense RNA leading to production of viral polypeptides and intact infectious virions. It has also been postulated that cornea itself may be extraneuronal site of latent infection.

Recurrence is common with genital (80%) and oral herpes (42% over 1 year) than with ocular herpes. The ocular herpes recurrence rate is 40% over a span of 5 years.

CLINICAL PRESENTATION

Ocular involvement by HSV occurs in three forms: Congenital and neonatal, primary, and recurrent; with following lesions:

A. Congenital and neonatal herpes

B. Primary ocular herpes

1. *Skin lesions:* Vesicles on the skin of lids and lid margin.
2. *Conjunctiva:* Conjunctivitis

3. *Corneal lesions*
   - Fine epithelial punctate keratitis
   - Coarse epithelial punctate keratitis
   - Dendritic ulcer

C. Recurrent ocular herpes

1. *Active epithelial keratitis*
   - Punctate epithelial keratitis
   - Dendritic ulcer
   - Geographical ulcer
2. *Stromal keratitis*
   - Disciform keratitis
   - Diffuse stromal necrotic keratitis
3. *Trophic keratitis (meta-herpetic)*
4. *Herpetic iridocyclitis and trabeculitis*
5. *HSV retinitis*

A. CONGENITAL AND NEONATAL HERPES

It occurs secondary to direct exposure to HSV II infected birth canal during late prenatal period or at birth.

Manifestations include:
- Conjunctivitis
- Epithelial keratitis
- Stromal immune reaction
- Cataract and necrotising chorioretinitis

Note: *Protective transplacental antibodies* are not sufficient to protect infants from development of ocular manifestations, though they might escape serious visceral involvement.

B. PRIMARY OCULAR HERPES

Primary infection (first attack) involves a non-immune person. It typically occurs in children after 6 months of age when the store of passively acquired maternal antibodies becomes depleted. 60% of all children by the age of 5 years become viral carrier. Initial infection occurs by direct contact of mucous membranes with infected secretions.

Clinical features

1. *Systemic features* include mild fever, malaise and non-suppurative lymphadenopathy. Rarely, severe morbidity can result from multisystem failure. Disease may be fatal when encephalitis develops.
2. *Skin lesions.* Vesicular lesions may occur involving skin of face, lips, lids, periorbital region and the lid margin (*vesicular blepharitis*).

3. *Ocular lesions.* Typically these occur unilateral blepharoconjunctivitis characterised by:

- *Acute follicular conjunctivitis* with regional lymphadenitis is the usual and sometimes the only manifestation of the primary infection.
- *Keratitis.* Cornea is involved in about 50% of the cases. The keratitis can occur as a coarse punctate or diffuse branching epithelial keratitis. Deeper involvement as stromal keratitis and uveitis are uncommon as the host is not immunologically sensitized against the virus.

Treatment

- *Primary infection is usually self-limiting* but virus travels up to the trigeminal ganglion and establishes the latent infection.
- *Treatment is recommended to limit corneal involvement.* Topical trifluridine or vidarabine, or oral acyclovir can be used. A cycloplegic (atropine) may be added for comfort from ciliary spasm.

C. RECURRENT OCULAR HERPES

The virus which lies dormant in the trigeminal ganglion, periodically reactivates and replicates. The reactivated virus in enveloped infectious form travels down along the trigeminal nerve to cause recurrent infection. The recurrent herpetic ocular infection is not associated with systemic features and typically is a unilateral disease.

These patients have developed both cellular and humoral immunity against the virus.

Predisposing stress stimuli which trigger an attack of herpetic keratitis include fever such as malaria, flu, exposure to ultraviolet rays, general ill health, emotional or physical exhaustion, mild trauma, menstrual stress following administration of topical or systemic steroids and immunosuppressive agents.

1. Epithelial keratitis

Symptoms

Symptoms of epithelial HSV keratitis include redness, pain, photophobia, tearing and decreased vision.

Signs

I. Corneal signs

Three distinct patterns of epithelial keratitis seen are: Punctate epithelial keratitis, dendritic ulcer and geographical ulcer.

1. *Punctate epithelial keratitis* (Fig. 25.17A and B). The initial epithelial lesions of recurrent herpes resemble those seen in primary herpes and may be either in the form of fine or coarse superficial punctate lesions due to swollen

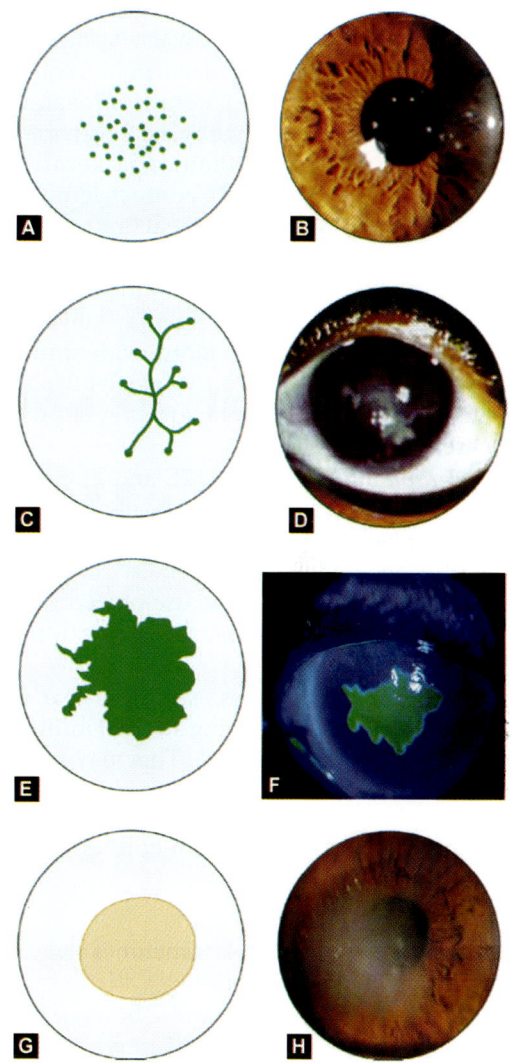

Fig. 25.17: *Lesions of recurrent herpes simplex keratitis; diagrammatic depiction and clinical photograph. A and B, Punctate epithelial keratitis; C and D, Dendritic ulcer; E and F, Geographic ulcer; G and H, Disciform keratitis*

opaque epithelial cells. The corneal vesicles coalesce and erupt to form dendritic or geographic ulcer.

2. *Dendritic ulcer* (Fig. 25.17C and D). Dendritic ulcer is a typical and most common lesion of recurrent epithelial keratitis. The ulcer is of an irregular, zigzag linear branching shape. The branches are generally knobbed at the ends. Floor of the ulcer stains with fluorescein and the virus-laden cells at the margin take up rose bengal associated mild subepithelial haze is typical. There is an associated marked diminution of corneal sensations.

Differential diagnosis of dendritic ulceration includes herpes zoster keratitis (pseudodendritis), toxic keratopathy, healing corneal abrasion, early Acanthamoeba keratitis, epithelial effects of soft contact lens and epithelial rejection in a corneal graft.

After healing of dendritic ulceration, a mild subepithelial haze may persist for weeks. In some cases, mild scarring may develop, which tends to become more evident often every recurrence. Since the lesions usually involve pupillary area, often vision in threatened substantially.

3. *Geographic ulcer* (Fig. 25.17E and F). Sometimes, the branches of dendritic ulcer enlarge and coalesce to form a large epithelial ulcer with a 'geographic' or 'amoeboid' configuration, hence the name. The use of steroids in dendritic ulcer hastens the formation of geographic ulcer.

Marginal ulcer, sometimes, can form near the limbus, that has an underlying stromal infiltrate and adjacent limbal infection. This may mimic a bacterial infection.

II. Other signs associated with epithelial keratitis

These include:

- *Eyelid vascular lesions*, may sometimes coincide with epithelial ulceration.
- *Follicular conjunctivitis*, may also be associated in some cases. Further, topical antiviral drugs may also cause this.
- *Anterior chamber reaction*, of mild intensity, may also be noticed in some cases.
- *Raised intraocular pressure*, is not uncommon.

Treatment

A. *Definitive treatment*

1. *Antiviral drugs* are the first choice presently. Any one of the following drugs may be given:

- *Acycloguanosine* (aciclovir) 3% ointment: 5 times a day for 14–21 days. It is least toxic and most commonly used antiviral drug. It penetrates intact corneal epithelium and stroma, achieving therapeutic levels in aqueous humour, and can therefore be used to treat herpetic keratitis.
- *Ganciclovir* (0.15% gel), 5 times a day until ulcer heals and then 3 times a day for 5 days. It is more toxic than aciclovir.
- *Trifluorothymidine* 1% drops: Two hourly until ulcer heals and then 4 times a day for 5 days.
- *Adenine arabinoside* (vidarabine) 3% ointment: 5 times a day until ulcer heals and then 3 times a day for 5 days.

2. *Mechanical debridement* of the involved area along with a rim of surrounding healthy epithelium with the help of sterile cotton applicator under magnification helps by removing the virus-laden cells. Before the advent of antiviral drugs, it was the treatment of choice. Now it is reserved for resistant cases, cases with noncompliance and those allergic to antiviral drugs.

3. *Systemic antiviral drugs* for a period of 10 to 21 days are increasingly being considered for recurrent and even acute cases in following doses:

- Acyclovir 400 mg p.o. tid to bid, or
- Famcyclovir 250 mg p.o. bid, or
- Valacyclovir 500 mg p.o. bid.

B. *Non-specific supportive therapy* and physical and general measures are same as for bacterial corneal ulcer (*see* page 396).

2. Stromal keratitis

It accounts for 20–48% of recurrent ocular HSV disease. Each episode of stromal keratitis increases the risk of future episodes. It may occur:

- *As immune response to viral antigens* (immune stromal keratitis—disciform and interstitial)
- *Secondary to direct viral invasion* of the cornea (necrotising).

Disciform keratitis

Pathogenesis. It occurs due to delayed hyper-sensitivity reaction to the HSV antigen. Both HSV-specific CD4 and CD8 T lymphocytes and anti-HSV antibodies have been implicated in pathogenesis of stromal keratitis. Cell-mediated immunity to corneal antigens appear to be upregulated by HSV infection and the bystander effects of proinflammatory cytokine secretion by infected corneal cells. Primarily, there occurs endotheliitis. Endothelial damage results in disciform corneal stromal oedema due to imbibition of aqueous humour.

Symptoms include photophobia, mild-to-moderate ocular discomfort, and a reduction in visual acuity.

Signs. Disciform keratitis is primarily endo-theliitis which presents as (Fig. 25.17G and H):

- *Focal disc-shaped patch* of stromal and epithelial oedema without necrosis, usually with an intact epithelium.
- *Folds in Descemet's membrane*, are often present.
- *Keratic precipitates* are seen under the area of stromal oedema.
- *Iridocyclitis* can be associated, and the disciform keratitis may be confused with uveitis with secondary corneal endothelial decompensation. However, in disciform keratitis, disc-shaped stromal oedema and keratic precipitates appear out of proportion to the degree of anterior chamber reaction.
- *Ring of stromal infiltrate* (Wessley immune ring) may be present surrounding the stromal oedema. It signifies the junction between viral antigen and host antibody.
- *Corneal sensations* are diminished.
- *Intraocular pressure* (IOP) may be raised despite only mild anterior uveitis due to trabeculitis. In severe cases, anterior uveitis may be marked.

> **Important note.** During active stage, diminished corneal sensations and keratic precipitates are the differentiating points from other causes of stromal oedema.

Disciform keratitis due to HSV and that due to VZV are clinically indistinguishable.

Treatment. *Definitive treatment* consists of:
- *Topical steroid eye drops* instilled 4–5 times a day, to be tapered over a period of several weeks.
- Antiviral cover (aciclovir 3%) twice a day, or oral acivir is must.
- *When disciform keratitis is present with an infected epithelial ulcer,* antiviral drugs should be started 5–7 days before the steroids.

Non-specific and supportive treatment (*see* page 396).

Interstitial keratitis

Interstitial keratitis may present as unifocal or multifocal interstitial haze or whitening of the stroma. It occurs in the absence of epithelial ulceration. Mild stromal oedema may occur but involvement of epithelium is uncommon. There are no significant extracorneal inflammatory signs such as conjunctival injection or anterior chamber cells and it may be difficult to identify active disease in an area of previous scar and thinning. Long-standing or recurrent HSV inter-stitial keratitis may lead to corneal vasculari-sation.

Stromal necrotic keratitis

Necrotising herpetic keratitis appears as suppurative corneal inflammation caused by active viral invasion and tissue destruction. It is probably the least common form of herpetic keratitis.

Symptoms. Pain, photophobia and redness are common symptoms.

Signs are as below:
- *Corneal lesions* (Fig. 25.18) include necrotic, blotchy, cheesy white infiltrates that may lie under the epithelial ulcer or may present independently under the intact epithelium.

  It is severe, rapidly progressive and may mimic fulminant bacterial or fungal keratitis. The epithelial defect may occur somewhat eccentric to the infiltrate.
- *Mild iritis* and keratic precipitates are usually associated (herpetic keratouveitis).
- *Stromal vascularization* may occur.

Treatment is similar to disciform keratitis but frequently the results are unsatisfactory.

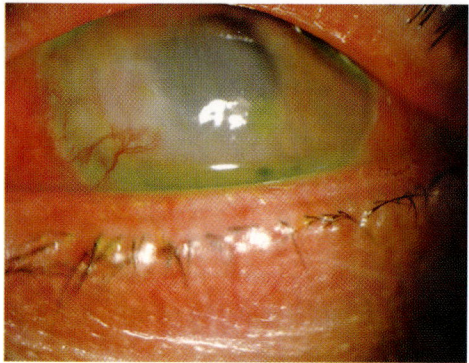

Fig. 25.18: *Necrotising herpetic keratitis*

- Systemic antiviral drugs for 10 to 21 days are being considered in recurrent cases and in those with associated herpetic uveitis.
- Keratoplasty should be deferred until the eye has been quiet with a little or no steroidal treatment for several months; because viral interstitial keratitis is the form of herpes which is most likely to recur in a new graft.

3. Metaherpetic (neurotrophic) keratitis

Metaherpetic keratitis (*epithelial sterile trophic ulceration*) is not an active viral disease, but is a mechanical healing problem due to persistent defects in the basement membrane of corneal epithelium (similar to recurrent traumatic erosions) which occurs at the site of a previous herpetic ulcer.

Clinical features. It presents as an indolent linear or ovoid epithelial detect. Margins of the ulcer are grey and thickened due to heaped up epithelium (Fig. 25.19).

Treatment is aimed to promote healing by use of lubricants (artificial tears), bandage soft contact lens and prolonged lid closure (tarsorrhaphy).

HSV iridocyclitis

- *Granulomatous or non-granulomatous irido-cyclitis* may accompany necrotising stromal keratitis or occur independently of corneal disease or with epithelial keratitis (Fig. 25.18).
- *Elevated intraocular pressure* (IOP) caused by trabeculitis or patchy iris transillumination defects may be found in patients with HSV iridocyclitis.

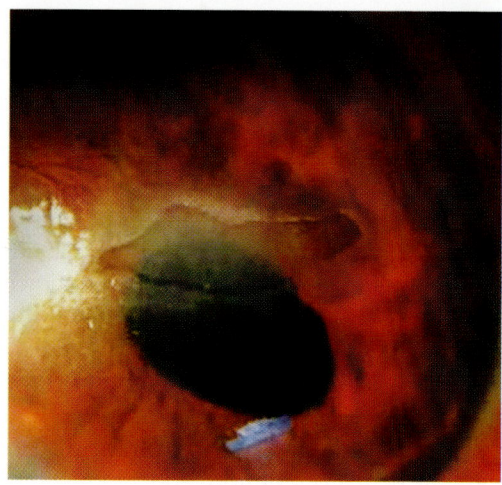

Fig. 25.19: *Neurotrophic ulcer—rolled out, thickened edges*

- *Infectious virus has been cultured* from the anterior chamber of such patients and its presence positively correlated with ocular hypertension.
- *Diagnosis of HSV iridocyclitis* is suggested by a unilateral presentation associated with an elevated IOP with or without focal iris transillumination defects. A history or clinical evidence of prior HSV ocular disease is suggestive.
- *HEDS trial suggested* the benefit of oral acyclovir (400 mg, 5 times daily) in treating HSV iridocyclitis in patients also receiving topical corticosteroids.

HEDS (HERPETIC EYE DISEASE STUDY)

- *Epithelial HSV responds* to topical antivirals and there is no role of systemic antivirals in resolution of such lesions.
- *Stromal keratitis.* Topical corticosteroids are effective in resolution of stromal keratitis. There is no role of oral steroids in reducing the inflammation in episodes of stromal keratitis. Topical antiviral agents are ineffective in necrotising keratitis and cause toxicity which may complicate the clinical picture.
- *HEDS showed no additional benefit of oral acyclovir* in treating active HSV stromal keratitis in patients receiving concomitant topical corticosteroids and trifluridine. When given briefly along with trifluridine during an

episode of epithelial keratitis, acyclovir also did not appear to prevent subsequent HSV stromal keratitis or iritis. (Available topical antiviral medications are not absorbed by the cornea through an intact epithelium, but orally administered acyclovir penetrates an intact cornea and anterior chamber.)

- *The HEDS showed no additional benefit when acyclovir was added to trifluridine and predni-solone* for the treatment of herpetic stromal keratitis, but **disciform keratitis was not analysed as a separate entity.** Long-term suppressive oral acyclovir therapy reduces the rate of recurrent HSV keratitis and helps preserve vision. Long-term antiviral prophy-laxis is recommended for patients with multiple recurrences of HSV stromal keratitis.

HERPES ZOSTER OPHTHALMICUS

Herpes zoster ophthalmicus is an acute infection of gasserian ganglion of the fifth cranial nerve by the varicella-zoster virus (VZV) involving first (ophthalmic) division. It constitutes approximately 10% of all cases of herpes zoster. Herpes zoster (*shingles*) occurs more commonly in immunocompromised individuals.

ETIOLOGY

Varicella-zoster virus. It is a DNA virus and produces acidophilic intranuclear inclusion bodies. It is neurotropic in nature.

Pathogenesis. The VZV infection is contracted in childhood, which manifests as chickenpox and the child develops immunity. The virus then remains dormant in the sensory ganglion of trigeminal nerve. It is thought that, usually in elderly people, though (can occur at any age) with depressed cellular immunity, the virus reactivates, replicates and travels down along one or more of the branches of the ophthalmic division of the fifth nerve to produce cutaneous and ocular lesions.

Risk factors. Then people, particularly prone to herpes zoster ophthalmicus, are elderly with depressed cellular immunity, for example, those suffering from, disseminated TB, cancer, leukemia, AIDS, immunocompromised organ transplant recipient and lymphoma (Hodgkin and non-Hodgkin).

CLINICAL FEATURES

- *Frontal nerve* is more frequently affected than the lacrimal and nasociliary nerves in herpes zoster ophthalmicus.
- *Ocular complications* occur in about 50% cases of herpes zoster ophthalmicus.
- *Hutchinson's rule,* which implies that ocular involvement is frequent if the side or tip of nose presents vesicles (cutaneous involvement of nasociliary nerve), is useful but not infallible.
- *Lesions are strictly limited* to one side of the midline of head.

Clinical phases of herpes zoster ophthalmicus are:

  I. *Acute phase lesions,* which may totally resolve within few weeks.

 II. *Chronic phase lesions,* which may persist for years.

III. *Relapsing phase lesions,* where acute or chronic lesions reappear sometimes years later.

I. Acute phase lesions

A. General features. The onset of illness is sudden with fever, malaise and severe neuralgic pain along the course of the affected nerve. The distribution of pain is so characteristic of zoster that it usually arouses suspicion of the nature of the disease before appearance of vesicles.

B. Cutaneous lesions. Cutaneous lesions (Fig. 25.20) in the area of distribution of the involved nerve appear usually after 3 to 4 days of the onset of disease. To begin with, the skin of lids

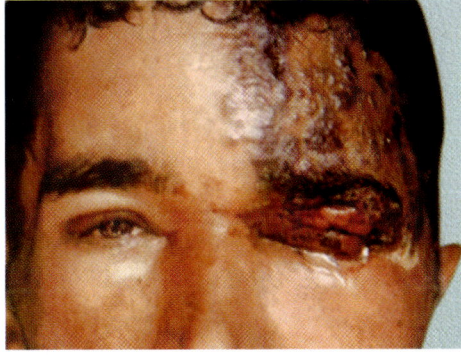

Fig. 25.20: *Cutaneous lesions of herpes zoster ophthal-micus*

and other affected areas become red and oedematous, maculopapular rash (mimicking erysipelas), followed by vesicle formation. In due course of time vesicles are converted into pustules, which subsequently burst to become crusting ulcers. When crusts are shed, permanent pitted scars are left. The active eruptive phase lasts for about 3 weeks. Main symptom is severe neuralgic pain which usually diminishes with the subsidence of eruptive phase.

Eyelid cutaneous lesions. They can lead to secondary bacterial infection, eyelid scarring, marginal notching, loss of cilia, trichiasis, cicatricial entropion or ectropion. Scarring and occlusion of lacrimal puncta or canaliculi may also occur.

C. Ocular lesions. Ocular complications occur in more than 70% of patients with herpes zoster ophthalmicus (HZO). These usually appear at the subsidence of skin eruptions and may present as a combination of two or more of the following lesions:

1. *Conjunctivitis* is one of the most common lesions of herpes zoster. It may occur as mucopurulent conjunctivitis with petechial haemorrhages or acute follicular conjunctivitis with regional lymphadenopathy. Sometimes, severe necrotising membranous inflammation may be seen.

2. *Zoster keratitis* occurs in 40% of all patients and sometimes may precede the neuralgia or skin lesions. Diminished corneal sensations develop in about 50% of patients. The zoster keratitis may occur in several forms (Fig. 25.21):

• *Epithelial keratitis.* To begin with there occurs fine or coarse punctate epithelial keratitis (Fig. 25.21A and B). It is followed by microdendritic epithelial ulcers (Fig. 25.21C and D) which unlike dendritic ulcers of herpes simplex are usually peripheral and stellate rather than exactly dendritic in shape. In contrast to herpes simplex dendrites, they have tapered ends which lack bulbs. So, also labelled as pseudodendritic keratitis.

• *Nummular keratitis* (Fig. 25.21E and F) characterised by anterior stromal infiltrates is seen in about one-third number of total cases. It typically occurs as multiple tiny granular

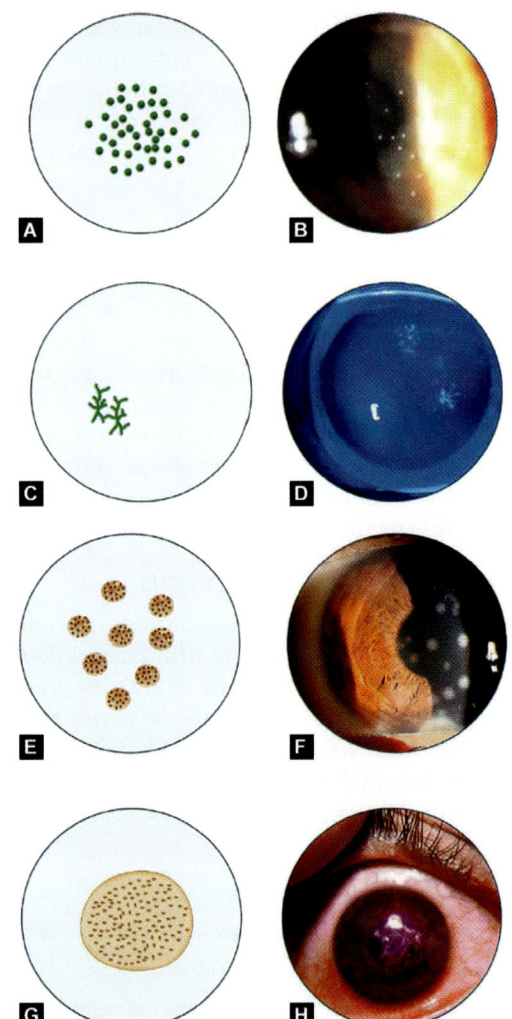

Fig. 25.21: *Types of zoster keratitis. Diagrammatic depictions and clinical photographs of: A and B, Punctate epithelial keratitis; C and D, Microdendritis epithelial ulcer; E and F, Nummular keratitis; G and H, Disciform keratitis*

deposits surrounded by a halo of stromal haze. After healing 'nummular scars' are left behind.

• *Disciform keratitis* (Fig. 25.21G and H) occurs in about 50% of cases and is always preceded by nummular keratitis.

• *Keratouveitis with endotheliitis* is of common occurrence. The endothelium is a favoured site of attack and acute endothelial cell loss occurs during herpes zoster keratouveitis.

• *Chronic corneal stromal inflammation* can lead to corneal vascularization, lipid keratopathy and corneal opacity. Neurotrophic keratopathy is common in such patients due to profound corneal anaesthesia.

3. *Episcleritis and scleritis* occur in about one-half of the cases. These usually appear at the onset of the rash but are frequently concealed by the overlying conjunctivitis. Episcleritis and scleritis associated with zooster may be nodular of diffuse.

4. *Iridocyclitis* is of a frequent occurrence and may or may not be associated with keratitis. There may be associated hypopyon and hyphaema (acute haemorrhagic uveitis).

5. *Focal choroiditis* is also reported in patients with HZO.

6. *Acute retinal necrosis* (ARN) and occlusive retinal vesculitis may occur in some cases.

7. *Secondary glaucoma.* It may occur due to trabeculitis in early stages and synechial angle closure in late stages.

8. *Anterior segment necrosis and phthisis bulbi,* may occur rarely as a result from zoster vasculitis and ischaemia.

D. Associated neurological complications. Herpes zoster ophthalmicus may also be associated with other neurological complications such as:

1. *Cranial nerve palsies* specially involving the third (most common), fourth, sixth or seventh nerves, occur in one-third of HZO cases.

2. *Optic neuritis* (papillitis or retrobulbar neuritis) occurs in about 1% of cases.

3. *Encephalitis* occurs rarely with severe infection.

II. Chronic phase lesions

Chronic phase lesions are basically sequelae of acute phase, which may persist for up to 10 years.

1. *Post-herpetic neuralgia* refers to persistence of pain even after subsidence of eruptive phase of zoster which occurs in about 10% of cases. Pain is mild to moderate in intensity, worsens at night and is aggravated by touch and heat. But sometimes, it may persist for years with a little diminution of intensity.

There occurs some anaesthesia of the affected skin which when associated with continued post-herpetic neuralgia is called *anaesthesia dolorosa.*

2. *Lid lesions,* which occur as sequelae of scarring include ptosis, trichiasis, entropion and notching.

3. *Conjunctival lesions* include chronic mucous secreting conjunctivitis.

4. *Corneal lesions* are:

- *Neuroparalytic ulceration* may occur as a sequelae of acute infection and gasserian ganglion destruction.

- *Exposure keratitis* may supervene in some cases due to associated facial palsy.

- *Mucous plaque keratitis* develops in 5% of cases between 3rd and 5th months and is characterised by sudden development of elevated mucous plaque which stains brilliantly with rose bengal.

5. *Scleritis and uveitis* may persist in chronic form.

III. Relapsing phase lesions

Relapsing phase lesions, which may recur even after ten years of acute phase, include nummular keratitis, mucous plaque keratitis, episcleritis, scleritis and secondary glaucoma.

TREATMENT

Therapeutic approach to herpes zoster ophthalmicus should be vigorous and aimed at preventing severe devastating ocular complications and promoting rapid healing of the skin lesions without the formation of massive crusts which result in scarring of the nerves and post-herpetic neuralgia. The following regime may be followed.

I. Systemic therapy for herpes zoster

1. *Oral antiviral drugs.* These significantly decrease pain, curtail vesiculation, stop viral progression and reduce the incidence as well as severity of keratitis and iritis. In order to be effective, the treatment should be started immediately after the onset of rash.

It has no effect on post-herpetic neuralgia.

- *Acyclovir* in a dose of 800 mg 5 times a day for 10 days, or

- *Valaciclovir* in a dose of 500 mg TDS for 10 days.

- *Famciclovir* in a dose of 500 mg TDS for 10 days.

2. *Analgesics.* Pain during the first 2 weeks of an attack is very severe and should be treated by analgesics such as combination of mephenamic acid and paracetamol or pentazocine or even pethidine (when very severe).

3. *Systemic steroids.* They appear to inhibit development of post-herpetic neuralgia when given in high doses. However, the risk of high doses of steroids in elders should always be taken into consideration. Steroids are commonly recommended in cases developing neurological complications such as third nerve palsy and optic neuritis.

4. *Cimetidine* in a dose of 300 mg QID for 2–3 weeks starting within 48–72 hours of onset has also been shown to reduce pain and pruritis in acute zoster—presumably by histamine blockade.

5. *Amitriptyline* should be used to relieve the accompanying depression in acute phase.

6. *Gabapentin or carbamazepine* may be required for neuralgia.

II. Local therapy for skin lesions

1. *Antibiotic-corticosteroid skin ointment or lotions.* These should be used three times a day till skin lesions heal.

2. *Capsaicin cream,* applied to the involved skin may be helpful in post-herpetic neuralgia.

Note. Cool zinc calamine application, as advocated earlier, is better avoided, as it promotes crust formation.

III. Local therapy for ocular lesions

1. *For zoster keratitis, iridocyclitis and scleritis*
- *Topical steroid* eye drops 4 times a day.
- *Cycloplegics* such as cyclopentolate eye drops BD or atropine eye ointment OD.
- *Topical acyclovir* 3% eye ointment should be instilled 5 times a day for about 2 weeks.

2. **To prevent secondary infections,** topical antibiotics are used.

3. *For secondary glaucoma*
- 0.5% timolol or 0.5% betaxolol drops, BD.
- Acetazolamide 250 mg, QID.

4. *For mucous plaques*, add topical mucolytics, e.g. acetylcysteine 5 to 10%, three times a day.

5. *For persistent epithelial defects* use:
- Lubricating artificial tear drops
- Bandage soft contact lens.

IV. Surgical treatment

For neuroparalytic corneal ulcer caused by herpes zoster:

1. *Lateral tarsorrhaphy* should be performed.
2. *Amniotic membrane transplantation* (AMT) or conjunctival flap should be considered for non-healing cases.
3. *Tissue adhesive* with bandage contact lens for corneal perforation.
4. *Keratoplasty.* It may be required for visual rehabilitation of zoster patients with dense scarring. However, these are high-risk patients.

CYTOMEGALOVIRUS: OCULAR LESIONS

PATHOGENESIS

Cytomegalovirus (CMV) is a ubiquitous herpesvirus that infects over 90% of humans. Spread of CMV occurs through the sharing of saliva, ingestion of breast milk, or sexual contact. CMV results in subclinical infection in children and a non-specific febrile illness lasting 1–3 weeks in adults. A viremia transmits the virus to the bone marrow, where it becomes latent in CD34+ myeloid progenitor cells until these cells are activated, which allows expression and shedding of the virus.

CLINICAL PRESENTATION

Epithelial and stromal CMV keratitis are rare. *Cases of endothelial rejection in keratoplasty* are now also shown to be due to CMV.

Anterior uveitis and endothelial. CMV has now been increasingly identified as a significant cause of anterior uveitis and corneal endotheliitis and is characterised by thin stellate keratic precipitates. Due to improved diagnostic tests such as PCR for AC tap, the previously undetected cases of anterior uveitis are being attributed to CMV and treated accordingly.

Anterior uveitis is characterised by an acute or chronic iritis, with moderate to severe rises in IOP that are variably responsive to topical corticosteroids. The addition of keratic precipitates, endothelial cell loss, and diffuse or local corneal oedema suggests CMV endotheliitis. These presentations are often misdiagnosed as HSV-related endotheliitis, trabeculitis, or Posner-Schlossman syndrome and can be distinguished only by their response to therapy and by results of laboratory investigation.

CMV retinitis. CMV has been most commonly associated with a sectoral, necrotising retinitis that is seen commonly in AIDS and other immunocompromised states.

LABORATORY EVALUATION

Laboratory confirmation of disease is usually accomplished through PCR testing of aqueous humour for CMV. Aqueous humour is obtained by an anterior chamber tap, which must be performed during an episode of active disease. Concomitant testing for other herpesviruses can also be performed. Serum samples may be tested to confirm that the viraemia is local rather than systemic. CMV may also be diagnosed through histologic examination of biopsy specimens.

MANAGEMENT

CMV-associated anterior segment disease is treated with ganciclovir and is not responsive to famciclovir, acyclovir, or its derivatives. Resistance of a presumed HSV infection to these agents should raise the suspicion of CMV. There has been no standard treatment of CMV associated anterior segment disease but treatment with oral valganciclovir 900 mg twice daily (with the possibility of lower maintenance dosing) has been shown to be effective. Valganciclovir may be poorly tolerated and recurrence of disease with withdrawal of the medication is common. Ganciclovir implants may be helpful. Topical ganciclovir has no role in anterior segment disease. The role of corticosteroids is controversial, as some reports suggest that steroid use may prolong or worsen CMV-associated anterior segment disease.

ADENOVIRUS KERATITIS

CLINICAL PRESENTATION

Each subgroup (A–F) of adenoviruses and each serotype possesses unique tissue tropisms that reveal the association of specific adenoviruses with distinct clinical syndromes. adenoviral eye disease may present clinically as:

- Simple follicular conjunctivitis (multiple serotypes)
- Pharyngoconjunctival fever (most commonly serotype 3 or 7)
- Epidemic keratoconjunctivitis (EKC; usually serotypes 8, 19, or 37, subgroup D).

Different adenoviral syndromes are indistinguishable in early phase and may be unilateral or bilateral.

Adenoviral follicular conjunctivitis is self-limited, not associated with systemic disease, and often so transient that patients do not seek care. Epithelial keratitis, if present, is mild and fleeting.

Pharyngoconjunctival fever is characterised by fever, headache, pharyngitis, follicular conjunctivitis, and preauricular adenopathy. The systemic signs and symptoms may mimic influenza. Any associated epithelial keratitis is mild.

Epidemic keratoconjunctivitis is the only adenoviral syndrome with significant corneal involvement. The infection is bilateral in most patients and may be preceded by an upper respiratory tract infection. One week to 10 days after inoculation, severe follicular conjunctivitis develops, associated with a punctate epithelial keratitis. The conjunctiva shows follicular reaction along with chemosis. Petechial haemorrhages or larger subconjunctival haemorrhages can occur. Preauricular adenopathy is common. Pseudomembranes occur predominantly on the tarsal conjunctiva and are specially common in children. Patients usually present tearing, light sensitivity, and foreign body sensation.

Within 7–14 days after onset of eye symptoms, multifocal subepithelial (stromal) corneal infiltrates become apparent on slit-lamp examination. Photophobia and reduced vision from adenoviral subepithelial infiltrates may persist for months to years. Epithelial keratitis occurs because of adenovirus replication within the corneal epithelium. Subepithelial infiltrates are caused by an immunological response of keratocytes to viral infection in the superficial corneal stroma. In severe cases, central geographic corneal erosions can develop and may persist for several days despite patching and lubrication. Chronic complications of conjunctival membranes include subepithelial conjunctival scarring, symblepharon formation, and dry eye due to alterations within the lacrimal glands or lacrimal ducts.

Viral shedding may persist for 10–14 days after the onset of clinical signs and symptoms. Transmission can be prevented by personal hygiene measures, including frequent handwashing; cleaning of towels, pillowcases, and handkerchiefs. Patients should be considered infectious if they are still hyperaemic and tearing. It is more difficult to assess transmissibility in patients treated with topical corticosteroids, as they may appear quiet but still shed virus.

TREATMENT

Because corticosteroids may prolong viral shedding from adenovirus-infected patients and can lead to worsening of HSV infections, their use should be reserved for patients with clinical signs of adenovirus infection who present with specific indications for treatment, including conjunctival membranes and reduced vision due to bilateral subepithelial infiltrates.

The use of topical corticosteroids does not affect the natural course of the disease, and it may be difficult to wean patients from them. Nonsteroidal anti-inflammatory drugs (NSAIDs) are ineffective for adenoviral subepithelial infiltrates, but they may be helpful in preventing recurrence following tapering of the corticosteroids. Topical cyclosporin 1% is considered in patients failing other therapy.

PROTOZOAL KERATITIS

INTRODUCTION

Protozoa are unicellular eukaryotes found ubiquitously in soil and water. They exist as free-living organisms and can rarely cause of microbial keratitis in individuals with coexisting morbid conditions.

Acanthamoeba species are protozoa that can cause an isolated infection of the human cornea as their primary disease in humans. Other systemic conditions such as disseminated dermatitis, visceral infestation, and encephalitis may also be caused by Acanthamoeba.

Microsporidia are obligate intracellular parasites and can cause myriad of conditions ranging from keratoconjunctivitis to endophthalmitis.

Toxoplasma gondii causes one of the most common parasitic infections of humans but commonly effects the posterior segment causing chorioretinitis.

ACANTHAMOEBA KERATITIS

Acanthamoeba keratitis has recently gained importance because of its increasing incidence, difficulty in diagnosis and unsatisfactory treatment.

ETIOPATHOGENESIS

Acanthamoeba castellani, the causative organism is a free-living genus of amoeba found in soil, fresh water, well water, sea water, sewage and air. It exists in trophozoite and encysted forms. Acanthamoeba life cycle includes a motile trophozoite form (15–45 µm in diameter) and a dormant cyst form (10–25 µm in diameter) which are formed under adverse conditions. The cysts are double-walled and resistant to most environmental extremes and toxins, including chlorine. The cysts transform into trophozoites under favourable conditions completing the life cycle. Acanthamoeba has tremendous capacity to survive in diverse conditions and in contrast to many other pathogenic amoeba, this organism is not naturally parasitic and does not require a host. In human, Acanthamoeba causes:

- Keratitis
- Granulomatous encephalitis
- Fulminant meningoencephalitis.

Risk factors

Corneal infection with Acanthamoeba results from direct corneal contact with any material or water contaminated with the organism.

Following risk factors of contamination have been described:

1. **Contact lens wearers** using home-made saline (from contaminated tap water and saline tablets) is the commonest situation recognised for Acanthamoeba infection in Western countries.

2. **Trauma associated** with contaminated matter such as vegetable matter, salt water diving, windblown contaminant and hot tub use forms the *non-contact lens-related situations*. Trauma with organic matter and exposure to muddy water are the major (90% cases) predisposing factors in developing countries.

3. **Opportunistic infection.** Acanthamoeba keratitis can also occur as opportunistic infection in patients with herpetic keratitis, bacterial keratitis, bullous keratopathy and neuro-paralytic keratitis.

Pathogenesis

Initial corneal epithelial adherence is mediated by a mannose-binding protein, with subsequent stromal invasion promoted by the expression of a mannose-induced protein (MIP-133) and various collagenases. Once attached to the stroma, systemic immune sensitisation by the organism seems ineffective at eliminating infection.

CLINICAL FEATURES

Symptoms

These vary from asymptomatic to foreign body sensation, mild pain to severe pain (out of proportion to the degree of inflammation), watering, photophobia, blepharospasm and blurred vision.

Signs

Acanthamoeba keratitis evolves over several months as a gradual worsening keratitis with periods of temporary remission. Presentation is markedly variable, making the diagnosis difficult.

Reported lesions of Acanthamoeba keratitis are as below:

1. **Epithelial lesions** occur initially and include:
- *Epithelial roughening* and irregularities, often mistaken for punctate epitheliopathy.

- *Epithelial ridges*, i.e. raised epithelial lines. Initially, typical reticular pattern is seen due to radial keratoneuritis.
- *Radial keratoneuritis* (Fig. 25.22A), reported in 50% of cases, seems to be pathognomonic early sign. It is thought to be the cause of severe pain disproportionate to inflammation.
- *Pseudodendrites* formation occurs and at this stage it is commonly mistaken for herpes simplex keratitis (Fig. 25.22B).
- *Epithelial and subepithelial* curvilinear opacities (usually fine).

2. **Limbal lesions** include limbitis which is reported in majority of cases in early stages of infection.

3. **Stromal lesions** occur over a period of week and include:
- *Stromal infiltrates* are seen grey-white super-ficial non-suppurative patchy and satellite in the central cornea.
- *Ring infiltrates*, central or paracentral, with overlying epithelial defects and underlying keratic precipitates (Fig. 25.22C).
- *Ring abscess* (Fig. 25.22D) associated with stromal necrosis and hypopyon may occur in late stages and mimic any suppurative keratitis.

  Note. There is remarkable absence of neo-vascularization in spite of chronic nature of disease.

4. **Scleritis,** usually anterior diffuse or nodular, can be contiguous with keratitis. Rarely posterior scleritis with optic neuritis is also reported.

5. Dacryoadenitis is also reported.

6. Intraocular extension has also been reported in untreated cases, but consecutive encephalitis has not been reported.

DIFFERENTIAL DIAGNOSIS

1. **Viral keratitis.** In early stages, both epithelial lesions and early infiltrates, especially pseudodendrites, are often mistaken for viral keratitis.

2. **Fungal keratitis** can also be misdiagnosed when ring infiltrates are associated with hypopyon.

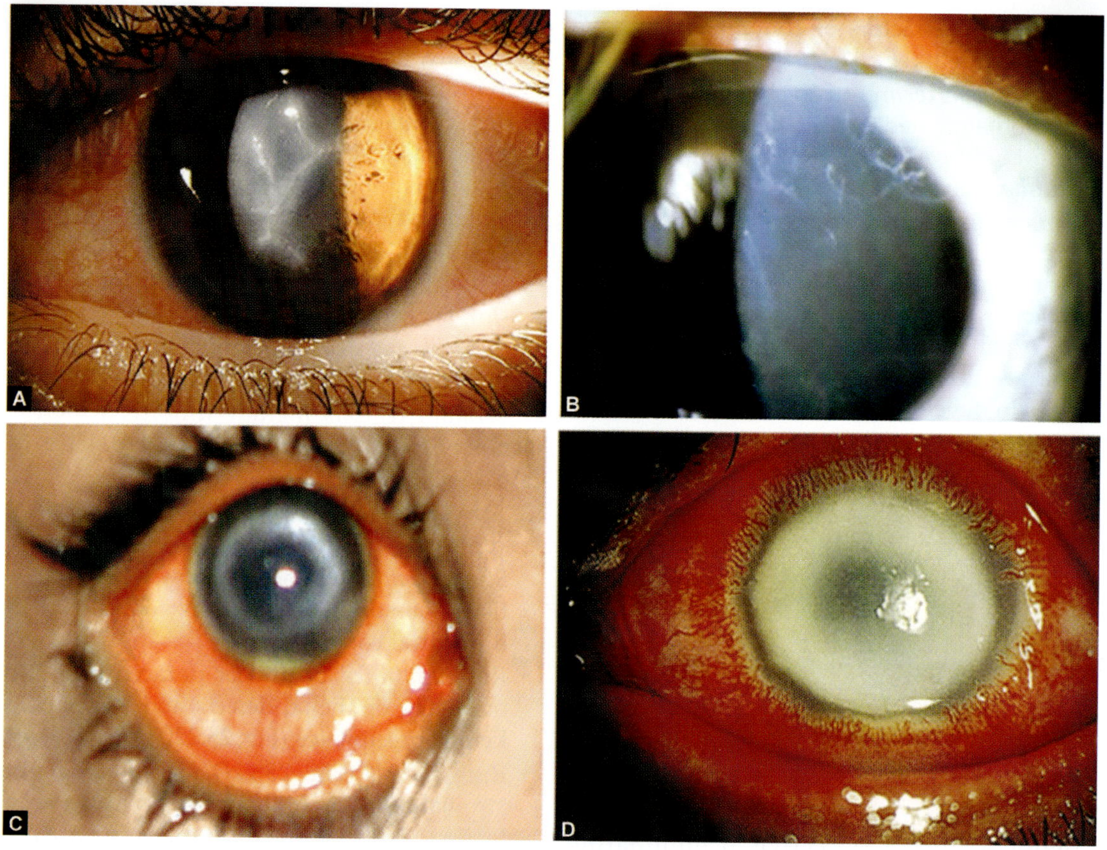

Fig. 25.22: *Acanthamoeba keratitis. A, Radial keratoneuritis; B, Acanthamoeba pseudodendrites; C, Ring infiltrate; D, Ring abscess*

3. *Suppurative keratitis* due to bacterial or other causes may be misdiagnosed in stage of stromal necrosis, and ring abscess formation.

DIAGNOSIS

1. *Clinical diagnosis.* It is difficult and usually made by exclusion with strong clinical suspicion out of the non-responsive patients being treated for herpetic, bacterial or fungal keratitis.

2. *Confocal microscopy,* when available allows direct visualization of the cysts in the cornea, which is diagnostic (Fig. 25.23).

3. *Laboratory diagnosis.* Corneal scrapings may be helpful in some cases as under:

Giemsa and PAS stain films may show trophozoites.

a. *Potassium hydroxide (KOH) mount* is reliable in experienced hands for recognition of Acanthamoeba cysts.

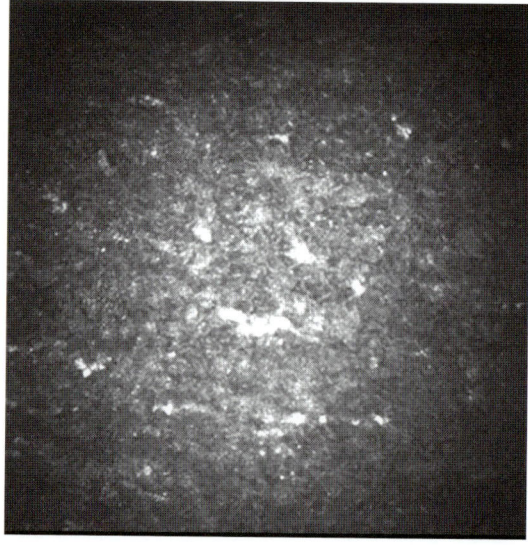

Fig. 25.23: *Acanthamoebal cysts as seen on confocal microscopy*

b. *Calcofluor white stain* is a fluorescent brightener which stains the cysts of Acanthamoeba bright apple green under fluorescence microscope.

c. *Lactophenol cotton blue stained* film is also useful for demonstration of Acanthamoeba cysts in the corneal scrapings.

d. *Culture on non-nutrient agar* (*E. coli* enriched) may show trophozoites within 48 hours in 35–50% of cases, which gradually turn into cysts.

e. *Polymerase chain reaction (PCR)* for amoebic DNA is reported to be useful.

f. *Corneal biopsy*, may be required in non-conclusive cases, may be positive for amoebic cyst.

TREATMENT

It is usually unsatisfactory.

1. *Non-specific treatment* is on the general lines for corneal ulcer (*see* page 396).

2. *Specific treatment.* Cases identified early, defined as *epithelial or anterior stromal*, have an excellent visual prognosis and generally respond well to *epithelial debridement*, followed by an *extended* (3–4 months) course of anti-amoebic therapy. The presence of deep stromal inflammation, a ring infiltrate, or extracorneal manifestations significantly worsen the prognosis with more stromal scarring and longer treatment (up to a year or more).

a. *Topical antiamoebic agents* include:
- *Diamidines:* Propamidine isethionate (0.1%), and hexamidine (0.1%).
- *Biguanides:* Polyhexamethylene biguanide (PHMB), 0.02% and chlorhexidine, 0.02%.
- *Aminoglycosides:* Neomycin and paromycin
- *Imidazoles:* Clotrimazole and miconazole.

Multiple drug therapy is needed for a long time (3–4 months) for early epithelial lesions and 6–12 months for stromal lesions. Any of the following combination may be choosen:
- Propamidine or hexamidine + PHMB (drug of choice), or
- Chlorhexidine + neomycin, or
- Paromycin + clotrimazole or miconazole or itraconazole.

Frequency of instillation: Hourly for a week, then taper slowly over 3–4 months for epithelial lesions and 6–12 months for stromal lesions.

b. *Oral ketoconazole* 200 mg BID, or itraconazole 100 mg BD may be added in advanced cases.

3. *Long-term prophylactic therapy* with PHMB, twice a day for a year is recommended.

4. *Penetrating keratoplasty* is frequently required in non-responsive cases. Surgery should be performed after a full course of maximum medical therapy and a quiescent phase of at least six months.

With effective anti-Acanthamoeba agents used as adjunctive therapy, keratoplasty now has a lower rate of recurrent infection and the primary risk factor for graft failure is inflammatory sequelae, including glaucoma. Collagen crosslinking is increasingly described as an adjunctive therapy for Acanthamoeba keratitis. Further studies are needed for its validation.

BIBLIOGRAPHY

1. Chin GN, Hydiuk RA, Kwasny GP, Schultz RO. Kerato- mycosis in Wisconsin. Am J Ophthalmol 1975;79:121-5.
2. Doughman DJ, Leavenworth NM, Campbell RC, Lindstrom RL. Fungal keratitis at the University of Minnesota: 1971-1981
3. Glynn RJ, Schein OD, Seddon JM, Poggio EC, Goodfellow JR, Scardino VA, et al. The incidence of ulcerative keratitis among aphakic contact lens wearers in New England. Arch Ophthalmol 1991;109:104-7
4. Hemady RK. Microbial keratitis in patients infected with the human immunodeficiency virus. Ophthalmology 1995;102:1026-30.
5. Jeffries DJ. Intrautrine and neonatal herpes simplex virus infection. Scand J Infect Dis Suppl 1991;80:21-6.
6. Jones DB, Sexton R, Rebell G. Mycotic keratitis in South Florida: A review of thirty-nine cases. Trans Ophthalmol Soc UK 1970;89:78-1797
7. Kaye S, Lynas C, Patterson A, et al. Evidence of herpes simplex viral latency in the human cornea. Br J Ophthalmol 1991;75:195-200.
8. Liesegang TJ. Epidemiology of ocular herpes simplex. Arch Ophthalmol 1989;107:1160-5.

9. Liesegang TJ, Forster RK. Spectrum of microbial keratitis in South Florida. Am J Ophthalmol 1980;90:38-47.

10. Lisegang TJ. Herpes simplex virus epidemiology and ocular importance. Cornea 2001;20:1-13.

11. Najjar DM, Aktan SG, Rapuano CJ, Laibson PR, Cohen EJ. Contact lens-related corneal ulcers in compliant patients. Am J Ophthalmol 2004;137:170-2.

12. Poggio EC, Abelson M. Complications and symptoms in disposable extended wear lenses compared with conventional soft daily wear and soft extended wear lenses. CLAO J 1993;19:31-9.

13. Radford CF, Minassian DC, Dart JK. Acanthamoeba keratitis in England and Wales: incidence, outcome, and risk factors. Br J Ophthalmol 2002;86:536-42.

14. Sharma S, Garg P, Rao GN. Patient characteristics, diagnosis, and treatment of noncontact lens related Acanthamoeba keratitis. Br J Ophthalmol 2000;84:1103- 8.

Allergic and Immunologic Keratitis

ALLERGIC KERATOCONJUNCTIVITIS

Atopy refers to hypersensitivity reaction in persons with hereditary background of allergic diseases. The most commonly recognized atopic conditions include eczema (atopic dermatitis), asthma, hay fever and allergic rhinitis. Atopy affects 28–32% of the population. Atopic ocular diseases include seasonal allergic conjunctivitis (SAC), perennial allergic conjunctivitis (PAC), vernal keratoconjunctivitis (VKC), atopic keratoconjunctivitis (AKC), and giant papillary conjunctivitis (GPC) and are described in Chapter 13. Few of these diseases affect only conjunctiva and some affect cornea as well as conjunctiva. VKC and AKC may cause significant corneal complications and may even lead to loss of vision.

VERNAL KERATOCONJUNCTIVITIS OR SPRING CATARRH

It is a recurrent bilateral, interstitial, self limiting allergic inflammation having a periodic seasonal incidence.

ETIOLOGY

Vernal keratoconjunctivitis (VKC) is considered as a hypersensitivity reaction to some exogenous allergens such as grass pollens. It is thought to be an atopic allergic disorder in which IgE mediated mechanisms play an important role. Such patients give personal or family history of other atopic diseases such as hay fever, asthma or eczema and their peripheral blood shows eosinophilia and increased serum IgE levels.

Vernal keratoconjunctivitis (VKC) is a seasonally recurrent, bilateral conjunctival inflammation of youth; boys are affected twice as often as girls. The most prominent symptom is itching, which can become worse toward evening and is exacerbated by rubbing. Tearing is characteristic and macerates the skin about the corner of the eye. A characteristic thick, mucoid, ropy discharge is noted.

PATHOPHYSIOLOGY

A personal or family history of atopy is seen in large proportion of VKC patients. VKC was originally thought to be due to IgE mediated reaction via mast cell release. A hereditary association has been suggested. Biopsy of tarsal conjunctival papilla in VKC reveals distinct findings. The epithelium contains large numbers of mast cells and eosinophils, neither of which are found in normal individuals. Human mast cells may be categorized based on the presence of neutral proteases. The epithelium of VKC patients contains mast cells predominantly containing the neutral proteases tryptase- and chymase-positive MCs (MCTC). Basophils are found in epithelium and may indicate delayed hypersensitivity reaction. Brush cytology of conjunctival epithelium from patients with VKC showed more eosinophils and neutrophils in patients with corneal erosion or ulcer than in those without. Goblet cell density is not elevated in the conjunctival epithelium of VKC. Eosinophil major basic protein is deposited diffusely throughout the conjunctiva of VKC patients, including the epithelium. Cornea and conjunctiva *in vivo* confocal microscopy confirms histology and offers an additional diagnostic aid.

CLINICAL PICTURE

Symptoms

Spring catarrh is characterised by marked burning and itching sensation which is usually intolerable and accentuated when patient comes in warm humid atmosphere. Itching is more marked with palpebral form of disease. Other associated symptoms include: Mild photophobia, lacrimation, stringy (ropy) discharge and heaviness of lids.

Vernal keratopathy

Corneal involvement in VKC may be primary or secondary due to extension of limbal lesions. Vernal keratopathy includes following 5 types of lesions.

1. Punctate epithelial keratitis

Punctate epithelial keratitis (Fig. 26.1) involving upper cornea is usually associated with the palpebral form of the disease. It is characterised by scattered fine punctuate corneal epithelial loss or damage. Symptoms are redness, lacrimation, photophobia and reduced vision. The

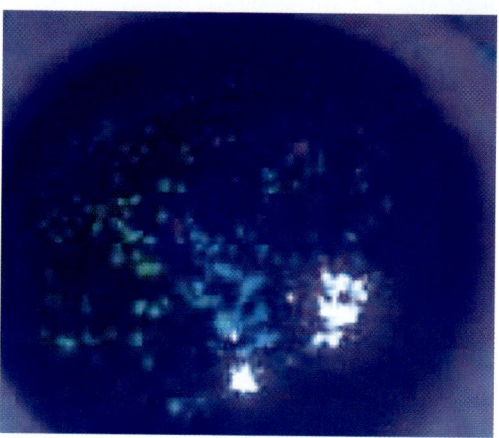

Fig. 26.1: *Punctate epithelial keratitis*

lesions always stain with rose bengal and invariably with fluorescein. Punctate epithelial erosions or keratitis can coalesce into macroerosions of the epithelium.

2. Ulcerative vernal keratitis (Shield ulcer)

Shield ulcer (Fig. 26.2) is an uncommon, incapacitating corneal manifestation that occurs in 3 to 11% of patients suffering from vernal keratoconjunctivitis.Vernal keratitis causes a discrete, horizontal oval, shallow, non-vascularized, indolent ulcer, generally in the superior half of the cornea. The ulceration results due to epithelial macroerosions. The edges are composed of shaggy, gray, dead epithelial cells, and infiltration of the underlying superficial stroma is present. It is a serious problem which may be complicated by bacterial keratitis. Cameron has graded Shield ulcer by severity.

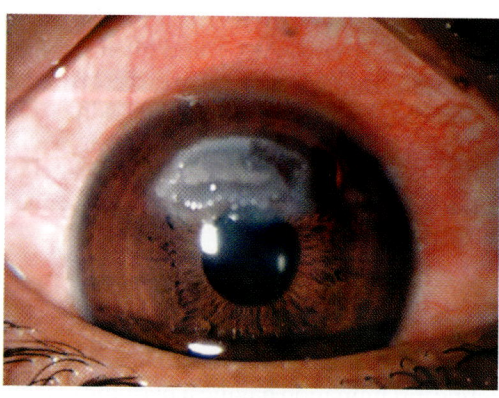

Fig. 26.2: *Shield ulcer*

Shield ulcers can be divided into 3 different grades.

- *Grade 1 ulcer* has a clear base and favourable outcome. These ulcers reepithelize with mild scarring on medical treatment.
- *Grade 2 ulcers* have inflammatory debris at the base and exhibit a poor response to medical therapy. The grade 2 ulcers are prone to infectious keratitis. Regular surgical debridement of these ulcers is necessary for rapid healing.
- *Grade 3 ulcers* have a large base and elevated plaque. These ulcers are generally refractive to medical treatment and surgical intervention in the form of AMT is necessary. The role of cyclosporin eye drops in low concentration (0.05%) along with standard medical treatment has been proven. After the ulcer heals, a mild corneal opacity may persist at the level of Bowman's layer. They may be indolent and persist for months.

3. Vernal corneal plaques

Vernal corneal plaques (Fig. 26.3) result due to coating of bare areas of epithelial macroerosions with a layer of altered exudates. When inflammatory debris accumulates at the base of an ulcer, an opaque plaque is formed. The composition of these plaques has not been resolved. However, Trocme et al have identified eosinophil major basic protein (MBP) in the plaques of VKC patients and suggested that MBP, a cytotoxic protein, may play a pathogenic role in the formation and/or persistence of

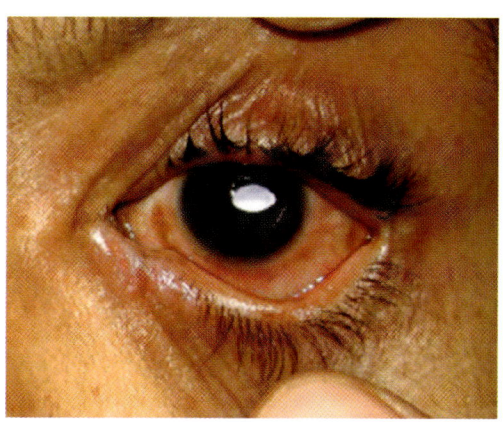

Fig. 26.3: *Vernal corneal plaques*

Shield ulcers. Shield ulcer plaques may not respond to the conventional topical treatment and may be complicated by amblyopia, strabismus, microbial keratitis, and corneal perforation. There is a paucity of literature on the management of nonhealing Shield ulcers and plaques.

4. Subepithelial scarring

It occurs in the form of ring scar.

5. Pseudogerontoxon

Pseudogerontoxon (Fig. 26.4) is characterised by classical 'cupid's bow' outline. The peripheral cornea may show a waxing and waning, superficial stromal, gray-white deposition termed pseudogerontoxon.

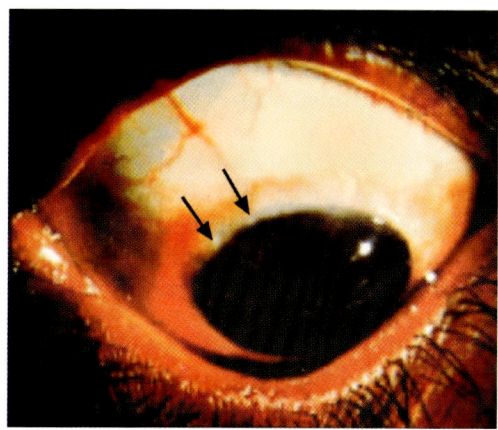

Fig. 26.4: *Pseudogerontoxon*

Clinical course

Disease is often self-limiting and usually burns out spontaneously after 5–10 years.

TREATMENT

A. Local therapy

1. **Topical steroids:** Topical corticosteroids are a critical component of VKC management, particularly in VKC exacerbations, but they have extensive side effect profiles including cataract and glaucoma. Initial treatment in an acute exacerbation should begin with steroids with low intraocular penetration such as loteprednol or fluorometholone to avoid complications associated with steroid use. More resistant cases should be treated with more potent steroids such as prednisolone acetate or dexamethasone.

2. **Mast cell stabilizers** such as sodium cromoglycate (2%) drops 4–5 times a day are quite effective in controlling VKC, especially atopic cases. It is a mast cell stabilizer. Azelastine eye drops are also effective in controlling VKC. Mast cell stabilizers are thought to prevent mast cell degranulation via inhibition of calcium channels, but their mechanism is not completely understood. There is increasing evidence that mast cell stabilizers act more broadly on inflammatory cell chemotaxis. Commonly used mast cell stabilizers include cromolyn sodium and lodoxamide, which are frequently used as first-line therapy. Lodoxamide has been shown to be superior to cromolyn sodium in relieving symptoms and clinical signs of VKC. The medications should be used 4–6 times daily and may take up to 2 weeks to show response in mild cases of VKC.

3. **Topical antihistaminics** are also effective. Antihistamines are sometimes used in the treatment of VKC: They are most often used in alleviating the symptoms of mild disease, but they have limited utility in severe cases. More recent medications that combine antihistamine properties with mast cell stabilization include ketotifen and olopatadine. Both have been shown to improve the signs and symptoms of VKC, and there is evidence that ketotifen may be more effective.[16] Some antihistamines may have a drying effect, which could exacerbate symptoms.

4. **Acetyl cysteine (0.5%)** used topically has mucolytic properties and is useful in the treatment of early plaque formation.

5. **Topical cyclosporine (1%)** drops have been recently reported to be effective in severe unresponsive cases. Cyclosporine is a calcineurin inhibitor that acts by inhibiting cytokine production by T-lymphocytes. It also has inhibitory effects on eosinophil and mast cell activation. Low-dose cyclosporine has emerged as an alternative to corticosteroids in some cases of VKC. It has an excellent side effect profile, limited to only a burning sensation and few systemic effects at the doses being used. Commercially available topical 0.05% cyclosporine A has been shown to improve clinical signs and symptoms of VKC, as well as decreasing tear cytokine concentration when used 4–6 times per day. Higher concentrations of 1–2% have been studied and shown to be safe and effective for even severe VKC, but the disadvantage is that they need to be extemporaneously compounded. More recent studies have shown even a dose of cyclosporine 0.05% 4 times per day may be effective in drug-resistant VKC in conjunction with topical corticosteroids.

B. Systemic therapy

1. **Oral antihistaminics** may provide some relief from itching in severe cases.

2. **Oral steroids** have been recommended for advanced, very severe, nonresponsive cases.

C. Treatment of large papillae

Very large (giant) papillae can be tackled either by:

- *Supratarsal injection* of long acting steroid: Injection of short- or long-acting steroids into the tarsal papilla has been shown to be effective in reducing their size.
- Cryoapplication: Cryoablation of upper tarsal cobblestones is reported to render short-term improvement. However, scar formation from this may lead to lid and tear film abnormalities. The risk of these adverse permanent changes is probably not warranted in this usually self-limiting disease.
- Surgical excision is recommended for extraordinarily large papillae: Surgical removal of the upper tarsal papilla in combination with forniceal conjunctival advancement or buccal mucosal grafting may result in obliteration of the fornix. Excision of upper tarsal papillae with or without adjunctive use of mitomycin C is also helpful.

D. General measures

These include:

- Dark goggles to prevent photophobia.
- Cold compresses and ice packs have soothing effects.

E. Desensitization

It has also been tried without much rewarding results.

F. Treatment of vernal keratopathy

- *Punctate epithelial keratitis* requires no extra treatment except that instillation of steroids should be increased.
- *A large vernal plaque* requires surgical excision by superficial keratectomy.
- *Severe Shield ulcer* resistant to medical therapy may need surgical treatment in the form of debridment, superficial keratectomy, excimer laser therapeutic keratectomy as well as amniotic membrane transplantation to enhance re-epithelialization.
- **Surgical intervention:** Persistent corneal complications such as non-healing Shield ulcers or corneal plaques may require surgical treatment. These interventions may range from scraping to superficial keratectomy. In rare cases of refractory giant papillae that do not respond to medical treatment, surgical interventions such as cryoablation may be employed. Therapies in conjunction with surgical excision to prevent recurrence include mitomycin C application, autologous conjunctival graft, or mucous membrane transplantation. Amniotic membrane transplantation in cases of refractory giant papillae has been shown to aid healing of corneal complications associated with giant papillae such as epitheliopathy and ulcers.

COMPLICATIONS

Severe vernal keratoconjunctivitis is most frequently a self-limiting disease; however, in some cases sight-threatening complications may develop. The corneal epithelium acts as a barrier to circulating pathogens, but may become damaged in severe disease both due to trauma from upper tarsal papillae and a complex array of inflammatory molecules. This combination of repeated trauma and inflammatory milieu may then lead to Shield ulcers and plaques. Shield ulcers usually form on the upper third of the cornea and can lead to sight-threatening complications in up to 6% of patients. They begin as punctate epithelial erosions which coalesce to form macroerosions which then develop into Shield ulcers which can be self-limiting or develop further consequences such as bacterial keratitis.[36] Plaques form when inflammatory debris accumulates at the base of a Shield ulcer. They are particularly resistant to topical therapy and may require surgical intervention.

PROGNOSIS

Generally VKC is a rather benign and self-limiting disease that may resolve with age or spontaneously at puberty. Complications typically arise from occasional corneal scarring.

ATOPIC KERATOCONJUNCTIVITIS (AKC)

It is regarded as an adult equivalent of vernal keratoconjunctivitis and is often associated with atopic dermatitis. Most of the patients are young atopic adults with male predominance.

EPIDEMIOLOGY

Atopic dermatitis is a chronic inflammatory skin disease that affects 15–20% of children and 1–3% of adults worldwide. It is estimated that 25–40% of patients with atopic dermatitis suffer from AKC.

ETIOLOGY

By definition, AKC is the chronic ocular surface inflammation suffered by patients with atopic dermatitis.

PATHOPHYSIOLOGY

The pathophysiology represents combination of type I (IgE mediated) and type IV (delayed) hypersensitivity reaction. This involves release of cytokines by mast cells, eosinophils, T cells and conjunctival epithelial cells. This release of allergic mediators leads to activation of T helper cells and chronic mast cell degranulation. AKC patients have also been shown to have decreased corneal sensitivity and conjunctival goblet cell density compared to controls.

Evidence of the pathologic process comes from histologic and immunohistochemical analysis of conjunctival biopsy specimens and from tear fluid analysis for mediators and cells. Mast cells and eosinophils are found in the conjunctival epithelium of AKC patients but not in normal individuals. Mast cells in the epithelium of AKC patients contain predominantly tryptase as the neutral protease. Goblet cell density and squamous metaplasia are then examined by impression cytology. The epithelium may become involuted, allowing pseudotubule structures to form. Antibodies to HLA-DR stain diffusely throughout the epithelium. This suggests an up-regulation of antigen presentation. There is an increase in the CD4:CD8 ratio in AKC over normal conjunctival epithelium. This increase of CD4 or helper T cells (Th) probably serves to amplify the immune response that is occurring. *In vivo* confocal microscopy reveals fewer basal epithelial cells in the cornea. Mucin proteins and mRNA are increased in the epithelium. Mast cells and eosinophils are found in the conjunctival epithelium of AKC patients but not in normal individuals. Mast cells in the epithelium of AKC patients contain predominantly tryptase as the neutral protease. This suggests an up-regulation of antigen presentation. The substantia propria in AKC has an increased number of mast cells compared to normal. Conjunctival inflammatory cell density showed a negative correlation with tear stability and corneal sensitivity and a positive correlation with the vital staining scores. Eosinophils, rarely found in normal structures, are present in the substantia propria in AKC. These eosinophils are found to have increased numbers of activation markers on their surface.

Risk factors

AKC is a multifactorial disease with genetic and environmental risk factors. The strongest associations are genetic predisposition for poor skin barrier function and dysregulation of immune system, asthma, allergic rhinitis and environmental allergens. The presence of food allergies and sensitivities in infancy and childhood is associated with more severe form of atopic dermatitis. Allergy and sensitivity to pollen, pets and dust mites have also been associated with AKC. Environmental factors such as climate, diet, urban living (including pollution exposure), tobacco smoke, duration of breastfeeding during infancy and obesity have been suggested as risk factors for AKC.

GENERAL PATHOLOGY

Histology of AKC typically shows proliferation of goblet cells, invasion of eosinophils and mast cells into epithelium as well as mononuclear cell infiltrate in substantia propria. Conjunctival epithelium of AKC patients shows increased levels of T cells, T-helper cells, macrophages and dendritic cells.

CLINICAL FEATURES

Symptoms

The chief symptom of AKC is intense, bilateral itching of conjunctiva, eyelids and periorbital skin. Tearing, burning, photophobia and blurry vision are commonly encountered symptoms.

Signs

1. *Eyelids and periorbita:* The eyelids and periorbital skin show evidence of eczematous dermatitis (erythematous, thickened dry skin with blistered patches). Eyelid findings include tylosis (thickening of the tarsal border of the eyelid) with crusting and scaling. Meibomian gland disease is very common in patients with AKC. Other lid findings often encountered are ectropion, trichiasis and madarosis.

2. *Conjunctiva:* The conjunctiva is hyperemic and edematous, with prominent tarsal papillae (papillary conjunctivitis). Mucoid discharge is often present. Severe conjunctival disease can result in scarring and symblepharon. Horner-Trantas dots may or may not be present.

3. *Cornea:* Corneal involvement is frequent, and can range from punctate epithelial erosions to ulcers and even perforation. Peripheral vascularization and pannus are common.

4. *Anterior segment:* Anterior and posterior subcapsular cataracts are common.

DIAGNOSIS

Clinical diagnosis is based mainly on history and ocular findings, though adjunctive diagnostic procedures and lab tests can aid in diagnosis and assessing severity of disease. Serum IgE and skin prick testing is non-specific, but can be helpful in establishing that a patient has atopic disease. IgE levels in tears have been shown to correlate with clinical severity of allergic eye disease. Brush cytology, which involves taking scrapings from tarsal conjunctiva can quantify levels of inflammatory cells such as eosinophils and neutrophils. It has been shown to correlate with amount of corneal damage. Conjunctival biopsy is rarely used to assist in diagnosing AKC.

Association may be keratoconus and atopic cataract.

TREATMENT

Treat facial eczema and lid margin disease. Sodium cromoglycate drops, steroids and tear supplements may be helpful for conjunctival lesions.

Primary prevention

Primary prevention involves reducing probability of disease in patients that do not have clinically evident disease. Breastfeeding has shown to be a protective factor, particularly before 3 months of age. Additionally, prenatal and postnatal probiotics could reduce the incidence of atopic disease by as much as 30%.

Management

The purpose of treatment in AKC is to improve symptoms, limit exacerbations and prevent complications/sequelae that lead to vision loss. It is also important to balance this with limiting side effects of treatment.

I. Medical therapy

Topical therapy: Mild disease can be treated similarly to other allergic eye disease, with emphasis placed on hand hygiene, cold compresses and topical mast cells stabilizers (olopatadine 0.1% or lodoxamide 0.1%) and antihistamines (zelastine 0.05%). Corticosteroid drops and ointments are commonly employed in the treatment of AKC, especially to achieve control of exacerbations and breakthrough inflammation. Steroid therapy should be tapered as quickly as possible while avoiding rebound inflammation. Calcineurin inhibitors (cyclosporine and tacrolimus) are an effective steroid-sparing therapy. Calcineurin is an enzyme involved in the activation of T cells, a key player in AKC. Tacrolimus is available as a 0.03% and 0.1% topical ointment for dermatologic use (Protopic). It has been used off label for

treatment of ophthalmic disease. Topical cyclosporine is available commercially in a 0.05% eye drop preparation (Restasis). Topical calcineurin inhibitors are safe and generally well tolerated, with stinging and eyelid skin maceration being the most common side effect.

Systemic medications: Systemic antihistamines are routinely used in atopic disease. Oral steroids and cyclosporine are generally reserved for severe/recalcitrant disease or for treatment of dermatologic disease, and are often employed in conjunction with the patient's dermatologist. Prolonged treatment with oral steroids is avoided due to unacceptable side effects. Systemic cyclosporine, given at dose of 5 mg/kg per day has been shown helpful in inducing remission of severe atopic disease.

II. Surgery

Amniotic membrane transplantation has been shown to be very effective for persistent corneal epithelial defects. Tectonic keratoplasty may be necessary for patients with severe corneal thinning or perforation. Penetrating keratoplasty (PK) may be indicated for corneal opacities or severe ulceration/thinning. Patients with AKC are at increased risk of cataract formation (especially anterior and posterior subcapsular), independent of steroid exposure. Postoperative care and final visual outcomes are impacted by ongoing ocular surface disease. Eyelid surgery may be necessary for correction of trichiasis, ectropion or entropion.

COMPLICATIONS

The clinical presentation of AKC can vary greatly, but in recalcitrant cases, it can cause severe and site threatening corneal complications. Corneal findings range from punctate epithelial erosions to ulcers (infectious or sterile), neovascularization and lipid keratopathy. Herpes simplex keratitis is more common in patients with AKC and often more severe. As with other ocular allergic diseases, patients with AKC are at increased risk of keratoconus due to chronic eye rubbing. Therefore, patients with AKC should be counselled to limit eye rubbing as much as possible, and should be provided with treatment to reduce or eliminate itching.

▪ PHLYCTENULAR KERATOCONJUNCTIVITIS

Phlyctenular keratoconjunctivitis is a characteristic nodular affection occurring as an allergic response of conjunctival and corneal epithelium to endogenous allergens to which they have become sensitized. Phlyctenular conjunctivitis is of worldwide distribution. However, its incidence is higher in developing countries. Phlyctenular keratoconjunctivitis, or phlyctenulosis, is thought to represent a delayed hypersensitivity reaction to a number of antigens, the most common being tuberculoprotein and staphylococcal antigen. The term phlyctenule is derived from the Greek word phlyctena, which means "blister." This was likely a reference to the appearance of a conjunctival or corneal nodule after undergoing necrosis and ulceration. The earliest description of phlyctenulosis is found in a textbook written by C. de St. Yves in 1722. In 1940s, Sorsby was the first to confirm the strong correlation with tuberculosis when he reported that 85% of patients with PKC tested positive to the tuberculin skin test versus 15% in a control group in the same hospital. Fritz et al and Philip et al later made similar observations in studies of impoverished Alaskan villages with high rates of tuberculosis, noting that the prevalence of PKC correlated directly with tuberculin skin sensitivity. There was also increased morbidity in children with PKC, who had greater odds of developing clinical tuberculosis.

ETIOLOGY

It is believed to be a delayed hypersensitivity (Type IV-cell mediated) response to endogenous microbial proteins.

PATHOPHYSIOLOGY

Immunologically, pathogenesis of PKC is presumed to be a cell-mediated type IV hypersensitivity reaction to microbial antigens. The histological findings in phlyctenule biopsies included predominance of monocyte-derived cells (macrophages and dendritic Langerhans cells) with moderate amount of T lymphocytes. These findings are comparable to what is seen in human skin tuberculin reaction, which is a classic example of delayed-type hypersensitivity. The inflammatory infiltrate is found just beneath the epithelium and also includes neutrophils that may be a response to necrosis that has occurred in these lesions. Aberrant HLA-DR4 antigen expression was present in basal epithelium of phlyctenule, and similar aberrant expression has been seen by keratinocytes in the tuberculin reaction. No microorganisms have been found in phlyctenule samples.

I. Causative allergens

1. *Tuberculous proteins* were considered, previously, as the most common cause.
2. *Staphylococcus proteins* are now thought to account for most of the cases.
3. *Other allergens* may be proteins of Moraxella Axenfeld bacillius and certain parasites (worm infestation).

II. Predisposing factors

1. *Age.* Peak age group is 3–15 years.
2. *Sex.* Incidence is higher in girls than boys.
3. *Undernourishment.* Disease is more common in undernourished children.
4. *Living conditions.* Overcrowded and unhygienic.
5. *Season.* It occurs in all climates but incidence is high in spring and summer seasons.

PATHOLOGY

1. *Stage of nodule formation.* In this stage there occurs exudation and infiltration of leucocytes into deeper layers of conjunctiva leading to a nodule formation. The central cells are polymorphonuclear and peripheral cells are lymphocytes. The neighbouring blood vessels dilate and their endothelium proliferates.

2. *Stage of ulceration.* Later on necrosis occurs at the apex of nodule and an ulcer is formed. Leucocytic infiltration increases with plasma cells and mast cells.

3. *Stage of granulation.* Eventually floor of ulcer becomes covered with granulation tissue.

4. *Stage of healing.* Healing occurs usually with minimal scarring.

CLINICAL PICTURE

Symptoms in simple phlyctenular conjunctivitis are few, like mild discomfort in the eye, irritation and reflex watering. However, usually there is associated mucopurulent conjunctivitis due to secondary bacterial infection.

Phlyctenular keratitis. Corneal involvement may occur secondarily from extension of conjunctival phlycten or rarely as a primary disease. It may present in two forms: The 'ulcerative phlyctenular keratitis' or 'diffuse infiltrative keratitis'.

A. Ulcerative phlyctenular keratitis

Ulcerative phlyctenular keratitis may occur in the following three forms:

1. *Sacrofulous ulcer* is a shallow marginal ulcer formed due to breakdown of small limbal phlycten. It differs from the catarrhal ulcer in that there is no clear space between the ulcer and the limbus and its long axis is frequently perpendicular to limbus. Such an ulcer usually clears up without leaving any opacity.

2. *Fascicular ulcer* (Fig. 26.5) has a prominent parallel leash of blood vessels. This ulcer usually remains superficial but leaves behind a band-shaped superficial opacity after healing.

3. *Miliary ulcer*. In this form multiple small ulcers are scattered over a portion of or whole of the cornea.

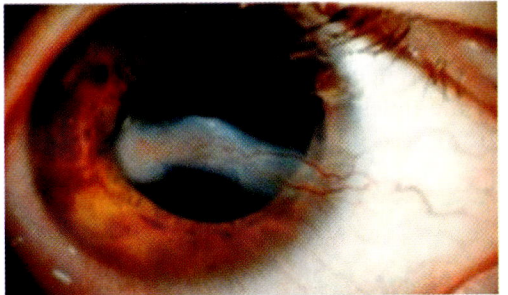

Fig. 26.5: *Fascicular corneal ulcer*

B. Diffuse infiltrative phlyctenular keratitis

Diffuse infiltrative phlyctenular keratitis may appear in the form of central infiltration of cornea with characteristic rich vascularization from the periphery all around the limbus. It may be superficial or deep.

Corneal phlyctenules typically appear at the limbus as a small white nodule with adjacent intense conjunctival injection. These phlyctenules often undergo necrosis, forming a marginal ulcer. The ulcer resolves, resulting in anterior stromal scarring, typically triangular in shape with the base of the triangle at the limbus. Superficial corneal neovascularization (pannus) can also develop. The pannus formation can be fascicular or broader, as seen in trachoma. Unlike trachoma, a broad pannus in PKC typically is inferiorly located and has an irregular border. Subsequent corneal phlyctenules can arise at the central edge of a pannus from prior attacks. This can happen multiple times such that the phlyctenule can appear to "wander" across the cornea. the phlyctenule can appear to 'wander' across the cornea. There are other less common corneal manifestations of PKC. Multiple small phlyctenular lesions may be distributed diffusely over the entire corneal surface (i.e. miliary phlyctenulosis). Corneal perforation secondary to phlyctenulosis is uncommon but can occur.

Clinical course is usually self-limiting and phlycten disappears in 8–10 days leaving no trace. However, recurrences are very common.

MANAGEMENT

It includes treatment of phlyctenular conjunctivitis by local therapy, investigations and specific therapy aimed at eliminating the causative allergen and general measures to improve the health of the child. All patients should be counseled on eyelid hygiene using baby shampoo or soap diluted in warm water on a washcloth or cotton tip applicator directed at the eyelash base and lid margins. This is primarily to address any underlying blepharitis. Artificial tears or lubricating ointments may be used for symptomatic relief as well. Antimicrobial therapy is generally tailored to the suspected organism. In cases of TB associated PED, patients should be screened for active or underlying infection, and treated with the appropriate medical therapy. Family members or close contacts should also be screened and treated.

Oral tetracycline has been effective in treating cases of *S. aureus* and *P. acnes* related disease. It has also been successfully used to treat patients with recurrent disease that has failed other therapeutic measures. Tetracycline should be administered for up to 3 weeks after patients become asymptomatic and then gradually tapered down over the course of weeks to months. Care should be taken when treating pediatric patients younger than 8 years old as potential side effects include discoloration and maldevelopment of teeth. Adults may additionally complain of gastrointestinal upset and photodermatitis.

Erythromycin can be used as an alternative.

Patients with helminthic infections should be treated with parasite-specific oral medication; mebendazole has been extremely effective. PED in these patients typically resolves quickly with therapy with a low rate of recurrence. Recurrence may be a sign of re-infection. Fungi related infections can be treated with appropriate antifungal therapy, and as with parasites, generally follow a successful course after treatment. Topical antibiotic agents are indicated for use in conjunction with anti-inflammatory medications such as corticosteroids or cyclosporine regardless of etiology. Topical therapy may be in the form of drops or ointments. Gatifloxacin, bacitracin, erythromycin, and azithromycin are all common choices.

Anti-inflammatory therapy is usually started early in the course of treatment. Topical corticosteroids are usually selected for this purpose. It is recommended to start patients on a q2–4 hour dosing regimen with a gradual taper once symptoms begin to resolve. Rapid tapers are associated with recurrence. In addition, topical corticosteroids are associated with ocular complications including increased intraocular pressure, cataract formation, and disturbance of accommodation amongst a list of others. Consequently, some ophthalmologists prefer to start patients on oral and topical antimicrobial therapy before initiating a steroid drop.

COMPLICATIONS

Phlyctenular nodules can lead to ulceration, scarring and mild to moderate vision loss. Although rare, corneal perforation can also occur.

PRIMARY INFECTION BY HERPES VIRUS TYPE I

Majority of patients infected during childhood are immunised. General symptoms of fever and malaise are apparent. In addition to numerous vescicles on the skin of the face and the eyelids. both corneas show myriads of small dendritic figures. The immunoglobulins against each of the viral antibodies have different protective effects.

Keratitis dendritica (Fig. 26.6): Keratitis dendritica is recurrence of herpetic disease in an already-immunised patient. Most patients have circulating anti-herpes immunoglobulins in their blood induced by primary infection during childhood. The herpesvirus has retired into nerve ganglion cells where it became latent. According to some studies the virus may also be latent inside cells of the cornea. The epithelial cells infected with active virus, however, display viral epitopes on their cell surface where they are presented in the cleft of HLA class I and class II molecules. In normal cornea most cells carry HLA class I molecules on their cell surface, but in the presence of herpes keratitis many cells in the cornea start expressing HLA class II complexes. In the epithelium active cells of basal layers in a large area surrounding dendritic ulcer acquire this surface marker. When a wandering T cell with anti-herpes receptors, a remnant of the primary infection, encounters such an infected cell, it becomes activated, secretes IL-2 and multiples. The daughter cells develop their cytotoxic equipment and start killing the

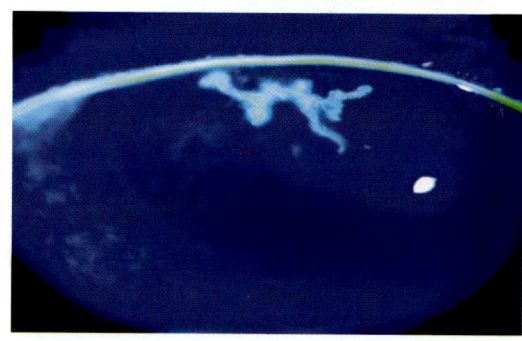

Fig. 26.6: *Herpetic dendritic keratitis*

infected cells by punching holes in their plasma membranes. Virus replication stops, the cell debris is eliminated and the epithelium heals. ADCC is also active in dendritic keratitis. The immunoglobulins A, G and M present in the tears bind to the exposed herpes antigen and mark the infected cells for destruction by polymorphs or especially macrophages. However, rather few lymphocytes wander on the corneal surface, and very few travel through the stroma. Replica histology of human dendritic lesions demonstrates paucity of leucocytes in lesion. The dendritic cells in the corneal epithelium do not seem to be particularly attracted by the virus-infected cells. It will take time before a T-lymphocyte with the required anti-herpes specific receptor stumbles on the tiny epithelial lesion. It will take even more time before an adequate attack against the virus is organised. As a consequence the natural history of keratitis dendritica runs over weeks and more; spontaneous healing is slow. The virus spilling out of the dying cells could infect other epithelial cells, but clinical observation shows that in most instances it fails to do so. Neither slow growth of the dendritic lesion nor the generation of additional dendrites as in primary infection, is seen. On the contrary, a dendritic figure usually attains its full size quickly, before the patient has time to see an ophthalmologist, and then it will remain stable until it fades away. The existence of immunoglobulins is one important reason, and their protective action has been demonstrated experimentally. In mice serum containing immunoglobulins or monoclonal immunoglobulins against herpes was injected simultaneously with the inoculation of the cornea with herpesvirus. This passive immunisation had no influence on the course of the epithelial keratitis, but reduces the spread of the virus to the deeper layers of the eye and the central nervous system. Similarly, in rabbits immunisation prior to ocular inoculation reduces, and immunosuppression.

DISCIFORM KERATITIS (Fig. 26.7)

This entity is characterised by a deep, central or peripheral disk-shaped stromal edema with minimal infiltrate and intact epithelium.

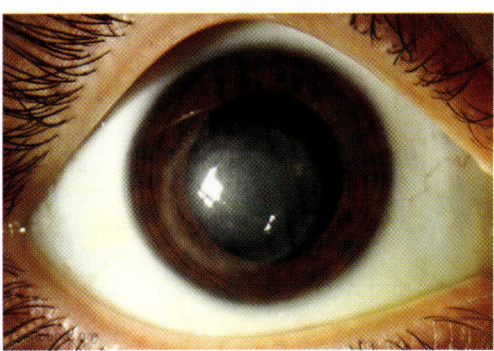

Fig. 26.7: *Disciform keratitis*

Multiple patches of oedema and circular immune rings develop. This entity represents a VZV viral infection of the endothelium or an immune reaction to soluble antigen or viral particles in the corneal stroma.

Disciform endotheliitis is far and away the most common presentation of endotheliitis. Patients with disciform endotheliitis present with photophobia and mild to moderate ocular discomfort. Limbal injection is usually seen, as these patients have an accompanying iritis. Visual acuity may range from normal to severely reduced, depending on the location and severity of the stromal edema. The most striking finding of disciform endotheliitis on slit lamp examination is a round or disc-shaped area of stromal edema. This oedema may be in central or paracentral cornea. The edema usually spans the entire stromal thickness, resulting in the usual ground-glass appearance seen with corneal edema from other entities of endothelial decompensation. Typically, in disciform endotheliitis, the edema is within a strikingly focal pattern with a definite demarcation between involved and uninvolved cornea. The epithelium shows microcystic edema overlying the areas of stromal edema. The accompanying edema from endothelial decompensation seen with disciform endotheliitis is in marked contrast to the lack of corneal edema seen in other causes of acute anterior uveitis. In addition, elevated intraocular pressure, which may be severe, is often present. The increased pressure may be due either to inflammatory cells blocking aqueous outflow or to a primary trabeculitis.

Disciform endotheliitis is normally exquisitely sensitive to topical corticosteroids, and early intervention usually leads to complete resolution of the edema and KP without stromal scarring or loss of vision. Many cases of disciform endotheliitis are self-limited and completely resolve even if left untreated. Severe cases, however, can lead to permanent edema, scarring, and neovascularization if untreated.

KERATITIS IN RHEUMATOID ARTHRITIS

Refer to Chapter 28.

KERATITIS ASSOCIATED WITH NON-RHEUMATOID COLLAGEN VASCULAR DISEASES

- Systemic lupus erythematosus (refer to Chapter 28)
- Relapsing polychondritis (refer to Chapter 28)
- Granulomatosis with polyangiitis (refer to Chapter 28)
- Polyarteritis nodosa (refer to Chapter 28)
- Churg-Strauss syndrome (refer to Chapter 28)
- Cogan syndrome
- Behçet disease
- Giant cell arteritis (refer to Chapter 28)
- Peripheral ulcerative keratitis (refer to Chapter 28)

CORNEAL ALLOGRAFT REJECTION

Corneal allograft rejection refers to the immunological response of the host to the donor corneal tissue without regard to the effect of the response on graft survival. Typically it is characterised by a period of graft clarity (about two weeks for a primary graft and one week for regraft) prior to the appearance of the sign of rejection.

Note: For details *see* page 610.

BIBLIOGRAPHY

1. American Academy of Ophthalmology. Staph phlyctenular keratoconjunctivitis. www.aao.org/image/staph-phlyctenular-keratoconjunctivitis-2 Accessed October 10, 2017.
2. AAO Basic and Clinical Science Course, External Disease and Cornea, 2010–2011
3. Buckley, R.J., Vernal keratoconjunctivitis. Int Ophthalmol Clin, 1988. 28(4): 303–8.
4. Culbertson WW, Huang AJ, Mandelbaum SH, Pflugfelder SC, Boozalis GT, Miller D. Effective treatment of phlyctenular keratoconjunctivitis with oral tetracycline. Ophthalmology. 1993; 100(9): 1358-1366.
5. De Smedt, S., G. Wildner, and P. Kestelyn, Vernal keratoconjunctivitis: an update. Br J Ophthalmol, 2013. 97(1): 9–14.
6. Herpetic Eye Disease Study Group. Acyclovir for the prevention of recurrent herpes simplex virus eye disease. N Engl J Med 1998;339:300-6.
7. Kumar, S., Vernal keratoconjunctivitis: a major review. Acta Ophthalmologica, 2009. 87(2): 133-147.
8. La Rosa, M., et al., Allergic conjunctivitis: a comprehensive review of the literature. Ital J Pediatr, 2013. 39: 18
9. Liesegang TJ, Melton LJ, 3rd, Daly PJ, Ilstrup DM. Epidemiology of ocular herpes simplex. Incidence in Rochester, Minn, 1950 through 1982. Arch Ophthalmol 1989; 107: 1155–9.
10. Thygeson P. Observations on nontuberculous phlyctenular keratoconjunctivitis. Transactions: American Academy of Ophthalmology and Otolaryngology. 1954; 58(1): 128–132.
11. Thygeson P. The etiology and treatment of phlyctenular keratoconjunctivitis. American Journal of Ophthalmology. 1951; 34(9): 1217–1236.
12. Wang JC. Keratitis, Herpes Simplex. Emedicine. Accessed online from: http://emedicine.medscape.com/article/1194268-overview. Updated 8/7/2009.

Trophic Corneal Ulcers

Trophic corneal ulcers develop due to disturbance in metabolic activity of epithelial cells. This group includes:

- Neurotrophic keratopathy
- Exposure keratopathy
- Atheromatous corneal ulcer.

NEUROTROPHIC KERATOPATHY

Neurotrophic keratopathy (neuroparalytic keratitis) occurs due to decreased corneal sensations owing to damage of sensory nerve supply of the cornea (trigeminal nerve).

CAUSES

A. Congenital

- Familial dysautonomia (Riley-Day syndrome).
- Congenital insensitivity to pain.
- Anhidrotic ectodermal dysplasia.

B. Acquired

- Following alcohol-block or electrocoagulation of Gasserian ganglion or section of the sensory root of trigeminal nerve for trigeminal neuralgia.
- A neoplasm (e.g. acoustic neuroma) pressing on Gasserian ganglion.
- Gasserian ganglion destruction due to acute infection in herpes zoster ophthalmicus.
- Acute infection of Gasserian ganglion by herpes simplex virus.
- Syphilitic (luetic) neuropathy.
- Involvement of corneal nerves in leprosy, diabetes.
- Injury to Gasserian ganglion.
- Drug toxicity.

PATHOGENESIS

Exact pathogenesis is not clear; the disturbances in the corneal sensations occur due to damage to sensory nerves and presumably as a consequence, metabolic activity of corneal epithelium is disturbed, leading to accumulation of metabolites; which in turn cause oedema and exfoliation of epithelial cells followed by ulceration. In such cases, corneal changes can occur even in the presence of a normal blink reflex and normal lacrimal secretions.

CLINICAL FEATURES

Typically neurotrophic keratitis is characterised by marked signs and minimal symptoms (due to decreased corneal sensation).

Symptoms

- Red eye, swollen eyelids and defective vision are common complaints.
- No pain and no tearing are characteristic features.

Signs

1. *Ciliary congestion* is marked.
2. *Corneal signs*

- *Sensations* are characteristically decreased, or absent
- *Sheen* is lost (dull sheen)
- *Punctate epithelial erosions* involving the interpalpebral area are initial lesions, which soon converts into epithelial defects.
- *Frank epithelial defects* occur due to exfoliation of corneal epithelium, later followed by corneal ulceration.
- *Corneal ulcer* is typically horizontally oval, located in the lower one-half of the cornea and have grey heaped-up epithelial borders (Fig. 27.1A).

Note. Relapses are very common, even the healed scars quickly breakdown again.

TREATMENT

- *Conventional treatment* with antibiotics, cycloplegics, lubricating drops and patching should be started immediately.
- *Topical nerve growth factor drops* and autologous serum drops may be helpful in addition to conventional treatment.
- *Topical collagenase inhibitors* such as N-acetyl-cysteine, tetracycline or medroxyprogesterone may be administered in the case of stromal melting.
- *Amniotic membrane transplantation* is recommended when patients present with large non-healing ulcers.
- *Lateral tarsorrhaphy* is usually required to promote healing and prevent relapses. It should be kept at least for one year along with

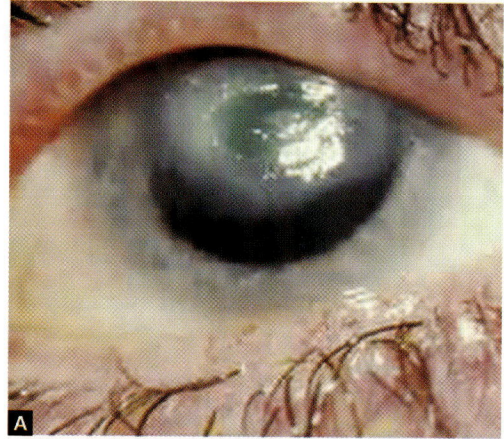

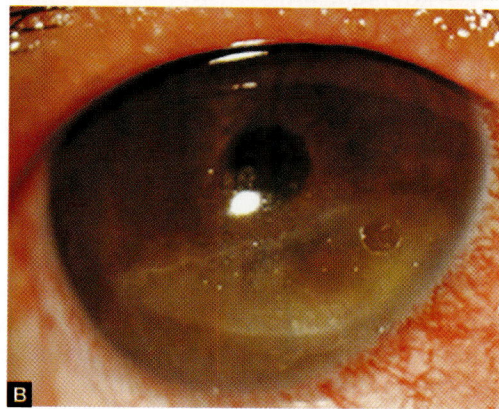

Fig. 27.1: *Trophic corneal ulcers. A, Neurotrophic; B, Exposure keratitis. (Note: Punctate epithelial defects in the lower third of cornea.)*

and prolonged use of artificial tears is also recommended.

- *Cyanoacrylate glue* and bandage soft contact lens are required in cases of small corneal perforation.
- *Lamellar or penetrating keratoplasty* may be required in large non-healing ulcers.

EXPOSURE KERATOPATHY

Normally, cornea is covered by *eyelids* during sleep and is constantly kept moist by blinking movements during awakening. When eyes are covered insufficiently by the lids and/or there is loss of protective mechanism of blinking, the condition of exposure keratopathy (keratitis lagophthalmos) develops.

CAUSES

Following factors which produce lagophthalmos may lead to exposure keratopathy:

1. *Extreme proptosis* due to any cause will allow inadequate closure of lids.
2. *Bell's palsy* or any other cause of facial palsy.
3. *Ectropion* of severe degree.
4. *Symblepharon* causing lagophthalmos.
5. *Deep coma* associated with inadequate closure of lids.
6. *Physiological lagophthalmos.* Occasionally, lagophthalmos during sleep may occur in healthy individuals.
7. *Thyroid ophthalmopathy* with lid retraction.
8. *Post-surgical lid retraction* following severe ptosis correction, eyelid reconstruction and large inferior rectus recession.

PATHOGENESIS

Due to exposure there occurs tear film unstability, decreased tear film break up time (TBUT) and the corneal epithelium dries up followed by desiccation. After the epithelium is cast off, invasion by infective organisms may occur.

CLINICAL FEATURES

Symptoms and signs of the causative disease are evident.

Symptoms of exposure keratopathy include ocular irritation, burning, foreign body sensation and redness. Symptoms are usually worse in the morning.

Signs of exposure keratopathy are:

- *Drying of cornea* occurs to begin with due to inadequate blinking or closure of the lids.
- *Punctate epithelial defects* develop in the lower third of cornea or as a horizontal band in the region of palpebral fissure (Fig. 27.1).
- *Corneal ulceration* may develop soon due to necrosis followed by bacterial superinfection. Typically the ulcer involves the inferior corneal area and is horizontally oval in shape. If neglected, corneal ulcer may even perforate soon.

MANAGEMENT

I. *Prophylaxis.* Once lagophthalmos is diagnosed following measures should be taken to prevent exposure keratitis.
- *Artificial tears* should be instilled frequently.
- *Instillation of ointment* and closure of lids by a tape or bandage during sleep.
- *Soft bandage contact lens* with frequent instillation of artificial tears is required in cases of moderate exposure.
- Treatment of the cause of exposure, e.g. proptosis, ectropion, symblepharon should be taken up.

II. *Treatment of the corneal ulcer* once developed is on the general lines (*see* page 393).
- *Tarsorrhaphy* is invariably required when it is not possible to treat the cause or when recovery of the cause (e.g. facial palsy) is not anticipated.

ATHEROMATOUS CORNEAL ULCER

Atheromatous corneal ulcer refers to corneal ulceration in an old leucomatous corneal opacity.

ETIOPATHOGENESIS

Long-standing leucoma undergoes degenerative changes with calcareous deposits. As the cornea is devitalised and insensitive a non-healy defect occurs in the centre of leucomatous corneal opacity, which is readily vulnerable to infections.

CLINICAL FEATURES

Symptoms and signs are similar to bacterial corneal ulcer (*see* page 390) with following special features:
- *Ulcer* is associated with old dense corneal opacity, which shows degenerative changes as lipid keratopathy and/or calcareous deposits.
- *Lipid keratopathy*, associated, is characterised by dense yellow or cream-coloured opacification or fan-like cholesterol crystals in the corneal stroma surrounding the corneal neovascular blood vessels.
- *Perforation of ulcer* occurs quietly and pan-ophthalmitis may supervene.

TREATMENT

- *Corneal ulcer* should be treated on the line of bacterial corneal ulcer (*see* page 393)
- *Copious lubricant* eye drops in the form of gel should be used frequently.
- *Bandage contact lens* may be required in non-healing epithelial defects.
- *Therapeutic keratoplasty* may be required in non-healing chronic cases.
- *Evisceration,* in blind eyes, relieves the patient of unnecessary agony.

BIBLIOGRAPHY

1. Aifa A, Gueudry J, Portmann A, Delcampe A, Muraine M. Topical treatment with a new matrix therapy agent (RGTA) for the treatment of corneal neurotrophic ulcers. Investigative ophthalmology and visual science
2. Albert, D. M. & Jakobiec, F. A. Principles and practice of ophthalmology. 2nd edn, (W.B. Saunders Co., 2000).
3. Bahn, R. S. Graves' ophthalmopathy. N Engl J Med 362, 726–738, doi:10.1056/NEJMra0905750 (2010).
4. Banerjee PJ, Chandra A, Sullivan PM, Charteris DG. Neurotrophic corneal ulceration after retinal detachment surgery with retinectomy and endolaser: a case series. JAMA ophthalmology 2014; 132: 750–2.
5. Bonini S, Lambiase A, Rama P, Caprioglio G, Aloe L. Topical treatment with nerve growth factor for neurotrophic keratitis. Ophthalmology 2000; 107: 1347–51; discussion 51–2.
6. Bonini S, Rama P, Olzi D, Lambiase A. Neurotrophic keratitis. Eye 2003; 17: 989–95.
7. Dart JK, Saw VP, Kilvington S. Acanthamoeba keratitis: diagnosis and treatment update 2009. American journal of ophthalmology 2009; 148: 487–99 e2.
8. Dawson, D. Development of a new eye care guideline for critically ill patients. Intensive Crit Care Nurs 21, 119–122, doi:10.1016/j.iccn.2005.01.004 (2005)
9. Ferrari G, Hajrasouliha AR, Sadrai Z, Ueno H, Chauhan SK, Dana R. Nerves and neovessels inhibit each other in the cornea. Investigative ophthalmology and visual science 2013; 54: 813–20.
10. Gerstenblith, A. T. & Rabinowitz, M. P. The Wills eye manual :office and emergency room diagnosis and treatment of eye disease. 6th edn, (Wolters Kluwer/Lippincott Williams & Wilkins, 2012).
11. Golebiowski B, Papas E, Stapleton F. Assessing the sensory function of the ocular surface: implications of use of a non-contact air jet aesthesiometer versus the Cochet-Bonnet aesthesiometer. Experimental eye research 2011; 92: 408–13.
12. Grixti, A., Sadri, M., Edgar, J. & Datta, A. V. Common ocular surface disorders in patients in intensive care units. Ocul Surf 10, 26–42, doi:10.1016/j.jtos.2011.10.001 (2012).
13. Hall, A. J. Some Observations on the Acts of Closing and Opening the Eyes. Br J Ophthalmol 20, 257–295 (1936).
14. Hersh PS, Rice BA, Baer JC, et al. Topical nonsteroidal agents and corneal wound healing. Archives of ophthalmology 1990; 108: 577–83.
15. Holland, E. J., Mannis, M. J. & Lee, W. B. Ocular surface disease : cornea, conjunctiva and tear film. (Elsevier/Saunders, 2013).
16. Holland, E. J., Mannis, M. J. & Lee, W. B. Ocular surface disease : cornea, conjunctiva and tear film. (Elsevier/Saunders, 2013).
17. Howitt, D. A. & Goldstein, J. H. Physiologic lagophthalmos. Am J Ophthalmol 68, 355 (1969).
18. Imanaka, H., Taenaka, N., Nakamura, J., Aoyama, K. & Hosotani, H. Ocular surface disorders in the critically ill. Anesth Analg 85, 343–346 (1997).
19. Jeng BH, Dupps WJ, Jr. Autologous serum 50% eyedrops in the treatment of persistent corneal epithelial defects. Cornea 2009; 28: 1104–8
20. Kauffmann T, Bodanowitz S, Hesse L, Kroll P. Corneal reinnervation after photorefractive keratectomy and laser *in situ* keratomileusis: an *in vivo* study with a confocal videomicroscope. German journal of ophthalmology 1996; 5: 508–12.
21. Krachmer, J., Mannis, M. J. & Holland, E. J. Cornea. Third edn, Vol. 1 (Mosby, 2011).
22. Kumar RL, Koenig SB, Covert DJ. Corneal sensation after descemet stripping and automated endothelial keratoplasty. Cornea 2010; 29: 13–8.
23. Kuruvilla, S., et al. Incidence and risk factor evaluation of exposure keratopathy in critically ill patients: a cohort study. J Crit Care 30, 400-404, doi:10.1016/j.jcrc.2014.10.009 (2015).
24. Lambiase A, Rama P, Bonini S, Caprioglio G, Aloe L. Topical treatment with nerve growth factor for corneal neurotrophic ulcers. The New England journal of medicine 1998; 338: 1174–80.

25. Lambiase A, Bonini S, Aloe L, Rama P, Bonini S. Anti-inflammatory and healing properties of nerve growth factor in immune corneal ulcers with stromal melting. Archives of ophthalmology 2000; 118: 1446–9.

26. Lawrence, S. and C. Morris (2008). Lagophthalmos Evaluation and Treatment. EyeNet. Accessed 2017.

27. Lin X, Xu B, Sun Y, Zhong J, Huang W, Yuan J. Comparison of deep anterior lamellar keratoplasty and penetrating keratoplasty with respect to postoperative corneal sensitivity and tear film function. Graefe's archive for clinical and experimental ophthalmology = Albrecht von Graefe's Archiv fur klinische und experimentelle Ophthalmologie 2014; 252: 1779–87.

28. Lockwood A, Hope-Ross M, Chell P. Neurotrophic keratopathy and diabetes mellitus. Eye 2006; 20: 837–9.

29. Mackie IA. Neuroparalytic keratitis. In: Fraunfelder F, Roy FH, Meyer SM, eds. Current Ocular Therapy. Philadelphia, PA: WB Saunders; 1995: 452–4.

30. Mantelli, F., et al. Cocaine snorting may induce ocular surface damage through corneal sensitivity impairment. Graefe's Arch Clin Exp Ophthalmol 253, 765–772, doi:10.1007/s00417-015-2938-x (2015).

31. McCulley, J.P. & Shine, W. A compositional based model for the tear film lipid layer. Trans Am Ophthalmol Soc 95, 79–88; discussion 88–93 (1997).

32. Mokhtarzadeh, A. & Bradley, E. A. Safety and Long-term Outcomes of Congenital Ptosis Surgery: A Population-Based Study. J Pediatr Ophthalmol Strabismus 53, 212–217, doi: 10.3928/01913913-20160511-02 (2016).

33. Mercieca, F., Suresh, P., Morton, A. & Tullo, A. Ocular surface disease in intensive care unit patients. Eye (London, England) 13 (Pt 2), 231–236, doi:10.1038/eye.1999.57 (1999).

34. Morishige N, Morita Y, Yamada N, Nishida T, Sonoda KH. Congenital hypoplastic trigeminal nerve revealed by manifestation of corneal disorders likely caused by neural factor deficiency. Case reports in ophthalmology 2014; 5: 181–5.

35. Netto MV, Mohan RR, Ambrosio R, Jr., Hutcheon AE, Zieske JD, Wilson SE. Wound healing in the cornea: a review of refractive surgery complications and new prospects for therapy. Cornea 2005; 24: 509–22.

36. Rajaii, F. and C. Prescott (2014). Management of Exposure Keratopathy. EyeNet Magazine. Accessed 2017.—rante le vita del subjecto.

37. Sacchetti M, Lambiase A. Diagnosis and management of neurotrophic keratitis. Clinical ophthalmology 2014; 8: 571–9.

38. Shaheen, B. S., Bakir, M. & Jain, S. Corneal nerves in health and disease. Surv Ophthalmol 59, 263–285, doi:10.1016/j.survophthal.2013.09.002 (2014).

39. Skibell, B. C., Soparkar, C.N., Tower, R. N. & Patrinely, J. R. Periocular anesthesia in aesthetic surgery. Semin Plast Surg 21, 37-40, doi:10.1055/s-2007-967746 (2007).

40. Tawfik, H. A., Abdulhafez, M. H. & Fouad, Y. A.Congenital upper eyelid coloboma: embryologic, nomenclatorial, nosologic, etiologic, pathogenetic, epidemiologic, clinical, and management perspectives. Ophthal Plast Reconstr Surg 31, 1–12, doi:10.1097/IOP.0000000000000347 (2015).

41. Tinley CG, Gray RH. Routine, single session, indirect laser for proliferative diabetic retinopathy. Eye 2009; 23: 1819–23.

42. Trussler, A. P. & Rohrich, R. J. MOC-PSSM CME article: Blepharoplasty. Plast Reconstr Surg 121, 1-10, doi:10.1097/01.prs.0000294667.93660.8b (2008)

43. Turkoglu E, Celik E, Alagoz G. A comparison of the efficacy of autologous serum eye drops with amniotic membrane transplantation in neurotrophic keratitis. Seminars in ophthalmology 2014; 29: 119–26.

44. Ueno H, Ferrari G, Hattori T, et al. Dependence of corneal stem/progenitor cells on ocular surface innervation. Investigative ophthalmology and visual science 2012; 53: 867–72

45. Vallabhanath, P. & Carter, S. R. Ectropion and entropion. Curr Opin Ophthalmol 11, 345–351 (2000).

46. Wasilewski D, Mello GH, Moreira H. Impact of collagen crosslinking on corneal sensitivity in keratoconus patients. Cornea 2013; 32: 899–902.

47. Wilson SE. Laser *in situ* keratomileusis-induced (presumed) neurotrophic epitheliopathy. Ophthalmology 2001; 108: 1082–7.

48. Wilson SE, Ambrosio R. Laser *in situ* keratomileusis-induced neurotrophic epitheliopathy. American journal of ophthalmology 2001; 132: 405–6.

Peripheral Ulcerative Keratitis

INTRODUCTION AND OVERVIEW

DEFINITION

Peripheral ulcerative keratitis (PUK) is a destructive disorder of the juxtalimbal cornea characterised by a crescent-shaped destructive inflammation of corneal stroma associated with an epithelial defect, the presence of inflammatory stromal cells and progressive stromal degradation and thinning[1-3] (Fig. 28.1).

OVERVIEW

PUK can be associated with various ocular and systemic infectious and noninfectious diseases. Various systemic autoimmune vasculitic diseases that can prove potentially fatal may present as PUK. Because of its association with a large number of disease, it is essential to diagnose the etiology of the PUK which often needs a battery of investigations.[1,2]

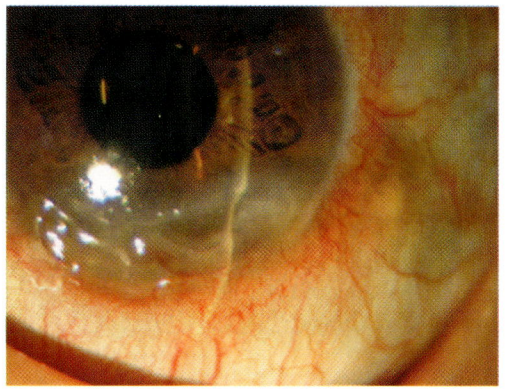

Fig. 28.1: *Peripheral ulcerative keratitis*

PUK often has involvement of adjacent structures like conjunctiva, episclera, and sclera. ***Potentially serious complications of PUK*** include corneal perforation and severe corneal scarring with thinning and vascularization. PUK-associated complications can be prevented with timely diagnosis, detection of the underlying systemic inflammatory disease, and proper treatment.

ETIOPATHOGENESIS OF PUKs

ETIOLOGICAL TYPES OF PUKs

PUKs can be associated with various ocular and systemic infectious and non-infectious diseases as described in Table 28.1.

Idiopathic PUKs. The most common form is the idiopathic variant known as Mooren's ulcer (MU) (Fig. 28.2).

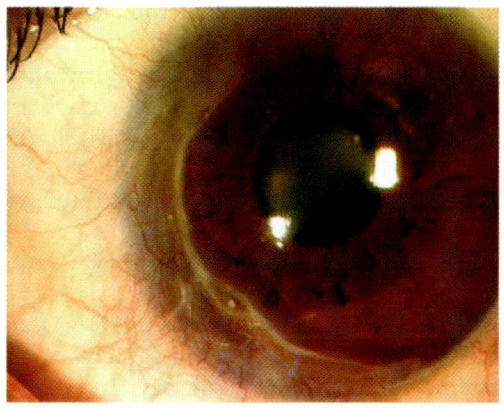

Fig. 28.2: *Mooren's ulcer*

PUKs associated with systemic collagen vascular diseases are the most common disorder associated with PUK, of which rheumatoid arthritis is the most common (Fig. 28.3), accounting for 34% of non-infectious PUK cases.[1,4] Approximately 50% of all non-infectious PUK cases have an associated collagen vascular disease.[1, 4, 5] Apart from rheumatoid arthritis, Wegener granulomatosis, relapsing poly-chondritis, systemic lupus erythematosus, classic polyarteritis nodosa, and its variants, microscopic polyangiitis or Churg-Strauss syndrome are other diseases that can be associated with PUK.[1–5] In more devastating immunologic conditions it may be associated with necrotizing scleritis (Fig. 28.4).

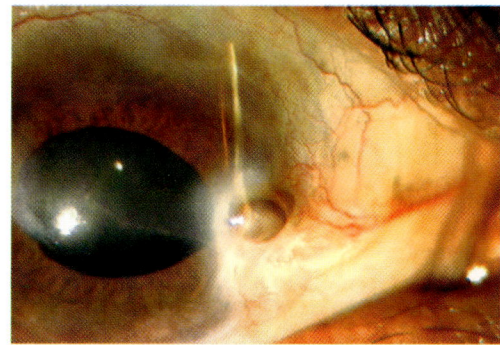

Fig. 28.3: *PUK due to rheumatoid arthritis*

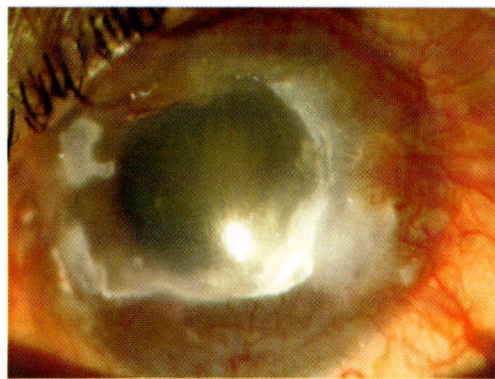

Fig. 28.4: *PUK with necrotizing scleritis*

Infectious PUKs. In our country PUK may be associated with infections (Fig. 28.5).

Degenerative PUKs include:
• Terrien's marginal degeneration
• Pellucid marginal degeneration

Table 28.1: *Causes of PUK*

Ocular causes		
	Bacterial	*Staphylococcus, Gonococcus, Moraxella, Haemophilus, Streptococcus*
	Viral	Herpes simplex, herpes zoster
	Amebic	*Acanthamoeba*
	Fungal	
	Traumatic	Chemical, thermal, radiation burn
	Local, autoimmune	Mooren's ulcer, allograft reaction
	Neurologic	Neurotrophic keratitis
Systemic causes		
	Autoimmune vasculitic diseases	Rheumatoid arthritis, Wegener's granulomatosis, relapsing polychondritis, systemic lupus erythematosus, polyarteritis nodosa, Sjögren's syndrome
	Dermatological disorders	Acne rosacea, cicatricial pemphigoid, Stevens-Johnson syndrome
	Inflammatory bowel disease	
	Malignancy	
	Bacterial	Tuberculosis, syphilis, gonorrhoea, borreliosis, bacillary dysentery
	Viral	Varicella zoster, acquired immune deficiency syndrome, hepatitis

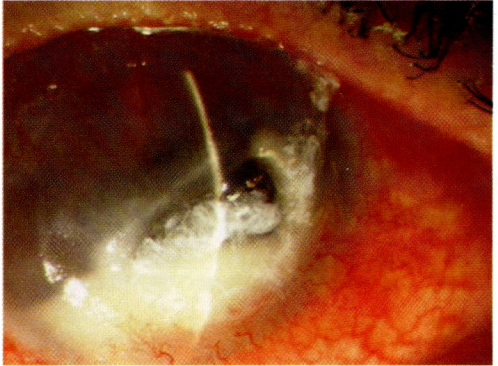

Fig. 28.5: *PUK with secondary bacterial infection*

PATHOGENESIS OF PUK

PATHOPHYSIOLOGIC MECHANISMS

The exact pathophysiologic mechanism of PUK remains unclear, but the same pathogenic mechanism is thought to occur in all forms of PUK.[6–8]

It has been postulated that both humoral-mediated and cell-mediated autoimmune processes are involved.[6–8]

Triggers for such response are believed to be trauma, surgery and systemic or local infections in genetically susceptible individuals.[7–9]

Reactions to corneal antigens, circulating immune complex deposition, and hypersensitivity reactions to exogenous antigens are some other hypothesized mechanisms involved in the pathogenesis of PUK.[6–9]

RISK FACTORS/TRIGGERS OF INFLAMMATION

Various factors that can trigger an acute attack of inflammation include the following:

1. *Peripheral cornea has typical morphologic and immunologic characteristics that predispose it to immune inflammation.* The limbus and the peripheral cornea get a portion of their nutrient supply from the capillary arcades, which extend only approximately 0.5 mm into the clear cornea. The vascular arrangement of the limbus is suitable for deposition of the first component of complement cascade C1, IgM, and other high molecular weight molecules and immune complexes in the limbus and corneal periphery.[6–9]

2. *Trauma or infection* may alter normal corneal antigens, which may lead to an autoimmune response. The altered antigen is taken up by macrophages that move through the conjunctival vessels to the peripheral lymph nodes, eventually resulting in T cell activation, differentiation, and proliferation.[10]

3. *Abnormal T cell responses* have been found in several studies on PUK.[6, 10, 11] It is hypothesized that T cells lead to antibody production and the formation of immune complexes that deposit in the peripheral cornea.[6]

4. *Deposition of these immune complexes lead to activation of the classical pathway of the complement system*, which causes the initiation in chemotaxis of inflammatory cells, predominantly neutrophils and macrophages in the peripheral cornea. The histopathologic examinations of cornea and conjunctiva from patients with PUK reveal a multitude of inflammatory cells including plasma cells, neutrophils, mast cells, and eosinophils.[6, 10] These cells release the various enzymes like collagenases and other proteases that destroy the corneal stroma.

5. *Apart from this, the release of proinflammatory cytokines* like interleukin 1 from the inflammatory cells causes stromal keratocytes to release matrix metalloproteinase 1 (MMP-1) and matrix metalloproteinase 2 (MMP-2), which result in accelerated destruction of the corneal matrix.[6, 12]

6. *Subconjunctival lymphatics and limbal capillaries in the peripheral cornea facilitate immunologically driven corneal inflammation.* Also, the limbus and conjunctiva that are surrounding the PUK have been thought to serve as a storehouse for various effector cells of the immune system and proinflammatory cytokines. Thus, it plays a critical role in the immunopathogenesis of PUK.[6, 10]

7. *Prior corneal surgery or trauma.* Corneoscleral incisions, particularly those related to extracapsular cataract extraction.[13, 14]

8. *Specific HLA haplotype.* Two recent studies demonstrated a strong connection between the HLA-DR17 haplotype and MU.[15, 16]

9. *Protein calgranulin C.* The calgranulins are a family of proteins secreted by neutrophils and monocytes that are involved in various immune responses. Calgranulin C has specifically been implicated in the immune response to filarial disease. In the human body, calgranulin C has been isolated in the corneal stroma also. It has therefore been suggested that a host-parasite interaction may lead to an autoimmune response to corneal calgranulin C, which in turns explains the development of MU.[17] This hypothesis may also explain why prior corneal trauma or surgery can increase one's risk of MU, in that the surgery or trauma might expose previously sequestered calgranulin C, lead-in to the cascade of events culminating in the development of MU.[18]

CLINICAL PROFILE OF PUKs

GENERAL CLINICAL FEATURES

SYMPTOMS

A case of PUK can present with the following features:

- *Ocular redness, pain, watering, and photophobia:* Pain is prominent and may be severe. Excruciating pain out of proportion to the severity of ulcer is often a characteristic feature of Mooren's ulcer. During the healing stage of the ulcer patients may get relief from the excruciating pain that has been present throughout the disease.

- *Decreased vision* secondary to induced astigmatism or corneal opacity in advanced cases.

SIGNS

A case of Mooren ulcer may present with the following signs:

- *Peripheral crescentic ulceration* with an epithelial defect, thinning and stromal infiltration at the limbus. It begins as a crescent-shaped gray-white infiltrate in the peripheral cornea later followed by epithelial defect and stromal thinning. Ulcer typically involving the superficial one-third of the stroma initially. The ulcer is concentric to limbus; the leading edges are undermined, infiltrated, and de-epithelialized. Spread is circumferential and occasionally central with variable epithelial loss and stromal thinning. As it progresses, it creates an overhanging edge at its central border. An undermined and infiltrated leading edge is characteristic. Probing of this edge may reveal a higher degree of stromal destruction in contrast to what it appears clinically.

- *Several distinct foci* may be present and subsequently coalesce.
- *Limbitis* may be present
- *Scleritis*, when present aids in distinguishing from systemic disease-associated PUK.
- *Vascularization involving the bed of the ulcer* up to its leading edge but not beyond.
- As the disease progresses, behind the advancing edge of the ulcer, healing may take place. The healing stage is characterised by thinning, vascularization and scarring. The healed area remains clouded.
- *In an advanced case of Mooren's ulcer* most of the cornea is lost, leaving behind a central island surrounded by the area of grossly thinned, scarred, and vascularized tissue.
- *Iritis and anterior chamber cells*, flares are not uncommon.
- *The adjacent conjunctiva and sclera* are usually inflamed and hyperemic.
- PUK associated with systemic autoimmune disease presents with *certain specific features that are often helpful* in differentiating from Mooren ulcer.
- In contrast to Mooren ulcer, *extension into the sclera* may occur.
- There is no separation between the ulcerative process and the limbus.

SPECIFIC CLINICAL PROFILE OF PUKs

Clinical profile of some etiological types of PUKs is described below.

MOOREN'S ULCER

Mooren's ulcer (MU) (Fig. 28.2) is a diagnosis of exclusion made for the case of PUK without any systemic association and scleritis. A typical case of MU takes 4–18 months for complete healing resulting in a scarred, vascularised cornea. Complications like iritis, hypopyon, glaucoma,

and cataract can be seen. Perforation may occur in 35 to 40% of cases, often associated with minor trauma to the weakened cornea.[1, 6]

Watson has classified the disease based on the clinical presentation and the low dose anterior segment fluorescein findings into:

- Unilateral Mooren's ulcer
- Bilateral aggressive Mooren's ulcer, and
- Bilateral indolent Mooren's ulcer.

Various characteristics are outlined in Table 28.2.

Unilateral Mooren's ulcer

It is a rare type that mainly affects patients aged above 60 years.

- Onset is rapid with redness and severe pain in the affected eye.
- *On examination*, the cornea will reveal the typical features of Mooren's ulcer, which may progress slowly or extremely rapidly form a single focal point. Over the period the central corneal stroma is removed completely and a thin layer of scar tissue covering an intact endothelium and covered by epithelium derived from conjunctiva remains.

Bilateral aggressive Mooren's ulcer

Bilateral Mooren's ulcer is commonly found in the Indian subcontinent and communities of Indian origin and parts of West Africa.

- *Age group* affected is usually between 14 and 40 years.
- *Usual presentation* includes unilateral typical lesion in one eye followed by the development of the lesion in the other eye (Fig. 28.3).
- *Angiography* reveals; changes in the architecture of episcleral vessels with some areas of closure, the breakup of the limbal arcade, leakage from the tips of these vessels and extension of the vessels into the bed of the ulcer.

Bilateral indolent Mooren's ulcer

- *Age group*. It usually affects patients in their fifth decade or older.
- *Presents as* bilateral indolent ulcers which progress slowly. Some may heal spontaneously.

Table 28.2: *Watson's classification of Mooren's ulcer and their comparative characteristic features*

Characteristics	Unilateral MU	Bilateral aggressive MU	Bilateral indolent MU
Age	Old	Young	Middle-aged or old
Gender	Usually female	Male	Male and female
Race	Usually White	Usually African/ Indian/Chinese	Usually Indian
Triggering factor	Minor trauma/infection	Trauma/infection	Chronic systemic infection. Minor ocular trauma or infection
Laterality	Unilateral	Bilateral	Bilateral
Pain	Excruciating	Painful	Less
Progression	Rapid	Slow	Slow
Anterior segment angiography	Vaso-obliteration of super-ficial vascular networks with leakage from large vessels. Intense deep leakage. Vascularization of ulcer, from superficial and deep vessels	Conjunctival and episcleral networks normal. Intense deep leakage. Ulcer vascularised from deep vessels	Superficial networks normal. Vasodilation of deep network.Ulcer vascularised from deep vessels
Treatment	Unsatisfactory	Immunosuppression	Local immunosuppressive therapy + supportive general treatment
Keratoplasty	Recurrence common	Recurrence common	Recurrence rare
Perforation	Very rare	Can occur	Rare

PUK ASSOCIATED WITH SYSTEMIC DISEASES

PUK may be associated with systemic conditions (Table 28.1) and can be an early manifestation of an underlying vasculitis. Most instances the systemic conditions are already known at the time of diagnosis, however, approximately in 25% cases, PUK precedes the systemic manifestations.[1, 6] Thus, a careful medical history, comprehensive review of systems, and appropriate laboratory testing are a must in a case of PUK.[5, 20] Some specific signs of causative systemic diseases associated with PUK may be noted (Table 28.3).

PUK with rheumatoid arthritis

Rheumatoid arthritis is the most common systemic disease associated with PUK. RA is observed in 34–42% of PUK cases.[6, 20]

Prevalence of PUK in patients with RA is around 3%.[6] Rheumatoid PUK frequently occurs in patients with destructive, often nodular, RA of long duration, often after 20 years of disease progression, and in patients with high titers of RF and anti-CCP antibodies.

Presentation. PUK can arise as a complication of scleritis or independently of this condition. The largest published series of patients with scleritis, comprising 500 patients, associated PUK was observed in 7.4% of scleritis cases, but in 35% of necrotizing scleritis cases[21] (Fig. 28.5).

- *Presentation of PUK may signify the trans-formation of RA into the systemic vasculitic phase.*[21–23] The presentation of PUK in a patient with RA suggests a life-threatening stage of the disease and should be treated as an emergent situation with immunosuppressants and cytotoxic therapy.[21–23]

- *Five years mortality rate for untreated RA with either PUK or scleritis is approximately 50%.*

Diagnosis. The patient's clinical profile and positive serologic studies help in establishing the diagnosis.

PUK with Wegener's granulomatosis

Wegener's granulomatosis (WG) is a rare disease, of unknown etiology, that is characte-rised by vasculitis of the upper and lower

Table 28.3: *Clinical signs of causative systemic diseases in peripheral ulcerative keratitis*

Clinical signs	Systemic disease
Saddle nose deformity	RP, WG
Auricular pinnae deformity	RP
Nasal mucosal ulcers	WG
Oral/lip/tongue mucosal ulcers	SLE, Sjög
Facial "butterfly" rash	SLE
Alopecia	SLE
Hypo-/hyper-pigmentation (scalp, face)	SLE, PSS, RP
Loss of facial expression	PSS
Facial telangiectasias	Rosacea, PSS
Rhinophyma	Rosacea
Facial/arms/legs rashes, ulcers	All vasculitic syndromes
Facial/arms/legs taut skin	PSS
Temporal artery erythema/tenderness	G-C
Raynaud's phenomenon (fingers)	PSS, SLE, G-C, Sjög
Ulcers in fingertips	All vasulitic syndromes
Subcutaneous nodules in arms and legs	RA, SLE, WG, CS, PAN
Arthritis in arms and legs	All vasculitic syndromes

SLE: Systemic lupus erythematosus; RA: Rheumatoid arthritis, RP: Relapsing polychondritis; PSS: Progressive systemic sclerosis; PAN: Polyarteritis nodosa; Sjög: Sjögren's disease; WG: Wegener's granulomatosis; CS: Churg-Strauss; G-C: Giant cell arteritis.

respiratory tracts, often in combination with glomerulonephritis.[1, 2, 24]

• *WG may affect multiple organs* including the skin, eye, heart, nervous system and gastro-intestinal tract and may cause a variety of ocular complications such as scleritis, proptosis, PUK, and conjunctivitis.

• *Peripheral ulcerative keratitis with WG* is a non-specific disease-causing conjunctival and scleral inflammation that eventually leads to corneal thinning if systemic therapy is not initiated. In contrast to RA, PUK often manifests at the onset of WG, leading to the diagnosis of the systemic condition. Ocular involvement occurs in up to 50 to 60%.[2, 24] The patients may present with conjunctivitis and scleritis that may progress to PUK or PUK may be present as an isolated finding. The sclera is usually involved in these cases, and this differentiates it from Mooren's ulcer in which sclera is generally not involved.[2]

Laboratory test, like serum anti-neutrophil cytoplasmic antibody (ANCA) test helps to establish the diagnosis, ANCA titres correlate with the severity and extent of the disease and tend to decrease in remission of the disease. Two patterns of staining are associated with this test—the c-ANCA (cytoplasmic anti-neutrophil cytoplasmic antibody) and the p-ANCA (perinuclear anti-neutrophil cytoplasmic antibody).

c-ANCA test has 99% specificity and 96% sensitivity.[24] This test also helps to follow the clinical response to therapy and chances of recurrence of PUK are more if these values have not normalized, despite apparent clinical remission when therapy has been tapered or discontinued. When the disease is limited, the sensitivity drops and fluctuation in the c-ANCA titre may correlate with the disease state.[2, 24]

PUK with polyarteritis nodosa

PAN is a rare multi-system disease with necrotizing vasculitis of the small- and medium-sized arteries.[25, 26] The etiology is unknown, and the diagnosis rests on the histopathology identification of typical vascular changes.

Ocular features. Scleritis, PUK, and retinal vasculitis are the predominant ocular inflammatory manifestations of this disease. PAN is a life-threatening disease with a death rate of 85% if untreated, a death rate of 50% if treated with corticosteroids only, and a death rate of only 5% if treated with cyclophosphamide and systemic corticosteroids with tapering of the corticosteroids.[26]

Clinical characteristics of PUK in this disease are similar to those of Mooren's ulcer.

• *Hepatitis B surface antigen is positive* in about 50% of patients with PAN.

Systemic immunosuppressive therapy is the key to retard the progression of PUK.[2, 26] Development of peripheral ulcerative keratitis or scleritis or retinal vasculitis in a patient with already diagnosed polyarteritis nodosa, on therapy, is indicative of a need for more vigorous therapy.[26]

PUK in other systemic diseases

Other systemic conditions associated with PUK include the ANCA associated vasculitides (Churg-Strauss syndrome, and microscopic polyangiitis), relapsing polychondritis (RP), systemic lupus erythematosus.[2, 6]

PUK IN OCULAR AND SYSTEMIC INFECTIONS

Ocular and systemic infections may also cause or be associated with PUK. Microbial pathogens implicated in the etiology of PUK include bacteria (*Staphylococcus* and *Streptococcus* species) (Fig. 28.6), spirochetes (*Treponema pallidum*), *Mycobacterium tuberculosis*, viruses (hepatitis C, herpes simplex virus, varicella-zoster virus), Acanthamoeba, and fungi.[2, 6, 10]

Marginal keratitis can present with the clinical appearance similar to PUK. The differentiation is often difficult during the active stage of ulceration. However, the signs are less severe and self-limited.

• *Marginal keratitis responds* rapidly to topical steroids, whereas PUK might worsen due to the lack of targeted systemic treatment.

• *Clear intervening zone between the infiltrate and limbus*, and the keratitis with associated with blepharitis can be seen in case of staphylococcal marginal keratitis.

• *Patients generally do not complain of severe pain* as seen in cases with MU.

Herpetic infections begin with an epithelial defect, followed by an infiltrate, which is the

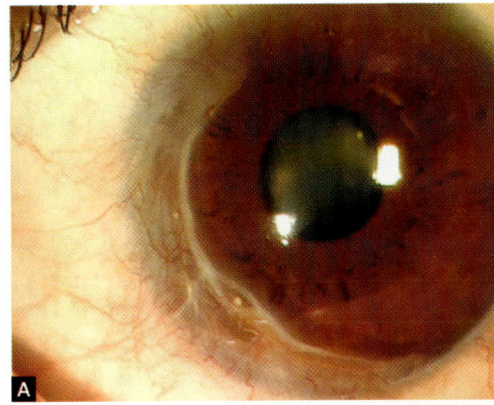
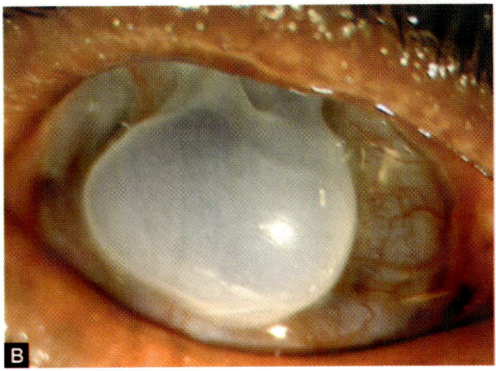

Fig. 28.6A and B: *Mooren's ulcer: Benign and malignant*

reverse order of that observed in marginal keratitis.

PERIPHERAL CORNEAL DEGENERATIONS

Terrien's marginal degeneration (TMD) can be confused with PUK due to associated progressive peripheral corneal thinning and superficial vascularization. However, unlike PUK and Mooren's ulcer, inflammation and epithelial defects are not hallmarks of TMD, TMD is typically painless, does not ulcerate. Demarcation from the central cornea with a gray line is characteristic of TMD. TMD begins superiorly as fine punctate stromal opacities, and a clear zone exists between the limbus and the infiltrate. Superficial vascularization is also present. The peripheral thinned zone is determined by a white lipid line at its central edge slowly progressive thinning spreads circumferentially and causes irregular astigmatism.[1, 2] Senile furrow degeneration is characterised by thinning in the lucid interval

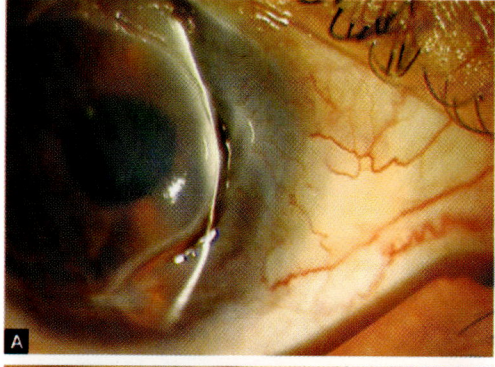

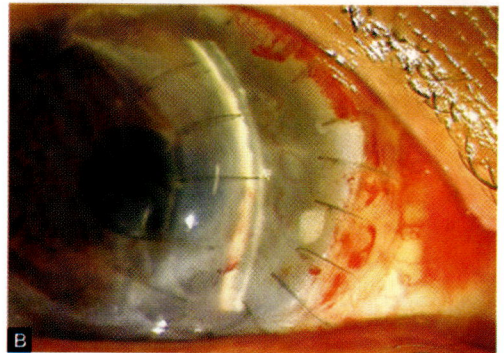

Fig. 28.7A and B: *Mooren's ulcer*

between an arcus and limbus may occur in the elderly.[2] However, the epithelium is intact, and there is no infiltrate or inflammation. The furrow is shallow and not vascularized, with sloping central and peripheral edges. Progression is extremely slow and has no risk of perforation.[1,2]

DIAGNOSIS OF PUKs

A thorough medical history and examination are mandatory for each suspected case of PUK. Clinical examination is often sufficient to diagnose a case of PUK, but a thorough investigation is often required to rule out the life-threatening systemic diseases that may be associated with it (Table 28.3).

Laboratory investigations. Following set of investigation are usually done to rule out systemic associations.

- *Complete blood cell count*, erythrocyte sedimentation rate, serum creatinine, blood urea nitrogen.
- *Rheumatoid factor* (RF) in cases of RA, Angiotensin-converting enzyme (ACE) which

may be elevated in sarcoidosis, antinuclear antibodies (ANA) which are positive in patients with SLE and RA, antineutrophil cytoplasmic antibodies (c-ANCA) for WG, anti-type II antibodies (positive in RP).

- *Complement C3 and C4, CH50*; in patients with SLE.
- *Hepatitis B surface antigen* (HBsAg); present in 40% of patients with PAN.
- *Chest X-ray* and *sinus CT scan* to exclude granulation disease like WG, sarcoidosis, and tuberculosis.
- *Routine scraping and culture* of the ulcer necessary in all cases to rule out any infectious etiology.

Imaging, i.e. anterior segment OCT and confocal microscopy. Peripheral anatomical changes of the cornea details can be measured and monitored with anterior segment OCT and *in vivo* confocal microscopy.[27]

Conjunctival resection/biopsy is not only helpful in identifying the various etiologic diagnoses in some cases but also helps in removing the limbal source of collagenases and other factors causing progressive ulceration.

- *Site for biopsies* is the bulbar conjunctiva adjacent to the ulcerating cornea. In a few cases, episcleral, scleral and corneal tissue may also be excised and analyzed.
- The cases where biopsy have been performed, should be seen any evidence of vasculitis, perivasculitis, granulomas, eosinophils, mast cells, and neutrophil and lymphocyte infiltrate to rule out the diagnosis of collagen vascular disease. However, vasculitis may be segmental and focal, and hence a single negative biopsy does not rule it out.

TREATMENT OF PUKs

The treatment of PUK depends upon two factors; the severity of corneal involvement and associated systemic disease.

- *Medical management aims at* reduction of inflammation, promote epithelial healing, and minimize stromal loss.
- *Surgery is indicated* in cases of corneal perforation, inadequate response to medical management and in advanced cases with

severe corneal scarring and thinning. Most experts would agree on a step-wise approach to the management of Mooren's ulcer, which is outlined below.[28–30]

MEDICAL THERAPY

TOPICAL THERAPY

Topical steroids are the treatment of choice for mild cases of Mooren's ulcer. Mild cases include; unilateral cases, less than 2 quadrants of peripheral corneal involvement, and less than 50% stromal loss.[29, 30] Initial therapy should include an intensive topical program: Prednisolone acetate or prednisolone phosphate 1%, hourly, in association with cycloplegics and prophylactic antibiotics. Such cases must be followed closely, every 2–3 days follow-up until healing occurs in the acute phase. If epithelial healing does not occur within 2 to 3 days, the frequency of topical steroid can be increased to every half hour. Once healing occurs, topical steroids can be tapered slowly over several months. Recurrence can occur with steroid taper hence these cases must be followed-up 3-monthly for six months following healing. Such management, especially in the unilateral, benign form, has yielded good results.

Preservative-free lubricating can be added to this regimen as a large number of patients with PUK also suffers from tear film abnormalities. Also, these artificial tear helps in removing or diluting harmful inflammatory proteins and mediators on the ocular surface. Collagenase inhibitors or collagenase synthetase inhibitors, such as topical 1% medroxyprogesterone and topical 20% acetylcysteine, helps in reducing additional stromal ulceration. The case of corneal involvement with the systemic association, topical corticosteroids should be avoided, because these drugs inhibit new collagen production and thereby increase the risk of perforation. Oral tetracycline derivatives may provide additional benefit in preventing further stromal loss by decreasing protease activity.[1,2]

ORAL/INTRAVENOUS GLUCOCORTICOIDS

Systemic corticosteroids are considered when topical therapy is ineffective after 7 to 10 days or in cases where topical steroids may be contraindicated because of precariously deep ulcer (more than 50% stromal loss) or infiltrate, large ulcers (more than two quadrants of peripheral corneal involvement) and bilateral cases.[29, 30] The usual starting dose is 1 mg/kg/day (maximum 60 mg/day), followed by a tapering schedule based on clinical response. Pulsed methylprednisolone 1 g/day for three consecutive days, followed by oral therapy, might be initiated in patients with imminent danger of vision loss.[29, 30] Example of such cases includes; bilateral cases, one-eyed, more than three quadrants of peripheral corneal involvement, >50% stromal loss, impending perforation.[2, 29, 30] Cases must be followed more frequently, e.g. alternate day follow-up in acute phase till healing starts.

It is essential to rule out any contraindication to steroid before starting oral steroids by appropriate history and investigations (e.g. history of peptic ulcer disease, blood pressure, fasting, and random blood sugar, Mantoux and chest X-ray for tuberculosis, any psychiatric illness, and osteoporosis). Preferably a thorough systemic evaluation by a physician to rule out any underlying systemic contraindications for steroid therapy should be done. Patients must be counseled regarding the long-term side effects of oral steroids. Regular evaluation to rule out any adverse effect of steroid must be carried out until systemic steroids are continued.

IMMUNOSUPPRESSIVE CHEMOTHERAPY/ IMMUNOMODULATORS

Immunosuppressive drugs or biologic agents are indicated in cases refractory to glucocorticoids or steroids need to be discontinued because of the steroid-induced side effects. There are, in general, four categories of immunomodulatory agents, used in cases of PUK. One single agent from one category can be combined with another single agent from a different category of immunomodulation. These categories are: (1) Calcineurin inhibitors, for example, cyclosporin and tacrolimus; (2) Myelosuppressive agents, for example, mycophenolate, azathioprine, methotrexate and cyclophosphamide; (3) Steroids, both oral and intravenous; (4) Biological therapies, for example, anti-TNF agents, rituximab and intravenous immunoglobulin.[28] A stepladder algorithm with oral methotrexate or cyclosporin at the base is useful, then stepping up to mycophenolate or azathioprine if there is intolerance to these agents or no response, then stepping up to cyclophosphamide, and finally stepping up to biologicals such as antitumour necrosis factor (anti-TNF) agents, rituximab or intravenous immunoglobulin.[28] Adding a short course of high-dose corticosteroids to any of these agents can help to control inflammation more rapidly.[28] Immunomodulators for PUK. The dosage, adverse reactions, and properties of commonly used immunomodulators are summarised in Table 28.4. Methotrexate and azathioprine are the two most commonly used.

SURGICAL TREATMENT

CONJUNCTIVAL RESECTION

The case where the steroid regimen is unable to stop the progression of the disease, the role of conjunctival resection come in to play. Conjunctiva surrounding to the peripheral corneal ulcer is supposed to have the reservoir for various inflammatory cells and cytokines. Thus, it plays a critical role in the immunopathogenesis of peripheral ulcerative keratitis. Under topical and subconjunctival anesthesia, the conjunctiva is excised to the bare sclera, extending at least two clock hours to either side of the peripheral ulcer, and about 4 mm posterior to the corneoscleral limbus and parallel to the ulcer.[2, 3, 30] The overhanging lip of ulcerating cornea may also be removed. Postoperatively, a firm pressure dressing should be used. Multiple resections may be needed.

Various authors have attempted to modify conjunctival resection to improve the outcome.

CRYOTHERAPY (KERATOEPITHELIOPLASTY)

Cryotherapy of limbal conjunctiva has been proposed for such cases.[2, 3] Kinoshita and colleagues reported success with a technique called *keratoepithelioplasty* in their series of 20 Mooren's patients.[31] In this procedure, donor corneal lenticules are sutured onto the scleral bed after conjunctival excision. It is postulated that the lenticules form a biological barrier between host cornea and the re-epithelializing conjunctiva and the immune components it may carry. In his study, 18 of 20 eyes (90%) showed prompt remission after surgery. Application of isobutyl cyanoacrylate, a tissue adhesive, may work in the same way but perhaps more simply and without the risk of epithelial rejection, glaucoma secondary to the chronic steroid use necessitated by keratoepithelioplasty and development of neurotrophic keratitis.[31]

AMNIOTIC MEMBRANE TRANSPLANTATION

The major problem associated with conjunctival resection is recurrence. Amniotic membrane transplantation (AMT) has been shown to be effective in eyes that do not respond to local medical therapy and conjunctival resection.[32, 33] AMT reduces the pain, the ocular surface inflammation is decreases, and the epithelialization occurs rapidly following surgery. Initial case reports showed good results with the use of AMT combined with conjunctival autografting or lamellar keratoplasty in cases of perforated or impending perforation.[32, 33] The case series by Ngan and Chau involving 18 eyes of 14 patients with PUK (7 recurrent episodes of ulceration, and 11 nonresponsive to medical therapy or conjunctival resection) showed a success rate of 89%.[34] However, in another series by Schallenberg et al, the results were poor in cases of severe progressive PUK.[35] Thus, the role of AMT in PUK needs further evaluation.

SUPERFICIAL LAMELLAR KERATECTOMY

Superficial lamellar keratectomy involves resection of the overhanging lip of the ulcerating cornea and application of tissue adhesive with bandage soft contact lens application or amniotic membrane. It has been shown to arrest the inflammatory process and allow healing.[36, 37] Superficial lamellar keratectomy may aid the removal of the corneal antigenic stimulus of the autoimmune process that causes stromal melting.[36, 37] It may also act by reducing activated keratocytes which may be a source of collagenase and polymorphonuclear neutrophils which have already invaded the corneal stroma as part of the pathological process.[38] In

Table 28.4: Immunomodulators used in PUK

Drug/agent	Group	Mode of action in PUK	Dose in PUK	ADR	Monitoring	Specific use
Methotrexate	Antimetabolite	Inhibits rapidly dividing cells, such as leukocytes	7.5 to 25 mg once per week in a single undivided dose (max. dose 25 mg/wk PO, SC, or IM)	Stomach upset, nausea, stomatitis, anorexia, hepatotoxicity, cytopenias, interstitial pneumonia, alopecia and rash Rarely cirrhosis	LFT, CBC to be obtained every 1 to 2 months	Often the 1st agent in the stepladder approach
Cyclosporin	T cell inhibitor	Affects immuno-competent T lympho-cytes that are in the G0 and G1 phase of their cell cycle, blocking replication, as well as their ability to produce lymphokines, such as IL	2 to 5 mg/kg/day in equally divided dose BD (max. dose 10 mg/kg/day)	Nephrotoxicity, hypertension, hepatotoxicity, gingival hyperplasia, myalgia, tremor, paresthesiae, hypomagnesaemia, hirsutism	BP at every visit and no less frequently then monthly initially and every 3 months for patients on long-term therapy. Serum creatinine should be checked every 2 weeks initially and monthly once dosage has stabilized	Treatment of severe, active RA that is poorly responsive to methotrexate
Azathioprine	Antimetabolite	Interferes with DNA replication and RNA transcription which in turn decrease the numbers of peripheral T and B lymphocytes, IL-2 synthesis and IgM production	1 to 3 mg/kg/day PO (max. dose 2.5–4 mg/kg/day)	Reversible bone marrow suppression, hepatotoxicity, gastrointestinal upset, nausea, and less commonly vomiting	CBC, and platelet count every 4 to 6 weeks, LFT every 12 weeks	RA, SLE. Often the 1st agent in the step-ladder approach

(Contd.)

Drug/agent	Group	Mode of action in PUK	Dose in PUK	ADR	Monitoring	Specific use
Mycophenolate	Antimetabolite	It prevents lymphocyte proliferation, suppresses antibody synthesis, interferes with cellular adhesion to vascular endothelium, and decreases recruitment of leukocytes to sites of inflammation	1 g twice daily PO (max. dose 1.5 gm BID	Pain, nausea, vomiting, diarrhoea, myalgia, fatigue, headache, nausea, leukopenia, lymphoma, non-melanoma skin cancers and opportunistic infections	CBC on a weekly basis for 4 weeks, then on a twice monthly basis for 2 months, with monthly testing thereafter	Graft rejection, RA
Cyclo-phosphamide	Nitrogen mustard-alkylating agent	Decreases the number of activated T lymphocytes, suppresses helper T lymphocyte functions, and decreases B lymphocytes, suppresses both primary and established cellular and humoral immune responses	1 to 3 mg/kg/day PO (max. dose 3 mg/kg/day)	Bone marrow suppression, myelodysplasias, haemorrhagic cystitis, teratogenicity, ovarian suppression, testicular atrophy, azoospermia, alopecia, nausea, vomiting, *P. carinii* pneumonia	CBC, platelet count, and urinalysis weekly initially and, when dosing is stable, at least every 4 weeks	Refractory cases of SLE, RA & WG
Prednisolone	Corticosteroids	Inhibits cytokine cascades, inhibits activation of T cells, decrease extravasation of inflammatory cells	1 mg/kg/day (60–80 mg/day) Maintenance dose—10 mg/day Tapering schedule	Cushingoid changes, delay of pubertal growth, infection, hypertension, fluid retention, diabetes mellitus, hyper-lipidemia, athero-sclerosis, peptic ulcer, osteoporosis, glaucoma, and cataracts, anxiety, sleeplessness, mood changes, easy bruising, and poor wound healing	BP and blood glucose should be monitored every 3 months. Bone mineral density evaluations, blood cholesterol and lipids should be monitored on an annual basis	Useful in acute inflammation

(Contd.)

Drug/agent	Group	Mode of action in PUK	Dose in PUK	ADR	Monitoring	Specific use
Infliximab	Chimeric anti-TNF-α antibody	Significantly reduces circulating MMPs which inhibit keratolysis	3–5 mg/kg body weight in an induction regimen at 0, 2 and 6 weeks, and thereafter every 8 weeks (max. dose 7.5 mg/kg)	Serious infections include TB and infections caused by viruses, fungi, or bacteria. Acute infusion reactions that include nausea, flushing, dizziness, dyspnoea, chest pain and hypotension or hypertension. Delayed infusion reactions include arthralgia, rash, myalgia and fatigue, myocardial infarction, pulmonary embolus, deep venous thrombosis, and retinal vein occlusion. Absolute contraindication is congestive heart failure	CBC, neutrophil and platelet count	In resistant cases of PUK when other agents have failed
Rituximab	Chimeric monoclonal antibody against the protein CD20	Decreases antibody-dependent cell-mediated cytotoxicity, complement-dependent cytotoxicity	Two 1000 mg infusions separated by 2 weeks every 24 weeks	Infusion reactions, infections, myocardial infarctions, abdominal pain, paraneoplastic pemphigus, lichenoid dermatitis, vesiculobullous dermatitis, SJS	Similar to infliximab	Refractory PUK

LFT: Liver function test; CBC: Complete blood count; IL: Interleukin; BP: Blood pressure; RA: Rheumatoid arthritis; SLE: Systemic lupus erythematosus; WG: Wegener granulomatosis; SJS: Stevens-Johnson syndrome a case series involving 17 eyes of 13 patients with Mooren's ulcer a combination therapy of local and systemic steroids, conjunctival resection, superficial keratectomy and application of cyanoacrylate tissue adhesive resulted in complete healing in 82.4% of cases while 17.6% failed to respond to treatment and either went into phthisis bulbi or healed with gross tissue distortion.[36] The healing time ranged from 4 to 24 weeks. The time taken for healing was directly related to the degree of severity at the time of the initial presentation. All cases of failure were in the advanced stage of ulceration at the initial examination. The authors concluded that application of cyanoacrylate tissue adhesive in the early stage of Mooren's ulcer is an effective therapy in controlling this devastating disease, but in advanced cases, failure chances are high and may require repeated application.[36]

KERATOPLASTY

Indications to perform keratoplasty in PUK arises in two conditions; PUK associated with perforation and in healed PUK with corneal scarring and thinning. In acute cases associated with perforation, it must be remembered that adequate control of inflammation is necessary before proceeding with surgery. Aggressive topical as well as systemic immunosuppression is required. Small perforations may be treated with the application of tissue adhesive and placement of a soft contact lens to provide comfort and to prevent dislodging of the glue. When a perforation is too large for tissue adhesive to seal the leak, some type of *patch graft* will be necessary.[2] *Lamellar keratoplasty is preferred,*[39] performing a full thickness graft should be avoided.[27] The ulcer is usually located at the peripheral cornea, forming an irregular morphology. This often leads to an irregular graft and graft-host mismatch. The surgery itself is a trauma that can lead to a flare-up of inflammation and allograft autolysis after surgery. In addition, peripheral graft, eccentric graft and proximity to limbus all lead to an increased risk of graft rejection. Lamellar keratoplasty (LK) can be complicated by chronic leakage at the graft-host interface which may lead to allograft autolysis and anterior iris synechia which may cause an oblique pupil, cannot be avoided.[27, 39–41] In advanced cases, two stages of surgery are done where initial lamellar tectonic grafting followed by central penetrating keratoplasty is done.

KERATOPROSTHESIS

Keratoprosthesis is *an option in patients with advanced PUK* in whom the corneal disease is severe, and attempts at grafting have failed. A recent case report by Basu et al reported excellent outcome with *Boston type 1 keratoprosthesis* in a patient with MU and the patient retained 20/30 vision after one year.[43]

RECENT ADVANCES IN PUKs

NEWER SYSTEMIC ASSOCIATIONS

Historically PUK has been associated with collagen vascular diseases such as rheumatoid arthritis, Wegener's granulomatosis, Churg-Strauss syndrome, and microscopic poly-angiitis), and relapsing polychondritis. *Recently PUK has been reported with* sarcoidosis,[44] Sweet syndrome,[45] acute myeloid leukaemia,[46] Behçet's disease,[47] pyoderma gangrenosum,[48] human immunodeficiency virus infection and low CD4 counts,[49] multiple myeloma,[50] helminthic infestation of the gastrointestinal tract.[51]

RECENT CONCEPTS OF PATHOMECHANISM

There has not been much research into the pathogenesis of PUK in recent times. In a recent study, Shinomiya et al performed immuno-histochemical staining of resected conjunctival tissues of four cases of PUK to identify the characteristics of the infiltrating cells in the conjunctival tissues. In all patients, infiltration of inflammatory cells was observed in the submucosal connective tissue of the conjunctiva. Inflammatory cell infiltration into the sub-mucosal layer of the conjunctiva was mainly composed of helper T lymphocytes and macro-phages (CD3 positive and CD45RO positive cells). Thus, suggesting that *helper T cells and macrophages contribute to the pathogenesis of Mooren's ulcer.*[52]

RECENT CONCEPTS IN THERAPY

Much advance has happened in the field of management of PUK. **Use of biological agents** such as rituximab, an antibody against CD20, and monoclonal antibodies against pro-inflammatory cytokine TNF-α (tumor necrosis factor α) is recently recommended as an alternative in resistant cases of PUK. Infliximab, the most commonly used agent, is a chimeric monoclonal antibody composed of the variable region of a mouse antibody joined to the constant region of human IgG1.[53]

Infliximab is directed against the pro-inflammatory cytokine TNF-α, which stimulates the production of the matrix metalloproteinases responsible for corneal stromal lysis in PUK. Infliximab binds with high affinity to both soluble and transmembrane forms of TNF-α. TNF-α is bound rapidly and irreversibly, and when infliximab is present in excess, it can block all 3 receptor-binding sites on TNF-α. A recent review including 22 patients from 12 reports on the use of infliximab in resistant cases of PUK found that in 77.27% of cases, keratolysis was halted.[53] In most of these reports, infliximab was administered in response to either corneal perforation or imminent corneal perforation because of severe inflammation and corneal thinning, despite previous systemic anti-inflammatory or immunosuppressive treatment.[53] The optimal frequency and dosing of infliximab for PUK is not established yet. Infliximab is associated with serious side effects that include opportunistic infections, myocardial infarction, pulmonary embolus, deep venous thrombosis, and retinal vein occlusion; thus, it is not indicated in the first instance for PUK treatment. However, in severe cases where all previous treatments have failed, the literature suggests that it may be a valuable elective option.

Adalimumab is a fully humanized recombinant IgG1 monoclonal antibody specific for TNF-α.[54] A recent case series by Cordero-Coma et al reported successful control of PUK with adalimumab in two cases where PUK was associated with immune-mediated systemic conditions.[54] Both the cases were resistant to steroids and other commonly used immuno-suppressive agents. Adalimumab (40 mg/2 weeks) could control the inflammation in both cases.

Modified lamellar keratoplasty and immuno-suppressive therapy guided by IVCM has been evaluated by Liu et al in 25 patients (31 eyes) with perforated Mooren's ulcer.[27] The modified LK consisted of patching the perforated with a thin, fresh posterior cornea containing the endothelium before a glycerin-preserved lamellar graft shaped like the defect was placed. Immunosuppressants and corticosteroids were used, and their dosages were adjusted following the density of dendritic cells in the corneal graft postoperatively as detected by IVCM. A large number of dendritic cells existed in the peripheral and central graft at one week postoperatively which significantly decreased at two months and became zero at six months following immunosuppressive therapy. Thus, IVCM can guide the immunosuppressive treatment and helps in the timely titration of the drug.

REFERENCES

1. Yagci A. Update on peripheral ulcerative keratitis. Clin Ophthalmol. 2012; 6: 747–54.
2. Garg P, Sangwan VS. Mooren's ulcer. In: Krachmer JH, Mannis MJ, Holland EJ, editors. In: Cornea: Fundamentals, Diagnostic, Management, 3rd ed. St Louis, MO: Elsevier; 2011.
3. Sharma N, Sinha G, Shekhar H, Titiyal JS, Agarwal T, Chawla B, Tandon R, Vajpayee RB. Demographic profile, clinical features and outcome of peripheral ulcerative keratitis: a prospective study. Br J Ophthalmol. 2015 Nov; 99(11): 1503–8.
4. Artifoni M, Rothschild PR, Brézin A, Guillevin L, Puéchal X. Ocular inflammatory diseases associated with rheumatoid arthritis. Nat Rev Rheumatol. 2014 Feb; 10(2): 108–16.
5. Tauber J, Sainz de la Maza M, Hoang-Xuan T, Foster CS. An analysis of therapeutic decision making regarding immunosuppressive chemotherapy for peripheral ulcerative keratitis. Cornea. 1990; 9: 66–73.
6. Galor A, Thorne JE. Scleritis and peripheral ulcerative keratitis. Rheum Dis Clin North Am. 2007; 33(4): 835–54.
7. Foster CS, Kenyon KR, Greiner J, et al. The immunopathology of Mooren's ulcer. Am J Ophthalmol 1979; 88: 149–59.

8. Martin NF, Stark WJ, Maumenee AE. Treatment of Mooren's and Mooren's-like ulcer by lamellar keratectomy: report of six eyes and literature review. Ophthalmic Surg 1987; 18: 564–9.

9. Zelefsky JR, Taylor CJ, Srinivasan M, et al. HLA-DR17 and Mooren's ulcer in South India. Br J Ophthalmol 2008; 92: 179–81

10. Dana M, Qian Y, Hamrah P. Twenty-five-year panorama of corneal immunology: emerging concepts in the immunopathogenesis of microbial keratitis, peripheral ulcerative keratitis, and corneal transplant rejection. Cornea 2000; 19(5): 625–43.

11. Mondino B. Inflammatory diseases of the peripheral cornea. Ophthalmology 1988; 95: 463–72.

12. Smith VA, Rishmawi H, Hussein H, Easty DL. Tear film MMP accumulation and corneal disease. Br. J. Ophthalmol. 2001; 85: 147–153.

13. Akpek EK, Demetriades AM, Gottsch JD. Peripheral ulcerative keratitis after clear corneal cataract extraction(1). J Cataract Refract Surg. 2000 Sep; 26(9): 1424–7.

14. Kiire CA, Srinivasan S, Inglis A. Peripheral ulcerative keratitis after cataract surgery in a patient with ocular cicatricial pemphigoid. Cornea. 2011 Oct; 30(10): 1176–8.

15. Taylor CJ, Smith SI, Morgan CH et al. HLA and Mooren's ulceration. Br J Ophthalmol. 2000; 84: 72–75.

16. Zelefsky JR, Taylor CJ, Srinivasan M et al. HLA-DR17 and Mooren's ulcer in South India. Br J Ophthalmol. 2008; 92(2): 179–181.

17. Gottsch JD, Li Q, Ashraf F et al. Cytokine-induced calgranulin C expression in keratocytes. Clin Immunol 1999; 91: 34–40.

18. Zelefsky JR, Srinivasan M, Cunningham Jr ET. Mooren's ulcer. Expert Rev Ophthalmol 2011; 6(4): 461–467.

19. Watson PG. Management of Mooren's ulceration. Eye (Lond). 1997; 11 (Pt 3): 349–56.

20. Sainz de la Maza M, Foster CS, Jabbur NS, Baltatzis S. Ocular characteristics and disease associations in scleritis-associated peripheral keratopathy. Arch Ophthalmol 2002; 120(1): 15–9.

21. Sainz de la Maza, M. et al. Clinical characteristics of a large cohort of patients with scleritis and episcleritis. Ophthalmology 2012; 119: 43–50.

22. Moreland LW, Curtis JR. Systemic nonarticular manifestations of rheumatoid arthritis: focus on inflammatory mechanisms. Semin. Arthritis Rheum 2009; 39: 132–143.

23. Zlatanoviæ G, Veselinoviæ D, Cekiæ S, Zivkoviæ M, Dorðeviæ-Jociæ J, Zlatanoviæ M. Ocular manifestation of rheumatoid arthritis-different forms and frequency. Bosn J Basic Med Sci. 2010 Nov; 10(4): 323–7.

24. Tarabishy AB, Schulte M, Papaliodis GN, Hoffman GS. Wegener's granulomatosis: clinical manifestations, differential diagnosis, and management of ocular and systemic disease. Surv Ophthalmol. 2010; 55: 430–444.

25. Akova YA, Jabbur NS, Foster CS. Ocular presentation of polyarteritis nodosa. Clinical course and management with steroid and cytotoxic therapy. Ophthalmology. 1993 Dec; 100(12): 1775–81.

26. Foster CS. Ocular manifestations of the potentially lethal rheumatologic and vasculitic disorders. J Fr Ophthalmol. 2013 Jun; 36(6): 526–32.

27. Liu J, Shi W, Li S, Gao H, Wang T. Modified lamellar keratoplasty and immunosuppressive therapy guided by in vivo confocal microscopy for perforated Mooren's ulcer. Br J Ophthalmol. 2015 Jun; 99(6): 778–83.

28. Saw VP. Immunotherapy for corneal inflammatory disorders: stepping up and down the ladder. Br J Ophthalmol. 2013 Nov; 97(11): 1364–7.

29. Ashar JN, Mathur A, Sangwan VS. Immunosuppression for Mooren's ulcer: evaluation of the stepladder approach—topical, oral and intravenous immunosuppressive agents. Br J Ophthalmol. 2013 Nov; 97(11): 1391–4.

30. Chow C, Foster CS. Mooren's Ulcer. Int Ophthalmol Clin 1996; 36: 1–13.

31. Kinoshuita S, Ohashi Y. Ohji M, Manabe R: Long-term results of keratoepithelioplasty in Mooren's ulcer. Ophthalmology 1991; 98: 438–445.

32. Lambiase A, Sacchetti M, Sgrulletta R, Coassin M, Bonini S. Amniotic membrane transplantation associated with conjunctival peritomy in the management of Mooren's ulcer: a case report. Eur J Ophthalmol. 2005 Mar-Apr; 15(2): 274–6.

33. Chen KH, Hsu WM, Liang CK. Relapsing Mooren's ulcer after amniotic membrane transplantation combined with conjunctival autografting. Ophthalmology. 2004 Apr; 111(4): 792–5.

34. Ngan ND, Chau HT. Amniotic membrane transplantation for Mooren's ulcer. Clin Experiment Ophthalmol. 2011 Jul; 39(5): 386–92.

35. Schallenberg M, Westekemper H, Steuhl KP, Meller D. Amniotic membrane transplantation

ineffective as additional therapy in patients with aggressive Mooren's ulcer. BMC Ophthalmol. 2013 Dec 17; 13: 81.

36. Agrawal V, Kumar A, Sangwan V, Rao GN. Cyanoacrylate adhesive with conjunctival resection and superficial keratectomy in Mooren's ulcer. Indian J Ophthalmol 1996; 44: 23–7.

37. Martin NF, Stark WJ, Maumenee AE. Treatment of Mooren's and Mooren's like ulcer by lamellar keratectomy: Report of six eyes and literature review. Ophth. Surg 1987; l8: 564–569.

38. Eiferman RA, Hynduik RA, Hensley JT. Limbal immunopathology of Mooren's ulcer. Ann Ophthalmol 1978; 10: 1203–1206.

39. Huang T, Wang Y, Ji J, et al. Evaluation of different types of lamellar keratoplasty for treatment of peripheral corneal perforation. Graefes Arch Clin Exp Ophthalmol 2008; 246: 1123–31.

40. Huang T, Wang YJ, Ji JP, et al. Lamellar keratoplasty for treatment of peripheral corneal perforation. Zhonghua Yan Ke Za Zhi 2008; 44: 104–10.

41. Cheng CL, Theng JT, Tan DT. Compressive C-shaped lamellar keratoplasty: a surgical alternative for the management of severe astigmatism from peripheral corneal degeneration. Ophthalmology 2005; 112: 425–30.

42. Vajpayee RB, Singhvi A, Sharma N, et al. Penetrating keratoplasty for perforated corneal ulcers: preservation of iris by corneal debulking. Cornea 2006; 25: 44–6.

43. Basu S, Taneja M, Sangwan VS. Boston type 1 keratoprosthesis for severe blinding vernal keratoconjunctivitis and Mooren's ulcer. Int. Ophthalmol. 2011; 31(3): 219–222.

44. Harthan JS, Reeder RE. Peripheral ulcerative keratitis in association with sarcoidosis. Cont Lens Anterior Eye. 2013 Dec; 36(6): 313–7.

45. Bilgin AB, Tavas P, Turkoglu EB, Ilhan HD, Toru S, Apaydin KC. An uncommon ocular manifestation of Sweet syndrome: peripheral

ulcerative keratitis and nodular scleritis. Arq Bras Oftalmol. 2015 Jan-Feb; 78(1): 53–5.

46. Morjaria R, Barge T, Mordant D, Elston J. Peripheral ulcerative keratitis as a complication of acute myeloid leukaemia. BMJ Case Rep. 2014 Oct 31; 2014.

47. Ji YS, Yoon KC. A rare case of peripheral ulcerative keratitis associated with Behçet's disease. Int Ophthalmol. 2014 Aug; 34(4): 979–81.

48. Imbernón-Moya A, Vargas-Laguna E, Aguilar A, Gallego MÁ, Vergara C, Nistal MF. Peripheral Ulcerative Keratitis with Pyoderma Gangrenosum. Case Rep Dermatol Med. 2015; 2015: 949840.

49. Soni ND, Ingole AB, Murade SM. An unusual case of peripheral ulcerative keratitis as a presenting feature in an otherwise healthy patient with undiagnosed human immunodeficiency virus infection and low CD4 counts. Indian J Ophthalmol. 2013 Mar; 61(3): 138–9.

50. Lim LT, Ramamurthi S, Collins CE, Mantry S. Peripheral ulcerative keratitis associated with multiple myeloma. Ann Acad Med Singapore. 2011 Dec; 40(12): 550–1.

51. Agarwal P1, Singh D, Sinha G, Sharma N, Titiyal JS. Bilateral Mooren's ulcer in a child secondary to helminthic infestation of the gastrointestinal tract. Int Ophthalmol. 2012 Oct; 32(5): 463–6.

52. Shinomiya K, Ueta M, Sotozono C, Inatomi T, Yokoi N, Koizumi N, Kinoshita S. Immunohistochemical analysis of inflammatory limbal conjunctiva adjacent to Mooren's ulcer. Br J Ophthalmol. 2013 Mar; 97(3): 362–6.

53. Huerva V, Ascaso FJ, Grzybowski A. Infliximab for peripheral ulcerative keratitis treatment. Medicine (Baltimore). 2014 Nov; 93(26): e176.

54. Cordero-Coma M, Méndez RS, Blanco AC, Corral AL, Calleja-Antolín S, de Morales JM. Adalimumab for refractory peripheral ulcerative keratitis. J Ophthalmic Inflamm Infect. 2012 Dec; 2(4): 227–9.

Non-ulcerative Keratitis: Superficial and Deep

Non-ulcerative keratitis can be divided into two groups: Non-ulcerative superficial keratitis and non-ulcerative deep keratitis.

SUPERFICIAL NON-ULCERATIVE KERATITIS

This group includes a number of conditions of varied etiology. Here, the inflammatory reaction is confined to epithelium, Bowman's membrane and superficial stromal lamellae. Non-ulcerative superficial keratitis may present in two forms:
• Superficial diffuse keratitis
• Superficial punctate keratitis.

SUPERFICIAL DIFFUSE KERATITIS

Diffuse inflammation of superficial layers of cornea occurs in two forms, acute and chronic.

1. Acute superficial diffuse keratitis

Etiology. Mostly of infective origin, may be associated with staphylococcal or gonococcal infections.

Clinical features. It is characterised by faint diffuse epithelial oedema associated with grey farinaceous appearance being interspersed with relatively clear area. Epithelial erosions may be formed at places. If uncontrolled, it usually converts into ulcerative keratitis.

Treatment. It consists of frequent instillation of antibiotic eye drops such as tobramycin or gentamicin 2–4 hourly.

2. Chronic superficial diffuse keratitis

It may be seen in rosacea, phlyctenulosis and is typically associated with pannus formation (Fig. 29.1). Another rare form, simply known as chronic superficial keratitis (CSK) is considered to be of immunological origin.

SUPERFICIAL PUNCTATE KERATITIS (SPK)

GENERAL CONSIDERATIONS

Superficial punctate keratitis is characterised by occurrence of multiple, spotty lesions in the

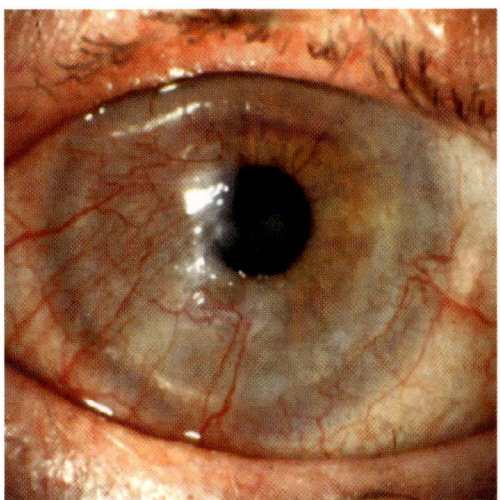

Fig. 29.1: *Superficial diffuse keratitis (rosacea keratitis)*

superficial layers of cornea (Fig. 29.2). It may result from a number of conditions, identification of which (causative condition) might not be possible most of the times.

CAUSES

Some important causes of superficial punctate keratitis are listed here.

1. *Viral infections* are the chief cause. Of these more common are: herpes zoster, adenovirus infections, epidemic keratoconjunctivitis, pharyngoconjunctival fever and herpes simplex.
2. *Chlamydial infections* include trachoma and inclusion conjunctivitis.
3. *Toxic lesions,* e.g. due to staphylococcal toxin in association with blepharoconjunctivitis.
4. *Trophic lesions,* e.g. exposure keratitis and neuroparalytic keratitis.
5. *Allergic lesions,* e.g. vernal keratoconjunctivitis.
6. *Irritative lesions,* e.g. effect of some drugs such as idoxuridine.
7. *Disorders of skin and mucous membrane,* such as acne rosacea and pemphigoid.
8. *Dry eye syndrome,* i.e. keratoconjunctivitis sicca.
9. *Specific type of idiopathic SPK,* e.g. Thygeson's superficial punctate keratitis and Theodore's superior limbic keratoconjunctivitis.
10. *Photo-ophthalmia* is a specific type of SPK.

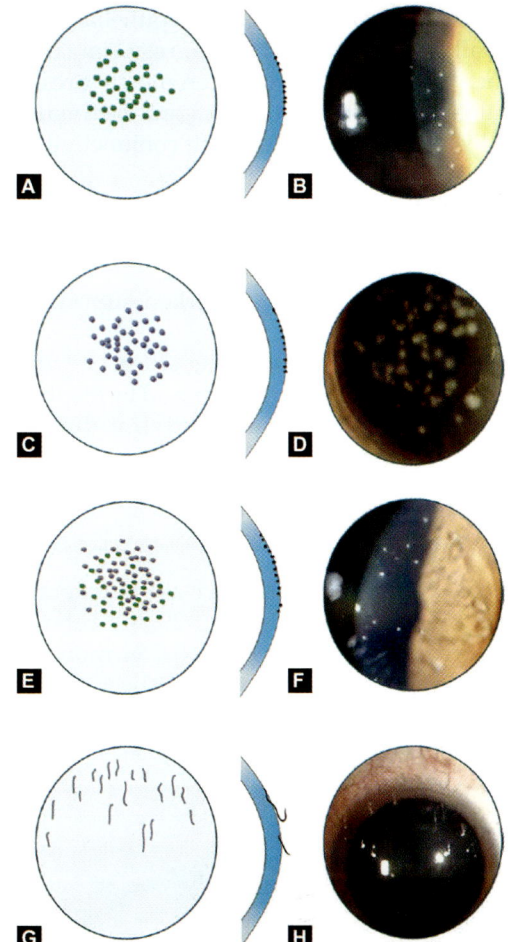

Fig. 29.2: *Morphological types of superficial punctate keratitis. Diagrammatic depictions and clinical photographs of: A and B, Punctate epithelial; C and D, Punctate subepithelial keratitis; E and F, Punctate combined epithelial and subepithelial keratitis; G and H, Filamentary keratitis*

MORPHOLOGICAL TYPES

1. Punctate epithelial erosions (multiple superficial erosions).
2. Punctate epithelial keratitis (Fig. 29.2A and B).
3. Punctate subepithelial keratitis (Fig. 29.2C and D).
4. Punctate combined epithelial and subepithelial keratitis (Fig. 29.2E and F).
5. Filamentary keratitis (Fig. 29.2G and H).

CLINICAL FEATURES

Superficial punctate keratitis may present as different morphological types (Fig. 29.2A to H) as enumerated above. Punctate epithelial lesions usually stain with fluorescein, rose bengal and other vital dyes. The condition mostly presents with acute pain, photophobia and lacrimation; and is usually associated with conjunctivitis.

TREATMENT

Treatment of most of these conditions is symptomatic.
1. *Topical steroids* have a marked suppressive effect.
2. *Artificial tears* have soothing effect.
3. *Specific treatment* of cause should be instituted whenever possible, e.g. antiviral drugs in cases of herpes simplex.

SPECIFIC TYPES OF SPK

PHOTO-OPHTHALMIA

Photo-ophthalmia also known as photokeratitis or ultraviolet keratitis (Fig. 29.3A) refers to occurrence of multiple epithelial erosions due to the effect of ultraviolet rays especially from 311 to 290 μm. A number of different terms, depending upon the cause, have been used to

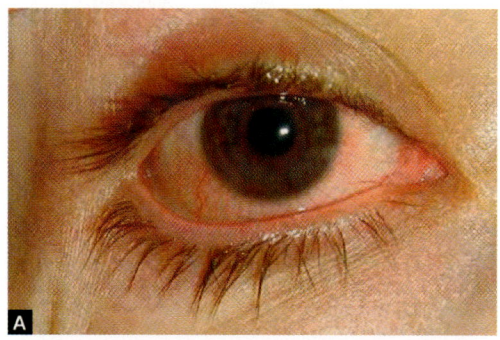

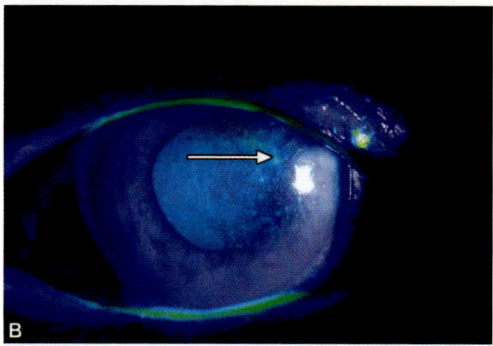

Fig. 29.3: *Photo-ophthalmia: A, Clinical photograph; B, As seen on fluorescein staining*

denote photokeratitis including arc-eye, snow blindness, welder's flash, bake eyes, corneal flash burns, sand man's eye, flash burns, niphablepsia, potato eye or keratoconjunctivitis photoelectrica.

Causes

Photokeratitis is caused by exposure of insufficiently protected eyes to the ultraviolet (UV) rays from either natural (e.g. intense sunlight) or artificial sources.

Common sources of exposure to UV rays are:
- *Exposure to bright light of a short circuit.*
- *Naked arc light exposure* as in industrial electric welding and cinema operators.
- *Exposure to UV lamps.*
- *Exposure to UV rays* from sun directly or indirectly, e.g. *snow blindness* due to reflected ultraviolet rays of sun from snow surface.

Pathogenesis

After an interval of 4–5 hours (latent period) of exposure to ultraviolet rays, there occurs desquamation of corneal epithelium leading to formation of multiple epithelial erosions.

Clinical features

Photokeratitis is akin to a sunburn of the cornea and conjunctiva, and is not usually noticed until several hours after exposure.

Characteristic features of photo-ophthalmia are:
- *Typically, patient presents* with severe burning pain, lacrimation, photophobia, blepharospasm, swelling of palpebral conjunctiva and retrotarsal folds.
- *History of exposure to ultraviolet rays* 4–5 hours earlier is positive.
- *On fluorescein staining* multiple spots are demonstrated on both corneas (Fig. 29.3B).

Prophylaxis

Crooker's glass (welding goggles) which cuts off all the infrared and ultraviolet rays should be used by those who are prone to exposure, e.g. welding workers, cinema operators, etc. Snow goggles should be used by people in snow bound areas.

Treatment

- *Cold compresses*, give soothing effect
- *Patching* with antibiotic ointment for 24 hours, heals most of the cases.
- *Oral analgesics* may be given if pain is intolerable.
- *Reassurance* to the patient is very important.
- *Single dose of tranquilliser* may be given to apprehensive patients.

SUPERIOR LIMBIC KERATOCONJUNCTIVITIS

Superior limbic keratoconjunctivitis of Theodore is the name given to inflammation of superior limbic, bulbar and tarsal conjunctiva associated with punctate keratitis of the superior part of cornea.

Etiology

Exact etiology is not known. It occurs with greater frequency in patients with hyperthyroidism and is more common in females.

Clinical features

Clinical course is chronic with remissions and exacerbations.

Symptoms include:
- Bilateral ocular irritation.
- Mild photophobia, and redness in superior bulbar conjunctiva.

Signs include (Fig. 29.4):
- *Congestion* of superior limbic, bulbar and tarsal conjunctiva.
- *Punctate keratitis* which stains with fluorescein and rose bengal stain is seen in superior part of cornea.
- *Corneal filaments* are also frequently seen in the involved area.

Treatment

- *Artificial tears* provide soothing effect.
- *Topical corticosteroids* in low doses may reduce the symptoms temporarily.
- *Faint diathermy of superior bulbar conjunctiva* in a checker board pattern gives acceptable results.
- *Recession or resection* of a 3–4 mm wide perilimbal strip of conjunctiva from the superior

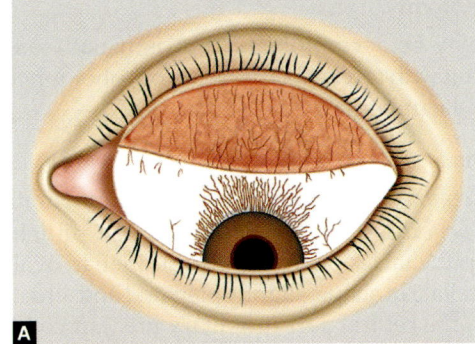

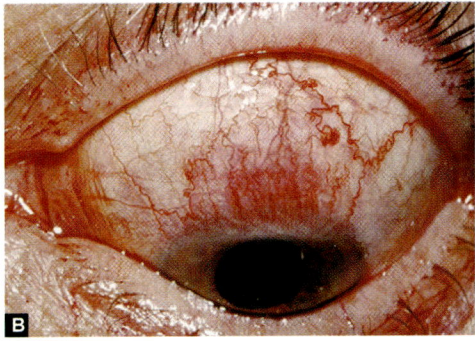

Fig. 29.4: *Superior limbic keratoconjunctivitis: A, Diagrammatic depiction; B, Clinical photograph*

limbus (from 10.30 to 1.30 o'clock position) may be helpful, if other measures fail.
- *Therapeutic soft contact lenses* for a longer period may be helpful in healing the keratitis.

THYGESON'S SUPERFICIAL PUNCTATE KERATITIS

It is a type of chronic, recurrent bilateral superficial punctate keratitis, which has got a specific clinical identity.

Etiology

Exact etiology is not known.
- *A viral origin* has been suggested without any conclusion.
- *An allergic or dyskeratotic nature* also has been suggested owing to its response to steroids.

Clinical features

- *Age and sex.* It may involve all ages with no sex predilection.
- *Laterality.* Usually bilateral.
- *Course.* It is a chronic disease characterised by remissions and exacerbations.

Symptoms

It may be asymptomatic, but is usually associated with foreign body sensation, photophobia and lacrimation.

Signs

- *Conjunctiva* is uninflamed (no conjunctivitis).
- *Corneal lesions*. There are coarse punctate epithelial lesions (snow flake) circular, oval or stellate in shape, slightly elevated and situated in the central part (pupillary area) of cornea. Each lesion is a cluster of heterogeneous granular grey dots.

Treatment

- *Disease is self-limiting* with remissions and may permanently disappear in a period of 5–6 years.
- *Topical steroids* during exacerbations the lesions and associated symptoms usually respond quickly to topical steroids (so, should be tapered rapidly).
- *Therapeutic soft contact lenses* may be required in steroid-resistant cases.

FILAMENTARY KERATITIS

It is a type of superficial punctate keratitis, associated with formation of corneal epithelial filaments (Fig. 29.2G and H).

Pathogenesis

Corneal filaments which essentially consist of a tag of elongated epithelium incorporated into the mucin strand attached to the surface. Any condition that leads to focal epithelial erosions may produce filamentary keratopathy, especially when there is an increase in tear film mucous to aqueous ratio.

Causes

Common conditions associated with filamentary keratopathy are:

1. Keratoconjunctivitis sicca (KCS).
2. Superior limbic keratoconjunctivitis.
3. Epitheliopathy due to radiation keratitis.
4. Following epithelial erosions as in herpes simplex keratitis, Thygeson's superficial punctate keratitis, recurrent corneal erosion syndrome and trachoma.

5. Prolonged patching of the eye particularly following ocular surgery like cataract.
6. Systemic disorders like diabetes mellitus, ectodermal dysplasia and psoriasis.
7. Idiopathic.

Clinical features

Symptoms

Patients usually experience moderate pain, ocular irritation, lacrimation and foreign body sensation.

Signs

Corneal examination reveals (Fig. 29.2G and H):

- *Filaments*, i.e. fine tags of elongated epithelium which are firmly attached at the base, intertwined with mucus and degenerated cells. The filament is freely movable over the cornea (Fig. 29.5).
- *Superficial punctate keratitis* of varying degree is usually associated with corneal filaments.

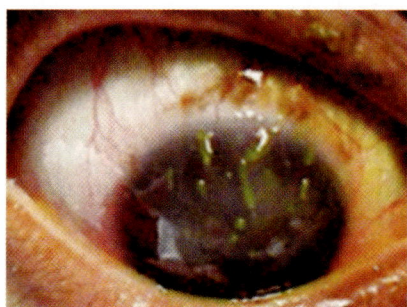

Fig. 29.5: *Filamentary keratitis*

Treatment

1. *Management of filaments* include their mechanical debridement and patching for 24 hours followed by lubricating drops.
2. *Therapeutic soft contact lenses* may be useful in recurrent cases.
3. *Treatment of the underlying cause* to prevent recurrence.

DEEP KERATITIS

INTRODUCTION

An inflammation of corneal stroma with or without involvement of posterior corneal layers constitutes deep keratitis, which may be non-suppurative or suppurative.

- *Non-suppurative deep keratitis* includes, interstitial keratitis, disciform keratitis, keratitis profunda and sclerosing keratitis.
- *Suppurative deep keratitis* includes central corneal abscess and posterior corneal abscess, which are usually metastatic in nature.

INTERSTITIAL KERATITIS

GENERAL CONSIDERATIONS

Interstitial keratitis denotes an inflammation of the corneal stroma without primary involvement of the epithelium or endothelium. It is non-suppurative inflammation, which is characterised by cellular infiltration of the corneal stroma.

Etiology

Inflammation may either be the direct result of an infectious process or, more commonly, secondary to an immunologic response to a specific foreign antigen. This immunologic response to a specific foreign antigen may take the form of antigen–antibody complex deposition, complement-mediated disease, or a delayed-type hypersensitivity reaction.

Causes of interstitial keratitis are:

- *Viral.* HSV, herpes zoster, EBV, mumps, measles.
- *Bacterial.* TB, syphilis (congenital more common than acquired), Lyme disease, lymphogranuloma venereum, leprosy.
- *Others.* Sarcoidosis, onchocerciasis, Cogan syndrome, rheumatoid arthritis, malaria.

A few important types of interstitial keratitis are described briefly.

SYPHILITIC (LUETIC) INTERSTITIAL KERATITIS

Syphilitic interstitial keratitis is associated more frequently (90%) with congenital syphilis than the acquired syphilis. The disease is generally bilateral in inherited syphilis and unilateral in acquired syphilis. In congenital syphilis, manifestations develop between 5 and 15 years of age.

Pathogenesis

It is now generally accepted that the disease is a manifestation of local antigen–antibody reaction. It is presumed that *Treponema pallidum* invades the cornea and sensitises it during the period of its general diffusion throughout the body in the foetal stage. Later, a small scale fresh invasion by Treponema or toxins excite the inflammation in the sensitised cornea. The inflammation is usually triggered by an injury or an operation on the eye.

Clinical features

Interstitial keratitis characteristically forms one of the late manifestations of congenital syphilis. Many times, it may be a part of Hutchinson's triad, which includes interstitial keratitis, Hutchinson's teeth and vestibular deafness.

The clinical features of interstitial keratitis can be divided into three stages: Initial progressive stage, florid stage and stage of regression.

1. *Initial progressive stage.* The disease begins with oedema of the endothelium and deeper stroma, secondary to anterior uveitis, as evidenced by the presence of keratic precipitates (KPs). There is associated pain, lacrimation, photophobia, blepharospasm and circum-corneal injection followed by a diffuse corneal haze *giving it a ground glass appearance.* This stage lasts for about 2 weeks.

2. *Florid stage.* In this stage, eye remains acutely inflamed. Deep vascularization of cornea, consisting of radial bundle of brush-like vessels develops. Since, these vessels are covered by hazy cornea, they look dull reddish pink which is called '*Salmon patch appearance*' (Fig. 29.6). There is often a moderate degree of superficial vascularization. These vessels arising from the terminal arches of conjunctival vessels, run a short distance over the cornea. These vessels and conjunctiva heap at the limbus in the form of *epulit.* This stage lasts for about 2 months.

3. *Stage of regression.* The acute inflammation resolves with the progressive appearance of vascular invasion. Clearing of cornea is slow and begins from periphery and advances centrally. Resolution of the lesion leaves behind some

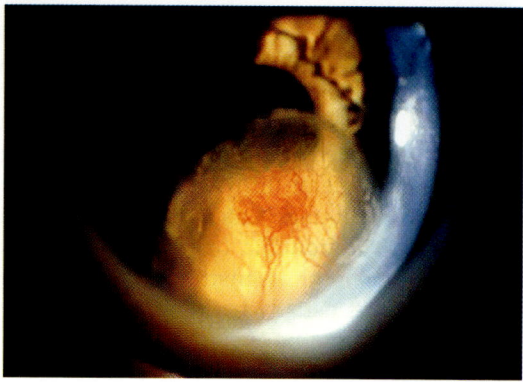

Fig. 29.6: *Interstitial keratitis: Salmon patch appearance*

opacities and *ghost vessels*. This stage may last for about 1 to 2 years.

Diagnosis

The diagnosis is usually evident from the clinical profile. A positive VDRL or *Treponema pallidum* immobilisation test confirms the diagnosis.

Treatment

The treatment should include topical treatment for keratitis and systemic treatment for syphilis.

1. *Local treatment* includes:
- *Topical corticosteroid drops,* e.g. dexamethasone 0.1% drops every 2–3 hours. As the condition is allergic in origin, corneal clearing occurs with steroids if started well in time and a useful vision is obtained.
- *Atropine eye ointment* 1% 2–3 times a day.
- *Dark goggles* to be used for photophobia.
- *Keratoplasty* is required in cases where dense corneal opacities are left.

2. *Systemic treatment* includes:
- *Penicillin* in high doses should be started to prevent development of further syphilitic lesions. However, an early treatment of congenital syphilis usually does not prevent the onset of keratitis at a later stage.
- *Systemic steroids* may be added in refractory cases of keratitis.

TUBERCULOUS INTERSTITIAL KERATITIS

The features of tubercular interstitial keratitis are similar to syphilitic interstitial keratitis except that it is more frequently unilateral and sectorial (usually involving a lower sector of cornea).

Treatment consists of systemic antitubercular drugs, topical steroids and cycloplegics.

COGAN'S SYNDROME

Cogan's syndrome comprises the interstitial keratitis of unknown etiology, acute tinnitus, vertigo, and deafness. It typically occurs in middle-aged adults and is often bilateral.

Treatment consists of topical and systemic corticosteroids. An early treatment usually prevents permanent deafness and blindness.

BIBLIOGRAPHY

1. Apple DJ and Rabb MF. Ocular Pathology. Clinical Applications and Self-Assessment. 4th ed. 1991.
2. Barron BA, Gee L, Hauck WW, et al:Herpetic eye disease study. A controlled trial of oral acyclovir for herpes simplex stromal keratitis. Ophthalmology 1994; 101: 1871–1882.
3. Braley AEK, Alexander RC: Superficial punctate keratitis: isolation of a virus, Arch Ophthalmol 50: 147, 1953.
4. Herpetic Eye Disease Study Group. Acyclovir for the prevention of recurrent herpes simplex virus eye disease. N Engl J Med. 1998 Jul 30; 339(5): 300–6.
5. Lemp MA, Chambers RW, Lurdy J: Viral isolation in superficial punctate keratitis, Arch Ophthalmol 91: 8, 1974.
6. Pepose JS, Margolis TP, LaRussa P, Pavan-Langston D.Ocular complications of smallpox vaccination. Am J Ophthalmol. 2003 Aug; 136(2): 343–52.
7. Thygeson P: Further observations on superficial punctate keratitis, Arch Ophthalmol 66: 158, 1962.
8. Thygeson P: Superficial punctate keratitis, JAMA 144: 1544, 1950.

Section
VI

Non-inflammatory Diseases of Cornea

Chapter

30

Keratoconus and other Ectatic Corneal Disorders

Chapter Outline

INTRODUCTION

The non-inflammatory ectatic corneal disorders include keratoconus, pellucid marginal degeneration (PMD), keratoglobus and posterior keratoconus.[1] All these conditions are associated with corneal thinning. The relation of the site of maximum corneal protrusion in relation to the area of corneal thinning helps in differentiating these conditions from each other (Table 30.1). Corneal topography and corneal tomography are the important investigative tools that help in arriving at an accurate diagnosis in such cases.

Keratoconus, pellucid marginal degeneration and keratoglobus share a relatively common treatment protocol in the early stage of the disease. Visual rehabilitation is done with non-surgical modalities like spectacles and contact lenses in these cases. In keratoconus patients, intra-stromal corneal ring segments can be used to improve the contact lens tolerance in some

cases. However, in advanced cases keratoplasty in the form of either deep anterior lamellar keratoplasty (DALK) or penetrating kerato-plasty (PK) may be warranted for visual rehabilitation. Corneal collagen crosslinking (CXL) has been described to arrest the progression of corneal ectasia in cases of progressive keratoconus.

Posterior keratoconus differs from the other three conditions in many aspects. A detailed description of this condition will follow in the discussion below.

The other ectatic conditions of the cornea include Terrein's marginal degeneration and post kerato-refractive surgery ectasia.

KERATOCONUS

Keratoconus is the most common ectatic corneal disorder. It is non-inflammatory, usually bilateral but may be asymmetric, ectatic corneal

Table 30.1: *Clinical presentation of common ectatic corneal disorders*

Characteristics	KC	PMD	Keratoglobus	Posterior KC	TMD
Frequency	Most common	Less common	Rare	Rare	Rare
Laterality	Usually bilateral	Bilateral	Bilateral	Unilateral	Bilateral
Age at onset	Puberty	20 to 40 years	Usually at birth	Birth	Middle-aged to elderly
Thinning	Inferior paracentral	Inferior band 1 to 2 mm wide	Maximum in periphery	Paracentral posterior excavation	Superior cornea
CCT	Reduced	Usually normal	May be normal	—	Usually normal
Protrusion	*Thinnest at apex*	Superior to band of thinning	Generalized	Usually none	Superior cornea
Rizutti's phenomenon Munson's sign	Present	Absent	Present	Absent	Absent
Fleischer ring	Present	Sometimes	None	Sometime	Absent
Scarring	Common	Only after hydrops	Mild	Common	Superior cornea with vascularization, lipid deposition and inflammation
Vogt's striae	Common	Sometimes	Sometimes	Absent	Absent

KC: Keratoconus; PMD: Pellucid marginal degeneration; TMD: Terrein marginal degeneration; CCT: Central corneal thickness

disorder associated with corneal thinning and steepening, wherein the area of maximum thinning coincides with the apex of the cone[1, 2] (Fig. 30.1). The location of maximum steepening (cone) usually lies inferior to the center of the cornea. The induced myopia and irregular astigmatism due to changes in corneal contour is the cause for decrease in visual acuity in these patients.

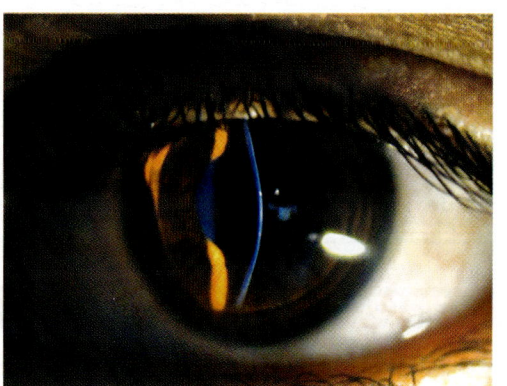

Fig. 30.1: *A case of KC with corneal ectasia and thinning*

EPIDEMIOLOGY, ASSOCAITED DISEASES AND GENETICS

EPIDEMIOLOGY

The prevalence of keratoconus varies from 54.5 to 230 per 1,00,000 population.[1] There is no gender predilection seen in this condition. Keratoconus has been reported in all the races, however, a higher rate has been reported in studies from Asian and Middle East countries. Although keratoconus usually has bilateral involvement, unilateral keratoconus has been observed in 2–4% of the cases.[1, 3] The onset of this condition is observed in puberty. Rapid progression is observed till the third decade of life following which the disease plateaus and by the fourth decade of life the progression stops.

ASSOCIATED DISEASES

Keratoconus is usually idiopathic in nature. However, there are certain systemic and ocular conditions associated with it.

Ocular associations include Leber's congenital amaurosis, retinitis pigmentosa, retinopathy of prematurity, cone-rod dystrophy, floppy eyelid syndrome, aniridia, granular corneal dystrophy, Fuchs endothelial corneal dystrophy, posterior polymorphous corneal dystrophy and vernal keratoconjunctivitis. Ocular allergy is the most common association noted in India.[4]

Systemic conditions associated with keratoconus include Down syndrome, atopy (asthma/eczema/hay fever), Marfan syndrome, Ehlers-Danlos syndrome, osteogenesis imperfecta, mitral valve prolapse and mental retardation.[2]

■ ETIOPATHOGENESIS

Genetics

There are multiple reports in literature which suggest the occurrence of keratoconus in monozygotic twins that suggest the genetic association of this condition. Family history is observed in 6% of the cases. Genetic associations observed with this condition include mutation of 17p13, variation in VSX1 gene, chromosome 7,11 translocation and, chromosome 13-ring abnormality. VSX1 is the most extensively studied gene in relation to keratoconus and is known to account 2–3% of cases of keratoconus.[2]

Environmental factors

Following environmental factors are reported to produce some molecular changes in cornea:

Eye rubbing has been implicated as one of the most important etiologic factors for development of keratoconus. Chronic rubbing of eyes results in corneal micro-trauma. This can result in the development of keratoconus. Chronic eye rubbing is often seen in cases of vernal keratoconjunctivitis and Down syndrome.

Other environmental factors include contact lens use (specially RGP), UV exposure, sleeping with face buried in pillow, atopy and some hormonal changes.

Inflammatory and immunological processes

Inflammatory and immunological processes are now being considered to play a role in pathogenesis of keratoconus. This is contrary to the long-established fact that keratoconus is a non-inflammatory disease. Raised systemic IgE levels, even I cases with no apparent associated ocular allergy indicates some role of immunological process in the pathogenesis of keratoconus.

Molecular changes in cornea

Molecular changes, being considered as precursors to the corneal thinning (by deranging corneal biomechanics) include:

- Defective formation/destruction of extracellular matrix
- Abnormal collagenase activity
- Increased levels of proteases and catabolic enzymes in the basal epithelial cells
- Decreased levels of proteinase inhibitors such as α_1 proteinase inhibitor and α_2 macroglobulin.

Histopathological changes in cornea

All the layers of cornea are involved in this condition.

- *Corneal epithelium* shows thinning with breaks in the basement membrane.
- *Z-shaped interruptions* are observed at the level of Bowman's layer with migration of the epithelium in the anterior corneal stroma and that of collagen into the corneal epithelium.
- *Corneal stroma*, although has normal collagen fibrils, has decreased number of collagen lamellae. There is reduced attachment between the collagen lamellae and the collagen lamellae with the Bowman's layer. This allows the collagen lamellae to slide over each other resulting in corneal thinning without collagenolysis.
- *Endothelial cell* pleomorphism and polymegathism has been reported in keratoconus. However, this is predominantly presumed to be because of the long-term contact lens use in these patients and not because of keratoconus *per se*.

Speculated pathogenesis of keratoconus

Based on the etiopathogenic factors described above, Khaled et al have proposed a model for pathogenesis of keratoconus (Fig. 30.2).

■ CLINICAL FEATURES

SYMPTOMS

A case of keratoconus can present with variable symptoms based on the stage of the disease.

- In the early stage, the patients usually complaints of *frequent change of glasses*.
- There may be symptoms of *progressive visual blurring and/or distortion* due to associated irregular astigmatism that is difficult to correct with spectacles alone.
- *Photophobia, glare, monocular diplopia*, and *ocular irritation* may also be associated.
- Rarely a patient may present with *symptoms of ocular allergy* and keratoconus is co-incidentally diagnosed.

SIGNS

Various signs can be seen on ocular examination based on the stage of the disease.

Mild keratoconus

- *Retinoscopy* reveals a scissoring of the red reflex.
- *Distant direct ophthalmoscopy* with +6 D lens placed in front of the patient's eye in dilated pupil reveals an oil droplet reflex also known as "Charleux sign". A dark reflex in the area of the cone with a central bright light is observed in the background of the red reflex from the fundus.

Moderate to severe keratoconus

- *Corneal thinning* is the most important corneal finding that often precedes corneal ectasia. The site of maximum thinning is usually inferior to the visual axis (infero-temporal > infero-nasal).
- *Ectatic protrusion of the cornea* is observed in these cases. The cone, like the area of thinning, is inferior to the visual axis. The thinnest point of the cornea corresponds to the site of maximum corneal protrusion (apex of cone). (Fig. 30.1) The cone can be of two types—nipple and oval cone.

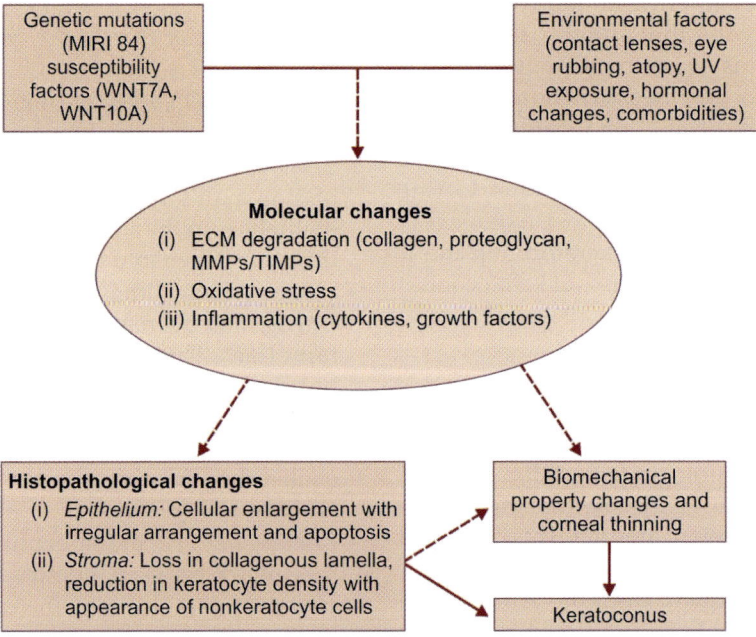

Fig. 30.2: *Flowchart depicting speculated pathogenesis of keratoconus. Source:* Khaled, et al. "Molecular and Histopathological Changes Associated with Keratoconus," BioMed Research International, vol. 2017, Article ID 7803029

- *The nipple-shaped cones* are round and smaller in diameter, while the oval cones are large may extend up to the limbus. The *oval cones* are often associated with difficulty in contact lens fitting.
- *Fleischer ring* is seen at the base of the cone. It occurs due to the deposition of haemosiderin (iron) at the basement membrane of the corneal epithelium. It appears brown in color and may be either partial or complete (annular). It is best observed in cobalt blue filter with a broad and oblique beam of light.
- *Sub-epithelial white fibrillary* lines may be observed just inside the Fleischer ring in some cases. These lines represent rupture or breaks in the Bowman's layer.
- *Sub-epithelial scarring* may be present in some cases (Fig. 30.3).

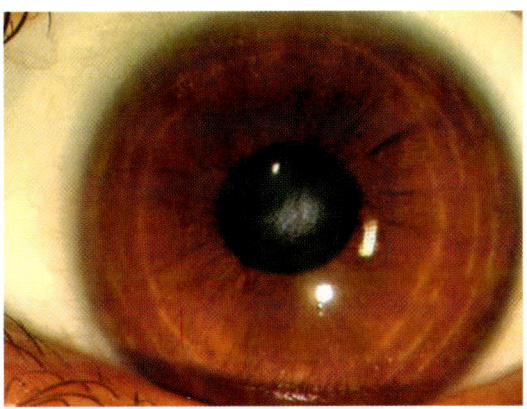

Fig. 30.3: *Sub-epthelial central corneal scarring*

- *Fine vertical lines* are also observed at the level of posterior corneal stroma and Descemet's membrane. These are called "*Vogt striae*" (Fig. 30.4). They disappear on transient increase in the intra-ocular pressure by gentle application of digital pressure over the globe.
- *Prominent corneal nerves* are often seen in these patients. The prominence of corneal nerves in these cases occur due to increased visibility of the nerves secondary to the corneal thinning and ectasia. In the early course of disease, the area of the cone shows hyperesthesia. However, the cone becomes less sensitive later.

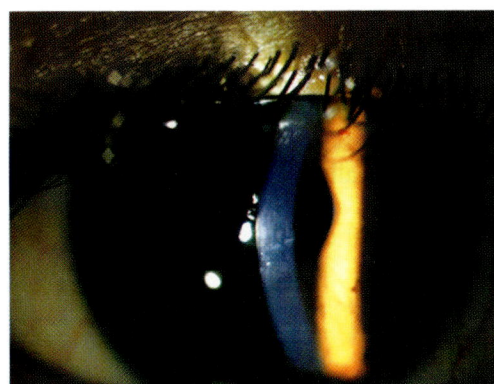

Fig. 30.4: *Slit-lamp photograph showing Vogt's striae and prominent corneal nerve*

Advanced stage keratoconus

In addition to the above described clinical features, cases of advanced keratoconus may demonstrate Rizzuti phenomenon, Munson sign and corneal scarring.

- *Rizzuti phenomenon.* When a penlight is projected on the cornea from the temporal aspect, a bright focus of light is seen at the nasal limbus. This is called Rizzuti phenomenon. It occurs due to the reflection of light from the apex of the cone.
- *Munson sign.* On downward gaze, a V-shaped angulation or anterior bowing of the lower lid is seen due to indentation of lid by the conical protrusion of the cornea. This is called Munson sign.
- *Acute corneal hydrops* may be seen in cases of advanced keratoconus (Fig. 30.5). It represents acute rupture of the Descemet's membrane

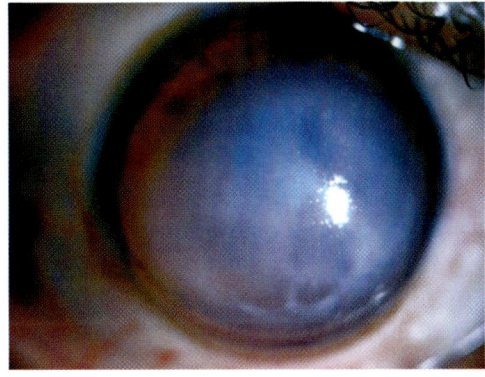

Fig. 30.5: *Slit-lamp photograph showing corneal oedema in a case of acute corneal hydrops*

with marked stromal oedema due to hydration of the corneal stroma by imbibition of aqueous. The patient complaints of sudden onset diminution of vision and clouding of the eye which may be associated with pain. Acute hydrops usually has a self-limiting course and resolves in few weeks to months but heals with residual corneal scarring. The eventual formation of corneal scar in these cases may result in flattening of the cone.

- *Deep corneal scarring* at the level of Descemet's membrane can be seen in some cases. This occurs secondary to an episode of acute hydrops.

CLASSIFICATION/GRADING

There are various classification systems for grading of keratoconus based on the cone morphology, stage of disease, ocular signs and certain index-based systems.

I. Morphological classification. Based on morphology of the cone, keratoconus can be classified into nipple, oval and globus cone.

- *Nipple cones* are usually small (diameter <5 mm), round and located either centrally or paracentrally (infero-nasal—most common). Visual rehabilitation in these cases can be easily done with contact lenses.
- *Oval cones* are large (diameter >5 mm) and usually paracentral or peripheral in location. Contact lens fitting is difficult in these cases.
- *Globus cones* involve >75% of the cornea and contact lens fitting in these cases is often challenging.

II. Keratometry based grading is as below:
- Mild keratoconus   <48 D
- Moderate keratoconus   48–54 D
- Severe keratoconus   >54 D

III. Amsler-Krumeich grading system, is the oldest and still the most widely used system by many for grading of keratoconus (Table 30.2). It is based on the evolution of the disease.

IV. ABCD grading system for keratoconus, introduced by Belin, incorporates the posterior corneal curvature, thinnest pachymetry and distance visual acuity in addition to the anterior corneal curvature[5] (Table 30.3). The measurement of the pachymetry and curvature is taken

Table 30.2: *Amsler-Krumeich classification of keratoconus*

Stage	Description
Stage 1	• Eccentric corneal steepening • Myopia and/or astigmatism <5 D • Mean keratometry ≤48 D
Stage 2	• Myopia and/or astigmatism >5 D but <8 D • Mean keratometry ≤53 D • Absence of corneal scarring • Minimum corneal thickness ≥400 μm
Stage 3	• Myopia and/or astigmatism >8 D but <10 D • Mean keratometry >53 D • Absence of corneal scarring • Minimum corneal thickness between 30 μm and 400 μm
Stage 4	• Refraction not possible • Mean keratometry >55 D • Central corneal scarring • Minimum corneal thickness <300 μm

at the thinnest point as opposed to apex of the cone in the ABCD grading system and therefore reflects the anatomic changes in various stages of the disease.

V. OCT based classification system has also been proposed based on the structural changes seen in the cornea during the course of the disease (Table 30.4). This is especially useful in cases of advanced ectasia wherein the corneal topography results are not reliable.

DIFFERENTIAL DIAGNOSIS

Keratoconus needs to be differentiated from the other ectatic corneal disorders like pellucid marginal degeneration, Terrein's marginal degeneration and keratoglobus. The differences based on the presentation and clinical features have been highlighted in Table 30.1.

INVESTIGATIONS

KERATOMETRY AND PACHYMETRY

Keratometry and pachymetry are the two most important parameters that are assessed while evaluating a case of keratoconus.

Keratometry mires in keratoconus are steep, irregular and often egg shaped. Various tools

Table 30.3: *The ABCD classification system for keratoconus*

ABCD criteria	A ARC	B PRC	C Thinnest pachy-metry (mm)	D BDVA	Scarring
Stage 0	>7.25 mm (<46.5 D)	>5.90 mm (<57.25 D)	>490	≥20/20	–
Stage I	>7.05 mm (<48.0 D)	>5.70 mm (<59.25 D)	>450	<20/20	–, +, ++
Stage II	>6.35 mm (<53.0 D)	>5.15 mm (<65.50 D)	>400	<20/40	–, +, ++
Stage III	>6.15 mm (<55.0 D)	>4.95 mm (<68.50 D)	>300	<20/100	–, +, ++
Stage IV	<6.15 mm (>55.0 D)	>4.95 mm (>68.50 D)	≤300	<20/400	–, +, ++

ARC: Anterior radius of curvature; PRC: Posterior radius of curvature; BDVA: Best corrected distance visual acuity; –: No corneal scarring; +: Corneal scarring with iris details visible; ++: Corneal scarring with iris details obscured.

Table 30.4: *ASOCT based classification of keratoconus*

Stage	Features	Other features
Stage 1	Thinning of epithelium and stromal layers at the cone	An annulus of thickened epithelium is seen surrounding the thin epithelium at the cone giving the characteristic "doughnut pattern"
Stage 2	Hyperreflective anomalies at the Bowman's layer level with a thickened epithelium at the cone	Variable amount of stromal opacities
Stage 3	Posterior displacement of the hyperreflective structures occurring at the Bowman's layer level with increased epithelial thickening and stromal thinning	Variable amount of stromal opacities
Stage 4	Pan-stromal scar	Thickened epithelium compensates for the stromal thinning.
Stage 5	Hydrops—large intra-stromal cysts communicating with anterior chamber through a tear in Descemet's membrane	• *Acute onset:* Descemet's membrane rupture and dilaceration of collagen lamellae with large fluid-filled intra-stromal cysts • *Healing stage:* Total corneal scarring with a remaining aspect of Descemet's membrane rupture

that can be used to assess keratometry include: Placido disc-based imaging (video-keratography), slit scanning-based imaging (Orbscan), combination of slit scanning and Placido disc-based imaging (Orbscan II), and Schiempflug imaging (Pentacam).

• The initial keratometric signs of keratoconus are absence of parallelism and inclination of the mires (Fig. 30.6).

• These can easily be missed in early cases. In keratoconic cornea, uneven spacing of the rings—especially inferiorly should be noted. The central rings may exhibit a tear-drop

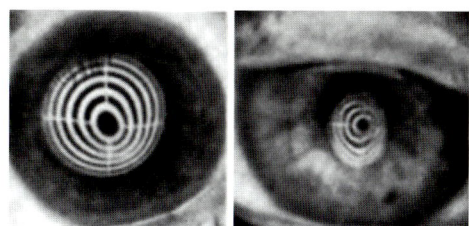

Fig. 30.6: *Keratometric ring showing absence of parallellism*

configuration, termed *'keratokyphosis'* (Fig. 30.7).

Pachymetry can be assessed by both ultrasonic as well as optical-based principles.

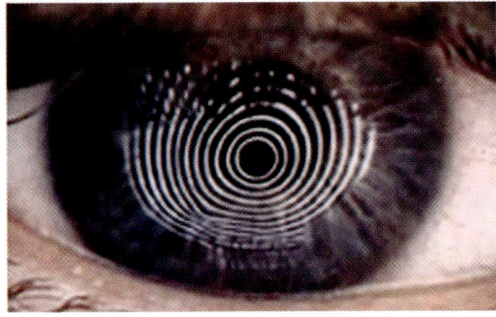

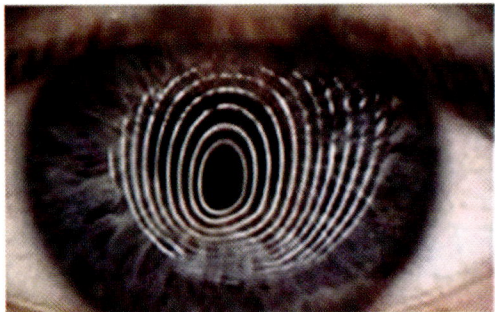

Fig. 30.7: *Tear drop configuration of keratometric mires in keratoconus*

Both keratometry and pachymetry are useful parameters for diagnosis, documenting progression and planning treatment for cases of keratoconus.

CORNEAL IMAGING

Topography and tomography

Various corneal imaging systems used for evaluation of keratoconus patients are described below.

Videokeratography

It is a *Placido disc-based imaging* system that provides useful information about the anterior corneal contour. However, it gives no information about the posterior corneal contour that is involved earlier in the course of the disease. The distance between the corneal rings is decreased with increased distortion of the rings in keratoconus.

Orbscan

It is based on *scanning slit beam-based imaging* and provides data for both the anterior as well as posterior corneal contour (keratometry and corneal elevation) along with a corneal pachymetry map. However, the data regarding the posterior corneal contour may not be absolutely accurate as it is based on certain assumptions.

Red flags on orbscan (Roush criteria) described to detect keratoconus are summarised in Table 30.5.

Table 30.5: *Red flags on Orbscan (Roush criterion)*	
Stage	*Findings*
Stage 1	A thinnest point of <470 mm on pachymetry
Stage 2	A difference of >100 mm from the thinnest point to the values of the 7 mm optic zone implies a steep gradient of thinning from midperiphery to the thinnest point
Stage 3	The thinnest point on the cornea should correspond with the highest point of elevation of the posterior corneal surface. On posterior elevations map, a posterior high point >50 mm above best-fit sphere (BFS). BFS power is greater than 55 D on the posterior profile.
Stage 4	Relative difference >100 mm between the highest and lowest point on the posterior elevation map. Keratometric mean power map >46 D. Bow-tie point or lazy C on the axial power map is suspect when the astigmatism shifts >20° from a straight line
Stage 5	A change within the central 3 mm optic zone of the cornea of more than 3 D from superior to inferior can be correlated to the presence of vertical coma (most common aberration seen in keratoconus)
Stage 6	Complete integrated information which includes highest point on the posterior elevation coincides with the highest point on the anterior elevation, the thinnest point on the pachymetry, and the point of steepest curvature on the power map

Pentacam

It is corneal tomography system based on Scheimpflug imaging and provides accurate data regarding both the anterior and posterior corneal contour (keratometry and corneal elevation), and pachymetry. The Pentacam also provides various special maps, graphs and scores that help in early detection of forme fruste keratoconus (FFKC) patients. The screening parameters on Pentacam for detection of keratoconus are highlighted in Table 30.6. The Scheimpflug imaging system provides data for wide area of the cornea making it an extremely useful tool for assessment of cases with peripheral corneal thinning disorder like in pellucid marginal corneal degeneration.

Table 30.6: *Screening parameters for keratoconus on Pentacam*

Sagittal map
- Kmax >48.7 D
- Superior–inferior difference (S-I) on the 5 mm circle ≥2.5 D
- Inferior–superior difference (I-S) ≥1.4 D
- Kmax–K2 difference >1 D
- Corneal astigmatism ≥6 D
- Km between both eyes >2 D
- SRAX >21°

Pachymetry map
- Thinnest location <470 μm with normal topography
- Thinnest location <500 μm with abnormal topography
- Y co-ordinate value of the thinnest location ≥ –500 μm
- Pachymetry apex—thickness at thinnest location ≥10 μm
- Superior–inferior at 5 mm circle ≥30 μm
- Difference in thickness between both eyes at thinnest locations ≥30 μm

Elevation maps
- Isolated focal island of ectasia (BFS mode) on either surface
- Values ≥12 μm within the central 5 mm on the anterior elevation map (BFTE mode)
- Values ≥15 μm within the central 5 mm on the posterior elevation map (BFTE mode)

Galilei

It is also based on Scheimpflug imaging system but has the advantage of using two Scheimpflug cameras for evaluation.

Sirius

It combines the Scheimpflug tomography with Placido disc-based corneal topography for evaluation of the anterior segment.

Anterior segment optical coherence tomography (ASOCT)

ASOCT can be used for assessment of changes in different layers of the cornea. It is hypothesized that the corneal epithelial changes occur in the early stages of keratoconus to compensate for the changes in corneal stroma. Hence, corneal epithelial mapping on ASOCT can be used for diagnosing early cases of keratoconus. It is extremely useful tool in assessing the depth of corneal scar that helps in surgical planning in these cases. An OCT based grading system for keratoconus has been proposed based on the structural changes observed in the cornea on ASOCT evaluation (Table 30.4). Also, in cases of acute hydrops ASOCT can help to delineate the area of Descemet's membrane tear and presence of intra-stromal fluid pockets.

Index-based system for keratoconus detection have been developed, based on corneal topography to define diagnostic criteria for keratoconus. Some of these include (Table 30.7):
- Rabinowitz/McDonnell system
- Maeda/Klyce
- Smolek/Klyce
- Rabinowitz/Rasheed
- McMahon et al

The data from Corvis and Pentacam have been combined to give two new indices which can help in detecting subclinical cases of keratoconus:
- Corvis Biomechanical Index (CBD), and
- Tomographic Biomechanical Index (TBC)

Role of corneal topography in keratoconus

Early/subclinical keratoconus

Forme fruste keratoconus (FFKC) is a clinical condition wherein the corneal topography shows signs of keratoconus in the absence of clinical signs of the same. Screening of patients with FFKC is especially useful when screening patients for cornea-based refractive surgery in order to avoid the risk of post-refractive surgery ectasia.

Topographic patterns of keratoconus

Corneal topography provides a colour-coded map of the corneal surface. The power in dioptres of the steepest and flattest meridians

Table 30.7: *Index-based systems for keratoconus detection. A higher value than the point of cut value suggests the presence of keratoconus*

Author	Index	Point of cut-off	Description
Rabinowitz/ McDonnell	K value I-S value	47.2 1.4	Diagnosis is performed based on central keratometry and the inferior–superior asymmetry in keratometric power
Maeda/Klyce	KPI KCI%	0.23 0%	KPI is derived from eight quantitative VKG indices. KCI% is derived form KPI and other four indexes
Smolek/Klyce	KSI	0.25	Keratoconus detection and the level of severity is assessed using an artificial intelligent system
Rabinowitz/ Rasheed	KISA%	100%	Diagnosis is derived from K value, I-S value, AST and SRAX
McMahon et al	KSS	0.5	Diagnosis is performed based on slit-lamp findings, corneal topography, corneal power and higher order first corneal surface wavefront root mean square error

I-S: Inferior–superior; KPI: Keratoconus prediction index; KCI: Keratoconus index; KSI: Keratoconus severity score; SRAX: Skewed radial axes; KISA: Keratoconus percentage index; AST: Keratometric astigmatism; VKG: Videokeratography

and their axes are calculated and displayed. Steep curvatures are marked orange or red, flat curvatures in blue or violet, and normal curvatures in green or yellow.

Various topographic patterns seen in keratoconus are depicted in Figs 30.8 to 30.14.

CORNEAL HYSTERESIS

The Ocular Response Analyzer (ORA; Reichert Ophthalmic Instruments, Buffalo, NY) and Corvis ST (Oculus, Wetzlar, Germany) are used for assessing the biomechanical changes of cornea. Various researches suggest that biomechanical weakening of the cornea is one of the earliest changes noted in keratoconus eyes. Both corneal hysteresis, which indicates the corneal viscoelasticity, and the corneal resistance factor are reduced in cases of corneal ectasia. However, because of the variability of results in these parameters, a definite cut-off could not

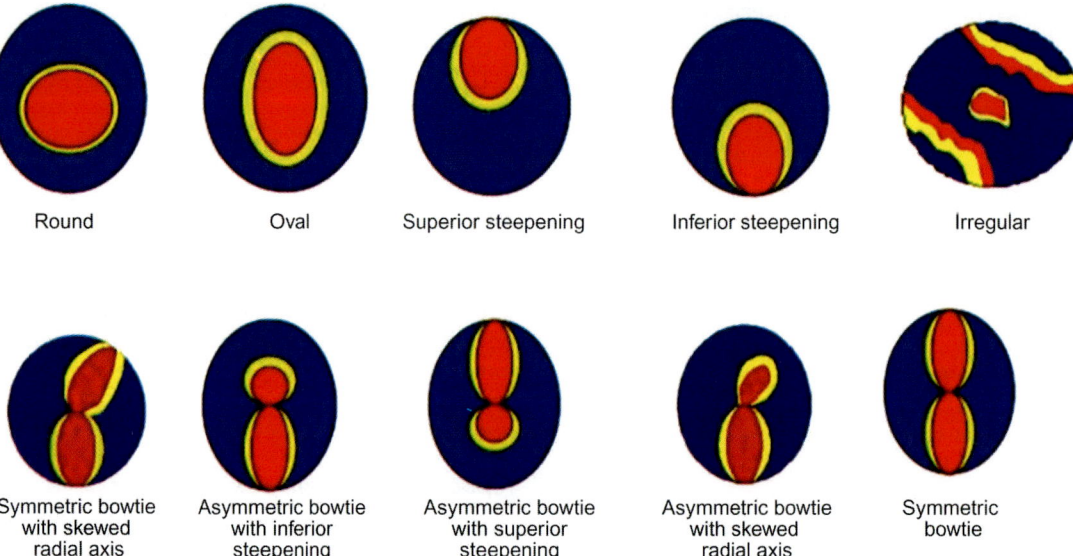

Round	Oval	Superior steepening	Inferior steepening	Irregular

Symmetric bowtie with skewed radial axis	Asymmetric bowtie with inferior steepening	Asymmetric bowtie with superior steepening	Asymmetric bowtie with skewed radial axis	Symmetric bowtie

Fig. 30.8: *Topographic patterns of keratoconus*

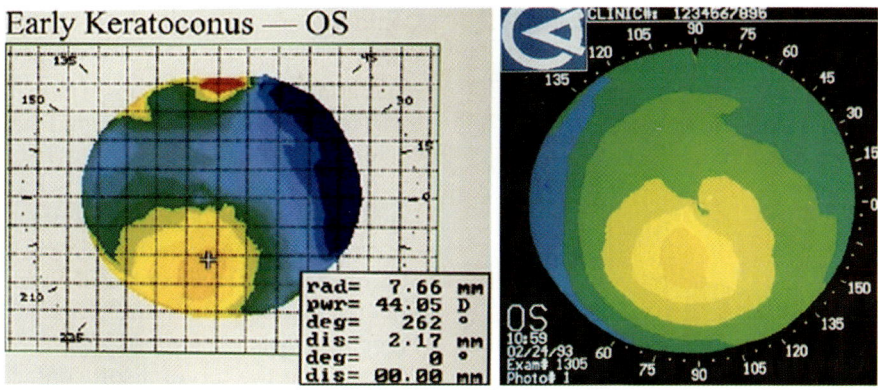

Fig. 30.9: *Keratoconus pattern: Inferior steepening without bowtie pattern especially more prominent temporally*

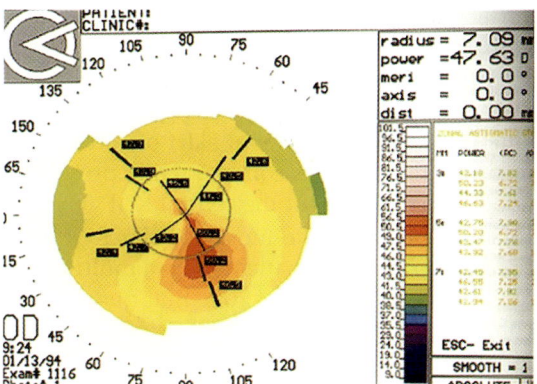

Fig. 30.10: *Keratoconus pattern: Asymmetric bowtie and inferior steepening*

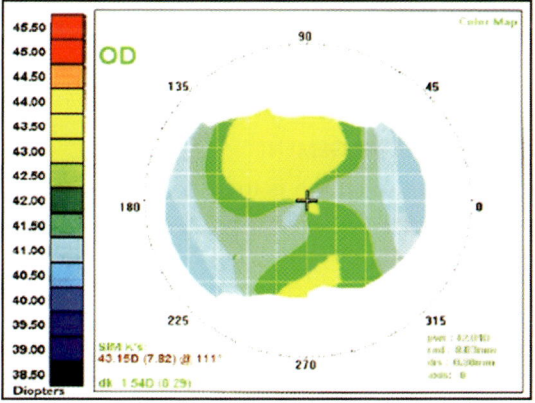

Fig. 30.11: *Keratoconus pattern: Asymmetric bowtie and superior steepening*

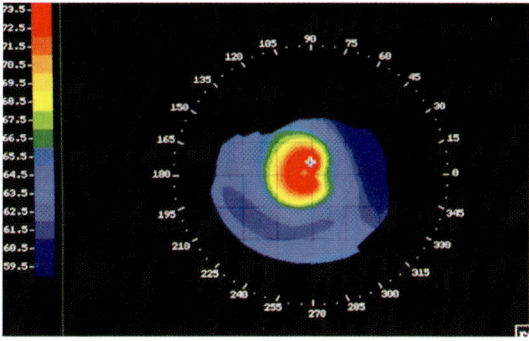

Fig. 30.12: *Keratoconus pattern: Central unusual steepening without bowtie*

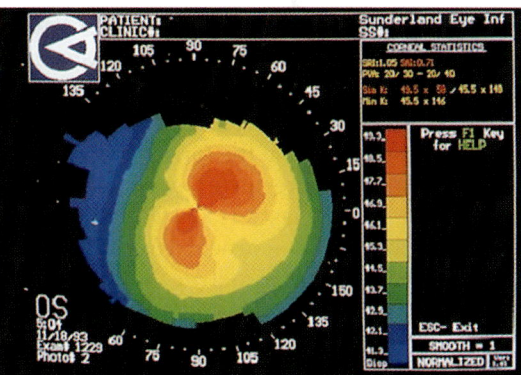

Fig. 30.13: *Keratoconus pattern: Central steepening superimposed with asymmetrical bowtie*

be established to diagnose keratoconus. Hence, these investigations should only be used in addition to the corneal tomography tests to assess the at-risk corneas.[6]

The other uses of corneal biomechanics can be to assess the biomechanical changes following corneal collagen cross-linking (CXL) and keratoplasty in patients with keratoconus. *In vitro* studies suggest that corneal biomechanical

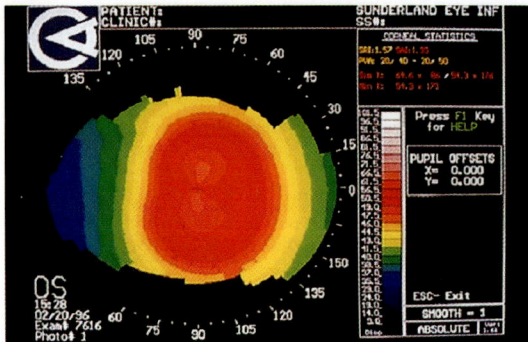

Fig. 30.14: *Keratoconus pattern: Globus topographic type of keratoconus*

strength increases by 300% following CXL. However, similar results could not be properly validated *in vivo* studies.

MANAGEMENT

MANAGEMENT STRATEGIES

The management of keratoconus primarily depends upon the stage of the disease and is primarily focused on:

I. **Arresting the progression of keratoconus.** Corneal collagen cross-linking is the gold standard treatment for arresting the progression of keratoconus.

II. **Visual rehabilitation.** In the early stages of disease visual rehabilitation can be done with *non-surgical modalities* like spectacles or contact lens.

Surgical intervention. Advanced cases require *corneal transplantation* in the form of either deep anterior lamellar keratoplasty (DALK) or penetrating keratoplasty (PK). *Other treatment options* include intra-corneal ring segments, topo-guided photorefractive keratectomy, phakic intra-ocular lens, and refractive lens exchange with toric intra-ocular lens implantation.

NON-SURGICAL MANAGEMENT

Spectacles

In the early course of the disease, visual rehabilitation can be achieved with spectacles. However, as the disease progresses, irregular astigmatism increases which is not amenable to spectacle correction. Such cases require contact lens for visual correction.

Contact lens

Various contact lenses are available for visual rehabilitation in keratoconus. These include soft toric lenses, standard bicurved hard lenses, custom-back toric lenses, piggyback systems, hybrid lenses, mini-scleral and scleral lenses.[2]

Rigid gas permeable (RGP). Contact lenses are the most commonly used lens in these patients. The *three-point touch* contact lens fitting is the preferred lens fitting in these cases (Fig. 30.15). *Piggyback lens* consists of a RGP contact lens that is fit on the top of a soft contact lens. The soft contact lens improves the patient's comfort and the RGP lens provides a uniform smooth surface to achieve adequate visual acuity (Fig. 30.16).

Hybrid contact lenses (SoftPerm, Solotica and Synergeyes) include a central rigid gas permeable lens with a peripheral skirt of soft lens to improve the patients comfort while providing good visual quality of the central RGP lens.

Rose K lenses are the most popular RGP lens used in keratoconus patients. It is a multi-curve lens with a small optical zone that fits over the cone (Fig. 30.17). It is often difficult to achieve a good contact lens fit in advanced cases and large cones.

Mini-scleral and scleral lens perform better in advanced cases with large cones. The scleral contact lens rests over the sclera and vaults over the cornea and the limbus (Fig. 30.18). These lenses are stable, maintain good centration and achieve good quality vision.

SURGICAL MANAGEMENT

Surgical intervention is to be considered when patients are not fully satisfied with non-surgical treatments are intolerant to contact lenses.

Corneal collagen crosslinking (CXL)

Wollensak introduced the concept of corneal collagen crosslinking and ever since it has become the gold standard for halting the progression of keratoconus. It utilizes *riboflavin (vitamin B_2)* and *UVA radiation* (365–370 nm) for inducing cross-linking of cornea and increasing the corneal rigidity and biomechanical strength of the cornea by inducing new chemical bonds[7] (Fig. 3.19). CXL has been reported to halt progression in 60–70% of the cases.

Contect Lens Management
Three-point Touch

Early Keratoconus
Three-point Touch Fitting Technique

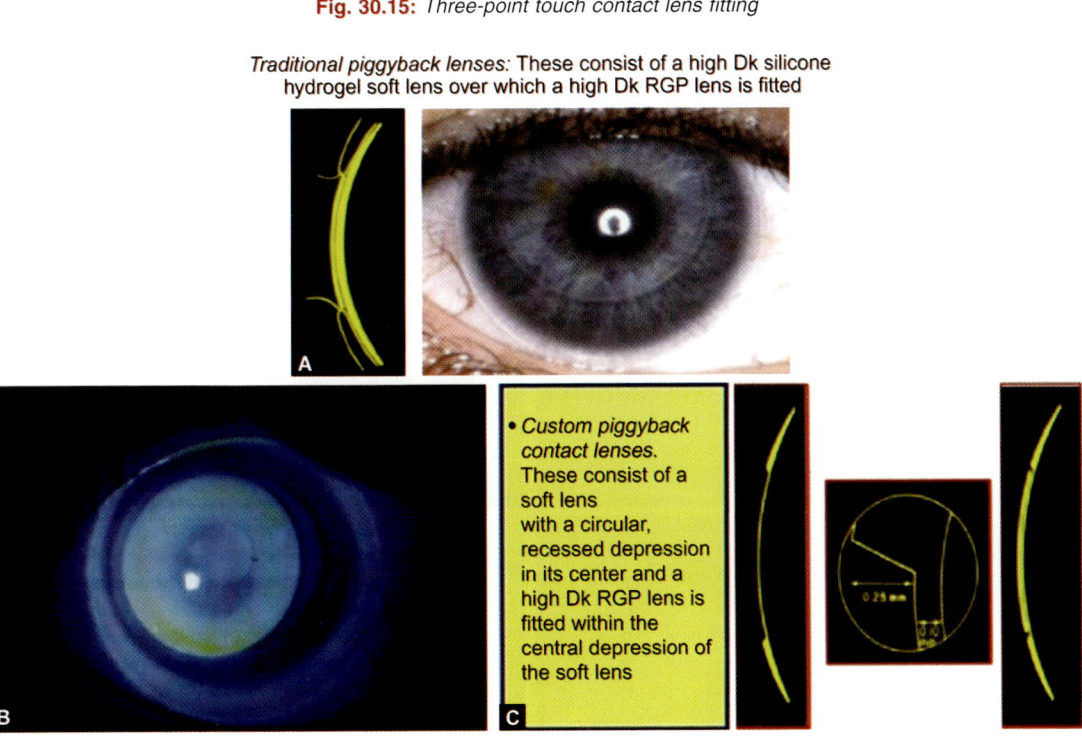

Four zones are created

- Slight apical touch
- Paracentral clearance
- Mid-peripheral bearing
- Peripheral clearance

Fig. 30.15: *Three-point touch contact lens fitting*

Traditional piggyback lenses: These consist of a high Dk silicone hydrogel soft lens over which a high Dk RGP lens is fitted

- *Custom piggyback contact lenses.* These consist of a soft lens with a circular, recessed depression in its center and a high Dk RGP lens is fitted within the central depression of the soft lens

Fig. 30.16: *Piggyback contact lenses in keratoconus. A and B, Traditional piggyback lenses; C, Custom piggyback lenses*

Procedure (Fig. 30.20) involves debriding the corneal epithelium in the central 8 mm zone. This is followed by application of riboflavin 0.1% every 2 minutes for 30 minutes. Subsequently UVA radiation is applied from a distance of 5 cm at 3 mW/cm^2 for 30 minutes (conventional CXL) with application of riboflavin every 2 minutes (Dresden protocol). At the end of the procedure

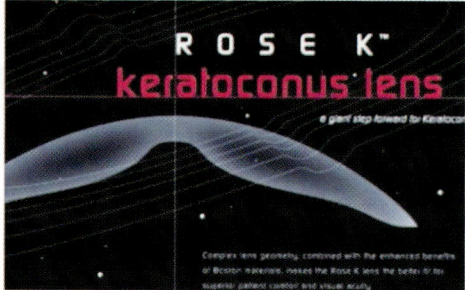

Fig. 30.17: *Rose K lens*

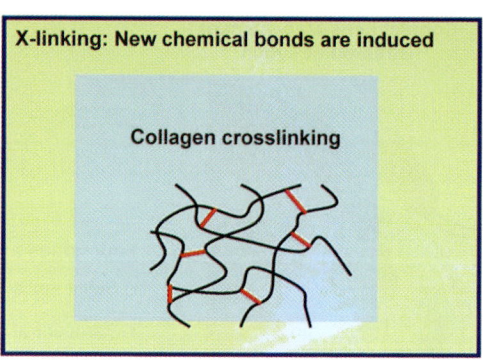

Fig. 30.19: *Principle of action of CCL or UVA-X*

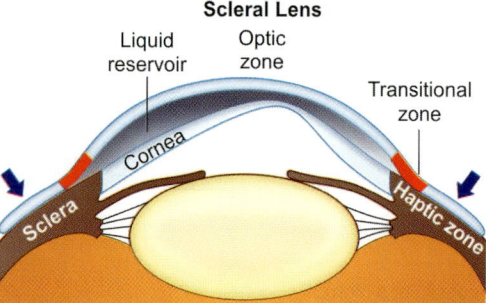

Fig. 30.18: *Scleral lenses used in keratoconus*

a bandage contact lens is applied. Riboflavin acts as a photosensitizer and increases the absorption of UVA radiation. UVA radiation induces release of reactive oxygen species that induces crosslinking between the collagen fibrils in the corneal stroma. According to the Bunsen Roscoe law, the effect of crosslinking remains the same if the total amount of energy delivered remains constant. This led to the concept of accelerated CXL.

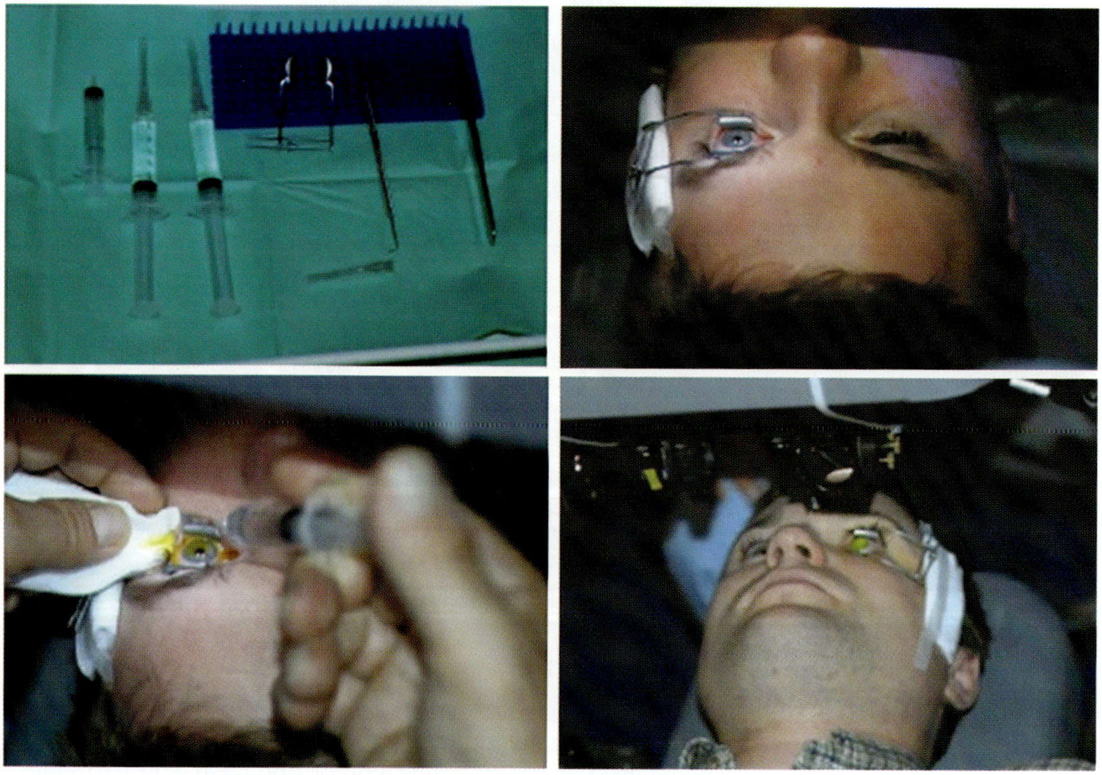

Fig. 30.20: *Procedure of collagen crosslinking*

Accelerated CXC. Herein keeping the total amount of delivered energy constant (5.4 mJ), UVA is delivered at 10 mW for 9 min, or 15 mW for 6 min, or 18 mW for 5 min, or 30 mW for 3 min. Accelerated CXL results in decrease in the total duration of the procedure, therefore increasing the patient's comfort.

CXL is not recommended in cases with thinnest pachymetry <400 µm as there is risk of corneal endothelial toxicity with UVA radiation. *Hypo-osmolar CXL, trans-epithelial CXL* and bandage contact lens assisted CXL are the treatment options in cases with pachymetry <400 µm.[7]

Complications associated with CXL include corneal haze, sterile infiltrate, progression of keratoconus and infective keratitis.[8]

Intra-corneal ring segments (ICRS)

ICRS is the treatment option for cases of mild to moderate keratoconus (K <58) who are intolerant to contact lenses, have a clear central cornea with thickness >400 microns.

- *It works on the principle* of hammock effect or arc shortening effect and improves the visual acuity by centering the cone, flattening the central cornea and reducing the astigmatism.
- *Target of implantation of ring segments* is to improve the contact lens fitting in these cases.
- *Commonly used ring segments* include Ferrara rings (Fig. 30.21) and INTACS. They are made of poly-methyl metha-acrylate (PMMA). The Intacs has a hexagonal shape on cross-section

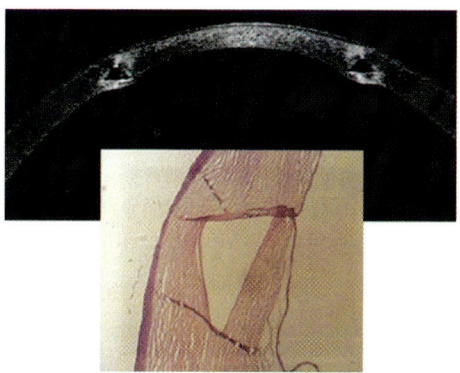

Fig. 30.21: *Ferrara ring implanted in the cornea of a patient with keratoconus. Note: The ring segments have a prism format; the flat posterior surface is implanted facing the corneal endothelium*

and is placed more peripherally (inner diameter of 6.8 mm) compared to Ferrara ring which appears triangular in cross-section and has an inner diameter of 5 mm.

- *INTACS SK* (SK—severe keratoconus) is used in more severe forms of keratoconus and has certain modifications in the design over the standard INTACS ring. It has a smaller inner diameter (6 mm Vs 6.8 mm) with an elliptical shape on cross-section.
- *A corneal thickness of 450 µm at the site of ICRS implantation is the cut-off to avoid complications.*
- *ICRS are implanted at 75–80% corneal* depth to achieve adequate effect.

Channel for implantation of the intracorneal ring segments (Fig. 30.22) can be created with the help of specialized lamellar dissectors or femtosecond laser.

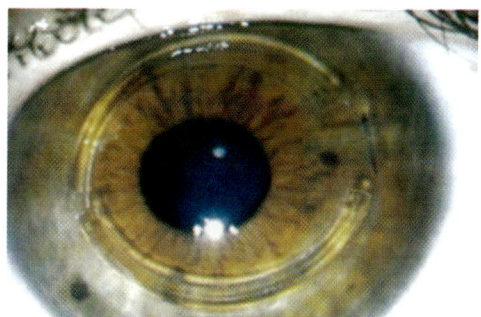

Fig. 30.22: *Intra-stromal tunnel made for implantation of intracorneal ring segments*

Under topical anaesthesia, a small corneal incision (1.8 mm in length) is made temporally at the edge of 7 mm optical zone. Then two intra-stromal tunnels (clockwise and counter-clockwise) are created. Special care is taken when making the inferior tunnel, where the cornea is relatively thinner. Selection of segments is based on the standard nomograms. In globus or central cone, 2 rings of equal thickness, and in asymmetrical cone, 2 rings thin in flatter and thick in steeper zone (usually inferior) are selected.

Complications associated with ICRS include corneal perforation at the time of implantation, ring extrusion, infective keratitis and epithelial ingrowth into the corneal channels.

Phakic IOLs

Phakic IOLs are used to correct high myopia and associated astigmatism of the keratoconus patients. Anterior chamber phakic IOLs can also be combined with INTACS. In such cases, the INTACS implantation is followed by toric phakic IOL implantation to correct the residual myopic and astigmatic refractive error.

Inclusion criteria include:

- Stable refractive error for more than 1 year
- Clear central cornea
- Central dioptic power <52 D

Exclusion criteria include:

- Central anterior chamber depth <2.8 mm
- Endothelial cell count <2000 per square mm
- Patients younger than 21 years of age

Keratoplasty

Penetrating keratoplasty is reserved for cases of keratoconus with central Descemet scarring (healed hydrops).[3] The success rate of PK in keratoconus is 90–95% with less risk of graft rejection, graft failure and postoperative complications compared to other indications for PK.

Deep anterior lamellar keratoplasty (DALK) is the most commonly performed and preferred corneal transplant procedure in cases of keratoconus since the host endothelium in these cases is healthy.[3]

- *Target in DALK* is to achieve a dissection plane as close to the Descemet's membrane as possible. Various agents have been described to achieve this dissection plane. These include air, fluid, viscoelastic, microkeratome and femtosecond laser.
- *Commonly used techniques for DALK include:* Layer-by-layer manual dissection, Air-assisted DALK (Archilla), big bubble DALK (Anwar), viscoelastic-assisted DALK (Melles et al), hydrodelamination (Sugita) and femtosecond-assisted DALK.[9]

Role of excimer laser ablation

- *Topography-guided photorefractive keratectomy* (T-PRK) followed by or combined with collagen crosslinking (c3R) has been reported to give promising but variable results.

- *Phototherapeutic keratectomy* (PTK) has been tried for keratoconus nodule.
- *Circular keratotomy* has been tried to reduce astigmatism and improve vision in stage 1 and stage 2 keratoconus.

SUMMARY OF TREATMENT

Treatment protocol of keratoconus is summarised in Fig. 30.23.

Role of thermokeratoplasty

Thermokeratoplasty is a rare procedure which involves placing a hot ring (holmium YAG laser, 2100 nm) along the base of the cone to heat and traumatize the cornea, resulting in corneal scar which reduces the corneal curvature. It allows a flatter contact lens to be fitted. Disadvantages of the procedure are transitory corneal haze and development of corneal scarring.

OTHER ECTATIC CORNEAL DISORDERS

PELLUCID MARGINAL DEGENERATION

INTRODUCTION

Pellucid marginal degeneration (PMD) is a non-inflammatory bilateral peripheral ectatic corneal disorder characterized by a narrow band of corneal thinning, extending from 4 to 8 o'clock position, separated from the limbus by a 1–2 mm wide band of uninvolved cornea with corneal ectasia superior to the band of corneal thinning[10] (Fig. 30.24). It is usually inferior in location, however, other locations have also been reported. The term "pellucid" means clear indicating absence of corneal scar, lipid deposition and vascularization in this clinical condition.

ETIOLOGY

The etiology of this condition is unknown and some researchers consider PMD, keratoconus and keratoglobus as different clinical presentations of the same disease.

CLINICAL FEATURES

Symptoms

- *Age.* The patients usually present between the second to fifth decade of life (later compared to keratoconus).

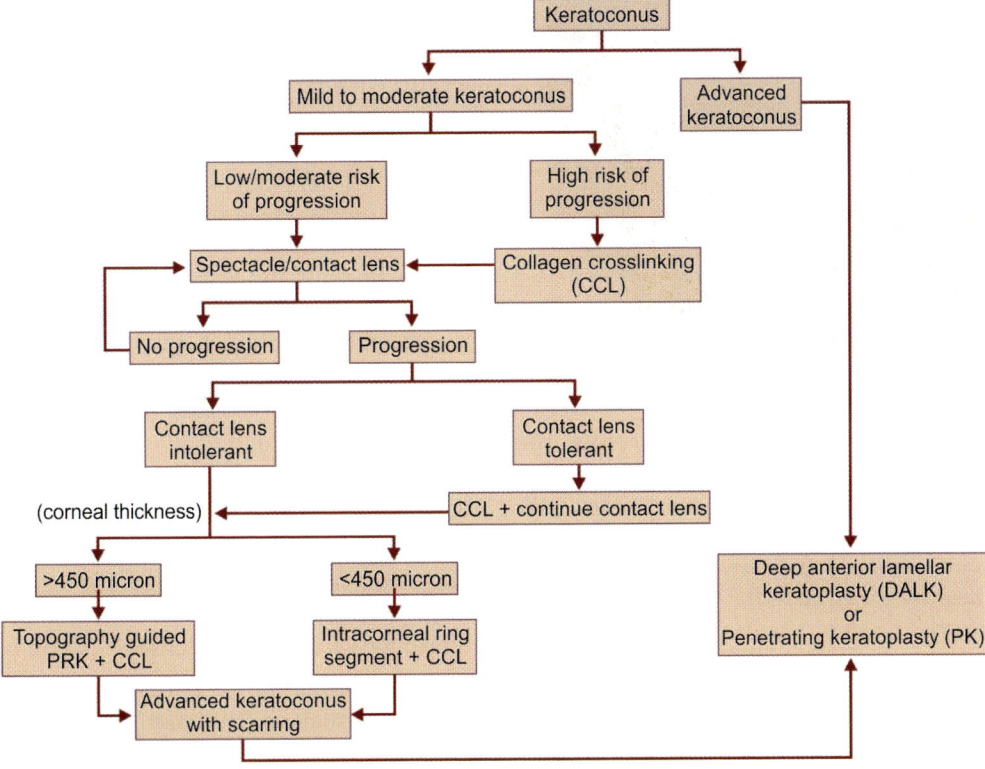

Fig. 30.23: *Flowchart summarising the treatment protocol of keratoconus*

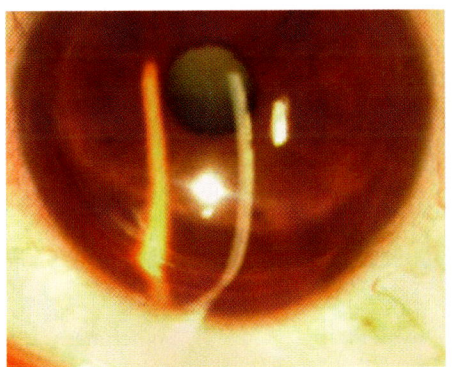

Fig. 30.24: *Pellucid marginal degeneration: Inferior corneal thinning extending from 4 to 8 o'clock position with a 1–2 mm width of cornea with normal thickness between the area of thinning and limbus*

- *Common presenting symptom.* Blurring of vision due to irregular astigmatism or frequent changes of glasses.[11]
- Rarely a patient may present with *sudden onset loss* of vision, pain, conjunctival injection, photophobia and glare (*acute hydrops*).[12]

Signs

- *Slit-lamp examination reveals* a narrow band of corneal thinning extending from 4 to 8 o'clock position.
- *The area of thinning is separated* from the limbus by a 1–2 mm wide band of uninvolved cornea of normal thickness (Fig. 30.24).
- *There is no scarring,* vascularization or lipid deposition.
- *The area of maximum corneal protrusion* is superior to the area of thinning unlike keratoconus wherein the area of maximum protrusion corresponds with the thinnest pachymetry (Fig. 30.25). Therefore, the resultant corneal contour on side profile is referred to as a "beer belly".
- *Corneal astigmatism* changes from against-the-rule in the superior cornea to with-the-rule near the point of maximum corneal protrusion.
- *Corneal scar* may occur at the level of Descemet's membrane with extension into the

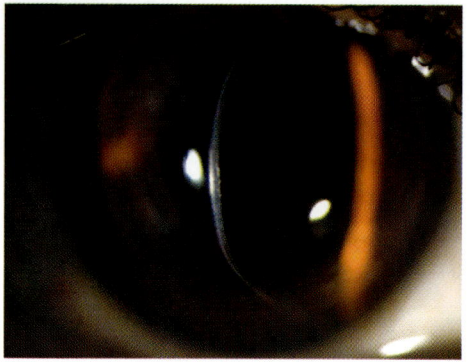

Fig. 30.25: *Corneal ectasia superior to area of thinning in PMD*

mid-stroma. It is usually located at the superior aspect of the corneal thinning.
• *Acute hydrops* may occur in these cases with resultant corneal oedema, scarring and vascularization. However, the occurrence of corneal hydrops in PMD is less common as compared to keratoconus.

INVESTIGATIONS

Corneal topography power maps represent a typical "crab claw" or "butterfly" or "lobster" or "kissing doves" appearance due to flattening of the superior cornea and steepening of the inferior cornea.[10] However, this appearance may also be seen in inferior keratoconus.

DIFFERENTIAL DIAGNOSIS

PMD needs to be differentiated from other ectatic corneal disorders like keratoconus, Terrien's marginal degeneration and kerato-globus. The clinical differences between these conditions have been highlighted in Table 30.1. Also, it needs to be differentiated from the peripheral corneal thinning disorders like furrow degeneration and Mooren ulcer. The differences between these clinical conditions have been highlighted in Table 30.8.

MANAGEMENT

Spectacles usually fail to achieve visual rehabilitation in these cases due to the presence of highly irregular astigmatism.

Contact lens fitting is also difficult in these cases due to the presence of peripheral corneal ectasia. Large diameter RGP can be tried initially but hybrid lenses and scleral lenses perform better.

Corneal transplantation is required in advanced cases for visual rehabilitation. Large diameter PK and eccentric PK have been described for management of PMD. However, both large graft and proximity of the graft to the corneal limbus increase the risk of graft rejection and subsequent graft failure.

Table 30.8: *Clinical features of peripheral corneal thinning disorder*

Features	PMD	TMD	Furrow degeneration	Mooren ulcer
Age of onset	2nd–5th decade	Middle age to elderly	Elderly	Adult to elderly
Laterality	Bilateral	Bilateral	Bilateral	Unilateral/bilateral
Sex	Male = Female	Male > Female	Male = Female	Male > Female
Astigmatism	Common	Common	Absent	Sometimes
Thinning	Inferior band 1–2 mm wide	Superior cornea	Occurs within arcus	Starts within lid fissure
Inflammation	Absent	May be present	Absent	Present
Epithelial defect	Absent	Usually absent	Absent	Present
Vascularization	Absent	Crosses area of thinning	Absent	Peripheral edge of thinning
Lipid deposition	Absent	Common; central to thinning	Absent	Rarely
Perforation	Can occur	Can occur	Never	Can occur

PMD: Pellucid marginal degeneration; TMD: Terrien's marginal degeneration

Other surgical options include:
- Large diameter DALK
- Tuck in lamellar keratoplasty (TILK)
- Combined lamellar keratoplasty with a small central PK
- Crescentic lamellar keratoplasty and crescentic wedge excision.[3, 13]
- *CXL* may be performed to halt the progression of the disease.[14]
- *Implantation of ICRS* has also been reported in PMD, but its role has not been well evaluated.

KERATOGLOBUS

Clinical features

Keratoglobus is an ectatic corneal disorder that is usually bilateral and non-progressive.
- It is characterised by generalised corneal thinning extending up to the limbus with globular corneal protrusion[15] (Figs 30.26 and 30.27).

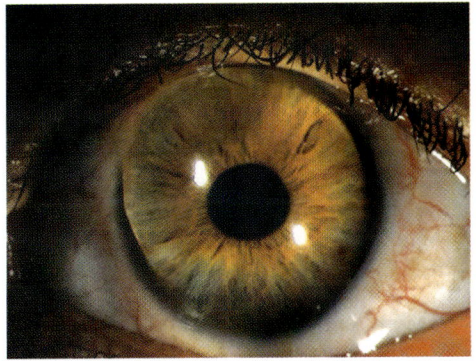

Fig. 30.26: *Globular corneal protrusion in keratoglobus*

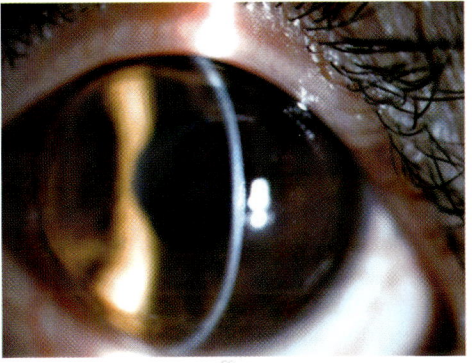

Fig. 30.27: *Limbus-to-limbus corneal thinning in keratoglobus*

- *Corneal diameter* is normal in these cases.
- *Minimal corneal* scarring may be present but Vogt striae and Fleischer ring are absent.
- Although *acute corneal hydrops* is less common in keratoglobus compared to keratoconus, the chances of corneal rupture and perforation is high in these cases.[16]
- *Association with various ocular* (Leber's congenital amaurosis, posterior polymorphous dystrophy, vernal keratoconjunctivits, chronic marginal blepharitis and idiopathic orbital inflammation) and systemic disorder (Ehlers-Danlos syndrome type VI, Marfan syndrome, Rubenstein-Taybi syndrome and osteogenesis imperfecta) has been observed in keratoglobus.[15,17]

Differential diagnosis

Other than ectatic corneal disorders like keratoconus and PMD, the other differentials for keratoglobus include congenital glaucoma and megalocornea.
- In contrast to congenital glaucoma, keratoglobus does not show signs of corneal oedema, Haab striae, raised intra-ocular pressure, optic disc changes, increased corneal diameter and globe size.
- In congenital megalocornea, the corneal diameter is >12 mm with a normal contour at birth while cases of keratoglobus have normal corneal diameter with globular corneal ectasia.

Investigations

Corneal topography maps reveal generalized corneal thinning with central and para-central corneal steepening.

Management

Management of keratoglobus involves initial rehabilitation with spectacles.

Contact lenses may be used in cases not improving with spectacles. However, it is difficult to achieve a good fitting of contact lens in these cases. Also, there is risk of inducing trauma to the eye while inserting and removing these lenses with risk of corneal perforation.

Surgical management in these cases is often challenging and is reserved for cases that fail achieve functional vision with other treatment modalities. The surgical treatment options include:

- *Large diameter* (limbus to limbus) PKP, epi-keratoplasty, epikeratoplasty with 360 host peripheral intra-stromal tucking, tuck-in lamellar keratoplasty, Pentacam-based deep anterior lamellar keratoplasty and epikeratoplasty/tectonic LK followed by second stage PK.

◼ POSTERIOR KERATOCONUS

Clinical features

Posterior keratoconus is a developmental anomaly that is non-progressive in nature and has a unilateral involvement.

- It is characterised by increased posterior corneal curvature with a relatively normal anterior corneal contour.
- There are *two clinical variants of posterior keratoconus*—keratoconus posticus circumscriptus and keratoconus posticus generalis.
  - *Keratoconus posticus circumscriptus* is characterised by a central or paracentral excavation in the posterior corneal surface and is associated with corneal scarring.
  - *Keratoconus posticus generalis* is characterised by a generalised increased curvature of the posterior corneal surface, however, the cornea remains clear.
- Posterior keratoconus is characterised by *mild diminution of vision*. The cause for diminution of vision is astigmatism and corneal scarring.
- *Corneal topography* shows corneal steepening in the area of the excavation with flattening of the peripheral cornea.

Acquired posterior keratoconus cases are reported following ocular trauma and interstitial keratitis.

Differential diagnosis

Some similarities have also been reported with Peter's anomaly, however, histopathologically Peter's anomaly is characterised by absence of Descemet's membrane and endothelium, while posterior keratoconus has a disorganised Descemet's membrane with an attenuated endothelium.

Treatment

Posterior keratoconus usually requires no treatment.

- *Spectacles*. Refractive error can be corrected with spectacles.
- *Contact lens* may be useful in cases with increased anterior corneal curvature in association with posterior keratoconus.
- *Penetrating keratoplasty* can be performed in cases with corneal scarring, however, amblyopia may limit the final visual acuity in these cases.

◼ REFERENCES

1. Krachmer JH, Feder RS, Belin MW. Keratoconus and related noninflammatory corneal thinning disorders. Surv Ophthalmol 1984; 28(4): 293–322.
2. Rabinowitz YS. Keratoconus. Surv Ophthalmol 1998; 42(4): 297–319.
3. Maharana PK, Dubey A, Jhanji V, Sharma N, Das S, Vajpayee RB. Management of advanced corneal ectasias. Br J Ophthalmol 2016; 100(1): 34–40.
4. Galvis V, Tello A, Carreño NI, Berrospi RD, Niño CA. Risk Factors for Keratoconus: Atopy and Eye Rubbing. Cornea 2017; 36(1): e1.
5. Belin MW, Duncan JK. Keratoconus: The ABCD Grading System. Klin Monbl Augenheilkd 2016; 233(6): 701–7.
6. Ambrósio R, Lopes BT, Faria-Correia F, Salomão MQ, Bühren J, Roberts CJ, et al. Integration of Scheimpflug-based Corneal Tomography and Biomechanical Assessments for Enhancing Ectasia Detection. J Refract Surg 2017; 33(7): 434–43.
7. Mohammadpour M, Masoumi A, Mirghorbani M, Shahraki K, Hashemi H. Updates on corneal collagen cross-linking: Indications, techniques and clinical outcomes. J Curr Ophthalmol 2017; 29(4): 235–47.
8. Maharana PK, Sahay P, Sujeeth M, Singhal D, Rathi A, Titiyal JS, et al. Microbial Keratitis After Accelerated Corneal Collagen Cross-linking in Keratoconus. Cornea 2018; 37(2): 162–67.
9. Seitz B, Cursiefen C, El-Husseiny M, Viestenz A, Langenbucher A, Szentmáry N. [DALK and penetrating laser keratoplasty for advanced keratoconus]. Ophthalmologe 2013 110(9): 839–48.

10. Jinabhai A, Radhakrishnan H, O'Donnell C. Pellucid corneal marginal degeneration: A review. Cont Lens Anterior Eye 2011; 34(2): 56–63.

11. Martínez-Abad A, Piñero DP. Pellucid marginal degeneration: Detection, discrimination from other corneal ectatic disorders and progression. Cont Lens Anterior Eye 2018.

12. Carter JB, Jones DB, Wilhelmus KR. Acute hydrops in pellucid marginal corneal degeneration. Am J Ophthalmol 1989; 107(2): 167–70.

13. Vajpayee RB, Jhanji V, Beltz J, Moorthy S. "Tuck in" lamellar keratoplasty for tectonic management of post-keratoplasty corneal ectasia with peripheral corneal involvement. Cornea 2011; 30(2): 171–74.

14. Mamoosa B, Razmjoo H, Peyman A, Ashtari A, Ghafouri I, Moghaddam AG. Short-term result of collagen cross-linking in pellucid marginal degeneration. Adv Biomed Res. 2016; 5: 194.

15. Keratoglobus. PubMed–NCBI [Internet]. [cited 2019 Feb 17]. Available from: https://www.ncbi.nlm.nih.gov/pubmed/23807384

16. Kiire C, Srinivasan S. Management of bilateral acute hydrops secondary to keratoglobus with perfluoroethane (C2F6) pneumodescemetopexy. Clin Experiment Ophthalmol 2009; 37(9): 892–94.

17. Fay J, Herzlich AA, Florakis GJ. Posterior Amorphous Corneal Dystrophy Associated with Keratoglobus: A Case Report. Cornea 2017; 36(12): 1562–66.

Corneal Dystrophies

GENERAL CONSIDERATIONS

INTRODUCTION

The term corneal dystrophy dates back to 1890 when it was first introduced by Groenouw in reference to two patients with "noduli corneae".[1] Thereafter, Biber,[2] Fuchs,[3] Uthoff[4] and Yoshida[5] described other such cases under the spectrum of corneal dystrophy. The word dystrophy has its origin in Greek literature (*dys* = wrong, difficult; *trophe* = nourishment). Corneal dystrophies are a heterogenous group of inherited corneal diseases that are typically bilateral, symmetric, non-inflammatory, slowly progressive, and usually bear no relationship to environmental or systemic factors.[6] However, there are exceptions to each of these characteristics. Clinically, the corneal dystrophies are divided into three groups based on the principal anatomical location of the abnormalities. Some affect primarily the corneal epithelium and its basement membrane or Bowman's layer and the superficial corneal stroma (anterior corneal dystrophies), the corneal stroma (stromal corneal dystrophies), or Descemet's membrane and the corneal endothelium (posterior corneal dystrophies). Most corneal dystrophies have no systemic associations and present with a variable degree of corneal involvement in a clear or cloudy cornea and affect visual acuity to different degrees.

PREVALENCE

Most of the published reports derive their prevalence data from the number of cases of corneal dystrophy undergoing keratoplasty.

Some of the recent reports are summarized in Table 31.1. While this may be an indicator of the prevalence of cases severe enough to warrant a corneal graft, it is not a true estimate of the prevalence of corneal dystrophy in the entire population. In a recent review of global distribution of indications for penetrating keratoplasty reported in peer-reviewed journals between 1980 and 2014, the percentage of cases undergoing keratoplasty for corneal dystrophies and degenerations (excluding keratoconus and FECD) were as follows: North America (3.9%), South America (1.5%), Europe (4.7%), Africa (8.6%), Middle East (5.9%), Asia (5.6%) and Australia (9.9%).[7] To the best of our knowledge, the only population-based prevalence of corneal dystrophy has been reported in the CORE study, wherein the prevalence was 0.04 % across all age groups.[8]

CLASSIFICATION OF CORNEAL DYSTROPHIES

The increasing availability of genetic studies over the last two decades highlighted the shortcomings of the phenotypic method of classification of corneal dystrophies. Abnormalities in different genes may produce a single phenotype, whereas various defects in a single gene can manifest as varying phenotypes.[16] The International Committee for Classification of Corneal Dystrophies (IC3D) was developed to incorporate the traditional classification of corneal dystrophies with new genetic, clinical, and pathologic information and was first published in 2008.[17] The anatomic classification continues to group dystrophies according to the corneal layers that are predominantly involved.

Evidence-based categories of corneal dystrophies

In order to indicate the level of evidence supporting the existence of a given dystrophy, four descriptive, evidential categories were created in the IC3D classification.[3]

Each dystrophy carries a template summarizing genetic, clinical and pathologic information. A category number from 1 through 4 is assigned depicting the level of evidence supporting the existence of the particular dystrophy. The most defined dystrophies belong to category 1 (a well-defined corneal dystrophy with a gene that has been mapped, identified and specific mutations are known) and the least defined belong to category 4 (a suspected dystrophy without substantial genetic evidence).[2]

Category 1: A well-defined corneal dystrophy in which the gene has been mapped and identified and specific mutations are known.

Category 2: A well-defined corneal dystrophy that has been mapped to one or more specific chromosomal loci, but the gene(s) remains to be identified.

Category 3: A well-defined corneal dystrophy in which the disorder has not yet been mapped to a chromosomal locus.

Category 4: This category is reserved for a suspected new, or previously documented, corneal dystrophy, although the evidence for it, being a distinct entity, is not yet established.

The category assigned to a specific corneal dystrophy can be expected to change over time as knowledge progressively advances. Eventually, all valid corneal dystrophies should attain the classification of category 1. Subsequently, this classification was updated over time and the revised edition was published in 2015.[18]

THE IC3D (2008) CLASSIFICATION[17] (C = CATEGORY)

Epithelial and subepithelial dystrophies

1. Epithelial basement membrane dystrophy (EBMD)—majority degenerative, some C1

Table 31.1: *Prevalence of corneal dystrophy in patients undergoing keratoplasty*							
	Iran[9] *1994–2004*	*Canada[10]* *1996–2004*	*India[11]* *1997–2003*	*Singapore[12]* *1991–2003*	*USA[13]* *1982–1996*	*USA[14]* *2001–2005*	*Italy[15]* *2002–11*
Total cases	19,668	794	2,022	901	4,217	1,162	3,615
No. of cases with corneal dystrophy	1,272 (6.47%)	101 (13%)	78 (3.85%)	64 (7.1%)	978 (23.2%)	126 (10.8%)	60 (1.8%)

2. Epithelial recurrent erosion dystrophy (ERED) C4 (Smolandiensis variant), C3
3. Subepithelial mucinous corneal dystrophy (SMCD) C4
4. Mutation in keratin genes: Meesmann corneal dystrophy (MECD) C1
5. Lisch epithelial corneal dystrophy (LECD) C2
6. Gelatinous drop-like corneal dystrophy (GDLD) C1

Bowman layer dystrophies
1. Reis-Bücklers corneal dystrophy (RBCD)—granular corneal dystrophy, type 3 C1
2. Thiel-Behnke corneal dystrophy (TBCD) C1, potential variant C2
3. Grayson-Wilbrandt corneal dystrophy (GWCD) C4

Stromal dystrophies
1. TGFBI corneal dystrophies
   A. Lattice corneal dystrophy
      i. Lattice corneal dystrophy, TGFBI type (LCD): Classic lattice corneal dystrophy (LCD1) C1, variants (III, IIIA, I/IIIA, and IV) are C1
      ii. Lattice corneal dystrophy, gelsolin type (LCD2) C1 (this is not a true corneal dystrophy but is included here for ease of differential diagnosis)
   B. Granular corneal dystrophy C1
      i. Granular corneal dystrophy, type 1 (classic) (GCD1) C1
      ii. Granular corneal dystrophy, type 2 (granular-lattice) (GCD2) C1
      iii. Granular corneal dystrophy, type 3 (RBCD): Reis-Bücklers C1
2. Macular corneal dystrophy (MCD) C1
3. Schnyder corneal dystrophy (SCD) C1
4. Congenital stromal corneal dystrophy (CSCD) C1
5. Fleck corneal dystrophy (FCD) C1
6. Posterior amorphous corneal dystrophy (PACD) C3
7. Central cloudy dystrophy of François (CCDF) C4
8. Pre-Descemet corneal dystrophy (PDCD) C4

Descemet membrane and endothelial dystrophies
1. Fuchs endothelial corneal dystrophy (FECD) C1, C2, or C3

2. Posterior polymorphous corneal dystrophy (PPCD) C1 or C2
3. Congenital hereditary endothelial dystrophy 1 (CHED1) C2
4. Congenital hereditary endothelial dystrophy 2 (CHED2) C1
5. X-linked endothelial corneal dystrophy (XECD) C2

CHANGES IN THE 2015 IC3D[18]

It was noted that majority of the corneal dystrophies involved more than one corneal layer, and therefore classifying dystrophies based solely on the commonly involved layer is not appropriate. As an example, previously classified Bowman layer dystrophies such as Reis-Bücklers corneal dystrophy (RBCD) and Thiel-Behnke corneal dystrophy (TBCD) involve not only the sub-epithelial layers but also the anterior stroma and deep stroma in late stages. Therefore, in the updated classification, genetics and primary cell of origin have been given more importance than the primary anatomical layer of involvement. The Bowman acellular layer and Descemet acellular membrane, as a result, have been excluded from the classification.

THE IC3D EDITION 2 (2015) CLASSIFICATION[18] (C = CATEGORY)

Epithelial and subepithelial dystrophies
1. Epithelial basement membrane dystrophy (EBMD)—majority degenerative, rarely C1
2. Epithelial recurrent erosion dystrophies (EREDs)—Franceschetti corneal dystrophy (FRCD) C3, Dystrophia Smolandiensis (DS) C3, and Dystrophia Helsinglandica (DH) C3
3. Subepithelial mucinous corneal dystrophy (SMCD) C4
4. Meesmann corneal dystrophy (MECD) C1
5. Lisch epithelial corneal dystrophy (LECD) C2
6. Gelatinous drop-like corneal dystrophy (GDLD) C1

Epithelial–stromal TGFBI dystrophies
1. Reis-Bücklers corneal dystrophy (RBCD) C1
2. Thiel-Behnke corneal dystrophy (TBCD) C1
3. Lattice corneal dystrophy, type 1 (LCD1) C1—variants (III, IIIA, I/IIIA, IV) of lattice corneal dystrophy C1

4. Granular corneal dystrophy, type 1 (GCD1) C1

5. Granular corneal dystrophy, type 2 (GCD2) C1

Stromal dystrophies

1. Macular corneal dystrophy (MCD) C1

2. Schnyder corneal dystrophy (SCD) C1

3. Congenital stromal corneal dystrophy (CSCD) C1

4. Fleck corneal dystrophy (FCD) C1

5. Posterior amorphous corneal dystrophy (PACD) C1

6. Central cloudy dystrophy of François (CCDF) C4

7. Pre-Descemet corneal dystrophy (PDCD) C1 or C4

Endothelial dystrophies

1. Fuchs endothelial corneal dystrophy (FECD) C1, C2, or C3

2. Posterior polymorphous corneal dystrophy (PPCD) C1 or C2

3. Congenital hereditary endothelial dystrophy (CHED) C1

4. X-linked endothelial corneal dystrophy (XECD) C2

Removed dystrophies

Grayson-Wilbrandt corneal dystrophy (GWCD) C4

Important facts of revised IC3D classification

- Grayson-Wilbrandt corneal dystrophy (GWCD) C4 is removed from revised classification.
- Revised IC3D classification has grouped dystrophies with a known common genetic basis, i.e. TGFB1 dystrophies together, although they affect multiple layers rather than confined to one corneal layer.
- Confocal microscopy also has emerged as a helpful tool to reveal *in vivo* features of several corneal dystrophies.
- Bowman acellular layer and Descemet acellular membrane have been excluded from revised classification.
- *As clinical manifestations vary widely with different entities, corneal dystrophies should be suspected* when corneal transparency is lost or corneal opacities occur spontaneously, particularly in both corneas, and especially in the

presence of a positive family history or in the offspring of consanguineous parents.

- *The management of corneal dystrophies* varies with the specific disease. Some are treated medically or with methods that excise or ablate the abnormal corneal tissue photo-therapeutic keratectomy (PTK). Corneal transplantation—penetrating or lamellar keratoplasty—may be required for visual rehabilitation in advanced cases. Other less debilitating or asymptomatic dystrophies do not warrant treatment. The prognosis varies from minimal effect on the quality and quantity of vision to corneal blindness, with marked phenotypic variability.

EPITHELIAL AND SUBEPITHELIAL DYSTROPHIES

EPITHELIAL BASEMENT MEMBRANE DYSTROPHY (EBMD)

CLINICAL PROFILE

Alternative names: Map-dot-fingerprint dystrophy, Cogan microcystic epithelial dystrophy, anterior basement membrane dystrophy, dystrophic recurrent erosion.

Epithelial basement membrane dystrophy is characterised by recurrent corneal erosions that occur as a result of abnormal epithelial-basement membrane adhesion complexes.[19] It is the most commonly encountered anterior corneal dystrophy in clinical practice.

Inheritance. Most cases have no definite hereditary pattern. Although autosomal dominant inheritance has been documented in a few cases it is now considered as a primarily degenerative disorder.[20]

Genetic locus. The genetic locus has been mapped to chromosome 5 (5q31); gene TGFBI has been isolated in a minority of cases.[21, 22]

Onset. The most common corneal dystrophy usually present in adult life, rarely in childhood.

Symptoms. The disease usually manifests in adult life around 30 years of age and has rarely been documented in childhood. Patients may remain asymptomatic or develop recurrent erosions with pain (Fig. 31.1), lacrimation, and blurred vision. Visual acuity, when affected is

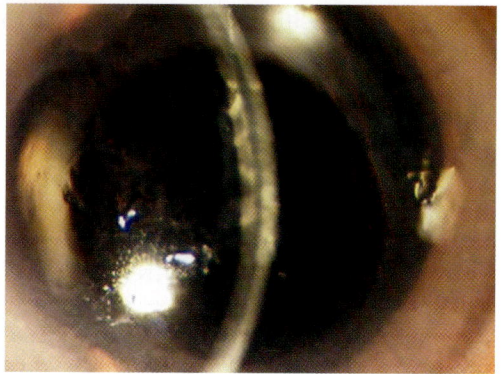

Fig. 31.1: *Recurrent corneal erosions in epithelial basement membrane dystrophy*

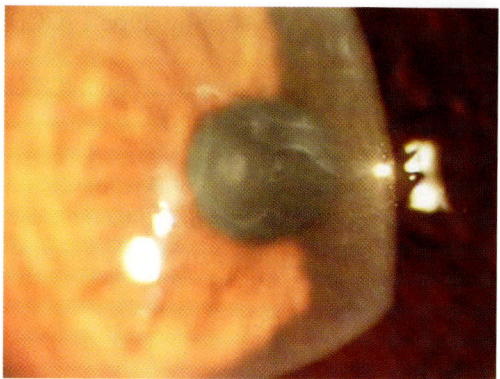

Fig. 31.3: *Map-like areas in epithelial basement membrane dystrophy*

usually a result of irregular astigmatism and an increase in higher-order aberration with resulting monocular diplopia and ghost images.

Signs

This disease is characterised by the appearance of maps, dots and fingerprint lines, which may occur in isolation or combination, the latter being a more common presentation (Figs 31.2 and 31.3).[23]

- *Maps* appear as gray geographical patches and are best observed on broad tangential illumination.
- *Dots (Cogan)* appear as irregular, round or comma-shaped gray-white intraepithelial opacities; assembled like an archipelago in the central cornea.
- *Dots (blebs of Bron and Brown)* are visualized as small clear round dots in a pebbled glass

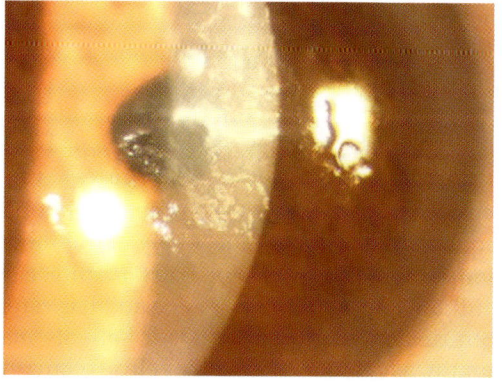

Fig. 31.2: *Map-like areas with dots in a case of epithelial basement membrane dystrophy*

pattern and are best appreciated on retro-illumination.

- *Fingerprint lines* appear as parallel, curvilinear, refractile, branching lines with club shaped terminations and are also best seen on retroillumination.

A combination of maps and dots is noted most frequently, followed by maps alone.

HISTOPATHOLOGY

- *Recurrent erosions* occur due to lack of hemi-desmosomal connections between the epithelial cells and the abnormal basement membrane, the primary pathology being the abnormal synthesis of the epithelial basement membrane.
- *Maps* are areas of projections of the abnormal multilamellar basement membrane into the epithelium.
- *Fingerprint lines* represent rib-like intra-epithelial extensions of basal laminar material.
- *Dots (Cogan)* are intraepithelial pseudocysts containing cytoplasmic debris.
- *Dots (blebs of Bron and Brown)* are irregular subepithelial accumulation of fibrillo-granular material.[23]

In vivo confocal microscopy images reveal abnormal epithelial basement membrane protruding into the corneal epithelium, epithelial cell abnormalities, and microcysts.[24] No abnormalities are observed in superficial epithelial cells or the stroma. Confocal microscopy has been reported to assist in the diagnosis of EBMD in patients suffering from recurrent erosion syndrome, particularly in patients with no corneal changes visible biomicroscopically.

MANAGEMENT

1. *Corneal scraping or debridement* may be performed in cases of recurrent corneal erosions. Following the procedure, a *soft contact lens* is placed for 24–48 hours and *topical antibiotics* and *lubricants* are given. A five-year cumulative probability of recurrence up to 44.7% has been reported following epithelial debridement for anterior basement membrane dystrophy.[25]

2. *Conservative therapy with hypertonic sodium chloride* that acts by dehydrating the epithelium and thus allowing it to adhere better, along with lubricating eye drops may be useful in reducing the frequency and severity of attacks.

3. *Stromal punctures.* It has been suggested that treatment of recurrent corneal erosions with debridement may be a better and safer option than stromal punctures with a 23- to 25-gauge needle.[26] *Anterior stromal puncture by Nd:YAG laser* has also been reported as a simple and effective procedure to treat recurrent corneal erosion with minimal complications.[27]

4. *Phototherapeutic keratectomy* using an excimer laser with low pulse energy and low number of pulses has been reported as an effective and minimal invasive treatment modality to achieve a fast and durable epithelial closure, prevent recurrent corneal erosions, and to increase visual acuity in most patients. A success rate of 84.6% to 100% has been reported by various authors.[28–31] Shallow ablations with mean ablation depth of 4.6 microns have been recommended by Zaidmman et al in view of decreased complications.[29, 30]

EPITHELIAL RECURRENT EROSION DYSTROPHY (ERED)

CLINICAL PROFILE

Alternative name: Franceschetti recurrent epithelial dystrophy.[32]

Variants include:
- Franceschetti corneal dystrophy (FRCD)
- Dystrophia Smolandiensis (DS)
- Dystrophia Helsinglandica (DH).

Inheritance. Inheritance pattern is autosomal dominant. The genetic locus remains unknown.[33]

Symptoms

Onset is usually in the first decade of life.

Presenting symptoms
- Most patients experience attacks of redness, photophobia, epiphora, and ocular pain due to corneal erosions that usually last a week (Fig. 31.4).
- *Attacks are recurrent*, often begin at night and may be precipitated by exposure to sunlight, dust, smoke and lack of sleep.
- *Some patients may present* with increased sensitivity of eyes for years or with visual impairment resulting from central corneal opacification that may occur in about half the patients.
- *Attacks generally decline* in frequency and intensity in the fourth and fifth decades of life and cease by the age of 50 years.

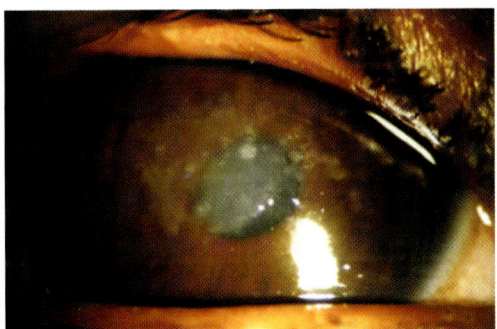

Fig. 31.4: *A case of gelatinous droplet corneal dystrophy with sub-epithelial, multiple, nodular lesions. Note the significant blepharospasm and photophobia*

Signs

- *Recurrent corneal erosions* appear typically at 4–6 years of age but occasionally, cases have been reported as early as 8 months of age. These may be precipitated by minimal trauma or may be spontaneous.
- *Biomicroscopically, evident changes* are usually absent during pain-free intervals, although the cornea may sometimes develop subepithelial haze or blebs between attacks. Diffuse, central, subepithelial opacification with subepithelial

fibrosis may be evident in advanced cases; formation of central corneal keloid like opacities is characteristic of the Smolandiensis variant (DS).[34]

HISTOPATHOLOGY

Light microscopic examination reveals irregular basal epithelium with enlarged intercellular spaces with intracellular and intercellular Alcian blue-positive deposits in FRCD. Partial destruction or even absence of the Bowman layer with intervening avascular connective tissue pannus between the basal epithelium and Bowman layer is also noted.

On the other hand, the keloid-like structure stains positive with Congo red in DS (negative in the former variant) indicating secondary amyloidosis.[34]

MANAGEMENT

- *Management of recurrent erosions* is on similar lines to that of epithelial basement membrane dystrophy.
- *Keratoplasty* is more commonly required in the DS variant with about a quarter of patients eventually requiring corneal grafts at mean age of 44 years. Recurrence has been noted at an average interval of 15 months; however, the opacities are mainly located in the graft periphery, sparing the central optical zone for many years.

▮ SUBEPITHELIAL MUCINOUS CORNEAL DYSTROPHY (SMCD)

CLINICAL PROFILE

Inheritance

This dystrophy has an autosomal dominant pattern of inheritance, although X-linked inheritance cannot be entirely excluded. The genetic locus and the gene remain unknown for this dystrophy.[35]

Symptoms

The onset is characterised by frequent, recurrent corneal erosions in the first decade, which usually subside during adolescence with subsequent formation of subepithelial opacities, causing progressive decreased vision.[35]

Signs

Bilateral, homogenous subepithelial haze is noted that is most dense centrally, and fades towards the periphery.

HISTOPATHOLOGY

Light microscopy reveals a subepithelial band of eosinophilic, periodic acid–Schiff-positive, Alcian blue-positive, Masson trichrome-positive hyaluronidase-sensitive material anterior to the Bowman layer. The overlying epithelium is thinned out. Immunohistochemistry staining is positive for combination of chondroitin-4-sulfate and dermatan sulfate.[35]

MANAGEMENT

Initial treatment includes management of recurrent corneal erosions. The superficial location of the pathology makes PTK a potential treatment modality.

▮ MEESMANN CORNEAL DYSTROPHY (MECD)

Alternate name: Juvenile hereditary epithelial dystrophy.
Variant: Stocker-Holt variant.

CLINICAL PROFILE

- This bilateral, diffuse corneal dystrophy involves the accumulation of intracyto-plasmic debris in the corneal epithelium, manifesting clinically with the formation of epithelial cysts.
- This dystrophy was first described clinically by Pameijer (1935).[36] The histopathological description was given by Meesmann (1938).[37]

Inheritance

Autosomal dominant inheritance with in-complete penetrance and variable expressibility is seen in a majority of cases. Autosomal recessive form has been reported by Stocker and Holt.[38]

Genetic locus has been mapped to chromosome 12q13 (KRT3); and the gene keratin K3 (KRT3) has been implicated.[39] Locus 17q12 (KRT12) and gene keratin K12 has been isolated in cases with the Stocker-Holt variant.[40] These genes are known to encode cytoskeletal proteins.

Symptoms

Onset of symptoms occurs in early childhood and clinical signs may be visible as early as 12 months of age. The dystrophy runs a slowly progressive course and majority of the patients may remain asymptomatic till the fourth or fifth decade of life.[41, 42]

Mild visual reduction, glare, light sensitivity or painful recurrent epithelial erosions may be present in some cases. Most patients retain good functional vision, although a few may complain of blurred vision secondary to corneal irregularity and scarring. Patients with the Stocker-Holt variant demonstrate more severe signs and symptoms with a relatively earlier onset.[38]

Signs

Corneal involvement is usually bilateral. Multiple, tiny epithelial vesicles are seen extending up to the limbus and are present most numerous in the interpalpebral area with clear surrounding epithelium. These appear as white spots on focal illumination and are seen as refractile cysts of retroillumination. Cysts may coalesce to form refractile linear opacities with intervening areas of clear cornea.

Stocker-Holt variant encompasses the entire cornea. Fine grayish, punctate epithelial opacities that take up fluorescein and fine linear opacities in whorl-like pattern are visible.[38]

HISTOPATHOLOGY

Light microscopy demonstrates thickened or disorganized epithelium filled with cysts containing periodic acid–Schiff-positive cellular debris. Variably thickened epithelium with vacuolated and degenerating cells along with thickened basement membrane that extends into the epithelium is seen in Stocker-Holt variant. Bowman's layer and anterior stroma are unaffected.

Transmission electron microscopy reveals intracytoplasmic "peculiar substance" representing a focal collection of fibrogranular material surrounded by tangles of cytoplasmic filaments. Tuft et al have reported hyporeflective areas in the basal epithelium ranging from 40 to 150 mm in diameter, with potential reflective spots in the center, that is visible on confocal microscopy.[43]

Associations

Cremona et al reported a rare case of bilateral and symmetric Meesmann corneal dystrophy concurrent with bilateral epithelial basement membrane dystrophy and bilateral but asymmetric posterior polymorphous corneal dystrophy in a patient of Armenian origin.[44]

MANAGEMENT

- *No treatment.* Most patients remain asymptomatic and may not require any treatment.
- *Palliative treatment* includes ocular lubricants, cycloplegics, and therapeutic contact lenses.
- *In severe cases*, management with epithelial debridement, phototherapeutic keratectomy, and lamellar keratoplasty has been advocated.[45] Yeung et al have suggested keratectomy with mitomycin C application in recurrent cases of Meesmann's dystrophy.[46]

LISCH EPITHELIAL CORNEAL DYSTROPHY (LECD)

Alternative names: Band-shaped and whorled microcystic dystrophy of the corneal epithelium.

Inheritance

X-chromosomal dominant inheritance with genetic locus at Xp 22.3 has been identified. The gene however remains unknown.[47, 48]

Clinical features

Symptoms. The typical onset is in childhood with a slowly progressive course. Most patients are asymptomatic, with few reporting blurred vision if the pupillary zone is involved.

Signs. Direct illumination reveals localized gray opacities of varying patterns: Whorl-like, radial, band shaped, flame or feathery shaped, or club shaped.[49–51] Indirect illumination reveals intraepithelial multiple, densely crowded microcysts with clear surrounding epithelium.

HISTOPATHOLOGY

Light microscopy documents diffuse cytoplasmic vacuolization of all cells in the affected area; the vacuoles are PAS positive, diastase labile, Luxol fast blue and Sudan black negative, consistent with presence of glycogen.

Confocal microscopy reveals highly hyper-reflective granular cytoplasm without any distinct deposits and hyporeflective nuclei. Uniform involvement of all epithelial layers within the affected areas along with well demarcated borders with adjacent normal epithelium and involvement of the limbal area are also noted.

MANAGEMENT

- The corneal abnormalities have been reported to recur after *corneal scrapping*.[52]
- Lisch et al reported that wearing *contact lenses* for a longer duration cause a significant regression of corneal opacities in LECD, the mechanism postulated as contact lens-induced thinning of corneal epithelium and reduction of epithelial layers.[53]

GELATINOUS DROP-LIKE CORNEAL DYSTROPHY (GDLD)

CLINICAL PROFILE

Alternative names: Subepithelial amyloidosis; primary familial amyloidosis.[54]

Inheritance

Inheritance pattern is autosomal recessive. The genetic locus has been isolated to 1p32; and tumor-associated calcium signal transducer 2 (TACSTD2, previously M1S1) gene has been implicated.[55, 56]

Symptoms

Onset is around first to second decade of life with patients presenting with significant decrease in vision, photophobia, irritation, redness, and lacrimation.

Signs

The lesions begin initially in the subepithelial layers and may even be confused with band-shaped keratopathy. They progress to form clusters of small multiple nodules and acquire a mulberry configuration (Fig. 31.4), which eventually may progress to development of stromal opacification or larger nodular

kumquat-like lesions in advanced stages (Fig. 31.5). The lesions show late staining with fluorescein, indicating hyperpermeability of the corneal epithelium. Superficial vascularization may be noted. This dystrophy is usually found in Japanese people, but has been reported in other regions of the world as well.[57]

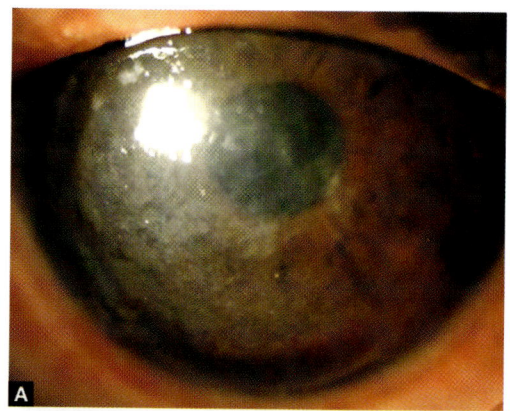

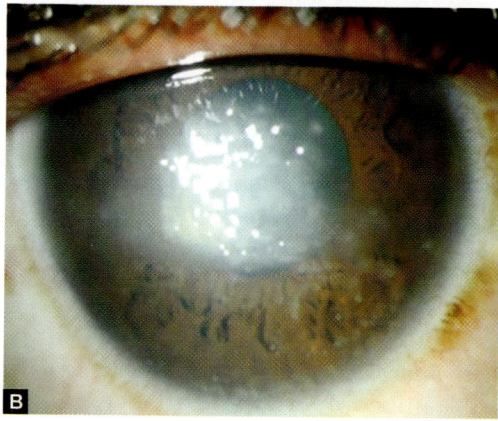

Fig. 31.5A and B: *Stromal opacification and larger nodular kumquat-like lesions in a case of gelatinous droplet corneal dystrophy*

Confocal microscopy

In vivo confocal microscopy reveals mild disorganization of the overall epithelial architecture with large accumulations of brightly reflective material within or beneath the epithelium and within the anterior stroma.

HISTOPATHOLOGY

Light microscopy demonstrates subepithelial and stromal amyloid deposits. Disruption of epithelial tight junctions in the superficial epithelium and the presence of amyloid in the basal epithelial layer is visible on transmission electron microscopy.

MANAGEMENT

Surgical management in the form of superficial keratectomy or corneal transplant procedures like lamellar keratoplasty or penetrating keratoplasty may be required for visual rehabilitation.[58,59]

- *Deep lamellar keratoplasty* has been reported to successfully treat gelatinous drop-like corneal dystrophy.[60] Recurrence is common after keratoplasty, typically within a few years and in nearly half the grafts. Lasram et al reported that the five cases of GDLD treated by them required multiple keratoplasties at a mean interval of five years because of recurrence of the disease on the corneal graft.[61]
- *Phototherapeutic keratectomy.* Ito et al reported that PTK may be a safe and useful modality to remove corneal opacities that recur after lamellar grafts.[62]

EPITHELIAL–STROMAL TGFBI DYSTROPHIES

This is a new subgroup added in the updated IC3D classification[15], which consists of previously classified Bowman layer dystrophies (namely Reis-Bücklers corneal dystrophy (RBCD) and Thiel-Behnke corneal dystrophy (TBCD)) and TGFBI stromal corneal dystrophies (namely lattice corneal dystrophy and its variants and granular corneal dystrophy and its variants). As mentioned earlier, this reclassification was done as it was noted that RBCD and TBCD, both involving TGFBI gene, affect the stromal layers in addition to Bowman's layer. Also, other TGBI dystrophies, LCD and GCD, which involve epithelium and stroma, were regrouped under this common heading. It is also important to note that Grayson-Wilbrandt corneal dystrophy that was previously classified as a Bowman layer dystrophy has now been removed from the updated classification as there is not enough evidence for it to be classified as a distinct clinical entity.

These dystrophies result from mutations in TGFBI gene encoding keratoepithelin. Transforming growth factor, beta-induced, 68kDa, also known as TGFBI (initially called BIGH3), is a protein which in humans is encoded by the TGFBI gene.[2] This gene encodes a protein that binds to types I, II and IV collagens. It is found in many extracellular matrix proteins modulating cell adhesion and serves as a ligand recognition sequence for several integrins. The protein is induced by transforming growth factor-beta and acts to inhibit cell adhesion.

REIS-BÜCKLERS CORNEAL DYSTROPHY (RBCD)

This dystrophy was first reported by Reis in 1917.[63] Detailed description was given by Bückler in 1949.[64] It primarily involves the Bowman's layer with secondary alterations in the epithelium and the stroma.

Alternative names include:
- Corneal dystrophy of Bowman layer, type I
- Geographic corneal dystrophy (Weidle)
- Superficial granular corneal dystrophy
- Atypical granular corneal dystrophy
- Granular corneal dystrophy, type 3
- Anterior limiting membrane dystrophy, type I.

CLINICAL PROFILE

Inheritance

Autosomal dominant inheritance with variable expressibility has been noted. Genetic locus lies at 5q31; Transforming growth factor beta-induced (TGFBI) gene has been implicated.[65–67]

Symptoms

Onset is in the first decade of life with recurrent corneal erosions manifesting as pain, redness, tearing and visual impairment. These attacks become less severe after the second decade, however, slowly progressive deterioration of vision owing to diffuse opacification is usually noted.

Signs

Irregular and coarse geographic opacities are noted at the Bowman's layer and superficial stromal level, secondary to generalised replacement of the Bowman's layer by irregular collagen fibres.[68] These are best seen with broad oblique illumination and may be linear, geographical, honeycomb or ring-like and are present in varying densities (Fig. 31.6). Peripheral cornea is usually spared, although a diffuse haze extending up to the limbus may be seen in advanced cases. Corneal sensations are decreased and prominent corneal nerves may be noted. Early cases may be confused with Thiel-Behnke corneal dystrophy.

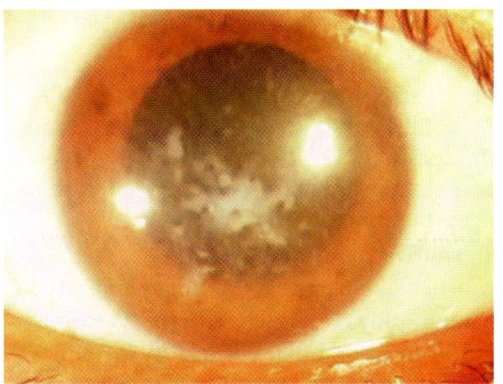

Fig. 31.6: *Reis-Bücklers corneal dystrophy showing irregular and coarse geographic opacities in the Bowman's layer and superficial stroma*

HISTOPATHOLOGY

- *Bowman's layer* is replaced by a sheet of irregularly placed collagen fibres, seen as granular deposits that stain with Masson trichrome red, which in advanced cases, can even extend to the subepithelial stroma.
- *Epithelial cells and anterior stromal keratocytes* show degenerative changes such as swelling of the endoplasmic reticulum and vacuole formation.
- *Posterior epithelial layer* shows a saw-tooth configuration.
- *Subepithelial electron-dense*, rod-shaped bodies that are immune-positive for transforming growth factor beta-induced protein (kerato-epithelin) are noted on electron microscopy. This is an important definitive distinguishing feature from TBCD where curly fibres are present.[69]

Confocal microscopy may also enable differentiation of TBCD and RBCD *in vivo*[70] with presence of epithelial basal cell layer deposits that display homogeneous reflectivity with round edges accompanying dark shadows in the former and similar deposits but with extremely high reflectivity from small granular materials without any shadows in the latter. Also, the reflectivity of materials that replace the Bowman's layer is reported to be much higher in Reis-Bücklers corneal dystrophy than in Thiel-Behnke corneal dystrophy.

MANAGEMENT

Conservative therapy. Recurrent corneal erosions are treated with conservative therapy in the initial stages.

- *PTK* has been reported to be an effective modality for the treatment, although recurrence is a common concern. Dinh et al reported that 47% of the eyes with Reis-Bücklers dystrophy developed clinically significant recurrence at an average of 21.6 months after PTK.[71]
- *Adjunctive application of topical mitomycin-C 0.02%* may be helpful in reducing the recurrence of the disease after PTK.[72] Corneal electrolysis has been reported to effectively treat subepithelial opacities in RBCD.[73] Keratoplasty may be required in severe cases.[74]

THIEL-BEHNKE CORNEAL DYSTROPHY (TBCD)

Alternative names include:

- Corneal dystrophy of Bowman layer, type II (CDB2)
- Honeycomb-shaped corneal dystrophy
- Anterior limiting membrane dystrophy, type II
- Curly fibers corneal dystrophy
- Waardenburg-Jonkers corneal dystrophy.

CLINICAL PROFILE

Inheritance

Autosomal dominant inheritance with genetic locus at 10q24 has been demonstrated; gene involved is TGFBI.[75]

Symptoms

Progressive erosions begin in childhood that diminish with time; however, slowly progressive deterioration of vision is noticed subsequently. The course of the disease is similar to RBCD but less severe and relatively later in onset as compared to RBCD.

Signs

- *Early stages reveal* solitary flecks with scattered opacities at the Bowman's level, followed later by symmetrical subepithelial reticular honeycomb like opacities, sparing the peripheral cornea.[76]
- *In advanced cases*, opacities can progress to deep stromal layers and corneal periphery.
- *Corneal sensations* are typically normal.
- It may be impossible to distinguish it clinically from Reis-Bücklers corneal dystrophy; however, presence of more irregular diffuse opacities with clear interruptions in RBCD as opposed to be multiple flecks with reticular formation in TBCD may help in clinical differentiation.

HISTOPATHOLOGY

- *A fibrillogranular material is deposited* under the epithelium and projects into the overlying cells in a "saw-tooth" configuration.
- *Alternating irregular thickening and thinning* of the epithelial layer to compensate for ridges and furrows of underlying stroma, with focal absence of the epithelial basement membrane is also noted.
- *Electron microscopy demonstrates* pathognomonic curly collagen fibres with a diameter of 9–15 nm and distinguishes this dystrophy from RBCD. These curly fibres demonstrate immunopositivity for TGFBI protein (keratoepithelin).[69]
- *The confocal microscopic images* may also enable differentiation from RBCD.[70]

▓ LATTICE CORNEAL DYSTROPHY

Alternative names: Biber-Haab-Dimmer[2].
Variants: Lattice corneal dystrophy (classic) and variants (IIIA, I/IIIA, IV)[77, 78, 79]

CLINICAL PROFILE

LCD was first described by Swiss ophthalmologist Hugo Biber in 1890.[2] Although the classic LCD is known to occur in numerous countries and is more common in the Western world, LCD variants are geographically restricted; LCD type IIIA and LCD type IV have been reported predominantly from Japan and Italy, and the two LCD type IV variants were reported to be derived from solitary founder mutations in Japan and Italy.

The previously designated lattice corneal dystrophy type 2 (LCD 2) or Meretoja syndrome,[80] is now known to be only an ocular manifestation of systemic amyloidosis, and is termed familial amyloidosis, Finnish type, or gelsolin type.[81]

Inheritance

Autosomal dominant with genetic locus and gene identified as 5q31 and TGFBI respectively. The LCD variants are caused by more than two dozen distinct heterozygous amyloidogenic mutations, nearly all of which are located in the fourth FAS1 domain of TGFBI.

Symptoms

Onset is usually in the first to second decade of life with symptoms of ocular discomfort and pain as a result of recurrent corneal erosions. Visual impairment is progressive and usually becomes significant around the fourth decade of life, but may be seen as soon as the first decade in some patients. LCD variants (previously designated types IIIA, I/IIIA, IV, and polymorphic amyloidosis) have a delayed onset compared with classic LCD.

Signs

- *Central superficial fleck-like opacities* are usually the first manifestations of the disease and become evident by the end of the first decade of life.
- *Retroillumination reveals* few isolated fine lattice lines, predominantly in the periphery and anterior stroma in initial stages.
- *Filamentous opacities* appear in the superficial layers of the cornea with intertwining delicate branching processes, particularly within the central corneal stroma, usually by the end of the first decade (Fig. 31.7).
- *Corneal sensation* is often diminished.

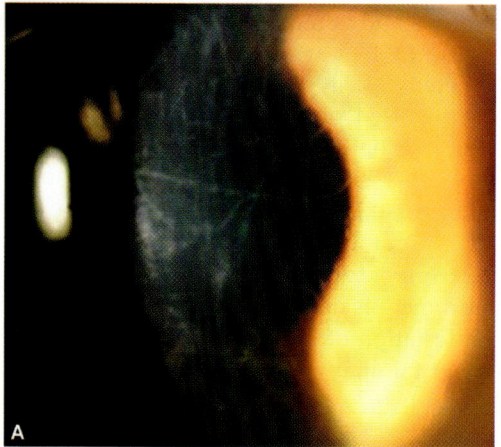

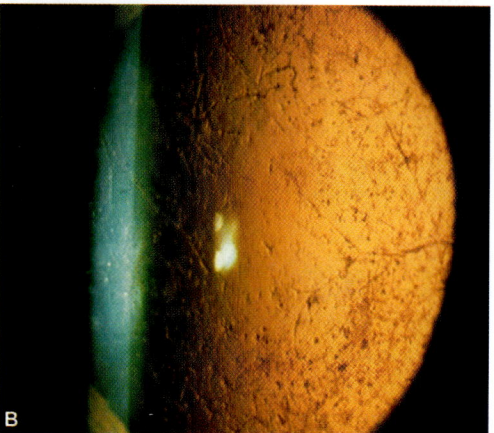

Fig. 31.7A and B: *Branching filaments in the corneal stroma, creating a lattice effect. A network of delicate, criss-cross filamentous opacities are seen within the cornea in lattice dystrophy. (Left: Direct illumination; Right: Retro-illumination)*

- *The interwoven linear opaque filaments* have some resemblance to nerves. Eventually, they spread centrifugally and to deeper layers, but the far peripheral stroma, Descemet membrane and endothelium remain un-involved.
- *Recurrent corneal erosions* may precede the corneal opacities and even appear in individuals lacking recognizable stromal disease. As the disease progresses, a diffuse subepithelial ground glass haze develops concurrently with the lattice lines in the central and paracentral cornea (Fig. 31.8).
- *Significant reduction in vision occurs* commonly by the fourth decade, although some cases

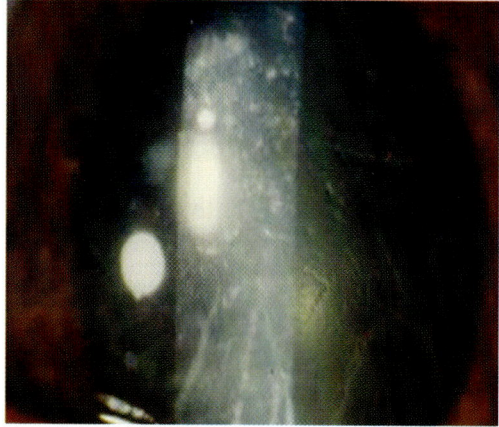

Fig. 31.8: *A case of lattice dystrophy with thick and opaque lattice lines that impart a ground glass haze to the cornea*

may require surgical intervention as early as second to third decade. Both corneas are usually symmetrically involved, but some-times one cornea remains clear or has discrete rather than the linear opacities.

There may be asymmetric involvement of both eyes and the number of lattice lines usually vary between two eyes of the same patient; unilateral cases have also been described.

The LCD IIIA variant commonly displays lattice lines that are thicker and more centrally placed as compared to classic LCD, whereas LCD IV variant is characterised by relatively deeper deposits without epithelial erosion.

HISTOPATHOLOGY

Light microscopy reveals atrophy and disruption of the epithelium along with degeneration of basal epithelial cells and focal thinning or absence of Bowman's layer that progressively increases with age.

- *Eosinophilic amyloid deposits* form a layer between epithelial basement membrane and Bowman's layer and distort the stromal architecture of corneal lamellae. Amyloid deposits stain positive with Congo red and display green birefringence with a polarizing filter and red-green dichroism when a green filter is added with this stain. Metachromasia is noted with crystal violet and fluorescence is noted with use of thioflavin T staining.
- Descemet's membrane and endothelium are essentially normal.

Transmission electron microscopy reveals extracellular masses of fine, electron-dense and uniformly sized fibrils with a diameter of 8 to 10 nm, arranged in a random pattern, that are characteristic of amyloid protein. Keratocytes in the areas of amyloid deposition are relatively lesser in number and are often degenerated with cytoplasmic vacuolization, whereas others appear metabolically active. Linear and branching structures in stroma with variable reflectivity and poorly demarcated margins can be seen on confocal microscopy.[82, 83]

Like nerves, the linear deposits of classic LCD are argyrophilic in silver impregnated preparations, but nerves have not been identified in relation to the eosinophilic amyloid deposits. Amyloid deposits occur throughout the corneal stroma[84] and coincide with the lattice pattern of lines and other opacities.[82] The amyloid seems to react mainly with antibodies to the N-terminal sequence of TGFBI protein and not with those to the C-terminal portion.[85]

The majority of cases of LCD1 throughout the world have been associated with a C→T transition at nucleotide 417 (417 C→T) in exon 4 of the TGFBI gene. This causes a p.Arg124Cys mutation in the affected codon.[86]

FAMILIAL AMYLOIDOSIS (FINNISH OR MERETOJA TYPE)

Previously designated as LCD 2, it has now been removed from the IC3D classification as this is now known to be systemic amyloidosis with corneal lattice lines. It is most commonly seen in Finland, where the disease was first discovered and most extensively studied.[80]

Clinical features. The condition first becomes apparent after 20 years of age with symptoms of dry eye and recurrent erosions.

- *Visual acuity* is usually normal until the sixth decade because the dystrophy progresses from the peripheral to central cornea.
- It has a slowly progressive course; the majority of affected individuals are in good health till the seventh decade. At around 40 years of age, some people may have sub-epithelial scarring resulting in corneal haze that can significantly obscure vision.

- *Bilateral involvement* with randomly scattered short fine glassy lines, which are less numerous, more delicate and more radially oriented than those in LCD1, affecting primarily the peripheral cornea and sparing the central cornea are usually seen. The cornea has fewer amorphous deposits than classic LCD and epithelial erosions are not a feature.
- *Finnish type amyloidosis* is a form of amyloidosis associated with gelsolin gene.[81] In persons homozygous for the relevant mutation in the GSN gene, the disorder begins earlier. Vision does not usually become significantly impaired before the age of 65 years.
- *Corneal abnormalities are accompanied by* a progressive and bilateral cranial and peripheral neuropathy, dysarthria, a dry and extremely lax, itchy skin with amyloid deposits.

Associated systemic conditions include cutis laxa and ataxia, a characteristic "mask-like" facial expression, protruding lips with impaired movement, pendulous ears and blepharochalasis.[87, 88]

Amyloid is composed of a mutated 71-amino acid long fragment of gelsolin and this protein accumulates in the corneal stroma, in addition to sclera, choroid and adnexal blood vessels as well as the lacrimal gland and perineurium of ciliary nerves. The amyloid is also found in the heart, kidney, skin, nerves, wall of arteries, and other tissues.[89]

Immunohistochemistry demonstrates deposition of mutated gelsolin in the conjunctiva, in the sclera, in the ciliary body, along the choriocapillaris, in the perineurium of ciliary nerves, in the walls of ciliary vessels, and in the optic nerve. Extraocular amyloid is found in arterial walls, peripheral nerves and glomeruli.

MANAGEMENT

Conservative treatment. Recurrent epithelial erosions are usually treated with preservative-free tear substitutes, along with ointments, eye patching or bandage contact lens. With effective care, these erosions usually heal within three days, although occasional sensations of pain may occur for the next six to eight weeks.

Amniotic membrane transplantation may be done for persistent epithelial defects.

Phototherapeutic keratectomy may be tried in all patients with superficially accentuated opacities in lattice dystrophy before undertaking a more invasive procedure, such as lamellar or penetrating keratoplasty. [90]

Corneal transplant is indicated in cases with visually significant epithelial scarring and corneal haze. Although people with lattice dystrophy have an excellent chance for a successful transplant, the disease may recur in the donor cornea as early as three years post-keratoplasty. A corneal graft is usually not indicated until after the fourth decade, but may be required as early as 20 years of age in some cases. The outcome of penetrating graft is excellent, but amyloid may deposit in the grafted donor tissue.

- *Anterior lamellar keratoplasty*, wherein partial removal of the diseased recipient stroma is done, has emerged as a good alternative to full thickness keratoplasty over the last few decades. Although there is no consensus regarding the better surgical option, few studies have shown that visual outcomes are slightly better with lamellar keratoplasty.

- *Recurrence of amyloidosis in the residual stroma is a concern.*[91] The results of the graft are generally good, but it is possible that the dystrophy may recur in the donor cornea within five to ten years. In one study, about half of the transplant patients with lattice dystrophy had a recurrence of the disease two to 26 years after the transplant. Of these, 15% required a second corneal transplant.[92]

- *Early lattice and recurrent lattice arising in the donor cornea responds well to treatment* with the excimer laser or anterior lamellar keratoplasty.

- *Possibility of a neurotrophic persistent epithelial defect* may be kept in mind when performing keratoplasty in cases of familial amyloidosis.

GRANULAR CORNEAL DYSTROPHY (GCD)

It has two variants: GCD type I (classic) and GCD type II.

Subtle differences in the clinical appearance of the discrete corneal opacities permit two types of GCD to be recognized: GCD type I (GCD1) and GCD type II (GCD2). GCD2 tends to have fewer corneal deposits than GCD1 and the corneal deposits in GCD2 sometimes resemble a combination of GCD and LCD.

GRANULAR CORNEAL DYSTROPHY TYPE I (GCD 1)

Former alternative names: Corneal dystrophy Groenouw type I.

It was first described by German ophthalmologist, Arthur Groenouw in 1890.[1] It has also been extensively studied in Denmark by Moller.[93]

Clinical profile

Inheritance. Autosomal dominant with genetic locus and gene identified as 5q31 and TGFBI respectively.

Symptoms. Onset is in the first decade with a few cases reporting features as early as 2–3 years of age. Glare and photophobia are early symptoms. Recurrent erosions occur frequently and visual acuity decreases as the opacification progresses with age. Homozygote affected individuals usually have more severe symptoms.

Signs. The clinical picture is characterised by multiple, small, white, discrete irregular-shaped, sharply demarcated spots that resemble breadcrumbs or snowflakes and become apparent beneath the Bowman's layer in the superficial central corneal stroma (Fig. 31.9). It

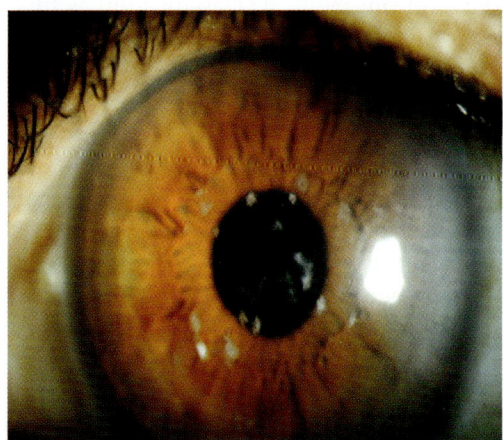

Fig. 31.9: *An early case of granular corneal dystrophy with granules composed of extremely small, translucent dots and opacities that do not extend to the corneal limbus*

begins as a vortex like pattern of brownish granules superficial to the Bowman's layer in children, and as the patient ages, well-defined white granules with clear intervening stroma are seen on direct illumination (Fig. 31.10). The size and number of granules gradually increase resulting in snowflake appearance. On retro-illumination, these granules appear as multiple extremely small, translucent dots and appear as vacuoles, glassy splinters, or crushed breadcrumbs. Opacities in GCD do not extend to the limbus. In later life, granules extend into the deeper stroma approaching the Descemet's membrane.

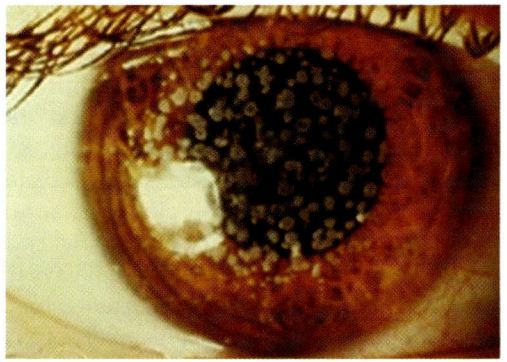

Fig. 31.10: *Intervening tissue between the opacities and the peripheral 2–3 mm of the cornea usually remains crystal clear in a case of granular corneal dystrophy*

Histopathology

The light microscopic and transmission electron microscopic (TEM) appearance along with the staining attributes of the corneal deposits in GCD are diagnostic. Eosinophilic deposits in GCD consist predominantly of an extracellular deposition of mutant TGFBI protein, which stains a brilliant red with the Masson trichrome stain. With the Wilder reticulin stain, the accumulations contain tangles of argyrophilic fibres. The deposits react with histochemical stains for protein as well as with antibodies to TGFBI protein. The granules stain positively with luxol fast blue and are reported to stain positively with antibodies to microfibrillar protein. By TEM, characteristic electron dense, discrete, rod-shaped or trapezoid bodies are evident.[94] Some rod-shaped structures appear homogeneous without a discernible inner

structure; others, however, are composed of an orderly array of closely packed filaments (70–100 nm in width) orientated parallel to their long axis, while others appear moth-eaten with variable-shaped cavities containing fine filaments. Descemet's membrane and the corneal endothelium are not affected, and so is the corneal tissue between the deposits. On confocal microscopy, multiple, hype-reflective opacities are evident. Confocal microscopy with anterior segment optical coherence tomography may provide sufficient diagnostic information to diagnose corneal granular dystrophies in a clinical setting.[95]

GRANULAR CORNEAL DYSTROPHY TYPE II (GCD 2)

Former alternative names: Avellino corneal dystrophy, combined granular-lattice corneal dystrophy.

For quite a long time, this dystrophy was considered as a mild GCD variant. Although Bücklers, as early as 1938, described and depicted a large family with this phenotype, it was only about 50 years later that Weidle published reporting the same patients and subdivided them according to subtle clinical differences and Folberg et al in 1988 described the histopathology of both amyloid and hyaline deposits in such patients.[96–98] The ancestry of some families with GCD2 have been traced to the Avellino district of Italy (hence the nomenclature Avellino corneal dystrophy). However, the global occurrence of this dystrophy is now recognized, making this synonym obsolete.

Clinical profile

Inheritance. Autosomal dominant with genetic locus and gene identified as 5q31 and TGFBI, respectively.

Symptoms.[99] Onset is in the first to second decade with homozygous patients having an earlier onset with dystrophy diagnosed, as early as 3 years of age. Most often, GCD 2 is diagnosed during teens or during early adulthood. Symptoms are similar to that of GCD 1. Homozygotes have an earlier onset and more severe disease course than heterozygotes. In most cases of GCD, visual acuity remains good until late in the course of the disease.

Signs. *Initial signs* are fine, tiny, whitish dots in the superficial corneal stroma, which typically have small spokes and may sometimes be arranged linearly like a string of pearls.

As the disease progresses, there is development of superficial white circular patches with moth-eaten centres with a ring-like appearance. Opacities do not extend to the corneal limbus. In children, there may be a vortex pattern of brownish granules superficial to the Bowman layer. In later life, granules may extend into the deeper stroma down to Descemet's membrane.

Most patients also develop fine projections that are anterior to the mid-stromal deposits and may be star, icicle, or spider-shaped and partially translucent in retroillumination, some display completely translucent short dash-like linear or dot-like deposits in the posterior stroma deep to the branching stromal opacities. The latter may be confused with lattice lines in LCD or its variants and are distinguished as follows:

- *Dashes in GCD 2 are relatively whiter* when compared to and lattice lines in LCD that are more refractile.
- *Dashes in GCD 2 rarely cross each other*, while lattice lines in LCD characteristically intersect to result in the pathognomonic lattice configuration.

Spontaneous extrusion of superficial granules has been noted in some cases after recurrent epithelial erosions which results in clearing of the central zone of opacity.

Recurrent attacks eventually lead to the formation of translucent flattened breadcrumb opacities in the sub-Bowman anterior stroma and increase in corneal thickness.

Phenotypic expressivity varies considerably with signs ranging from a few white dots to diffuse deposits throughout the stroma. Stromal opacities are usually less pronounced as compared to GCD 1.

Histopathology

On light microscopy, corneal opacities extend from the basal epithelium to the deep stroma. Although there is deposition of both typical GCD 1 deposits and amyloid; individual opacities stain with either Masson trichrome or Congo red. Homozygotes demonstrate more severe findings. On TEM, anterior stromal rod-shaped, electron-dense deposits composed of extracellular masses of fine, electron-dense, highly aligned fibrils are noted. An extremely common ultrastructural finding is the presence of randomly aligned fibrils of amyloid. Confocal microscopy demonstrates features of both GCD 1 and LCD. Reflective, breadcrumb-like round deposits with well-delineated borders or highly reflective, irregular trapezoidal deposits are present in the anterior stroma (similar to GCD 1). Additionally, linear and branching deposits with changing reflectivity are also observed (similar to LCD).

Management

Keratoplasty. Until relatively recently, a penetrating keratoplasty had been the traditional method for treating GCD, but postoperative recurrent disease can be detected in the donor tissue and even along the suture tracts within several years, particularly in GCD 2.[96] After a penetrating keratoplasty, the graft usually remains free of recurrence for at least 30 months, but the opacities may recur in the grafts, sometimes as early as within a year, usually superficial to the donor tissue, even with lamellar grafts, or at the host-graft interface.

Phototherapeutic keratectomy has been advocated as an initial therapy for GCD, but recurrent disease is still a common complication. Similarly, *deep anterior lamellar keratoplasty* (DALK) using the Melles technique[100] and automated lamellar keratoplasty[101] can restore and preserve useful visual function for a significant period in these patients in spite of recurrence.

Intralase femtosecond assisted lamellar kerato-plasty has also been described recently to treat Avellino dystrophy.[102]

Note: Injury to the central cornea may result in exacerbation of the corneal dystrophy. GCD 2 may also be exacerbated by laser epithelial keratomileusis (LASEK) and radial keratotomy (RK).[103] LASIK,[104] LASEK and other forms of refractive surgery are hence contraindicated in individuals with GCD 2.

STROMAL DYSTROPHIES

As discussed earlier, previously classified TGFBI corneal dystrophies, namely lattice corneal dystrophy (and variants) and granular corneal dystrophy (and variants) have been reclassified under epithelial–stromal TGFBI dystrophies in the updated IC3D classification.[15] Table 31.2 summarizes characteristic features of epithelial-stromal TGFBI dystrophies and stromal corneal dystrophies. Various stromal corneal dystrophies are described here briefly.

Table 31.2: *Epithelial–stromal TGFBI dystrophies and stromal corneal dystrophies and their characteristics*

Stromal corneal dystrophy	Inheritance	Onset	Clinical features	Histopathological features
Lattice type I	AD5q31 TGFBI	First decade	Subepithelial dots coalesce into typical, branching lattice lines—corneal haze	Amyloid; Congo red
Meretoja syndrome	AD9q34 GSN	Middle age with progressive facial palsy	Systemic features—progressive facial palsy; renal and cardiac failure	Amyloid deposits (corneal stroma and renal glomeruli)
Granular type I	AD5q31 TGFBI	First decade	Superficial and central white, crumb-like opacities become confluent and progress deeper and peripherally—spare limbus	Amorphous hyaline deposits—stain with Masson trichrome
Granular type II (Avellino)	AD	Late in life	Few, superficial discrete, ring-shaped, white, crumb-like opacities	Amorphous hyaline deposits + amyloid deposits
Macular dystrophy	AR16q22 CHST6	2nd decade	Progressive, generalized, corneal haze with focal, poorly delineated opacities; reduced corneal thickness	Abnormal closely packed collagen; lack of proteoglycans; aggregations of dermatan and chondroitin sulfate
Congenital stromal dystrophy	AD 12q13.2 DCN	Before birth	Moderate to severe visual loss; diffuse corneal clouding with flake-like opacities throughout stroma	–
Fleck dystrophy	AD 2q35 PIP5K3	At birth	Normal small discrete dandruff or ring-shaped, fleck-like opacities	–
Posterior amorphous corneal dystrophy	AD unknown	Infancy or childhood	Mildly affected diffuse sheet-like opacities especially in posterior corneal stroma	–

■ MACULAR CORNEAL DYSTROPHY (MCD)

CLINICAL PROFILE

Former alternative names and eponyms: Groenouw corneal dystrophy type II, Fehr speckled dystrophy.

Inheritance

MCD is inherited in autosomal recessive fashion and is thought to be caused by the lack or abnormal configuration of keratan sulfate (KS). KS is one of the major glycosaminoglycans of the corneal stroma and plays an important role in corneal transparency. Most cases of MCD are caused by mutations in CHST6 (carbohydrate sulfotransferase 6) gene with locus at chromosome 16q22.[105] The most frequent abnormalities are missense and nonsense single nucleotide polymorphisms in CHST6 that alter a conserved amino acid.

Symptoms

MCD has a childhood onset with a slowly progressive course. Visual impairment occurs early, between 10 and 30 years of age. Corneal sensitivity is reduced; pain from recurrent corneal erosions can occur but is much less common than in patients with lattice or granular dystrophies.

Signs

It is characterized by multiple, gray-white opacities in the corneal stroma that extend out into the peripheral cornea. These stromal opacities are distributed throughout the cornea without clear spaces (Figs 31.11 and 31.12). Initially, diffuse stromal haze develops extending to the limbus; later, superficial, central, elevated, irregular whitish opacities (macules) develop and give the condition its name. Unlike granular dystrophy, there are no clear areas between the corneal opacities. The cornea is thinner than normal in early disease. In the advanced stage, the corneal endothelium is affected and Descemet's membrane develops guttate excrescences. In addition, the stroma thickens from the imbibition of water from endothelial decompensation. Macular corneal dystrophy involves the entire thickness of the cornea and is more superficial centrally and

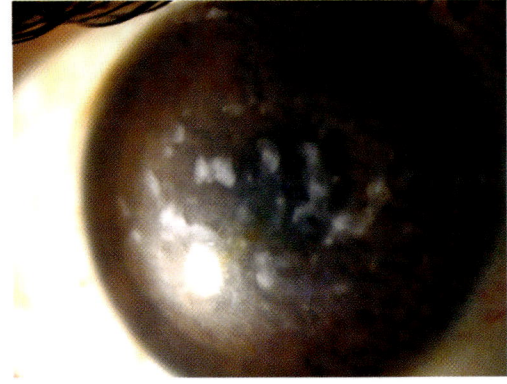

Fig. 31.11: *Macular corneal dystrophy with stromal opacities distributed throughout the cornea. Note that even in early cases, intervening stroma displays mild to moderate haze*

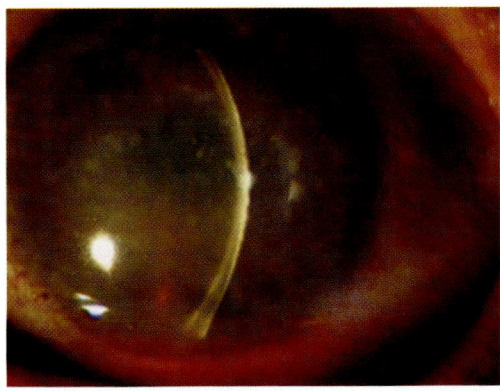

Fig. 31.12: *Macular corneal dystrophy with stromal opacities distributed throughout the cornea without clear spaces*

deeper peripherally. The first signs are usually noticed in the first decade of life that progress afterwards, with opacities developing in the cornea. Over time, the non-transparent areas progressively merge as the entire corneal stroma gradually becomes cloudy, causing severe visual impairment.

HISTOPATHOLOGY

It is characterized by an intracellular storage of glycosaminoglycans (GAGs) within the keratocytes and the corneal endothelium combined with an extracellular deposition of similar material in the corneal stroma and Descemet's membrane. Breaks in Bowman's layer are noted; Descemet's membrane and endothelium are also involved, as evidenced by Descemet's thickening and guttata plus endothelial staining with

Hale colloidal iron or Alcian blue, which also stains the deposits.

On TEM, numerous randomly distributed electron-lucent lacunae are noted throughout the cornea and some of these are filled with clusters of abnormal sulfated proteoglycan filaments. The extracellular matrix contains focal and diffuse fibrillogranular GAGs. The collagen fibrils have a normal diameter, but the interfibrillar spacing of collagen fibrils in affected corneas is less than that in the normal cornea. This close packing of collagen fibrils seems to be responsible for the reduced corneal thickness in MCD. The posterior non-banded portion of Descemet's membrane contains numerous corneal guttae.

Three immunophenotypes of MCD are recognized,[106] on the basis of immunoreactivity of specific sulphated epitopes of antigen keratan sulphates (AgKS) in the cornea and serum.

- *MCD type I* has no detectable antigen keratan sulfate (AgKS) in the serum or cornea.
- *MCD type II* has normal amounts of AgKS in the serum and cornea.
- *MCD type IA* lacks detectable antigenic keratan sulfate in the serum, but has stainable AgKS in the keratocytes.

Because keratan sulfate in the serum appears to be predominantly derived from the normal turnover of cartilage, these studies strongly suggest that the defect in keratan sulfate synthesis in macular corneal dystrophy is not restricted to corneal cells and that this condition may be a manifestation of a systemic disorder of keratan sulfate.[107]

Confocal microscopy reveals limited accumulations of highly reflective deposits in the basal epithelium and anterior and mid-stroma.

MANAGEMENT

In MCD, vision can be restored by corneal grafting, but the disease may recur in the graft after many years. Conventionally, the condition affects the entire corneal stroma, Descemet's membrane and the corneal endothelium; a lamellar keratoplasty will not excise all of the pathologic tissue. However, DALK with the big-bubble technique (Fig. 31.13) can be considered for visual rehabilitation in cases with no

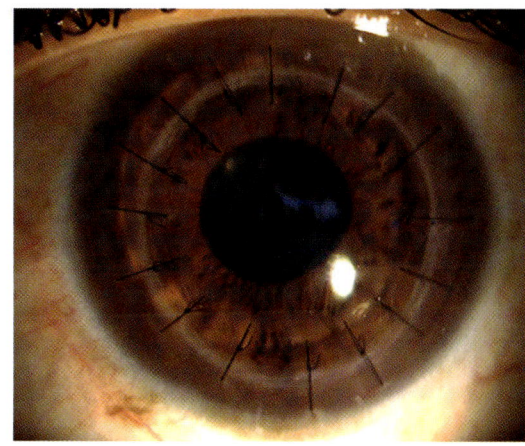

Fig. 31.13: *Deep anterior lamellar keratoplasty in a case of macular dystrophy*

significant Descemet's membrane and endothelial involvement.[108]

▉ FLECK CORNEAL DYSTROPHY (FCD)

CLINICAL PROFILE

Former alternative names and eponyms: François-Neetens speckled corneal dystrophy.

Inheritance

It is an autosomal dominant disease caused by mutations in phosphoinositide kinase, FYVE finger containing—PIKFYVE gene (previously known as PIP5K3 gene) which has been localized to chromosome 2q34.

Symptoms

It is either congenital or occurs in the first few years of life. The disease is non-progressive and, in most cases, asymptomatic, with mild photophobia reported by some patients.

Signs

Multiple symmetric minute opacities, some of which resemble "flecks", are scattered in the stroma of affected patients. Other opacities look more like snowflakes or clouds with distinct borders in the central and peripheral cornea with intervening portions of the cornea being normal. The corneal epithelium, Bowman's layer, and Descemet's membrane are unremarkable. Corneal sensation is usually normal.[109, 110]

HISTOPATHOLOGY

Swollen vacuolated keratocytes, which contain GAGs (staining with Alcian blue and colloidal iron) and complex lipids (demonstrated by Sudan black and Oil Red O) can be seen on light microscopy. TEM shows keratocytes with membrane-based inclusions with delicate granular material. Confocal microscopy reveals accumulation of hyperreflective 2–18 mm dot-like material in the normal-sized and enlarged stromal keratocyte nuclei.

MANAGEMENT

FCD is non-progressive, does not affect vision and is usually asymptomatic and does not require treatment, but mild photophobia has been reported. LASIK does not stimulate visually significant exacerbation of Fleck corneal dystrophy.[110]

CONGENITAL STROMAL CORNEAL DYSTROPHY (CSCD)

CLINICAL PROFILE

Former alternative names and eponyms: Congenital hereditary stromal dystrophy.

Inheritance

It has an autosomal dominant inheritance with the genetic locus at 12q21.33 involving Decorin (DCN) gene. This protein is a component of connective tissue, binds to type I collagen fibrils, and plays a role in matrix assembly protein.

Symptoms

It is an extremely rare, congenital non-progressive or slowly progressive form of corneal dystrophy. There is moderate to severe visual loss. Corneal erosions, photophobia and corneal vascularization are usually absent. Associated strabismus and glaucoma has been noted in some of the affected patients.

Signs

The main features of the disease are numerous bilateral opaque flaky or feathery areas of clouding in the stroma that multiply with age and eventually preclude visibility of the endothelium. Thickness of the corneal stroma is increased with diffuse involvement, but the fibrils of collagen that constitute stromal lamellae are reduced in diameter; Descemet's membrane and endothelium are relatively unaffected.[111]

HISTOPATHOLOGY

Light microscopy shows a peculiar arrangement of tightly packed lamellae having highly aligned collagen fibrils of an unusually small diameter,[111] suggesting a disturbance in collagen fibrogenesis. TEM reveals amorphous areas consisting of thin filaments randomly arranged in an electron-lucent ground substance that separate normal appearing lamellae; changes appear at all levels of stroma with broadening of abnormal areas in posterior stromal layers. The keratocytes and endothelium are normal, although absence of the anterior banded zone of Descemet's membrane has been reported. Accumulation of Decorin is found in the amorphous areas as determined by immuno-electron microscopy.

MANAGEMENT

Keratoplasty may be required in cases with visually disabling opacities.

POSTERIOR AMORPHOUS CORNEAL DYSTROPHY (PACD)

Former alternative names and eponyms: Posterior amorphous stromal dystrophy.

Inheritance. It demonstrates an autosomal dominant inheritance with genetic locus at 12q21.33 involving deletion of keratocan (KERA), lumican (LUM), decorin (DCN), and epiphycan (EPYC) genes.

CLINICAL PROFILE

Symptoms

Onset is often in the first decade with some cases occurring within a few months of life indicating a genetic origin. Visual acuity is usually minimally impaired and is usually better than 20/40.

Signs

It is characterized clinically by irregular, amorphous sheet-like opacities in posterior corneal stroma and Descemet's membrane. The abnormalities are observed in infancy and childhood and, in contrast to the traditional corneal dystrophies, non-corneal manifestations have been reported including abnormalities of the iris (irido-corneal adhesions, corectopia, and pseudopolycoria). Transparent corneal stroma between opacities is characteristic, while the Descemet's membrane and the corneal endothelium may show focal abnormalities.[112]

HISTOPATHOLOGY

Disorganized posterior stromal collagen lamellae, and an attenuated corneal endothelium have been observed.[112] A zone of collagen fibres may interrupt the Descemet's membrane beneath the anterior banded layer.

MANAGEMENT

Conservative management with *refractive correction* usually suffices with *keratoplasty* being required only in very few cases.

CENTRAL CLOUDY DYSTROPHY OF FRANÇOIS

INHERITANCE

It is unknown, although autosomal dominant inheritance has occasionally been reported. The gene and genetic locus also remain unknown.

CLINICAL PROFILE

Symptoms

With onset in the first decade of life, this condition is mostly asymptomatic.

Signs

Usually incidentally discovered, cloudy central polygonal or rounded stromal opacities that fade anteriorly and peripherally that are surrounded by clear tissue are noted. It may be phenotypically indistinguishable from posterior crocodile shagreen, which is a corneal degeneration.[113]

HISTOPATHOLOGY

Faint undulating appearance of the deep stroma and positive staining for GAGs may be seen. Extracellular vacuoles, often containing fibrillo-

granular material and electron-dense deposits may be seen on TEM.

PRE-DESCEMET CORNEAL DYSTROPHY (PDCD)

INHERITANCE

It is unknown in cases of isolated PDCD, although autosomal dominant inheritance has been reported in one pedigree in the punctiform/polychromatic subtype. The gene and genetic locus remain unknown in isolated cases. This condition may be associated with X-linked ichthyosis, in which case the steroid sulfatase (STS) gene is involved that has been localized to Xp22.31.

CLINICAL PROFILE

Symptoms

Onset is usually after 30 years of age, although the punctiform and polychromatic. Pre-Descemet's dystrophy has been reported in the first decade of life. The condition is asymptomatic and vision is usually unaffected.

Signs

Focal, fine, polymorphic gray opacities are seen located in the deep stroma immediately anterior to Descemet's membrane. They may be central, annular, or diffuse. Features are more uniform and polychromatism in an otherwise normal cornea are seen in the punctiform and polychromatic subtype. Similar opacities have been noted in association with other ocular and systemic diseases such as pseudoxanthoma elasticum, X-linked ichthyosis, keratoconus, posterior polymorphous dystrophy, epithelial basement membrane dystrophy and central cloudy dystrophy of François.[114]

HISTOPATHOLOGY

Normal cornea is seen except for enlarged keratocytes in the posterior stroma that contain vacuoles and intracytoplasmic inclusions of lipid-like material. Membrane-bound intracellular vacuoles containing electron-dense material suggestive of secondary lysosomes and inclusions of a lipofuscin-like lipoprotein consistent with a degenerative process may be seen on TEM.

ENDOTHELIAL DYSTROPHIES

The previously classified Descemet's membrane (DM) and endothelial dystrophies are now simply called endothelial dystrophies in the updated IC3D classification.[15]

FUCHS ENDOTHELIAL CORNEAL DYSTROPHY (FECD)

Fuchs endothelial dystrophy is a bilateral, progressive disease involving the corneal endothelium manifesting as corneal oedema and progressive deterioration of vision.

The condition was first described by Austrian Ernst Fuchs (1851–1930),[115] after whom it is named.

Inheritance

The inheritance is unknown in most of the cases, although some autosomal dominant cases have been reported. The genetics of FECD is complex demonstrating variable expressivity and incomplete penetrance.[116] Genetic and environmental factors also play a role and there is increased prevalence in the elderly and in females.

Genetic loci involved in Fuchs endothelial corneal dystrophy have been isolated at 13pTel –13q12.13, 15q and18q21.2 –q21.32.[117–119]

- *Early-onset variant Fuchs endothelial corneal dystrophy* may involve locus 1p34.3–p32 (FECD1) and the gene affecting collagen type VIII, alpha 2—COL8A2.
- *Late-onset FECD* has been reported to occur in association with 13pter–q12.13 (FECD2), 18q21.2–q21.3 (FECD3), 20p13–p12 (FECD4), 5q33.1–q35.2 (FECD5), 10p11.2 (FECD6), 9p24.1–p22.1 (FECD7), and 15q25 (FECD8).

Some authors have disputed the role of these genes in the pathogenesis of FCD and the genetic basis of this disease remains to be fully elucidated.

Associations

Fuchs dystrophy has been reported to be associated with cardiovascular disease, keratoconus, age-related macular degeneration, short axial length, narrow anterior chamber angles and open angle glaucoma.[120, 121]

CLINICAL PROFILE

Onset. Most cases have a reported onset in the fourth decade or later but the early variant can present in the first decade.[120]

Gender. Most studies suggest that FECD, both early and late variants, more commonly affect females, with as high as 4:1 female preponderance. The increased incidence in females has led to speculation about the role of hormones in the pathogenesis of FED.

Symptoms

- *Diminution of vision*, initially occurs intermittently and is more common in the morning; as the disease advances, progressive visual loss may occur.
- *Pain, foreign body sensation, photophobia, watering* can all result from epithelial edema and bullae.

Signs

Stage 1: Stage is cornea guttata. It occurs in the fourth or fifth decade of life when slit lamp examination by specular reflection reveals cornea guttata in the central part of the corneal endothelium. Pigment dusting of the endothelium may be noted. The condition spreads from the centre toward the periphery. The patient is asymptomatic and the corneal thickness and visual acuity remain unaffected, although there may be decrease in contrast sensitivity. Corneal guttae are often larger in size in late-onset FECD.

Stage 2: Stage of endothelial decompensation. This stage is characterised by deterioration in vision caused by incipient oedema of the corneal stroma. The excrescences of corneal guttata increase in number and may become confluent, resulting in a beaten metal appearance of the endothelial surface. As the stroma becomes edematous, the cornea acquires a ground glass appearance (Fig. 31.14). The patients complain halos around lights, blurred vision and glare. Vision may improve as the day progresses owing to evaporation and subsequent corneal deturgescence.

Stage 3: Stage of bullous keratopathy. The oedema progresses to involve the epithelium. Epithelial microcysts manifest as bedewing on

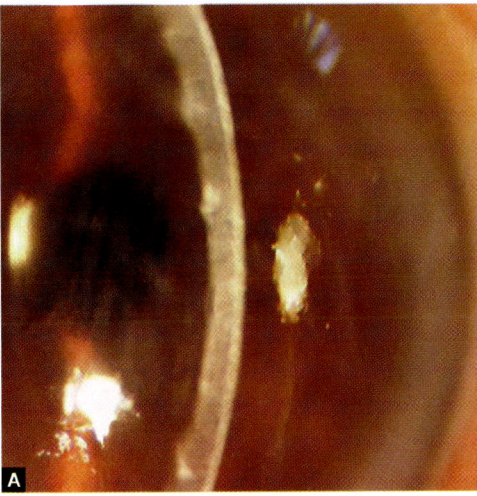

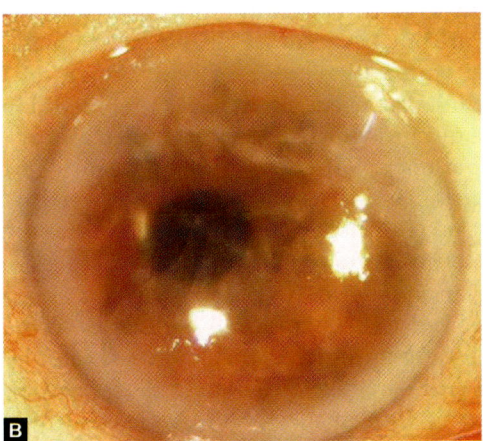

Fig. 31.14A and B: *Fuchs dystrophy with increased corneal thickness due to endothelial decompensation*

retroillumination. As these cysts enlarge and coalesce, they form larger intraepithelial or subepithelial bullae. When these bullae rupture, they cause significant pain and discomfort owing to exposure of the corneal nerves.

Stage 4: Stage of scarring. Eventually there is corneal scarring following long-standing oedema and rupture of bullae, which causes further diminution of vision, while ameliorating the pain. Sub-epithelial fibrosis and peripheral vascularization are also noted.

Specular microscopy

Following 5 stages on specular microscopic evaluation may be seen, as described by Laing et al[122]:

- *Stage 1:* The guttate excrescences are seen as dark structures with sharply defined single bright spots at their centre. They are smaller in size than a single endothelial cell and do not lie near the boundary wall of the cell.
- *Stage 2:* The excrescence is almost the size of the endothelial cell. The surrounding cells have a stretched appearance.
- *Stage 3:* The excrescence is considerably larger, and many cells are involved in one lesion. The dark structure is 5–10 times the size of an endothelial cell. The adjacent cells are abnormal and have missing boundaries. Many lesions are seen close to each other, but they do not coalesce. The excrescences are of two types, a smooth round shape or a rough excrescence.
- *Stage 4:* The individual excrescences have coalesced. The net result is multilobed, rather than a round outline. The dark areas have many bright spots. The multilobulated structures cover considerable area. The cells between the excrescence masses tend to become abnormal. Coalesced areas contain both the smooth and the rough varieties of excrescences.
- *Stage 5:* An organized mosaic of endothelial cells is difficult to see. Many stages may be observed in different areas of the same eye.

Confocal microscopy

In vivo confocal microscopy reveals polymegathism and pleomorphism of the endothelial cells. Subepithelial bullae formation may be seen on the anterior corneal surface. Subepithelial fibrosis may be seen subsequent to rupture of bullae. The Bowman membrane is normal, unless it has been involved in ulcer formation and keratitis, after the rupture of a bulla.

HISTOPATHOLOGY

Light microscopy reveals diffuse thickening and lamination of Descemet's membrane with hyaline excrescences on thickened Descemet's membrane (guttae). Endothelial cells are significantly reduced in number and those present may be atrophic or degenerated.

Transmission electron microscopy demonstrates degeneration of endothelial cells along with a severely disorganized and thickened stroma displaying a distorted architecture. While in early-onset FECD, there is thickening of the anterior banded layer of DM, multiple layers of basement membrane-like material are seen on the posterior non-banded part of DM in late-onset FECD.

MANAGEMENT

Conservative treatment

Patients of FCD with clear corneas (stage 1) do not require treatment. When corneal decompensation sets in medical therapy may be initiated and can be continued till good functional vision is maintained; beyond which keratoplasty is necessary.

Dehydrating agents are useful in early oedematous stage:

- *Sodium chloride 5%* eye drops especially in the early hours of the day; sodium chloride ointment is used at bedtime.
- *Glycerine* can be used for diagnostic purposes such as fundus evaluation as it causes rapid dehydration and clearing of the cornea.
- *Warm air* blown on the eyes (e.g. hair dryer) may help in reducing oedema.

Anti-glaucoma agents need to be administered in cases with concomitant glaucoma. Topical carbonic anhydrase inhibitors may be avoided as they hinder with the activity of the endothelial pump.

Supportive treatment for ruptured bullae

- *Anterior stromal punctures*, as indicated
- *Soft therapeutic contact lenses*
- *Cycloplegics*, local antibiotics with bandaging of the affected eye
- *Excimer laser phototherapeutic keratectomy*, amniotic membrane graft, or a conjunctival flap can also be considered for patients not willing for keratoplasty or in those with a poor visual prognosis.[123–126]

Keratoplasty: Changing trends

Corneal transplantation remains the definitive treatment for advanced cases of FCD.

Penetrating keratoplasty (PK) has been performed for many years to restore vision in patients with FCD. Chung et al suggested in patients with insufficient endothelial cell density like in FCD, a large trephine size could reduce chronic endothelial cell loss.[127]

Endothelial keratoplasty (EK) which selectively replaces the posterior layers of the cornea is now an established modality of treatment and has emerged as a successful alternative to penetrating keratoplasty for patients with endothelial diseases, including Fuchs endothelial dystrophy.[128] EK provides distinct advantages over PK, in that it is a less invasive procedure and leads to earlier recovery of vision. Additionally, this procedure does not require long-term corneal sutures, eliminating problems with suture breakage, suture abscesses, astigmatism, and wound dehiscence. Disadvantages of EK include the need for specially prepared donor tissue and additional surgeon training or experience. Patients with significant corneal scarring and vascularization (stage 4) may also not be amenable to DSAEK and require a full thickness graft.

Refractive ametropia and astigmatism are reported to be significantly less in Descemet's stripping automated endothelial keratoplasty (DSAEK)-treated eyes than in PK-treated eyes, even after suture removal and arcuate keratotomy.[129] DSAEK seems to be superior to PK in treating Fuchs endothelial keratoplasty in terms of faster visual recovery and decreased dependence on contact lenses and glasses. DSAEK, however, has a significant learning curve and may have initial endothelial cell loss greater than the conventional full thickness graft.[130]

Cataract extraction may be required in many of the patients of FCD. Anticipating the correct intraocular lens power for a patient undergoing cataract surgery alone followed by DSAEK or combined cataract surgery with DSAEK requires understanding the hyperopic shift that can occur with DSAEK and incorporating this correction preoperatively in the intraocular lens power selection.[131]

Descemet's membrane endothelial keratoplasty (DMEK) has been reported to effectively restore physiologic pachymetry and clarity, but donor preparation and attachment currently are slightly more challenging than with DSAEK.[132]

POSTERIOR POLYMORPHOUS CORNEAL DYSTROPHY (PPCD)

Former alternative names: Posterior polymorphous dystrophy, Schlichting dystrophy.[133]

In posterior polymorphous corneal dystrophy, dystrophic endothelial cells acquire epithelial characteristics, leading to secondary abnormalities in the Descemet's membrane.[134]

Inheritance

Autosomal dominant inheritance with low penetrance and variable expression is seen.[135–139] Isolated unilateral cases, without any family history, but with similar phenotype have also been reported. There are three types:

- **PPCD 1**—genetic locus isolated to 20p11.2–q11.2; gene remains unknown.
- **PPCD 2**—genetic locus mapped to 1p34.3–p32.3; gene collagen type VIII alpha 2, COL8A2 is involved.
- **PPCD 3**—genetic locus localized to 10p11.2; gene zinc-finger E box-binding homeobox (ZEB1) is implicated.

Associations

Associations with Alport syndrome, keratoconus and keratoglobus have been reported.[140–142]

Symptoms. The onset of this dystrophy is usually in the early childhood; the disease usually follows a non-progressive or slowly progressive course. Endothelial alterations occur; although often asymptomatic and unchanged over years, may cause visual disturbance. Rarely extensive and progressive visual impairment may occur due to stromal clouding. Vision loss may also be secondary to iridio-corneal adhesions and glaucoma.

Signs. Asymmetric involvement is common. Descemet's membrane and endothelial involvement in the form of geographic gray opacities, single or grouped vesicular lesions that are often surrounded by gray circular opacities and parallel gray-white endothelial bands with white "flaky" material (railroad tracks) that may involve the entire cornea are characteristic

(Fig. 31.15). Deep corneal lesions of various shapes including nodular, vesicular (isolated, in clusters, or confluent) and blister-like lesions are also observed.[143] Although keratoconus is a known association, non-keratoconic corneal steepening is also commonly seen. Stromal and epithelial oedema due to endothelial decompensation is rarely seen. Peripheral iridocorneal adhesions have been reported in about 25% of cases, and elevated intraocular pressure in 15% of cases.[143] Lipid deposition or band keratopathy have been reported in advanced cases. A congenital variant may manifest with corneal oedema at birth.

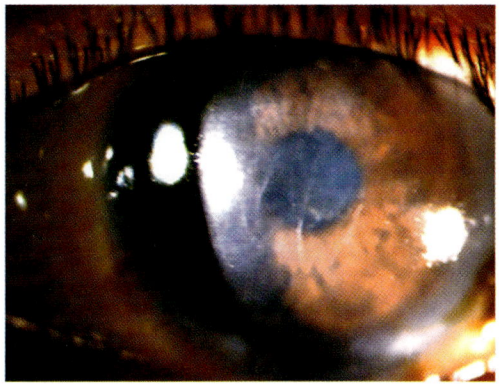

Fig. 31.15: *Posterior polymorphous corneal dystrophy*

Histopathology

"Epithelialization" of endothelial cells occurs and they are seen to acquire characteristics like cytoplasmic keratin, desmosomal junctions and microvilli. Metaplastic fibroblast-like endothelial cells have also been reported.[144] The altered endothelial cells are capable of migrating over the trabecular meshwork, thereby producing glaucoma. The posterior non-banded layer of the Descemet's membrane is abnormal in cases of PPMD, thickened with deposition of abnormal collagen, as seen on TEM. Rare cases of the congenital variant may involve the anterior banded layer. Stromal and epithelial changes may occur secondary to oedema due to endothelial dysfunction. Cases of PPCD1 display positive reactivity with anti-CK7, CK8, CK18, and CK19 antibodies.

Confocal microscopy demonstrates vesicular and linear abnormalities along with bright nucleus like structures in the endothelial cells.[145,146] Vesicular lesions appear as rounded dark areas with some cell detail apparent in the middle giving a doughnut-like appearance. Railroad track appearance of band-like dark area with irregular edges enclosing some smaller lighter cells resembling epithelium-like cells may be noted.

Management

Most cases are asymptomatic and may not require any treatment. Corneal transplantation may be required in severe cases. In a series of 120 cases of PPMD, 10% were reported to require a corneal graft. Co-existing glaucoma and iridio-corneal adhesions may compromise graft survival in these cases.

CONGENITAL HEREDITARY ENDOTHELIAL DYSTROPHY (CHED)

Congenital hereditary endothelial dystrophy was previously classified as type 1 (autosomal dominant, AD CHED) and type 2 (autosomal recessive, AR CHED).[147,148] However, due to lack of substantial evidence to support the autosomal dominant CHED as a separate clinic-patho-logical entity and due to an overlapping clinical, histopathologic, and electron microscopic picture with PPCD, the former has been removed from the classification in IC3D, 2015. The previously classifies AR CHED or type 2 is now considered as CHED.

Former alternative name and eponyms: Maumenee corneal dystrophy.[146]

Inheritance

Autosomal recessive inheritance pattern is seen. Genetic locus has been localized to 20p13 (telomeric portion); the solute carrier family 4, sodium borate transporter, member 11 (SLC4A11) gene has been implicated.[150–152]

Associations

It has not been consistently associated with any systemic disease. However, mutations in the SLC4A11 are also responsible for Harboyan syndrome,[153] a disorder with progressive post-lingual sensorineural hearing loss along with features of CHED.

Clinical features

Symptoms

The onset is at birth with a bilateral asymmetric involvement with a stationary to slowly progressive course. Parents often complain of diffuse corneal clouding along with history suggestive of photophobia. There can be associated poor vision associated with inability to fixate on objects and involuntary eye movements.

Signs

Corneal clouding ranging from diffuse haze to ground glass milky appearance with occasional focal gray spots are seen (Figs 31.16 and 31.17). Classically, the cornea is thickened to 2–3 times the normal thickness and endothelial cell count

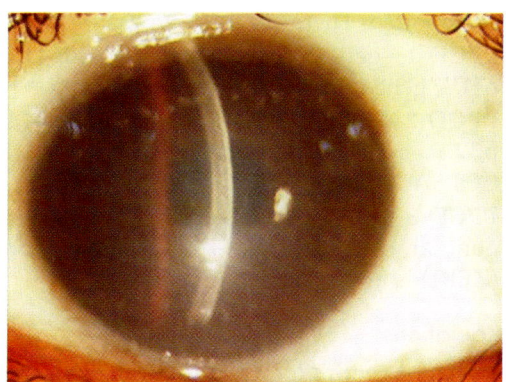

Fig. 31.16: *Milder form of congenital hereditary endothelial dystrophy. The hazy cornea does not preclude iris details completely*

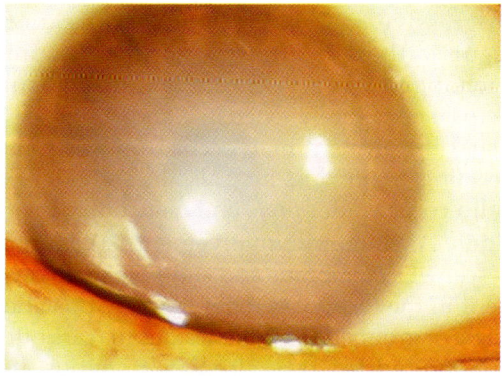

Fig. 31.17: *Diffuse corneal clouding in a case of congenital hereditary endothelial dystrophy. Note the ground glass appearance of the cornea*

is reduced significantly (about 10-fold as compared with age-matched controls). Nystagmus is usually present, possibly secondary to the severe visual impairment.[36] Congenital glaucoma, an important differential, may co-exist, but falsely elevated intraocular pressure measurement due to stromal oedema may lead to misdiagnosis.[154,155] Long-standing cases may display band keratopathy and subepithelial amyloidosis.[156, 157]

Histopathology

Diffuse thickening and lamination of Descemet's membrane with deposition of multiple layers of basement membrane-like material on the posterior part of Descemet's membrane has been noted. Endothelial cells can be degenerated, multinucleate, sparse or even atrophic. Diffuse epithelial and stromal oedema along with defects in Bowman's layer are other features. Transmission electron microscopy reveals multiple layers of BM-like material on posterior DM along with degenerated endothelial cells and a disorganised stroma.

Management of CHED

Corneal transplantation remains the definitive treatment for CHED. Paediatric keratoplasty, however, is a surgically challenging procedure and demands intensive postoperative monitoring and therapy. The timing of the surgery remains controversial in view of the possible challenges and complications. While some recommend early surgery, others suggest delaying the procedure as long as the patient demonstrates good fixation and normal alignment.[158,159]

Schaumberg et al reported 2-year survival rate of first grafts performed for CHED at a median age of 40 months to be 71%.[160] However, just four of the 10 eyes attained a visual acuity of 20/200 or better. They concluded that penetrating keratoplasty for CHED in children has a reasonable chance of surgical success when performed at a young age; however, the prognosis for improved visual acuity in children appears to be more guarded as compared to adults. Javadi et al reported the absence of a relationship between postoperative visual outcome and age at keratoplasty, and advocated a conservative approach and careful risk-benefit ratio evaluation in patients with CHED.[161]

DSAEK has emerged as a viable alternative to PK for treatment of CHED. Technical difficulties during Descemet's membrane scoring and stripping and poor visualization along with a shallow anterior chamber in a phakic patient are the major concerns.[162]

X-LINKED ENDOTHELIAL CORNEAL DYSTROPHY (XECD)

Inheritance

X-chromosomal dominant inheritance with genetic locus at Xq25 has been reported; the gene remains unknown.

Clinical features

Symptoms

Males may complain of clouding of cornea from birth with slowly progressive blurred vision while females are asymptomatic.

Signs

Congenital clouding ranging from a diffuse haze to a ground glass appearance is noted; milky appearance has been reported in male patients with advanced involvement.[52] Moon crater-like endothelial changes along with secondary subepithelial band keratopathy are also noted. Nystagmus is often associated.

In females, moon crater-like endothelial changes are the only clinical findings.

Histopathology

Light microscopy reveals irregular thickening of Descemet's membrane with small excavations and pits (corresponding to moon crater endothelial changes). There may be associated thinning of epithelium and Bowman's membrane along with irregularly arranged collagen lamellae.

Transmission electron microscopy reveals thickening of Descemet's membrane (20–35 mm) with presence of an abnormal anterior and posterior banded zone, the latter may even be completely absent in some cases. Discontinuous endothelial layer with partly normal and partly degenerative appearing cells. Subepithelial accumulations of an amorphous granular material are noted.[163]

Management

Refractive correction and medical management may suffice in early cases. Corneal transplantation may be required in advanced cases.

REFERENCES

1. Groenouw A. Knoetchenfoermige Hornhauttruebungen (Noduli corneae). Arch Augenheilkd. 1890; 21: 281–289.
2. Biber H. Ueber einige seltene Hornhauterkrankungen: die oberflaechliche gittrige Keratitis [Inaugural Dissertation]. A Diggelmann Zuerich. 1890.
3. Fuchs E. Dystrophia epithelialis corneae. Arch Ophthalmol. 1910; 76: 478–508.
4. Uthoff W. Ein Fall von doppelseitiger zentraler, punktfoermiger, supepithelialer knoetchenfoermiger Keratitis, Groenouw mit anatomischem Befunde. Klin Monatsbl Augenheilkd. 1915; 54: 377–383.
5. Yoshida Y. Ueber eine neue Art der Dystrophia corneae mit histologischem Befunde. Albrecht von Graefes Arch Clin Exp Ophthalmol. 1924; 114: 91–100.
6. Afshari NA, Bouchard CS, Colby KA, de Freitas D, Rootman DS, Tu EY, Weisenthal RW. Corneal dystrophies and ectasias. In: Weisenthal RW, ed. 2014–2015 Basic and Clinical Science Course, Section 8: External Disease and Cornea. San Francisco; American Academy of Ophthalmology; 2014: 253–287.
7. Matthaei M, Sandhaeger H, Hermel M, Adler W, Jun AS, Cursiefen C, Heindl LM. Changing Indications in Penetrating Keratoplasty: A Systematic Review of 34 Years of Global Reporting. Transplantation. 2017 Jun; 101(6): 1387–1399.
8. Gupta N, Vashist P, Tandon R, Gupta SK, Dwivedi S, Mani K. Prevalence of corneal diseases in the rural Indian population: the Corneal Opacity Rural Epidemiological (CORE) study. Br J Ophthalmol. 2015 Feb; 99(2): 147–52.
9. Kanavi MR, Javadi MA, Sanagoo M. Indications for penetrating keratoplasty in Iran. Cornea. 2007 Jun; 26(5): 561–3.
10. Dorrepaal SJ, Cao KY, Slomovic AR. Indications for penetrating keratoplasty in a tertiary referral centre in Canada, 1996–2004. Can J Ophthalmol. 2007 Apr; 42(2): 244–50.
11. Sony P, Sharma N, Sen S, Vajpayee RB. Indications of penetrating keratoplasty in northern India. Cornea. 2005 Nov; 24(8): 989–91.
12. Tan DT, Janardhanan P, Zhou H, et al. Penetrating keratoplasty in Asian eyes: the Singapore Corneal Transplant Study. Ophthalmology. 2008 Jun; 115(6): 975–982.
13. Dobbins KR, Price FW Jr, Whitson WE. Trends in the indications for penetrating keratoplasty in the midwestern United States. Cornea. 2000 Nov; 19(6): 813–6.
14. Ghosheh FR, Cremona F, Ayres BD, et al. Indications for penetrating keratoplasty and associated procedures, 2001–2005. Eye Contact Lens. 2008 Jul; 34(4): 211–4.
15. de Sanctis U, Alovisi C, Bauchiero L, Caramello G, Girotto G, Panico C, Vinai L, Genzano F, Amoroso A, Grignolo F. Changing trends in corneal graft surgery: a ten-year review. Int J Ophthalmol. 2016 Jan 18; 9(1): 48–52.
16. Gupta SK, Hodge WG. A new clinical perspective of corneal dystrophies through molecular genetics. Curr Opin Ophthalmol. 1999 Aug; 10(4): 234–41.
17. Weiss JS, Møller HU, Lisch W, et al. The IC3D classification of the corneal dystrophies [in English and Spanish]. Cornea. 2008; 27(suppl 2): S1–S83.
18. Weiss JS, Møller HU, Aldave AJ, et al. The IC3D classification of the corneal dystrophies – Edition 2 [in English and Spanish]. Cornea. 2015; 34: 117–157.
19. Bron AJ, Tripathi RC. Cystic disorders of the corneal epithelium II. Pathogenesis. Br J Ophthalmol. 1973; 57: 361–375.
20. Laibson PR, Krachmer JH. Familial occurrence of dot (microcystic), map, fingerprint dystrophy of the cornea. Invest Ophthalmol Vis Sci. 1975; 14: 397–399.
21. Boutboul S, Black GCM, Moore JE, et al. A subset of patients with epithelial basement membrane corneal dystrophy have mutations in TGFBI/BIGH3. Hum Mutat. 2006; 27: 553–557.
22. Munier FL, Korvatska E, Djemai A, et al. Kerato-epithelin mutations in four 5q31-linked corneal dystrophies. Nat Genet. 1997; 15: 247–251.
23. Rodrigues MM, Fine BS, Laibson PR, et al. Disorders of the corneal epithelium. A clinicopathologic study of dot, geographic, and

fingerprint patterns. Arch Ophthalmol. 1974; 92: 475–482.

24. Labbé A, Nicola RD, Dupas B et al. Epithelial basement membrane dystrophy: evaluation with the HRT II Rostock Cornea Module. Ophthalmology. 2006 Aug; 113(8): 1301–8.

25. Itty S, Hamilton SS, Baratz KH et al. Outcomes of epithelial debridement for anterior basement membrane dystrophy. Am J Ophthalmol. 2007 Aug; 144(2): 217–221.

26. Torres Pérez JD, Herreras Cantalapiedra JM, Jiménez Benito FJ, et al. Anterior stromal puncture for recurrent corneal erosion. Arch Soc Esp Oftalmol. 2002 May; 77(5): 257–62.

27. Tsai TY, Tsai TH, Hu FR, et al. Recurrent corneal erosions treated with anterior stromal puncture by neodymium: yttrium-aluminum-garnet laser. Ophthalmology. 2009 Jul; 116(7): 1296–300.

28. Pogorelov P, Langenbucher A, Kruse F, et al. Long-term results of phototherapeutic keratectomy for corneal map-dot-fingerprint dystrophy (Cogan-Guerry). Cornea. 2006 Aug; 25(7): 774–7.

29. Zaidman GW, Hong A. Visual and refractive results of combined PTK/PRK in patients with corneal surface disease and refractive errors. J Cataract Refract Surg. 2006 Jun; 32(6): 958–61.

30. Chow AM, Yiu EP, Hui MK, et al. Shallow ablations in phototherapeutic keratectomy: long-term follow-up. J Cataract Refract Surg. 2005 Nov; 31(11): 2133–6.

31. Bourges JL, Dighiero P, Assaraf E, et al. Photo-therapeutic keratectomy for the treatment of Cogan's microcystic dystrophy. J Fr Ophtalmol. 2002 Jun; 25(6): 594–8.

32. Franceschetti A. Hereditaere rezidivierende Erosion der Hornhaut. Z Augenheilk. 1928; 66: 309–316.

33. Wales HJ. A family history of corneal erosions. Trans Ophthalmol Soc NZ. 1956; 8: 77–78.

34. Hammar B, Lagali N, Ek S, et al. Dystrophia Smolandiensis: a novel morphological picture of recurrent corneal erosions. Acta Ophthalmol. 2010 Jun; 88(4): 394–400

35. Feder RS, Jay M, Yue BY, et al. Subepithelial mucinous corneal dystrophy. Clinical and pathological correlations. Arch Ophthalmol. 1993; 111: 1106–1114.

36. Pameijer JK. Ueber eine Fremdariege Familiere ObrflEchliche Hornhaurtver Enderung (German) Klin Monatsbl Augenheilkd. 1935; 95: 516.

37. Meesmann A. Uber eine bisher nicht beschriebene dominant vererbte Dystrophia epithelialis corneae. Ber Zusammenkunft Dtsch Ophthalmol Ges. 1938; 52: 154–158.

38. Stocker FW, Holt LB. Rare form of hereditary epithelial dystrophy. Arch Ophthalmol. 1955; 53: 536.

39. Szaflik JP, O³dak M, Maksym RB, et al. Genetics of Meesmann corneal dystrophy: a novel mutation in the keratin 3 gene in an asymptomatic family suggests genotype-phenotype correlation. Mol Vis. 2008 Sep 15; 14: 1713–8.

40. Seto T, Fujiki K, Kishishita H, et al. A novel mutation in the cornea-specific keratin 12 gene in Meesmann corneal dystrophy. Jpn J Ophthalmol. 2008 May-Jun; 52(3): 224–6.

41. Burns RP. Meesmann's corneal dystrophy. Trans Am Ophthalmol Soc.1968; 66: 530–635.

42. Fine BS, Yanoff M, Pitts E, et al. Meesmann's epithelial dystrophy of the cornea. Am J Ophthalmol. 1977; 83: 633–642.

43. Tuft S, Bron AJ. Imaging the microstructural abnormalities of Meesmann corneal dystrophy by *in vivo* confocal microscopy. Cornea. 2006; 25: 868–870.

44. Cremona FA, Ghosheh FR, Laibson PR, et al. Meesmann corneal dystrophy associated with epithelial basement membrane and posterior polymorphous corneal dystrophies. Cornea. 2008 Apr; 27(3): 374–7.

45. Jalbert I, Stapleton F. Management of Symptomatic Meesmann Dystrophy. Optom Vis Sci. 2009 Sep 7. [Epub ahead of print]

46. Yeung JY, Hodge WG. Recurrent Meesmann's corneal dystrophy: treatment with keratectomy and mitomycin C. Can J Ophthalmol. 2009 Feb; 44(1): 103–4.

47. Charles NC, Young JA, Kunar A, et al. Band-shaped and whorled microcystic dystrophy of the corneal epithelium. Ophthalmology. 2000; 107: 1761–1764.

48. Lisch W, Buttner A, Offner F, et al. Lisch corneal dystrophy is genetically distinct from Meesmann corneal dystrophy and maps to Xp22.3. Am J Ophthalmol. 2000; 130: 461–468.

49. Butros S, Lang GK, Alvarez de Toledo J, et al. The different opacity patterns of Lisch corneal dystrophy. Klin Monbl Augenheilkd. 2006 Oct; 223(10): 837–40.

50. Alvarez-Fischer M, de Toledo JA, Barraquer RI et al. Lisch corneal dystrophy. Cornea. 2005 May; 24(4): 494–5.

51. Robin SB, Epstein RJ, Kornmehl EW. Band-shaped, whorled microcystic corneal dystrophy. Am J Ophthalmol. 1994; 117: 543–544.

52. Lisch W, Steuhl KP, Lisch C, et al. A new, band-shaped and whorled microcystic dystrophy of the corneal epithelium. Am J Ophthalmol.1992 Jul 15; 114(1): 35–44.

53. Lisch W, Wasielica-Poslednik J, Lisch C, et al. Contact lens-induced regression of Lisch epithelial corneal dystrophy. Cornea. 2010 Mar; 29(3): 342–5.

54. Klintworth GK, Valnickova Z, Kielar RA, et al. Familial subepithelial corneal amyloidosis —a lactoferrin-related amyloidosis. Invest Ophthalmol Vis Sci. 1997; 38: 2756–2763.

55. Ren Z, Lin PY, Klintworth GK, et al. Allelic and locus heterogeneity in autosomal recessive gelatinous drop-like corneal dystrophy. Hum Genet. 2002; 110: 568–577.

56. Tsujikawa M, Kurahashi H, Tanaka T, et al. Identification of the gene responsible for gelatinous drop-like corneal dystrophy. Nat Genet. 1999; 21: 420–423.

57. Ide T, Nishida K, Maeda N, et al. A spectrum of clinical manifestations of gelatinous drop-like corneal dystrophy in Japan. Am J Ophthalmol. 2004; 137: 1081–1084.

58. Toshida H, Uesugi Y, Nakayasu K, et al. Keratoplasty for gelatinous drop-like corneal dystrophy. Jpn J Clin Ophthalmol. 1995; 49: 449.

59. Huo YN, Yao YF. Current advances in gene diagnosis and therapy of gelatinous drop-like corneal dystrophy. Zhejiang Da Xue Xue Bao Yi Xue Ban. 2006 Mar; 35(2): 228–32.

60. Higaki S, Hori Y, Maeda N, et al. Long-term results of deep lamellar keratoplasty using grafts with endothelium. Acta Ophthalmol. 2008 Feb; 86(1): 49–52.

61. Lasram L, Rais C, el Euch M, et al. Gelatinous dystrophy of the cornea. Apropos of 5 cases. J Fr Ophtalmol. 1994; 17(1): 24–8.

62. Ito M, Takahashi J, Sakimoto T, et al. Histological study of gelatinous drop-like dystrophy following excimer laser photo-therapeutic keratectomy. Nippon Ganka Gakkai Zasshi. 2000 Jan; 104(1): 44–50.

63. Reis W. Familiare, fleckige Hornhautentartung. Dtsch Med Wochenschr. 1917; 43: 575.

64. Bücklers M.U. ber eine weitere familiare Hornhaut-dystrophie (Reis). Klin Monatsbl Augenkeilkd. 1949; 114: 386–397.

65. Wheeldon CE, de Karolyi BH, Patel DV, et al. A novel phenotype-genotype relationship with a TGFBI exon 14 mutation in a pedigree with a unique corneal dystrophy of Bowman's layer. Mol Vis. 2008 Aug 18; 14: 1503–12.

66. Konishi M, Yamada M, Nakamura Y, et al. Immunohistology of keratoepithelin in corneal stromal dystrophies associated with R124 mutations of the BIGH3 gene. Curr Eye Res. 2000; 21: 891–896.

67. Small KW, Mullen L, Barletta J, et al. Mapping of Reis-Bücklers corneal dystrophy to chromosome 5q. Am J Ophthalmol. 1996; 121: 384–390.

68. Jones ST, Stauffer LH. Reis-Bücklers corneal dystrophy. Trans Am Acad Ophthalmol Otolaryngol. 1970; 74: 417.

69. Kuchle M, Green WR, Volcker HE, et al. Reevaluation of corneal dystrophies of Bowman's layer and the anterior stroma (Reis-Bücklers and Thiel-Behnke types): a light and electron microscopic study of eight corneas and a review of the literature. Cornea. 1995; 14: 333–354.

70. Kobayashi A, Sugiyama K. *In vivo* laser confocal microscopy findings for Bowman's layer dystrophies (Thiel-Behnke and Reis-Bücklers corneal dystrophies). Ophthalmology. 2007; 114: 69–75.

71. Dinh R, Rapuano CJ, Cohen EJ, et al. Recurrence of corneal dystrophy after excimer laser photo-therapeutic keratectomy. Ophthalmology. 1999 Aug; 106(8): 1490–7.

72. Miller A, Solomon R, Bloom A, et al. Prevention of recurrent Reis-Bücklers dystrophy following excimer laser phototherapeutic keratectomy with topical mitomycin C. Cornea. 2004 Oct; 23(7): 732–5.

73. Kamoi M, Mashima Y Kawashima M, et al. Electrolysis for corneal opacities in a young patient with superficial variant of granular corneal dystrophy (Reis-Bücklers corneal dystrophy). Am J Ophthalmol. 2005 Jun; 139(6): 1139–40.

74. Pandrowala H, Bansal A, Vemuganti GK, et al. Frequency, distribution, and outcome of keratoplasty for corneal dystrophies at a tertiary eye care center in South India. Cornea. 2004 Aug; 23(6): 541–6.

75. Yee RW, Sullivan LS, Lai HT, et al. Linkage mapping of Thiel-Behnke corneal dystrophy (CDB2) to chromosome 10q23-q24. Genomics. 1997; 46: 152–154.

76. Thiel HJ, Behnke H. Eine bisher unbekannte subepitheliale hereditare Hornhautdystrophie. Klin Monatsbl Augenheilkd. 1967; 150: 862–874.

77. Stock EL, Feder RS, O'Grady RB, et al. Lattice corneal dystrophy type IIIA. Clinical and histopathologic correlations. Arch Ophthalmol. 1991; 109: 354–358.

78. Tsujikawa K, Tsujikawa M, Yamamoto S, et al. Allelic homogeneity due to a founder mutation in Japanese patients with lattice corneal dystrophy type IIIA. Am J Med Genet. 2002; 113: 20–22.

79. Fukuoka H, Kawasaki S, Yamasaki K, et al. Lattice corneal dystrophy type IV (p.Leu527Arg) is caused by a founder mutation of the TGFBI gene in a single Japanese ancestor. Invest Ophthalmol Vis Sci. 2010; 51: 4523–4530.

80. Meretoja J: Familial systemic paramyloidosis with lattice dystrophy of the cornea, progressive cranial neuropathy, skin changes and various internal symptoms. A previously unrecognized heritable syndrome. Ann Clin Res. 1969, 1:314–324.

81. Chapelle A, Kere J, Sack GH, et al. Familial amyloidosis, Finnish type: G654-a mutation of the gelsolin gene in Finnish families and an unrelated American family. Genomics. 1992; 13: 898–901.

82. Klintworth GK: Lattice corneal dystrophy. An inherited variety of amyloidosis restricted to the cornea. Am J Pathol 1967, 50: 371–399.

83. Hida T, Proia AD, Kigasawa K, et al. Histopathologic and immunochemical features of lattice corneal dystrophy type III. Am J Ophthalmol. 1987; 104: 249–254.

84. Eifrig DE Jr, Afshari NA, Buchanan HW IV, Bowling BL, Klintworth GK. Polymorphic corneal amyloidosis: a disorder due to a novel mutation in the TGFBI (BIGH3) gene. Ophthalmology. 2004, 111: 1108–1114.

85. Konishi M, Yamada M, Nakamura Y, Mashima Y: Immunohistology of keratoepithelin in corneal stromal dystrophies associated with R124 mutations of the BIGH3 gene. Curr Eye Res. 2000, 21: 891–896.

86. Hotta Y, Fujiki K, Ono K, Fujimaki T, Nakayasu K, Yamaguchi T, Kanai A. Arg124Cys mutation of the betaig-h3 bene in a Japanese family with lattice corneal dystrophy type I. Jpn J Ophthalmol. 1998; 42: 450–455.

87. Kiuru-Enari S, Keski-Oja J, Haltia M.Cutis laxa in hereditary gelsolin amyloidosis. Br. J. Dermatol. 2005; 152 (2): 250–7.

88. Tanskanen M, Paetau A, Salonen O, et al. Severe ataxia with neuropathy in hereditary gelsolin amyloidosis: a case report". Amyloid 2007; 14 (1): 89–95.

89. Meretoja J: Comparative histopathological and clinical findings in eyes with lattice corneal dystrophy of two different types. Ophthalmologica. 1972, 165: 15–37.

90. Das S, Langenbucher A, Seitz B. Excimer laser phototherapeutic keratectomy for granular and lattice corneal dystrophy: a comparative study J Refract Surg. 2005 Nov-Dec; 21(6): 727–31.

91. Yao YF, Jin YQ, Zhang B, Zhou P, Zhang YM, Qiu WY, Mou SL, Wu LQ. Recurrence of lattice corneal dystrophy caused by incomplete removal of stroma after deep lamellar keratoplasty Cornea. 2006 Dec; 25(10 Suppl 1): S41–6.

92. Marcon AS, Cohen EJ, Rapuano CJ, Laibson PR. Recurrence of corneal stromal dystrophies after penetrating keratoplasty. Cornea. 2003 Jan; 22(1): 19–21.

93. Moller HU: Granular corneal dystrophy Groenouw type I. Clinical aspects and treatment. Acta Ophthalmol (Copenh). 1990; 68: 384–389.

94. Akiya S, Brown SI: Granular dystrophy of the cornea. Characteristic electron microscopic lesion. Arch Ophthalmol. 1970; 84: 179–192.

95. Dalton K, Schneider S, Sorbara L, Jones L Confocal microscopy and optical coherence tomography imaging of hereditary granular dystrophy. Cont Lens Anterior Eye. 2010; 33(1): 33–40. Epub 2009 Nov 28.

96. Holland EJ, Daya SM, Stone EM, Folberg R, Dobler AA, Cameron JD, Doughman DJ: Avellino corneal dystrophy. Clinical manifestations and natural history. Ophthalmology. 1992, 99: 1564–1568.

97. Bücklers M. Die erblichen Hornhautdystrophie. Klin Monatsbl Augenheilkd. 1938;3:1–135.

98. Folberg R, Alfonso E, Croxatto JO, et al. Clinically atypical granular corneal dystrophy with pathologic features of lattice-like amyloid deposits: a study of three families. Ophthalmology. 1988; 95: 46–51.

99. Han KE, Chung WS, Kim T, et al. Changes of clinical manifestation of granular corneal deposits because of recurrent corneal erosion in granular corneal dystrophy types 1 and 2. Cornea. 2013; 32: e113–e120.

100. Salouti R, Hosseini H, Eghtedari M, Khalili MR. Deep anterior lamellar keratoplasty with Melles technique for granular corneal dystrophy. Cornea. 2009 Feb; 28(2): 140–3.

101. Chen W, Qu J, Wang Q, Lu F, Barabino S. Automated lamellar keratoplasty for recurrent granular corneal dystrophy after photo-therapeutic keratectomy. J Refract Surg. 2005 May-Jun; 21(3): 288–93.

102. Agarwal A, Brubaker JW, Mamalis N, Kumar DA, Jacob S, Chinnamuthu S, Nair V, Prakash G, Meduri A, Agarwal A. Femtosecond-assisted lamellar keratoplasty in atypical Avellino corneal dystrophy of Indian origin. Eye Contact Lens. 2009 Sep; 35(5): 272–4.

103. Feizi S, Pakravan M, Baradaran-Rafiee AR, Yazdani S: Granular corneal dystrophy manifesting after radial keratotomy. Cornea. 2007; 26: 1267–1269.

104. Lee WB, Himmel KS, Hamilton SM, Zhao XC, Yee RW, Kang SJ, Grossniklaus HE. Excimer laser exacerbation of Avellino corneal dystrophy. J Cataract Refract Surg. 2007; 33(1): 133–8.

105. Klintworth G.Corneal dystrophies Orphanet J Rare Dis. 2009; 4: 7.

106. Thonar EJ, Meyer RF, Dennis RF, Lenz ME, Maldonado B, Hassell JR,Hewitt AT, Stark WJ Jr, Stock EL, Kuettner KE, Klintworth GK: Absence of normal keratan sulfate in the blood of patients with macular corneal dystrophy. Am J Ophthalmol 1986,102: 561–569.

107. Akama TO, Nishida K, Nakayama J, Watanabe H, Ozaki K, Nakamura T, Dota A, Kawasaki S, Inoue Y, Maeda N, Yamamoto S, Fujiwara T, Thonar EJ, Shimomura Y, Kinoshita S, Tanigami A, Fukuda MN: Macular corneal dystrophy type I and type II are caused by distinct mutations in a new sulphotransferase gene. Nat Genet 2000; 26: 237–241.

108. Patel AK, Nayak H, Kumar V. Comparative evaluation of big-bubble deep anterior lamellar keratoplasty and penetrating keratoplasty in a case of macular corneal dystrophy. Cornea. 2009 Jun; 28(5): 583–5.

109. Purcell JJ Jr, Krachmer JH, Weingeist TA. Fleck corneal dystrophy Arch Ophthalmol 1977, 95: 440–444.

110. Banning CS, Larson PM, Randleman JB. Outcome of LASIK in fleck corneal dystrophy. Cornea. 2006 Dec; 25(10): 1262–4.

111. Bredrup C, Knappskog PM, Majewski J, Rodahl E, Boman H: Congenital stromal dystrophy of the cornea caused by a mutation in the decorin gene. Invest Ophthalmol Vis Sci 2005, 46: 420–426.

112. Carpel EF, Sigelman RJ, Doughman DJ. Posterior amorphous corneal dystrophy. Am J Ophthalmol 1977, 83: 629–632.

113. Bramsen T, Ehlers N, Baggesen LH. Central cloudy corneal dystrophy of François. Acta Ophthalmol (Copenh). 1976; 54: 221–226.

114. Curran RE, Kenyon KR, Green WR. Pre-Descemet's membrane corneal dystrophy. Am J Ophthalmol. 1974; 77: 711–716.

115. Fuchs E. Dystrophia epithelialis corneae. Albrecht von Graefes Arch Clin Exp Ophthalmol. 1910; 76: 478–508.

116. Hemadevi B, Srinivasan M, Arun Kumar J, et al. Genetic analysis of patients with Fuchs endothelial corneal dystrophy in India. BMC Ophthalmol. 2010 Feb 10; 10(1): 3.

117. Riazuddin SA, Eghrari AO, Al-Saif A. Linkage of a mild late-onset phenotype of Fuchs corneal dystrophy to a novel locus at 5q33.1-q35.2. Invest Ophthalmol Vis Sci. 2009 Dec; 50(12): 5667–71.

118. Krachmer JH, Purcell JJ Jr, Joung CW, et al. Corneal endothelial dystrophy. A study of 64 families. Arch Ophthalmol. 1978; 96: 2036–2039.

119. Sundin OH, Jun A, Broman KW, et al. Linkage of late-onset Fuchs corneal dystrophy to a novel locus at 13ptel-13q12.13. Invest Ophthalmol Vis Sci. 2006; 47: 140–145.

120. Hogan MJ,Wood J, Fine M. Fuchs' endothelial dystrophy of the cornea. Am J Ophthalmol. 1974; 78: 363–383.

121. Waring GO III, Rodrigues MM, Laibson PR. Corneal dystrophies. II. Endothelial dystrophies. Surv Ophthalmol. 1978; 23: 147–168.

122. Laing RA, Leibowitz HM, Oak SS, et al. Endo-thelial mosaic in Fuchs dystrophy. A qualitative evaluation with the specular microscope. Arch Ophthalmol. Jan 1981; 99(1): 80–3.

123. Sharma N, Prakash G, Sinha R, et al. Indications and outcomes of phototherapeutic keratectomy in the developing world. Cornea. 2008 Jan; 27(1): 44–9.

124. Pires RT, Tseng SC, Prabhasawat P, et al. Amniotic membrane transplantation for symptomatic bullous keratopathy. Arch Ophthalmol. 1999 Oct; 117(10): 1291–7.

125. Alino AM, Perry HD, Kanellopoulos AJ, et al. Conjunctival flaps. Ophthalmology. 1998 Jun; 105(6): 1120–3.

126. Zemba M.Palliative treatment in bullous keratopathy. Oftalmologia. 2006; 50(2): 23–6.

127. Chung SH, Kim HK, Kim MS. Corneal Endothelial Cell Loss after Penetrating Keratoplasty in Relation to Preoperative Recipient Endothelial Cell Density. Ophthal-mologica. 2009 Oct 28; 224(3): 194–198.

128. Rose L, Kelliher C, Jun AS. Endothelial keratoplasty: historical perspectives, current techniques, future directions. Can J Ophthalmol. 2009 Aug; 44(4): 401–5.

129. Hjortdal J, Ehlers N. Descemet's stripping automated endothelial keratoplasty and penetrating keratoplasty for Fuchs endothelial dystrophy. Acta Ophthalmol. 2009 May; 87(3): 310–4.

130. Price MO, Gorovoy M, Benetz BA, et al. Descemet's Stripping Automated Endothelial Keratoplasty Outcomes Compared with Penetrat ing Keratoplasty from the Cornea Donor Study. Ophthalmology. 2010 Mar; 117(3): 438–444.

131. Eghrari AO, Daoud YJ, Gottsch JD. Cataract surgery in Fuchs corneal dystrophy. Curr Opin Ophthalmol. 2010 Jan; 21(1): 15–9.

132. Price MO, Giebel AW, Fairchild KM, et al. Descemet's membrane endothelial kerato-plasty: prospective multicenter study of visual and refractive outcomes and endothelial survival. Ophthalmology. 2009 Dec; 116(12): 2361–8.

133. Schlichting H. Blasen und dellenformige Endotheldystrophie der Hornhaut. Klin Monatsbl Augenkeilkd. 1941; 107: 425–435.

134. Rodrigues MM, Waring GO, Laibson PR, et al. Endothelial alterations in congenital corneal dystrophies. Am J Ophthalmol. 1975; 80: 678–689.

135. Hosseini SM, Herd S, Vincent AL, et al. Genetic analysis of chromosome 20-related posterior polymorphous corneal dystrophy: genetic heterogeneity and exclusion of three candidate genes.Mol Vis. 2008 Jan 16; 14: 71–80.

136. Aldave AJ, Yellore VS, Principe AH, et al. Candidate gene screening for posterior polymorphous dystrophy. Cornea. 2005; 24: 151–155.

137. Shimizu S, Krafchak C, Fuse N, et al. A locus for posterior polymorphous corneal dystrophy (PPCD3) maps to chromosome 10. Am J Med Genet. 2004; 130: 372–377.

138. Heon E, Mathers WD, Alward WL, et al. Linkage of posterior polymorphous corneal dystrophy to 20q11. Hum Mol Genet. 1995;4:485–488.

139. Krafchak CM, Pawar H, Moroi SE, et al. Mutations in TCF8 cause posterior poly-morphous corneal dystrophy and ectopic expression of COL4A3 by corneal endothelial cells. Am J Hum Genet. 2005; 77: 694–708.

140. Bower KS, Edwards JD, Wagner ME, et al. Novel corneal phenotype in a patient with alport syndrome. Cornea. 2009 Jun; 28(5): 599–606.

141. Harissi-Dagher M, Dana MR, Jurkunas UV. Keratoglobus in association with posterior polymorphous dystrophy. Cornea. 2007 Dec; 26(10): 1288–91.

142. Cremona FA, Ghosheh FR, Rapuano CJ, et al. Keratoconus associated with other corneal dystrophies. Cornea. 2009 Feb; 28(2): 127–35.

143. Cibis GW, Krachmer JA, Phelps CD, et al. The clinical spectrum of posterior polymorphous dystrophy. Arch Ophthalmol. 1977; 95: 1529–1537.

144. Krachmer JH. Posterior polymorphous endo-thelial dystrophy: a disease characterized by epithelial like endothelial cells which influence management and prognosis. Trans Am Ophthalmol Soc. 1985; 83: 413–475.

145. Patel DV, Grupcheva CN, McGhee CNJ. In vivo microscopy of posterior polymorphous dystrophy. Cornea. 2005; 24: 550–554.

146. Szaflik JP, Kolodziejska U, Udziela M, et al. Posterior polymorphous dystrophy—changes in corneal morphology in confocal microscopy. Klin Oczna. 2008; 110(7–9): 252–8.

147. Pearce WG, Tripathi RC, Morgan G. Congenital endothelial corneal dystrophy. Clinical, pathological, and genetic study. Br J Ophthalmol. 1969; 53: 577–591.

148. Judisch GF, Maumenee IH. Clinical differences of recessive congenital hereditary endothelial dystrophy and dominant hereditary endo-thelial dystrophy. Am J Ophthalmol. 1978; 85: 606–612.

149. Maumenee AE. Congenital hereditary corneal dystrophy. Am J Ophthalmol. 1960; 50: 1114–1124.

150. Toma NMG, Ebenezer ND, Inglehearn CF, et al. Linkage of congenital hereditary endothelial dystrophy to chromosome 20. Hum Mol Genet. 1995; 4: 2395–2398.

151. Callaghan M, Hand CK, Kennedy SM, et al. Homozygosity mapping and linkage analysis demonstrate that autosomal recessive congenital hereditary endothelial dystrophy (CHED) and autosomal dominant CHED are genetically distinct. Br J Ophthalmol. 1999; 83: 115–119.

152. Jiao X, Sultana A, Garg P, et al. Autosomal recessive corneal endothelial dystrophy (CHED2) is associated with mutations in SLC4A11. J Med Genet. 2007; 44: 64–68.

153. Siddiqui S, Zenteno JC, Rice A, et al. Congenital hereditaryendothelial dystrophy caused by SLC4A11 mutations progresses to Harboyan syndrome. Cornea. 2014; 33: 247–251.

154. Ramamurthy B, Sachdeva V, Mandal AK, et al. Coexistent congenital hereditary endothelial dystrophy and congenital glaucoma. Cornea. 2007 Jul; 26(6): 647–9.

155. Khan AO, Al-Shehah A, Ghadhfan FE. High measured intraocular pressure in children with recessive congenital hereditary endothelial dystrophy. J Pediatr Ophthalmol Strabismus. 2010 Jan-Feb; 47(1): 29–33.

156. Akhtar S, Bron AJ, Meek KM. Congenital hereditary endothelial dystrophy and band keratopathy in an infant with corpus callosum agenesis. Cornea. 2001 Jul; 20(5): 547–52.

157. Mahmood MA, Teichmann KD. Corneal amyloidosis associated with congenital hereditary endothelial dystrophy. Cornea. 2000 Jul; 19(4): 570–3.

158. Graham MAR, Azar NF, Dana MR. Visual rehabilitation in children with congenital hereditary endothelial dystrophy. Int Ophthalmol Clin. 2001; 41: 9–18.

159. Sajjadi H, Javadi MA, Hemmati R, et al. Results of penetrating keratoplasty in CHED: congenital hereditary endothelial dystrophy. Cornea. 1995; 14: 18–25

160. Schaumberg DA, Moyes AL, Gomes JA, et al. Corneal transplantation in young children with congenital hereditary endothelial dystrophy. Multicenter Pediatric Keratoplasty Study. Am J Ophthalmol. 1999 Apr; 127(4): 373–8.

161. Javadi MA, Baradaran-Rafii AR, Zamani M, et al. Penetrating keratoplasty in young children with congenital hereditary endothelial dystrophy. Cornea. 2003 Jul; 22(5): 420–3.

162. Pineda R 2nd, Jain V, Shome D, et al. Descemet's stripping endothelial keratoplasty: Is it an option for congenital hereditary endothelial dystrophy? Int Ophthalmol. 2009 Jul.

163. Schmid E, Lisch W, Philipp W, et al. A new, X-linked endothelial corneal dystrophy. Am J Ophthalmol. 2006; 141: 478–487.

Chapter
32

Corneal Degenerations

GENERAL CONSIDERATIONS

INTRODUCTION

Degenerations are defined as the gradual decomposition and deterioration of a tissue that was previously normal with frequent loss of its functional activity.

Degenerations of the ocular surface may result from physiologic changes associated with ageing, be related to a specific disease, or follow chronic environmental insults to the eye, such as exposure to ultraviolet (UV) light, continuous oxidative stress triggers degenerative processes.[1, 2]

Degenerations are late in onset, may be associated with specific local diseases and mostly unilateral or be related simply with ageing process and usually bilateral but often asymmetric and peripherally located. They uncommonly exhibit an inheritance pattern. Changes caused by inflammation, maturity or systemic diseases result in deposition, thinning or vascularization of corneal tissue. It is important to differentiate corneal degenerations from corneal dystrophies.

Corneal degenerations have been classified as; anterior/posterior, involutional/noninvolutional with material or pigments deposition, and eccentric/marginal degenerations. To simplify our understanding, we can classify corneal degeneration into involutional, i.e. primarily related age while noninvolutional, i.e. related with local or systemic condition.[3, 4]

CLASSIFICATION

Involutional corneal degenerations
- White limbal girdle of Vogt
- Arcus senilis
- Hassall-Henle bodies

Non-involutional corneal degenerations

Degenerations of epithelium and Bowman's membrane

- Coats' white ring
- Iron deposits
- Corneal verticillata
- Band-shaped keratopathy
- Spheroidal degeneration

Degenerations of corneal stroma

- Salzmann's nodular degeneration
- Lipid kerotopathy
- Amyloid degeneration
- Anterior/posterior crocodile shagreen
- Cornea farinata
- Corneal keloid
- Senile furrow degeneration
- Dellen
- Terrien's marginal degeneration
- Pellucid marginal degeneration

Degenerations of endothelium

- Peripheral corneal guttae/Hassall-Henle bodies.

INVOLUTIONAL CORNEAL DEGENERATIONS

Various age-related changes cannot be classified under any specific heading. As a result of ageing, the cornea gradually becomes flatter in the vertical meridian inducing astigmatism, decrease in thickness. Its refractive index increases, and Descemet membrane becomes thicker. Occasional peripheral endothelial guttae, sometimes known as Hassall-Henle bodies, can form with age. Age-related attrition of corneal endothelial cells results in a cell loss. The average rate of decrease in endothelial cell density throughout adult life is approximately 0.6% per year. Corneal luster also diminishes with age.

WHITE LIMBAL GIRDLE OF VOGT

Clinical features. Limbal girdle of Vogt is a narrow, crescentic, chalky white opacity in the nasal and temporal limbal areas of the cornea within the interpalpebral fissure.[5] It occurs more frequently in the nasal limbus than in the temporal limbus but is often symmetric.[5] With exposure, the inferior limbus may be involved as well. There are two types of limbal girdle:

Type 1 is thought to represent early calcific band keratopathy and is characterized by a white band that contains multiple holes separated from the limbus by a clear area.

Type 2 is the more common true limbal girdle. It is a chalky band without holes that is contiguous to the conjunctiva. No lucent zone is present. Fine white lines that run radially in type 2 limbal girdle are best seen using retroillumination and sclerotic scatter.

Incidence of Vogt's limbal girdle increases with age.

It has not been found before age 20. The incidence rises to approximately 55% in the 40–60-year age group and 100% in those over 80.[5]

Histopathologically, the lesion is subepithelial and may have overlying epithelial atrophy. Destruction and calcification of Bowman's layer have been observed in type 1.

Although calcium also has been identified at the level of Bowman in type 2. Elastotic degeneration similar to that seen in pinguecula has been found.

Treatment. This degeneration is an incidental finding and is asymptomatic. No treatment is required.

ARCUS SENILIS

Arcus senilis is considered the most common involutional corneal degeneration in elderly, with a prevalence of almost 100% in over 90-year-old subjects.

It is also known as *gerontoxon* in the aged and *arcus juvenilis* or anterior embryotoxon in the young population. It is a degenerative change involving lipid deposition in the peripheral cornea.

Clinical features

- *Location.* It first appears in the inferior cornea, followed by the superior cornea, and then encircles the entire cornea.[6,7]
- *Appearance.* Arcus senilis is an annular lipid infiltration of corneal periphery (Fig. 32.1). There is a clear interval between the sharply demarcated peripheral edge of the arcus and

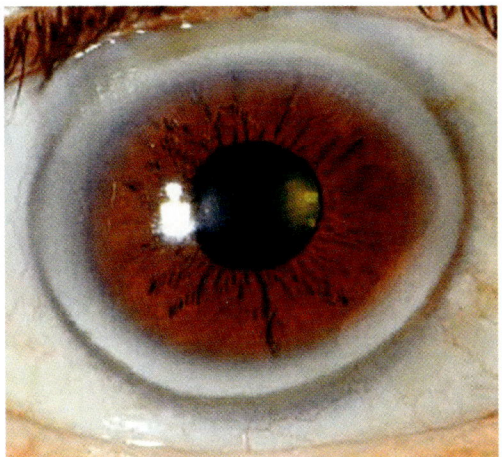

Fig. 32.1: *Arcus senilis*

the limbus that is approximately 0.3 to 1.0 mm (*lucid interval of Vogt*). The central edge is usually indistinct and the central cornea is never involved.

- *Laterality.* Typically it occurs symmetrically and bilaterally but can also occur unilaterally. Unilateral arcus senilis has been associated with unilateral carotid artery occlusion and also associated with ocular hypotony due to surgery or trauma.
- *Age and race.* It is found more commonly in men than in women, and is more common in blacks than in any other race.[8, 9]

Pathological features

Pathologically, deposits are composed of extracellular cholesterol, cholesterol esters, phospholipids, and triglycerides.[10, 11] These lipids, particularly low-density lipoproteins (LDL) of vascular origin, leak across the limbal capillaries into the cornea.[12] Corneal arcus preferentially forms in areas of increased vascularity.[8]

In the warmer regions of the cornea there is increased vascular permeability resulting in preferential lipid deposition. Because the inferior and superior portions of the cornea are the warmest regions of the cornea, whereas the central cornea is the coolest, arcus preferentially forms peripherally. Lipid deposits are first seen in the the deep stroma in proximity to the Descemet's membrane to extend to the sub-Bowman's superficial stroma, ending abruptly

with the termination of this structure. In advanced stages deposition is seen between the stromal lamellae, sparing the limbus.

- *Symptoms.* Patients with arcus senilis are asymptomatic and do not require treatment.

Etiopathogenesis

- *Aging.* Arcus senilis is generally a consequence of ageing.
- *Hyperlipoproteinaemia.* Patients under the age of 40 with corneal arcus have an increased risk of coronary artery disease and should be evaluated for hyperlipoproteinaemia.
- *Hyperlipoproteinaemia* types IIa and IIb are associated with premature corneal arcus formation, the most commonly observed being type IIa hyperlipoproteinaemia,[13] and should be referred to physician to undergo lipid and cardiovascular evaluation.

NON-INVOLUTIONAL CORNEAL DEGENERATIONS

There are various local and systemic causes for non-involutional corneal degenerations. *Depending upon the site of involvement,* these can be grouped as below.

- Degenerations of epithelium and Bowman's membrane
- Degenerations of corneal stroma
- Degenerations of endothelium

DEGENERATIONS OF EPITHELIUM AND BOWMAN'S MEMBRANE

COATS' WHITE RING

Coats first described a small (1 mm or less in diameter) circle or oval-shaped area of discrete gray-white dots sometimes seen at the level of Bowman's layer secondary to iron deposition. The overlying epithelium remains intact. It is usually located in the inferior cornea. The rings are secondary to corneal trauma and may in fact represent remnants of old metallic foreign bodies. Coats' rings are incidental findings and do not require treatment.

IRON DEPOSITS

Iron deposits occur due to abnormalities of tear pooling occurring as a consequence to surface irregularities. It shows variety of configurations including lines, rings, or diffuse depositions. Oftenly, they can be seen only by using red-free or cobalt blue illumination.

Histologically, iron (ferritin) is found intracellularly and extracellularly in the basal epithelial layer of the cornea, regardless of the type of iron line.

Source and etiology of the iron have been very controversial. The source has been attributed to the tears, aqueous humor, cellular breakdown, blood breakdown, or blood plasma. The most common theory attributes the deposition to localized trauma at the site of contour change or to a pooling of tears at this site.[14,15]

Hudson-Stähli line. The most common iron depositions are the Hudson-Stähli lines located in the deep corneal epithelium at the line of eyelid closure at the junction of the middle and lower thirds of the cornea. The line curves downward at its centre, is approximately 0.5 mm wide, 1 to 2 mm long, and is usually yellow, green, brown in colour. It occurs most commonly in patients over the age of 50, but decrease in frequency after the age of 70.[16–18] There is no sex predilection.

Other iron lines include:
- *Fleischer rings* around a cone in keratoconus,[17]
- *Ferry lines* near filtering blebs,[15] and
- *Stocker-Busacca lines* in front of pterygia.[19]

Iron lines can occur superficial corneal scars, after corneal transplants,[20] and surrounding refractive corneal procedures.[21, 22] Iron lines are asymptomatic and do not require treatment.

CORNEAL VERTICILLATA

Corneal verticillata, also called *vortex keratopathy*, was first described by Fleischer in 1910 as a whorl-shaped corneal dystrophy characterised by stippling of the corneal epithelium in patients with Fabry's disease.[23] Corneal verticillata consists of fine lines that swirl from a point below the centre of the cornea and radiate to the peripheral cornea in a vortex-like pattern (Fig. 32.2). Corneal verticillata consists of deposits at the level of the epithelium that usually do not alter visual acuity.

Vortex keratopathy is caused by side effects of certain drugs inducing deposits which results

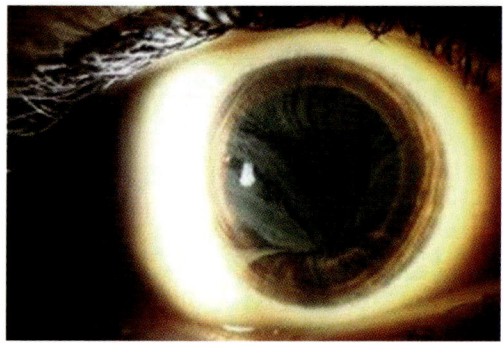

Fig. 32.2: *Cornea verticillata*

from chronic prolonged systemic therapies with amiodarone, chloroquine, hydroxychloroquine, tamoxifen, indomethacin, and phenothiazine with deposition in the cornea of phospholipids not metabolized by lysosomal phospholipases. Theses deposits are usually dose-dependent higher doses cause vortex keratopathy. The deposits are generally reversible and disappear on discontinuation of the systemic medication. *The vortex keratopathy is also seen in lipid storage disorder* called Fabry disease caused by inherited enzymatic deficiency. Corneal lipid depositions are localized in the basal epithelial cells.[24–26] Recent confocal investigation showed deeper stromal deposits in advanced forms, suggesting a higher toxicity than was thought until now in long-term treated patients.[27]

BAND-SHAPED KERATOPATHY

Calcific band keratopathy is characterised by deposition of calcium salt, hydroxyapatite, within the anterior cornea in epithelial basement membrane, Bowman's layer, most typically in the interpalpebral fissure.

Etiopathogenesis

Causes for band-shaped keratopathy mainly are:
- *Hypercalcaemic states*: Hypercalcaemia, hyperphosphataemia, chronic liver disease.
- *Chronic ocular disease*: Chronic keratitis, long-standing glaucoma, chronic uveitis or pthisis bulbi.
- *Chemicals (eye drops)*: Pilocarpine with mercurial preservatives, intraocular silicone oil, older viscoelastics with high phosphate

concentrations, and phosphate forms of corticosteroids.

- *Inherited diseases*: Hypophosphatasia, Norrie's disease.
- *Systemic disease:* Hyperparathyroidism, milk-alkali syndrome, sarcoidosis, vitamin D toxicity, and metastatic neoplastic disease.
- *Idiopathic*

Pathophysiology. Precipitation of calcium can occur due to alteration in tear osmolality, increase in pH from corneal tissue metabolism, increase in the concentration of either calcium or phosphate, or tear evaporation from exposure within the interpalpebral fissure. The pH of the interpalpebral fissure is higher than that of the rest of the ocular surface because of carbon dioxide release from the exposed zone. This also enhances calcium precipitation.

Symptoms. Band keratopathy is typically asymptomatic. Visual acuity decreases with the advancement of deposits. In the advanced stages, the density of calcium deposition might create a severe visual impairment, the deposits become elevated and produce considerable discomfort because of the ocular surface alterations and foreign body sensation.

Clinical features

Signs. Band keratopathy typically starts in the peripheral cornea at the 3 and 9 o'clock positions (Fig. 32.3) and encroaches to central cornea gradually. In advanced cases, the calcium deposits involve the entire cornea (Fig. 32.4). The peripheral edge is usually sharply demarcated and separated from the limbus by a clear zone.

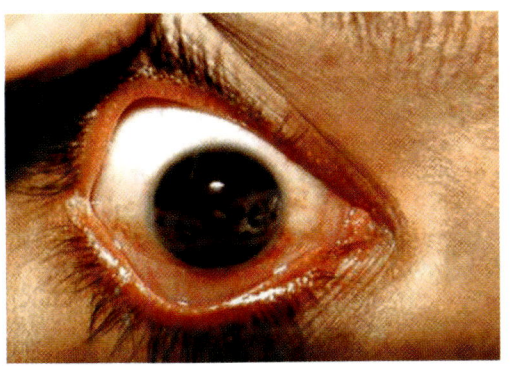

Fig. 32.3: *Band keratopathy*

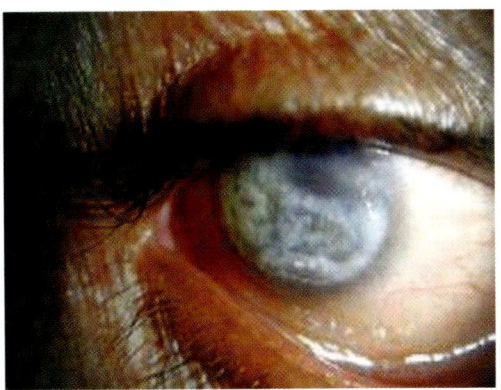

Fig. 32.4: *Advanced case of band keratopathy*

The clear zone may be due to the termination of Bowman's layer in the peripheral cornea.[28] The central edge of the deposit tends to be less sharply demarcated with a feathery appearance.

In early stage, calcium deposition is hazy and grey and progresses to become chalky white and opaque in later stage. Small translucent holes scattered throughout the band keratopathy represent the corneal nerves penetrating Bowman's layer, giving the deposit a **"Swiss cheese"** appearance.

Investigations

Investigations should include serum calcium, phosphorus, uric acid, and renal function measurements. If hyperparathyroidism or sarcoid is suspected, parathyroid hormone (PTH) can be obtained.

Treatment

Early stages of band keratopathy are asymptomatic. Later stages can be symptomatic with decreasing vision, foreign body sensation, tearing, or photophobia. When the patient becomes symptomatic, treatment is required.

1. Chelation. The mainstay of treatment is the application of ethylenediaminetetra-acetic acid (EDTA) 0.5–1.5%.

Epithelium is removed after instillation of topical anaesthetic since EDTA will not penetrate the epithelium. EDTA is then applied to the calcific areas, any cylindrical tube that approximates the corneal diameter (e.g. corneal trephine, or well) can facilitate the process by acting as a reservoir to confine the chelating solution to the desired treatment area; however, this is not always necessary. With the reservoir in place, very gentle surface agitation with a truncated cellulose sponge may further enhance the release of the impregnated calcium. If used at all, scraping should be gentle so as to prevent damage to the Bowman's layer. A diamond burr or No. 15 blade can be used to remove any residual calcium and to produce a smooth corneal surface.

2. Phototherapeutic keratectomy. Band keratopathy has been treated successfully using excimer laser phototherapeutic keratectomy.[29–32] The excimer laser has been used to clear the visual axis and improve vision. Laser therapy may be performed directly on smooth band keratopathy. Rough surface keratopathy requires scalpel removal of large plaques and a masking fluid to ablate tissue and leave a smooth surface.[29–32]

3. Amniotic membrane transplantation has been used after the primary surgical removal of band keratopathy to quickly restore a stable ocular surface.

4. Keratoplasty may be required in advanced cases.

SPHEROIDAL DEGENERATION

Spheroidal corneal degeneration is also known as corneal elastosis, Labrador keratopathy, climatic droplet keratopathy, Bietti's nodular dystrophy, proteinaceous corneal degeneration, elastotic degeneration, Fisherman's keratopathy, and Eskimo's corneal degeneration.

It was described by Bietti in 1955 and is characterised by oil-like, amber-coloured, spheroidal deposits at the limbus and in the peripheral interpalpebral cornea. This degeneration can affect both cornea and conjunctiva.

Etiology

Etiology and risk factors include ultraviolet radiation, ageing, low humidity, welding, prior corneal inflammation, extremes of temperature, and microtrauma from wind, sand.[33, 34] Its incidence increases with age. A high incidence of open angle glaucoma has been reported spheroidal degeneration.[35] It has male preponderance because of occupational exposure differences.

Classification

Spheroidal degeneration has been classified into three types:
- *Type 1* is a primary corneal degeneration that occurs bilaterally in corneas without ocular pathology.
- *Type 2* is a secondary corneal degeneration that occurs in association with other ocular pathology.
- *Type 3* is the conjunctival form that may coexist with either type 1 or 2 disease.[36, 37]

Primary spheroidal degeneration

Primary spheroidal degeneration has been further classified from trace to grade 4.

Trace: Small numbers of deposits in either one or both eyes with one end of the interpalpebral space.

Grade 1: Asymptomatic, fine shiny droplets in the peripheral cornea, best seen with retroillumination. These golden yellow droplets occur within the interpalpebral fissure in areas of exposure and are found beneath the conjunctival and corneal epithelium, within Bowman's layer in the cornea, or in the superficial corneal stroma.

Grade 2: It has central corneal involvement with larger deposits in the anterior stroma and concomitant decreased vision to the 20/100 level.

Grade 3: Large corneal nodules that elevate the epithelium and reduce vision to the 20/200 level or worse.

Grade 4: Larger deposits form elevated nodules and also involves deeper till anterior stroma and reduce vision.

Secondary spheroidal degeneration

Secondary spheroidal degeneration does not follow this grading system and tends to occur only in areas of scarring. Type 2 spheroidal degeneration occurs in patients with ocular disease such as chronic corneal edema, traumatic corneal scars, herpetic keratitis, glaucoma, and lattice corneal dystrophy.

The conjunctival form of spheroidal degeneration develops within the interpalpebral fissure and is generally associated with pingueculae.[36, 37]

Clinical features

Clinically on slit lamp, clear to yellow-gold spherules are seen in the subepithelium, within Bowman's layer or in the superficial corneal stroma (Fig. 32.5). They measure from 0.1 to 0.4 mm. In the early stages of type 1, they appear at the limbus in the interpalpebral zone at 3 and 9 o'clock. In type 2 the spherules may be diffuse or begin centrally. The conjunctival form also occurs interpalpebrally in the 3 and 9 o'clock positions.

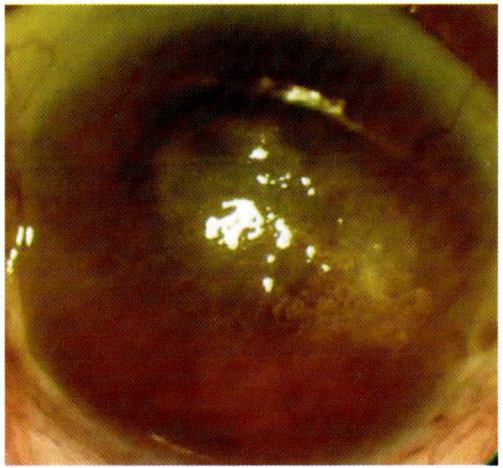

Fig. 32.5: *Spheroidal corneal degeneration*

Histopathogensis

Histopathogenesis of spheroidal degeneration is the deposition of advanced glycation end products of sugars and proteins that diffuse from limbal and conjunctival blood vessels on anterior corneal stroma which is degraded by ultraviolet radiation and the ageing process, inducing oxidative stress and molecular damage. Deposits demonstrate extracellular, proteinaceous, hyaline deposits with characteristics of elastotic degeneration. The composition is not lipid, despite its **"oil droplet"** appearance.

Advanced lesions may be nodular and break through the epithelium, causing irritation or foreign body sensation. It might cause focal, sterile ulceration may lead to a descemetocele or perforation. The lesions are often hypoesthetic or anesthetic. Sometimes superadded infection may occur.

Treatment

No medical therapy is of much value, although lubrication is recommended to address uneven layering of the tear film over affected areas.

Excimer laser phototherapeutic keratectomy[38] may be beneficial for milder form of degeneration.

Lamellar or penetrating keratoplasty is used to treat the severe advanced degenerations corneal form to restore vision.

■ DEGENERATIONS OF CORNEAL STROMA

SALZMANN'S NODULAR DEGENERATION

Salzmann's nodular degeneration (SND), first described in 1925, is a non-inflammatory, slowly progressive disease characterised by single or multiple grey or blue-grey subepithelial corneal nodules (Fig. 32.6). The nodules elevate the epithelium, often in a circular array at areas of corneal scarring or at the junction of old corneal scars and clear cornea. Nodules are often annular in location and in the mid-periphery. Each nodule is separated from other nodules by clear cornea, and iron lines may outline each nodule.[39] The nodules are not vascularized. A degenerative process that follows episodes of keratitis and commonly associated with a history of phlyctenular disease but was also observed after vernal keratoconjunctivitis, trachoma, measles, scarlet fever, exposure keratopathy, keratitis sicca, Thygeson's superficial punctate keratitis or interstitial keratitis.

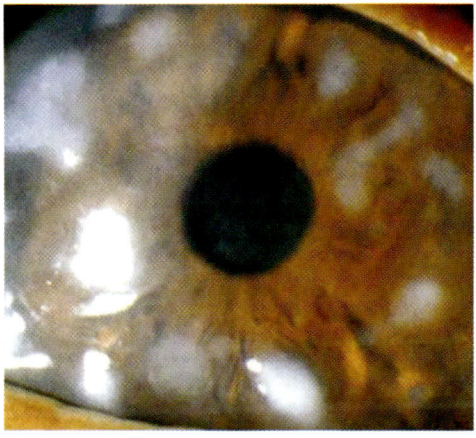

Fig. 32.6: *Salzmann's nodular degeneration*

These lesions are found more often in women than in men[40] and may be either unilateral or bilateral.

Main symptoms are visual disturbances and photophobia, ocular discomfort, mainly characterised by dryness, and foreign body sensation. In severe forms, characterised by elevated nodules, painful epithelial lesions can occur. Visual impairment is progressive and due to high irregular astigmatic defect produced by the nodules.

Diagnosis

The diagnosis of Salzmann's degeneration is based on clinical findings, several investigations such as corneal topography, anterior segment optical coherence tomography, and confocal microscopy are useful to provide a better understanding of the corneal alterations and to quantify the amount of visual impairment.

Corneal topography demonstrates the irregularities of the corneal shape produced by corneal nodules, and the induced surface alteration depends on their number and localization.

AC-OCT allows the evaluation of the nodules' dimension and depth of the stromal extension of the nodules that can help decide the surgical approach.[41]

Confocal microscopy shows an increased reflectivity of the anterior stroma with abnormal and activated keratocytes and marked stromal scatter corresponding to the nodules as a result of the presence of fibrosis.[42-44]

Histopathologically, dense collagen plaques with hyalinization are located between epithelium and Bowman's layer but may extend to one-third of the anterior stroma.

Frequently, there is an excessive secretion of basement membrane-like material, Bowman's layer is absent under the lesion replaced by fibrosis, and the overlying epithelium may be atrophic or absent,[45, 46] and also disorganization of the underlying stromal collagen.

Increased expression of matrix metalloproteinase 2 (MMP-2) was recently detected in patients affected by Salzmann's degeneration, and this may be responsible for the induction of the basement membrane and Bowman's layer disruption.[42, 44, 47, 48]

Treatment

Conservative therapy. In early forms, treatment is aimed with conservative therapy concerning eyelid hygiene, lubricants, and anti-inflammatory eye drops sufficiently to eliminate dry eye symptoms and foreign body sensation.

Surgical treatment. These patients usually present to outpatient department with varying degree of visual loss. Visual loss is an indication for surgical treatment, which consists of the removal of the nodules and the restoration of corneal surface regularity.

Excimer laser PTK. In superficial nodules, less than 100 micron the excimer laser PTK is usually performed to smoothen the surface.

Anterior lamellar kertoplasty in case of deep extension up to 140 micron superficial anterior lamellar kertoplasty (SALK) is sufficient to provide uniform smooth ocular surface. In the case of deeper ingrowth deep anterior lamellar keratoplasty (DALK) becomes necessary.

Recurrence of Salzmann's nodules after surgical removal can occur with varying prevalence rates (18–21.9%) and periods of time to recurrence (1 month to 6 years).[49–51]

LIPID KERATOPATHY

Lipid keratopathy (lipid degeneration, fatty degeneration of the cornea) is characterized by the deposition of grey to yellow-white lipids in the posterior corneal stroma, typically around abnormal blood vessels. The infiltrate is usually dense and yellowish white with feathery edges.

Pathophysiology

The lipid deposits tend to follow the distribution of vessels within the cornea and often has a fan-shaped appearance.

The lipids are similar to those seen in arcus senilis and consist of intracellular and extracellular cholesterol, cholesterol esters, phospholipids, and triglycerides.[52, 53] The cause of lipid keratopathy is unknown. Increased permeability of the newly formed vessels which are fragile and has weak intercellular junctions and altered metabolic activity of dying keratocytes may result in the release of lipids into the stroma. Lipid keratopathy is more common in women than men, with a ratio of 70 : 30.[54]

Clinical profile

Lipid keratopathy occurs in two forms: primary and secondary.

Primary lipid keratopathy is rare and is not associated with trauma or corneal neovascularization, family history of similar condition. No known disorders of lipid metabolism.[55, 56]

Primary lipid keratopathy is bilateral and is thought to be an extension of arcus senilis into the central cornea, decreasing vision when it extends into the visual axis. Patients with primary lipid keratopathy have serum lipids in the normal range.

Secondary lipid keratopathy can be seen with any condition that causes corneal neovascularization, including trauma, interstitial keratitis, herpetic keratitis, trachoma, corneal hydrops, corneal ulceration, and diffuse anterior scleritis.

Its onset is sudden and may cause a rapid decrease in vision.

The degeneration may be sea fan-shaped with feathery edges or as a dense discoid lesion. The discoid lesion occurs in areas of active inflammation, whereas the sea fan appears in areas of post-inflammatory inactive neovascularization. Sometimes crystals can be seen at edges of lesion.

Several rare autosomally inherited disorders deposit lipid in the cornea. These diseases are autosomally inherited and include familial LCAT deficiency, apolipoprotein A-1 deficiency, Tangier disease, and fish eye disease.[57] Patients with primary lipid keratopathy should be referred for screening of these disorders.

Treatment

In primary lipid keratopathy penetrating keratoplasty can be done for compromised cosmetic appearance or decreased vision. It may recur in graft.

For secondary lipid keratopathy treatment should focus on the underlying disease first. Successively, abnormal vascularization should be eliminated by argon laser photocoagulation or needle point cautery to induce the absorption of the lipids through the destruction of the feeder vessels. Corneal grafting remains the last treatment option, but it needs a relative quiescence,

and the clinical outcome is rather poor because of the corneal thinning, hypesthesia, and persistent vascularization.[58, 59]

AMYLOID DEGENERATION

The term amyloid applies to a group of fibrillar hyaline proteins including amyloid P protein (AP), prealbumin or transthyretin (AF), immunoglobulin light chains (AL), and acute phase reactants (AA) are deposited in a variety of target tissues[60] that were originally discovered because of starch like staining characteristics.

These serum proteins are found in various body tissues including the eye. Amyloidosis may be local or systemic, and each form may be primary or secondary. There are familial and nonfamilial forms of primary amyloidosis.

Secondary amyloidosis occurs in association with trauma or prolonged inflammatory conditions and is the most common cause of amyloidosis of the cornea.

Polymorphic amyloid degeneration is a bilaterally symmetric, slowly progressive corneal degeneration that appears late in life. The corneal opacities emerge as either stellate flecks in mid- to deep stroma or irregular filaments.

Histopathologically, amyloid stains metachromatically with crystal violet or methyl violet, produces secondary fluorescence with thioflavine, and shows red-green birefringence following Congo red staining when viewed under a polarizing microscope.

Clinical features

Amyloidosis can be primary or secondary, each of which can be systemic or localized.

Systemic amyloidosis

Primary systemic nonfamilial amyloidosis typically involves amyloid deposition in the tongue, heart, gastrointestinal tract, peripheral nerves, and kidney, leading to macroglossia, cardiomyopathy, malabsorption, neuropathy, and nephrotic syndrome. This form may be responsible for polyneuropathies and may cause ophthalmoplegia, ptosis, vitreoretinal veils and glaucoma.[4, 60] Meretoja syndrome, an example of a familial form of primary systemic amyloidosis, presents with lattice corneal dystrophy and cranial neuropathies.

Systemic amyloidosis rarely has ocular manifestations.

Secondary systemic amyloidosis is the most commonly encountered form of amyloidosis. It is typically found in association with malignancies, tuberculosis, syphilis, rheumatoid arthritis, and other chronic inflammatory conditions.[61] In secondary systemic amyloidosis, amyloid deposits accumulate in the liver, spleen, and kidney. Ocular involvement is rare, but can include immunoglobulin deposits in the cornea and conjunctiva in association with multiple myeloma and paraproteinemia.[62]

Localised amyloidosis

In contrast to systemic amyloidosis, localized amyloidosis commonly has ocular manifestations. Localized amyloidosis can also be primary or secondary. Primary localized amyloidosis encompasses disorders such as lattice corneal dystrophy, polymorphic amyloid degeneration (PAD), and gelatinous drop-like corneal dystrophy.

- *In lattice dystrophy* amyloid is typically deposited beneath the corneal epithelium in the anterior stroma. It may be large and filamentous, cause decreased vision and recurrent erosions, and are inherited and begin early in life.
- *PAD* is a common condition in elderly individuals in which bilateral amyloid deposition occurs in the central posterior corneal stroma and causes indentation of Descemet's membrane.[63,64] The deposits appear as punctate or filamentous opacities in the stroma that appear grey with direct illumination and may look crystalline on retroillumination. The lesions may branch with intervening clear stroma, similar in appearance to the deposits of lattice dystrophy. PAD deposits are usually not associated with any other conditions, are not inherited, do not affect vision, and do not require treatment.

Primary localized amyloidosis can be manifested yellow-pink masses located on the palpebral conjunctiva.

Secondary localized amyloidosis can also be found in the cornea, most commonly occurring in association with local eye disease such as ocular trauma, uveitis, keratoconus, retinopathy of prematurity, and trachoma.[65, 66] It has been found histologically in a subepithelial nodule or pannus, in deep corneal stroma, or in association with corneal neovascularization.[61]

Diagnosis

Diagnosis is typically made pathologically rather than clinically. In pathologic series, the incidence of amyloid corneal deposition was 3.5%, although the clinical significance of this finding is uncertain.[61] In patients with chronic keratitis or inflammation, large amyloid deposits can accumulate in the subepithelial anterior cornea and cause a foreign body sensation or interfere with vision. Such "**cobblestone**" amyloid degeneration can result in thinning of the epithelium and destruction of Bowman's layer.

Treatment

Treatment usually requires a penetrating keratoplasty.

ANTERIOR/POSTERIOR CROCODILE SHAGREEN

Crocodile shagreen, resemble as crocodile skin or cobblestone with mosaic pattern within the cornea, consists of grayish, white, sawtooth opacities separated by clear spaces.[67] Crocodile shagreen is typically seen bilaterally.

The opacities are most commonly seen in the anterior cornea but can also be seen in the posterior cornea. Both forms are usually seen in elderly patients.

Histopathologically, it shows folds in stroma either at Bowman's layer in anterior crocodile shagreen or at Descemet's membrane in posterior crocodile shagreen. The mosaic or sawtooth pattern of irregularly arranged collagen corresponds with the grayish opacity. Calcium may be deposited at the peaks of the sawtooth. Ridges form, indenting the epithelium and producing the mosaic pattern. Collagen lamellae that results in alternating clear and opaque areas.

Anterior crocodile shagreen is an age-related degeneration primarily. It has also been associated with band keratopathy, hypotony, trauma, X-linked megalocornea, and in kerato-conus patients wearing hard contact lenses. Generally anterior crocodile shagreen is visually insignificant, but rarely can reduce visual acuity.

Posterior crocodile shagreen is always age-related. Opacities are at the level of the deep corneal stroma. Central cloudy dystrophy of François has an autosomal-dominant inheri-tance pattern and is clinically similar to posterior crocodile shagreen.[68] In contrast to anterior crocodile shagreen, the opacities in posterior shagreen are mainly central, when peripherally located they may resemble arcus senilis. These opacities are usually visually insignificant and do not require treatment.

CORNEA FARINATA

Cornea farinata appears with fine tiny, grayish, comma-shaped, dust-like, flour-like opacities scattered in the posterior corneal stroma near Descemet's membrane. Cornea farinata has an appearance similar to pre-Descemet's dys-trophies, but the opacities are smaller and occur later in life.[69] These opacities occur bilaterally in elderly patients, are usually in the pupillary area, and are seen best on retroillumination. The deposits may consist of lipofuscin, a degene-rative pigment that appears in old ageing cells. The condition does not affect vision and has no clinical significance, except that it is sometimes mistaken for a progressive dystrophy.

CORNEAL KELOID

Corneal keloids are white, superficial but may extend up to stroma, and sometimes protuberant glistening corneal masses that can eventually involve the entire corneal surface. They are thought to be secondary to a vigorous fibrotic response to corneal injury or chronic ocular surface inflammation. Keloids can be congenital or primary, and they have been reported in association with many congenital conditions, such as Lowe syndrome. They have sometimes been confused with hypertrophic scars, Salzmann's degeneration, or dermoids. Keloids are usually seen in a younger age group than Salzmann's degeneration and occur more frequently in men.[70]

Histopathologic examination demonstrates fibroblastic proliferation intermixed with hyalinized collagen bundles. AS-OCT is helpful to determine its boundries and depth into cornea for surgical planning. Treatment with superficial keratectomy or lamellar or penetrating keratoplasty may be performed for visually significant lesions.

SENILE FURROW DEGENERATION

Senile furrow degeneration is a rare condition found in older individuals in which the lucent area peripheral to corneal arcus undergoes minimal thinning. The epithelium is intact. There is no inflammation, vascularization, or tendency to perforate. Patients are typically asymptomatic and do not require treatment.

DELLEN

Dellen is a localized area of corneal thinning in the periphery close to the limbus. It is located in proximity to the areas of tissue swelling or inflammation when correct spreading of the tear layer is highly disturbed. It is seen commonly in temporal part of peripheral cornea. Dellen are usually transient, lasting only 24 to 48 hours, but in rare cases can last several weeks and lead to scarring. Clinically, dellen are saucer-like depressions in the corneal surface. They are more commonly adjacent to elevated areas of conjunctival chemosis from pterygia, epi-scleritis, conjunctivitis, or after cataract, glaucoma filtering, or strabismus surgery, penetrating keratoplasty. Dellen are also seen after anaesthetic use, particularly with cocaine. Histopathologically, there is thinning of the corneal epithelium, Bowman's layer, and the superficial stroma. This relatively common condition is reversible. In fact, the restoration of the normal film layer spreading and intense lubrication. Recently, the use of a large-diameter soft contact lens was proven to be an effective therapeutic solution to treat the dellen that arose after a pterygium removal.[71]

TERRIEN'S MARGINAL DEGENERATION

It was first described by Terrien in 1900, as painless, noninflammatory, unilateral or asymmetrically bilateral, slowly progressive thinning of the peripheral cornea. The degenerative etiology being unknown but commonly seen in those between 20 and 40 years of age. Male to female ratio is 3:1 and can occur in the second eye decades after the first.[72]

Clinical profile (Fig. 32.7). It starts superonasally or superotemporally with fine punctate stromal opacities separated from the limbus by a clear cornea. Superficial vascularization from limbal vessels differentiating it from corneal arcus. Peripheral stroma thins out gradually over period of times with epithelium remains intact. Peripheral progressive thinning extends in a circumferentially involving the whole corneal periphery, and in the advanced forms, the degeneration becomes circumferential. A yellow-white zone of lipid deposition can be seen central to the advancing edge.

Spontaneous perforation is rare, although it can easily occur with minor trauma. Ruptures in Descemet's membrane can result in interlamellar fluid or even a hydrops.

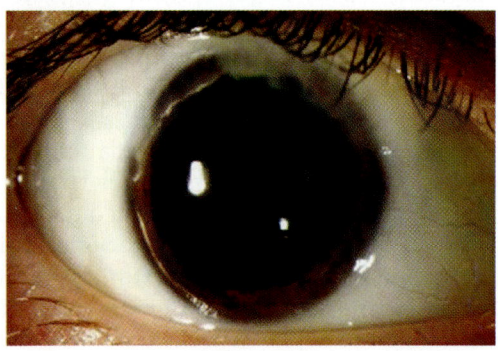

Fig. 32.7: *Terrien's marginal degeneration*

Histopathology, shows fibrillar degeneration of collagen. Epithelium is normal; Bowman's layer is fragmented or absent. Breaks in Descemet's membrane may be seen in thinned areas with aqueous pockets occasionally can be seen on slit lamp examination and also on AS-OCT. The lipid deposits consist of cholesterol crystals.

Corneal topography reveals flattening of the peripheral thinned cornea, with steepening of the corneal surface approximately 90° away from the midpoint of the thinned area. This pattern usually results in high against-the-rule or oblique astigmatism. Topography shows

typical lobster claw appearance. The AC-OCT might be helpful in the evaluation of the peripheral thinning and in differential diagnosis with other peripheral corneal disorders. Recent AC-OCT findings report the stromal cavity formation in the peripheral cornea probably due to the collagen phagocytosis.[73]

Differential diagnosis should consider the peripheral corneal melt, Mooren's ulcer, pellucid marginal degeneration, and dellen.

Treatment

Patients may present with decreased vision from the induced astigmatism or with episodes of painful inflammation, episcleritis, or scleritis. However, there is no treatment to prevent the progression of the disease, patients are treated with rigid gas permeable contact lenses or semi-scleral contact lenses for the astigmatism. Banana, crescent-shaped lamellar or eccentric penetrating corneo-scleral patch grafts may be used in impending perforation or perforation; they have been reported to arrest the progression of severe against-the-rule astigmatism. Annular lamellar keratoplasty grafts may be required in severe cases of 360° marginal degeneration.

PELLUCID MARGINAL DEGENERATION

Pellucid (meaning, transparent) is nonhereditary, bilateral, peripheral thinning of cornea, commonly inferior in the absence of inflammation. The etiology is unknown. This entity usually located inferiorly from 4 to 8 o'clock position. There is 1–2 mm area of band of thinning with some uninvolved area between thinning and limbus. Unilateral cases have also been reported.[74, 75] Pellucid marginal degeneration is seen in most patients between 20 and 40 years of age, and men and women are affected equally.

Pellucid marginal degeneration versus keratoconus. In contrast to keratoconus, protrusion of the cornea occurs above the band of thinning. The central protruding cornea is usually of normal thickness (Fig. 32.8).

In early cases, a clear distinction between pellucid marginal degeneration and keratoconus is not possible. A cornea with keratoconus will

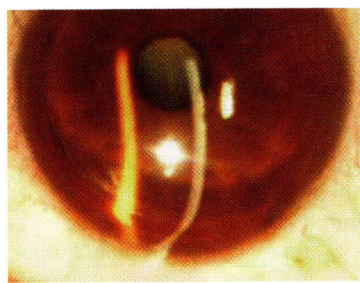

Fig. 32.8: *Pellucid marginal degeneration*

show protrusion at the point of maximal thinning, but pellucid marginal degeneration can inferior and will show protrusion above the area of maximum thinning. In moderate cases, pellucid marginal degeneration can easily be differentiated from keratoconus by slit-lamp evaluation because of the classical location of the thinning.

Advanced pellucid marginal degeneration may be difficult to distinguish from keratoconus because the thinning may progress to involve most of the inferior cornea.

Investigation with pentacam, videokeratography is very useful to make the distinction. Pellucid marginal degeneration (PMD) has a classical "crab-claw" or "butterfly" appearance and demonstrates abnormal corneal contour induces a shift in the axis of astigmatism from against-the-rule, superiorly, to with-the-rule, near the point of maximal protrusion.

PMD can be differentiated from other ectatic and peripheral thinning disorders in terms of no vascularization, lipid deposition, infiltrates, no iron rings occur, but posterior stromal scarring has been noted within the thinned area.

Histopathologic examination shows the epithelium, Descemet's membrane, and the endothelium are normal. Rodrigues et al found normal or focal disruption of Bowman's layer.[76] Stromal scars have been described at the level of Descemet's membrane extending into the mid-stroma, located at the superior aspect of the thinned area. Cameron reported such scars in 39% of PMD patients.[77] Subtle Descemet's folds, which are occasionally seen concentric to the inferior limbus, may disappear with external pressure. While the cornea can become quite thin, rupture rarely occurs. Acute hydrops has

been reported, and, though rare, spontaneous corneal perforation has also occurred.

Treatment

Decreased vision due to high against the astigmatism. Spectacle correction will not be of much help.

Contact lenses

In early and mild cases, overall large diameter mini-scleral or scleral contact lenses with high gas permeability can be attempted, although lens fitting is more difficult in pellucid marginal degeneration than in keratoconus. Hybrid (gas permeable contact lenses with a soft lens "skirt") may be options.

In patients in whom contact lenses do not adequately correct vision or in patients who are contact lens intolerant, surgery may be considered.

Surgical treatment

Wedge resection or crescentic lamellar tectonic keratoplasty is a useful initial surgical procedure in patients with pellucid marginal degeneration. This approach often reduces the astigmatism and in some instances makes the patient contact lens tolerant.

Penetrating keratoplasty. In contact lens failures, large-diameter or eccentric penetrating keratoplasty may be necessary to encompass the area of peripheral thinning. PK may be required to restore vision. Because of the location of the thinning, the grafts tend to be large and close to the limbus, making surgery technically more difficult and the graft more prone to rejection. Kremer et al described a two-stage procedure in which a large-diameter lamellar keratoplasty is followed by a smaller central penetrating keratoplasty.[78]

Collagen crosslinking may also be considered for some of these patients.

■ DEGENERATIONS OF ENDOTHELIUM

PERIPHERAL CORNEAL GUTTAE/ HASSALL-HENLE BODIES

It is an involutional change wherein peripheral cornea guttae (Hassall-Henle bodies) are small, wart-like excrescences that appear in the peripheral portion of Descemet's membrane. A normal ageing change, they result from the thickening of Descemet's membrane that happens throughout life; they occur on the posterior part of the membrane and protrude toward the anterior chamber. On slit lamp examination, Hassall-Henle bodies (Fig. 32.9) have the appearance of small, dark dimples within the endothelial mosaic; these are best seen by specular reflection. Rarely seen before age 20, they then increase steadily in number with age. When they appear in the central cornea, they are pathologic and are called cornea guttae. Central cornea guttae associated with progressive stromal and eventually epithelial edema represent Fuchs endothelial dystrophy.[79]

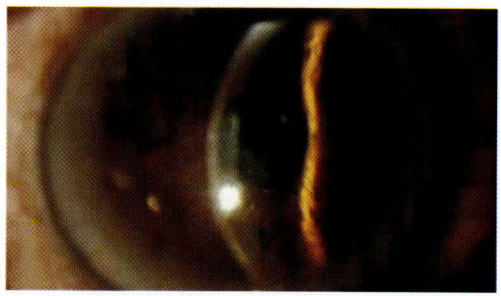

Fig. 32.9: *Peripheral corneal guttae/Hassall-Henle bodies*

REFERENCES

1. Friedlaender MH, Smolin G. Corneal degenerations. Ann Ophthalmol. 1979; 11(10): 1485–95.
2. Saccà SC, Roszkowska AM, Izzotti A. Environmental light and endogenous antioxidants as the main determinants of non-cancer ocular diseases. Mutat Res 2013; 752(2): 153–71.
3. Duke-Elder S, Leigh AG. System of ophthalmology. In: Diseases of the outer eye. Vol 8. St Louis: Mosby; 1965.
4. Sugar A. Corneal and conjunctival degenerations. In: Kaufman HE, et al. (Eds). The cornea. New York: Churchill Livingstone; 1988.
5. Sugar HS, Kobernick S. The white limbus girdle of Vogt. Am J Ophthalmol 1960; 50: 101–107.
6. François J, Feher J. Arcus senilis. Doc Ophthalmol 1973; 34: 165–182.
7. Rifkind BM. Corneal arcus and hyperlipoproteinemia. Surv Ophthalmol 1972; 16: 295–304.
8. Barchiesi BJ, Eckel RH, Ellis PP. The cornea and disorders of lipid metabolism. Surv Ophthalmol 1991; 36: 1–22.
9. Cooke NT. Significance of arcus senilis in Caucasians. JR Soc Med 1981; 74: 201–204.
10. Cogan DG, Kuwabara T. Arcus senilis: Its pathology and histochemistry. Arch Ophthalmol 1959; 61: 553–560.
11. Andrews JS. The lipids of arcus senilis. Arch Ophthalmol 1962; 68: 264–266.
12. Walton KW. Studies on the pathogenesis of corneal arcus formation: the human corneal arcus and its relation to atherosclerosis as studied by immunofluorescence. J Pathol 1973; 111: 263–274.
13. Crispin S. Ocular lipid deposition and hyperlipoproteinaemia. Prog Retin Eye Res. 2002; 21: 169–224.
14. Barraquer-Somers E, Chan CC, Green WR. Corneal epithelial iron deposition. Ophthalmology 1983; 90: 729–734.
15. Ferry AP. A 'new' iron line of the superficial cornea. Arch Ophthalmol 1968; 79: 142–145.
16. Norn MS. Hudson-Stähli line of the cornea. Acta Ophthalmol (Copenh) 1968; 46: 106.
17. Gass JDM. The iron lines of the superficial cornea. Arch Ophthalmol 1964; 71: 348–358.
18. Rose GE, Lavin MJ. The Hudson–Stähli line. I. An epidemiologic study. Eye 1987; 1: 466.
19. Stocker FW. Demonstrationen: eine pigmentierte Hornhautlinie bei Pterygium. Schweiz Med Wochenschr 1939; 20: 19.
20. Mannis MJ. Iron deposition in the corneal graft. Another corneal iron line. Arch Ophthalmol 1983; 101: 1858–1861.
21. Koenig SB, Mc Donald MB, Yamaguchi T, et al. Corneal iron lines after refractive keratoplasty. Arch Ophthalmol 1983; 101: 1862–1865.
22. Vongthongsri A, Chuck RS, Pepose JS. Corneal iron deposits after laser *in situ* keratomileusis. Am J Ophthalmol 1999; 127: 85–86.
23. Collyer RT. Amyloidosis of the cornea. Can J Ophthalmol 1968; 3: 35–38.
24. D'Amico DJ, Kenyon KR, Ruskin JN. Amiodarone keratopathy: drug-induced lipid storage disease. Arch Ophthalmol 1981; 99(2): 257–61.
25. Hollander DA, Aldave AJ. Drug-induced corneal complications. Curr Opin Ophthalmol 2004; 15(6): 541–8.
26. Falke K, Büttner A, Schittkowski M, Stachs O, Kraak R, Zhivov A, Rolfs A, Guthoff R. The microstructure of cornea verticillata in Fabry disease and amiodarone-induced keratopathy: A confocal laser-scanning microscopy study. Graefes Arch Clin Exp Ophthalmol 2009; 247(4): 523–34.

27. Ciancaglini M, Carpineto P, Zuppardi E, Nubile M, Doronzo E, Mastropasqua L. *In vivo* confocal microscopy of patients with amiodarone-induced keratopathy. Cornea 2001; 20(4): 368–73.

28. O'Connor GR. Calcific band keratopathy. Trans Am Ophthalmol Soc 1972; 70: 58.

29. O'Brart DPS, et al. Treatment of band keratopathy by excimer laser phototherapeutic keratectomy: surgical techniques and long-term follow up. Br J Ophthalmol 1993; 77: 702–708.

30. Amano S, Oshika T, Tazawa Y, et al. Long-term follow-up of excimer laser phototherapeutic keratectomy. Jpn J Ophthalmol 1999; 43: 513–516.

31. Dogru M, Katakami C, Miyashita M, et al. Ocular surface changes after excimer laser phototherapeutic keratectomy. Ophthalmology. 2000; 107: 1144–1152.

32. Rapuano CJ. Excimer laser phototherapeutic keratectomy: long-term results and practical considerations. Cornea 1997; 16(2): 151–157.

33. Garner A, Fraunfelder FT, Barras TC, et al. Spheroidal degeneration of the cornea and conjunctiva. Br J Ophthalmol 1976; 60: 473.

34. Norn M, Franck C. Long-term changes in the outer part of the eye in welders. Acta Ophthalmol (Copenh) 1991; 69: 382.

35. Hanna C, Fraunfelder FT. Spheroidal degeneration of the cornea and conjunctiva. 2. Pathology. Am J Ophthalmol 1972; 74: 829–839.

36. Fraunfelder FT, Hanna C. Spheroidal degeneration of the cornea and conjunctiva. 3. Incidence, classification, and etiology. Am J Ophthalmol 1973; 76: 41.

37. Fraunfelder FT, Hanna C, Parker JM. Spheroidal degeneration of the cornea and conjunctiva. 1. Clinical course and characteristics. Am J Ophthalmol 1972; 74: 821–828.

38. Ayres BD, Rapuano CJ. Excimer laser phototherapeutic keratectomy. Ocul Surf 2006; 4(4): 196–206.

39. Reinach NW, Baum J. A corneal pigmented line associated with Salzmann's nodular degeneration. Am J Ophthalmol 1981; 91: 677.

40. Severin M, Kirchhof B. Recurrent Salzmann's corneal degeneration. Graefe's Arch Clin Exp Ophthalmol 1990; 228: 101–104.

41. Humeric V, Yoo SH, Karp CL, Galor A, Vajzovic L, Wang J, Dubovy SR, Forster RK. *In vivo* morphologic characteristics of Salzmann nodular degeneration with ultra-high-resolution optical coherence tomography. Am J Ophthalmol 2011; 151: 248–56.

42. Meltendorf C, Bühren J, Bug R, Ohrloff C, Kohnen T. Correlation between clinical *in vivo* confocal microscopic and *ex vivo* histopathologic findings of Salzmann nodular degeneration. Cornea 2006; 25: 734–8.

43. Ku JY, Grupcheva CN, McGhee CN. Microstructural analysis of Salzmann's nodular degeneration by *in vivo* confocal microscopy. Clin Experiment Ophthalmol 2002; 30: 367–8.

44. Roszkowska AM, Aragona P, Spinella S, Pisani A, Puzzolo D, Micali A. Morphological and confocal investigation on Salzmann nodular degeneration of the cornea. Invest Ophthalmol Vis Sci 2011; 52: 5910–9.

45. Wood TO. Salzmann's nodular degeneration. Cornea 1990; 9: 17–22.

46. Werner LP, Issis K, Werner LP, et al. Salzmann's corneal degeneration associated with epithelial basement membrane dystrophy. Cornea 2000; 19(1): 121–123.

47. Stone DU, Astley RA, Shaker RP, Chodosh J. Histopathology of Salzmann nodular corneal degeneration. Cornea 2008; 27: 148–51.

48. Vannas A, Hogan MJ, Wood I. Salzmann's nodular degeneration of the cornea. Am J Ophthalmol 1975; 79: 211–9.

49. Sinha R, Chhabra MS, Vajpayee RB, Kashyap S, Tandon R. Recurrent Salzmann's nodular degeneration: Report of two cases and review of literature. Indian J Ophthalmol 2006; 54: 201–2.

50. Severin M, Kirchhof B. Recurrent Salzmann's corneal degeneration. Graefes Arch Clin Exp Ophthalmol 1990; 228: 101–4.

51. Yoon KC, Park YG. Recurrent Salzmann's nodular degeneration. Jpn J Ophthalmol. 2003; 47: 401–4.

52. Jack RL, Lase SA. Lipid keratopathy, an electron microscopic study. Arch Ophthalmol 1970; 83: 678.

53. Friedlaender MH, Cavanagh HD, Sullivan WR, et al. Bilateral central lipid infiltrates of the cornea. Am J Ophthalmol 1977; 84: 781.

54. Crispin S. Ocular lipid deposition and hyperlipoproteinaemia. Prog Retin Eye Res 2002; 21: 169–224.

55. Fine BS, Townsend WM, Zimmerman LE, et al. Primary lipoidal degeneration of the cornea. Am J Ophthalmol 1974; 78: 12.

56. Baum JL. Cholesterol keratopathy. Am J Ophthalmol 1969; 67: 372.

57. Rifkind BM. Corneal arcus and hyperlipo-proteinemia. Surv Ophthalmol 1972; 16: 295–304.

58. Croxatto JO, Dodds CM, Dodds R. Bilateral and massive lipoidal infiltration of the cornea (secondary lipoidal degeneration). Ophthalmology 1985; 92(12): 1686–90.

59. Levy J, Benharroch D, Lifshitz T. Bilateral severe progressive idiopathic lipid keratopathy. Int Ophthalmol 2005; 26: 181–4.

60. Blodi FC, Apple DJ. Localized conjunctival amyloidosis. Am J Ophthalmol 1979; 88: 346–350.

61. McPherson SD, Kiffney GT. Corneal amyloidosis. Am J Ophthalmol 1966; 62: 1025–1033.

62. Gorevic PE, et al. Lack of evidence for protein AA reactivity in amyloid deposits of lattice corneal dystrophy and amyloid corneal degeneration. Am J Ophthalmol 1984; 98: 216–224.

63. Mannis MJ, Krachmer JH, Rodrigues MM, et al. Polymorphic amyloid degeneration of the cornea: a histopathologic study. Arch Ophthalmol 1981; 99: 1217–1223.

64. Nirankari V, Rodrigues MM, Rajagopalan S, et al. Polymorphic amyloid degeneration. Arch Ophthalmol 1989; 107: 595.

65. Collyer RT. Amyloidosis of the cornea. Can J Ophthalmol 1968; 3: 35–38.

66. Garner A. Amyloidosis of the cornea. Br J Ophthalmol 1969; 53: 73–81.

67. Vogt A. Textbook and atlas of slit lamp microscopy of the living eye. Bonn: Wayenborgh Editions, 1981.

68. Bramsen T, Ehlers N, Braggesen LH. Central cloudy corneal dystrophy of François. Acta Ophthalmol (Copen) 1976; 54: 221–226.

69. Curran RE, Kenyon KR, Green WR. Pre-Descemet's membrane corneal dystrophy. Am J Ophthalmol 1974; 77: 711–716.

70. Mullaney PB, Teichmann K, Huaman A, et al. Corneal keloid from unusual penetrating trauma. J Pediatr Ophthalmol Strabismus. 1995; 32: 331–334.

71. Kymionis GD, Plaka A, Kontadakis GA, Astyrakakis N. Treatment of corneal dellen with a large diameter soft contact lens. Cont Lens Anterior Eye 2011; 34(6): 290–2.

72. Goldman KN, Kaufman HE. Atypical pterygium: a clinical feature of Terrien's marginal degeneration. Arch Ophthalmol. 1978; 96: 1027–1029.

73. Hattori T, Kumakura S, Mori H, Goto H. Depiction of cavity formation in Terrien marginal degeneration by anterior segment optical coherence tomography. Cornea 2013; 32(5): 615–8.

74. Rosenthal P, Cotter JM. Clinical performance of a spline-based apical vaulting keratoconus corneal contact lens design. CLAO J 1995; 21: 42–46.

75. Yeung K, Egbahli F, Weissman BA. Clinical experience with piggyback contact lens systems on keratoconic eyes. J Am Optom Assoc 1995; 66: 539–543.

76. Rodrigues MM, Newsome DA, Krachmer JH, Eiferman RA. Pellucid marginal corneal degeneration: a clinicopathologic study of two cases. Exp Eye Res 1981; 33: 277–288.

77. Cameron JA. Deep corneal scarring in pellucid marginal corneal degeneration. Cornea 1992; 11: 309–310.

78. Kremer I, Sperber LT, Laibson PR. Pellucid marginal degeneration treated by lamellar and penetrating keratoplasty. Arch Ophthalmol 1993; 111: 169–170.

79. Yanoff M, Fine BS. Ocular pathology. 5th ed. St. Louis: Mosby. 2002.

Iridocorneal Endothelial Syndrome

GENERAL CONSIDERATIONS AND PATHOGENESIS

GENERAL CONSIDERATIONS

Iridocorneal endothelial (ICE) syndrome is characterised by an abnormal corneal endothelium associated with iris atrophy, corneal oedema and secondary angle-closure glaucoma. Originally, it was described that ICE includes three clinical entities, viz. progressive iris atrophy, Chandler's syndrome and Cogan-Reese (iris naevus) syndrome, which were distinguished on the basis of changes in the iris. However, presently it is considered that the three clinical variants represent a spectrum of ICE syndrome rather than distinct clinical entities.

PATHOGENESIS

Formation of endothelial membrane

The characteristic features of ICE syndrome is the presence of corneal endothelial cells which proliferate to form a membrane which covers the angle of the anterior chamber and to some extent the anterior surface of the iris. Contraction of this membrane leads to the following changes:

- *Secondary angle-closure glaucoma*, due to the formation of PAS.
- *Iris defects,* such as correctopia, stretch holes and iris nodules.
- *Ischaemia of iris* may occur secondary to contraction, which may lead to the 'melt holes'.

Theories of endothelial membrane formation

What causes the abnormal corneal endothelium is still not clear. Absence of positive family history and the presence of postnatal layer of Descemet's membrane suggest that it is an acquired disorder. Following views were put forward:

- *Abnormal proliferation of neural crest cells* has been held responsible for abnormal endothelial cells by some workers.
- *Viral theory*, blaming HSV has been put forward based on the electron micrographic,

immunohistochemical and serological studies while in some studies Epstein-Barr virus has been blamed. The viral theory is attractive and might explain the unilaterality of the syndrome in majority of the patients.

CLINICAL PROFILE AND MANAGEMENT

CLINICAL FEATURES

General features

Age and sex. ICE syndrome typically affects middle-aged females (20–40 years) more often.
Laterality. The condition is almost always unilateral. However, subclinical abnormalities of corneal endothelium are reported in the fellow eye.

Clinical presentation

Presenting features include reduced visual acuity, pain, corneal oedema, abnormalities of iris and raised IOP.
Glaucoma occurs in about 50% of cases.

Signs

1. *Corneal signs* include:
- *Fine hammered silver appearance* of the posterior cornea, similar to Fuchs endothelial dystrophy is seen on slit-lamp examination.
- *Abnormal endothelial cells* on specular microscopy appear dark with a light central spot and light peripheral zone with varying degree of pleomorphism in shape and size and less of clear hexagonal margins.
- *Corneal oedema* occurs when IOP is raised.

2. *Iris signs* are pathognomonic of various clinical variants of ICE syndrome as described below.

3. *Lens signs.* The retrocorneal membrane may grow over the anterior surface of the lens. It simulates anterior lens capsule and may create confusion while creating a capsulorrhexis during cataract surgery.

4. *Peripheral anterior synechiae* (PAS), usually extending to or beyond the Schwalbe's line seen on gonioscopy, are characteristic feature of ICE syndrome.

5. *IOP* rises when PAS becomes extensive. On occasion, IOP may be raised despite open-angle

due to pretrabecular membrane before contraction.

CLINICAL SPECTRUM OF ICE SYNDROME

Depending upon the characteristic features, the three clinical variants (now considered to be the spectrum of ICE syndrome) are as below.

1. Progressive essential iris atrophy

In progressive essential iris atrophy, the iris features predominate (Fig. 33.1) with:
Marked correctopia, iris atrophy and ectropion uveae that usually occur toward the quadrant with most prominent PAS.
Iris holes which are of two types:
- *Stretch holes,* caused by traction, occur in the quadrant away from the direction of pupillary displacement.
- *Meet holes,* ischaemic in nature, occur without correctopia.

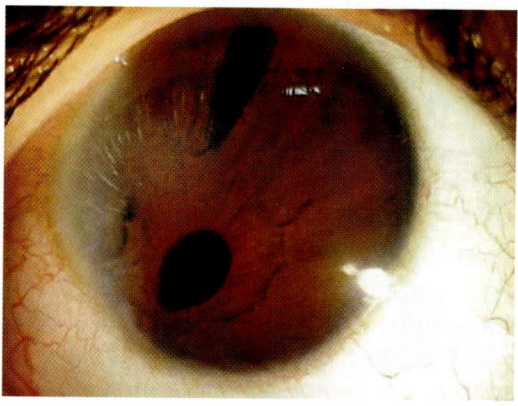

Fig. 33.1: *Essential iris atrophy*

2. Chandler's syndrome

It is characterised by:
- *Iris changes* are minimal to absent.
- *Corneal changes* are marked and oedema may occur even at normal IOP.

3. Cogan-Reese syndrome

It is characterised by nodular or diffuse pigmented lesions of the iris. Therefore, it is called iris naevus syndrome. Ultrastructure of the iris nodules is similar to that of the underlying iris stroma and is always surrounded by the continuation of the retrocorneal membrane. Corneal oedema may or may not be associated.

MANAGEMENT

A. Treatment of glaucoma

1. Medical therapy with aqueous suppressants may be effective in early cases. However, failure with medical therapy is common.

2. Surgical therapy is often required.

i. *Trabeculectomy with mitomycin C use* may be useful. Failure of trabeculectomy with endothelialization of the filtering bleb is not uncommon. Repeat trabeculectomy may be considered. The success rates for repeated trabeculectomies are comparable to those of the initial procedure and similar to repeat procedures in patients with POAG.

ii. *Glaucoma drainage devices* may be tried in cases with failure of repeat trabeculectomy.

iii. *Cyclodestructive procedures* are last resort considerations.

B. Treatment of corneal oedema

1. *Lowering of IOP*, as described above, clears the corneal oedema in most of the cases.

2. *Hypertonic saline* solution may be used for early clearance of corneal oedema.

3. *Penetrating keratoplasty* is required in non-responsive cases.

C. Treatment of underlying mechanism

1. *Role of antiviral drugs* needs to be evaluated, if the viral theory of etiology is proved.

2. *Role of immunotoxin drugs* is being evaluated to inhibit the proliferation of human corneal endothelium in tissue culture.

Prognosis

Overall prognosis of ICE syndrome is not good inspite of the best efforts.

BIBLIOGRAPHY

1. Bourgeois J, Shields MB, Thresher R: Open-angle glaucoma associated with posterior polymorphous dystrophy: A clinicopathologic study. Ophthalmology 1984:91;420.

2. Rodrigues MM, Phelps CD, Krachmer JH, Weingeist TA. Glaucoma due to endothelialization of the anterior chamber angle: A comparison of posterior polymorphous dystrophy of the cornea and Chandler's syndrome. Arch Ophthalmol 1980;98:688.

3. Shields MB. Progressive essential iris atrophy, Chandler's syndrome, and the iris nevus (Cogan-Reese) syndrome: A spectrum of disease. Surv Ophthalmol 1979;24:3.

Abnormalities of Corneal Transparency

INTRODUCTION

Normal cornea is a transparent structure. Any condition which upsets its anatomy or physiology causes loss of its transparency to some degree.

CAUSES

Common causes of loss of corneal transparency are:
• Corneal oedema
• Drying of cornea
• Depositions on cornea
• Inflammations of cornea
• Corneal degenerations
• Dystrophies of cornea
• Vascularization of cornea
• Scarring of cornea (corneal opacities).

Note. Most of the conditions responsible for decreased transparency of cornea have been described earlier.

However, some important *symptomatic conditions of the cornea* such as corneal oedema, corneal opacity and vascularization of cornea are described here.

CORNEAL OEDEMA

The water content of normal cornea is 78%. It is kept constant by a balance of factors which draw water in the cornea (e.g. intraocular pressure and swelling pressure of the stromal matrix = 60 mm of Hg) and the factors which draw water out of cornea (viz. the active pumping action of corneal endothelium, and the mechanical barrier action of epithelium and endothelium).

Disturbance of any of the above factors leads to corneal oedema, wherein its hydration becomes above 78%, central thickness increases and transparency reduces.

CAUSES

1. *Raised intraocular pressure* is a common cause of corneal oedema.

2. *Endothelial damage*
   • *Due to injuries,* such as birth trauma (forceps delivery), surgical trauma during intraocular operation, contusion injuries and penetrating injuries.
   • *Endothelial damage associated with corneal dystrophies* such as Fuchs dystrophy,

congenital hereditary endothelial dystrophy and posterior polymorphous dystrophy.

- *Endothelial damage secondary to inflammations* such as uveitis, endophthalmitis and corneal graft infection.

3. *Epithelial damage* due to:
   - Mechanical injuries
   - Chemical burns
   - Radiational injuries
   - Thermal injuries
   - Inflammation and infections.

CLINICAL FEATURES

Initially, there occurs stromal haze with reduced vision. In long-standing cases with chronic endothelial failure (e.g. in Fuchs dystrophy) there occurs permanent oedema with epithelial vesicles and bullae formation (*bullous keratopathy*).

This is associated with marked loss of vision, pain, discomfort and photophobia, due to periodic rupture of bullae.

TREATMENT

1. *Treat the cause* wherever possible, e.g. raised IOP and ocular inflammations.
2. *Dehydration of cornea* may be tried by use of:
   - Hypertonic agents, e.g. 5% sodium chloride drops or ointments or anhydrous glycerine may provide sufficient dehydrating effect.
   - Hot forced air from hair dryer may be useful.
3. *Therapeutic soft contact lenses* may be used to get relief from discomfort of bullous keratopathy.
4. *Penetrating keratoplasty* is required for long-standing cases of corneal oedema, non-responsive to conservative therapy.

CORNEAL OPACITY

The word *'corneal opacification'* literally means loss of normal transparency of cornea, which can occur in many conditions. Therefore, the term *'corneal opacity'* is used particularly for the loss of transparency of cornea due to scarring.

CAUSES

1. *Congenital opacities* causes can be remembered by the *mnemonic* STUMPED:
   - **S**clerocornea
   - **T**ear in Descemet's membrane, congenital glaucoma, birth trauma.
   - **U**lcer: HSV, bacterial, neurotropic.
   - **M**ucopolysaccharidosis, mucolipidosis, tyrosinosis.
   - **P**osterior corneal defect: Peter's anomaly, posterior keratoconus.
   - **E**ndothelial dystrophy: Congenital hereditary posterior polymorphous.
   - **D**ermoid
2. *Healed corneal wounds* and *healed corneal ulcers* are common causes of corneal opacities.

CLINICAL FEATURES

Corneal opacity may produce loss of vision (when dense opacity covers the pupillary area) or blurred vision (due to astigmatic effect).

Types of corneal opacity

Depending on the density, corneal opacity is graded as nebula, macula and leucoma.

1. *Nebular corneal opacity.* It is a faint opacity which results due to superficial scars involving Bowman's layer and superficial stroma (Figs 34.1A and 34.2A).

   A thin, diffuse nebula covering the pupillary area interferes more with vision than the localised leucoma away from pupillary area. Further, the nebula produces more discomfort to patient due to blurred image owing to irregular astigmatism than the leucoma which completely cuts off the light rays.

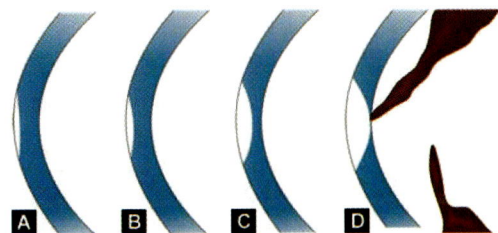

Fig. 34.1: *Diagrammatic depiction of corneal opacity: A, Nebular; B, Macular; C, Leucomatous; D, Adherent leucoma*

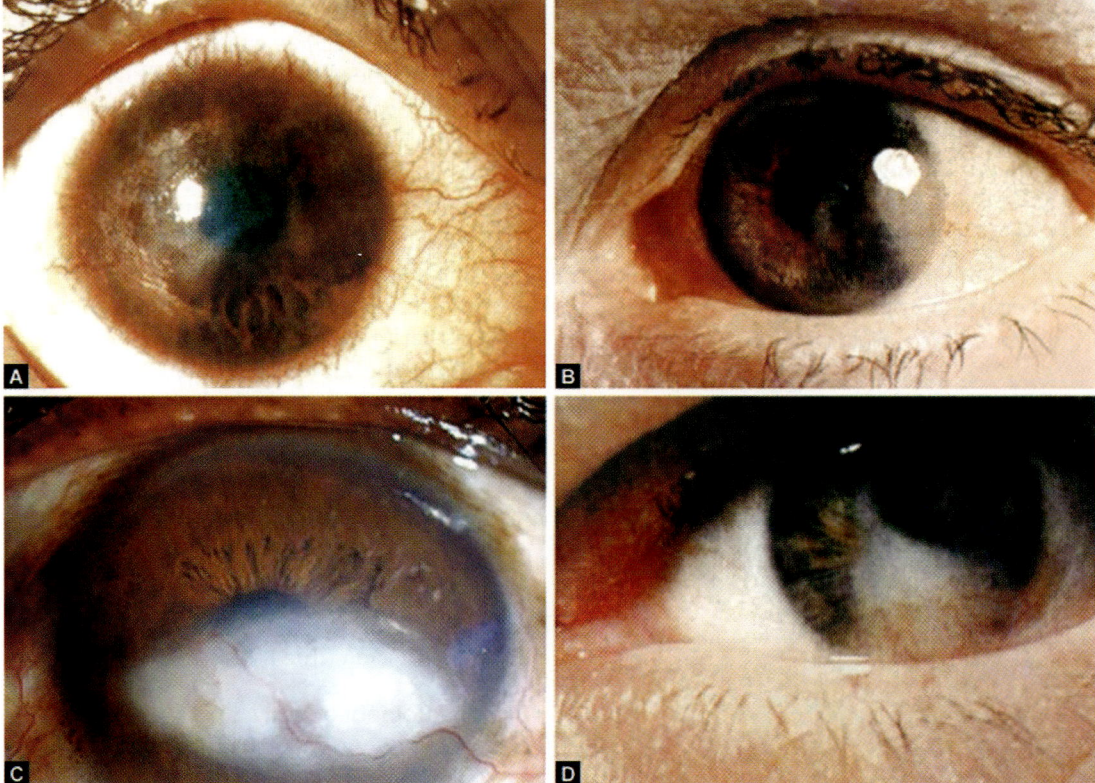

Fig. 34.2: *Clinical photographs of corneal opacity. A, Nebular; B, Macular; C, Leucomatous; D, Adherent leucoma*

2. *Macular corneal opacity.* It is a semi-dense opacity produced when scarring involves about half the corneal stroma (Figs 34.1B and 34.2B).

3. *Leucomatous corneal opacity* (leucoma simplex). It is a dense white opacity which results due to scarring of more than half of the stroma (Figs 34.1C and 34.2C).

4. *Adherent leucoma.* It results when healing occurs after perforation of cornea with incarceration of iris (Figs 34.1D and 34.2D).

5. *Corneal facet.* Sometimes, the corneal surface is depressed at the site of healing (due to less fibrous tissue); such a scar is called facet.

6. *Kerectasia.* In this condition, corneal curvature is increased at the site of opacity (bulge due to weak scar).

7. *Anterior staphyloma.* An ectasia of pseudo-cornea (the scar formed from organised exudates and fibrous tissue covered with epithelium) which results after total sloughing of cornea, with iris plastered behind it is called *anterior staphyloma* (Fig. 34.3A and B).

Secondary changes in corneal opacity which may be seen in long-standing cases include: Hyaline degeneration, calcareous degeneration, pigmentation and atheromatous ulceration.

TREATMENT

1. *Optical iridectomy.* It may be performed in cases with central macular or leucomatous corneal opacities, provided vision improves with pupillary dilatation.

2. *Phototherapeutic keratectomy (PTK)* performed with excimer laser is useful in superficial (nebular) corneal opacities.

3. *Keratoplasty provides good visual results* in uncomplicated cases with corneal opacities, where optical iridectomy is not of much use.

4. *Cosmetic-coloured contact lens* gives very good cosmetic appearance in an eye with

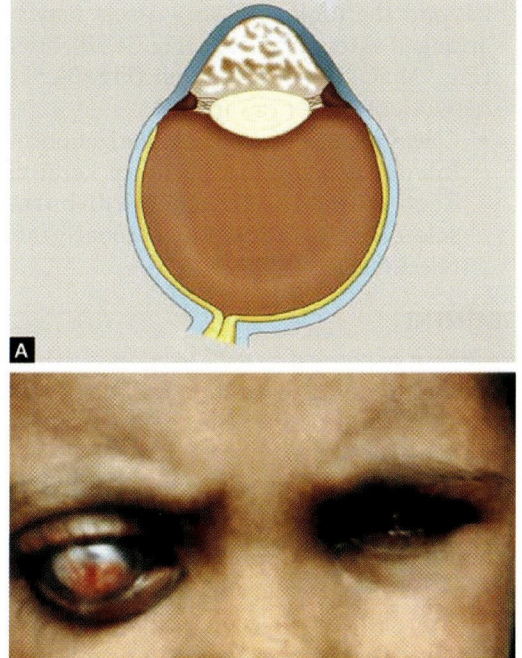

Fig. 34.3: *Anterior staphyloma. A, Diagrammatic cross-section; B, Clinical photograph*

ugly scar having no potential for vision. Presently, this is considered the best option, even over and above the tattooing for cosmetic purpose.

5. *Tattooing of scar.* It was performed for cosmetic purposes in the past. It is suitable only for firm scars in a quiet eye without useful vision. For tattooing Indian black ink, gold or platinum may be used. To perform tattooing, first of all, the epithelium covering the opacity is removed under topical anaesthesia (2% or 4% Xylocaine). Then a piece of blotting paper of same size and shape, soaked in 4% gold chloride (for brown colour) or 2% platinum chloride (for dark colour) is applied over it. After 2–3 minutes, the piece of filter paper is removed and a few drops of freshly prepared 2% hydrazine hydrate solution are poured over it. Lastly, eye is irrigated with normal saline and patched after instilling antibiotic and atropine eye ointment. Epithelium grows over the pigmented area.

CORNEA VERTICILLATA

- This is a whorl-like opacity in the corneal epithelium seen in patients on long-term treatment with medications such as amiodarone, chloroquine, phenothiazines and indomethacin (Fig. 34.4).
- It is also seen in patients with Fabry disease and its carrier state.
- The whorl-like pattern shows the direction of migration of corneal epithelial cells. Occasionally, the condition had been known to cause glare and surface discomfort which responds to topical lubricants.
- The condition is generally asymptomatic, harmless and reversible on stopping the drug.

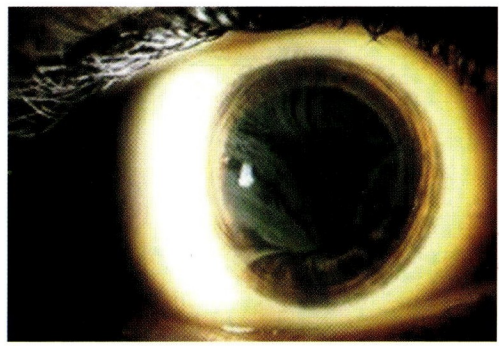

Fig. 34.4: *Cornea verticillata*

CORNEAL VASCULARIZATION

Normal cornea is avascular except for small capillary loops which are present in the periphery for about 1 mm. In pathological states, it can be invaded by vessels as a defence mechanism against the disease or injury. However, vascularisation interferes with corneal transparency and occasionally may be a source of irritation.

PATHOGENESIS

Pathogenesis of corneal vascularization is still not clear. It is presumed that mechanical and chemical factors play a role.

Vascularization is normally prevented by the compactness of corneal tissue. Probably, due to some vasoformative stimulus (*chemical factor*) released during pathological states, there occurs proliferation of vessels which invade from the limbus; when compactness of corneal tissue is loosened (*mechanical factor*) due to oedema (which may be traumatic, inflammatory, nutritional, allergic or idiopathic in nature).

CLINICO-ETIOLOGICAL FEATURES

Clinically, corneal vascularization may be superficial or deep.

1. *Superficial corneal vascularization.* In it, vessels are arranged usually in an arborising pattern, present below the epithelial layer and their continuity can be traced with the conjunctival vessels (Fig. 34.5A).

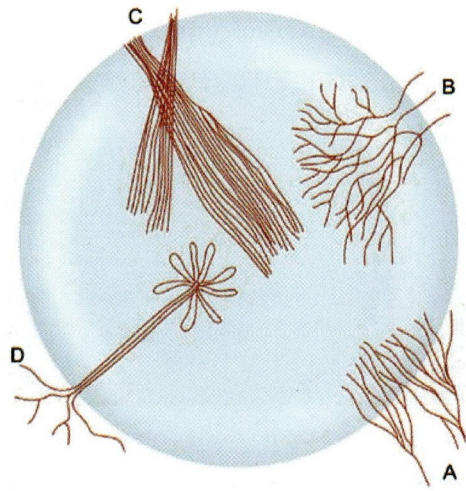

Fig. 34.5: *Corneal vascularization: A, Superficial; B, Terminal loop type; C, Brush type; D, Umbel type*

- *Common causes* of superficial corneal vascularization are: Trachoma, phlyctenular keratoconjunctivitis, superficial corneal ulcers, contact lens users and rosacea keratitis.
- *Pannus.* When extensive superficial vascularization is associated with white cuff of cellular infiltration, it is termed pannus. In progressive pannus, corneal infiltration is ahead of vessels while in *regressive pannus,* it lags behind.

2. *Deep vascularization.* These vessels are generally derived from anterior ciliary arteries and lie in the corneal stroma. These vessels are usually straight, not anastomosing and their continuity cannot be traced

beyond the limbus. Deep vessels may be arranged as terminal loops (Fig. 34.5B), brush (Fig. 34.5C), parasol, umbel (Fig. 34.5D), network or interstitial arcade.

- *Common causes* of deep vascularization are: Interstitial keratitis, disciform keratitis, deep corneal ulcer, chemical burns, sclerosing keratitis and corneal grafts rejection.

TREATMENT

Treatment of corneal vascularization is usually unsatisfactory. Vascularization may be prevented by timely and adequate treatment of the causative conditions.

- Corticosteroids may have vasoconstrictive and suppressive effect on permeability of capillaries.
- Application of irradiation is more useful in superficial than the deep vascularization.
- Surgical treatment in the form of peritomy may be employed for superficial vascularization.

BIBLIOGRAPHY

1. Afshari, N.A., Li Y.J., Pericak-Vance M.A, et al. Genome wide linkage scan in Fuchs endothelial corneal dystrophy. IOVS, 1–14.
2. Afshari, N.A., Mullally, M.S., Afhsari M.A., et al. Survey of patients with Granular, Lattice, Avellino, and Reis-Bücklers corneal dystrophies for mutations in the BIGH3 and Gelsolin genes. Archives of Ophthalmology 119, 16–22.
3. Ashton, N.: Corneal vascularization, in Duke-Elder, W. S., and Perkins, E. S., editors: The transparency of the cornea, Oxford, 1960
4. Bron, A.J. Genetics of the corneal dystrophies: What we have learned in the past twenty-five years. Cornea 19, 699–711.
5. Chang KC, Kwon JW, Han YK, Wee WR, Lee JH. The epidemiology of cosmetic treatments for corneal opacities in a Korean population. Korean J Ophthalmol. 2010; 24(3): 148–54.
6. Ciralsky J, Colby K. Congenital corneal opacities: a review with a focus on genetics. Semin Ophthalmol. 2007; 22(4): 241–246.
7. Comer RM, Daya SM, O'Keefe M. Penetrating keratoplasty in infants. J AAPOS. 2001; 5(5): 285–90.

8. Cook, C, and Langham, M.: Corneal thickness in interstitial keratitis, Brit. J. Ophth. 37: 301, 1953.

9. Cotran PR, Bajart AM. Congenital corneal opacities. Int Ophthalmol Clin. 1992; 32(1): 93–105.

10. Dada T, Sharma N, Vajpayee RB. Indications for pediatric keratoplasty in India. Cornea. 1999; 18(3): 296–8.

11. Dinh, R. Rapuano, C.J., Cohen E.J. et al. Recurrence of corneal dystrophy after excimer laser phototherapeutic keratectomy. Ophthalmology 106, 1490-97

12. Eghrari AO, Gottsch JD. Fuchs' corneal dystrophy. Expert Rev Ophthalmol. 2010; 5: 147–59.

13. Gagnon MM, Boisjoly HM, Brunette I, Charest M, Amyot M. Corneal endothelial cell density in glaucoma. Cornea. 1997; 16: 314–8.

14. Heydenreich, A.: Das Verhalten der Hornhautvaskularisation im Tierversuch, Klin.Monatsbl. Augenh. 127: 465, 1955.

15. Maurice DM. The structure and transparency of the cornea. J Physiol. 1957; 136: 263–86.

16. Piatigorsky J. Review: A case for corneal crystallins. J Ocul Pharmacol Ther. 2000; 16: 173–80.

Section
VII

Surgical Procedures for Ocular Surface and Cornea

Chapter

35

Pterygium Surgery and Conjunctival Flaps

PTERYGIUM

INTRODUCTION

The term "Pterygium" is derived from the Greek word "pterygion" meaning "small wing". It is a triangular-shaped growth of bulbar conjunctival epithelial and subconjunctival fibrovascular tissue encroaching the cornea centripetally from either the medial or lateral side or infrequently from both sectors simultaneously. This is accompanied by ocular surface inflammation and potential vision impairment. Apart from being cosmetically unacceptable, it is known to cause tear film instability, irregular astigmatism and may eventually progress to obscure the visual axis. Described as early as 1000 BC by Sushruta and Hippocrates, pterygium is a common ocular condition particularly in hot equatorial climates and in outdoor working population.

EPIDEMIOLOGY AND RISK FACTORS

Studies and various surveys from worldwide have suggested that countries near the equator have a higher prevalence for this condition. Talbot et al were the first to suggest in 1948 about the association between ultraviolet radiation and pterygium occurrence. Cameron in 1965 described the "**pterygium belt**" to be within the latitudes of 37 degrees north and south of the equator. The prevalence in India ranges from 9.5 to 13%. Prevalence rate is seen to increase with age and the condition is more common in males working outdoors as compared to females. Those exposed to chronic irritation from airborne particulate matter and those in occupations such as farming and welding are particularly prone to the condition. Hereditary factors may play a role in the development of pterygium. Corneal curvature and ocular prominence have been seen to influence the concentration of ultraviolet light exposure over the conjunctival surface particularly on the nasal side.

MORPHOLOGY AND CLASSIFICATION

Pterygium may be **primary or recurrent**. While primary pterygium arises *de novo* in the conjunctiva, recurrent pterygium occurs weeks to months after excision of a primary pterygium and is usually more aggressive than the former. Pterygium more commonly occurs nasally in the interpalpebral fissure. This was demonstrated and attributed to the "**albedo**" effect on the eye wherein UV light from the temporal side is focused on the nasal limbus secondary to reflection from the nose. Temporal pterygium may also occur and is usually present along with nasal pterygium and such a condition is referred to as "**double pterygium**". Primary pterygium may be unilateral or bilateral. Bilateral pterygium is often asymmetric.

A fully developed pterygium presents a well formed "**apex**" or "**head**" (cornea), a "**body**" (conjunctiva extending between the limbus and the canthus), and a "**neck**" (limbus) (Fig. 35.1). The head is usually preceded by an avascular cap at the leading edge. Scalloped and irregular advancing margin of the cap is referred to as "**Fuchs islets**" or "**Fuchs islands**". An epithelial iron line "**Stocker's line**" encircles the cap. Head and body of the pterygium may be indistinguishable morphologically.

Pterygium may be "**Progressive**" or "**Regressive**". A progressive pterygium is thick, fleshy and vascular with zone of infiltration ahead of vascularization while a regressive pterygium is thin and atrophic with a little or no vascularization.

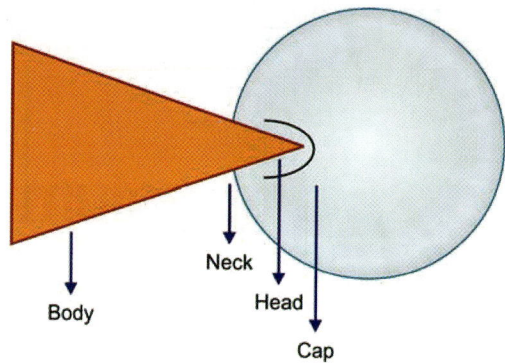

Fig. 35.1: *Anatomical parts of a pterygium*

A pterygium must be distinguished from a "**Pseudopterygium**" which is essentially a pannus or fibrovascular scar post-mechanical or chemical injury or a sequelae of peripheral corneal degenerations (Fig. 35.2). Contrary to a true pterygium a pseudopterygium can occur at any age and at any site in the eye. It is usually stationary and can be distinguished from a true pterygium by a probe test wherein a probe can be passed under the neck of a pseudopterygium unlike in a true pterygium.

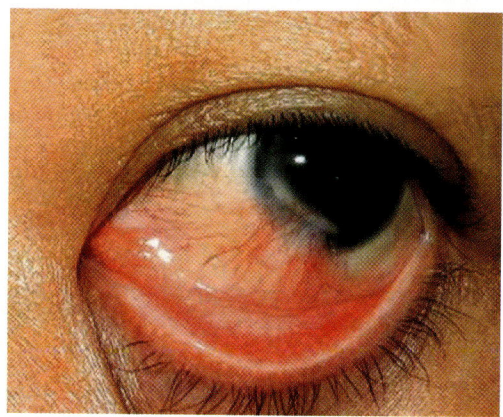

Fig. 35.2: *Pseudopterygium*

Morphological classification

Tan et al classified pterygium according to the morphology into three grades (Fig. 35.3).

Grade T1 (mild pterygium or atrophic) refers to a pterygium in which episcleral vessels underlying the body of the pterygium are unobscured and clearly distinguished (Fig. 35.3A).

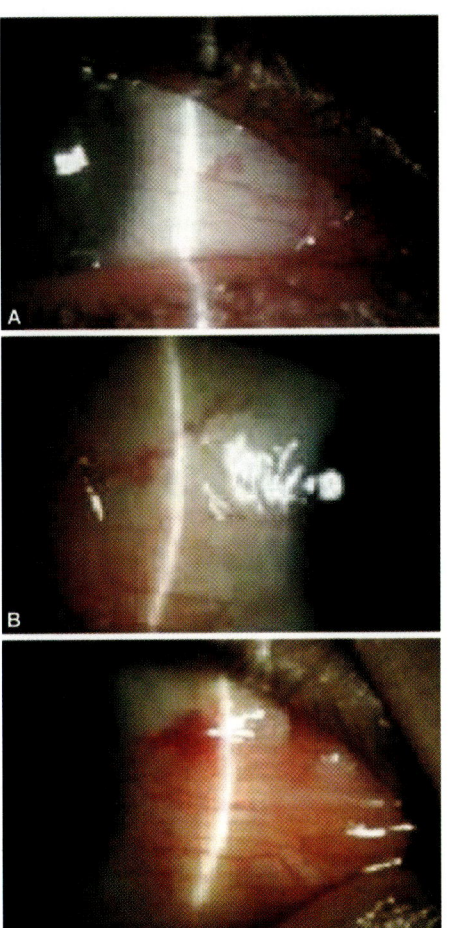

Fig. 35.3: *Pterygium morphological (Tan's) classification. A, Grade T1 (mild pterygium)—underlying episcleral vessels unobscured; B, Grade T2 (moderate pterygium)—underlying vessels partially obscured; C, Grade T3 (severe pterygium)— underlying episcleral vessels completely obscured*

Grade T2 (moderate pterygium or intermediate) refers to a pterygium in which underlying vessels are partially obscured (Fig. 35.3B).

Grade T3 (severe pterygium or fleshy) refers to a thick pterygium in which episcleral vessels underlying the body of the pterygium are totally obscured (Fig. 35.3C).

PATHOGENESIS

Duke Elder described the condition as a "triangular-shaped degenerative and hyperplastic process". Classically described as an elastotic degeneration of the subconjunctival tissue, it is characterised by an altered basal epithelial cell proliferation, vascularization, and invasion of the adjacent corneal epithelium. Matrix metalloproteinases at the advancing pterygium edge have been hypothesized to be responsible for destruction of Bowman's layer and invasion into the cornea. It has also been suggested by many researchers that UV light causes focal destruction of limbal stem cells. The resultant limbal stem cell deficiency causes the conjunctiva to migrate across the limbus leading to fibrous in growth and vascularization. Laboratory studies have suggested overexpression of p53 tumour suppressor gene in the basal epithelial layer of pterygium. Oncogenic viruses such as Epstein-Barr virus, herpes simplex virus and cytomegalovirus have also been implicated in the development of pterygium. A large set of pro-inflammatory cytokines such as IL-1 and IL-6, lipid mediators, growth factors and their receptors have been described to be associated in the development of pterygium. Cyclooxygenases (COX), LOX and cytochrome P450 monooxygenases (CYP) derived eicosanoids have also been found to be increased in excised pterygium tissue. The expression of VEGF, TGF-β and PGE_2 using immunohistochemical assays have been studied . VEGF and PGE_2 have been shown to be significantly increased in the epithelial cells while TGF-β has been shown to have moderate expression in the epithelium and stroma of primary pterygium.

CLINICAL FEATURES

Usually an asymptomatic condition, pterygium may cause **foreign body sensation** or **grittiness** due to tear film instability. It may have occasional episodes of associated redness over the mass, a condition commonly referred to as "**inflamed pterygium**". It may be associated with regular or irregular astigmatism due to mechanical distortion and flattening of the cornea which is directly correlated with the extent and total area involved. Pterygia commonly induce with the rule astigmatism followed by against the rule and oblique astigmatism. A pterygium larger than 3 mm is seen to cause over 1 diopter of astigmatism. In advanced stages when they cross the pupillary axis, they may **obscure vision. Diplopia** arising due to limitation of ocular movements may also occur. It is often considered a **cosmetic blemish** which remains the leading indication for its removal.

SURGICAL MANAGEMENT

Early in the disease process, often a conservative approach, limiting therapy to lubricating medications and use of protective eyewear is taken.

Indications for pterygium surgery

- Visually significant induced astigmatism
- Involvement or impending threat of involvement of the visual axis
- Severe symptoms of foreign body sensation
- Cosmesis
- Diplopia

Historical landmarks in pterygium surgery

Earliest evidence of pterygium surgery dates back to Sushruta (1000 BC) who used a threaded needle or sharp hook for its removal. He also described using a powdered salt for loosening the pterygium before excision.

Variety of pterygium excision procedures by various surgeons over the past have been compositely illustrated in 1950 by King (Fig. 35.4).

Primary aim of all techniques is however, excision of pterygium and prevention of recurrence. Recurrence rates have been reported from 0 to 80% as per various studies and are directly correlated with the type and adequacy of surgery (Table 35.1).

COMMON SURGICAL TECHNIQUES

- Bare sclera excision
- Excision and closure with conjunctival flaps
  - Direct conjunctival flap
  - Rotational conjunctival flap
  - Gundersen conjunctival flap
  - Conjunctival autograft
  - Conjunctival limbal autograft
- Excision with antimitotic therapy
- Amniotic membrane transplantation
- Lamellar corneal transplant

Table 35.1: *Recurrence rate of various therapeutic modalities for pterygium*

Treatment modality	Recurrence rate
Bare sclera excision	20–80%
Excision with conjunctival closure	25–40%
Excision with conjunctival autograft	<3%
Excision with antimitotic therapy	3–43%
Conjunctival limbal autograft	3–5%
Amniotic membrane transplantation	10–15%
Mini simple limbal epithelial transplant (mini SLET)	Long-term results awaited
PERFECT surgery	<1%

- Mini simple limbal epithelial transplant (mini SLET)
- PERFECT surgery

BARE SCLERA EXCISION

Described first by D'Ombrain in 1946, this technique involves excising the head and body of the pterygium (Fig. 35.5A and B) and laying the sclera bare which subsequently re-epithelizes presumably after re-epithelization of bare cornea (Fig. 35.5C). This technique however reported recurrence of pterygium between 20 and 89% and the recurrent pterygium is often more aggressive than the primary lesion often associated with development of symblepharon and restriction of ocular motility leading to diplopia.

EXCISION WITH DIRECT CONJUNCTIVAL FLAP

Post-excision of pterygium, conjunctival margins are pulled forward to cover the bare sclera and approximated with either fibrin glue or sutures (10–0 nylon). This technique is useful for grade 1 pterygium. Care must be taken to completely excise the pterygium to prevent recurrence. Relaxing incisions may be given to help in pulling forth the conjunctiva.

EXCISION WITH ROTATIONAL CONJUNCTIVAL FLAP

After completely excising the pterygium, the area of bare sclera is measured with calipers. Peritomy is done at superior and inferior conjunctiva and pedicle flaps are fashioned. The pedicle flaps are then rotated and transposed

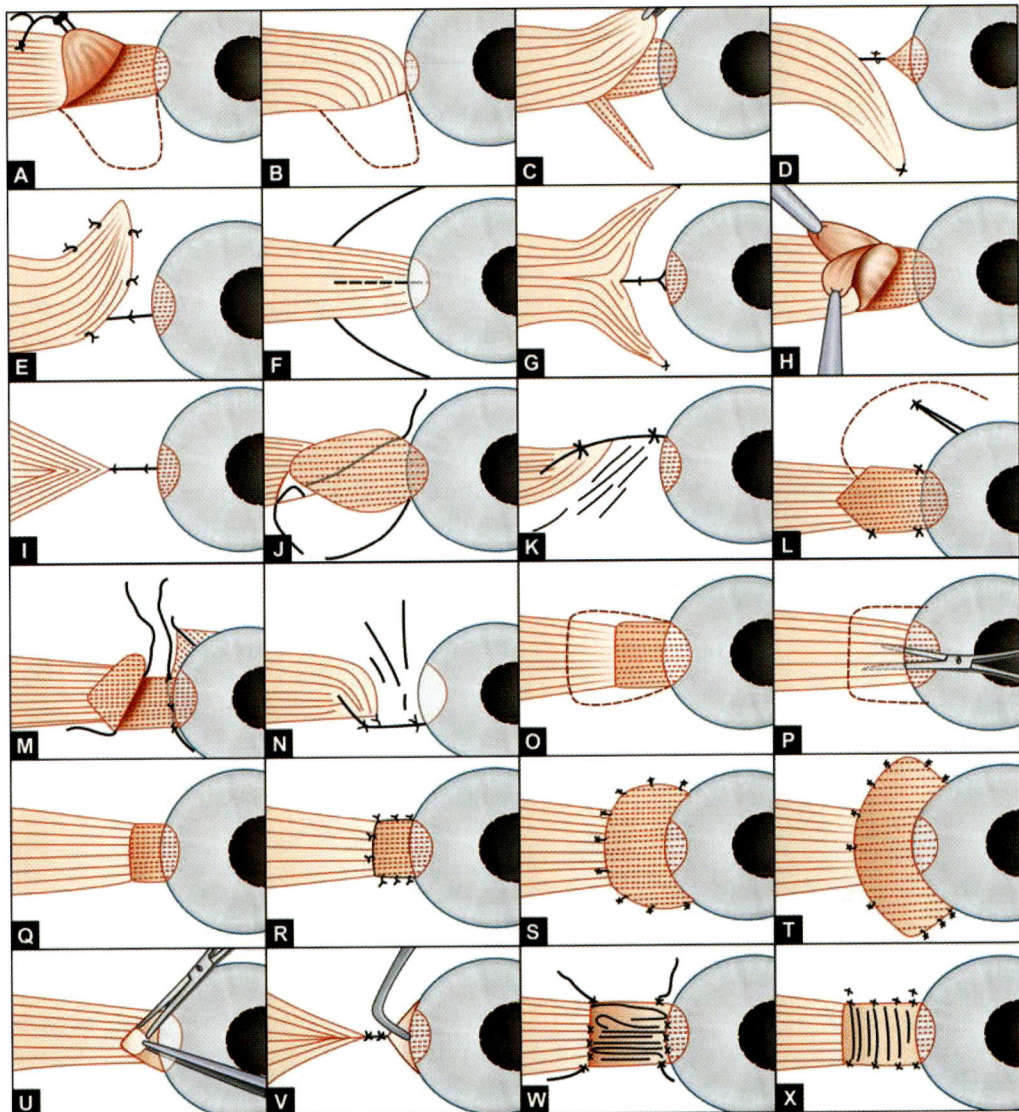

Fig. 35.4A to X: *Variety of pterygium surgery (Arch Ophthal, 1950; 44: 856)*

towards the bare sclera and sutured with 10–0 nylon sutures. Recurrence rates in this method range from 29 to 37% as per some studies.

EXCISION WITH GUNDERSEN CONJUNCTIVAL FLAP

Subconjunctival injection of lidocaine with epinephrine may be given in the desired area of harvesting the flap to delineate the plane of dissection and reduce bleeding. The dissection can be commenced from either the limbus or superior fornix. Dissection of conjunctiva from underlying Tenon fascia is performed. After the flap has been dissected, peritomy in the area of dissection is performed. The flap is further undermined and pulled forth to cover the bare sclera without traction or tension. The flap is then sutured with episcleral bites with 10–0 nylon sutures.

EXCISION WITH CONJUNCTIVAL AUTOGRAFT (CAG)

This technique is considered the procedure of choice in management of pterygium. The graft

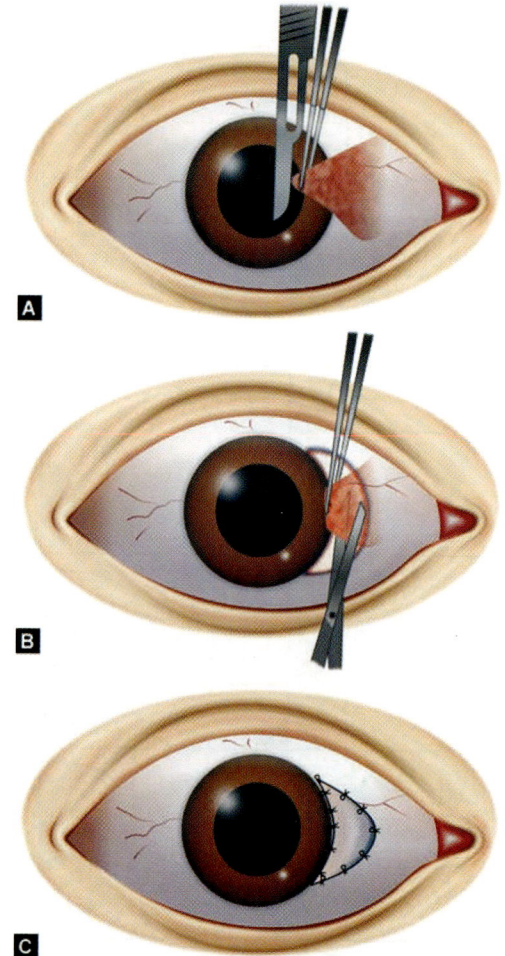

Fig. 35.5: *Surgical technique of pterygium excision. A, Dissection of the head from the corner; B, Excision of the pterygium tissue under the conjunctiva; C, Conjunctival autograft*

is preferably taken from the superior temporal bulbar conjunctiva which is shielded from actinic damage from the upper lid and also because of the technical ease of harvesting the graft from this area as compared to the inferior bulbar conjunctiva. The head of the pterygium can either be **avulsed** by grasping the head with a forceps or it can be removed by **superficial keratectomy**. In the latter, a small incision is made adjacent to the head of the pterygium. Once the plane is defined, the pterygium head is easily dissected from the corneal surface using a No. 15 Bard-Parker blade. The body of the

pterygium is then excised with blunt dissection without damaging the overlying conjunctiva and underlying horizontal rectus muscle. The exposed scleral surface is measured using Castroviejo calipers and the dimensions are marked onto the superotemporal conjunctiva. Conjunctival plane is identified and the graft is excised using Vannas scissors. The conjunctival graft is then slid onto the cornea and moved onto the scleral bed using non-toothed forceps with the limbal side aligned. The graft is secured using interrupted 10–0 nylon sutures with episcleral bites or application of **fibrin glue** (Fig. 35.5C). Autologous serum or patient's own blood may be used as an adhesive instead of sutures or glue. The donor area is covered by pulling the forniceal conjunctiva forward which is either sutured with 10–0 nylon suture or apposed with fibrin glue. Postoperatively, topical steroid eye drops in tapering doses, topical antibiotics and tear substitutes are prescribed. Suture removal is done at 4 weeks. The recurrence rates with this technique are as low as 2%.

EXCISION WITH CONJUNCTIVAL LIMBAL AUTOGRAFT (CLAG)

This technique was first described by Kenyon in 1985. This procedure is similar to conjunctival autografting except that the graft is dissected further to include the limbal epithelium. In a series from India, Rao et al reported the outcomes of this procedure in 53 eyes with 36 primary and 17 recurrent pterygia, with a mean follow-up of 18.9 + 12.1 months. The recurrence rate in their series was 3.8%. The procedure is similar to conjunctival autografting except that while harvesting the graft dissection is extended to include the limbal epithelium. This technique addresses the etiology of focal limbal stem cell deficit but has the disadvantage of causing surgical trauma to donor site limbal stem cells.

EXCISION WITH ANTIMITOTIC THERAPY

Beta irradiation: Strontium 90 which emits beta irradiation is a safe and effective method that inhibits the mitosis of actively dividing cells such as fibroblasts. Doses varying from 2000 to

6000 rads as a single dose or weekly dose up to 6 weeks has been used. It however may lead to cataract formation and scleral necrosis.

Mitomycin C (MMC): MMC is an antibiotic anticancer agent used either intraoperatively or as eyedrops. It inhibits DNA synthesis and cell proliferation. Intraoperative single application of MMC (0.02%) over the bare sclera for 3–5 minutes is recommended. MMC eyedrops (0.01%) twice a day for 5 days postoperatively are infrequently used. Recurrence rate for intraoperative application with MMC range from 3 to 43%. Its use has however been associated with complications such as scleral melting, iritis, limbal ischaemia, secondary glaucoma, corneal perforation and cataract.

EXCISION WITH AMNIOTIC MEMBRANE TRANSPLANTATION (AMT)

Amniotic membrane in place of an autograft can be used after pterygium excision. Amniotic membrane is known to help in epithelial cell migration, differentiation and basal cell adhesion. It has the additional advantages of preventing scarring and fibrosis and has anti-angiogenic properties as well. This technique can be used for primary as well as recurrent pterygium. It also eliminates harvesting autografts and disturbing the ocular surface.

Prabhasawat et al first reported using AMT in pterygium surgery. They reported a recurrence rate of 10.9% for primary pterygium following excision with AMT and concluded that AMT could serve as a useful alternative to conjunctival grafts especially in cases of large conjunctival defect such as primary double-headed pterygia. They are a good surgical option in cases where bulbar conjunctiva needs to be preserved such as in those patients who may require a glaucoma surgery in future. Combining AMT with CLAG may be employed in the management of recurrent pterygia.

A combined approach including pterygium excision, AMT, CLAG and application of mitomycin C has reported to be beneficial in the management of chronically recurring pterygium in young patients. AMT as a first-line measure for recurrent pterygia however is less favourable in comparison to CAG.

EXCISION WITH MINI SIMPLE LIMBAL EPITHELIAL TRANSPLANT (MINI SLET)

Mini simple limbal epithelial transplantation can be carried out in recurrent pterygia after failed conjunctival autografts, AMT or MMC application. In this procedure limbal biopsies are placed only over affected limbal area after removal of pterygium. Successful outcomes of this technique have been reported. Mini SLET can also be a good choice for management of primary pterygium.

EXCISION WITH LAMELLAR KERATOPLASTY

Technically challenging, this procedure is carried out in cases of recurrent pterygium wherein the bare cornea is covered by a lamellar corneal graft and the bare sclera is covered with conjunctival autograft.

EXCISION WITH PERFECT SURGERY

PERFECT, which stands for 'pterygium extended removal followed by extended conjunctival transplant' is a technique described by Hirst et al from Australia. In this approach, an extensive conjunctival autografting (15 mm by 12 mm) is done after hooking extraocular muscles. This technique has reported less recurrence (0.1%) and a better cosmetic outcome as graft edge lie hidden in the fornices. This is however a time-consuming and technically challenging procedure.

COMPLICATIONS FOLLOWING PTERYGIUM SURGERY

- Corneal thinning or perforation
- Scleral thinning or perforation
- Recurrence
- Displacement of graft
- Retraction of graft
- Inappropriately sized graft
- Graft necrosis
- Damage to medial rectus muscle
- Pyogenic granuloma
- Endophthalmitis

RECENT ADVANCES

Subconjunctival injections with anti-VEGF agent such as **Bevacizumab**, a recombinant humanized monoclonal antibody, is being used to manage neovascularization and preventing the pterygium recurrence. It can be supplemented with argon laser phototherapy to obliterate specific feeder vessels.

Cyclosporine A, an immunosuppressive drug that prevents T-helper cells activation and inhibits angiogenic factors, is recently being used in the treatment of pterygium to prevent recurrence. A 1% solution is administrated twice a day for over several weeks.

CONJUNCTIVAL FLAPS IN OCULAR SURFACE DISEASES

INTRODUCTION

Conjunctival flaps are a good modality of treatment for various conditions of the ocular surface. They are a valuable technique in a surgeon's armamentarium to restore the integrity of ocular surface and eventually help in visual rehabilitation of patients. Over the years, advances in ophthalmic science such as bandage contact lenses, amniotic membrane grafting, tissue adhesives and better lubricating drops have diminished the use of this technique. Nevertheless, they are a useful modality in improving the quality of ocular surface. It is a reversible technique and relatively easy to master. It requires less resources and expertise and significantly improves the health of ocular surface. Described as early as a century ago, the technique was made popular in 1958, by Gundersen. It ameliorates the inflammation of the ocular surface and helps to thus improve the results of subsequent keratoplasty as well. The purpose of a conjunctival flap is to help provide metabolic support in terms of vascularization to the host bed and help in providing ambient environment to a chronically compromised corneal surface for healing.

MECHANISM OF ACTION, OBJECTIVES AND INDICATIONS

Mechanisms of action and objectives achieved by a conjunctival flap are, namely:
- *Restoration of integrity* of a chronically compromised ocular surface

- *Provision of metabolic and mechanical support* for corneal healing
- Conjunctival flap acts as biological patch, conferring a trophic effect because of the nutritional and immunologic supply by its vascular connective tissue.
- Improvement in cosmetic appearance and providing a base for fitting of cosmetic prosthesis.
- Reduction in ocular inflammation and promotion of healing.
- Reduction in pain.

Indications for conjunctival flap include:
1. Persistent corneal epithelial defects. Sterile defects resulting from neurotrophic ulceration, exposure keratitis post-facial nerve palsy, corneal anaesthesia following herpes zoster ophthalmicus, metaherpetic ulcers due to chronic herpes simplex keratitis and chemical burns.
2. Bullous keratopathy.
3. Microbial keratitis. Bacterial, fungal, Acanthamoebic keratitis and microbial keratitis post-keratoplasty.
4. Corneal abscess.
5. Post-cataract surgery wound infection.
6. Corneal thinning and perforation.
7. Descemetocele.
8. Pterygium surgery.
9. Necrotising scleritis.
10. Leaking blebs post-glaucoma surgery.
11. Exposed glaucoma drainage devices.
12. Surface preparation for a cosmetic scleral shell for patients in painful blind eye or phthisis bulbi.
13. Impending perforations where donor corneal tissue for kertoplasty is not available.

SURGICAL TECHNIQUES

ANAESTHESIA

The procedure is performed under peribulbar anaesthesia in cooperating adults. General anaesthesia is reserved for children and uncooperative adults.

Common types of conjunctival flaps include:
- Total conjunctival flap or Gundersen's flap

- Advancement flap
- Single pedicle flap
- Bipedicle bridge flap

TOTAL CONJUNCTIVAL FLAP (GUNDERSEN FLAP)

The most commonly utilized total conjunctival flap is the pedicle bridge flap described by Gundersen. The surgical steps are as follows:

1. *Inspection of the ocular surface.* Before undertaking any conjunctival flap, it is important for the surgeon to evaluate the mobility of the conjunctiva. Scarring of the conjunctiva may limit performing this technique. Any symblepharon if present must be released before attempting mobilization of conjunctiva.

2. *Removal of corneal epithelium.* Brimonidine eye drop can be administered two to three times 15 minutes before the procedure to minimise bleeding. After placement of a speculum, the corneal epithelium is removed by mechanical debridement using surgical blade, Weckcel sponge or cautery. The blade when used to scrape off the epithelium is kept parallel to the surface. Care should be taken to avoid any injury to the underlying cornea or limbus.

3. *Mobilization of the conjunctival flap is carried out as below:*

- A 6–0 silk traction suture is placed at the 12 o'clock limbus (Fig. 35.6A) to infraduct the eye to gain exposure of the superior bulbar conjunctiva and fornix. If an inferior advancement flap is planned the eye can be supraducted with traction suture at inferior limbus.
- *Local anaesthetic such as* 2% lidocaine can be injected into subconjunctival space to balloon up the conjunctiva and separate it from Tenon's capsule facilitating dissection (Fig. 35.6B).
- A 360-degree peritomy is performed using Westcott scissors (Fig. 35.6C) to increase the mobility of the conjunctiva and minimise tension.
- *Blunt dissection of superior conjunctivitis* is carried out from the fornix to limbus (approximately 14 mm) to be able to get sufficient length of tissue to cover entire cornea (Fig. 35.6D and E). Non-toothed forceps and blunt-tipped scissors should be used when handling the conjunctiva in order to avoid trauma (Fig. 35.6E). Care must be

taken to avoid deep or superficial dissection. Deep dissection leads to inclusion of Tenon's capsule and superficial dissection leads to buttonholing.

- *Conjunctival flap* is then mobilized and slid onto the debrided corneal surface. Relaxing incisions may be given at 3 and 6 o'clock positions to minimise tension (Fig. 35.6F).

4. *Conjunctival flap suture.* The flap is then sutured into place with interrupted 10–0 nylon or 8–0 vicryl sutures. The superior conjunctiva is left bare which heals by subsequent re-epithelialization (Fig. 35.6F).

ADVANCEMENT FLAP

This technique is used for juxtalimbal lesions. After measuring the lesion to be covered, limbal incision is given and limited peritomy is done (Fig. 35.7A). Relaxing incisions are given as per requirement (Fig. 35.7B). The conjunctiva is then dissected to create a flap without tension and is pulled forward to cover the corneal lesion (Fig. 35.7C). This technique can be employed over a lamellar corneal graft, corneal patch graft or scleral patch graft. Interrupted nylon or vicryl sutures are used to secure the flap in place (Fig. 35.7D). This flap may retract with time.

Single pedicle flap (racquet flap)

This type of flap is used for perilimbal corneal lesions that are not large enough to require a total flap. After removal of corneal epithelium, the area of conjunctiva (which is 20–30% larger than the corneal lesion) to be mobilized is marked (Fig. 35.8). A thin flap is dissected and rotated to cover the desired area. It is then secured with interrupted nylon sutures (Fig. 35.8). This type of flap is less prone to retraction than the advancement flap.

Bipedicle bridge flap

This type of flap is used for small central or paracentral corneal lesions. The surgical procedure is similar to that of Gundersen flap except that it is less in width and does not cover entire cornea. After removal of corneal epithelium careful blunt dissection is performed from periphery to the limbus on either side of the cornea. The thin flaps are then mobilized over the corneal lesion and sutured in place with

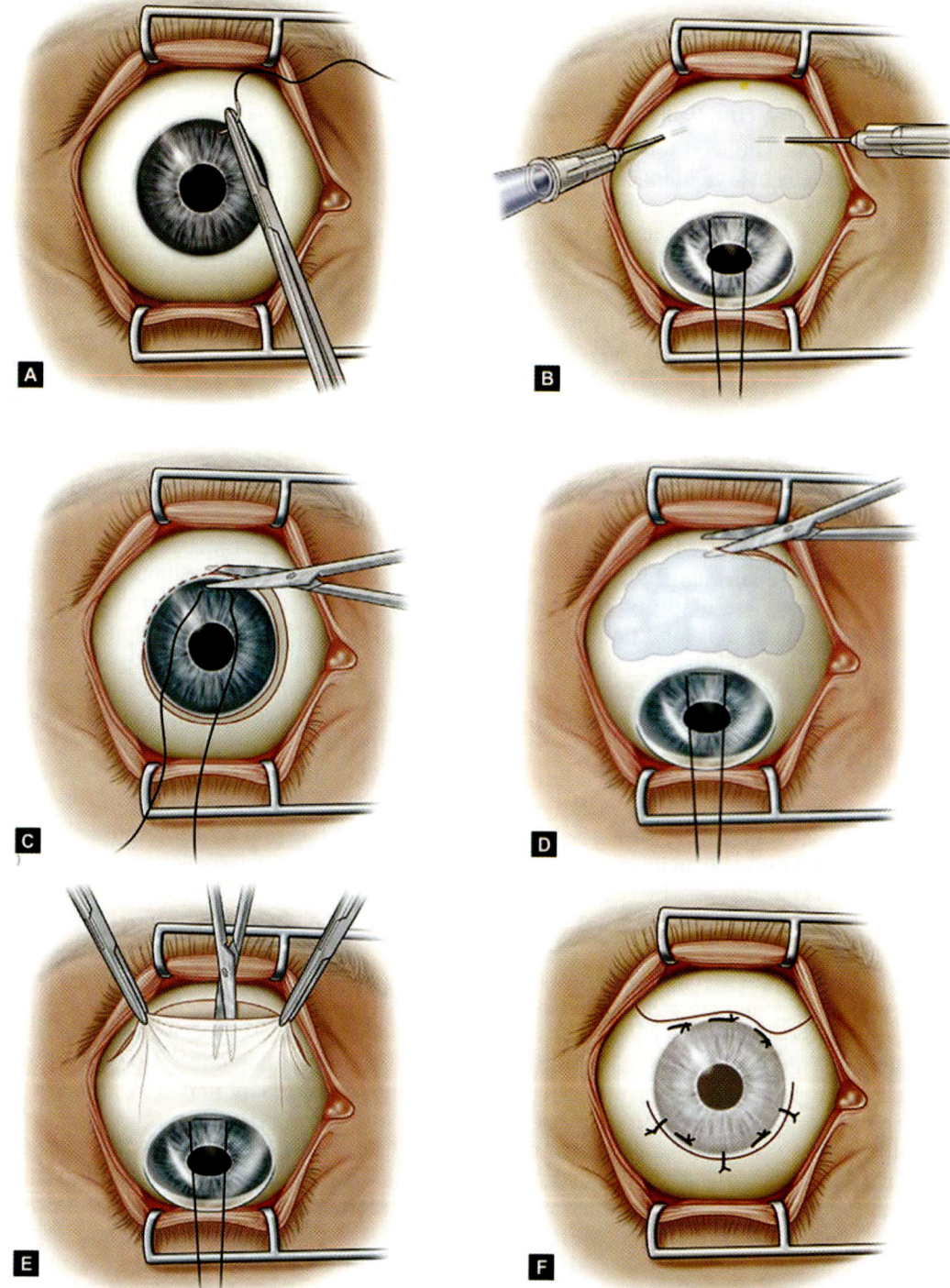

Fig. 35.6: *Surgical steps of total conjunctival (Gundersen) flap. A, Traction suture at 12 o'clock position; B, Ballooning of conjunctiva by subconjunctival lidocaine; C, Peritomy; D and E, Dissection of conjunctiva from superior fornix to limbus; F, Conjunctival flap mobilised over the debrided corneal surface and sutured with interrupted sutures*

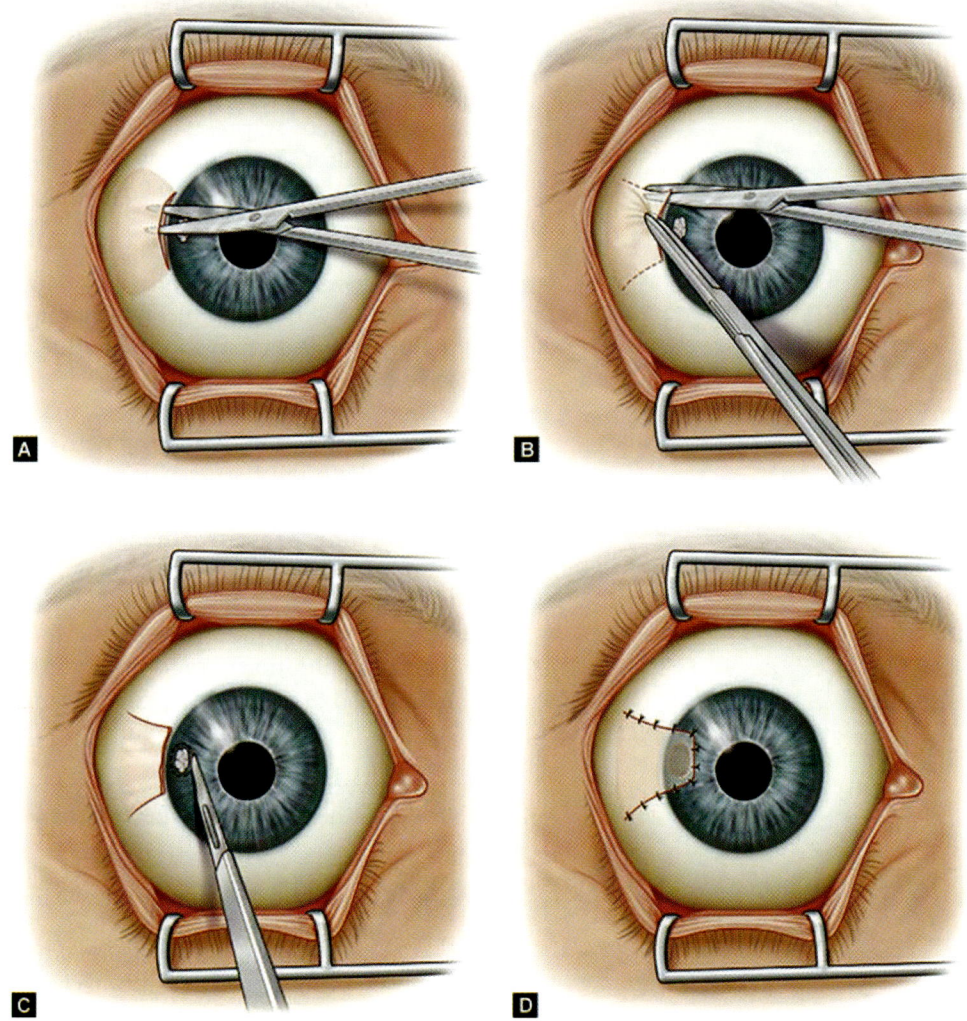

Fig. 35.7: *Advancement conjunctival flap. A and B, Conjunctival dissection and relaxing incision; C, Debridement of involved cornea; D, Conjunctival flap advanced and sutured at the margin of corneal debrided area*

interrupted nylon sutures (Fig. 35.9). The width of the flap should be measured 20–30% larger than the diameter of the corneal lesion to ensure adequate coverage without tension.

◼ COMPLICATIONS

INTRAOPERATIVE COMPLICATIONS

1. *Bleeding:* This can be minimized with preoperative use of brimonidine eye drops and good anaesthesia and cauterisation.

2. *Dissection of an inadequate flap:* Preoperative assessment about flap size is a prerequisite to

avoid this complication. Absence of scarring and free movement of the conjunctiva should be looked for. If dissection is not adequate to cover the desired area, it can modified to a bipedicle bridge flap by mobilizing conjunctiva from the opposite side.

3. *Buttonhole formation:* Care must be taken to use blunted scissors and non-toothed forceps for dissection. Attention must be paid to the depth of dissection. Any buttonhole must be sutured with 10–0 or 11–0 nylon suture immediately to avoid their enlargement.

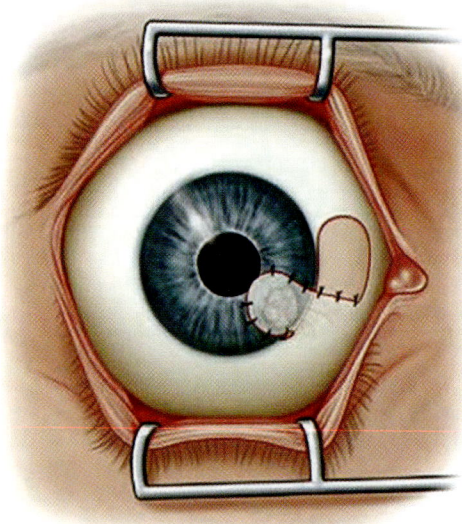

Fig. 35.8: *Single pedicle conjunctival flap*

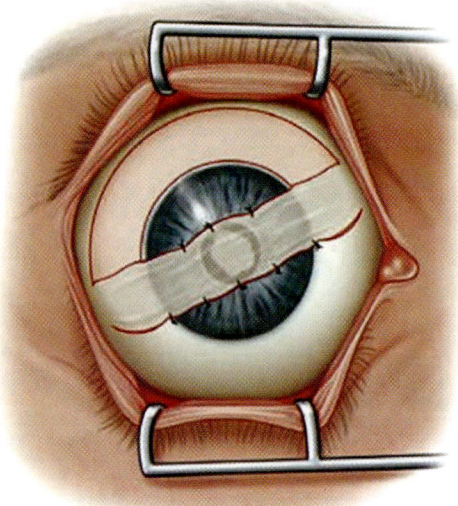

Fig. 35.9: *Bridge or bipedicle conjunctival flap*

POSTOPERATIVE COMPLICATIONS

1. *Retraction of the flap.* This occurs mainly due to inadequate mobilization of the conjunctiva and tension on the flap. These may require readvancement and suturing without minimal tension.

2. *Necrosis of flap.* This may occur in setting of infection or inflammation. Appropriate medical management with antibiotic and steroid eye drops must be done.

3. *Cysts.* Epithelial cysts may form under the flap if underlying corneal epithelium is not completely removed.

4. *Suture granuloma.* A rare complication which can be avoided by prescribing antibiotic and steroid eye drops post surgery. Non-absorbable sutures must be removed by 2 weeks.

LIMITATIONS

- Conjunctival flap should be used with caution in patients with active ulcer as monitoring of the ulcer beneath flap is difficult due to poor visibility.
- Vision is obscured when the visual axis is completely covered with conjunctival flap. In cases where the flap is performed for peripheral disease vision is not affected.
- Intraocular pressure measurement and monitoring is difficult over conjunctival flaps.
- Large areas of healthy conjunctiva is mobilized rendering them unsuitable for future glaucoma filtration surgery if required.
- It may lead to poor cosmetic appearance if the cornea is completely covered.

BIBLIOGRAPHY

PTERYGIUM

1. Asokan R, Venkatasubbu RS, Velumuri L, Lingam V, George R. Prevalence and associated factors for pterygium and pinguecula in a South Indian population. Ophthalmic Physiological Optics 2012; 32: 39–44.
2. Cameron M. Ultraviolet radiation. Pterygium throughout the world 1965; 41–54.
3. Cardillo JA, Alves MR, Ambrosio LE, Poterio MB, Jose NK. Single intraoperative application versus postoperative mitomycin C eye drops in Pterygium Surgery. Ophthalmology 1995; 102(12): 1949–52.
4. Chalkia AK, Spandidos DA, Detorakis ET. Viral involvement in the pathogenesis and clinical features of ophthalmic pterygium (Review). Int J Mol Med 2013; 32: 539–43.
5. Coroneo M. Albedo concentration in the anterior eye: A phenomenon that locates some solar diseases. Ophthalmic surgery 1990; 20: 60–66.
6. Das S, Ramamurthy B, Sangwan VS. Deep lamellar keratoplasty for recurrent advanced pterygium. Ophthalmic surgery, lasers and imaging 2009; 40: 43–45.

7. D'Ombrain A. The surgical treatment of pterygium. British journal of ophthalmology 1948; 65–71.

8. Dorland's illustrated medical dictionary. In: Illustrated medical dictionary. Philadelphia, PA: Saunders, 2007.

9. Duke-Elder S. Diseases of the outer eye. System of Ophthalmology 1965; 8: 573–85.

10. Hernández-Bogantes E, Amescua G, Navas A, et al. Minor ipsilateral simple limbal epithelial transplantation (mini SLET) for pterygium treatment. British Journal of Ophthalmology 2015; 99: 1598–1600.

11. Hirst LW. Recurrent pterygium surgery using pterygium extended removal followed by extended conjunctival transplant: recurrence rate and cosmesis. Ophthalmology 2009; 116: 1278–86.

12. Karai I, Horiguchi S. Pterygium in welders. British Journal of Ophthalmology 1984; 68: 347–49.

13. Kenyon KR, Wagoner MD, Hettinger ME. Conjunctival autograft transplantation for advanced and recurrent pterygium. Ophthalmology 1985; 92: 1461–70.

14. King JH. The pterygium—brief review and evaluation of certain methods of treatment. Archives of Ophthalmology 1950; 4: 854–69.

15. Kria L, Ohira A, Amemiya T. Immunohistochemical localization of basic fibroblast growth factor, platelet derived growth factor, transforming growth factor-beta and tumor necrosis factor-alpha in the pterygium. Acta Histochem 1996; 98: 195–201.

16. Kwok LS, Coroneo MT. A model for pterygium formation. Cornea 1994; 13: 219–24.

17. Ma DH, See LC, Hwang YS, Wang SF. Comparison of amniotic membrane graft alone or combined with intraoperative mitomycin C to prevent recurrence after excision of recurrent pterygia. Cornea 2005; 24: 141–15.

18. Nuzzi R, Tridico F. Efficacy of subconjunctival bevacizumab injections before and after surgical excision in preventing pterygium recurrence. J Ophthalmol, 2017.

19. Perez-Rico C, Pascual G, Sotomayor S, Asunsolo A, Cifuentes A, et al. Elastin development-associated extracellular matrix constituents of subepithelial connective tissue in human pterygium. Invest Ophthalmol Vis Sci 2014; 55: 6309–18.

20. Prabhasawat P, Barton K, Burkett G, Tseng SCG. Comparison of conjunctival autografts, amniotic membrane grafts and primary closure for pterygium excision. Ophthalmology 1997; 104(6): 974–85.

21. Rao SK, Lekha T, Mukesh BN, Sitalakshmi G, Padmanabhan P. Conjunctival-limbal autografts for primary and recurrent pterygia: Technique and results. Indian Journal of Ophthalmology 1998; 46: 203–9.

22. Rosenthal JW. Chronology of pterygium therapy. American Journal of Ophthalmology 1953; 36: 1601–6.

23. Sangwan VS, Murthy SI, Bansal AK, Rao GN. Surgical treatment of chronically recurring pterygium. Cornea 2003; 22: 63–65.

24. Singh G, Wilson MR, Foster CS. Mitomycin eye drops as treatment for pterygium. Ophthalmology 1988; 95: 813–21.

25. Talbot G. Pterygium: prevalence, demography and risk factors. Ophthlmic Epidemiology 1999; 6(3): 219–28.

26. Tan DT, Chee SP, Dear KB, Lim AS. Effect of pterygium morphology on pterygium recurrence in a controlled trial comparing conjunctival autografting with bare sclera excision. Arch Ophthalmol 1997; 115: 1235–40.

27. Tan DTH, Lim ASM, Goh HS, Smith DR. Abnormal expression of the p53 tumor suppressor gene in the conjunctiva of patients with pterygium. American Journal of Ophthalmology 1997; 123(3): 404–5.

28. Tseng SCG, Lee S-B, Lee D-Q. Limbal stem cell deficiency in the pathogenesis of pterygium. In: Taylor HR, editor. Pterygium. The Netherlands Kugler Publications, 2000: 41–56.

29. Yalcin Tok O, Burcu Nurozler A, Ergun G, Akbas Kocaoglu F, Duman S. Topical cyclosporine A in the prevention of pterygium recurrence. Ophthalmologica 2008; 222: 391–96.

30. Zhang J-D. An investigation of etiology and heredity of pterygium. Report of 11 cases in a family. Acta Ophthalmologica 1987; 65: 413–16.

CONJUNCTIVAL FLAPS IN OCULAR SURFACE DISORDERS

1. Alino AM, Perry HD, Kanellopoulos AJ, et al. Conjunctival flaps. Ophthalmology 1998; 105: 1120–23.

2. Anduze AL. Conjunctival flaps for pterygium surgery. Ann Ophthalmol (Skokie) 2006 Fall; 38(3): 219–23.

3. Brown DD, McCulley JP, Bowman RW, et al. The use of conjunctival flaps in the treatment of herpes keratouveitis. Cornea 1992; 11: 44–46.

4. Buxton JN, Fox ML. Conjunctival flaps in the treatment of refractory Pseudomonas corneal abscess. Ann Ophthalmol 1986; 18(11): 315–18.

5. Cheng KC, Chang CH. Modified Gundersen conjunctival flap combined with an oral mucosal graft to treat an intractable corneal lysis after chemical burn: a case report. Kaohsiung J Med Sci 2006; 22(5): 247–51.

6. Cies W. The racquet conjunctival flap. Ophthalmic Surg 1976; 7: 31–32.

7. Cosar CB, Cohe EJ, Rapuano CJ, et al. Clear corneal wound infection after phacoemulsification. Arch Ophthalmol 2001; 119(12): 1755–59.

8. Davidson RS, Erlanger M, Taravella M, et al. Tarsoconjunctival pedicle flap for the management of a severe scleral melt. Cornea 2007; 26(2): 235–37.

9. Geria RC, Wainsztein RD, Brunzini M, et al. Infectious keratitis in the corneal graft: treatment with partial conjunctival flaps. Ophthalmic Surg Lasers Imaging 2005; 36(4): 298–302.

10. Godfrey D, Merritt J, Fellman R, et al. Interpolated conjunctival pedicle flaps for the treatment of exposed glaucoma drainage devices. Arch Ophthalmol 2003; 121: 1772–75.

11. Gundersen T, Pearlson HR. Conjunctival flaps for the corneal disease: Their usefulness and complications. Trans Am Ophthalmol Soc 1969; 67: 78–95.

12. Gundersen T. Conjunctival flaps in the treatment of corneal disease with reference to a new technique of application. Arch Ophthalmol 1958; 60: 880–87.

13. Madhusudhan S, Chandra KP. Forniceal conjunctival pedicle grafts. Eye 2007; 21: 283–84.

14. Mauger TF, Craig E. Combined Acanthamoeba and *Stenotrophomonas maltophilia* keratitis treated with a conjunctival flap followed by penetrating keratoplasty. Cornea 2006; 25: 631–33.

15. Rosenfeld SI, Alfonso EC, Gollamudi S. Recurrent herpes simplex infection in a conjunctival flap. Am J Ophthalmol 1993; 116(2): 242–44.

16. S Wadhwani RA, Bellows AR, Hutchinson BT. Surgical repair of leaking filtering blebs. Ophthalmology 2000; 107(9): 1681–87.

17. Sandinha T, Zaher SS, Roberts F, et al. Superior forniceal conjunctival advancement pedicles (SFCAP) in the management of acute and impending corneal perforations. Eye 2006; 20: 84–89.

18. Sugar HS. The use of Gundersen flaps in the treatment of bullous keratopathy. Am J Ophthalmol 1964; 57: 977–83.

Limbal Stem Cell Transplantation

INTRODUCTION

The management of severe ocular surface diseases such as chemical and thermal burns, congenital abnormalities, vascularised scars with conjunctivalisation and cicatrizing diseases is a challenging scenario. Various procedures were proposed in the past without successful results due to the limitation in knowledge about limbal stem cells.

LIMBAL STEM CELL MIGRATION

Following hypothesis has been put forward to describe limbal stem cell migration: Thoft's XYZ hypothesis.

Limbal stem cells are now believed to be the prime source of daughter transient amplifying cells that migrate centripetally onto the cornea.[1–7]

Post-mitotic suprabasal cells from their division migrate to the epithelial surface as described by Thoft's XYZ hypothesis of corneal epithelial cell maintenance.[8] As per the hypothesis, X represents proliferation of basal epithelial cells, Y represents centripetal migration of stem cells and Z represents the epithelial cell loss which must be equal to the sum of X and Y (Fig. 36.1).

Niche hypothesis has been proposed by Schofield in 1983, according to which, stem cells reside in an optimal niche whereby only one of the daughter cells can re-enter the niche and all other daughter cells enter the pathway of terminal differentiation.[9] The corneal epithelial cells which are constantly being desquamated are replaced by proliferating basal epithelial cells from the periphery. This is a state of dynamic equilibrium which is maintained by the stem

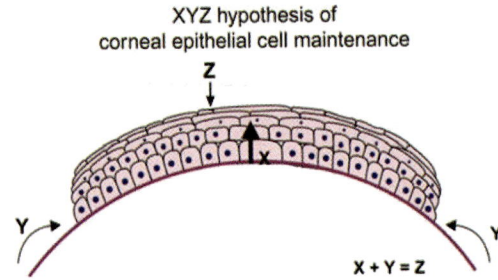

XYZ hypothesis of
corneal epithelial cell maintenance

$$X + Y = Z$$

Fig. 36.1: *XYZ hypothesis of Thoft and Friend*

cells residing within the palisades of Vogt at the limbus (niche).[10] Cell cycle for the stem cells is slow and they have a long lifespan.[11]

Corneal epithelial stem cells lack plasticity and are developmentally committed to give rise only to cells of their own particular tissue type unlike haematopoietic stem cells which may trans-differentiate into different body tissue types.[12]

LIMBAL STEM CELL DEFICIENCY

Limbal stem cell deficiency (LSCD) is characterised by a loss or deficiency of stem cells which are responsible not only for corneal epithelial renewal and regeneration but also function as a barrier, preventing conjunctival epithelium from growing onto the cornea, referred to as conjunctivalisation.[13,14]

In LSCD, the corneal epithelium is unable to repair and renew itself. This results in epithelial breakdown and persistent epithelial defects, corneal conjunctivalisation, neovascularisation, corneal scarring and chronic inflammation.

CLASSIFICATION OF LSCD

Limbal stem cells are indispensable for regeneration and maintenance of a smooth ocular surface. LSCD can be classified based on the etiology and extent of damage.

I. Etiological classification

Conditions leading to deficiency of limbal stem cells can be either primary or secondary.[1]

- *LSCD is primary:* Characterised by the absence of identifiable external factors causing deficiency. These conditions are associated with an unfavourable environment for the stem cells to survive.

- *LSCD is secondary:* Characterised by destruction of limbal stem cells by external factors.

Etiological factors for both primary and secondary LSCD are enumerated in Table 36.1.

Table 36.1: *Etiological classification of LSCD*

Primary
- Aniridia
- Multiple endocrine deficiency
- Ectodermal dysplasia (keratitis-ichthyosis-deafness or KID syndrome)
- Dyskeratosis congenita

Secondary
- Chemical/thermal/radiation injury
- Stevens-Johnson syndrome
- Mucous membrane pemphigoid
- Post-surgical excision of pterygium, limbal tumour
- Post-infectious keratitis
- Neurotrophic keratitis
- Severe vernal keratoconjunctivitis
- Contact lens wear
- Pterygium
- Vitamin A deficiency
- Antimetabolites (mitomycin C, 5-fluorouracil)
- Idiopathic

II. Classification based on extent of damage

Depending on the extent of damage LSCD may be either:
- *Partial LSCD*, wherein only a part of the limbus is damaged, and
- *Total LSCD*, wherein there is 360 degrees damage to the limbal stem cells.

CLINICAL FEATURES

Symptoms

Presenting symptoms of LSCD are pain (due to recurrent erosions) decreased vision, redness, watering, photophobia, blepharospasm, and contact lens intolerance.

Signs

Signs to look for in a patient of LSCD include:
Hallmark triad of LSCD comprises:[13, 14]
- Conjunctivalisation,
- Neovascularisation, and
- Chronic inflammation

Other signs include:[15]
- Progressive epitheliopathy with hazy translucent epithelium extending from the limbus, most commonly superior limbus.
- Recurrent and persistent epithelial defects
- Stippled appearance of fluorescein-stained conjunctivalised cornea[6,18]
- Loss of palisades of Vogt
- Superficial vascularization
- Scarring
- Fibrovascular pannus
- Ulceration
- Corneal melt
- Corneal perforation

Confocal microscopy in vivo may show absence of palisade of Vogt in the affected sector, metaplastic wing, and basal epithelial cells with significantly decreased basal epithelial cell density and sub-basal nerve density and replacement of normal limbal epithelium by vascular fibrotic tissue in late stage.

LABORATORY WORKUP

While the diagnosis of LSCD is mainly clinical, laboratory tests such as impression cytology, immunocytochemistry, histopathology and fluorophotometry may aid in determining LSCD.

Impression cytology of the perilimbal area by pressing nitrocellulose acetate paper on the ocular surface and subsequent staining with periodic acid–Schiff (PAS) or Alcian blue stain demonstrates goblet cells on the cornea in cases of LSCD. Severe ocular inflammation or squamous metaplasia may render this negative.[20, 21]

Immunocytochemistry from areas of LSCD may demonstrate cytokeratin 19 (CK19), a marker for conjunctival epithelium. The cytokeratin markers for corneal suprabasal corneal epithelial cells being cytokeratins 3 and 12 (CK3 and CK12).

Histopathology examination of the resected pannus is confirmatory.

Fluorophotometry quantifies the corneal barrier dysfunction at the subclinical level.

MANAGEMENT

Limbal stem cell transplantation is currently the treatment of choice for LSCD. Careful evaluation and management of dry eye, adnexal and systemic diseases is important for favourable outcomes of limbal stem cell transplantation. Medical management is limited to mild disease.

MEDICAL MANAGEMENT

Asymptomatic or patients with mild symptoms especially in iatrogenic cases may not require therapy. Medical management is aimed at restoring the limbal microenvironment with a stepwise approach:

1. *Stopping traumatic or toxic* insults to the limbus by withholding the typical toxic drugs, and discontinuation of contact lens.
2. *Aggressive lubrication* with preservative-free artificial tear.
3. *Topical steroids* help alleviate symptoms and cause regression in clinical signs in patients with chronic low grade inflammation. Inflammation and vascularization are seen to regress with topical steroids.
4. *Topical retinoic acid and interferon α-2b* has been shown by some researchers to promote regression and prevent progression in mild to moderate disease.[23]
5. *Autologous serum drops* may stimulate healing of corneal surface.
6. *Oral doxycycline* is useful in patients with rosacea.

SURGICAL MANAGEMENT

A true limbal stem cell deficiency often needs surgical replacement of stem cells. The limbal stem cells may be drawn either from the fellow eye (**autograft**), a cadaver (**allograft**) or a living relative (**Lr-allograft**). The limbal stem cells are harvested with a carrier which may be either the conjunctiva (conjunctival-limbal auto- or allograft) or cornea (keratolimbal allograft). Choice of appropriate surgical technique depends on the *laterality* and *extent* of LSCD. The algorithm for management of LSCD depends on whether the condition is unilateral or bilateral and involves some or all of the limbal stem cells (Fig. 36.2).

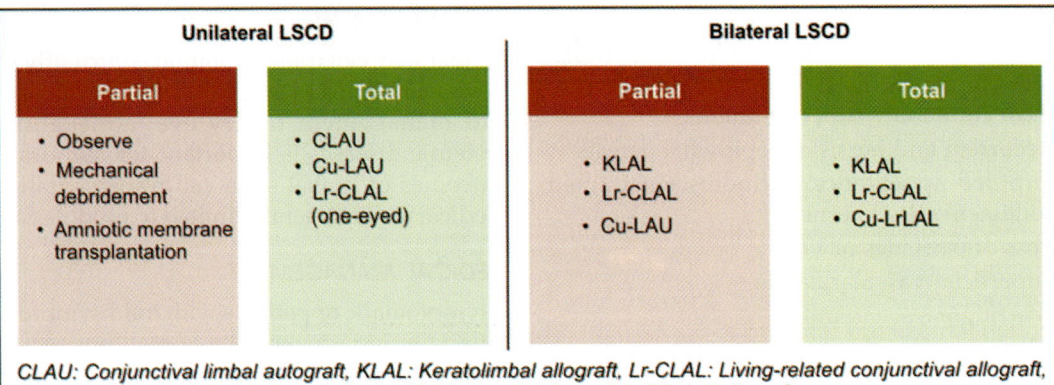

Fig. 36.2: *Treatment algorithm for limbal stem cell deficiency*

SURGICAL OPTIONS

Treatment options based on the laterality and extent of the disease.

A. Unilateral cases with partial LSCD

1. *Sequential sector conjunctival epitheliectomy (SSCE)* or repeated mechanical debridement, described by Dua et al.[24]
2. *Amniotic membrane transplantation* provides a scaffold for the growing epithelium. It also promote transdifferentiation of conjunctiva like epithelium into corneal epithelium and possesses anti-inflammatory properties.

B. Unilateral cases with total LSCD

1. *Conjunctival limbal autograft* (CLAU) from fellow eye.
2. *Transplantation of cultured limbal stem cells* from the fellow eye or from a living-related donor in a one-eyed patient.

C. Bilateral cases with total LSCD

1. Conjunctival-limbal allograft living (CLAL) related
2. Keratolimbal allograft living (KLAL) related
3. Transplantation of cultured limbal stem cells.

SURGICAL TECHNIQUES

Choice of anaesthesia: Depending on the age and systemic condition of the patient, this procedure can be performed under local peribulbar or general anaesthesia.

Preparation of recipient bed

Pannus dissection is a crucial initial step. Conjunctival peritomy is done 4–5 mm parallel from the limbus. The pannus is then completely dissected off the cornea using a bevel-up Beaver blade. Wet-field cautery or dilute adrenaline (1:10,000) is used to achieve hemostasis. Symblephera if any are resected.

Conjunctival-limbal autograft (CLAU)

In this procedure donor tissue is harvested from the fellow eye. Transplantation of more than six clock hours is not recommended to avoid iatrogenic stem cell deficiency in the fellow eye. Often the fellow eye may be carrying the same disease or may have had exposure to the same insult as the affected eye and may thus be harboring a subclinical LSCD.

A conjunctival flap 3 to 4 mm from the limbus and 6 clock hours in length, without the underlying Tenon's capsule is reflected forwards onto the cornea until the vascular arcades are reached. Donor tissue is then excised and sutured in limbus to limbus orientation at the host site with interrupted 10-0 monofilament nylon sutures. Kenyon and Tseng first described this technique in a series of 26 patients.[25] The cases comprised patients of chemical and thermal injuries in 22 (84.6%), contact lens induced keratopathy in 3 (11.5%) and stem cell deficiency following multiple surgeries in 1 (3.8%). In 10 (38.5%) patients with persistent epithelial defects for 3 weeks to 4 years, there was rapid re-epithelialisation (1–4 weeks). Failure of epithelialisation was seen in 3 (11.5%) eyes.

Keratolimbal allograft (KLAL)

This procedure involves lamellar dissection of the peripheral rim of corneal tissue to 1/3–1/2 depth from a donor cadaveric tissue which acts as a carrier for limbal stem cells. If the whole globe is used, a vacuum trephine may be used centrally, set to a depth of 150 µm and the dissection of the peripheral cornea and limbus may be carried out with a diamond knife. The donor lenticule is then placed proper anatomical position overlying the recipient limbus. This edge should lie flush with the cornea. Two corneoscleral rims placed end to end can cover 360° of the host limbus. This however is a time consuming and technically demanding procedure with the risk of damage to the limbal stem cell in the process. Published results describe the success of this technique in restoring ocular surface integrity to be between 57 and 83.3%.[26–28]

Conjunctival-limbal allograft (CLAL)

This procedure is done in one-eyed patients with total LSCD, or those with bilateral LSCD. Conjunctival-limbal allograft is taken preferably from an HLA-matched living-related donor. Donor preparation is similar to that for conjunctival limbal autograft. The tissue is stored either in balanced salt solution or in Ringer's lactate solution. This is immediately followed by host bed preparation as described earlier. Donor tissue is then placed in the correct orientation and sutured with nonabsorbable monofilament sutures. As with CLAU, harvesting of tissue from a healthy eye has the potential risk of inducing iatrogenic LSCD in the same. However, experiments have proved that the yield of limbal stem cells cultured from a live donor is much higher than that from cadaveric tissue.[29] It also requires need for immunosuppression post-surgery for a long period of time despite HLA matching. Kwitko and co-authors were among the first to describe the technique and reported a success rate of 91.6% (11/12) with an improvement in visual acuity of 5/11 (45.5%).[30]

Cultured corneal epithelial or limbal stem cell transplantation (CLET)

The major limitation for conjunctival-limbal auto- and allografts are availability of normal healthy epithelium from the contralateral eye or related donor and the potential for LSCD at donor site. The basic principle is to be able to culture stem cells using a small amount of tissue thereby minimising the damage to the donor surface. Incidence of rejection may also be reduced as practically only epithelial cells without blood vessels are used. Limbal biopsy from the donor, approximately 1 mm is taken. There are two types of culture techniques, namely:

1. *Suspension culture technique*—the limbal cells are trypsinised and supported by the feeder cells (Mouse NIH3T3-J2 fibroblasts).

2. *Explants culture technique*—the limbal biopsy specimen is transported to laboratory in modified human corneal epithelium (HCE) medium and shredded into multiple pieces onto the human amniotic membrane (HAM) and cultured in HCE medium with 10% autologous serum at 37°C, 5% CO_2 and 95% air.

- *Medium is changed on alternate days* and the growth of limbal stem cells is monitored daily under an inverted phase contrast microscope.
- *Culture system is maintained for 14–28 days* and then transferred to the recipient bed and sutured to the limbus with 10–0 nylon sutures.

Pellegrini et al first described the results of cultured autologous corneal epithelial cells in two patients and reported stabilization of ocular surface with no recurrence of conjunctivalisation in both the cases.[31]

Simple limbal epithelial transplantation (SLET)

Sangwan et al first described this novel procedure for patients with unilateral LSCD.[32] In this procedure a small limbal biopsy (2 mm × 2 mm) from the contralateral healthy superior limbus is dissected (Fig. 36.3A). Sub-conjunctival dissection is carried out until the limbus is reached. A shallow dissection is then carried out 1 mm into the clear cornea (Fig. 36.3B and C). The donor tissue is placed in balanced salt solution. After dissection of pannus (Fig. 36.3D)

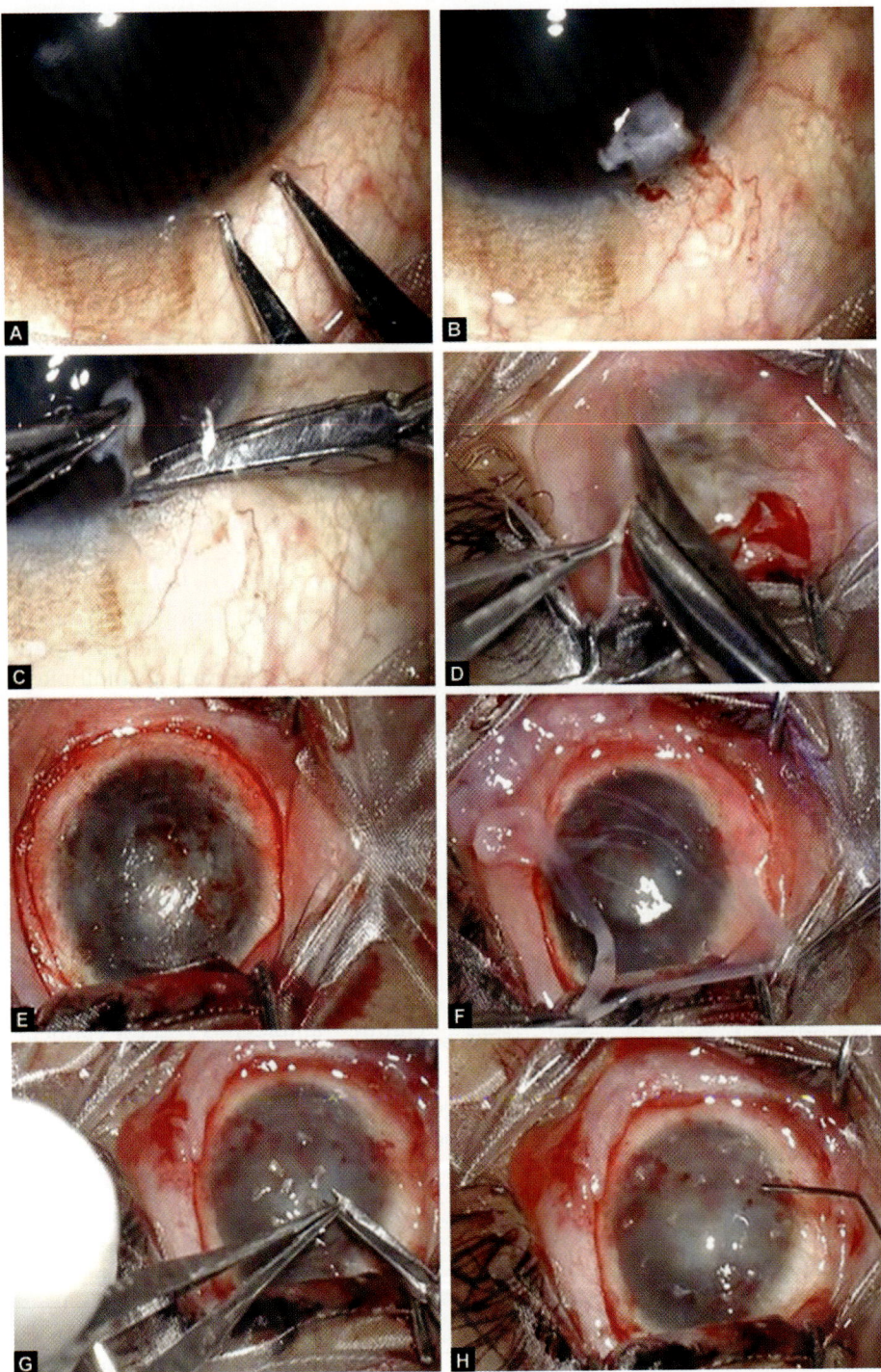

Fig. 36.3: *Surgical technique for simple limbal epithelial transplantation (SLET). A, 2 x 2 mm donor site marked on contralateral eye before harvesting graft; B, Conjunctival–limbal flap raised; C, Limbal biopsy excised; D, Pannus dissection on affected done; E, 360 degrees peritomy done; F, Amniotic membrane graft (AMG)spread over ocular surface; G, Limbal biopsy divided into 8–10 small explants with Vanna's scissors; H, Explants secured with fibrin glue on the AMG and BCL placed*

and preparation of the recipient bed (Fig. 36.3D and E) as described earlier, human amniotic membrane is glued to the diseased ocular surface with fibrin glue (Fig. 36.3F). The donor tissue previously harvested is divided into 8–10 smaller pieces with Vannas scissors (Fig. 36.3G). The tiny limbal transplants are then placed on top of the secured amniotic membrane in a circular fashion (Fig. 36.3H). It has been shown that amniotic membrane promotes the differentiation of limbal stem cells and itself has healing and regenerative properties.[33,34]

In the study by Sangwan et al, after surgery, a completely epithelialised, avascular and stable corneal surface (Fig. 36.4) was seen in all recipient eyes by 6 weeks, and this was maintained at a mean ± SD follow-up of 9.2 ± 1.9 months. Visual acuity improved from worse than 20/200 in all recipient eyes before surgery to 20/60 or better in four (66.6%) eyes, while none of the donor eyes developed any complications. Long-term outcomes of SLET in 125 eyes, published by Basu et al revealed that at a median postoperative follow-up of 1.5 years, 95 of 125 eyes (76%) maintained a successful outcome.[35] Two-line improvement in visual acuity was seen in 75.2% of the cases and 67% of successful cases attained 20/60 or better vision (P <0.0001). Success rates for SLET were comparable when performed either by faculty or trainees (P= 0.71).

Advantages of SLET over other procedures

- Rapid
- Easy technique
- Easily reproducible
- Low cost
- Utilizes minimal donor tissue
- Does not need a sophisticated laboratory for cell expansion
- Does not need an interval of 2 weeks to grow stem cells in laboratory and transplantation as in CLET.

Comparison of different techniques of autologous limbal stem cell transplantation

Table 36.2 describes the comparison of different techniques of autologous limbal stem cell transplantation.

Modification of SLET

Various modifications and applications of SLET have been described since it was first described by Sangwan et al.

- SLET has been successfully used in paediatric cases of uniocular burns.[36]
- In treatment of extensive **ocular surface squamous neoplasia**.[37]
- Live-related **Allo SLET** wherein biopsy from live-related donor is taken,[38] and
- **Mini-SLET** in which limbal biopsies are placed only over affected limbal area in cases

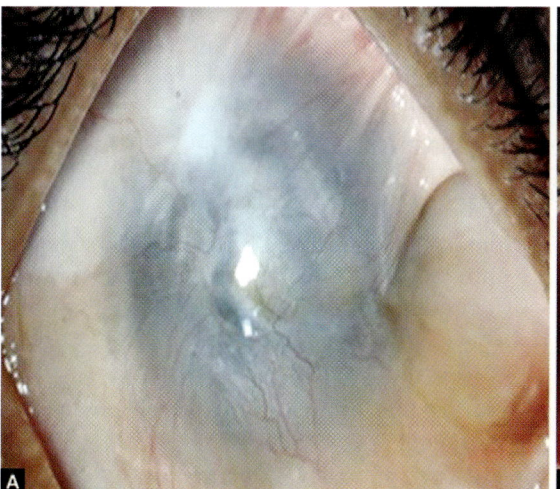
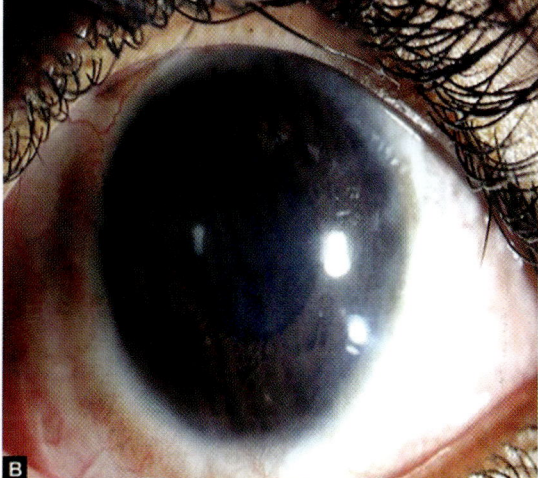

Fig. 36.4: *A, In a patient with total limbal stem cell deficiency post-chemical injury; B, Clear cornea with stable ocular surface was achieved post-SLET*

Table 36.2: *Comparison of different techniques of autologous limbal stem cell transplantation*

Parameters	SLET	CLET	CLAU
Stages	One	Two	One
Interval between stages	None	2 weeks	None
Need for stem cell laboratory	No	Yes	No
Need for human amniotic membrane	Yes	Yes	No
Donor tissue size (mm)	2	2	20
Time to epithelialisation	4–6 weeks	0	4–6 weeks
Repeatability	Yes	No	No
Donor eye LSCD	No	No	Yes
Long-term success	76%	50–100%	77–100%

of pterygium have been described to have successful outcomes.[39]

POSTOPERATIVE CARE

Treatment

Postoperative treatment for all of the above mentioned procedures includes:

- *Topical antibiotics preferably preservative-free* are prescribed until healing of the conjunctival and corneal epithelial defects.
- *Topical corticosteroids* in tapering doses are prescribed and continued long-term on a low maintenance dose.
- *Judicious use of preservative-free tear substitutes* is recommended.
- *Immune suppression* with topical cyclosporine A has been used in allolimbal transplantation.
- *Systemic immunosuppressants* commonly used after limbal stem cell transplantation include cyclosporine A (3–12 mg/kg), cyclophosphamide (1–2 mg/kg daily), mycophenolate mofetil (2 g/day), tacrolimus (0.1–0.2 mg/kg/day) and prednisolone (1 mg/kg/day) after proper physician evaluation.

Follow-up

- *In the immediate postoperative period* patients are kept under a close follow-up until the epithelium heals.
- *On subsequent follow ups,* recurrence of LSCD, clarity of the cornea and signs of rejection (in cases of allograft) if any are noted. Dosage of immunosuppression is monitored and systemic blood tests are conducted at regular intervals to detect drug-induced side effects.

COMPLICATIONS

Intraoperative complications include:

- Bleeding
- Corneal perforation
- Thick donor lenticule dissection
- Insufficient harvesting of limbal stem cells
- Wrinkled or damaged grafts
- Loss of graft

Postoperative complications include:

- Epithelial breakdown
- *Limbal allograft rejection.* Clinical features include appearance of epithelial defect, ischaemia of the graft and engorgement of limbal blood vessels. In case of rejection hourly steroid eye drops is administered. Subconjunctival or sub-Tenon's depot corticosteroids in the section of rejection may be required. The survival of stem cells post-rejection is debatable.
- Infection
- Secondary glaucoma

OUTCOME OF LSCT

Limbal stem cell transplantation by various techniques is an effective method in restoration of ocular surface in a variety of challenging diseases. The outcome of the procedure is influenced by:

- *Nature and duration* of underlying ocular pathology
- Presence of ocular inflammation
- Primary causes of limbal stem cell deficiency
- Quantity and quality of tear film.

- *Innovations such as SLET* which is a low cost novel procedure for stem cell transplantation has brought hope in treating challenging cases in remote corners of developing world.
- *With reported successful outcomes,* limbal stem cell transplantation has modified the course of morbidity in difficult case scenarios.

REFERENCES

1. Kruse EF. Stem cells and corneal regeneration. Eye 1994; 8: 170–83.
2. Kuwabara T, Perkins DG, Cogan DG. Sliding of epithelium in experimental corneal wounds. Invest Ophthalmol 1976; 15: 4–14.
3. Buck RC. Cell migration in repair of mouse corneal epithelium. Invest Ophthalmol Vis Sci 1979; 18: 767–84.
4. Kinoshita S, Friend J, Thoft RA. Sex chromatin of donor corneal epithelium in rabbits. Invest Ophthalmol Vis Sci 1981; 21: 434–41.
5. Buck RC. Measurement of centripetal migration of normal corneal epithelial cells in the mouse. Invest Ophthalmol Vis Sci 1985; 26: 1296–99.
6. Dua HS, Forrester HV. The corneo-scleral limbus in human corneal epithelial wound healing. Am J Ophthalmol 1990; 110: 646–56.
7. Lemp MA. Corneal epithelial cell movement in humans. Eye 1989; 3: 438–45.
8. Thoft RA, Friend J. The XYZ hypothesis of corneal epithelial cell maintenance [letter]. Invest Ophthalmol Vis Sci 1983; 24: 1442–43.
9. Schofield R. The stem cell system. Biomed Pharmacother 1983; 37: 375–80.
10. Davanger M, Evensen A. Role of pericorneal papillary structure in renewal of corneal epithelium. Nature 1971; 229: 560–61.
11. Slack JMW. Stem cells in epithelial tissues. Science 2000; 287: 1431–33.
12. Jackson KA, Majka SM, Wulf GG, Goodell MA. Stem cells: A mini-review. J Cell Biochem (Suppl) 2002; 38: 1–6.
13. Huang AJ, Tseng SC. Corneal epithelial wound healing in the absence of limbal epithelium. Invest Ophthalmol Vis Sci 1991; 32: 96–105.
14. Ebato B, Friend J, Thoft RA. Comparison of limbal and peripheral human corneal epithelium in tissue culture. Invest Ophthalmol Vis Sci 1988; 29: 1533–37.
15. Chen JJ, Tseng SC. Corneal wound healing in partial limbal deficiency. Invest Ophthalmol Vis Sci 1990; 31: 1301–14.
16. Kruse FE, Chen JJ, Tsai RJ, Tseng SC. Conjunctival transdifferentiation is due to the incomplete removal of limbal basal epithelium. Invest Ophthalmol Vis Sci 1990; 31: 1903–13.
17. Dua HS, Azuara-Blanco A. Limbal stem cells of the corneal epithelium. Surv Ophthalmol 2000; 44: 415–25.
18. Dua HS, Gomes JA, Singh A. Corneal epithelial wound healing. Br J Ophthalmol 1994; 78: 401–8.
19. Kinoshita S, Adachi W, Sotozono C, Nishida N, Yokoi N, Quantock AJ, Okubo K. Characteristics of human ocular surface epithelium. Prog Ret Eye Res 2001; 20: 639–73.
20. Egbert PR, Lauber S, Maurice DM. A simple conjunctival biopsy. Am J Ophthalmol 1977; 84: 798–801.
21. Puangsricharern V, Tseng SC. Cytologic evidence of corneal disease with limbal stem cell deficiency. Ophthalmology 1995; 102: 1476–85.
22. Revoltella RP, Papini S, Rosellini A, Michelini M. Epithelial stem cells of the eye surface. Cell Prolif 2007; 40(4): 445–61.
23. Tan JC, Tat LT, Coroneo MT. Treatment of partial limbal stem cell deficiency with topical interferon α-2b and retinoic acid. Br J Ophthalmol 2016; 100(7): 944–48.
24. Dua HS. The conjunctiva in corneal epithelial wound healing. Br J Ophthalmol 1998; 82: 1407–11.
25. Kenyon KR, Tseng SCG. Limbal autograft transplantation for ocular surface disorders. Ophthalmology 1989; 96: 709–23.
26. Tsai RJF, Tseng SCG. Human allograft limbal transplantation for corneal surface reconstruction. Cornea 1994; 13: 389–400.
27. Dua HS, Azuara-Blanco A. Allo-limbal transplantation in patients with limbal stem cell deficiency. Br J Ophthalmol 1999; 83: 414–19.
28. Tsubota K, Satake Y, Kaido M, Shinozaki N, Shimmura S, Bissen-Miiyajima H, Shimazaki J. Treatment of severe ocular surface disorders with corneal epithelial stem cell transplantation. N Eng J Med 1999; 340: 1697–703.
29. Kwitko S, Marinho D, Barcaro S, Bocaccio F, Rymer S, Fernandes S, Neumann J. Allograft conjunctival transplantation for bilateral ocular surface disorders. Ophthalmology 1995; 102: 1020–51.
30. Vemuganti GK, Kashyap S, Sangwan VS, Singh S. The proliferative potential of stem cells from fresh versus cadaveric limbal tissues. Invest Ophthalmol Vis Sci 2002; 43: S1623.

31. Pellegrini G, Traverso CE, Franzi AT, Zingirian M, Canced da R, DeLuca M. Long-term restoration of damaged corneal surfaces with autologous cultivated corneal epithelium. Lancet 1997; 349: 990–93.

32. Sangwan VS, Basu S, MacNeil S, Balasubramanian D. Simple limbal epithelial transplantation (SLET): A novel surgical technique for the treatment of unilateral limbal stem cell deficiency. Br J Ophthalmol 2012; 96 (7): 931–34.

33. Pires RT, Chokshi A, Tseng SC. Amniotic membrane transplantation or conjunctival limbal autograft for limbal stem cell deficiency induced by 5-fluorouracil in glaucoma surgeries. Cornea 2000; 19: 284–87.

34. Anderson DF, Ellies P, Pires RR TF, Tseng SCG. Amniotic membrane transplantation for partial limbal stem cell deficiency. Br J Ophthalmol 2001; 85: 567–75.

35. Basu S, Sureka SP, Shanbhag SS, Kethiri AR, Singh V, Sangwan VS. Simple limbal epithelial transplantation: Long-term clinical outcomes in 125 cases of unilateral chronic ocular surface burns. Ophthalmology 2016; 123: 1000–10.

36. Mittal V, Jain R, Mittal R, et al. Successful management of severe unilateral chemical burns in children using simple limbal epithelial transplantation (SLET). British Journal of Ophthalmology 2016; 100: 1102–8.

37. Mittal V, Narang P, Menon V, Mittal R, Honavar S. Primary simple limbal epithelial transplantation along with excisional biopsy in the management of extensive ocular surface squamous neoplasia. Cornea 2016; 35(12): 1650–52.

38. Iyer G, Srinivasan B, Agarwal S, Tarigopula A. Outcome of allo simple limbal epithelial transplantation (allo SLET) in the early stage of ocular chemical injury. Br J Ophthalmol 2017; 101(6): 828–33.

39. Hernández-Bogantes E, Amescua G, Navas A, et al. Minor ipsilateral simple limbal epithelial transplantation (mini SLET) for pterygium treatment. British Journal of Ophthalmology 2015; 99: 1598–1600.

Amniotic Membrane Transplantation and Mucous Membrane Grafting

AMNIOTIC MEMBRANE TRANSPLANTATION

INTRODUCTION

Human amniotic membrane is a semi-transparent innermost layer of placenta. Amniotic membrane (AM) was first used as skin graft in 1910 by Davis. Since then it was used as graft substrate in various procedures. First ophthalmological use of amniotic graft was done in 1940. However, its use was abandoned for decades till 1990 and after that amniotic membrane is used in a variety of ophthalmological procedures.

HISTOLOGY OF AMNIOTIC MEMBRANE

Human placenta consists of three layers:
1. *Innermost layer* surrounding the fetal side is amnion.
2. *Middle layer* is allantois.
3. *Outermost layer* surrounding the endometrium is chorion.

Amnion

Histologically, amnion layer is 0.2–0.5 mm thick and consists of three layers (Fig. 37.1):

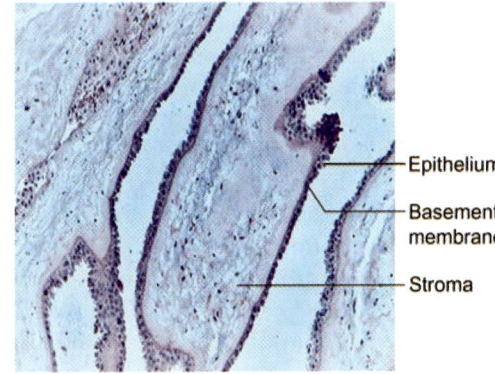

Fig. 37.1: *Histology of amniotic membrane (20X view; Courtesy: Ocular Pathology Lab, SCEH)*

Epithelial monolayer consists of single layer of polygonal cells with large number of microvilli on apical surface.

Basement membrane is the thickest membrane of the human tissue. The structural integrity, elasticity and transparency makes it the ideal substrate for the growth of epithelial progenitor cells. The basement membrane of AM, cornea and conjunctiva contain collagen types IV, V, VII, fibronectin and laminin.

Stromal matrix is avascular and hypocellular, rich in fetal hyaluronic acid. It has a compact layer that gives tensile strength. It suppresses TGF-β signaling, proliferation and myofibroblastic differentiation of normal fibroblast. Thus, it helps to reduce scarring.

It also suppresses expression of inflammatory cytokines which originate during inflammation such as IL-1a, IL-2, IL-8, interferon-γ, TNF-β, PDGF and FGF. This explains anti-inflammatory property of AM.

PROCESSING AND STORAGE

Amniotic membrane is processed from placenta after elective caesarean section.

- *Screening of donor.* Before collection of the amniotic membrane, donor is screened for HIV, HBsAg, HCV, syphilis and again after 6 months post-harvesting.
- *Placenta is collected in balanced salt solution* (BSS) in sterile environment and sent for processing at 4°C. After collection it is washed thoroughly.
- *Amniotic membrane (AM) is separated from placenta along with chorion.* Debris is removed from the surface and amniotic membrane is thoroughly cleaned in BSS and again washed several times with sterile phosphate buffer saline (PBS) containing antibiotic cocktail.
- *Storage of AM:* The AM is placed over nitrocellulose filter paper with epithelial side up. Amniotic membrane is stored in 50% glycerol in Dulbeco's modified Eagle Medium (DMEM, Gibco) or TC-199 (Fig. 37.2). Currently two main types of amniotic membrane which in use are cryopreserved and dehydrated.
- *Cryopreserved AM:* It includes preservation of amniotic membrane in DMEM/glycerol media at –80°C, slow freezing is done without ice formation. This retains extracellular matrix components which promote anti-inflammatory effects and healing. The tissue is stored at –80°C and brought to room temperature 15 minutes before use.
- *Dehydrated AM:* It is preserved using vacuum with low temperature heat to retain devitalized cellular components. However, FDA claimed its limited role in wound healing. It is kept at room temperature but it is being rehydrated before its use.

PROPERTIES OF AMNIOTIC MEMBRANE

- *Amniotic membrane is a non-toxic and immunologically inert material,* i.e. it does not induce any immunologic reaction when used as a graft material.
- *It provides platform for epithelial growth and migration.* It also reinforces basal cell adhesion and induces epithelial differentiation. Thus, promotes epithelialization.
- *It has anti-inflammatory, anti-microbial, anti-fibrotic, anti-angiogenic property* that helps to prevent or modulates scarring.

INDICATIONS OF AMNIOTIC MEMBRANE TRANSPLANTATION (AMT)

Amniotic membrane transplantation has made a important place in ocular surface diseases. Because of the above mentioned properties of amniotic membrane, it has been widely used in ophthalmology nowadays. Due to low immunogenicity, safety, low complication rate it can be used as bandage or graft for ocular surface disorders. Besides this, a lot of research is going on for the role AM extract eye drops in ocular surface reconstruction.

Common indications of AMT include:
- Pterygium surgery
- Chemical burns
- Shield ulcers
- Bullous keratopathy and band keratopathy
- Infectious keratitis
- Conjunctival tumours
- Glaucoma
- Neurotrophic ulcer
- Ocular surface reconstruction

SURGICAL TECHNIQUES OF AMT

There are three different surgical techniques by which amniotic membrane can be implanted onto the ocular surface (Fig. 37.3). In AMT, the amniotic membrane graft is attached to ocular surface with the help of either sutures or tissue adhesives preferably fibrin glue (Fig. 37.2).

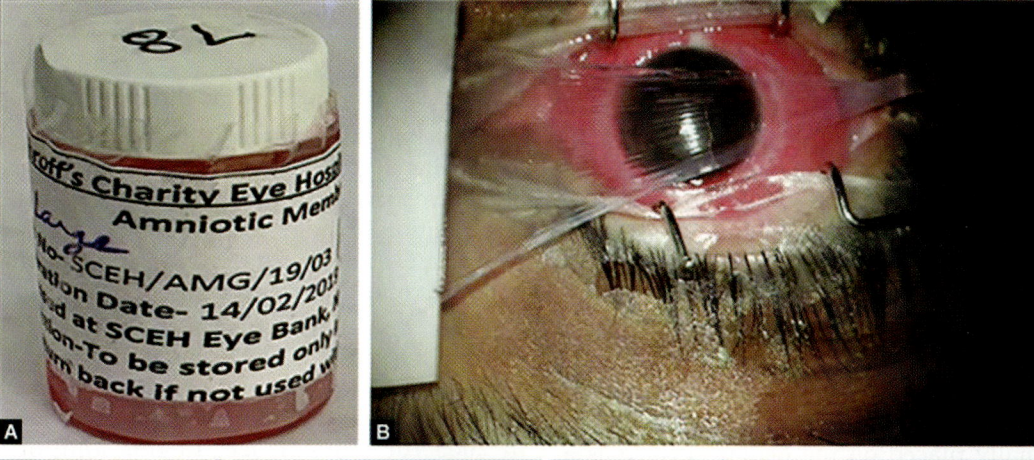

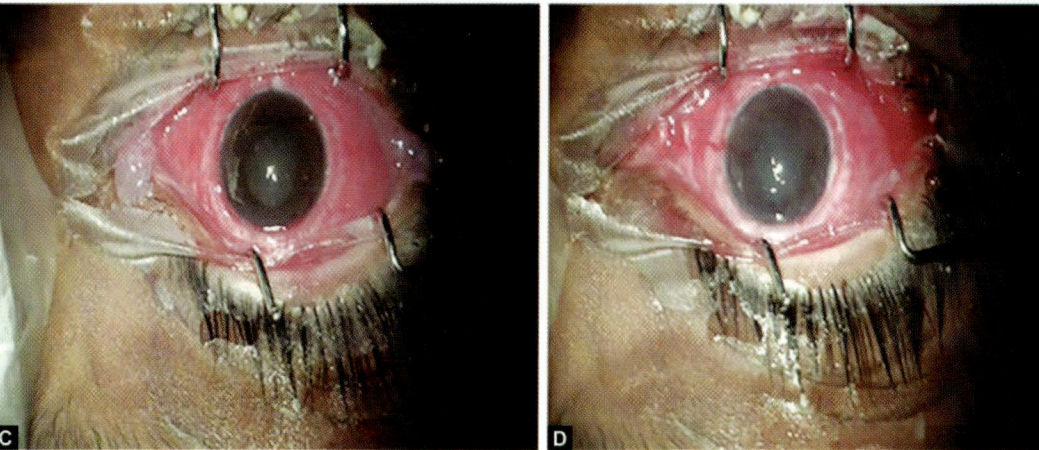

Fig. 37.2: *A, Amniotic membrane graft in bottle containing DMEM culture media; B, Amniotic membrane present over nitrocellulose membrane; C, Amniotic membrane is placed over raw ocular surface (patch technique) with stromal side up to help in healing of corneal epithelium along with entire coverage of conjunctiva in case of acute Stevens-Johnson syndrome; D, Amniotic membrane attached to the surface with fibrin glue and edges of membrane is excised with corneal scissors*

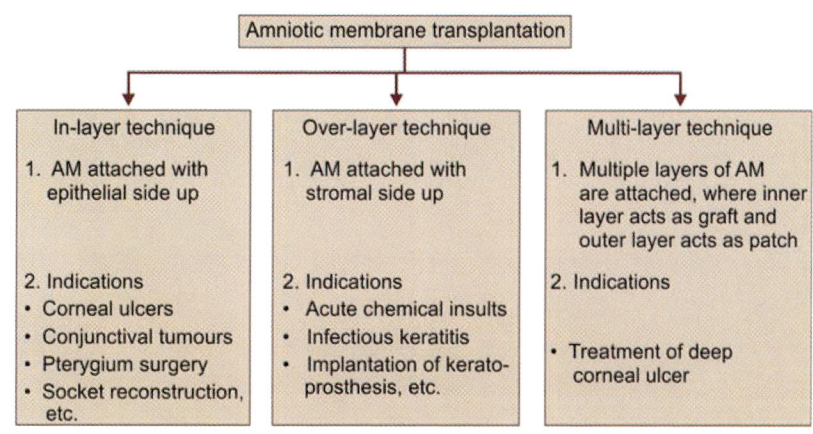

Fig. 37.3: *Types of amniotic membrane transplantation*

1. Graft or inlay technique

AM is attached to ocular surface with epithelial surface up as the permanent basement membrane substitute that helps to grow epithelial cells acting as a platform (Fig. 37.4). This technique is used for deficient or destroyed ocular surface caused by some disease or surgery. Examples are persistent epithelial defects, corneal ulceration, and conjunctival tumours, pterygium surgery, socket reconstruction, etc.

2. Patch or overlay technique

In patch or overlay technique, the AM is provisionally placed on the ocular surface as a "biological bandage" (Fig. 37.2C), i.e. stromal side is placed up to save the fragile epithelium and promote epithelial healing with minimal or no scarring. Examples are acute chemical insults, infectious keratitis, implantation of keratoprosthesis, etc.

3. Combined or multilayer technique

In this technique, multiple layers are used where the smaller inner layer acts as a graft and larger outer layer acts as a patch. This technique is the combination of inlay technique and overlay technique and is generally done for the treatment of deep corneal ulcers.

ProKera—a sutureless AM graft

ProKera (Bio-tissue) is a form of cryopreserved amniotic membrane that is approved by FDA in 2003 for clinical use. In this amniotic membrane is secured around a elastomeric band or polycarbonate ring. It does not require any assembly and can be directly used as a contact lens placement. In the stromal side, it acts as a

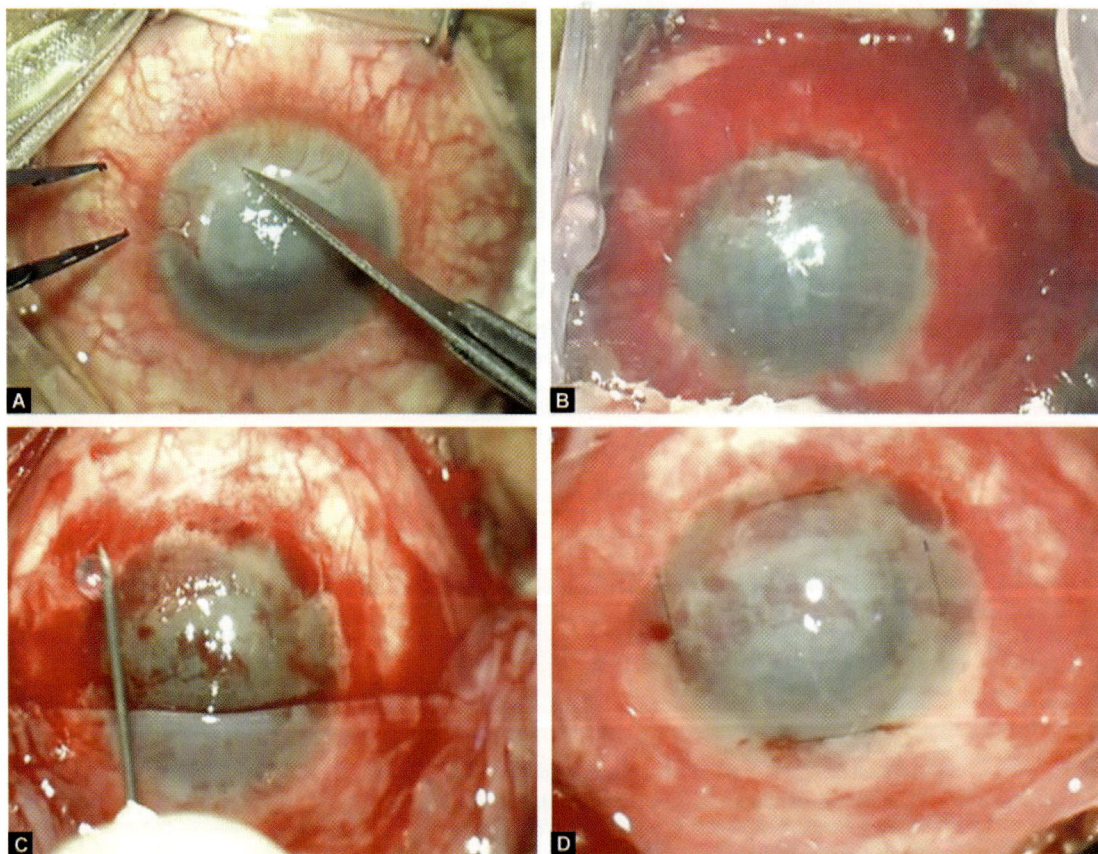

Fig. 37.4: *Amniotic membrane transplantation: A, Pannus dissection around persistent epithelial defect (PED); B, AMG spread over ocular surface; C, AMG secured with fibrin glue; D, AMG secured with intrastromal 10-0 nylon sutures*

biological bandage in contact with the cornea. However, ProKera device is an easier, less time consuming and economical procedure than other surgical techniques of the AM.

MUCOUS MEMBRANE GRAFTING

HISTORY

The first report on the application of oral mucosa as a substitute for conjunctiva dates back to 1873, when Stellwag von Carion used lip mucosa to treat conjunctival defects.

Van Milligen (1880) and Portmann (1900) transplanted oral mucosal strips to treat trichiasis.

In the early 20th century, oral mucosa was often transplanted in ophthalmic surgery. Wolff (1905) used it to treat a symblepharon, Denig (1910) to correct scarring after burns. Morton (1898), De Voe (1945), and Stallard (1946) transplanted it to the orbit prior to placement of orbital prostheses.

Today oral mucosa is used as a substitute for tarsal and conjunctival tissues.

Other than ophthalmology, oral mucosal grafts are used in maxillofacial and urological reconstructive surgeries.

APPLIED ANATOMY

Conjunctiva

The conjunctiva is the mucous membrane of eye that begins at the mucocutaneous junction (MCJ) of both the lids, covers the inner surface of tarsal plate, cover the anterior sclera and ends at the limbus. Broadly it is divided into three parts, palpebral or tarsal, forniceal and bulbar.

Histology: Conjunctiva begins as 150–200 μm wide parakeratinized squamous epithelium and 100–150 μm wide squamous transition zone; together forming the MCJ. It is followed by 0.3–1.5 mm wide area known as lid wiper zone which consists of stratified cuboidal epithelium and high density of goblet cells. It is believed that this lid wiper zone is in contact with the ocular surface and plays major role in spreading tear film during blinking. This zone is followed by subtarsal fold and tarsal conjunctiva which consists of pseudostratified columnar epithelium. Fornix is the junction of palpebral and bulbar conjunctiva. Bulbar conjunctiva comprises stratified cuboidal epithelium. Mucoussecreting goblet cells constitute 5–10% of the conjunctival epithelial basal cells. The highest density of goblet cells occurs in the inferonasal bulbar conjunctiva and tarsal conjunctiva.

Table 37.1: *Tissue options for fornix reconstruction*

Graft material	Stiffness	Stability	Goblet cells	Epithelial stem cells	Availability[1] included	Source/cosmesis
Conjunctiva	–	+	+	+	–	Autologous Excellent
Tarsus	+	++	+	+	–	Autologous Excellent
Buccal mucosa						Autologous
Full thickness	+	++	–	+	++	Poor
Split thickness	+	++	–	+	++	Good
Hard palate	++	++	–	+	+	Autologous Good
Nasal septal cartilage	++	++	+	+	+	Autologous Fair
Nasal turbinate mucosa	+	+	++	+	+	Autologous Fair
Amniotic membrane	–	–	–	–	+++	Heterolgous Excellent

Oral mucosa

Oral mucosa begins at the vermillion border and extends posteriorly till the beginning of oropharynx. It is a stratified squamous epithelium consisting of cells tightly attached to each other and arranged in a number of distinct layers or strata. Based on the appearance in histological sections and staining with specific markers such as keratin antibodies, oral epithelium can be divided into two types: Keratinized epithelium, covering areas of masticatory mucosa, such as hard palate and gingiva, and non-keratinized epithelium, covering areas of lining mucosa such as cheeks, soft palate, and floor of mouth.

The oral mucosa varies considerably in its firmness and texture. The lining mucosa of the lips and cheeks, for example, is soft and pliable, whereas the gingiva and hard palate are covered by a firm, immobile layer. These differences have important clinical implications when it comes to giving local injections of anaesthetics or taking biopsies of oral mucosa. Fluid can be easily introduced into loose lining mucosa, but injection into the masticatory mucosa is more difficult and can be painful for the patient. Lining mucosa gapes when surgically incised and frequently requires suturing, whereas masticatory mucosa, being more firmly attached, may not. Similarly, the accumulation of fluid with inflammation is obvious and painful in masticatory mucosa, but in lining mucosa the fluid disperses, and inflammation may not be so evident or as painful.

GRAFTS FOR CONJUNCTIVAL DEFECTS

An ideal epithelial graft tissue should have the following properties:

1. Same cosmetic appearance as conjunctiva,
2. Result in the formation of normal tissue and cell types, including goblet cells, and
3. Prevent postoperative cicatrization.

Choice of graft depends on the extent of conjunctival deficiency (Table 37.1).
- For small defects, conjunctival autograft is favourable.
- For larger defect, amniotic membrane grafting can be performed.

- For areas involving larger areas, fornix and lid margin, mucous membrane grafting can be done.

Mucous membrane grafts

Full-thickness oral mucous membrane graft is the simplest graft to use if conjunctiva or tarsus is not available.

Split-thickness mucosal grafts contract more than full-thickness grafts, and are therefore less suitable for fornix reconstruction, but are less bulky and pink than full-thickness grafts, and therefore should be used on the globe.

Hard palate grafts are the thickest oral mucosal grafts and contract the least. They are more difficult to harvest than other oral mucosal grafts, but are useful where sufficient buccal or labial mucosa is not available or when it is particularly desirable to avoid contracture. Oral mucosa does not contain goblet cells and therefore does not supplement the tear film.

Nasal mucosal grafts contain goblet cells that may contribute mucous to the tear film. This is maximized in turbinate mucosal grafts, which can relieve discomfort in extreme dry eye situations. Nasal septal cartilage contains fewer goblet cells, but is useful in the reconstruction of the posterior lamella when the tarsus is lacking; the graft replaces the rigidity of the tarsus, and its attached mucoperichondrium provides a mucosal binding which does not shrink and can be wrapped around the skin of the reconstructed eyelid to form a stable eyelid margin.

INDICATIONS OF MMG

- Lid margin keratinization (LMK)
- Surface preparation for LVP keratoprosthesis
- As a part of minor salivary gland transplant
- Refractory giant papillary conjunctivitis
- Contracted socket
- As posterior lamellar graft in lid reconstruction
- Cicatricial entropion
- Conjunctival insufficiency following glaucoma filtration surgery.

- *For lid margin keratinization in SJS:* Lid-related keratopathy in SJS can occur in acute/sub-acute stages due to recurrent conjunctival ulcerations and in chronic stages due to lid margin keratinization. The 'sand paper effect' caused by the roughened lip wiper region leads to corneal complications like corneal erosions, persistent epithelial defects, infectious keratitis, corneal melts and perforations. Replacing the keratinized area (Figs 37.5A and 37.6A) with a smooth mucosal surface (Figs 37.5B and 37.6B) restores the barrier function of the mucocutaneous junction and prevents crossover of the keratinized epithelium.

- *Preoperative assessment:* Lid margins of all the lids should be assessed for the extent of keratinization. Presence of any other pathology like extensive symblephara, entropion, and severe ocular surface cicatrisation, which would necessitate additional surgical procedures, should be noted and managed accordingly.

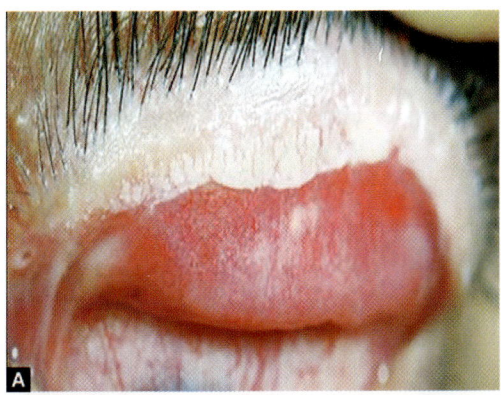

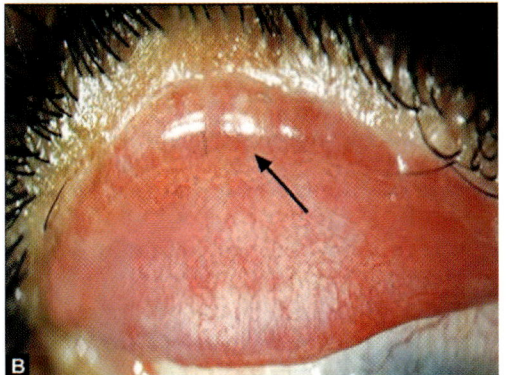

Fig. 37.5: *Mucous membrane graft. A, Keratinised lid in a case of Stevens-Johnson syndrome; B, MMG in situ after removal of keratinization*

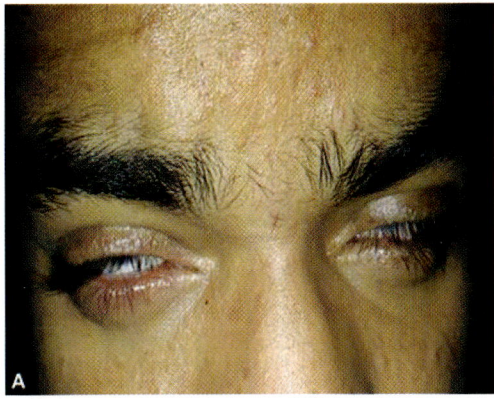

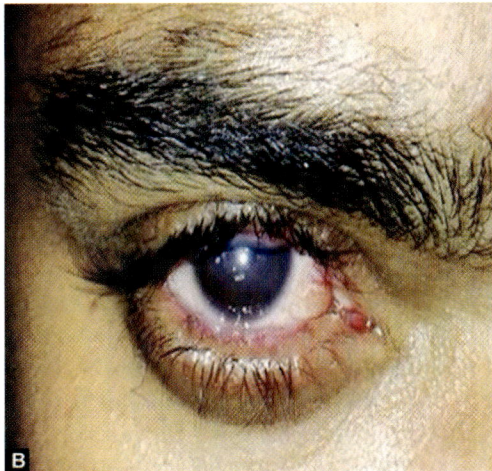

Fig. 37.6: *Clinical case. A, Severe photophobia, foreign body sensation and discomfort due to lid keratinization in a case of Stevens-Johnson syndrome; B, MMG in situ with marked decrease in ocular discomfort*

Health of oral mucosa should be assessed to rule out active ulcerations and extensive cicatrization so as to preclude surgery.

SURGICAL STEPS OF MMG

Anaesthesia

General anaesthesia is always preferred for following reasons:
- It is comfortable for both the surgeon and the patient
- All four lids can be planned in a single sitting
- Hypotensive anaesthesia can be given to control bleeding to a great extent.

Endotracheal tube is to be kept away from the intended site of graft harvest. Nasal intubation can be tried for lower lip grafts and is avoided for upper lip grafts as lip eversion becomes difficult.

Lid margin dissection

1. 2–3 traction sutures/lid using 4–0 silk are passed on skin away from lash line, parallel to lid margin and deep enough to include part of tarsus into the bite to prevent cheese-wiring.
2. Lid is everted using lid spatula or buds. Cotton buds when used provides hemostasis as they are flexible and can indent from underneath the everted lids.
3. Incision is given at the grey line using 15 no. blade on BP handle. It is always advisable to be liberal enough to include all the kerati-nization by placing the incision as anterior as required.
4. Canthus to canthus incision is preferred unless keratinization is localized to a small part. In general, the incision length should be around 20–25 mm.
5. Using 15 no. blade or a crescent knife, posterior lid margin is dissected including the meibomian orifices and making a pocket above the tarsus plate up to a width of 5 mm. Care should be taken to include all the keratinized lid margin and not to leave any tags of conjunctiva in the bed. Tarsus plate should not be included in the dissection as it can lead to floppy lid and ectropion post-surgery.

Oral mucosa harvesting

1. It is always preferable to give submucosal infiltration of lignocaine and adrenaline injection (1:1,600,000) before initiating lid margin dissection to have a good hemostasis during graft harvesting.
2. Lower lip is the preferred site for graft harvesting, followed by upper lip and buccal mucosa.
3. Two full-thickness stay sutures are used to evert the lip. Alternatively a hemostasis clamp can also be used.
4. Graft site is identified and marked. Frenulum and areas of submucosal fibrosis are avoided.

5. Dissection is done using Westcott's scissors and graft is made as thin as possible without causing a buttonhole. In case buttonhole occurs, graft should always be sutured using 8–0 vicryl sutures before placing the graft on the lid margin. Figure 37.7A shows the nicely harvested MMG.
6. Mucosal wound is either sutured using interrrupted 6–0 vicryl sutures or AMG is applied using fibrin glue. After 6 weeks the donor site becomes healthy (Fig. 37.7B).

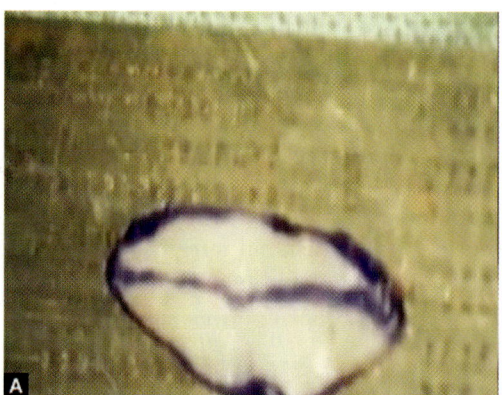

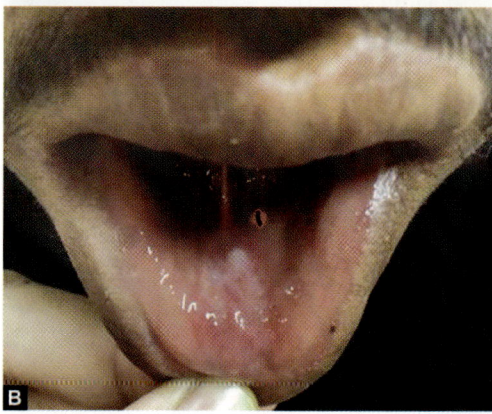

Fig. 37.7: *Mucous membrane graft. A, Harvested mucous membrane graft from lip (size 30 mm × 10 mm); B, Healthy lip mucosa at donor site 6 weeks postoperatively*

Graft debulking: The most important step that determines graft survival is graft preparation. Dissected graft is kept moist and stretched over the finger and using a Westcott's scissor all the fat, minor salivary glands and submucosal tissue is dissected. Buttonholing should be avoided. Achieving a transparent enough graft to see the colour of underlying glove should be the end point of dissection. The graft is then divided as per requirement into 2 or 4 pieces.

Suturing the graft

1. The graft is stretched out well after placing it at the lid margin achieving edge to edge approximation.
2. Anterior edge of the graft is sutured using 8–0 vicryl sutures. Continuous interlocking technique is preferred over interrupted technique.
3. Suture bites are passed through the tarsus and knots are pulled towards eyelashes in case of interrupted sutures.
4. Posterior part of the graft is glued using fibrin glue.

Postoperative management

Postoperative management includes the use of topical antibiotic eye drop 4 times daily for a week along with frequent application of lubricants.

Topical steroids may be used if required.

Postoperative chlorhexidine mouthwash is continued for a week after surgery.

Patients are examined on day 1, weeks 1 and 6, and subsequently every 3 months.

Iyer et al studied the cytokine profile post-MMG and concluded that there is reversal of most of the cytokine profile following MMG, correlating with the clinical improvement. They also noted an increase in goblet cell density following MMG, the exact underlying mechanism of which is yet to be elucidated as oral mucosa is devoid of goblet cells.

MMG FOR LVP KERATOPROSTHESIS

Visual rehabilitation in chronics SJS depends on the wetness of ocular surface. Type 1 Boston keratoprosthesis is preferred in wet eyes, whereas MOOKP, type 2 Boston kerato-prosthesis and modifications of type 1 device are preferred in dry eyes. One such modification is LVP Kpro, which consists of a design of the Boston type I keratoprosthesis but with slightly elongated optical cylinder. This design allows the MMG to be tucked underneath the front plate.

Surgical steps

1. In the first stage, 360° peritomy is done and the dermalised pannus is excised, exposing the underlying de-epithelised ocular surface.
2. A 30 × 30 mm labial mucosal graft is obtained from the lower lip as mentioned previously.
3. Graft is sutured over the ocular surface with 6–0 vicryl sutures, including four anchoring sutures passed through each rectus muscle to provide vascular supply to the graft.
4. The second stage involves placement of LVP Kpro three months after MMG. The mucosa is lifted as an inferior fornix-based flap; appropriately sized LVP Kpro is assembled and sutured in place; the mucosal flap is repositioned and sutured using continuous interlocking 6–0 vicryl sutures; finally, a central cruciate opening is made in the mucosa overlying the optical cylinder and the edges of the mucosal opening are tucked under the front plate of the LVP Kpro.

Postoperative management

Topical antibiotics and lubricants are given after stage 1. Topical steroid drops are usually added after stage 2 of the procedure.

MMG FOR REFRACTORY GIANT PAPILLARY VKC

The standard of care in the management of GPC includes topical antihistamines, mast cell stabilizers, intralesional steroids, topical and systemic steroids, and topical immunomo-dulators. Cases refractory to medical management have been addressed by cryotherapy and in extreme cases by surgical excision of the giant papillae. MMG has been tried with good results to prevent corneal complications and freedom from long-term steroid use.

Surgical steps

Most of the steps remain identical as described for lid margin MMG.

1. The extent of GPC on the tarsal surface of the everted lid is marked. A subconjunctival incision is made posterior to the lid margin, 1 to 2 mm from the edge of the papillae, and the tarsal conjunctiva along with the giant papillae is excised, taking care to avoid any damage to the tarsal plate.

2. Labial mucosal graft is harvested and prepared.
3. Anterior edge is sutured to the conjunctival edge; graft glued to bare tarsus using fibrin glue; posterior edge is sutured with interrupted sutures.

Postoperative management

Same as lid margin MMG.

No recurrence of GPC leading to corneal complications was observed in any of the 11 eyes in the study conducted by Iyer et al. However, reactivation of the allergic activity in the bulbar conjunctiva requiring a short course of topical steroids was noted in all the eyes.

COMPLICATIONS OF MMG

Intraoperative complications

1. Bleeding during lid margin dissection is common in chronically inflamed eyes. Extra measures are generally not required and cautery should be used judiciously as over-cauterization leads to postoperative entropion formation. Blood coagulates in the interim period of oral mucosa harvesting.
2. Dissection involving the tarsal plate can occur if eyelids are not properly everted and if view is obscured because of bleeding.
3. Piecemeal dissection can occur especially at the subtarsal fold. Keratinized conjunctiva should be identified and dissected.
4. Bleeding from oral harvesting site. It can be avoided by preoperative use of Xylocaine and adrenaline infiltration.
5. Buttonhole formation of graft.
6. Thicker grafts lead to bulky looking tissue in the late postoperative period.
7. Inadequate graft sizing. Labial grafts are elastic and can be stretched little bit during suturing. If width is inadequate, another oral mucosal strip should be excised and sutured. Deficiency in length is usually not a cause of concern if the entire keratinized conjunctiva is excised.

Postoperative complications

1. Graft dehiscence.
2. Necrosis.

3. Infection.
4. Granuloma formation.
5. Recurrence of keratinization. Keratinization beyond the graft not in contact with the ocular surface can be left alone. MMG should be augmented for keratinization significant enough to cause ocular surface inflammation.
6. Complications at donor site include submucosal fibrosis leading to contracture, granuloma formation and infection.

BIBLIOGRAPHY

1. Adinolfi M, Akle CA, McColl I. Expression of HLA antigens, β_2-microglobulin and enzymes by human amniotic epithelial cells. Nature 1982; 295: 325–27.
2. Azuara-Blanco A, Pillai CT, Dua HS. Amniotic membrane transplantation for ocular surface reconstruction. Br J Ophthalmol 1999; 83: 399–402.
3. Basu S, Nagpal R, Serna-Ojeda JC, Bhalekar S, Bagga B, Sangwan V. LVP keratoprosthesis: anatomical and functional outcomes in bilateral end-stage corneal blindness. Br J Ophthalmol 2018; pii: bjophthalmol-2017-311649
4. Batmanov IE, Egorova KS, Kolesnikova LN. Use of fresh amnion in the treatment of corneal diseases. Vestn Oftalmol 1990; 106: 17–19.
5. Bennett JP, Matthews R, Faulk WP. Treatment of chronic ulceration of the legs with human amnion. Lancet 1980; 1: 1153–56.
6. Bose B. Burn wound dressing with human amniotic membrane. Ann R Coll Surg Engl 1979; 61: 444–47.
7. Bourne GL. The microscopic anatomy of the human amnion and chorion. Am J Obstet Gynecol 1960; 79: 1070–73.
8. Colocho G, Graham WP III, Greene AE. Human amniotic membrane as a physiologic wound dressing. Arch Surg 1974; 109: 370–73.
9. Danforth DN, Hull RW. The microscopic anatomy of the fetal membranes with particular reference to the detailed structure of the amnion. Am J Obstet Gynecol 1958; 75: 536–50.
10. Davis JW. Skin transplantation with a review of 550 cases at the Johns Hopkins Hospital. Johns Hopkins Med J 1910; 15: 307.
11. de Rotth A. Plastic repair of conjunctival defects with fetal membranes. Arch Ophthalmol 1940; 23: 522–25.

12. Fernandes M, Sridhar MS, Sangwan VS, et al. Amniotic membrane transplantation for ocular surface reconstruction. Cornea 2005; 24: 643e53.

13. Filipas D, Wahlmann U, Hohenfellner R. History of Oral Mucosa. Eur Urol 1998; 34: 165–68.

14. Gurumurthy S, Iyer G, Srinivasan B, Agarwal S, Angayarkanni N. Ocular surface cytokine profile in chronic Stevens-Johnson syndrome and its response to mucous membrane grafting for lid margin keratinization. Br J Ophthalmol. 2018; 102(2): 169–76.

15. Hao Y, Ma DH, Hwang DG. Identification of antiangiogenic and anti-inflammatory proteins in human amniotic membrane. Cornea 2000; 19: 348–52.

16. Henderson HW, Collin JR. Mucous membrane grafting. Dev Ophthalmol 2008; 41: 230–42.

17. Iyer G, Agarwal S, Srinivasan B. Outcomes and Rationale of Excision and Mucous Membrane Grafting in Palpebral Vernal Keratoconjunctivitis. Cornea 2018; 37(2): 172–76.

18. Iyer G, Pillai VS, Srinivasan B, Guruswami S, Padmanabhan P. Mucous membrane grafting for lid margin keratinization in Stevens-Johnson syndrome: results. Cornea 2010; 29(2): 146–51.

19. Kim JC, Tseng SC. The effects on inhibition of corneal neovascularization after human amniotic membrane transplantation in severely damaged rabbit corneas. Korean J Ophthalmol 1995; 9: 32–46.

20. Kim JC, Tseng SCG. Transplantation of preserved human amniotic membrane for surface reconstruction in severely damaged rabbit corneas. Cornea 1995; 14: 473–84.

21. King AE, Paltoo A, Kelly RW, et al. Expression of natural antimicrobials by human placenta and fetal membranes. Placenta 2007; 28: 161e9.

22. Kurpakus-Wheater M. Laminin-5 is a component of preserved amniotic membrane. Curr Eye Res 2001; 22: 353–57.

23. Lee SB, Li DQ, Tan DT, Meller DC, Tseng SC. Suppression of TGF-β signaling in both normal conjunctival fibroblasts and pterygial body fibroblasts by amniotic membrane. Curr Eye Res 2000; 20: 325–34.

24. Lee SH, Tseng SC. Amniotic membrane transplantation for persistent epithelial defects with ulceration. Am J Ophthalmol 1997; 123: 303–12.

25. Murri MS, Moshirfar M, Birdsong OC, Ronquillo YC, Ding Y, Hoopes PC. Amniotic membrane extract and eye drops: a review of literature and clinical application. Clin Ophthalmol 2018; 12: 1105–12.

26. Ni J, Abrahamson M, Zhang M, et al. Cystatin E is a novel human cysteine proteinase inhibitor with structural resemblance to family Z cystatins. J Biol Chem 1997; 272: 10853e8.

27. Niknejad H, Peirovi H, Jorjani M, et al. Properties of the amniotic membrane for potential use in tissue engineering. Eur Cell Mater 2008; 15: 88e99.

28. Sangwan VS, Burman S, Tejwani S, et al. Amniotic membrane transplantation: A review of current indications in the management of ophthalmic disorders. Indian J Ophthalmol 2007; 55: 251e60.

29. Shimazaki J, Yang HY, Tsubota K. Amniotic membrane transplantation for ocular surface reconstruction in patients with chemical and thermal burns. Ophthalmology 1997; 104: 2068–76.

30. Shimmura S, Shimazaki J, Ohashi Y, Tsubota K. Anti-inflammatory effects of amniotic membrane transplantation in ocular surface disorders. Cornea 2001; 20: 408–13.

31. Tseng SC, Li DQ, Ma X. Suppression of transforming growth factor-beta isoforms, TGF-β receptor type II, and myofibroblast differentiation in cultured human corneal and limbal fibroblasts by amniotic membrane matrix. J Cell Physiol 1999; 179: 325–35.

32. Wolf H, Desoye G. Immunohistochemical localization of glucose transporters and insulin receptors in human fetal membranes at term. Histochemistry 1993; 100: 379–85.

33. Woo HM, Kim MS, Kweon OK. Effects of amniotic membrane on epithelial wound healing and stromal remodelling after excimer laser keratectomy in rabbit cornea. Br J Ophthalmol 2001; 85: 345–49.

Chapter

38

Management of Perforated Corneal Ulcer

Chapter Outline

INTRODUCTION
- Descemetocele
- Causes

CLINICAL PROFILE
- Symptoms
- Signs

TREATMENT MODALITIES
- Tissue adhesives/glue
- Patch graft
- Therapeutic keratoplasty
- Other modalities

INTRODUCTION

Infective corneal ulcer is one of the most common etiologies of corneal perforation followed closely by trauma. This may be due to direct microbial invasion of corneal stroma or from collagenases released by the leucocytes from host chemotaxis.

Descemetocele refers to a lesion where destruction and thinning of corneal stroma has lead to only Descemet's membrane (DM) and endothelium remaining for support (Fig. 38.1).

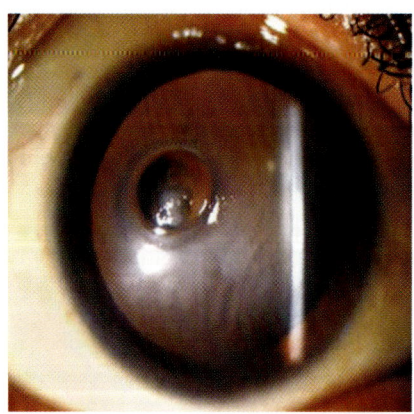

Fig. 38.1: *Large descemetocele in a case of viral keratitis*

It is as grave as a perforation and warrants urgent attention to preserve ocular integrity.

Causes of perforated corneal ulcer include:
- *Bacterial keratitis* is the most common cause of microbial keratitis leading to perforation.
- *Viral infections* may lead to corneal perforation during active recurrences or neurotrophic keratopathy.
- *Fungal keratitis,* albeit slowly progressive in nature, may still lead to perforation unless managed timely.

CLINICAL PROFILE

SYMPTOMS

Patients with corneal ulcers, after perforation, may complain of:

- *Sudden gush of fluid* or discharge from the eye and may experience slight decrease in pain.
- *Severe pain* secondary to haemorrhagic choroidal detachment from sudden decrease in intraocular pressure (IOP) may also occur.
- Sometimes patients may notice *autoeviscerated ocular contents* and may report relief of symptoms despite decreased visual acuity.

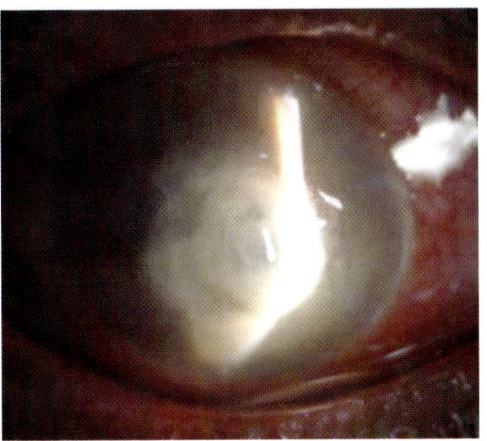

Fig. 38.2: *Flat anterior chamber and relatively clear central cornea seen in case of perforated corneal ulcer*

Note: At risk patients should be warned about these symptoms and given protective eyewear whenever feasible.

SIGNS

Clear central zone in presence of a large and dense surrounding infiltrate and sudden clearing of hypopyon should arise suspicion of a corneal perforation in eyes with microbial keratitis (Fig. 38.2).

Most commonly appreciated signs on slit-lamp examination are shallow or flat anterior chamber (AC), positive Seidel test, uveal tissue prolapse and hypotony.

Pluging of the defect sometime may occur by uveal tissue or pseudocornea leading to reformed AC, negative Seidel test and normal or raised IOP. A negative Seidel test may also be seen in completely flat AC, where aqueous production and outflow are hampered.

Fistula formation is common in centrally perforated ulcers.

Descemetocele, an impending perforation, may be diagnosed by presence of radiating folds in DM emanating from base of the ulcer.

■ TREATMENT MODALITIES

Various treatment modalities available for dealing with corneal perforations include tissue adhesives or lamellar patch grafting, lamellar or penetrating keratoplasty (PKP), sclerocorneal

patch, tarsorrhaphy and conjunctival flap depending on the size and response of perforation. The primary goals of therapy are to maintain the integrity of the globe and eradicate the infective process. A failure to do so will result in progression of the infection that will jeopardize the eye in both structure and function. Without therapeutic surgery, these eyes may become unsalvageable secondary to phthisis or endophthalmitis thereby requiring enucleation. The secondary aim of these therapeutic procedures is visual rehabilitation. In most of the conditions, the current practices and available options consider ambulatory vision as a satisfactory outcome and reasonable therapeutic benefit.

Various modalities available are discussed below.

TISSUE ADHESIVES/GLUE

Tissue adhesives also known as 'glue' are biocompatible compounds which have adhesive properties and can be used for repair of tissue defects by local application. They are minimally invasive, sutureless, and easy to use with no additional training or instructions required. In the field of ophthalmology, these substances help the surgeon secure ocular tissues or protect them from further damage. The two types of glue of commercially available ophthalmic purpose glues include cyanoacrylate glue (Fig. 38.3) and fibrin glue.

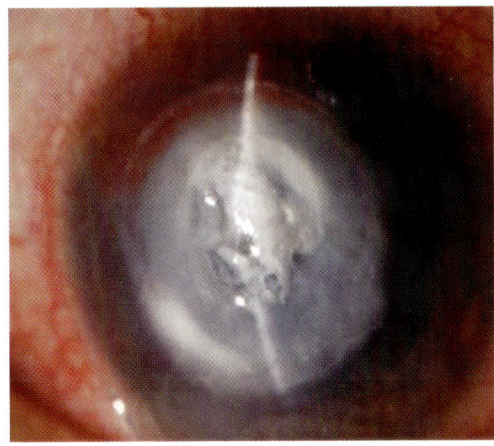

Fig. 38.3: *Cyanoacrylate glue applied in a case of perforated pseudomonas ulcer*

Cyanoacrylate glue

Cyanoacrylates belong to a family of strong fast-acting adhesives with industrial, medical, and household uses. These have a short shelf-life, if not used, about one year from manufacture, if unopened, one month once opened. They have some minor toxicity. The modified compound with reduced toxicity has been approved by US FDA for medical use. The cyanoacrylate has a property of immediate solidification when in touch with water. They exist in low viscosity liquid form in their packaging and become a hard solid when in contact with water containing body tissues. These compounds are cheap, easily available, have inherent bacterio-static property and can effectively seal smaller perforations (up to 3 mm in size). Method of application is described in Table 38.1. Ideally, the cyanoacrylate glue with the bandage contact lens should be left *in situ* until spontaneous sloughing occurs. Duration of glue adherence ranges from a few days to an average of more than 2 months.

Table 38.1: *Method of application of cyanoacrylate glue*

- Instill topical anaesthetic into affected eye
- Apply eyelid speculum
- Dry cornea with cotton bud or other similar absorbent
- Debride surrounding epithelium
- Form AC with air or viscoelastic whenever needed
- Place a small amount of cyanoacrylate glue onto a sterile plastic drape or the inside of sterile, glove wrapping paper and draw into a 30-gauge needle on a tuberculin syringe.
- Apply minimal quantity of glue directly onto the cornea
- Wait till the glue hardens
- Apply soft bandage contact lens for a smooth surface

Fibrin glue

Fibrin glue is composed of two components, namely fibrinogen (in lyophilized pooled human concentrate form) and thrombin (bovine). The enzymatic action facilitated by thrombin converts fibrinogen into fibrin monomers in a time frame of 10 to 60 seconds giving rise to a three-dimensional gel. This gives rise to a fibrin clot with good attachment to biological tissues. Method of application begins in a way similar to cyanoacrylate glue except that the two components are applied to the corneal defect individually using 27 G needle. The Duplojet injection system (supplied with Tissel glue, Baxter) can also be used for application. Although the glue sets in about 30 seconds, it is advisable to let the glue stabilise for several minutes before performing Seidel test and bandage contact lens application. Amniotic membrane can also be used concurrently for better sealing and scaffold.

Polyethylene glycol hydrogel

Polyethylene glycol hydrogel also known as PEG hydrogel is a different material from cyano-acrylate or fibrin glue. It comes as two separate materials, a polyethylene glycol solution and a trilysine amine solution, which, when mixed together by the user, form the sealant that can be applied with the aid of an applicator provided with the kit. The procedure is similar to the fibrin glue application. However, the solidification time is shorter requiring the mixing process to be done near the tissue to be sealed.

Use of cyanoacrylate glue requires removal of the glue at a later date which is a cumbersome task. However, the other two adhesives are biodegradable and are cleared by the enzymatic processes of the body. Cyanoacrylate glue is the choice when the procedure is done to cover the interval period up to a definitive corneal procedure.

PATCH GRAFT

A large corneal defect more than 3 mm in size not amenable to glue can be effectively sealed with patch graft. Corneal patch graft is indicated primarily in corneal perforations or desce-metocele which spare the central host cornea (Fig. 38.4). The donor tissue may be preserved in McCarey Kaufman or Optisol or glycerine in extreme circumstances. The tissues generally selected are those unsuitable for conventional keratoplasty with good graft clarity and healthy stroma. Use of a non-optical grade donor tissue and repair being performed on the peripheral region of the host cornea make patch grafts a

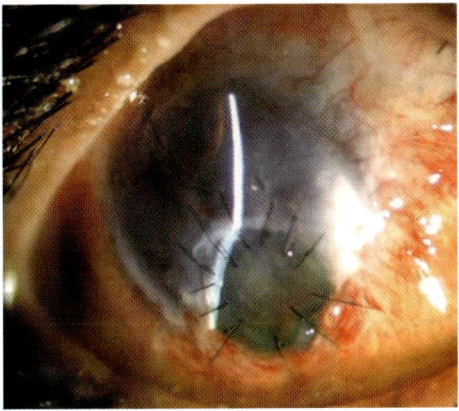

Fig. 38.4: *Peripheral corneal perforation managed by a corneal patch graft*

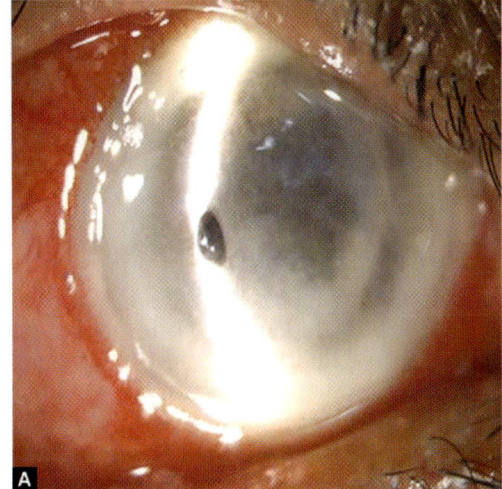

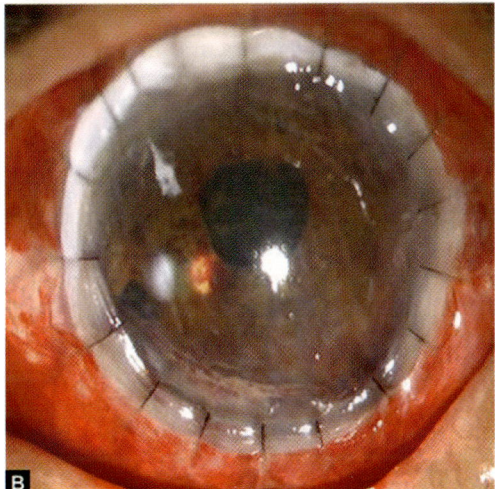

Fig. 38.5: *A, A case of large corneal perforation with surrounding infiltrate; B, Managed by a large therapeutic penetrating keratoplasty*

successful mode of management. This maintains the optical viability of the host cornea for longer duration with good scope of visual rehabilitation. However, the eccentricity of the repair itself subjects to a lot of shear forces causing larger degrees of astigmatism. Although the proximity to the host limbus increases the chances of graft rejection, a lesser amount of tissue transplanted compared to complete penetrating keratoplasty, nullifies the increased risk. About 80 to 85% achieve successful infection control with about 50% receiving an optical keratoplasty subsequently. The involved area of the host cornea is marked and the margins refreshed. The AC is washed and all exudative material removed. The patch graft is harvested from the donor tissue of the desired size with the alignment synchronous to the host tissue. The donor tissue is placed over the host and approximated with interrupted nylon 10–0 sutures. Recently, use of tissue adhesives has also been described for keeping patch grafts in place. This avoids various suture-related complications.

THERAPEUTIC KERATOPLASTY

Usually indicated for non-healing infectious corneal ulcers or perforated corneal ulcers more than 5 mm in size, therapeutic PKP form a major type of keratoplasty in developing countries (Fig. 38.5). If performed early with an optical grade corneal tissue, it may result in an excellent visual outcome, however, there exists larger

chances of rejection, re-infection and failure. The decision of therapeutic keratoplasty should be taken and executed before the peripheral host cornea is involved by the infectious agent. This gives a better margin for application of sutures. In eyes where the infectious process has involved the limbus circumferentially, the chances of visual recovery is reserved. Non-optical grade tissue may also be used in emergency situations. The size of the graft should be large enough to incorporate the corneal defect and the ulcer margin with the infiltrates. Donor button is recommended to be oversized by 01 mm to keep the AC formed and account for the oedema of the host cornea and sutured in place with 16 interrupted 10–0 monofilament nylon sutures. Continuous suture increases the chance of wound dehiscence after the oedema subsides and make the suture replacement difficult.

OTHER MODALITIES

Amniotic membrane grafting and tarsorrhaphy are contraindicated in active infection and, therefore, play a little role in emergency management of perforated corneal ulcers. However, these form useful methods of salvaging eyeball in persistent epithelial defect or neurotrophic phase of microbial keratitis. Conjunctival flaps provide no corneal support and are more prophylactic than therapeutic in management of perforated corneal ulcers.

CONCLUSION

A corneal perforation resulting from an infectious cause is an emergency threatening the integrity of the globe. The surgeon is expected to respond with the quickest modality possible. The clinical decision of the modality is made with due consideration of the possibility of visual rehabilitation on a later date and all ophthalmic surgeons should be well-versed with the different options available for this condition.

BIBLIOGRAPHY

1. Balabanov C, Murgova S, Parashkevova B. Treatment of perforated infectious corneal ulcers with penetrating 2007; 13: 35–39.
2. Boujemaa C, Souissi K, Daghfous F, Marrakchi S, Jeddi A, Ayed S. [Urgent penetrating keratoplasty in perforated infectious corneal ulcers.] J Fr Ophtalmol [Internet]. 2005 Mar [cited 2017 Feb 22]; 28(3): 267–72. Available from: http://www.ncbi.nlm.nih.gov/pubmed/15883491.
3. Carley FM. Double drape tectonic patch with cyanoacrylate glue in the management of corneal perforation with iris incarceration. 2013; 32(5): 137–38.
4. Chenault HK, Bhatia SK, DiMaio WG, Vincent GL, Camacho W, Behrens A. Sealing and healing of clear corneal incisions with an improved dextran aldehyde-PEG amine tissue adhesive. Curr Eye Res [Internet]. 2011 Nov 14 [cited 2017 Feb 22]; 36(11): 997–1004. Available from: http://www.ncbi.nlm.nih.gov/pubmed/21999226.
5. Degoricija L, Johnson CS, Wathier M, Kim T, Grinstaff MW. Photo cross-linkable bio-dendrimers as ophthalmic adhesives for central lacerations and penetrating keratoplasties. Investig Opthalmology Vis Sci [Internet]. 2007 May 1 [cited 2017 Feb 22]; 48(5): 2037. Available from: http://www.ncbi.nlm.nih.gov/pubmed/17460258.
6. Duchesne B, Tahi H, Galand A. Use of human fibrin glue and amniotic membrane transplant in corneal perforation. Cornea [Internet]. 2001 Mar [cited 2017 Feb 22]; 20(2): 230–32. Available from: http://www.ncbi.nlm.nih.gov/pubmed/11248838.
7. Hirst LW, Smiddy WE, De Juan E. Tissue adhesive therapy for corneal perforations. Aust J Ophthalmol [Internet]. 1983 May [cited 2017 Feb 22]; 11(2): 113–18.
8. Huang T, Wang Y, Ji J, Gao N, Chen J. Evaluation of different types of lamellar keratoplasty for treatment of peripheral corneal perforation. Graefe's Arch Clin Exp Ophthalmol [Internet]. 2008 Aug 30 [cited 2017 Feb 22]; 246(8): 1123–31. Available from: http://www. ncbi.nlm.nih.gov/pubmed/18446359.
9. Jhanji V, Young AL, Mehta JS, Sharma N, Agarwal T, Vajpayee RB. Management of Corneal Perforation. Surv Ophthalmol [Internet]. 2011; 56(6): 522–38. Available from: http://dx.doi.org/10.1016/j.survophthal. 2011.06.003.
10. Letko E, Stechschulte SU, Kenyon KR, Sadeq N, Romero TR, Samson CM, et al. Amniotic membrane inlay and overlay grafting for corneal epithelial defects and stromal ulcers. Arch Ophthalmol (Chicago, Ill 1960) [Internet]. 2001 May [cited 2017 Feb 22]; 119(5): 659–63. Available from: http://www.ncbi.nlm.nih.gov/pubmed/11346392.
11. Oelker AM, Berlin JA, Wathier M, Grinstaff MW. Synthesis and characterization of dendron cross-linked PEG hydrogels as corneal adhesives. Biomacromolecules [Internet]. 2011 May 9 [cited 2017 Feb 22]; 12(5): 1658–65. Available from: http://www.ncbi.nlm.nih.gov/pubmed/21417379.
12. Portnoy SL, Insler MS, Kaufman HE. Surgical management of corneal ulceration and perforation. Surv Ophthalmol [Internet]. [cited 2017 Feb22]; 34(1): 47–58. Available from: http://www.ncbi.nlm.nih.gov/pubmed/2678553

13. Sony P, Sharma N, Vajpayee RB, Ray M. Therapeutic keratoplasty for infectious keratitis: a review of the literature. CLAO J [Internet]. 2002 Jul [cited 2017 Feb 22]; 28(3): 111–18. Available from: http://www.ncbi.nlm.nih.gov/pubmed/12144228.

14. Sukhija J, Jain AK. Outcome of therapeutic penetrating keratoplasty in infectious keratitis. Ophthalmic Surg Lasers Imaging [Internet]. [cited 2017 Feb 22]; 36(4): 303–09. Available from: http://www.ncbi.nlm.nih.gov/pubmed/16156147.

15. Villa-Camacho JC, Ghobril C, Anez-Bustillos L, Grinstaff MW, Rodríguez EK, Nazarian A. The efficacy of a lysine-based dendritic hydrogel does not differ from those of commercially available tissue sealants and adhesives: an *ex vivo* study. BMC Musculoskelet Disord [Internet]. 2015 Dec 13 [cited 2017 Feb 22]; 16(1): 116. Available from: http://www.ncbi.nlm.nih.gov/pubmed/25968126.

16. Vote BJ, Elder MJ. Cyanoacrylate glue for corneal perforations: A description of a surgical technique and a review of the literature. Clin Experiment Ophthalmol [Internet]. 2000 Dec [cited 2017 Feb 22]; 28(6): 437–42. Available from: http://www.ncbi.nlm.nih.gov/pubmed/11202468.

17. Weiss JL, Williams P, Lindstrom RL, Doughman DJ. The use of tissue adhesive in corneal perforations. Ophthalmology [Internet]. 1983 Jun [cited 2017 Feb 22]; 90(6): 610-15. Available from: http://www.ncbi.nlm.nih.gov/pubmed/6888854.

Chapter

39

Keratoplasty

GENERAL CONSIDERATIONS

DEFINITION

Keratoplasty, also called corneal grafting or corneal transplantation, is an operation in which the patient's diseased cornea is replaced by the healthy clear cornea. Broadly, keratoplasty can be classified as follows:

A. Autokeratoplasty which can be:

1. *Rotational autokeratoplasty*, in which patient's own cornea is trephined and rotated to transfer the pupillary area having a small corneal opacity to the periphery.

2. *Contralateral autokeratoplasty*, in which diseased cornea of one eye of the patient with potential vision is exchanged with the normal clear cornea of the second eye (which is blind due to some posterior segment disease, e.g. optic atrophy, old case of central retinal artery occlusion, etc.).

B. Allografting or allokeratoplasty, in which patient's diseased cornea is replaced by the donor's healthy cornea. It can be broadly divided into penetrating keratoplasty and lamellar keratoplasty and small patch graft.

CORNEA AND IMMUNE SYSTEM

Corneal allograft is one of the most successful forms of solid organ transplantation. Normally, HLA typing and systemic immunosuppressive drugs are not utilized, yet 90% of corneal allografts survive.[1,2] The better acceptance of corneal allografts compared to other categories of allografts is due to the unique immunological property of cornea, coined by Medawar as immune privilege. This immune privilege is abolished in conditions such as inflammation, neovascularization, or trauma to cornea.

Mechanisms of immune privilege

Immune privilege of corneal allografts is sustained by one or more of the following: (1) blocking the induction of immune responses; (2) deviating immune responses down a tolerogenic pathway; or (3) blockade of immune effector elements.[1,2]

1. Blocking the Induction of Immune Responses. The most widely accepted explanation for corneal allograft survival is the absence of blood and lymph vessels in the non-inflamed cornea and graft bed. Earlier the concept was that absence of blood vessels is more important for immune privilege. However, recent study suggests that absence of lymph vessels is primarily responsible for immune privilege. It has recently been reported that corneal epithelial and stromal cells secrete a soluble form of vascular endothelial growth factor (VEGF) receptor 2 (VEGFR-2), which blocks and inhibits lymphangiogenesis in the cornea.[3]

2. Role of Immune Deviation and T Regulatory Cells. Antigens introduced into the anterior chamber (AC) induce a unique spectrum of systemic immune responses that are characterized by the antigen-specific suppression of delayed-type hypersensitivity responses and the preferential production of non-complement-fixing antibody isotypes (i.e. IgG1) and the exclusion of complement-fixing antibodies.[1,2,4] This form of immune deviation is termed anterior chamber-associated immune deviation (ACAID). After surgery, corneal endothelial cells are sloughed from corneal allografts and enter the AC, where they induce ACAID. The aqueous humor also contains numerous anti-inflammatory and immunosuppressive molecules, in turn, suppresses alloimmune responses and promotes corneal allograft survival.

3. Blockade of Immune Effector Elements. The cornea expresses a number of cell membrane-bound molecules that neutralize immune response. FasL (CD95L) is expressed on the cell membranes on many cells within the eye, including the corneal endothelium, and induces apoptosis of neutrophils and lymphocytes that encounter the cornea during inflammation. Programmed death ligand-1 (PD-L1) is expressed on the cornea and when it engages its receptor (PD-1) on lymphocytes, it inhibits T-lymphocyte proliferation, induces T-lymphocyte apoptosis, and prevents T-lymphocyte production of interferon-γ (IFN-γ). Tumor necrosis factor-related apoptosis-inducing ligand (TRAIL) is expressed on the corneal endothelium and induces apoptosis of activated T cells expressing its receptor (TRAIL-R2). Cell membrane-bound complement regulatory proteins (CRP) expressed on corneal epithelial cells and the soluble CRP present in the aqueous humor buffers the capacity of complement-fixing antibodies to produce corneal allograft rejection. Macrophage migration inhibitory factor (MIF) and transforming growth factor-β (TGF-β) are present in the aqueous humor at concentrations that are known to produce profound inhibition of NK cell-mediated cytolysis.

Thus, the cornea and the underlying aqueous humor have the capacity to not only block, but also eliminate immune effector elements from both the adaptive and innate immune systems. This "sword and shield" strategy provides immune privilege to the corneal allograft.

Loss of immune privilege

The corneal immune privilege is lost or compromised following certain events or in certain conditions leading to an increased risk of graft rejection.[1,2] These are described below.

1. Post-transplant Local Events: These events are a loose suture, suture associated infection, or herpetic infection recurrence. These lead to recruitment of alloreactive cells, angiogenesis, lymphangiogenesis, and up-regulation of MHC molecules on the graft cells.

2. Vascularization of the Graft Recipient Bed: Corneal vascularization due to any cause such as keratitis, trauma or surgery lead to loss of immune privilege.

3. Rejected Previous Transplant: Whether corneal allograft rejection is accompanied by vascularization or not, there is heightened risk of rejection of a subsequent allograft.

4. Inflammation at the Time of Transplant: A high antigen presenting cells (APC) count is seen in excised recipient cornea in inflamed eyes.

Cornea transplantation is avoided in actively inflamed eyes and every attempt is made to obtain the best possible control of corneal inflammation before transplantation.

5. Atopy: Perioperative or sustained local conjunctival or corneal inflammation can increase the allograft rejection risk by breaching the immune privilege.

EYE BANKING AND DONOR CORNEA

Eye banks retrieve and store eyes for cornea transplants and research. The first Eye Bank in India was established in Madras in 1945. Donor corneas are retrieved through two modalities of eye donation, which are voluntary eye donation (VED) and hospital corneal retrieval program (HCRP). In VED, the family member of the deceased informs the eye bank and the eye bank staff registers the details. Once the details are registered, the eye bank team headed by the doctor reaches the destined place to retrieve the eye. In HCRP, eye donation counselor (EDC) also called grief counselors are stationed in the hospital premises to motivate the family member of the deceased and to enlighten them about the importance of eye donation.

A team consisting of the doctor assisted by the technician retrieves the corneo-scleral button and transfers it to cornea preservation media (e.g. McKarey-Kaufman or Optisol). Blood sample of 5 ml is taken from the jugular or femoral vein for serological testing. The donor eye is treated with 5% betadine (povidone iodine) and with antibiotic. Thereafter the post-antibiotic corneal swabs are taken and sent for bacterial and fungal culture in the transport media.

Biomicroscopic examination of donor tissue is done on a slit lamp (Fig. 39.1). The endothelium cell count is done using Konan KSS-EB10 specular microscope (Fig. 39.2). There are different grading systems for donor cornea tissue. *Cornea Donor Study grading system* is the most commonly followed system worldwide.

Note: Details about eyebanking and donor cornea are described in Section VIII.

TYPES OF CORNEAL TRANSPLANTATION

Corneal transplantation procedures can be classified in two ways: (A) depending upon the

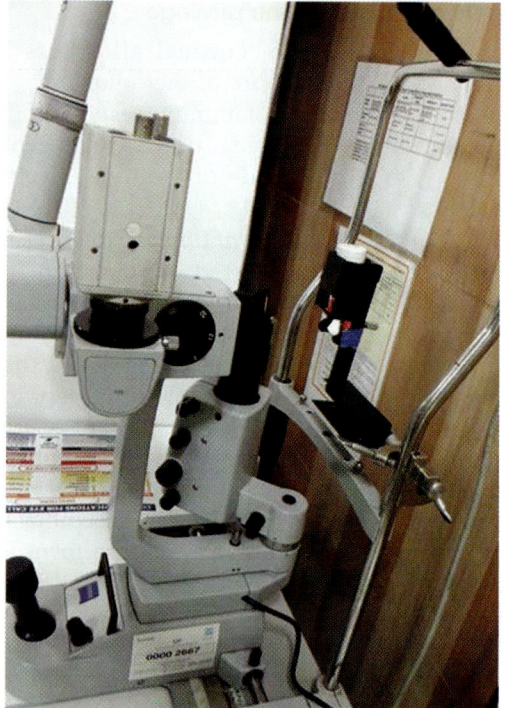

Fig. 39.1: *Donor tissue evaluation on slit lamp*

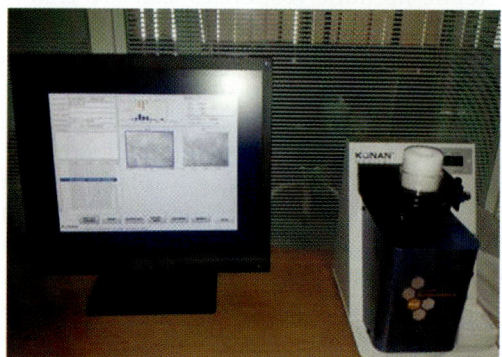

Fig. 39.2: *Konan KSS-EB10 specular microscope*

indication for which it is done and (B) depending upon the surgical technique[5, 6] (Table 39.1).

A. Depending upon the indication

i. *Optical keratoplasty* (Fig. 39.3A): In this, the keratoplasty is performed for visual rehabilitation.

ii. *Therapeutic keratoplasty* (Fig. 39.3B): In this keratoplasty is performed for treatment of an underlying disease and the primary aim is to achieve the cure but never the visual

Table 39.1: *Types of keratoplasty*

1. **Lamellar keratoplasty** (optical, therapeutic, tectonic indications)
    i. *Anterior lamellar keratoplasty*
        • *Superficial anterior lamellar keratoplasty (SALK)*—dissection depth less than 160 µm.
        • *Deep anterior lamellar keratoplasty (DALK)*—dissection depth more than 160 µm: Manual layer by layer, air assisted (big bubble, double bubble), viscoelastic assisted, diamond blade assisted, femtosecond assisted.
    ii. *Posterior lamellar keratoplasty*
        • *Descemet stripping endothelial keratoplasty (DSEK)/Descemet stripping automated endothelial keratoplasty (DSAEK).*
        • *Descemet membrane endothelial keratoplasty (DMEK).*
2. **Penetrating keratoplasty** (optical, therapeutic, tectonic indications)

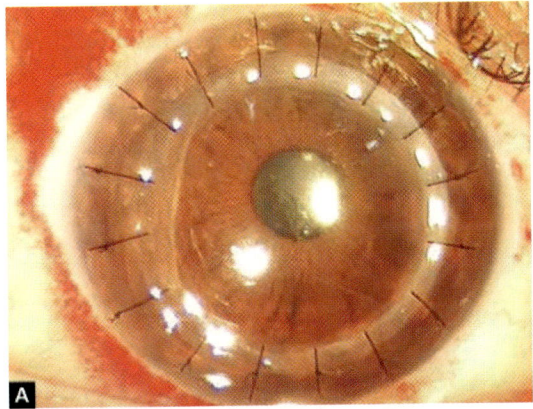

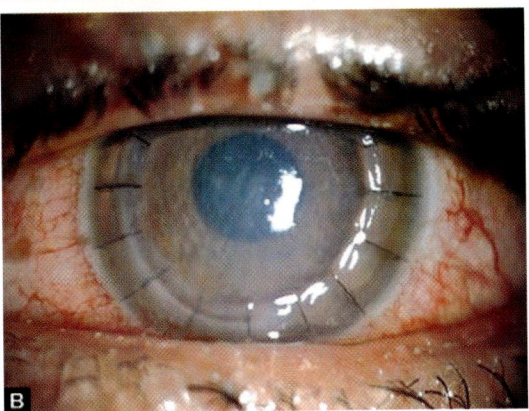

Fig. 39.3: *Postoperative appearance after penetrating keratoplasty. A, Optical; B, Therapeutic*

improvement. Example includes keratoplasty for control of infection in cases of infective corneal ulcers.

iii. *Tectonic keratoplasty:* In this keratoplasty is performed to enhance corneal strength, e.g. crescentic lamellar keratoplasty performed for advanced cases of pellucid marginal degeneration.

B. Depending upon the technique (Fig. 39.4)

1. **Penetrating keratoplasty:** In this, a full thickness graft replaces the host cornea.
2. **Lamellar keratoplasty:** In this, only a part of donor corneal is transplanted instead of the full thickness graft. It can be classified into two broad categories
    a. *Anterior lamellar keratoplasty:* This includes all the procedure where Descemet membrane-endothelial layer and/or a part of posterior corneal stroma of the host cornea are spared. This includes the following procedures:
        i. *Superficial anterior lamellar keratoplasty,* where epithelium-basement membrane and a part of anterior stroma are replaced.
        ii. *Deep anterior lamellar keratoplasty (DALK),* where the donor cornea up to deeper stroma or up to Descemet membrane is replaced.
    b. *Posterior lamellar keratoplasty:* This includes all procedure where Descemet-endothelial layer with or without a part of deeper stroma is replaced. It includes the following techniques:
        i. *Descemet stripping endothelial keratoplasty (DSEK),* wherein Descemet-endothelium complex along with a part of deeper stroma of variable thickness is transplanted and the graft preparation is done manually.
        ii. *Descemet stripping automated endothelial keratoplasty (DSAEK):* It is similar to DSEK, the difference being use of a microkeratome for donor preparation.
        iii. *Descemet membrane endothelial keratoplasty (DMEK):* In this technique, only descemet-endothelium complex is transplanted without any stroma.

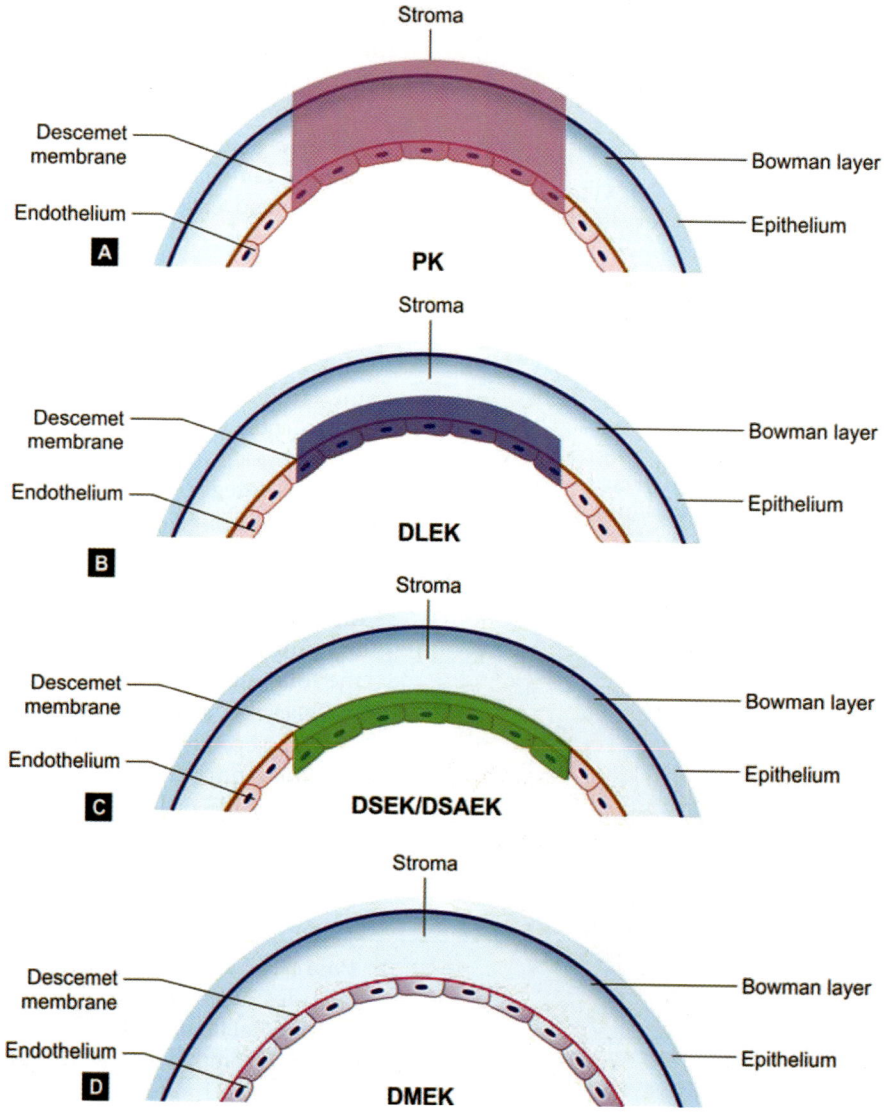

Fig. 39.4: *Different surgical techniques of keratoplasty. A, Penetrating keratoplasty (PKP); B, Anterior lamellar keratoplasty (ALK); C, Deep anterior lamellar keratoplasty (DLK); D, Endothelial keratoplasty*

iv. *Hybrid techniques*, which consist of a combination of two or more techniques, e.g. central DMEK and peripheral DSAEK.

LAMELLAR KERATOPLASTY

Lamellar keratoplasty (LK) is the partial replacement of host cornea with lamella of a healthy donor cornea.[6–8] The differences between LK and PKP are summarized in Table 39.2. LK can be divided into two types depending upon the level of replacement of diseased cornea, i.e. anterior lamellar keratoplasty (ALK) and posterior lamellar keratoplasty (PLK).

PREOPERATIVE INVESTIGATIONS

The following investigations (Table 39.3) are done before proceeding for lamellar keratoplasty.

I. Visual potential assessment: Preoperative evaluation of visual potential is important before

Table 39.2: *Differences between lamellar and penetrating keratoplasty*

Characteristics	Lamellar keratoplasty	Penetrating keratoplasty
Level of transplant	Lamellar	Full thickness
Risk associated with open globe procedures (e.g. expulsive haemorrhage)	No risk	Risk present
Wound strength	Weak	Stronger
Suture removal	Early	Delayed
Duration of topical steroid use	Short duration	Prolonged duration
Postoperative astigmatism	Less	More
Risk of endothelial rejection	No risk (except in DSAEK)	Risk present
Risk of interface haze	Present	No risk
Chances of getting 6/6 vision	Less chances as compared to PK	More chances as compared to LK
Use of single cornea in multiple cases	Possible	Not possible
Risk of intraocular complication	No risk (except DSAEK)	Risk present
Visual outcome	Inferior than PK	Better than LK

Table 39.3: *Preoperative work up for lamellar surgeries*

Visual potential assessment	Refraction and BCVA with contact lens
	Laser interferometer (LI)
	Potential acuity meter (PAM)
	Visually evoked response (VER)
Ocular surface evaluation	Tear break up time (TBUT)
	Schirmer test
Endothelium assessment	Specular microscopy
Posterior segment evaluation	Ophthalmoscopy
	Ultrasonography
Corneal topography and pachymetry	
	ASOCT
	Ultrasonic videokeratography
	Orbscan
	Pentacam

proceeding for surgery. This is important in decision making as well as explaining the prognosis to the patient.

a. *Refraction and contact lens corrected visual acuity:* Best corrected visual acuity with spectacles or with contact lenses often can give an idea about the visual potential, especially in case of keratoconus. However, in presence of corneal opacity these are not reliable.

b. *Laser interferometer (LI):* It uses the coherent white light or helium neon generated inter-ference stripes or fringes projected on retina through some clearer portion within the corneal opacity. The ability of the patient to identify the orientation of fringes gives an idea about the visual potential.

c. *Potential acuity meter (PAM):* PAM is a simple visual test where a tiny beam of light is directed through the patient's pupil onto the retina. This light beam actually contains a visual acuity chart with letters for the patient to read.

d. *Visually evoked response (VER):* VER measures the electrical potential generated in response to visual stimulus. It represents the integrity of visual pathway from retina to occipital lobe, but it cannot differentiate between macula, optic nerve, occipital lobe pathology. The amplitude and latency of the visual stimulus is recorded. Decreases in amplitude or increases latency of stimulus suggest the poor visual potential. VER is an invaluable tool in visual potential assessment of pediatric patients.

II. Ocular surface evaluation: Evaluation of ocular surface is essential before LK. Tear break up time (TBUT) and Schirmer test are usually done to assess the tear film status. A poor ocular surface or presence of dry eye predisposes to postoperative persistent epithelial defect. Hence, ocular surface must be stabilised before proceeding for LK.

III. Endothelial function: Normal functioning endothelium is a must for any anterior lamellar graft. Specular microscopy is used for evaluation of endothelial function.

IV. Anterior segment optical coherence tomography (ASOCT): ASOCT is a new imaging system that gives high-resolution cross-sectional images of the cornea and anterior chamber. ASOCT is an invaluable tool before proceeding for anterior LK. It provides a number of useful information such as level of the scarring, location and depth of lesion in the cornea, corneal thickness, and anterior chamber details (Fig. 39.5).

V. Ultrasonography (USG): The role ultrasonography (USG) is important in cases where posterior segment visualization is difficult. USG can help to rule out condition like retinal detachment, vitreous haemorrhage, or glaucomatous optic atrophy.

VI. Pachymetry: Corneal thickness can be measured with ultrasonic pachymeter or instruments based on optical principle such as Orbscan, Pentacam and specular microscopy. While ultrasonic method is the gold standard, pentacam provides the most accurate values. Corneal thickness has got both diagnostic and therapeutic values. Prior to any LK it provides the surgeon the most important information of thinnest point on the cornea. Pachymetry also helps in deciding the surgical procedure especially in cases of keratoconus. For example, when corneal thickness is >350 μm in a case of keratoconus anterior lamellar therapeutic keratoplasty (ALTK) is planned while thickness >250 μm warrants DALK and <250 μm warrants a manual LK.

VII. Corneal topography: Videokeratography, Orbscan, or Pentacam can be used for corneal topography. Corneal topography is useful in diagnosis of diseases such as keratoconus. The purpose of topography before proceeding for surgery is to identify the areas of maximum steepness and thinnest location. These areas are to be taken care of, while performing lamellar dissection as these are the areas where chances of corneal perforation is maximum.

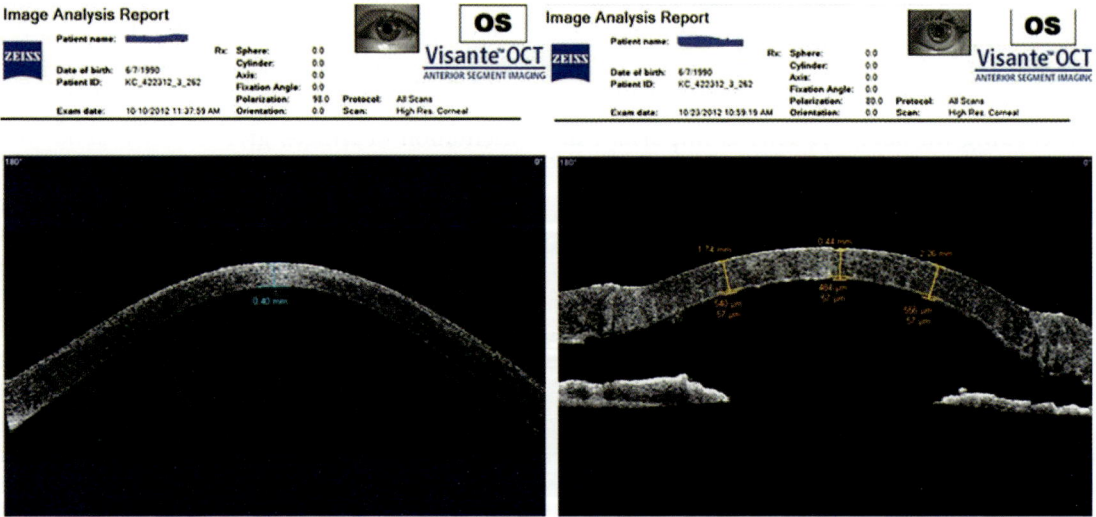

Fig. 39.5: *Pre- and postoperative ASOCT picture of a patient with keratoconus who underwent DALK*

◼ ANTERIOR LAMELLAR KERATOPLASTY (ALK)

Anterior lamellar surgery can be further sub-classified into two procedures: Superficial anterior lamellar keratoplasty (SALK), with dissection depth less than one-third or 160 µm and deep anterior lamellar keratoplasty (DALK), with a dissection depth greater than one-third or 160 µm.[7] ALTK is a type of ALK where both donor and host lamellar dissection is carried out with the help of a microkeratome and it can be used for corneal opacities extending up to 250 µm depth.[8,9]

INDICATIONS AND CONTRAINDICATIONS OF ALK

Indications for ALK

i. For visual rehabilitation. Various conditions involving superficial corneal stroma causing decreased vision are ideal candidates for ALK, provided endothelium of involved cornea is still healthy and functioning. Following are such conditions.

a. *Ectatic disorders:* Keratoconus (Fig. 39.6A), keratoglobus (Fig. 39.6B), pellucid marginal degeneration, Terrien's marginal degeneration, post-LASIK ectasias.

b. *Superficial corneal scar* of various etiologies such as post-trauma, corneal ulcer, post-surgical injury, post-chemical injury.

c. *Corneal dystrophies* where corneal endothelium is not affected like epithelial basement membrane dystrophy, Reis-Bücklers' dystrophies, map-dot fingerprint dystrophy with recurrent erosions, and stromal dystrophies.

d. *Degenerations* like Salzmann's nodular degeneration, spheroidal degeneration, band-shaped keratopathy (Fig. 39.7).

e. *Ocular surface diseases:* ALK has also been described in various ocular surface disorders such as Stevens-Johnson syndrome, ocular cicatricial pemphigoid, chemical/thermal burns and vernal keratoconjunctivitis (VKC) with stromal opacity.

ii. Therapeutic indication: Another emerging indication for DALK is infectious keratitis where infectious process has not progressed beyond DM or descematocele. Its use has been described in advanced cases of bacterial, fungal, or

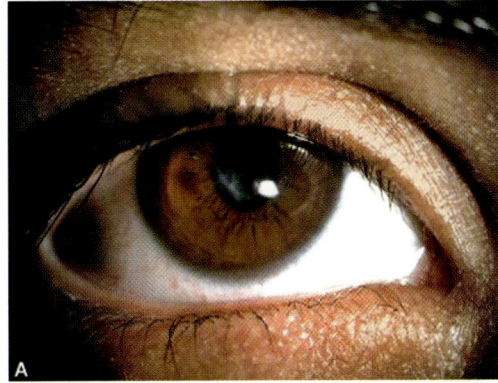
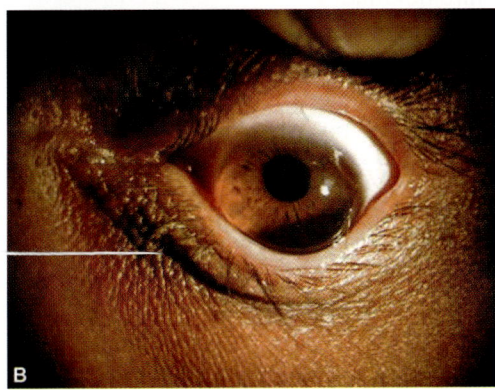

Fig. 39.6: *Ectatic disorders. A, Advanced keratoconus with corneal scarring; B, Keratoglobus*

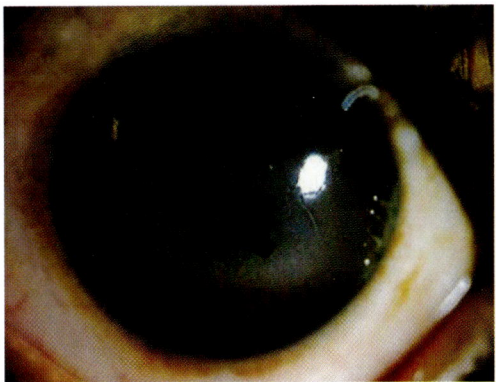

Fig. 39.7: *Band-shaped keratopathy*

Acanthamoeba keratitis, non-perforated microsporidial, post-LASIK mycobacterial and gonococcal keratitis.[8]

iii. Surgical complications like post-LASIK ectasia, persistent folds in the LASIK flap, intracorneal ring segment complications.

iv. Tectonic support: To provide the strength to the globe using corneal patch graft. The size of the patch is taken according to the size of corneal defect. Various lesions like:

- Descemetocele
- Pellucid marginal degeneration and Terrien's marginal degeneration
- Peripheral corneal ulcers related to auto-immune disorders
- Following dermoid and some tumors excision
- Perforations repairs

Contraindications

ALK is contraindicated in all corneal condition which have unhealthy endothelium. Also pre-existing Descemet's membrane tear is contra-indication for the ALK.

SUPERFICIAL ANTERIOR LAMELLAR KERATOPLASTY (SALK)

In procedures like SALK, microkeratome such as the Moria ALTK system is used. Diseases where superficial anterior lamellar keratoplasty can be useful include those characterised by superficial irregular opacities such as Reis-Bücklers, granular, and lattice corneal dystrophies. Use of SALK in such cases helps in replacement of the anterior cornea with a smooth donor tissue, improve vision and reducing the recurrent erosions that may be associated with these conditions. In cases of the recurrence of dystrophy in the graft replacement of superficial graft is possible easily. Superficial scars that are depressed, however, are not amenable to this technique because the microkeratome cut follows the surface profile and would lead to the same defect on the stromal bed. These cases are best treated with the technique described for DALK.

Technique

This procedure is two stages procedure. In the stage one, preoperative pachymetry is done. It is important to have a minimum corneal thickness of 400 µm. A large, hinged 160 µm flap is made (using the Moria ALTK system), and repositioned similar to a conventional LASIK procedure. In the second stage, at least 6 weeks later, under topical anaesthesia, a vacuum trephine is used to make a partial-thickness cut

through the LASIK-style flap, 7.5 to 8.5 mm in diameter, ideally leaving a 1 mm flap rim. The trephined flap is easily peeled away from the patient. It is then replaced by a same-sized donor tissue that is created using the Moria ALTK system with a 130 µm microkeratome head (initially completely excising a donor cap, and then cutting the cap with a trephine). The donor cap is placed on the recipient bed, without suturing, and a bandage contact lens is applied. Intraoperative keratometry can help in the positioning of the donor tissue to reduce post-operative astigmatism. These grafts clear almost immediately, but, as with penetrating kerato-plasty, irregular astigmatism may limit best-corrected acuity.

Sutureless Femtosecond Laser-assisted Anterior Lamellar Keratoplasty (FALK) is another technique of SALK. Anterior segment OCT (ASOCT) is used for assessing the depth of corneal involvement. The lamellar cut in the recipient with donor corneas is made using femtosecond laser. Donor cornea is cut according to the depth of the lesions with an additional 10–20% thickness. This extra thickness is to compensate for donor tissue swelling. The scarring in recipients corneal tissue is removed and replaced with the corneal donor lenticule. The incision is dried, and flap adhesion is checked. A bandage soft contact lens is placed over the cornea.

DEEP ANTERIOR LAMELLAR KERATOPLASTY (DALK)

DALK is a surgical procedure that involves removing the corneal stroma down to Descemet's membrane and replacing it with a donor cornea, with or without the Descemet membrane. DALK can be performed in virtually all cases of anterior cornea pathology (epithelium, Bowman's layer and stroma) that do not involve the corneal endothelium. Although different surgical techniques vary in their details, the basic surgery consists of the following steps.

Recipient eye preparation

The goal of DALK is to achieve a depth of dissection as close as possible to DM. Various agents have been used to create a plane of separation between DM and the deep stromal layers. These include air, fluid, viscoelastic, microkeratome and a femtosecond laser.[8]

Common techniques of DALK are described below (Fig. 39.8).

1. Layer by layer manual dissection

This is one of the earliest techniques described. This is a very useful technique in cases such as keratoconus with scar due to previous corneal hydrops, advanced keratoconus, presence of deep stromal scarring, or in presence of extreme thinning. In this technique, after an initial partial trephination of variable depth ranging from 50–70% of corneal thickness, the stroma is removed using either a crescent knife or various types of lamellar dissectors by layer by layer stromal removal. The major limitations of this technique are poor visual outcome due to residual stroma and interface haze. In addition, it is a very time consuming process.[8]

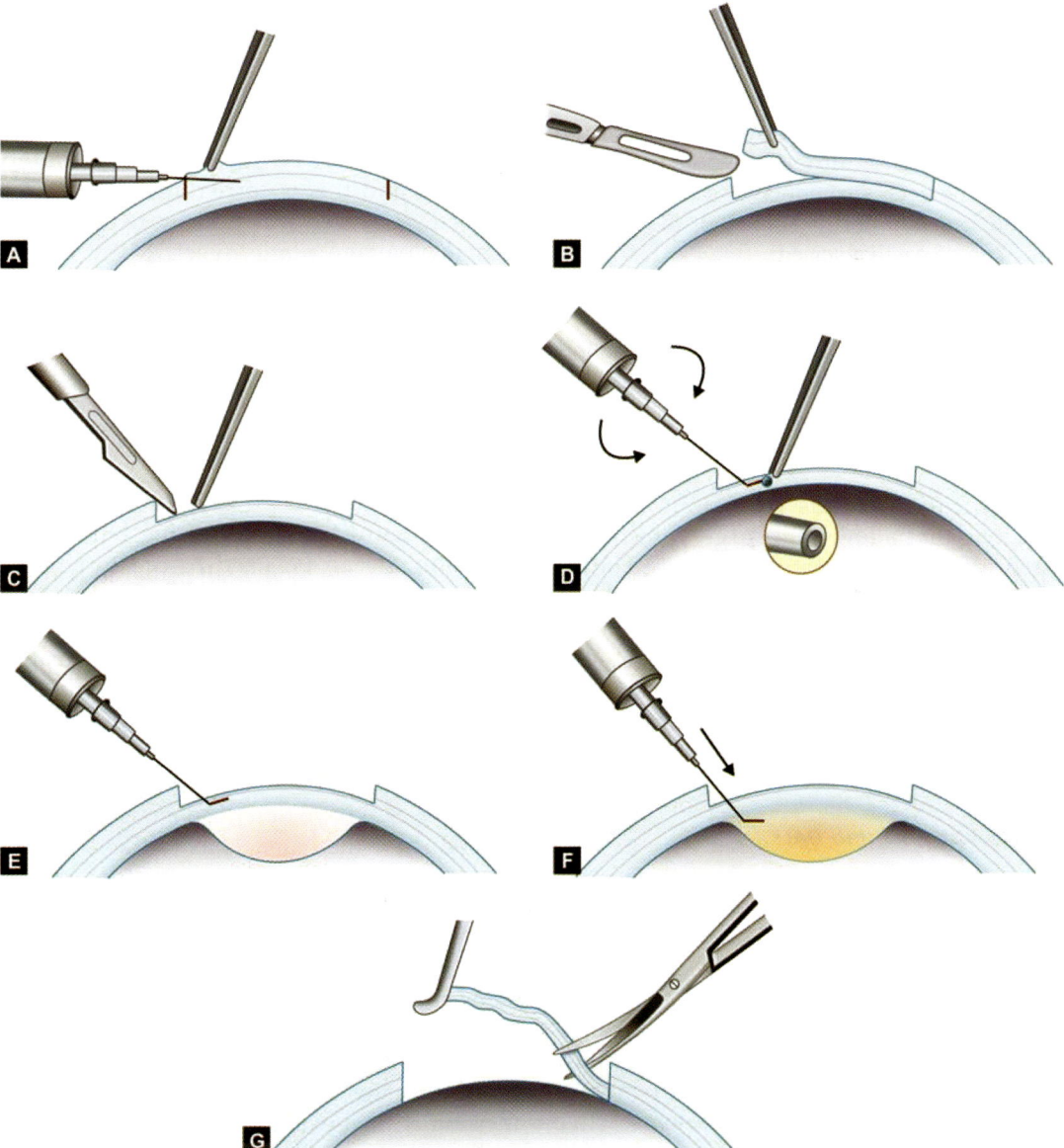

Fig. 39.8A to G: *Surgical technique of deep anterior lamellar keratoplasty*

2. Air-assisted DALK

Air-assisted lamellar keratoplasty involves injection of air into the corneal stroma that helps to achieve dissection as close as possible to DM. Archila first described the technique of air assisted deep lamellar keratoplasty.[10,11] Over a period, many modifications of air-assisted DALK were tried. The big-bubble technique, by Anwar and Teichmann in 2002, became popular and it continues to be the most widely used technique of DALK.

Big bubble DALK. The basic step of this technique involves injecting air into the corneal stroma deep into a groove, which is created by trephining 60 to 80 percent of the stromal thickness. The air infiltrates the potential space between the deep stromal layer and DM. Once a plane of separation is achieved, the stromal tissue can be easily excised.

The main advantage of this technique is that the quality of vision achieved is as good as PK. However, the learning curve associated with this technique is very steep. Inadvertent DM perforation can occur at any stage of the surgery. This often requires the surgeon to convert to PK.[6,8]

A modification to this is 'Double Bubble' technique that allows the surgeon to immediately identify the formation of an adequate big bubble.[12] In this technique, air is injected into the anterior chamber before it is injected into the stroma to achieve big bubble formation. A shift of the bubble in the anterior chamber into the periphery acts as an indicator of successful DM separation by a mechanism similar to small bubble technique.[6,8]

3. Viscoelastic-assisted DALK

Melles et al described a technique that uses a viscoelastic injection rather than air to achieve a cleavage plane between DM from stroma.[13,14] In this technique, the anterior chamber is completely filled with air. An initial stromal pocket is created with the depth of stromal dissection guided by the "air to endothelium" interface, which is seen by a specular light reex localized at the tip of the blade. The non-reactive dark band between the blade tip and the light reex represents the non-incised corneal tissue,

which becomes thinner with advancement of the blade into the deeper stromal layers. Thus, the corneal depth of the blade could be judged from the thickness of the dark band. A viscoelastic injection is injected through the scleral incision into the stromal pocket. Once the plane is achieved, the superficial stroma is removed using trephine and lamellar dissection.

4. Hydrodelamination

In this technique, saline solution is injected into the cornea, which enhances the identification and removal of the deep stromal fibres. The solution penetrates between the collagen bars, which whiten and swell. Stroma that was not apparent will swell up and can be safely removed and this is carried out until DM is reached. However, it is difficult to achieve an actual cleavage plane over DM by hydro-delamination.

5. Femtosecond-assisted DALK

The femtosecond laser computer-guided cuts allow precise, accurate and reproducible placement of incisions at desired depths in the corneal stroma.[15] Hence, it can be used to create the initial cut at the desired depth to inject air for the successful formation of big bubbles. In addition, it can be used to create corneal incisions with customized graft edges and lamellar planes for both donor and recipient corneas. Thus, FSL can be utilized for creating customized graft host interfaces, such as mushroom or zigzag-shaped DALK.

6. Diamond-knife assisted DALK

Vajpayee et al have described a new technique of DALK for the management of keratoconus that is easy to perform, provides visual outcomes comparable to those of big-bubble DALK, and can be performed in cases of extreme corneal thinning or corneal scars.[16] The essential steps of this technique involve the use of a diamond knife set at a depth of 30 µm less than the pachymetry reading is to make a 2.0 mm incision at the 11 to 12 o'clock position. This incision is then extended circumferentially as well as centripetally to take out the anterior leaving a thin stromal bed.

7. Tuck in lamellar keratoplasty

Tuck in lamellar keratoplasty (TILK) technique is useful for cases with advanced corneal ectasia involving corneal periphery such as advanced keratoconus, keratoglobus, post-PK corneal ectasia and pellucid marginal degeneration. A routine DALK cannot be the procedure of choice in these cases, as the peripheral cornea needs to be supported. In this technique, the central anterior stromal disc is removed and a centrifugal lamellar dissection is performed using a crescent knife to create a peripheral intrastromal pocket extending 0.5 mm beyond the limbus. The donor cornea is prepared in such a way that it has a central full thickness graft with a peripheral partial thickness flange. The flange of the graft is tucked into the peripheral intrastromal pocket of the host and the graft is sutured. The major limitation of this technique is its technical difficulty and the chance of leaving behind residual stroma that can affect the final visual acuity.

Donor tissue selection and preparation

Donor selection for DALK is not as stringent as for PK. Even non-optical grade tissue can be used for DALK provided the stroma is clear, devoid of any scar and the arcus is not that wide. This is of great help in countries like India where the demand far exceeds the availability of donor cornea. The recipient trephine size is usually larger compared to PK. For a normal diameter cornea, it ranges between 7.75 and 8.5 mm. For keratoconus cases the donor is usually oversized by 0.25 mm than the host bed. The surgeons past experience and axial length of the eye should guide the final decision regarding the disparity between recipient and donor trephine size. A few authors prefer same size donor, however we believe same-size or undersized donor tissue may be associated with problems such as flat graft surface, shallow angles, difficult contact lens fitting and severe interface wrinkling, hence it is better avoided.[8]

The retention or removal of donor DM during preparation of donor tissues is controversial. Retained donor DM can delay wound healing at the recipient-donor interface, and the donor endothelium may present potential antigens for rejection. Therefore, it is better to remove the DM during donor tissue preparation. Descemet's membrane and endothelium are removed by gently swabbing the posterior corneal surface of the donor corneoscleral rims with dry cellulose sponges. Then a corneal button is punched out from the tissue. Suturing technique (interrupted, running or combined interrupted-running 10.0 nylon sutures) can be done according to the surgeon's preference in DALK.

Postoperative care

Topical corticosteroids, antibiotics and lubricants are administered postoperatively. Overall, patient compliance is better compared to PK due to a shorter course of corticosteroids and early suture removal.

Complications

1. Stromal rejection. Stromal rejection manifested as acute stromal oedema and/or stromal neovascularization. Most of these rejections occurs within 12 months. The inflammatory process and presumed graft rejection can be rapidly reversed with topical steroid therapy.

2. DM perforation. Chances of DM perforation range from 4 to 39.2%.[8] One of the major problems with DALK is the risk of DM perforation, especially with inexperienced surgeons. It can occur at any step of surgery, including trephination, stromal excision and donor suturing. The risk of DM perforation is significantly higher in cases with inexperienced surgeons, corneal scarring near the DM due to healed hydrops or healed keratitis, and advanced ectasias with corneal thickness less than 250 µm. The perforation may be a micro-perforation (a small defect that allows a small output of aqueous material) or macroperforation (a rupture that leads to the collapse of the anterior chamber). A small perforation can be managed with air injection and converting to careful stromal dissection, whereas in the case of a macroperforation, the procedure needs to be converted to PK.

3. Pseudoanterior chamber. Breaks in DM usually cause the pseudo-anterior chamber. A shallow pseudochamber may be self-limited and may resolve after a few days. However, large pseudochambers may persist for weeks and surgical correction of pseudo anterior chambers may be performed by injection of air or expandable gases such as sulphur hexafluoride (SF6).

4. Fixed dilated pupil (Urrets-Zavalia syndrome). This complication was first reported by Urrets-Zavalia in six patients following PKP in keratoconus who developed fixed dilated pupil with iris atrophy up to 6 weeks after surgery. It is commonly associated with other features such as iris ectropion, pigment dispersion, posterior synechiae, and anterior subcapsular lens opacities. The exact pathogenesis is still not known however; the proposed mechanism includes pupillary block and iris ischemia. Rise in IOP during the management of DM perforation in DALK by intracameral air/gas injection has been related to this complication. Although uncommon, it can have serious long-term consequences such as decreased BCVA and halo at night.

5. Interface wrinkling. Folds in the DM following DALK are usually due to a mismatch between the donor button and the recipient bed size or localized corneal tissue expansion that may occur in advanced keratoconus. Majority of such folds are transient and disappear over time.

6. Interface vascularization. Interface vascularization can occur due to inflammatory, infective, and traumatic episodes or loose sutures after DALK. Recently, few reports have suggested the intrastromal injection of bevacizumab can be considered for management of intrastromal vascularization after DALK.

7. Interface keratitis. Interface keratitis is often a serious complication of DALK. Various organisms have been reported such as *Klebsiella*, non-tuberculous mycobacteria and *Candida*. *Candida* accounts for most of the cases. Graft infection can be acquired at any time following surgery, but most of it occurs during the first 6 months postoperatively. The organism primarily comes from the donor tissue or from ocular flora of the conjunctiva and ocular adnexa. The interface acts as a potential dead space and once the organism gains access to the space it proliferates without a host immune response. Moreover, postoperative steroid therapy can further complicate the process. Conservative treatment is usually unsuccessful due to difficulty in obtaining specimens for microbiology or inadequate penetration of topical, intraocular and systemic antibiotics. Interface irrigation with amphotericin may help, however, most cases need a therapeutic PK.

Outcomes

The outcomes of DALK are excellent, success rate of up to 90–99% have been reported in cases of keratoconus. Excellent outcomes have been reported with stromal dystrophies other than macular dystrophy. Recurrence of original disease in the graft is of concern, however, it is rare.

POSTERIOR LAMELLAR KERATOPLASTY (ENDOTHELIAL KERATOPLASTY)

Endothelial keratoplasty (EK) has emerged as the surgical procedure of choice for the treatment of corneal oedema from endothelial dysfunction.[17,18] It allows selective replacement of diseased host endothelium with a healthy donor endothelium. The cornea remains in a state of deturgescence, maintained by endothelial cell Na/K ATPase and by tight junctions between endothelial cells that limit entrance of fluid into the stroma. Various diseases like pseudophakic bullous keratopathy, Fuchs' endothelial keratopathy can lead to endothelial functional abnormalities leading to corneal oedema with resultant diminution of vision, and painful bullae. In posterior lamellar keratoplasty, this disease or abnormal endothelium is replaced with healthy endothelium graft.

INDICATIONS, CONTRAINDICATIONS AND PREOPERATIVE WORKUP

Indications

i. Endothelial dystrophies
  a. Fuchs' endothelial dystrophy (FED)
  b. Posterior polymorphous corneal dystrophy (PMCD)
  c. Congenital hereditary endothelial dystrophy (CHED) (Fig. 39.9)
  d. Irido-corneal endothelial syndrome (ICE)

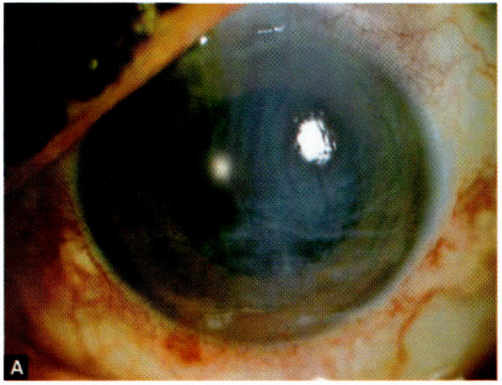

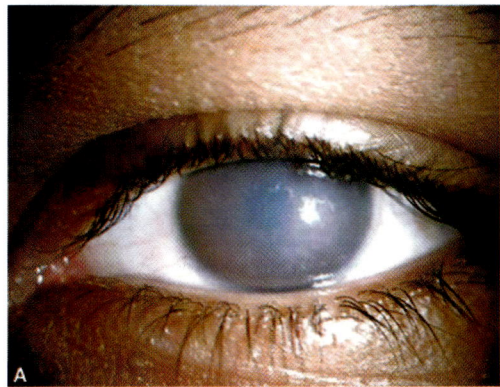

Fig. 39.9: *Indications of endothelial keratoplasty. A, Pseudophakic corneal decompensation; B, Endothelial dystrophies like CHED*

ii. Pseudophakic or aphakic bullous keratopathy

iii. Endothelial decompensation from trauma

iv. Post-glaucoma surgery or other intraocular surgery

v. Failed keratoplasty

vi. Aniridia with corneal decompensation

Contraindications

Any corneal scar which involves the anterior corneal stroma along with endothelial involvement should not be considered for the posterior lamellar keratoplasty. In the presence of high astigmatism (≥6D) also EK is better avoided. In such cases penetrating keratoplasty should be considered.

Preoperative workup

Preoperative workup for posterior lamellar keratoplasty is similar to anterior lamellar keratoplasty. When severe corneal oedema is present confocal scanning can give the details about endothelial cells. ASOCT is an invaluable tool before surgery as it gives the details of anterior segment.

SURGICAL TECHNIQUE

DSEK AND DSAEK

The technique for the DSEK and DSAEK are similar except that the donor corneal dissection is done manually in DSEK, and with automated microkeratome assisted approach in DSAEK.[17]

Technique involves 3 principal steps (Fig. 39.10):

• donor preparation,
• host preparation, and
• graft insertion.

Donor tissue can be prepared during surgery or "pre cut" by an Eye Bank facility. Pre-cut tissue is prepared using either a microkeratome (Fig. 39.11) or a femtosecond laser. The microkeratome cutting depth is adjustable to a depth of 350 μm, which generally prepares a donor tissue of 150–200 μm in thickness.

Host preparation includes creating a limbal or corneoscleral incision of a 4–5 mm. Descemet stripping is the next step performed within a diameter of 8.0 mm. Reverse-bent Sinskey hook or Descemet scrapper is used for stripping the Descemet membrane.

Insertion of donor tissue. The donor tissue is trephined to the appropriate size, most commonly 8.0–8.5 mm. Donor tissue is inserted into the anterior chamber using several methods such as forceps, Busin glide, cystotome, suture pull-through, and a variety of new inserters designed to provide a more delicate method. Once inserted, the graft is unfolded with a combination of balanced salt solution and air and then positioned. Interface fluid is removed with gentle external compression of the corneal surface with the Cindy sweeper, and the anterior chamber is completely filled with air. The main wound can be sutured. The tissue is left undisturbed for 10 minutes to promote adherence. After 10 minutes, nearly all of the intracameral air is exchanged for balanced salt solution to leave a 5 to 9 mm freely mobile air

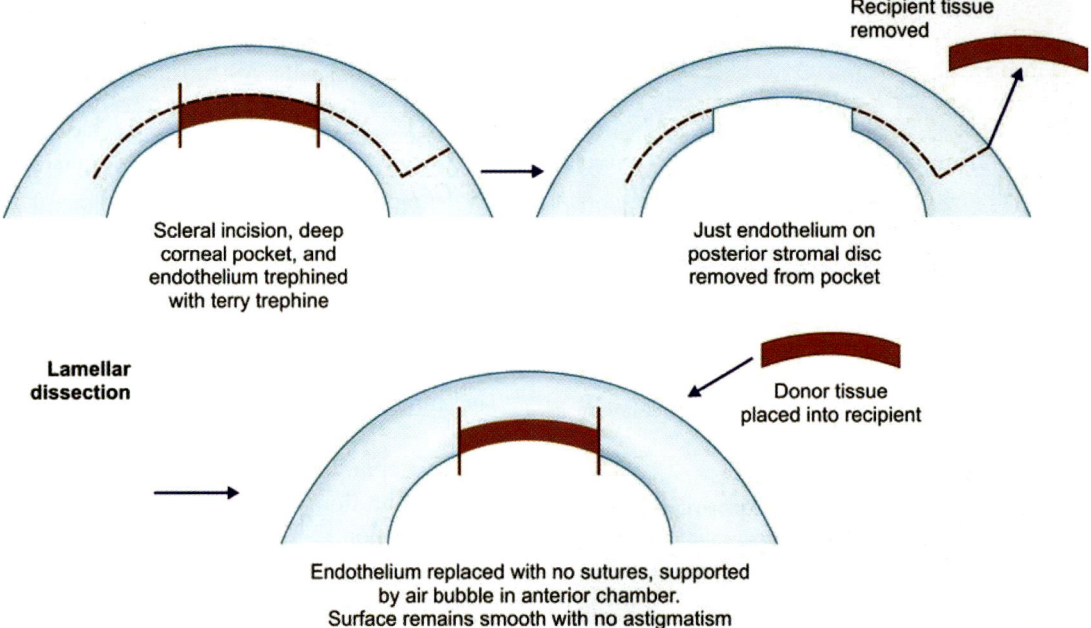

Fig. 39.10: *Principal surgical steps of endothelial keratoplasty (Descemet's stripping endothelial keratoplasty, i.e. DSEK, Descemet's stripping automatic endothelial keratoplasty, i.e. DSAEK, and Descemet's membrane keratoplasty, i.e. DMEK)*

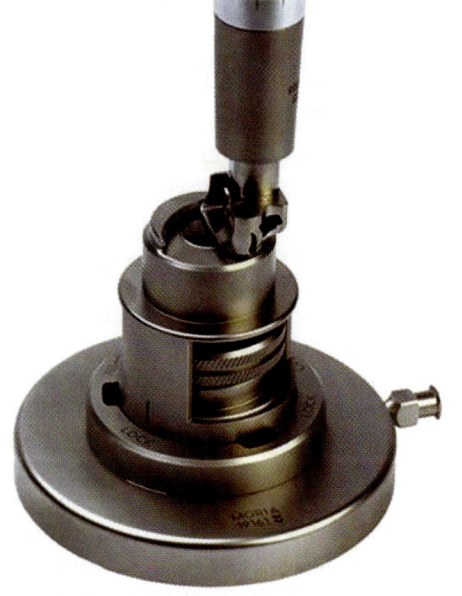

Fig. 39.11: *Moria artificial anterior chamber with micro-keratome*

bubble in anterior chamber. The patient remains supine for one hour at the hospital and then as much as possible at home until the postoperative day 1 examination.

Double pass technique

In this technique an initial debulking cut is performed using a microkeratome with a 300 µm head.[19] A second cut (refinement cut) is carried out from the direction opposite to the one of the first cut. The size of the head used for this step is selected such that a residual bed with a central thickness of approximately 100 µm is left. The aim is to achieve a thinner graft that will improve the visual outcome.

DESCEMET MEMBRANE ENDOTHELIAL KERATOPLASTY (DMEK)

More recent modifications of endothelial keratoplasty have attempted to transplant only donor DM and have been named Descemet membrane endothelial keratoplasty (DMEK).[20–22] Different techniques have been described. In general the corneoscleral buttons are mounted on a suction trephine, then endothelium is gently marked with an 8.0 mm trephine and stained with 0.06% trypan blue. The DM peripheral to the mark is incised with a sharp blade. The central edge is first lifted with a round blade and then grasped with 2 forceps. An incomplete detachment of the DM is done through a simultaneous centripetal movement of the 2 forceps. After this trephination with an 8.0 mm trephine is done. Transfer of the graft into the patient's eye and the unfolding is achieved by placing the DM into a customized glass injector, or a variety of modified intraocular lens injectors. Recipient preparation is done through a small corneal incision (approximately 2.5 mm), and the patient's DM is removed under air using an inverted hook. The graft is injected into the AC. The DM is then positioned centrally using short bursts of balanced salt solution and injecting a series of small air bubbles. Once the donor is completely and properly unfolded, air is then injected underneath the graft until the AC is completely filled. The air is left in place for 30 minutes. On completion of the procedure, air is aspirated, leaving behind 50% of the AC volume.[21, 22]

COMPLICATIONS

1. Primary graft failure

Primary graft failure is characterized by the clinical situation in which a corneal graft does not clear as expected after surgery usually by two months. Primary graft failures indicate a lack of endothelial function. It can result from poor quality donor tissue, unhealthy recipient circumstances (blood, interface foreign bodies, infection, flat chamber), or poor surgical technique. The reported incidence is <1% in DSAEK.

2. Graft detachment and dislocation

Early postoperative graft detachment/dislocation remains one of the most common complications of DSAEK surgery. It manifests as interface fluid, significant graft displacement or a graft that is completely dislocated into the anterior chamber. A partially detached DSAEK graft may reattach spontaneously, hence can be observed. However large, central or complete detachments need a combination of an injection of an AC air bubble (rebubbling) with re-positioning or refloating of the graft.

3. Graft rejection

The incidence of graft rejection following DSAEK is relatively less compared to PKP. The reported rates ranges from 0 to 45.5% with an average rate of 10% with follow-up ranging from 3 months to 2 years. Most of the rejection episodes are reversible with topical steroids.

4. Glaucoma

Glaucoma following DSAEK can occur due to pupillary block, inflammation, or steroid use. The reported incidence of glaucoma after DSAEK ranges from 0 to 15%, with an average rate of 3.0%. Topical or oral intraocular pressure-lowering medications are usually successful in controlling IOP. The management of pupillary block includes release of anterior chamber air via a paracentesis, which can be performed at the slit lamp or in the operation theatre.

5. Endothelial loss

The ranges of endothelial loss reported from larger series (involving ≥100 eyes) ranges from 14.9 to 59% with follow-up ranging from six months to three years. Most of the loss occurs intra-operatively or in the immediate post-operative stage.

6. Infectious keratitis

Bacterial, fungal, and herpetic, all forms of keratitis have been reported following DSAEK. The most commonly isolated causative organism is *Candida albicans*.

7. Interface haze

Interface abnormalities can occur due to blood, retained ophthalmic viscosurgical device, inflammatory cells, debris, irregular cut of the donor tissue by the microkeratome, retained fragments of DM, microkeratome-generated plastic particles and epithelial cells.

PENETRATING KERATOPLASTY

Penetrating keratoplasty (PKP) is the operative procedure where the full thickness host cornea is replaced with a full thickness donor corneal graft.[5,23,24] With the advent of lamellar keratoplasty, the preference for PKP has come down dramatically. However, in inexperienced hands and where the facilities for LK are lacking, PKP is still the most commonly performed procedure.

INDICATIONS

PKP can be performed in any case of corneal opacity due to any cause. Common indications include:

- Pseudophakic corneal oedema
- Aphakic corneal oedema
- Keratoconus and corneal ectasias
- Corneal degenerations
- Corneal dystrophies
- Healed keratitis
- Congenital opacities
- Chemical injury sequelae
- Mechanical trauma
- Failed graft

PREOPERATIVE INVESTIGATIONS

Preoperative indications include ocular surface evaluation, visual potential assessment and evaluation of posterior segment as described under lamellar keratoplasty. However, more sophisticated investigations like specular microscopy, ASOCT and confocal scanning are not routinely done.

SURGICAL PROCEDURE

Surgical steps vary among surgeons, but three fundamental goals are mandatory in penetrating keratoplasty surgery:

- Obtain good wound alignment with minimal astigmatism,
- Avoid endothelial cell damage, and
- Avoid the complications associated with vitreous up-thrust.[5]

Achieving preoperative hypotony with mannitol (1 g/kg) is a must to avoid serious complications like expulsive haemorrhage.

Surgical steps of penetrating keratoplasty are briefly described:

1. *Insertion of lid speculum.* The lid speculum is sized and positioned to minimize pressure against the eye, either from the speculum itself or indirectly from the lids. A lateral canthotomy may be helpful to reduce pressure in case of narrow palpebral aperture.

2. *Placement of scleral fixation ring.* A scleral fixation ring is sutured with four interrupted 5/0 Dacron or 7/0 Vicryl sutures with half-thickness scleral bites. It maintains scleral support, exerting its influence once the eye is opened if scleral rigidity is insufficient.

3. *Marking of host cornea.* The donor graft is usually centred on the host cornea or over the pupillary axis.

4. *Trephination of donor cornea.* The donor cornea is trephined with the endothelial side facing up using a sharp disposable blade in a Teflon block apparatus (Fig. 39.12A). The donor trephine is routinely sized 0.25 mm larger than the host trephine because, using current techniques, donor corneal tissue cut with a trephine from the endothelial surface measures approximately 0.25 mm less in diameter than host corneal tissue cut with the same diameter trephine from the epithelial surface.

5. *Host trephination.* Sizing of the host trephine depends on several factors, including host corneal size, pathology, and risk of rejection. The host cornea is trephined using a hand-held disposable trephine held perpendicular to the cornea (Fig. 39.12B). Minimal pressure is exerted against the cornea as the trephine is progressively rotated, allowing its sharp edges to penetrate gently to pre-Descemet's membrane or until the anterior chamber is entered. For patients with a larger-than-average corneal horizontal diameter (limbal white-to-white measurement ≥12.5 mm), an 8.25 or 8.5 mm host trephine is often used, and for patients with a smaller-than-average corneal diameter (white-to-white measurement ≤11.5 mm), a 7.5 or 7.75 mm trephine is often used.[5] When partial thickness incision is made with trephine, it is completed with the help of corneo-scleral scissors (Fig. 39.12C).

6. *Placement of viscoelastic material in the anterior chamber.* The anterior chamber is filled with a viscoelastic. This helps maintain donor button orientation for accurate suture placement and provides inexpensive endothelial protection.

7. *Placement of the donor corneal tissue in the host bed.* The tissue is gently grasped with fine-toothed forceps at the junction of the epithelium and stroma and transferred on to the recipient bed, where it rests on viscoelastic material.

8. *Placement of four cardinal sutures* (Fig. 39.12D). The first 10/0 nylon interrupted suture

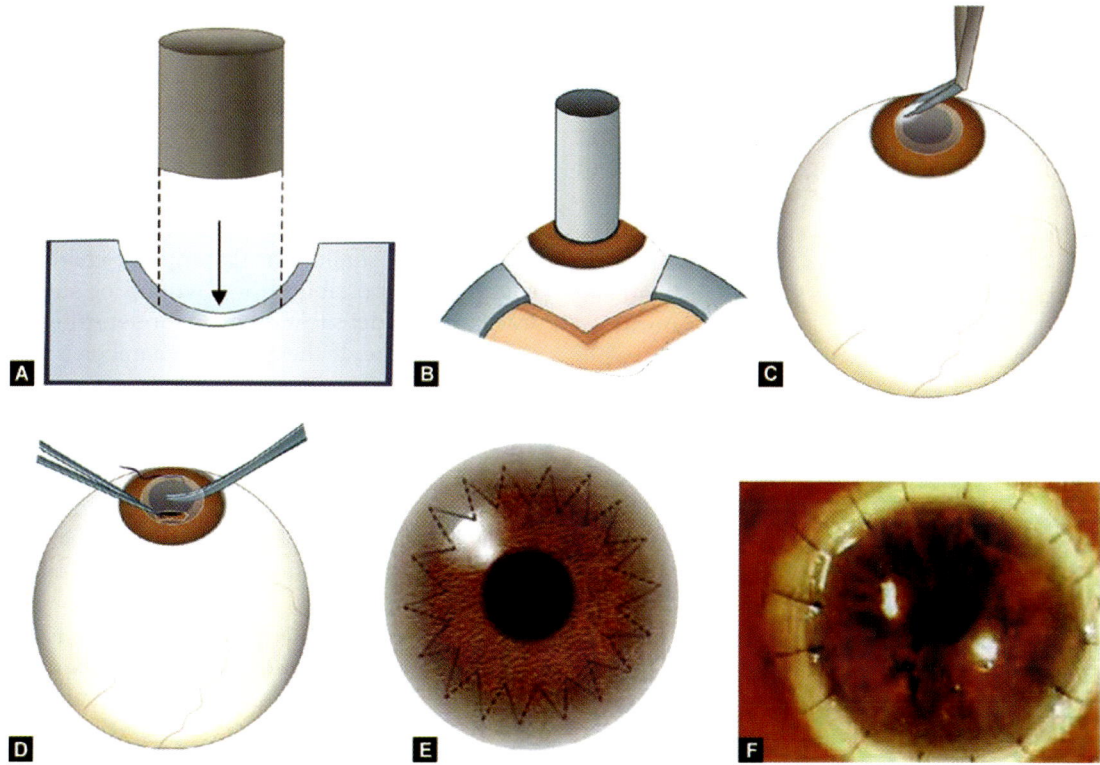

Fig. 39.12A to F: *Surgical steps of penetrating keratoplasty*

is placed in the 12 o'clock position. Suture depth is approximately 90% to prevent wound gape. The second suture, placed 180° away at 6 o'clock. It should be placed so that an equal amount of tissue is distributed on either side. The 3 o'clock suture is placed and tied, followed by the 9 o'clock suture. Formation of a uniform diamond shape on the donor cornea after putting 4 cardinal sutures suggests proper suture positioning.

9. *Completion of suturing.* Twelve additional radial interrupted 10/0 nylon sutures are placed snugly to ensure adequate tissue apposition (Fig. 39.12E). The anterior chamber is reformed balanced salt solution as needed. A variety of suturing techniques exist: Interrupted sutures only, running suture only (Fig. 39.12F), combined interrupted and running sutures, and double running sutures, all of which are valid approaches to wound closure.

Interrupted sutures are indicated for pediatric grafts, therapeutic grafts and for inflamed and vascularized beds due to rapid wound healing that may occur differentially in these cases warranting early suture removal in some areas.

10. *At the end of the procedure* subconjunctival dexamethasone, 4 mg; subconjunctival gentamicin, 20 mg; and subconjunctival cefazolin, 25 mg, or another suitable antibiotic are injected.

Note: Penetrating keratoplasty may be combined with cataract surgery, secondary intraocular lens implantation, glaucoma surgery and retinal surgery.

POSTOPERATIVE MEDICATIONS

- *Pressure patch and shield* should be placed.
- *Analgesics.* Treatment of postoperative pain should be undertaken with acetaminophen and oral nonsteroidal anti-inflammatory medications and, in more severe cases, with narcotic medication.[5]
- *Antibiotics* should be given to prevent infection. The newer generation of fluoro-

quinolone, moxifloxacin 0.5% or gatifloxacin 0.3% is preferred.

- *Topical steroid* treatment is initiated with prednisolone acetate 1% or prednisolone sodium phosphate 1% drops. These are administered at a dosage of 4 to every hour depending upon the grade of inflammation.
- *Prophylactic antiglaucoma medications* should be given if simultaneous cataract surgery, vitrectomy, or lysis of synechiae has been done, and in cases with preoperative inflammation, glaucoma, and use of larger amounts of viscoelastic material.[5]

COMPLICATIONS

The various complications are described below.[5, 23–27]

Intraoperative complications

1. Improper trephination. If the trephines are inadvertently reversed and the donor button is smaller than the recipient site, it may be difficult to suture the button in place and secure a watertight wound.

2. Eccentric trephination. Improper, eccentric placement of the trephine can result in large amounts of postoperative astigmatism and increased risk of graft rejection.

3. Damaged donor button. Donor corneas must be handled with extreme care to prevent damage to the endothelium.

4. Retained Descemet's membrane. Retained Descemet's membrane is often difficult to see. The iris should be gently picked up and identified with forceps or trypan blue staining can delineate the retained descemet's membrane. In addition, viscoelastic placed behind retained Descemet's membrane will elevate it from the iris and facilitate removal.

5. Posterior capsule tear. During combined keratoplasty and cataract extraction, the posterior capsule may be torn. Small tears without vitreous loss are usually of little significance, and careful placement of a posterior chamber intraocular lens with sulcus or in-the-bag fixation is possible. A large tear needs proper anterior vitrectomy.

6. Expulsive choroidal haemorrhage. The incidence of expulsive haemorrhage has been reported from 0.47[18] to 3.3%. Predisposing factors are hypertension, glaucoma, or previous trauma. Pre-operative hypotony is necessary to avoid this complication.

Postoperative complications

1. Wound leaks. During the early postoperative period, low intraocular pressure and/or the presence of a shallow or flat anterior chamber suggests the possibility of a wound or suture track leak. Seidel's test is useful for detecting an area of leakage. If the anterior chamber is flat and a wound or suture track leak is present, immediate surgical repair is indicated. If the anterior chamber remains formed despite the wound or suture track leak, a pressure patch may be used to re-appose the wound, and seal the leak. If nonsurgical attempts fail to seal the leak after 24 to 48 hours, surgical repair is recommended.

2. Persistent epithelial defects. During the early postoperative course of penetrating keratoplasty, re-epithelialization and the maintenance of an intact epithelium is critical for postoperative wound healing, improved visual acuity, graft transparency, graft survival, and protection of the stroma against infection and melting. Normally it takes 5–7 days for complete re-epithelialization.

Risk factors include:

- Any lid or lash abnormalities including trichiasis, ectropion, entropion, and lagophthalmos
- Ocular surface disease secondary to dry eye, alkali burn, Stevens-Johnson syndrome, ocular cicatricial pemphigoid
- Decreased preoperative corneal sensation
- Longer donor storage time, and increased recipient age
- Herpetic keratitis
- Systemic diseases; Diabetes, chronic liver disease, malnutrition.

Management: Postoperative medications should be modified to minimize epithelial toxicity. Since topical corticosteroids inhibit corneal epithelial wound healing, their use should be kept to a minimum. Preservative-free lubricants should be prescribed. Pressure patching avoids trauma from the eyelid motion over the healing surface.

Bandage soft contact lenses have also been used to prevent and treat postoperative epithelial defects. If all these measures fail, a temporary tarsorrhaphy is done. Amniotic membrane transplantation is also an effective treatment modality. The possibility of active herpes virus infection must always be considered when an epithelial defect does not respond to treatment.

3. Filamentary keratitis. Filaments consist of abnormal collections of mucus and epithelial cells on the corneal surface. Patients with minimal symptoms should be treated with hypotonic artificial tears and with severe symptoms; the filaments should be carefully removed with a forceps followed by treatment with hypotonic tears and/or topical acetyl-cysteine, which has a mucolytic action.

4. Suture-related complications include:

i. Suture exposure. When suture knot or tip exposure occurs, suture rotation should be attempted at the slit lamp. If rotation is not possible, removal of the exposed suture should be performed as early as wound healing permits. Any suture that is broken, loose, or associated with stromal vascularization across the wound, however, should be removed immediately.

ii. Suture-related infection. Exposed sutures are often associated with the accumulation of mucus and debris that may act as a nidus for microbial colonization. The suture must be removed and sent for culture. Broad-spectrum fortified antibiotics should be initiated until an organism is identified and antibiotic sensitivities are known. The use of topical corticosteroids should be temporarily discontinued in the early stages of treatment. During this period, systemic corticosteroids may be used in order to protect against an associated rejection episode. Once the infection is controlled, topical corticosteroids may be cautiously resumed.

iii. Suture-related immune infiltrates. Suture-related immune infiltrates may also occur in the early postoperative period. The frequency of topical corticosteroids should be increased to at least every 2 hours, and the addition of a corticosteroid ointment at bedtime should be considered.

iv. Kaye dots. The dots are found primarily in the depressed zone central to the swollen donor cornea edge. Their formation may be a non-specific response of the epithelium to an area of tissue angulation.

5. Elevated intraocular pressure. The measurement of intraocular pressure in the early postoperative period is important. Pressure readings obtained by Goldmann applanation tonometry are inaccurate. The use of a pneumotonometer or an electronic tonometer is recommended.

6. Pupillary block. The presence of a flat or shallow anterior chamber and a securely closed wound, suggests the presence of pupillary block. Medical management includes the repeated application of mydriatic and cycloplegic agents in a vigorous attempt to dilate the pupil. Peripheral iridectomy should be performed if there is no response to medical treatment.

7. Postoperative inflammation. Postoperative inflammation can usually be controlled with topical corticosteroids. If fibrin membrane forms, hourly topical corticosteroids and mydriatics should be used to prevent the development of posterior synechiae and pupillary block. If the condition fails to improve, the use of periocular and/or systemic corticosteroids is recommended.

8. Hyphaema. Although rare it can occur if extensive synechiolysis, iridoplasty, or iridectomy has been performed. If the haemorrhage fails to clear spontaneously, irrigation/aspiration, aspiration with vitrectomy or manual expression of the clot through a limbal incision can be done.

9. Fixed dilated pupil. The development of a fixed, dilated pupil following penetrating keratoplasty for keratoconus has been observed as part of a syndrome associated with iris atrophy, scattered pigment on the lens capsule and corneal endothelium, and secondary glaucoma with posterior synechia.

10. Postoperative infection. Bacterial or fungal keratitis in the early postoperative period may result from contamination of donor material, incomplete excision of an infected host cornea, or acquisition of microorganisms from the environment. Graft infection usually manifests within 24 to 48 hours with ciliary injection, graft oedema, mucopurulent discharge, and occasionally an infiltrate in the graft or around a suture. Gram stain and culture with sensitivities should be performed. Broad-spectrum topical antibiotics should be initiated until culture results are obtained. Should a graft become extensively involved with infection, it should be replaced to prevent the development of endophthalmitis.

11. Primary donor failure. Primary donor failure results in irreversible oedema of the corneal graft in the immediate postoperative period. It is due to inadequate endothelial cell function of an unhealthy donor endothelium, inadequate tissue preservation, or surgical trauma. Once a diagnosis of primary donor failure is made, regrafting may be performed as soon as the eye is no longer inflamed. Cases of suspected primary graft failure should be observed for at least 3 weeks for signs of graft clearing before regrafting.

12. Postkeratoplasty astigmatism. Visual acuity, binocular visual function, and patient satisfaction can be severely limited by postoperative astigmatism and anisometropia. Average postkeratoplasty astigmatism has been cited to be in the range of 4 to 6 diopters.[5] Various factors that contribute include; corneal thinning, eccentric trephination of the donor or host tissue, and failure to excise peripheral pathology in keratoconus or pellucid marginal degeneration, quality of wound healing, and the tension, length, depth, and configuration of corneal suture placement. Corneal topography provides the most useful and complete information regarding corneal shape. A technique for reducing postkeratoplasty astigmatism includes spectacles or contact lens wear, selective suture removal, relaxing incisions, compression sutures, wedge resection, laser vision correction, and toric lens implantation. Repeat keratoplasty can be done when these measures fail.

13. Corneal allograft rejection. Corneal allograft rejection is the leading cause of corneal graft failure.

Risk factors. Collaborative Corneal Transplantation Studies (CCTS) has shown that failed graft and more than two quadrants of deep stromal vascularization are the major risk factors of graft rejection. Other risk factors include young recipient age (less than 40 years), large-diameter corneal grafts, eccentric graft, loose sutures in the graft, presence of pre-existing inflammation in the eye, recent anterior segment surgery, pre-existing glaucoma and anterior synechiae (Table 39.4).

Table 39.4: *Risk factors for corneal allograft rejection*

Donor factors: HLA and ABO incompatibility *(controversial)*, storage method and duration

Host factors:
- *Preoperative:* Young age, bilateral graft, previous rejected grafts, history of recent anterior segment surgery, vascularized and inflamed bed, limbal stem cell deficiency, poor ocular surface, dry eye, chemical burns, pre-existing anterior synechia, glaucoma, herpetic eye disease
- *Intraoperative:* Large, eccentric graft, iris incarceration at graft host junction
- *Postoperative:* Loose sutures, anterior synechia, exposed knots, suture removal, anterior segment surgery

Clinical features: Appreciation of the clinical features of corneal allograft rejection is critical to early recognition of rejection, and is the first step toward effective therapy.

Symptoms of redness of the eye, decreased vision, light sensitivity, or discomfort in the eye that lasts longer than a few hours requires evaluation to exclude an episode of graft rejection.

Clinical signs of graft rejection include ciliary congestion (often the earliest sign of rejection), anterior chamber flare, anterior chamber cells, discrete subepithelial infiltrates Krachmer's lines, endothelial keratic precipitates. Linear deposit of keratic precipitates on endothelium referred, as Khodadoust line is the hallmark of corneal allograft rejection. Often, there is associated graft oedema overlying the area that has been traversed by the advancing keratic precipitates while the rest of the graft is clear, known as differential oedema. Ultrasonic corneal pachymetry showing an isolated increase in corneal thickness can be a sign of allograft rejection. Elevated intraocular pressure, or sudden onset of an epithelial defect in a previously healed corneal graft can also be manifestations of corneal allograft rejection.

Graft rejection can be three types—epithelial rejection, stromal rejection (Fig. 39.13) and endothelial rejection. Endothelial rejection is the most common of the three types, with reported rates from 8 to 37% of cases undergoing rejection.

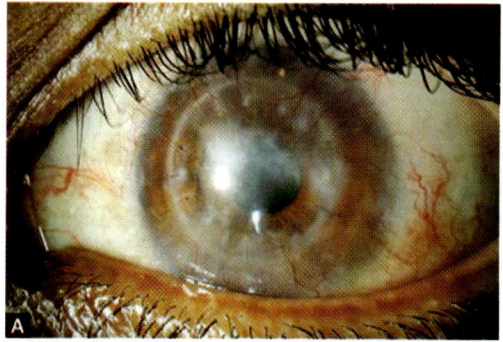

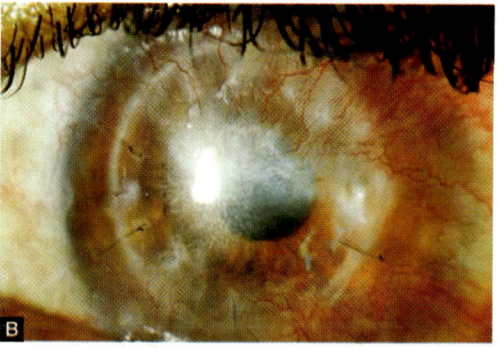

Fig. 39.13A and B: *Stromal rejection*

Differential diagnosis of graft rejection includes:

• *An episode of rejection can confuse with herpes simplex keratouveitis.* The clue to differentiate is the observation that the endothelial keratic precipitates in herpetic inflammation are not confined to the graft but involve as well the peripheral host endothelium.

• When *epithelial downgrowth* presents with inflammatory response, the differentiation becomes difficult. Steroid therapy will ultimately differentiate the conditions, since the epithelial down growth will not respond to steroid therapy.

• A *low-grade corneal infection* can masquerade as corneal allograft rejection.

Treatment of corneal allograft rejection. Fortunately, most episodes of corneal allograft

rejection reaction can be reversed if therapy is initiated early and aggressively.

• *Corticosteroid therapy* by topical, periocular, or systemic administration is the treatment of choice for acute corneal allograft rejection reaction. Intravenous methylprednisolone pulse therapy (3–5 mg/kg IV push) may be considered in severe graft rejection. Immuno-suppression by long-term corticosteroid therapy is associated with unacceptable ocular and systemic side effects.

• *Immunosuppressive agents* such as cyclosporine, tacrolimus, and mycophenolate mofetil can be used as steroid sparing agent.

14. Graft failure. A corneal graft is considered to be failed if it fails to serve the purpose for which it was done. It may be *primary* due to progressive endothelial loss or it may be *secondary* to graft infection, recurrence of the disease or repeated graft rejection episodes. Repeated graft rejection is the most common cause of graft failure.

Management of graft failure is by repeat corneal graft. In cases where the graft failure is only due to endothelial, failure endothelial keratoplasty is a better alternative than a full thickness graft.

THERAPEUTIC KERATOPLASTY

Therapeutic keratoplasty (TPK) is a surgical procedure where the primary purpose is either to restore the structural integrity of the eye (tectonic keratoplasty), or to resolve an infectious or inflammatory keratitis that is refractory to conventional medical therapy.

INDICATIONS

The indications of TPK includes the following:

• Infectious keratitis not responding to medical management

• Impending corneal perforation

• Descematocele

• Perforated corneal ulcer

Therapeutic keratoplasty helps for complete removal the infection and decrease the organism's load in the cornea to a level at which antibacterial agents and the patient's host defense mechanisms can be effective. For cases of perforated or impending corneal ulcer and descemetoceles, it is an effective procedure to maintain the integrity of globe.

SURGICAL TECHNIQUE

The technique is more or less similar to PKP. *Special considerations* include:

- At the time of therapeutic keratoplasty, the size of the graft should be carefully determined by placing the appropriate trephine over the cornea. The main aim of surgery is to excise all necrotic or infected tissue during the trephination. If possible, a 1 mm rim of healthy corneal tissue should be removed to leave a stable, non-infected recipient bed. After measuring the host cornea to be removed, the donor cornea can be trephined and is usually 0.5–1.0 mm larger than the host trephine.
- *Care should be taken not to place pressure on the globe*, which can cause extrusion of the intra-ocular contents or an expulsive choroidal haemorrhage.
- *Administration of 20% mannitol*, 1 hour before surgery at a dose of 1 gm/kg is necessary to reduce the vitreous up-thrust.
- *A self-retaining lid speculum* or lid sutures are very helpful to prevent pressure on the globe.
- *The loss of scleral rigidity with decreased intraocular pressure* can make host trephination difficult.
- When there is vitreous in the perforation, an anterior vitrectomy is performed through the limbal incision.
- When there is significant chamber shallowing with vitreous pressure, a pars plana vitrectomy can be considered.
- If cyanoacrylate adhesive can be applied preoperatively or intra-operatively, the anterior chamber can be re-formed with visco-elastic, and the host trephination can be performed under a more controlled environment.

POSTOPERATIVE MANAGEMENT

Anti-infectious therapy should be maintained until the corneal epithelium has healed. Duration of treatment depends on the severity of the infection and the causative organism.

Care should be taken for promotion of epithelial healing, by use of preservative free lubricant eye drops and avoid injudicious use of epithelial toxic medication like fortified antibiotic eye drops.

In postoperative period patients with a therapeutic keratoplasty for herpes simplex keratitis on acyclovir 400 mg twice daily or valacyclovir, 500 mg once a day for 6 months after surgery should be maintained.

Cycloplegics are given in case of severe anterior chamber inflammation is present.

The use of topical corticosteroids following a therapeutic keratoplasty for an infectious organism is controversial. There is controversy regarding the use of corticosteroids after therapeutic keratoplasty involving infections that do not respond readily to treatment, such as fungal or Acanthamoeba corneal ulceration. Ideally, steroid should be started if the culture report of the excised host cornea comes out to be negative or the margins are free. When there is any sign of active fungal or Acanthamoeba infection following a therapeutic keratoplasty, corticosteroids should be avoided.

Postoperatively, the patient's intraocular pressure should be followed carefully. Approximately 50% of keratoplasties develops glaucoma in postoperative period.

CORNEA TRANSPLANTATION IN INDIA

AN OVERVIEW

National Program for Control of Blindness (NPCB) was introduced in India in 1976. Since implementation, there is significant reduction in burden of blindness due to various causes. For the cases of corneal blindness approach is not only involves the increased in numbers of corneal transplant but also to reduce the burner of corneal blindness. There are also measures taken to increase the awareness of the eye donation. Considering current population 122 crores of India as per the census of 2011, and 1% of population (vision 6/60 or less than 6/60), i.e. approximately 1.22 crores are blind. As per RAAB (rapid assessment of avoidable blindness) conducted by MOH & FW 2006–07, 1% of total blindness constituting 1.22 lakhs are bilaterally corneal blind out of which only 60000 can be provided the visual rehabilitation by keratoplasty.[28] Rest 50% was not able to rehabilitate because of some posterior segment pathology. In addition, of above 20000 new cases of corneal blindness are added every year. Considering the maximum of collected corneas, backlog of corneal blindness and annual addition of fresh cases of corneal blindness, it can be concluded that India needs approximately 1.40 lakh corneas per year as of today.[28] Thus, every effort must be made to improve the eye donation rate in India.

REFERENCES

1. Niederkorn JY, Larkin DF. Immune privilege of corneal allografts. Ocul Immunol Inflamm. 2010; 18: 162–71.
2. Streilein JW. Ocular immune privilege: therapeutic opportunities from an experiment of nature. Nat Rev Immunol. 2003; 3(11): 879–889.
3. Albuquerque RJ, Hayashi T, Cho WG, et al. Alternatively spliced vascular endothelial growth factor receptor-2 is an essential endogenous inhibitor of lymphatic vessel growth. Nat Med. 2009; 15(9): 1023–1030.
4. Niederkorn JY. Anterior chamber-associated immune deviation and its impact on corneal allograft survival. Curr Opin Organ Transplant. 2006; 11: 360–365.
5. Keratoplasty, part XI. Cornea, 3rd Edition: Krachmer, Mannis & Holland, Elsevier.
6. Arenas E, Esquenazi S, Anwar M, Terry M. Lamellar corneal transplantation. Surv Ophthalmol. 2012 Nov; 57(6): 510–29.
7. Tan DT, Anshu A. Anterior lamellar keratoplasty: 'Back to the Future'- a review. Clin Experiment Ophthalmol. 2010 Mar; 38(2): 118–27.
8. Maharana PK, Agarwal K, Jhanji V, Vajpayee RB. Deep anterior lamellar keratoplasty for keratoconus: a review. Eye Contact Lens. 2014 Nov; 40(6): 382–9.
9. Vajpayee RB, Vasudendra N, Titiyal JS, Tandon R, Sharma N, Sinha R. Automated lamellar therapeutic keratoplasty (ALTK) in the treatment of anterior to mid-stromal corneal pathologies. Acta Ophthalmol Scand. 2006 Dec; 84(6): 771–3.
10. Archila EA. Deep lamellar keratoplasty dissection of host tissue with intra-stromal air injection. Cornea 1984; 3: 217–218.
11. Anwar M, Teichmann KD. Deep lamellar keratoplasty; surgical techniques for anterior lamellar keratoplasty with and without baring of Descemet's membrane. Cornea 2002; 21: 374–383.
12. Jhanji V, Beltz J, Sharma N, Graue E, Vajpayee RB. "Double bubble" deep anterior lamellar keratoplasty for management of corneal stromal pathologies. Int Ophthalmol. 2011; 31: 257–62.
13. Melles GR, Remeijer L, Geerards AJ, Beekhuis WH. A quick surgical technique for deep, anterior lamellar keratoplasty using visco-dissection. Cornea. 2000; 19: 427–32.
14. Sugita J, Kondo J. Deep lamellar keratoplasty with complete removal of pathological stroma for vision improvement. Br J Ophthalmol 1997; 81: 184–8.
15. Buzzonetti L, Laborante A, Petrocelli G. Standardized big-bubble technique in deep anterior lamellar keratoplasty assisted by femtosecond laser. J Cataract Refract Surg. 2010; 36: 1631–1636.
16. Vajpayee RB, Maharana PK, Sharma N, Agarwal T, Jhanji V. Diamond knife assisted deep anterior lamellar keratoplasty to manage keratoconus. J Cataract Refract Surg. 2014; 40: 276–82.
17. Anshu A, Price MO, Tan DT, Price FW Jr. Endothelial keratoplasty: a revolution in evolution. Surv Ophthalmol. 2012 May-Jun; 57(3): 236–52.
18. Lee WB, Jacobs DS, Musch DC, et al. Descemet's stripping endothelial keratoplasty: Safety and outcomes: A report by the American Academy of Ophthalmology. Ophthalmology. 2009; 116: 18–30.
19. Hsu M, Hereth WL, Moshirfar M. Double-pass microkeratome technique for ultra-thin graft preparation in Descemet's stripping automated endothelial keratoplasty. Clinical Ophthalmology 2012; 6: 425–432.
20. Price FW Jr, Price MO. Descemet's stripping with endothelial keratoplasty in 50 eyes: a refractive neutral corneal transplant. J Refract Surg. 2005; 21: 339–345.
21. Ang M, Wilkins MR, Mehta JS, Tan D. Descemet membrane endothelial keratoplasty. Br J Ophthalmol. 2015 May 19.
22. Tourtas T, Laaser K, Bachmann BO, Cursiefen C, Kruse FE. Descemet membrane endothelial keratoplasty versus descemet stripping automated endothelial keratoplasty. Am J Ophthalmol. 2012 Jun; 153(6): 1082–90.

23. Güell JL, El Husseiny MA, Manero F, Gris O, Elies D. Historical Review and Update of Surgical Treatment for Corneal Endothelial Diseases. Ophthalmol Ther. 2014 Feb 18.

24. Ple-Plakon PA, Shtein RM. Trends in corneal transplantation: Indications and techniques. Curr Opin Ophthalmol. 2014 Jul; 25(4): 300–5.

25. Mozayan E, Lee JK. Update on astigmatism management. Curr Opin Ophthalmol. 2014 Jul; 25(4): 286–90.

26. Qazi Y, Hamrah P. Corneal Allograft Rejection: Immunopathogenesis to Therapeutics. J Clin Cell Immunol. 2013 Nov 20; 2013 (Suppl 9).

27. Young AL, Kam KW, Jhanji V, Cheng LL, Rao SK. A new era in corneal transplantation: paradigm shift and evolution of techniques. Hong Kong Med J. 2012 Dec; 18(6): 509–16.

28. Managing Corneal Blindness. NPCB India news letter April-June 2012.

Chapter

40

Keratoprosthesis

GENERAL CONSIDERATIONS

INTRODUCTION

The basic concept of using an artificial cornea or keratoprosthesis to replace a damaged and opaque cornea is as obvious as placing a window on a house to be able to see out. This possibility first occurred to the French doctor Guillaume Pellier de Quengsy, who published the feat in the times of the French Revolution (18th century).[1-3]

Keratoprosthesis is a surgical procedure wherein a diseased cornea is replaced with an artificial cornea. Traditionally, keratoprosthesis is recommended after a person has had a failure of one or more donor corneal transplants. While conventional cornea transplant uses donor tissue for transplant, an artificial cornea is used in the keratoprosthesis procedure. The surgery is performed to restore vision in patients suffering from severely damaged cornea due to congenital birth defects, infections, injuries and burns.

Keratoprotheses are made of clear plastic with excellent tissue tolerance and optical properties. They vary in design, size and even the implantation techniques may differ across different treatment centres.

During the 19th century there were scattered surgeons who attempted to follow on Quengsy's footsteps, but with equally disastrous outcomes (endophthalmitis, extrusion, and loss of the eye). Thus, it was not until the 1950s with the introduction of new materials, such as transparent non-toxic plastics, that some measure of success began to be reported.[4-7] The good results of these new designs has to be also attributed to the discovery of antibiotics and steroids, which improved the postoperative management significantly.

Prosthetic corneas form the last resort for corneal blindness, especially in eyes with end-stage ocular surface disorders and in those at a high risk for conventional penetrating kerato-plasty.[8,9] The choice of keratoprosthesis (K-Pro) depends on the underlying etiology, the anatomy of the ocular surface and the tear film status.

INDICATIONS

K-Pros are performed for bilateral corneal blindness not amenable to conventional penetrating keratoplasty.

- Stevens-Johnson syndrome
- Ocular cicatricial pemphigoid (stages 3 and 4)
- Chemical injuries
- Trachoma (stage C0 according to WHO) with severe dry eye
- Vascularized corneas with complete stem cell loss and dryness
- Multiple failed penetrating keratoplasty/ amniotic membrane or stem cell grafting.

TYPES/DESIGNS OF KERATOPROSTHESIS

The design of a K-Pro can be likened to some extent to that of an intraocular lens consisting of an optic and a haptic.

Optic, which forms the central part of the K-Pro responsible for viewing, in most types is a cylinder made of polymethyl methacrylate (PMMA)—creating an optically clear window.

Haptic of the K-Pro determines the type of the prosthesis. Based on the type of haptic material it can be:

- *Biocompatible*—usually a PMMA skirt with the corneal graft as in the Boston type 1 and 2 K-Pro
- *Biointegrated*—as in the Dacron mesh that forms the skirt around the PMMA optic in the Pintucci K-Pro
- *Biological*—tooth or the bone that forms an autologous biological tissue that supports the optical cylinder in the osteo-odonto and the osteo-K-Pro, respectively.

Basic types of K-Pro

Keratoprosthesis designs have primarily been variations of 3 main types (Fig. 40.1):

- *First type* PMMA stem with skirt embedded within the cornea (Fig. 40.1A)
- *Second type* Transparent membrane with porous edges inserted into the cornea (Fig. 40.1B)

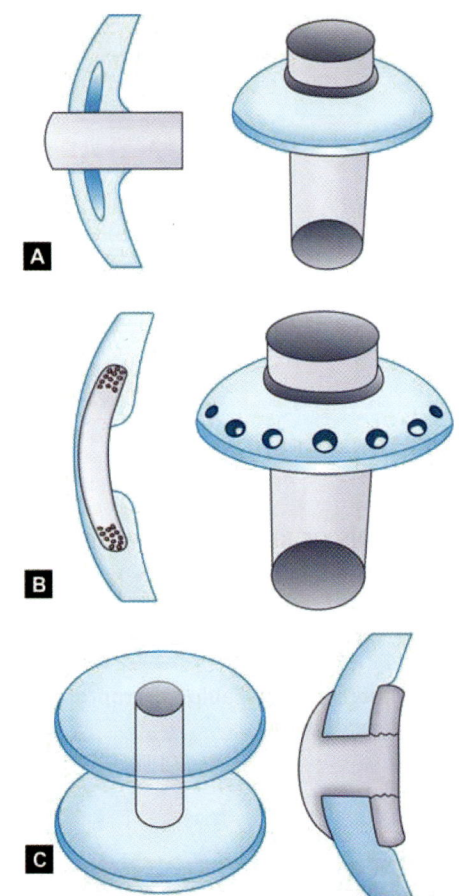

Fig. 40.1: *Basic keratoprosthesis designs: A, First type— PMMA stem with skirt embedded within the cornea; B, Second type—transparent membrane with porous edges inserted into the cornea; C, Third type—PMMA collar button with cornea between*

- *Third type* PMMA 'collar button' with cornea between the plates (Fig. 40.1C).

Types of supporting cover tissue/material of K-Pro

Supporting cover tissue/material adds to the K-Pro complex and is important fact to be considered.

Common supporting tissues/materials used are:

- *Bandage contact lens* is used in Boston type 1 K-Pro. It prevents the carrier graft desiccation.
- *Skin of eyelids* is used as supporting cover in Boston type 2 K-Pro.
- *Buccal mucosa* is used as supporting tissue for the osteo-odonto and Pintucci K-Pros.

SOME COMMERCIALLY AVAILABLE KERATOPROSTHESIS

BOSTON KERATOPROSTHESIS

Also known as Boston K-Pro, consists of two plates with a cylinder in one plate (Fig. 40.2). It takes the shape of collar stud button when fitted. It is fixed using the donor corneal graft. Boston K-Pro is of two types:

Boston type I keratoprosthesis is currently the most commonly used keratoprosthesis device in the US. It consists of a clear plastic polymethyl-methacrylate (PMMA) optic and back plate sandwiched around a corneal graft and secured with a titanium locking ring. After the device is assembled, a partial-thickness trephination is performed on the host cornea. Full-thickness resection of the patient's cornea is then completed using curved corneal scissors. The keratoprosthesis is then secured to host tissue using interrupted or running sutures.

It is used in patients with an adequate wet ocular surface with good blink reflex.

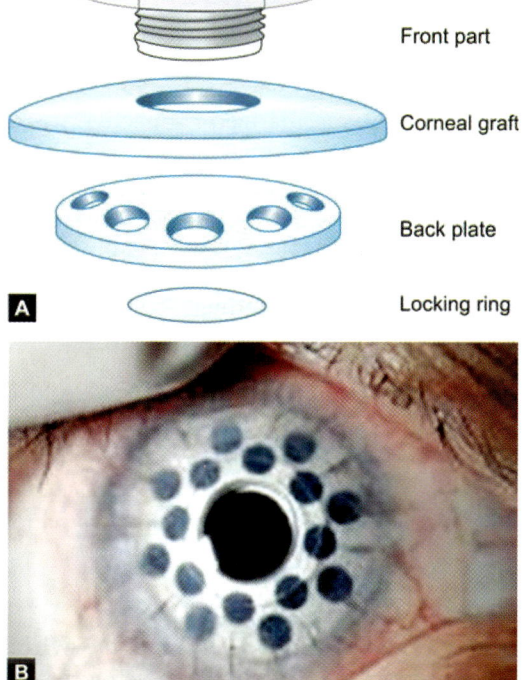

Fig. 40.2: *Boston K-Pro. A, Diagrammatic depiction of parts; B, Fitted in a patient*

Front part

Corneal graft

Back plate

Locking ring

Boston K-Pro type II is used in patients with significant conjunctival scarring, dry eye and exposure. It is fitted through the lids.

MODIFIED OSTEO-ODONTO KERATOPROSTHESIS

The use of osteo-dental tissue for kerato-prosthesis was first described by Strampelli in the early 1960.[10] The modified osteo-odonto keratoprosthesis (MOOKP) (Fig. 40.3) is fixed with the patient's own tooth root and alveolar bone. There is long-term retention of the implant.

Surgery is multi-staged and requires cross speciality experience consisting of:

Stage I: Preparation of globe with buccal mucous membrane graft and preparation of osteo-odonto acrylic lamina (OOAL).

A monocuspidate tooth is removed along with the adjacent maxillary bone and a thin section is cut from the tooth. An optical cylinder made up of PMMA is inserted through a hole made in the section. A pocket is created in the lower eyelid into which the entire prosthesis is inserted and left for 3 months. During this time soft tissue grafts to the bone to which the tooth is attached.

Stage II: Implantation of OOAL: Part of the oral mucosa is stripped off the cornea and sclera to make space for the final implantation of prosthesis. The prosthesis is detached from the eyelid pocket and implanted, with the optical cylinder protruding through a hole in the mucosa.

CHIRILA (ALPHACOR KERATOPROSTHESIS)

It is the newest keratoprosthetic device (Fig. 40.4). It was FDA-approved in August 2002 for patients at high risk for donor penetrating keratoplasty (PKP).

Design

The implant is a 7 mm diameter, one-piece, non-rigid synthetic cornea. It is composed of an outer skirt, that is an opaque, porous, high-water PHEMA (poly[2-hydroxyethyl methacrylate]), with a transparent central optic core of gel PHEMA. An interpenetrating polymer network (IPN) which is junction between skirt and central optic zone and serves as a permanent bond. It has a refractive power close to that of human cornea.

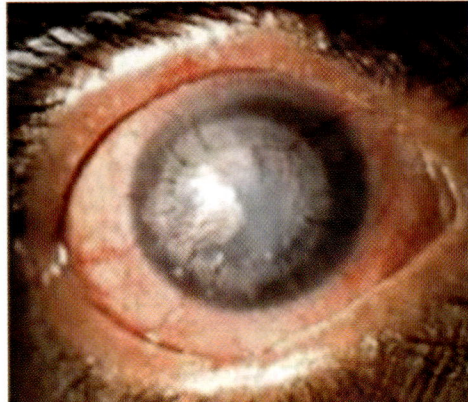

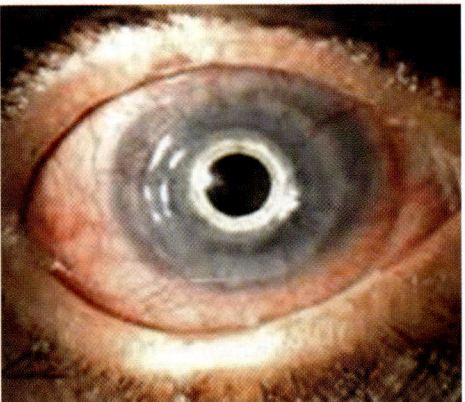

Fig. 40.3: *Modified osteo-odonto keratoprosthesis*

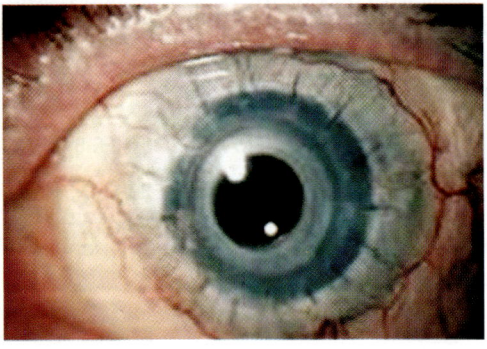

Fig. 40.4: *AlphaCor keratoprosthesis*

Surgical procedure

In Stage I, an intrastromal trephine is used to remove the central posterior corneal lamellae for insertion of the device. A corneal incision is made and dissection instruments are used to continue the corneal dissection throughout the circumference of the corneal graft, thereby creating an intralamellar pocket. An AlphaCor sizer, used to test the size and centration, is inserted into the intralamellar pocket followed by removal of the posterior disc via a 3.5 mm intrastromal trephine. After insertion of the device and closure of the limbal incision, the surface is often covered with a Gundersen conjunctival flap. If the Gundersen flap is inadequate to cover the cornea an amniotic membrane graft may be required.

In Stage II, performed approximately 2 months after Stage I, the overlying conjunctiva created by the Gundersen flap is removed and trephination of the central 4 mm of the conjunctival flap and anterior corneal lamellae is done.

Note: It is used less frequently because it requires 2-stage procedure and there are problems with the retention as well.

PINTUCCI KERATOPROSTHESIS

The Pintucci keratoprosthesis (KP) can be implanted in thinned or perforated corneas, in corneas with stromal melting, and in eyes that have undergone several procedures including penetrating keratoplasty, other KP implantations, and glaucoma, cataract and vitreoretinal surgery.

Design. The supporting element of the Pintucci KP is made of a biointegrated Dacron fabric skirt that allows three-dimensional colonization by newly formed vascularized connective tissue. This fabric is soft and pliable, can be easily cut into the desired shape and sutured, and is chemically inert and not subject to resorption. The Dacron fabric support is fixed to the PMMA optical cylinder with a specific reliable method (international patent pending).

CHONDRO-KERATOPROSTHESIS

It is fixed with patient's own cartilage. Not in use nowadays.

ONYCHO KERATOPROSTHESIS

It is fixed with the help of patient's own nail. It is also not in much use.

STANFORD KERATOPROSTHESIS

It is a recently introduced device which incorporates the grafting of bio-active factors with a change in the bulk material design. Still not popular.

SINGH AND WORST COLLAR-STUD KERATOPROSTHESIS

It is fixed with stainless steel sutures. It has been used and popularised by the designer late Prof. Daljit Singh from India. Presently it is also not popular due to the available better options.

COMPLICATIONS, FUTURE PROSPECTS AND CONCLUSION

COMPLICATIONS

Though the rate of success with keratoprosthesis is high, in rare cases, certain serious complications could occur.

- *Necrosis of tissue around the keratoprosthesis* (which if unchecked can lead to leak, infection, extrusion).
- *Postoperative uveitis*—can lead to the following:
  - Retroprosthetic membrane
  - Vitreous opacities
  - Retinal detachment
  - Macular oedema
  - Epiretinal membrane, etc.
- *Glaucoma*—especially in Stevens-Johnson syndrome, pemphigoid, chemical burns.
- *Infection*—endophthalmitis—now rare
- *Extrusion of the implant* is a serious complication that could occur.
- *Sudden vitritis* can cause a drastic reduction in vision. However, it is possible to treat this condition through antibiotics or by a minor laser surgery.

FUTURE PROSPECTS

Keratoprosthesis is continuously evolving with newer generation materials that seek to improve treatment outcomes. The advances shown herein are only a small sample of the boiling point in which the field of keratoprostheses has recently turned into. Current research is aimed at improving, on the one hand, the anatomical results by using more biocompatible materials that provide better integration with the host tissue, and on the other hand, at providing optimal long-term and sustained visual acuity to our patients. However, postoperative complications remain the great enemy to beat (mainly glaucoma, infection, and extrusion).

Future designs will have to incorporate newer materials that provide excellent optical properties, while at the same time become biointegrated with the ocular tissue. In short, the perfect keratoprosthesis has yet to be discovered, although every day the goal gets closer and closer.

CONCLUSION

Keratoprosthesis carries a somewhat greater burden postoperatively than standard keratoplasty. Successful outcome requires patient compliance, more frequent follow-up and more demands on physician time. However, in cases where keratoplasty appears futile, keratoprosthesis can be most rewarding.

REFERENCES

1. Mannis, M.J.; Dohlman, C.H. The Artificial Cornea: A Brief History. In Corneal Transplantation: A History in Profiles; Mannis, M.J., Mannis, A.A., Eds.; Hirschberg History Ophthalmology; Wayenborgh Press: Oostende, Belgium, 1999; pp. 321–335.
2. Chirila, T.V.; Hicks, C.R. The origins of the artificial cornea: Pellier de Quengsy and his contributions to the modern concept of keratoprosthesis. Gesnerus 1999, 56, 96–106.
3. Keeler, R.; Singh, A.D.; Dua, H.S. Guillaume Pellier de Quengsy: A bold eye surgeon. Br. J. Ophthalmol. 2014, 98, 576–578.
4. Franceschetti, A. Corneal grafting. Trans. Ophthalmol. Soc. UK 1949, 69, 17–35.
5. Györffy, I. Acrylic corneal implant in keratoplasty. Am. J. Ophthalmol. 1951, 34, 757–758.
6. Stone, W.J.; Herbert, E. Experimental study of plastic material and replacement of the cornea; A preliminary report. Am. J. Ophthalmol. 1953, 36, 168–173.
7. Wünsche, G. Versuche zur totalen Keratoplastie und zur cornea arteficialis. Arztliche Forsch. 1947, 1, 345–356.
8. Khan B, Dudenhoefer EJ, Dohlman CH. Keratoprosthesis: An update. Curr Opin Ophthalmol 2001; 12: 282–7.
9. Saeed HN, Shanbhag S, Chodosh J. The Boston keratoprosthesis. Curr Opin Ophthalmol 2017; 28: 390–6.
10. Strampelli B: Osteo Odonto Keratoprosthesis, Ann Ottalmol Clin Ocul.1963; 89: 1039.

Surgical Repair of Corneo-scleral Injuries

CORNEO-SCLERAL TEARS

INTRODUCTION

Corneo-scleral injury is one of the most important causes of unilateral vision loss in developing countries. It represents not only a cause of severe visual loss but also a profound psychological and economic trauma to patients and their families. These injuries are more common in the younger age groups since nearly half of patients are under 40 years of age and majority are males. Corneoscleral injuries, being a major cause of visual morbidity, therefore, urgent and appropriate measures are necessary in these cases to improve the visual outcome.

Although the terminology and classification of trauma have been dealt in Chapter 1, but before going into the details of corneoscleral injuries let us discuss these briefly. The need for a standardized terminology of the types of eye injury has led to the new widely accepted classification designed by the Ocular Trauma Group based on the "Birmingham Eye Trauma Terminology" (BETT).

CLASSIFICATION

Classification of open globe injuries

Type
- a. Rupture
- b. Penetrating
- c. Intraocular foreign body (IOFB)
- d. Perforating
- e. Mixed

Grade (visual acuity)
- a. $\geq 20/40$
- b. 20/50 to 20/100
- c. 19/100 to 5/200
- d. 4/200 to light perception
- e. Absence of light perception

Pupillary response
- a. Positive relative afferent pupillary defect in injured eye
- b. Negative relative afferent pupillary defect in injured eye.

Zone
- i. Cornea and limbus

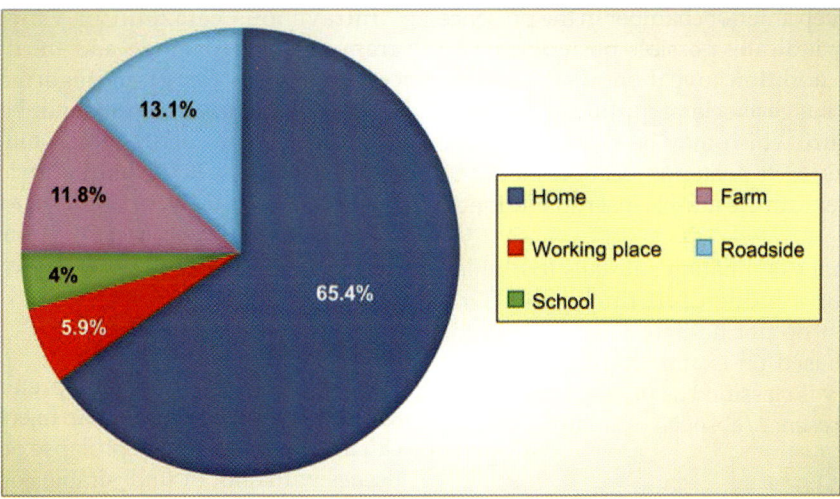

Fig. 41.1: *Distribution of place of injury in cases of ocular trauma*

ii. Limbus to 5 mm posterior into sclera

iii. Posterior to 5 mm from the limbus

EPIDEMIOLOGY

- *Incidence.* Rate of corneo-scleral involvement with serious injuries is 10%.
- *Age.* Younger age group are more commonly involved. Mean age of involvement is 32 years.
- *Sex.* Males are five times more likely to be involved than females.
- *Place.* As per one study, the place of injury has been reported as in Fig. 41.1: 65.4% home, 13.1% roadside, 11.8% farm, 5.9% working place, and 4% school.
- *Cause* of corneo-scleral injuries reported are: 33% blunt object, 13% sharp object, 12% fall, and 12% roadside accidents.

EVALUATION OF A CASE OF CORNEO-SCLERAL TEAR

HISTORY

The foremost step in the management of any corneo-scleral injury repair is detailed history with regards to mode, duration, time and the object of injury. The mechanism of injury makes the examiner vigilant to identify the possibility of unsuspected or occult globe injury, such as globe perforation and posterior scleral rupture. The mode and type of injury alerts the surgeon about the possibility of concomitant microbial contamination and intraocular foreign body. Duration is important since the time elapsed between injury and presentation of the case determines the ultimate prognosis of vision. In addition, the associated life-threatening injuries need to be explored since these will take precedence over ocular injury. Nevertheless corneo-scleral injuries should be addressed as early as possible in order to avoid the devastating complication, like endophthalmitis.

OPHTHALMIC EXAMINATION

The preliminary examination may be carried out by naked eye and direct ophthalmoscope on the bedside of the patient, however, a complete and thorough ocular examination should be done preferably with slit-lamp and 90D fundus examination whenever possible. At no point of time, pressure should be exerted on the eyeball in a suspected case of globe rupture. Best corrected visual acuity and relative afferent pupillary defect are most important prognostic factors. Signs, such as diffuse chemosis; massive subconjunctival haemorrhage; corneal laceration (partial thickness, full thickness), asymmetrical depth of anterior chamber; peaked pupil (the apex of the peak is often aligned with the meridian of the rupture), should be recorded.

Intraocular pressure measurement is contra-indicated in a suspected open globe injury.

However, deep anterior chamber in the presence of hypotony indicates possible posterior scleral rupture. In addition, uveal shows under the conjunctiva suggests scleral rupture and the one scleral rupture which may be trying to escape detection due to its posterior location should be suspected beneath the muscle insertion (thinnest sclera).

If the initial examination still fails to exclude a rupture or a hidden full thickness scleral wound, then do not hesitate to explore in the OT. Thus, based on examination, the corneo-scleral injury is classified as per the type, grade, zone and presence/absence of relative afferent pupillary defect.

INVESTIGATIONS

After assessment of the anterior segment and extent of the injury, several investigations are must in a case of corneo-scleral injury.

- *X-ray orbit* both AP and lateral views to rule out presence of any foreign body and bony fractures.
- *CT scan* is the imaging modality of choice, if we are suspecting an open globe injury. Especially in cases of occult globe rupture, retained intraocular foreign bodies (RIOFBs) and orbital wall fractures.
- *MRI* is contraindicated, if we are suspecting a magnetic foreign body.
- *Cultures* should be sent from the margins of the wound, in case the wound is infected.
- *Ultrasonography* for assessment of posterior segment and any defect in the posterior layer of sclera is contraindicated till the primary repair is completed, otherwise pressure of transducer can extrude intraocular contents in an open globe injury.

MANAGEMENT

PREOPERATIVE MANAGEMENT

The patient should be asked to stay empty stomach for 4–6 hours. If not recently inoculated, patient should receive tetanus vaccine particularly in case of roadside accident or injury by organic matter. Patient should be started on intravenous antibiotics having broad-spectrum coverage.

Intravenous cefazolin or vancomycin for gram-positive coverage and third generation cephalosporin for gram-negative coverage. Open globe injury case must not be prescribed eyedrops or ointments which may permeate through open wound and be toxic to tissues. Finally the anxiety of patient and his/her relatives must be allayed by counselling and prognosis of vision may be explained on the basis of ocular trauma score.

ANAESTHESIA

General anesthesia is usually preferred, and to avoid retrobulbar/peribulbar injections which can induce or aggravate prolapse of intraocular tissues with a lot of undesirable consequences.

GOALS AND PRINCIPLES OF WOUND REPAIR

Goals in the management of corneo-scleral injury include:
- Restoration of the integrity of the globe.
- Avoidance of further injury to ocular tissues.
- Prevention of corneal scarring and astigmatism.

Principles of wound repair are
- *Primary aim*: Complete water-tight closure of the globe with restoration of structural integrity.
- *Secondary aim*: Restoration of normal anatomic relationships, avoidance of uveal tissue and vitreous incarceration in the wound, removal of necrotic tissue debris, removal of disrupted lens, removal of foreign bodies.

SURGICAL PRINCIPLES

Scleral wounds

Anterior scleral wounds (Fig. 41.2) are mostly obvious, however, posterior ones may be difficult to diagnose. Scleral ruptures can sometimes be missed since they can be hidden by the intact conjunctiva and/or large subconjunctival hematoma. In case of any doubts, globe exploration under general anaesthesia should be done. If necessary, a 360-degree peritomy is made so as to retract the conjunctiva and provide good exposure of the sclera. Special attention is given to the areas of muscle insertions as the area beneath them is one of the most common sites for a rupture.

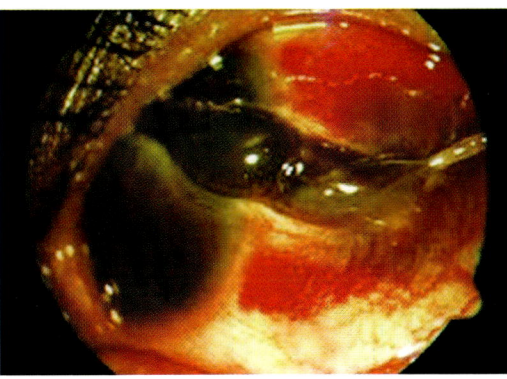

Fig. 41.2: *Corneo-scleral laceration*

Suturing techniques are as below:
- Full thickness scleral wounds are generally apposed with interrupted sutures with "8–0" silk or nylon. A micropoint needle with a spatulated end should be used since it is least traumatic.
- A complete 360-degree periotomy is done to ensure good exposure. The posterior extent, margins and depth of the wound should be identified. If limbus is involved, then first suturing of the limbus to reconstruct it should be done. Scleral wounds are generally closed from anterior to posterior direction.
- Also, unlike the closure of the corneal laceration, in order to prevent prolapse of intraocular contents, the sclera should be closed in a stepwise fashion the so-called "close as you go" technique. This technique involves a limited anterior dissection, exposure of a small portion of the scleral defect, and closure of the visible anterior defect prior to further posterior dissection.
- Prolapsed uveal tissue is gently reposited to avoid incarceration in the wound. If vitreous is present in the wound, then vitrectomy should be done at the scleral surface with the help of vitreous cutter. Prolapsed retinal tissue is gently reposited, if possible.
- If the scleral wound extends under an extraocular muscle, an assistant can retract the muscle gently using a muscle hook to aid in exposure. If more exposure is needed especially if the laceration is under the insertion of the muscle, the same may need to be temporarily disinserted so as to allow the

suturing. Following the closure of the scleral defect, the muscle may be reinserted.

CORNEAL WOUNDS

Suturing techniques

As cornea forms the major refractive surface of the eye, there is a need of restoration of the optically clear, smooth surface and curvature of the cornea. The idea is to appose the edges of the laceration with properly placed sutures at landmarks, such as limbus, sharp angles of laceration and pigmentation lines in epithelium (Fig. 41.3).

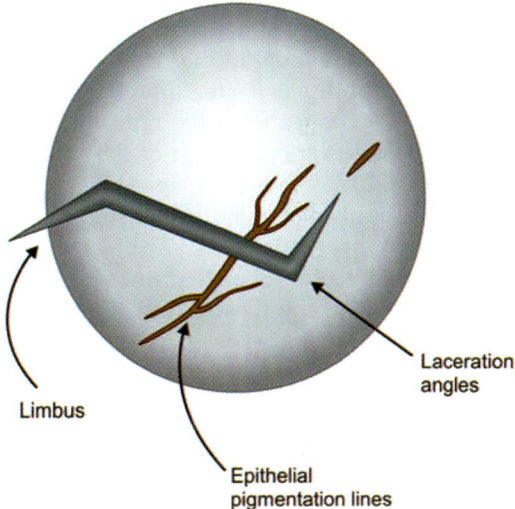

Fig. 41.3: *Landmarks where sutures should be applied*

a. Basic suturing technique. Suturing with interrupted sutures with 10–0 monofilament nylon sutures and micropoint spatulated needles is the preferred method of wound apposition. Suture passes should be approximately 1.5 to 2 mm length in total, i.e. 0.75 to 1 mm on either side. The depth of the sutures should be 85–90% of full thickness, which would mean that the needle passes over the Descemet's membrane. Full thickness corneal lacerations generally have one of the following configurations:
- *Vertical/perpendicular laceration*: The distance from the wound margin to the entry site is the same as the distance from the wound margin to the exit site as shown in Fig. 41.4.

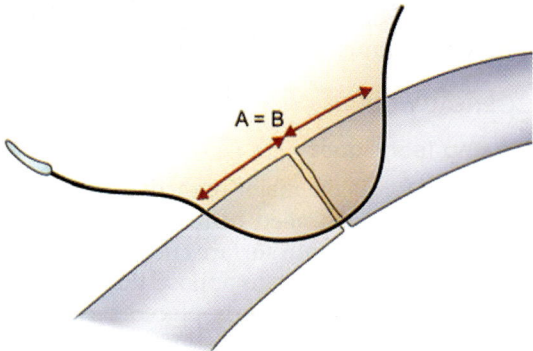

Fig. 41.4: *Corneal suturing technique in a vertical laceration*

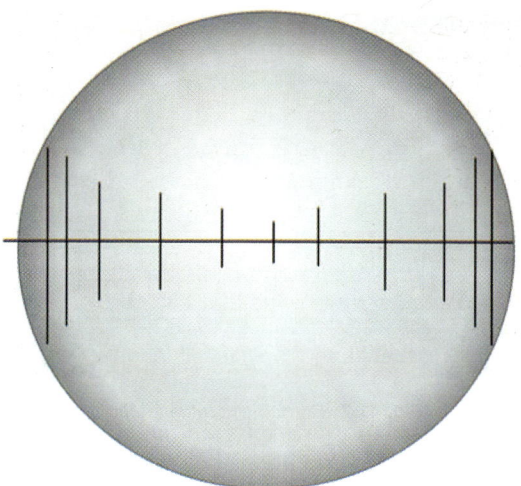

Fig. 41.6: *Rowsey-Hays technique of corneal suturing in a horizontal wound*

- *Oblique/bevelled laceration*: The distance from the anterior margin of the wound to the suture entry site is not equal to that from the same point to the suture exit site. But what matters here is the distance from the entry and exit sites to the posterior margin of the wound, which is equal as shown in Fig. 41.5. Sutures should be applied perpendicular to the surface of the wound to prevent slippage of the wound. Tightening of the suture will cause compression of the tissues, but if correctly done there will not be any eversion or inversion of the edges.

c. Stellate wounds. This is the most difficult problem in corneal wound repair. Techniques useful for a stellate laceration include multiple interrupted sutures, bridging sutures and purse string suture as shown in Fig. 41.7. The centre of a stellate laceration is difficult to appose,

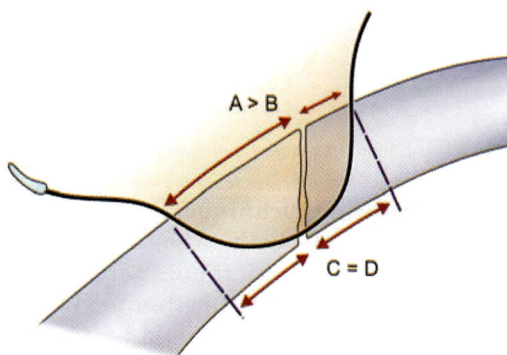

Fig. 41.5: *Corneal suturing technique in an oblique laceration*

b. Rowsey-Hays technique of corneal suturing. The periphery of the wound is closed with long tight compression suture bites. This results in flattening of periphery and compensatory steepening of the corneal centre. The centre is then closed with short, spaced, minimally compressive suture bites to preserve the central steepening as shown in Fig. 41.6. This will result in flattened periphery with a spherical centre.

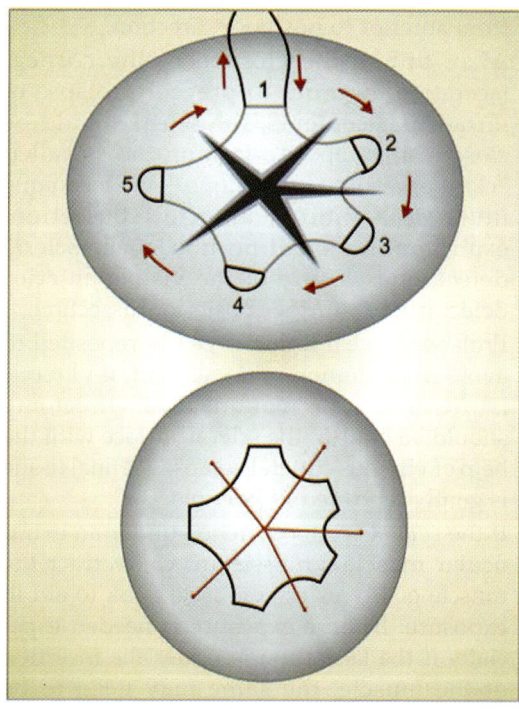

Fig. 41.7: *Corneal suturing technique in a stellate wound*

therefore, requires bandage contact lens application, tissue adhesive or patch grafting.

Profile of corneal wound repair

i. Corneal lacerations without incarceration. It comprises the wound which does not have iris and vitreous incarceration and it does not extend beyond the limbus (Fig. 41.8). Any wound less than 2 mm can be managed with glue with or without bandage contact lens (BCL). Glue to be used can be synthetic or natural, i.e. it can be cyanoacrylate or fibrin glue. Wounds more than 2 mm which are not self-sealing require repair in the operating room by one of the surgical techniques discussed above.

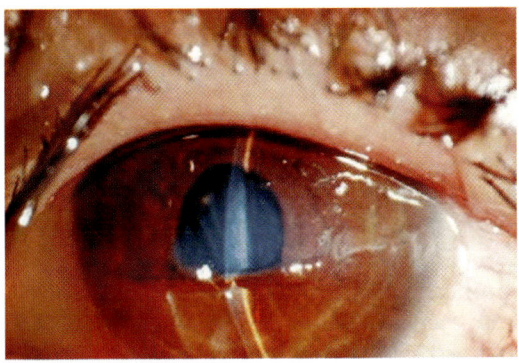

Fig. 41.8: *Corneal laceration without iris incarceration*

ii. Corneal laceration with iris incarceration. Corneal wound is sutured after separating iris from the posterior surface of the wound by sweeping with help of iris repositor and reconstructing the anterior chamber after injecting viscoelastic substance in AC. If iris prolapse is present, then the prolapsed tissue, is assessed for its viability (Fig. 41.9). It is important to resect the prolapsed tissue, if it is more than 24 hours old to prevent any early infection and delayed epithelial ingrowth. Viability of the iris tissue is checked and if it is not necrotic and is not contaminated by discharge and exudates, then repositioning is preferred and iridoplasty is done; whereas if iris tissue is dead, then iris is abscised.

iii. Laceration with vitreous loss/incarceration. Complete vitreous removal from the anterior chamber by bimanual anterior vitrectomy is must. The pupil should be circular, round

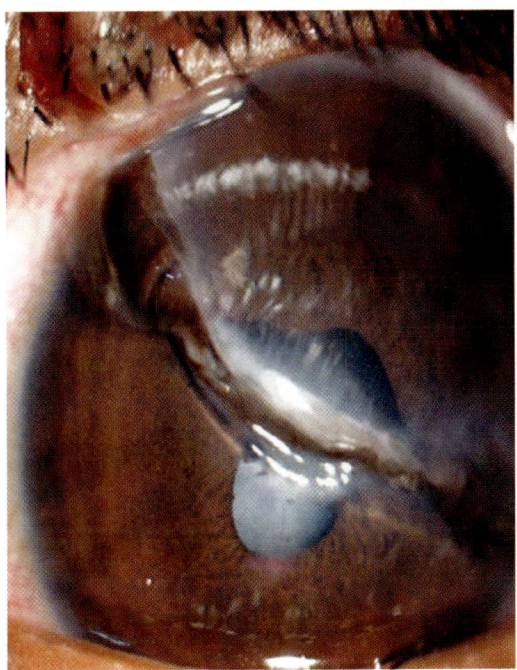

Fig. 41.9: *Corneal wound by glass injury with incarcerated iris tissue*

without peaking. The injury with total lens extrusion and vitreous loss are bad prognosis injuries, especially those in association with intraocular haemorrhage. Such injuries should be assessed regarding the expected postoperative visual gain and if the eyes have no visual potential, then it is better to counsel the patient and his relatives regarding the poor visual prognosis before posting for primary repair.

iv. Loss of tissue. Tissue loss exceeding 5 mm in diameter, a corneal patch graft is usually required. A lamellar patch graft is effective and may be performed with a corneal autograft or donor sclera. These grafts are often located outside of the visual axis; therefore, graft clarity may not be essential for good postoperative vision.

Corneo-scleral wounds

It is common to see corneoscleral ruptures in the superonasal area with a blunt force coming from the unprotected inferotemporal quadrant due to countercoup injury (Fig. 41.10). Here we need to combine the principles of corneal and scleral

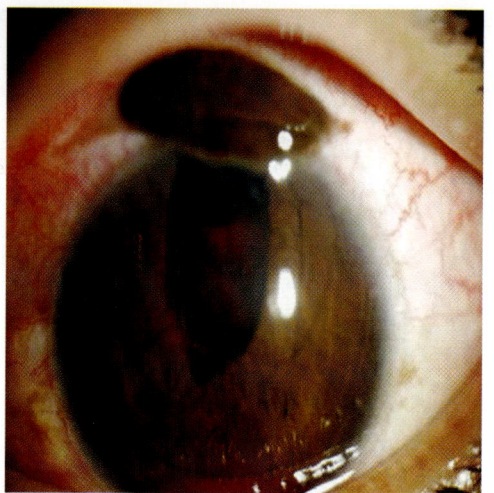

Fig. 41.10: *Corneal scleral tear with iris prolapse and hyphaema*

wound repair. Commonsense dictates that the major landmark here is the limbus which must be apposed and sutured first as shown in Fig. 41.11. Next continue with repair of the corneal aspect followed by the scleral aspect.

INTRAVITREAL ANTIBIOTICS

Injection of 1.0 mg of vancomycin and 2.25 mg of ceftazidime intravitreally may be considered

in contaminated wounds and in injuries with organic matter.

POSTOPERATIVE MANAGEMENT

- *Broad-spectrum antibiotics* topically like moxifloxacin 0.3%. If wound seems to be infected, then fortified cefazolin 5% and tobramycin 0.3% can be added.
- *Intravenous antibiotics* are to be continued as given preoperatively.
- *Cycloplegic drugs,* like 2% homatropine/1% atropine should be given twice daily.
- *Antiglaucoma drugs* may be added, if there is rise of IOP.
- *Topical corticosteroids* are withheld and started 48 hours later after assessing the wound in the postoperative period. In such cases, oral corticosteroids can be given immediately.

Corneal scar

Good apposition of the cut edges with deeply placed corneal sutures leaves a fine scar which gradually thins over a period of 6–9 months. Corneal scars in the pupillary axis which are significantly causing deterioration of vision can be treated by optical penetrating keratoplasty after assessing the posterior segment.

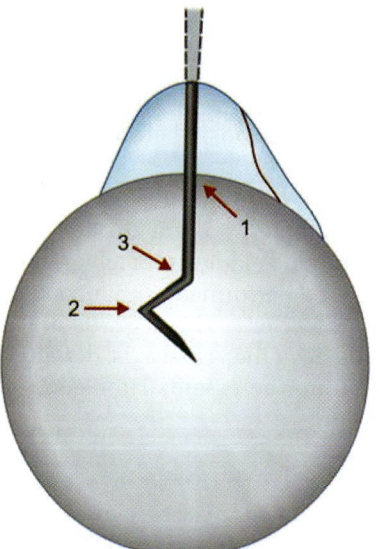

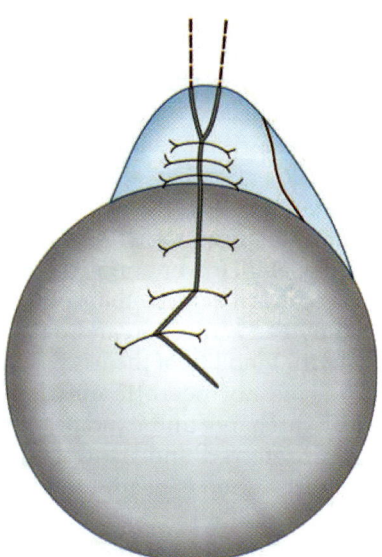

Fig. 41.11: *Suturing technique in a corneo-scleral tear, the first suture should be applied at the limbus. Left side figure shows the anatomic landmarks identified in the corneo-scleral wound. These are limbus (1) and the angles of the wound (2, 3). So, first suture at (1), then corneal part and then scleral part*

Prognosis

The main factors indicating good visual prognosis (6/18 or better) are following:
- Presenting acuity after injury of 6/60 or better,
- Wound location anterior to the pars plana,
- Wound length of 10 mm or less
- A sharp mechanism of injury.

It is seen that wounds longer than 20 mm, which extend posterior to the equator, will lead to poor final vision and subsequent enucleation in the overwhelming majority of cases.

SUMMARY

Conjunctiva and cornea are frequently injured anterior segment ocular structures. Conjunctival injuries are mostly innocuous but may conceal the presence of more serious ocular injury. Corneal injuries frequently are not isolated and are usually sight-threatening and, therefore, require timely and appropriate management. The care of patients sustaining corneo-scleral injuries calls for an approach which should be systematic and methodical. Corneo-scleral lacerations are an important cause of vision loss and should be dealt diligently on an emergency basis so as to improve both structural and functional outcome. Main cause of error is non-identification of true extent of the wound so a proper examination needs to be done. The globe must be closed so that it is water-tight with the restoration of the original anatomy. Long corneal wounds are closed utilizing the Rowsey-Hays technique, whereas scleral wounds extending posteriorly are closed in a stepwise fashion, proceeding posteriorly only after the anterior portion has been sutured. Timely intervention and meticulous evaluations can salvage vision in these compromised eyes.

BIBLIOGRAPHY

1. Fukuyama JI, Hayasaka S, Yamada K, Setogawa T. Causes of subconjunctival hemorrhage. Ophthalmologica 1990; 200: 63–7.
2. Heier JS, Enzenauer RW, Wintermayer SF, et al. Ocular injuries and disease at a combat supported hospital in support of operation desert shield and desert storm. Arch Ophthalmol 1993; 111: 795–8.
3. Hersh SP, Zagelbeum BM. Anterior segment trauma. In: Principles and Practice of Ophthalmology by Albert and Jakobiec. Philadelphia. 2001; 372: 5201–21.
4. McCormack P. Penetrating injury of the eye [editorial]. Br J Ophthalmol 1999; 83: 1101–2.
5. Ocular Trauma Principles and Practice-Ferenc Kuhn, Dante j Pieramici. 2002: Thieme NY 10001.
6. Scott IU, Mccabe CM, Flynn HW, et al. Local anesthesia with intravenous sedation for surgical repair of selected open globe injuries. Am J Ophthalmol 2002; 134: 707–11.
7. Setlik DE, Seldomridge DL, Adelman RA, Semchyshyn TM, Afshari NA. The effectiveness of isobutyl cyanoacrylate tissue adhesive for the treatment of corneal perforations. Am J Ophthalmol 2005; 140(5): 920–1.
8. Sharma A, Kaur R, Kumar S, Gupta P, Pandav S, Patnaik B, Gupta A. Fibrin glue versus N-butyl-2-cyanoacrylate in corneal perforations. Ophthalmology 2003; 110(2): 291–8.
9. Wiedemann P, Konen W, Heimann K. Reconstruction of the anterior and posterior segment of the eye after massive injury. Ger J Ophthalmol 1994; 3: 1–6.

Newer and Evolving Therapeutic Concepts in Corneal Diseases

FEMTOSECOND LASER-ASSISTED KERATOPLASTY

The name Femto is derived from the Danish word for number 15. One femtosecond is equal to 10 to the power minus 15. The femtosecond laser is a focussable, near-infrared (1053 nm) laser that generates ultrashort pulses in the femtosecond (10^{-15} second) range. This is similar to Nd:YAG laser, which uses pulses in the nanosecond (10^{-9} second) duration. When pulse duration is shortened from nanosecond to femtosecond time domain, the energy required for producing tissue breakdown is also reduced. It minimizes collateral tissue damage, inflammation and thermal damage to surrounding tissues. Femtosecond laser vapourizes small volumes of tissue by photodisruption, generating a plasma of rapidly expanding hot ionic gases. The resulting shock wave is followed by formation of a cavitation bubble (CO_2 and H_2O), which in the cornea, eventually escapes through the surrounding stromal tissue. It operates in the infrared wavelength range at 1053 nm. A unique feature of the femtosecond laser is its ability to produce tissue disruption at very low energy settings. This is due to the very short pulse width or pulse duration, associated with the laser (600 to 800 fs), and to the very rapid pulse repetition or speed of the laser (15,000 to 60,000 pulses per second). Because power = energy/time, femtosecond pulses allow energy settings to be low, yet retain high peak power. Consequently, postoperative inflammation can be reduced, especially when pulse repetitions become faster. The increased speed of the laser decreases suction time for enhanced safety and patient comfort and decreases the time of procedure. Tighter spot placement produces better dissection quality and a smoother corneal interface and facilitates flap elevation. There are several uses for the femtosecond laser:

- Penetrating keratoplasty
- Creating corneal flaps for LASIK
- Deep lamellar keratoplasty
- Femtosecond-assisted anterior lamellar keratoplasty (FALK)
- Femtosecond-assisted endothelial keratoplasty (FLEK)
- Creating a channel for INTACS

FEMTOSECOND LASER-ASSISTED PENETRATING KERATOPLASTY

In femtosecond laser-assisted keratoplasty (Fig. 42.1), the donor tissue is cut after mounting it on an artificial anterior chamber with preset parameters—the power, spot separation and line separation. The pattern of trephination can

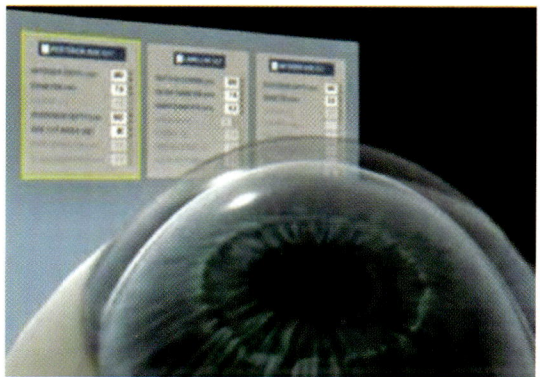

Fig. 42.1: *Femtosecond laser-assisted keratoplasty*

be chosen. For the recipient, the procedure may be performed under topical anaesthesia. As the femtosecond laser is usually located outside the operating room in most settings, and the patient requires subsequent additional preparation for surgery, it is usually desirable not to go full thickness with the host trephination. Leaving a small bridge of uncut corneal tissue ensures globe integrity until the patient is shifted to the operating room. Side cut bridges are generally stronger than lamellar bridges. Once the laser trephination has been performed, the patient can be shifted for surgery, preferably, with the eye shielded. The laser trephination incision may be explored with a blunt instrument like Sinskey hook. The wound edges usually separate easily. Some sharp dissection may be needed in areas of dense corneal scarring. The posterior bridge of uncut corneal tissue may be cut with scissors after entering anterior chamber. Software upgradation with orientation teeth allows greater precision with suture placement.

FEMTOSECOND LASER-ASSISTED DEEP ANTERIOR LAMELLAR KERATOPLASTY (FDALK)

The procedure of deep anterior lamellar keratoplasty or DALK is indicated for pathologies affecting the stroma but sparing the endothelium. These include pathologies like keratoconus, post-refractive surgery, keratectasia, stromal dystrophies and even infectious keratitis. Besides giving a tectonically more stable globe, the procedure completely elimnates the possibility of endothelial rejection. The big-bubble technique for baring of Descemet's membrane is the most popular for preparation of the host bed. However, the technique of DALK is technically challenging. Intraoperative perforation of the Descemet's membrane requiring conversion to a penetrating graft are common. The use of the femtosecond laser may make the procedure simpler, reducing the rate of complications.

A preoperative pachymetry of the cornea is essential to determine the depth of laser trephination. The depth is set about 70–100 μm lesser than the thinnest pachymetry value in the trephination zone. This gives a residual stromal bed with a minimal thickness without posing the risk of perforation. Further refinement of the bed may be done by manual dissection or big-bubble techniques. Laser trephination patterns similar to those in penetrating keratoplasty are used. In case of an inadvertent perforation, the case may be easily converted to a penetrating graft.

FEMTOSECOND LASER-ASSISTED ANTERIOR LAMELLAR KERATOPLASTY (FALK)

It aims at removing the anterior diseased stromal tissue. It is usually indicated for superficial corneal scars and superficial dystrophies, although it has also been performed for keratoconus.

Preoperative considerations

A preoperative anterior segment OCT imaging is required to assess the depth of involvement of the stroma by the pathologic process as well as to determine the total corneal thickness. FALK may not be performed, if the total corneal pachymetry is below 300 μm or the residual bed of clear stroma is estimated below 120 μm.

Operative procedure

The procedure is performed in two steps. First, the donor corneal tissue is prepared, mounted over an artificial anterior chamber. Next, the recipient cornea is treated. An oversizing of about 0.2 mm prevents corneal flattening, especially if sutures are required. For superficial stromal pathologies, FALK can be performed without sutures. This has the potential to greatly limit postoperative astigmatism and enhance visual rehabilitation. FALK can usually be performed even with dense corneal scars by increasing the laser energy and reducing spot separation. However, for extremely dense pathology that limits visualization of the anterior segment, it is advisable not to perform this procedure.

FEMTOSECOND LASER-ASSISTED ENDOTHELIAL KERATOPLASTY (FLEK)

The femtosecond laser has also been used to cut donor endothelial discs for Descemet's stripping endothelial keratoplasty (DSEK). The donor is prepared after mounting on an artificial anterior chamber. After the lamellar cut is made, a trephine is used to punch a required diameter of the donor disc. The recipient is prepared by scoring the Descemet's membrane, following which the donor can be inserted by any chosen technique. FLEK requires deep lamellar cuts, at about 400 μm, within the corneal stroma. At such depths, microkeratomes have been found to give smoother interfaces and better cut quality. For this reason, FLEK has not gained as much popularity as the other techniques of femtosecond laser-assisted keratoplasty.

ADVANTAGES AND DISADVANTAGES OF FEMTOSECOND LASER OVER MICROKERATOMES

Advantages of femtosecond laser over microkeratomes

- Ability to create predictable flap diameter and thickness as compared to mechanical microkeratome.
- Ability to create flaps in eyes with different corneal and/or orbital configuration.
- It is free from complications like decentred and free flaps, irregular edges and surface, epithelial abrasions, button hole perforations, cap lacerations and inadequate diameter for a given correction.
- Reoperation can be done after waiting period of 45 minutes unlike microkeratome systems which require at least 3 months before reoperations can be attempted.
- Can be performed in opaque corneas
- It has less incidence of induced optical aberrations as compared to microkeratome created flaps.
- Greater accuracy of flap creation
- Lesser intraocular pressure rise during suction
- Fewer higher order aberrations
- Less dry eye
- Better contrast sensitivity.

Disadvantages of flaps produced by femtosecond laser

- Incomplete flaps
- Suction breaks
- Granular bed
- Transient light sensitivity

DESCEMET MEMBRANE ENDOTHELIAL TRANSFER

Since its introduction in 2002, Descemet membrane endothelial keratoplasty (DMEK) has increasingly become the globally preferred surgical treatment option for patients with corneal endothelial disorders. More recently, 'Descemet membrane endothelial transfer' (DMET) has been reported, in which descemetorhexis is followed by insertion of an almost completely free-floating Descemet roll (i.e. with the graft contacting the posterior cornea only at the corneal incision) aiming to obtain corneal clearance by endothelial cell migration. Currently, the preferred treatment option for corneal endothelial diseases, such as Fuchs endothelial corneal dystrophy and pseudo-phakic bullous keratopathy, is endothelial keratoplasty in order to restore corneal clarity. DMEK provides excellent and rapid visual recovery in these cases. However, DMET technique is technically more simple but that has also given us more insight into the processes involved in endothelial cell wound healing. Although the mechanisms for cell migration and endothelialization are not still completely clear, DMET may provide corneal clearance in difficult cases where, after descemetorhexis, the complete unfolding and/or attachment of the graft would be not achieved, and the surgery would otherwise be considered unsuccessful. By converting from DMEK to DMET, the cornea may still clear eventually without the need for a re-surgery and a new donor graft.

DMET consists of the implantation of a Descemet roll that is mostly 'free floating' in the anterior chamber being attached only to the corneal incision. DMET is a simplified version of DMEK. As in DMEK surgery, DMET technique involves performing three side ports, a 9 mm descemetorhexis with a reversed Sinskey hook and a 3.0 mm tunnel incision at the limbus for the insertion of the graft. The donor graft is stained with a 0.06% Trypan Blue solution sucked into a custom-made injector and placed into the recipient anterior chamber as a roll. In contrast to DMEK, there is no need to unfold the Descemet roll or to completely attach the

graft onto the recipient corneal surface. However, contact between the donor Descemet roll and the host posterior stroma is ensured by fixating the proximal edge of the graft within the corneal tunnel incision. To do so, once the graft is injected through the main incision, the proximal end should be kept within the tunnel incision (but the graft should not protrude on the surface). The fixation can be done by pushing gently with the tip of the cannula until the end of the graft is in place.

DMET technique represents a tremendous simplification from DMEK. The challenging steps of DMEK (unfolding and attaching the graft to the stroma) can be circumvented with the DMET technique because it eliminates the most technically difficult parts of DMEK and also the need for an intraocular air bubble to induce and maintain graft attachment. Removing the need for an air bubble tamponade significantly shortens the duration of the surgical procedure and also removes the risk of pupillary block glaucoma because no air bubble is left in the anterior chamber.

As in DMEK, postoperative medication includes chloramphenicol and dexamethasone 0.1% changed to fluorometholone 0.1% at 1 month after surgery. It has been suggested that endothelial cell migration and proliferation are possible mechanisms by which corneal clearance might be achieved. Endothelial cell proliferation in human corneas is, however, thought to be rare since the mitotic activity of endothelial cells *in vivo* is arrested in G1 phase and inhibited by several different factors, such as the presence of transforming growth factor β in aqueous humor or the lack of effective growth factor stimulation. However, the potential for human corneal endothelial cells to migrate in normal human eyes had been previously also suggested by the spontaneous resolution of corneal oedema following large persistent Descemet membrane detachments following cataract surgery and, even more important, after descemetorhexis without endothelial graft implantation. In these last cases where the descemetorhexis was not followed by the implantation of the graft, confocal images of the central cornea showed an almost complete repopulation of the bare areas with irregular endothelial cells. However, despite the presence of endothelial cells in the area of the descemetorhexis, not all patients achieved complete corneal clearance.

RHO KINASE INHIBITION IN CORNEAL DISEASES

RHO KINASES

Rho kinase is a serine/threonine protein kinase involved in the modulation and regulation of cell size and shape by acting on cytoskeleton. They are involved in regulation of calcium independent smooth muscle contraction, control of cytoskeletal dynamics, actomyosin contractile forces, cell adhesion, cell stiffening, extracellular matrix reorganization and cell morphology.

History of Rho kinase inhibitors

Research on Rho kinase started from late 1990s and has continued till present. The majority of research has emphasized on intraocular pressure (IOP) lowering effect of Rho kinase (ROCK) inhibitors. Fewer studies have dealt with effect of Rho kinase inhibitor on diabetic retinopathy and healing effects on corneal endothelium. In 1998, Alan Hall elucidated the relationship between Rho pathway and actin cytoskeleton functions. He showed that Rho kinase pathway was an important regulator of actin cytoskeleton. In 2001, studies began at University of Tokyo in Japan and Duke University in North Carolina to investigate the effects of Rho kinase inhibitors on lowering of IOP. They were designed to discover how aqueous humor outflow facility was increased by ROCK inhibitors. In 2014, Ripasudil, a ROCK inhibitor, gained approval in Japan to be specifically used for treatment of ocular hypertension and glaucoma. As recently as December 18th, 2017, Rhopressa, a Rho kinase inhibiting drug consisting of Netarsudil, gained FDA approval.

Rho kinase signalling pathway

Rho kinase is a downstream effector of Rho A protein, a small GTPase. GTPases alternate between two conformations: A guanosine triphosphate (GTP) bound active conformation and a guanosine diphosphate (GDP) bound inactive conformation. This GTPase activation regulation is controlled by guanine nucleotide exchange factors (GEFs), GTPase activating proteins (GAPs), and guanine nucleotide dissociation inhibitors (GDIs). After activation of Rho A, the coiled-tail serine/threonine kinase, the downstream effector Rho kinase, becomes active. The Rho kinase has two isoforms—ROCK 1 and ROCK 2. Rho kinase phosphorylates various intracellular substrates, the myosin light chain and the LIM kinase. These substrates interact to control actomyosin contractility, membrane permeability, cellular adhesion, cell stiffening, cell morphological changes, extracellular matrix organization as well as DNA synthesis.

Corneal endothelium

The innermost layer of cornea is the corneal endothelium, which controls corneal hydration. It is formed by a single layer of flattened cells. The corneal endothelium, through its pump and leak barrier functions, maintains corneal transparency by regulating amount of water inside corneal stroma. One characteristic of corneal endothelial cell is poor regenerative ability. Consequently, any damage to the corneal endothelium is repaired by compensatory migration and spreading of the residual CECs to cover the wounded area, with a resultant drop in CEC density. This density is typically 2000–2500 cells/mm^2 in a normal subject, and a drop below a critical level, usually less than 500–1000 cells/mm^2 can cause corneal oedema due to decompensation of corneal endothelium. The only current therapeutic choice for treating corneal endothelial decompensation is keratoplasty. Penetrating keratoplasty, in which a whole-thickness cornea is replaced with a donor cornea, has been performed since 1906. Descemet's stripping endothelial keratoplasty (DSEK) was introduced to reduce the invasiveness of penetrating keratoplasty and improve clinical outcomes. The further introduction of Descemet's membrane endothelial keratoplasty (DMEK) is now resulting in higher recovery of visual quality even in comparison to DSEK. The evolution of surgical procedures has enabled less invasive treatment of corneal endothelial decompensation with better clinical outcomes. However, these surgeries still have associated issues, such as the difficulty of the actual surgical technique, graft rejection, acute and chronic cell loss and the shortage of donor corneas. Thus, Rho kinase (ROCK) inhibitors can be used for both pharmaceutical and tissue engineering treatment. Due to varied cellular responses controlled by Rho kinase signaling pathway, Rho kinase inhibitors increase cell adhesion and proliferation in corneal endothelium. It allows preservation of corneal endothelial cells and slowing of apoptosis. Thus, Rho kinase inhibitors help with acute corneal endothelial damage, that can potentially occur in cataract surgery.

ROLE OF RHO KINASE INHIBITORS IN CORNEAL ENDOTHELIAL DISEASES

Healing of corneal endothelium

Inactivation of Rho kinase blocks serum stimulated DNA synthesis, whereas activation of Rho A induces G1/S progression in fibroblasts. Inhibition of Rho/ROCK signaling pathway suppresses cell cycle progression in various cells, including lung carcinoma, melanoma and kidney tumor cells. Treatment of endothelial cells with Rho kinase inhibitor increases cyclin D levels and suppresses phosphorylation of p27kip1 by activation of phosphatidylinositol 3-kinase signaling. Cyclin D and p27 are regulators of G1/S progression. Effect of ROCK inhibition can vary depending on the status of the cornea. They cause increased proliferation and decreased apoptosis. In general, the corneal endothelium has a very limited proliferating capacity. Thus, any structural damage is repaired by migration of remaining corneal endothelial cells to afflicted area with resultant drop in endothelial density. There have been two proposed methods of delivery of ROCK inhibitors to heal the corneal endothelium, including topical eye drops and anterior chamber injection with cultured endothelial cells.

Cell division

Cells in the corneal endothelium are frozen in the cell cycle. They cannot divide due to inhibiting factors in their surroundings and the tightly packed pattern of the corneal endothelium. Furthermore, ROCK inhibitors, when used to treat corneal endothelial cells, allow for increased cyclin D levels and suppression of phosphorylation of cyclin-dependent kinase inhibitor 1B, p27kip1, which are regulators of cell division in corneal endothelial cells.

Slowing of cellular apoptosis

Rho kinases are directly related to apoptosis due to cellular responses associated with its pathway. The actin cytoskeleton contractile force, regulated by Rho kinase, allows for cellular contraction, membrane blebbing, and nuclear disintegration. Apoptosis in the corneal endothelium can be inhibited using ROCK inhibitors, which stop this contractile force from killing the cells. It has been shown that apoptosis can be slowed within a day of using Rho kinase inhibitors.

Increased cell adhesion

Cellular adhesion is a key component in healing of corneal endothelium. One method of healing the corneal endothelium is an anterior chamber injection of cultured endothelial cells and a Rho kinase inhibitor. Cellular adhesion allows for successful propagation of these cells. ROCK inhibitors allow for increased cellular adhesion due to the enhancement of actomyosin contractility. Therefore, there is a greater potential for healing of corneal endothelial trauma using injection of cultured endothelial cells and Rho kinase inhibitors.

Fuchs' corneal dystrophy

Fuchs' endothelial corneal dystrophy is a progressive disease resulting in corneal endothelial cell loss. Cell death is one of the major contributing factors for disease progression. The current mainstay method of treatment for Fuchs is keratoplasty. Another treatment option is the use of Rho kinase inhibitors as an intracameral injection of cultured corneal endothelial cells. This procedure consists of injecting a combination of cultured corneal endothelial cells and an ROCK inhibitor in the anterior chamber of the eye and then allowing the patient to lie face down to allow the cells to be directed towards the corneal endothelium. The ROCK inhibitor facilitates increased adhesion of the cultured cells to the substrate, leading to an increase in corneal endothelial regeneration and restoration of corneal transparency.

Acute corneal trauma

Acute corneal trauma can lead to corneal degeneration. The risk for corneal degeneration increases with decreasing density of corneal endothelial cells. ROCK inhibitors can be used to increase the proliferation rates of these cells to allow for greater density in this layer. This allows for increased healing and migration of corneal endothelial cells to cover the afflicted area.

INTRACAMERAL INJECTION OF CULTIVATED ENDOTHELIAL CELLS

The human corneal endothelium is non-regenerative *in vivo*. Because endothelial cell loss due to dystrophy, trauma or surgery is followed by a compensatory enlargement of the remaining endothelial cells which results in permanent corneal endothelial dysfunction. Penetrating keratoplasty for corneal endothelial dysfunction is not risk free and alternative methods for replacing the endothelium without corneal trephination and sutures have been developed, including posterior lamellar keratoplasty, deep lamellar endothelial keratoplasty, and Descemet's stripping endothelial keratoplasty. Fresh donor corneas are necessary to treat corneal endothelial dysfunction and because their availability is limited, replacement of endothelial cells with cultivated corneal endothelial cells (CECs) constitutes an important alternative treatment method for corneal endothelial dysfunction.

The human corneal endothelium (CE) plays a critical role in regulation of corneal hydration, maintaining corneal thickness and keeping cornea transparent. The human CE has a very limited propensity to proliferate *in vivo*. Hence, in order to replace dead or damaged corneal endothelial cells (CECs), the existing cells spread out to maintain functional integrity and sustain corneal deturgescence. In a situation whereby an individual experiences accelerated or acute corneal endothelial cell loss due to either accidental or surgical trauma, endothelial dysfunction may occur. This results in their inability to pump fluid out of the stroma, causing stromal and epithelial oedema, loss of corneal clarity and visual acuity and eventually bullous keratopathy. Arrested in phase G1 of the cell cycle, HCECs do not regenerate *in vivo*, and further cell loss by accidental or surgical trauma, or genetic dystrophies leads to loss of endothelial function.

In vitro expansion of HCECs using a two-step peel-and-digest culture method faces the challenge of endothelial to mesenchymal transition (EnMT). This transformation of canonical, hexagonal-shaped HCECs toward a fibroblastic fate becomes evident after only a few passages and leads to the disruption of the cellular monolayer, loss of tight junctions and cell-cell contact inhibition, as well as changes in the extracellular matrix composition, cell morphology, and function.

STABILISING MEDIA COMPONENTS

Table 42.1 depicts the stabilising media components.

Significant efforts have been garnered for the development of tissue-engineered cultured endothelial cells that may potentially

Table 42.1: *Stabilising media components*

	Stabilising media 1	Stabilising media 2
Base media	Human endothelial serum free media	OPTI-MEM media
Base media composition	Artificial liquid media; sodium selenite	Artificial liquid media; sodium selenite ammonium metavandate
FBS	4%	4%
Antibiotics	50 µg/ml gentamicin, IX antibiotic anti-mycotic solution	50 µg/ml gentamicin, IX antibiotic anti-mycotic solution

circumvent the shortage of transplant grade donor corneas. To facilitate the development of a tissue-engineered endothelium, the ability to cultivate the human corneal endothelial cells (CECs) in an *in vitro* culture system is critical. HCEnCs have a capacity to proliferate *in vitro*. Therefore, cultured HCEnCs could be a prospective alternative treatment for corneal endothelial diseases. Several methods to define the media, conditions, isolation techniques, etc. for cultivation of HCEnCs have been successfully investigated.

GENE THERAPY IN CORNEAL DISEASES

INTRODUCTION

Gene therapy is a technique that uses genes for treatment or prevention of diseases. It allows treatment of a disorder by inserting a gene into patient's cells. Several approaches have been tried for gene therapy.

- Replacing a mutated gene with healthy copy of gene.
- Introducing a new gene into body
- Inactivating, or 'knocking out', a mutated gene that is not functioning properly.

Gene therapy is the term applied to any treatment that mediates its therapeutic effect via application of a nucleic acid based product be it DNA, RNA or various synthetic analogues. It modifies gene expression within the target cell, either by directly correcting a deleterious mutation or to mediate a more beneficial effect such as promotion of cell survival. All cells in human body contain genes making them potential targets for gene therapy. Gene therapy introduces genetic material into cells to compensate for abnormal genes or to make a beneficial protein. If a mutated gene causes a necessary protein to be faulty or missing, gene therapy may be able to introduce normal copy of gene to restore protein function. These cells can be divided into somatic cells and germ cells. Gene therapy using germ cells results in permanent changes that are inherited to subsequent generations. It produces permanent transmissible modifications in phenotype by modifying the gametes or embryo in early stages of development. Somatic gene therapy is the modification of specific cells of body confined to that patient. It is more conservative and safe approach as it affects only targeted cells and is not passed to further generations and its effects are short lived.

TYPES OF SOMATIC GENE THERAPY

Ex vivo

- Genes are transferred to the cells grown in culture, transformed cells are selected, multiplied and then introduced into the patient.
- The use of autologous cells avoids immune system rejection of introduced cells.
- The cells are sourced initially from the patient to be treated and grown in culture before being reintroduced into same individual.

In vivo

- It involves the transfer of cloned genes directly into tissues of the patient.
- It is done in case of tissues whose individual cells cannot be cultured *in vitro* in sufficient numbers.
- Liposomes and certain viral vectors are employed for this purpose.

CORNEAL TISSUE FOR GENE THERAPY

The cornea is an ideal tissue for gene therapy due to ease of access and relative immune-privilege. Several gene transfer vectors have been evolved. Next generation viral and nano-particle vectors, characterization of delivered gene levels, localization have propelled gene therapy towards establishing gene-based therapies for corneal blindness. Gene therapy to the cornea can potentially correct inherited and acquired diseases of the cornea.

GENE THERAPY VEHICLES FOR CORNEA

A carrier, i.e. vector, is genetically engineered to deliver the gene. Vectors can be divided into viral and non-viral delivery systems. Certain viruses are often used as vectors because they can deliver the new gene by infecting the cell. The vector can be injected or given intravenously directly into a specific tissue in the body where it is taken up by individual cells.

Major considerations in determining the optimal vector and delivery system are (1) the target cells and its characteristics, i.e. the ability to be virally transduced *ex vivo* and reinfused to the patient, (2) the longevity of expression required, and (3) the size of the genetic material to be transferred.

VIRAL VECTORS

Viruses can be used to deliver genes into different cells and tissues. Viruses can be used as vector in 70% cases (Fig. 42.2A and B). The most commonly used viral vectors are derived from retrovirus, adenovirus, and adenoassociated virus (AAV). Other viral vectors that have

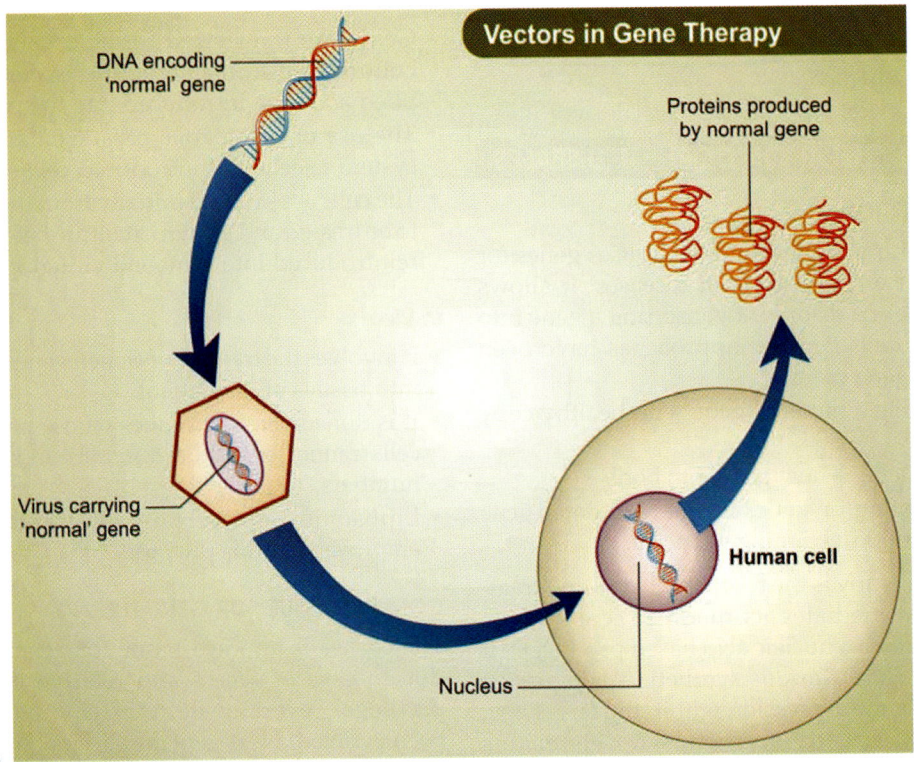

A

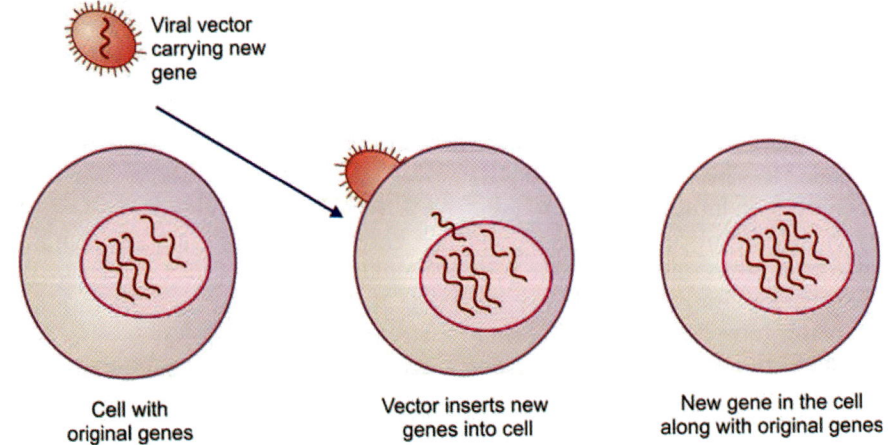

B

Fig. 42.2A and B: *Viral vectors for gene therapy*

been less extensively used are derived from herpes simplex virus 1 (HSV-1), vaccinia virus, or baculovirus. Nonviral vectors can be either plasmid deoxyribonucleic acid (DNA), which is a circle of double-stranded DNA that replicates in bacteria or chemically synthesized compounds that are or resemble oligodeoxynucleotides. Among viral vectors, AAV appears promising for corneal gene therapy because of their potency and safety profile. Recombinant AAV vectors have shown great promise for ocular gene therapy and restoration of vision in patients with no major side effects.

Advantages of viral vectors
- They have high transfection efficiency.
- Target specific type of cells.
- Very good at targeting and entering cells.

Disadvantages of viral vectors
- High immunogenicity
- High cost of production
- Low packaging capacity
- Carry lesser amount of genetic material

NON-VIRAL VECTORS

Introduction of plasmid DNA expressing therapeutic genes into target cells without use of viruses constitute non-viral gene transfer methods. Non-viral gene therapy is safer than viral due to low toxicity, immunogenicity and pathogenicity. Additionally, plasmid vector production is cost effective. The chief advantage to non-viral methods is that they are usually completely non-immunogenic, however, they also present with several substantial disadvantages, most significant of these being their limited efficacy *in vivo*. Effective gene delivery by non-viral methods is hampered by many factors including vector instability *in vivo*, loss of vector to interaction with non-target tissues, intracellular processing leading to mislocalisation or destruction of the transgene and loss of transgenic construct upon cell division. Whilst much progress has and continues to be made, non-viral methods currently lag behind the alternative of virally mediated gene therapy, with inspiration for improvements of non-viral

systems often being gleaned from viruses themselves.

Microinjection technique

Introduction of plasmid via microinjection has led to successful delivery of genes including GFP, interleukin (IL)18, Flt23k and endostatin into various cells of cornea. Microinjection targeting different layers of cornea has been performed including intrastromal, subconjunctival and directly into the anterior chamber (Fig. 42.3).

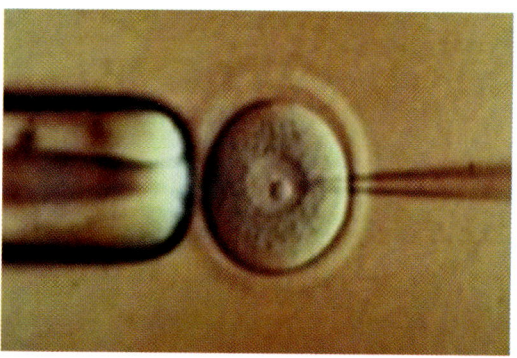

Fig. 42.3: *Microinjection technique*

Electroporation

Electroporation (Fig. 42.4), also known as electrogenetherapy or electropermeabilization, makes use of high-intensity electrical pulses to form transient pores in the cell membrane and is useful for gene delivery in both cultured eye cells and ocular surface tissues *in vivo*. An advantage is that large DNA constructs can be transported into cells although specialized equipment is necessary.

Sonoporation

Sonoporation (Fig. 42.5) employs ultrasound waves to create pores in the plasma membrane in order to deliver DNA to the nucleus. Ultrasound is effective for cell transfection *in vitro* and *in vivo*. Transfection efficiency of this approach is dependent on the transducer frequency, acoustic pressure, output strength, and pulse duration of ultrasound treatment in addition to the use of contrast agents such as microbubbles. Microbubbles were generated as contrast agents to not only enhance imaging but

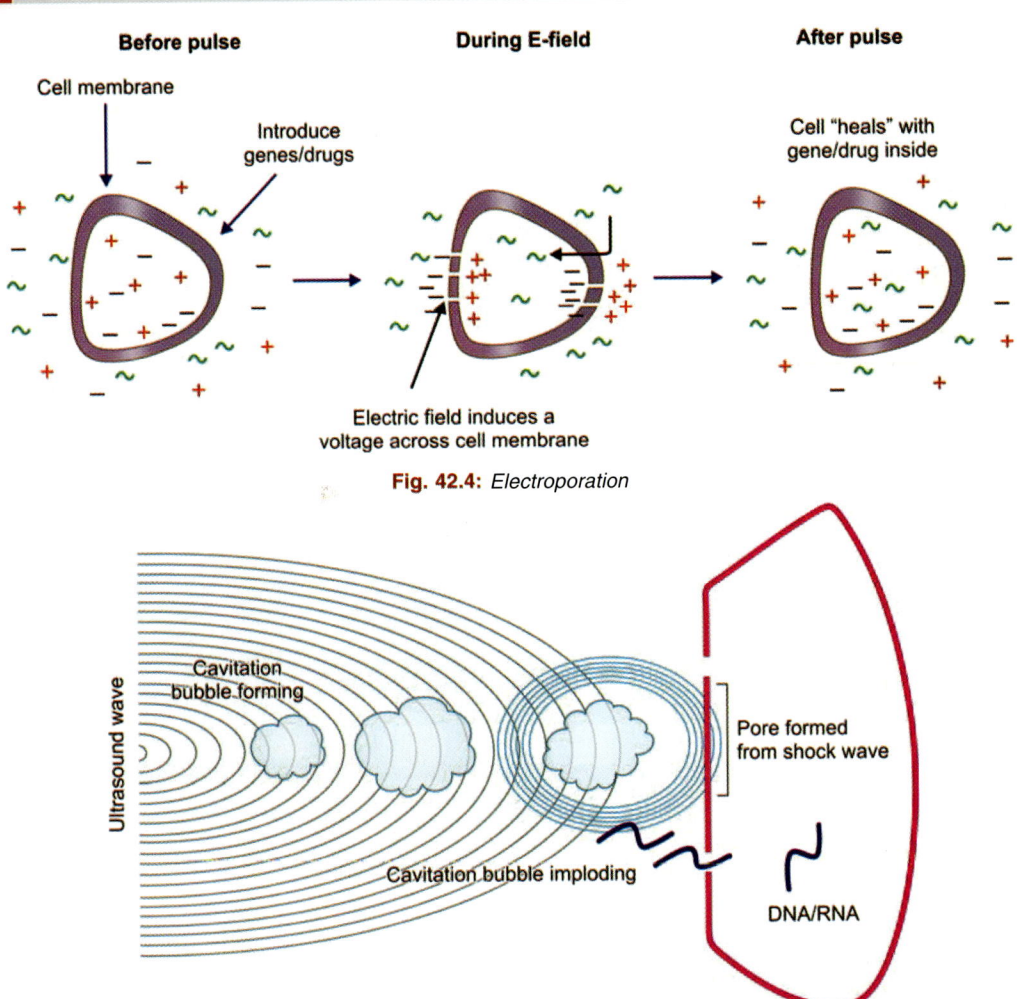

Fig. 42.4: *Electroporation*

Fig. 42.5: *Sonoporation*

also improve gene delivery efficiency by boosting cell permeability.

Gene gun

Gene gun (Fig. 42.6) is a ballistic (also called bioballistic) gene transfer method. It utilizes microsized biologically inert heavy metal (gold, silver or tungsten) particles and mechanical or macroprojectile (centripetal, magnetic or electrostatic) force. The bombarding of DNA-coated particles on cells/tissues with high velocity results in gene transfer. Gene delivery with gene gun depends on many factors such as amount of DNA-coated on particles, temperature, amount of cells, amount of force, number of DNA-coated particles, etc. Shallow penetration of particles, substantial cell damage, uncontrolled gene transfer, high cost, access to internal organs, etc. are a few among many limitations of this method. The successful gene delivery in the cornea with gene gun has been reported. Genes such as IL-4 and IL-10 plasmid DNA and opioid growth factor receptor (OGFr) have been introduced into the corneal epithelium with this method.

Laser

Recently, a stromal pocket technique involving the use of the femtosecond laser to introduce genes into the pig cornea *ex vivo* was reported.

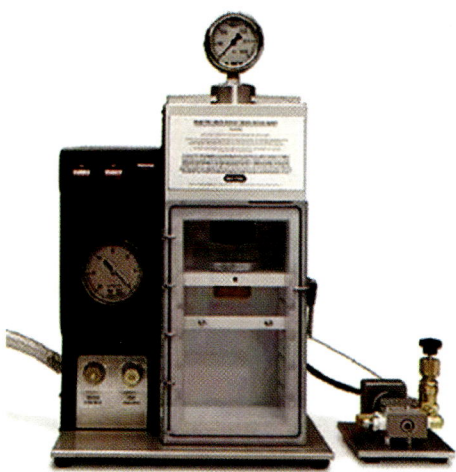

Fig. 42.6: *Gene gun*

A stromal pocket 110 µm in depth was produced with a femtosecond laser and lentiviral vector expressing GFP was injected. Histology of corneal tissue performed 5 days after vector application showed wound closure and marker gene expression in the cells (most likely keratocytes) around the corneal pocket. Interestingly, the levels of transgene expression noted at day 5 remained up to 3 weeks. This method facilitates gene delivery into cells in a specific, targeted corneal region. However, femtosecond laser is known to induce intense wound healing and infiltration of inflammatory cells in the rabbit cornea.

Chemicals

Scores of natural and synthetic chemicals have been tested to introduce genes into corneal cells. Among many lipids dioleoyltrimethylammonium chloride (DOTMA), dioleoylphosphatidylethanolamie (DOPE), 1,2-dioleoyl-3-trimethylammonium-propane (DOTAP), dimethyldioctadecylammonium bromide (DDAB), 3β-[N-(N,N-dimethylaminoethane) carbamoyl)cholesterol (DC-cholesterol), and N-methyl-4(dioleyl) methylpyridinium chloride (SAINT-2) have shown promise for corneal gene therapy.

Advantages of non-viral vectors

- Better safety profile
- Lower cost of production

Disadvantages of viral vectors

- Low transfection efficiency
- Insufficient cellular uptake
- Poor targeted delivery

ROLE OF GENE THERAPY IN CORNEAL DISEASES

Corneal disorders are the 3rd leading cause of blindness in the world according to the World Health Organization. Eight million people in the world, including 1.5 million children, are blind due to corneal abnormalities. Gene therapy holds great promise for treating as well as preventing corneal diseases and disorders.

Corneal graft rejection

Keratoplasty is currently used for treating many corneal diseases. Corneal graft rejection due to immunological reaction is the chief cause of failure despite the cornea enjoying an immune privilege status. Postoperative complications and lack of good quality donor corneas are the other concerns. Gene therapy approaches have been tested to improve allograft survival by delivering various therapeutic genes to modulate cellular transport, apoptosis, angiogenesis, and wound healing *in vivo*.

Corneal scarring and wound healing

Wound healing plays a central part in the maintenance of corneal transparency and thus normal vision. Corneal injury, regardless of cause, may ignite a dysregulated wound healing response that commonly leads to corneal fibrosis and loss of visual function. Corneal wound healing is an extremely intricate process under the regulation of several cytokines and growth factors. Among several cytokines, transforming growth factor beta (TGF-β) has been identified as a chief player in the formation of myofibroblasts and opacity in the cornea. Thus, it has become a prime target for gene therapy aimed at preventing corneal scarring and other corneal disorders caused by TGF-β. Many investigators share the thought that impeding TGF-β or its signal transduction represents a powerful strategy to modulate uncontrolled corneal healing and prevent or even cure corneal scarring.

Corneal neovascularization

Neovascularization may occur in any of the layers of the cornea following ocular trauma, infection, injury, etc. and leads to corneal opacity. The sprouting of new blood vessels in the cornea from the limbus is closely linked to the inflammatory response and poses a major risk for corneal allograft rejection. The mechanism of neovascular formation and regression is tremendously complex involving cytokines, growth factors, and cell types. However, it is widely accepted that vascular endothelial growth factor (VEGF) plays a pivotal role in the development of new blood vessels. Gene therapy strategies using endostatin have also shown promise in treating CNV. Endostatin, a naturally occurring fragment of collagen type XVIII, blocks endothelial cell adhesion, migration and proliferation, and inhibits apoptosis.

Corneal alkali burn

Alkali burn injury to the cornea is a major clinical entity that leads to sight-threatening sequelae such as corneal scarring, neovessel formation, and ulceration. In 2007, the Saika group outlined the use of adenovirus to introduce peroxisome proliferator-activated receptor γ (PPARγ) to keratocytes in a mouse alkali burn model. Gene therapy employing PPARγ, a nuclear hormone receptor with immunomodulatory functions, has been evaluated extensively for non-ocular tissues. In the cornea, a faint expression of PPARγ was noted via immunohistochemistry in the undamaged corneal epithelium as well as corneas subjected to NaOH and treated with Cre-adenovirus.

Herpes simplex keratitis

Corneal inflammation due to ocular herpes simplex virus (HSV) infection, or herpes stromal keratitis (HSK), is a leading cause of infectious blindness worldwide particularly in more developed nations including US recurrent infections often lead to corneal scarring, neovascularization and thinning resulting in visual abnormalities and blindness. Many studies have shared the common goal of developing a vaccine using gene transfer technology to enhance protection against ocular HSV. These studies have used individual HSV-1 glycoproteins (i.e. gD) as well as a cocktail of glycoproteins and have shown variable success in controlling HSV keratitis. The recent development of a humanized HLA-Tg rabbit model will hopefully assist in the design of future vaccines for HSV-1 keratitis as it demonstrates spontaneous HSV reactivation leading to recurrent HSK comparable to what is seen clinically. Moreover, this rabbit model expresses human, rather than rabbit, HLA class I proteins.

Corneal dystrophy

Necessary requirements for attempts at gene therapy for a corneal dystrophy are:
- The genetic defect must have been identified and mapped.
- Vision must be significantly impaired or likely soon to be impaired.
- No better or equivalently effective treatment must be available.
- Treatment must be capable of modulating existing corneal pathology.
- Delivery of the genetic manipulation material must be practicable and safe.

BIBLIOGRAPHY

1. Byrne SM, Mali P, Church GM. Genome editing in human stem cells. Methods Enzymol 2014; 546: 119–38.
2. Chamberlain WD, Rush SW, Mathers WD, et al. Comparison of femtosecond laser-assisted keratoplasty versus conventional penetrating keratoplasty. Ophthalmology 2011; 118: 486–91.
3. Dapena I, Ham L, Melles GR. Endothelial keratoplasty: DSEK/DSAEK or DMEK-the thinner the better? Curr Opin Ophthalmol. 2009; 20: 299–307.
4. Engelmann K, Friedl P. Optimization of culture conditions for human corneal endothelial cells. *In Vitro* Cell Dev Biol 1989; 25: 1065–72.
5. Jonas JB, Rank RM, Budde WM. Immunologic graft reactions after allogeneic penetrating keratoplasty. Am J Ophthalmol 2002; 133: 437–43.
6. Klausner EA, Zhang Z, Wong S, Chapman RL, Volin MV, Harbottle RP. Corneal gene delivery: chitosan oligomer as a carrier of CpG rich, CpG free or S/MAR plasmid DNA. J Gene Med 2012; 14: 100–8.

7. Koizumi N, Sakamoto Y, Okumura N, et al. Cultivated corneal endothelial cell sheet transplantation in a primate model. Investigative Ophthalmology & Visual Science 2007; 48(10): 4519–26.

8. Mian SI, Shtein RM. Femtosecond laser-assisted corneal surgery. Current Opinion in Ophthalmology 2007; 18(4): 295–99.

9. Mosca L, Fasciani R, Tamburelli C, et al. Femtosecond laser assisted lamellar keratoplasty: early results. Cornea 2008; 27: 668–72.

10. Okumura N, Kinoshita S, Koizumi N. Cell-based approach for treatment of corneal endothelial dysfunction. Cornea 2014; 33(Suppl 11): S37–S41.

11. Okumura N, Kinoshita S, Koizumi N. The role of Rho kinase inhibitors in corneal endothelial dysfunction. Current Pharmaceutical Design 2016; 23(4): 660–66.

12. Rao R, Borkar DS, Colby KA, et al. Descemet membrane endothelial keratoplasty after failed Descemet stripping without endothelial keratoplasty. Cornea 2017; 36: 763–66.

13. Slade SG. Applications for the femtosecond laser in corneal surgery. Current Opinion in Ophthalmology 2007; 18(4): 338–41.

14. Stewart RM, Hiscott PS, Kaye SB. Endothelial migration and new Descemet membrane after endothelial keratoplasty. Am J Ophthalmol 2010; 149: 683.

15. Wang J, Quake SR. RNA-guided endonuclease provides a therapeutic strategy to cure latent herpes viridae infection. Proc Natl Acad Sci USA. 2014; 111: 13157–62.

16. Zhou J, Wang J, Shen B, et al. Dual sgRNAs facilitate CRISPR/Cas9-mediated mouse genome targeting. FEBS J 2014; 281: 1717–25.

Section
VIII

Corneal Blindness and Eye Banking

Chapter
43

Corneal Blindness: An Overview

INTRODUCTION

Blindness continues to be one of the major public health problems in developing countries. Using World Health Organization (WHO) definition of blindness as a visual acuity of 3/60 or less, it is estimated that currently there are 45 million individuals worldwide who are bilaterally blind and another 135 million who have severely impaired vision in both the eyes. Cataract and corneal diseases are the major causes of blindness in developing countries. Figure 43.1 shows the estimates of corneal blindness worldwide. In India, it is estimated that there are approximately 6.8 million people who have vision less than 6/60 in at least one eye due to corneal diseases; of these, about a million have bilateral involvement. It is expected that the number of individuals with unilateral corneal blindness in India will increase to 10.6 million by 2020. According to estimate there is addition of 50,000 corneal blindness cases every year in the country. The burden of corneal diseases in our country is reflected by the fact that 90% of the global cases of ocular trauma and corneal ulceration leading to corneal blindness occur in developing countries.

CAUSES OF CORNEAL BLINDNESS

The epidemiology of corneal blindness is complicated and includes a variety of infectious and inflammatory eye diseases that cause corneal scarring, which ultimately leads to functional blindness. It is highly dependent on the ocular diseases that are endemic in each geographical area.

Causes of corneal blindness include a wide variety of infections and inflammatory eye diseases, ranging from keratitis, xerophthalmia, eye trauma, trachoma, congenital diseases and traditional eye medicines or home remedies, which often harm the eye rather than relieve pain or improve eyesight. The causal factors responsible for corneal blindness vary with age.

- *In adults*, residing in countries with less developed economies, significant causes of corneal blindness (based on indications of keratoplasty) are corneal traumatic scars , non-traumatic scars and active keratitis.

- *In children*, common causes of corneal blindness are xerophthalmia and ophthalmia neonatorum. It is estimated that approximately half of all childhood blindness in India is preventable or treatable, to which vitamin A associated corneal blindness is a significant contributor. Each year there are half a million new cases, 70% of which are due to vitamin A deficiency which leads to xerophthalmia.

PREVENTION OF CORNEAL BLINDNESS

Objectives regarding corneal blindness under 'Vision 2020', in India are:
- To reduce prevalence of preventable and curable corneal blindness.
- To identify the infants at risk in cooperation with RCH programme.

Nearly 80% of all corneal blindness is avoidable. Prevention is more cost-effective than surgical intervention, as demonstrated by success in reducing corneal blindness from trachoma, vitamin A deficiency, and onchocerciasis. Preventing corneal blindness in the community involves action by the community itself, as well as actions by government and non-governmental organisations in the form of health and development services.

LEVELS OF PREVENTION

Prevention of corneal blindness takes place at three levels:
1. **Primary prevention:** Actions or interventions taken to prevent the onset of disease.
2. **Secondary prevention:** Actions taken to prevent complications and/or the development of visual disability due to an existing disease.
3. **Tertiary prevention:** After the immediate problem has been addressed by surgery or other treatment, actions to restore function or reduce existing disability from disease complications, i.e. corneal transplantation.

1. PRIMARY PREVENTION

There are many social factors associated with corneal diseases, such as poverty, inadequate water supply, sanitation, poor nutrition and dangerous agricultural practices. A good programme should support the community to obtain the health care and other services it needs, either by mobilising the community's own resources or by lobbying government for help. To address the immediate medical causes and risk factors, the programme should provide health education about risk factors and how to avoid them, as well as information about what to do and where to go for help if an eye problem develops.

2. SECONDARY PREVENTION

Many health and community development programmes already in existence, such as measles immunisation, perinatal care, nutrition, water supply, and sanitation, make a significant contribution in reducing the most common causes of corneal blindness. It is important to support these programmes by informing policy makers and funding agencies of their impact on the prevention of blindness, as this will increase the motivation of those involved and may improve the prospects for continued political and financial support.

3. TERTIARY PREVENTION

Tertiary prevention consists of keratoplasty but it is not always possible or suitable.

STRATEGIES FOR CONTROL OF CORNEAL BLINDNESS

GENERAL STRATEGIES

1. Identification of infants at risk in cooperation with RCH programmes to take appropriate measures.
2. Identification of preschoolchildren at risk by door to door survey.
3. Identification of schoolchildren through school health services.
4. Identification of senior citizens with pseudophakic or aphakic bullous keratopathy.
5. To ensure supply of essential drugs required for primary eye care—tetracycline eye ointment, antibiotic eye drops and vitamin A supplements.
6. A total ban should be placed on the ophthalmic practice by quacks and sale of

harmful eye medicines especially various 'surmas'.

7. The eyes of industrial workers and agriculturists should be given protection by goggles and eye shades.

8. The use of traditional eye medicines (TEM) is a public health problem that exists throughout the developing world. Educating traditional healers and eliciting their co-operation in directing patients to appropriate health care facilities is a first step in preventing complications leading to blindness from the use of traditional medicines.

DISEASE SPECIFIC STRATEGIES

1. Eye infections including ophthalmic neonatorum

Ocular prophylaxis at birth with broad spectrum antibiotics is very important. Efforts to decrease the incidence of ophthalmia neonatorum include prevention of sexually transmitted diseases in adults, antenatal screening of pregnant women, ocular prophylaxis at birth and early diagnosis and treatment of ocular infections in neonates.

- Studies have shown that a 2.5% solution of aqueous *povidone iodine* applied to the eyes of neonates is just as effective and cheaper than erythromycin ointment or 1% silver nitrate (Crede's prophylaxis) in preventing the majority of cases of chlamydial and gonorrhoeal ophthalmia neonatorum. Tetracycline ointment may also be used.

- If *topical prophylaxis fails*, a single intramuscular injection of cefataxime (100 mg/kg) is effective against gonorrhoea in newborn, and a two-week course of erythromycin orally (50 mg/kg daily in four divided doses) is recommended for the treatment of Chlamydia.

- *Health education and improvement* in personal hygiene will reduce the incidence of conjunctivitis, corneal ulcer and other eye infections.

- *Early treatment of eye infections* will prevent corneal blindness.

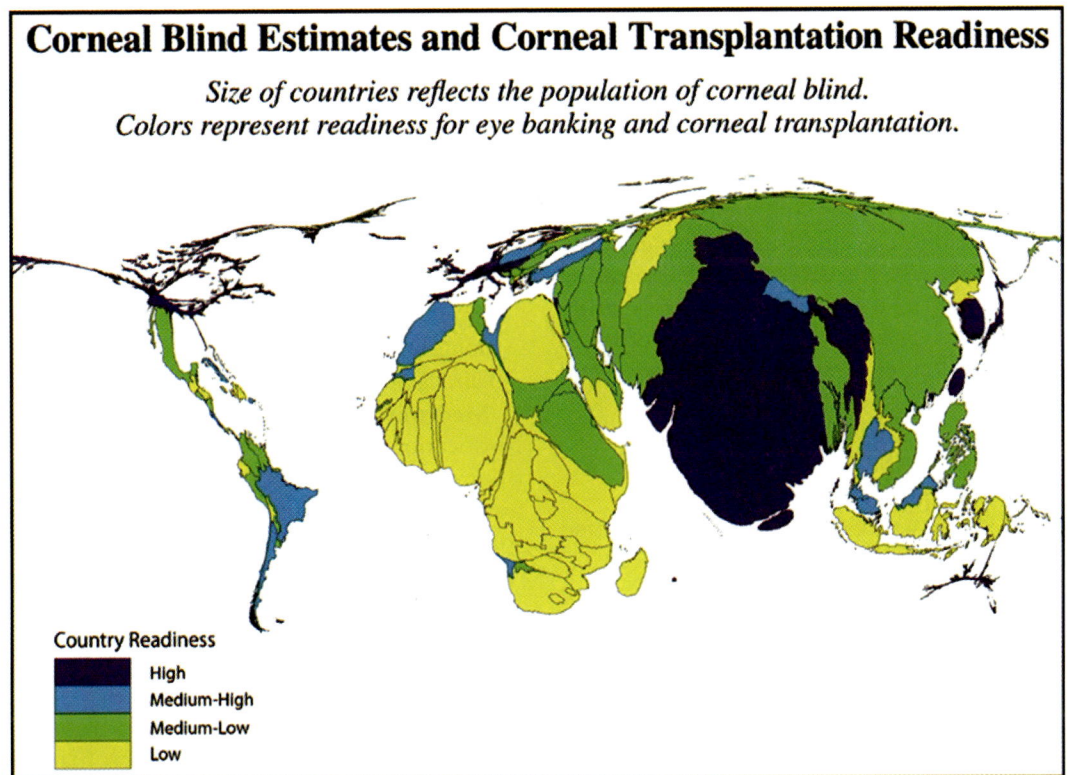

Corneal Blind Estimates and Corneal Transplantation Readiness

Size of countries reflects the population of corneal blind.
Colors represent readiness for eye banking and corneal transplantation.

Country Readiness

- High
- Medium-High
- Medium-Low
- Low

Fig. 43.1: *Corneal blind estimates worldwide*

2. Eye injuries

Health education regarding *avoidance of ocular trauma* like blast, industrial accidents, road accidents and other trauma should be provided thus reducing permanent corneal blindness.

- *Ocular trauma cases should be immediately referred* to specialists for effective management. There should be facilities for administration of general anaesthesia for ocular trauma patients at secondary eye care level.

3. Measles

Primary prevention consists of measles immunisation. *Secondary prevention* consists of vitamin A treatment for children with measles and treatment of corneal ulcers.

4. Trachoma blindness

Trachoma is a leading cause of preventable blindness worldwide with an estimated 5.9 million persons blind or at immediate risk because of trichiasis. The disease accounts for nearly one-sixth of the global burden of blindness. In India, corneal blindness due to trachoma (0.39% WHO-NPCB, 1986–88) is on decline when compared with previous figures (20% ICMR, 1975). However, in isolated pockets (focal) blindness related to trachoma continues to be important. The emphasis on prevention is essential because the outcome of penetrating keratoplasty in trachoma patients is often disappointing due to extensive corneal vascularization, ocular surface problems, and the invariable presence of entropion and trichiasis.

Prevention of trachoma blindness

Effective interventions have been demonstrated in developing nations using **SAFE** strategy:
- **S**urgery to correct lid deformity and prevent blindness,
- **A**ntibiotics for acute infections and community control,
- **F**acial hygiene, and
- **E**nvironmental change including improved access to water and sanitation and health education.

Elimination of blindness due to trachoma is considered feasible, eradication of trachoma is not. Trachoma has disappeared from North America and Europe because of improved socio-economic conditions and hygiene. Research needs include validation of rapid community assessment techniques, identification of barriers to the acceptance of preventive surgical procedure, studying effectiveness of annual treatment cycles and cost effective studies. WHO has organized an Alliance for Global Elimination of Trachoma by the year 2020 (GET, 2020).

5. Prevention of xerophthalmia

Prevention of xerophthalmia will strongly decrease number of corneal blinds.

Prophylaxis against xerophthalmia

The three major known intervention strategies for the prevention and control of vitamin A deficiency are:

a. **Short-term approach.** It comprises periodic administration of vitamin A supplements. WHO recommended universal distribution schedule of vitamin A for prevention is depicted in Table 43.1.

A revised schedule of vitamin A supplements being followed in India since August 1992, under the programme named 'Child Survival and Safe Motherhood (CSSM)' is as follows:

First dose (1 lakh IU)—at 9 months of age along with measles vaccine.
Second dose (2 lakh IU)—at 18 months of age along with booster dose of DPT/OPV.
Third dose (2 lakh IU)—at 2 years of age.

b. **Medium-term approach.** It includes food fortification with vitamin A.

c. **Long-term approach.** It should be the ultimate aim. It implies promotion of adequate intake of vitamin A rich foods such as green leafy vegetables, papaya and drumsticks. Nutritional health education should be included in the curriculum of children in schools.

6. Onchocerciasis (river blindness)

Onchocerciasis leads to blindness through an inflammatory response to the microfilaria of *Onchocerca volvulus* in the retina and the cornea. Control programmes have been very effective in preventing blindness through the mass distribution of ivermectin and measures to control the Simulum fly. With the administration of one tablet of ivermectin twice a year to all individuals in endemic areas, it is estimated that there will be no new cases of onchocerciasis by the year 2020.

7. Traumatic corneal abrasion

Traumatic corneal abrasion is a common event and is the major risk factor for microbial keratitis in low and middle income countries. Simple topical antibiotic prophylaxis for a few days while the epithelium heals can protect the eye from developing potentially blinding infection.

KERATOPLASTY AND EYE BANKING

There is a need of around 2 lakh corneas per year for transplantation to clear the backlog of corneal blindness in India. Currently we are collecting around 60,000 eyes per year. As keratoplasty operation can restore vision in a significant number of coarneal blinds, an intensive publicity and cooperation of government and non-government agencies is needed to enhance the voluntary eye donations. Under NPCB, eye donation fortnight is organized from 25th August to 8th September every year to promote eye donation. More eye banks should be established and more ophthalmic surgeons should be trained for corneal grafting. *Under Vision 2020: Indian initiative* emphasis is on hospital retrieval system to get better donor material. Death certificates should bear one line on eye donations.

ORGANIZATIONS DEVOTED TO CORNEAL BLINDNESS

NATIONAL PROGRAM FOR CONTROL OF BLINDNESS AND VISUAL IMPAIRMENT

National policies and programmes on corneal blindness have focused almost entirely on sustaining infrastructure for eye banking by providing grants for setting up of eye banks and eye donation centres, reimbursing processing fees for cornea collection and keratoplasty surgeries done free of cost with a little to no

investment in prevention programmes. From being a 100% centrally sponsored scheme, there has been a shift in budget allocation to 60:40 (NPCB: States) except in the North East States where it is 90:10. Despite the change in funding pattern, states continue to reserve maximum funds for cataract surgery and refractive error. For example, in the state of Uttar Pradesh which has the highest prevalence of blindness in the country, nearly 60% of the state NPCB budget for 2018–2019 has been carved out for cataract surgery. Similar trends are noticed in most other states, leaving the epidemic of preventable corneal blindness unaddressed.

RECOMMENDATIONS

National government

- Realign national policy response to shift focus solely from eye banking and corneal transplants to cost-effective, quality screening prevention programmes that prevent future corneal blindness.
- Integrate and scale-up prevention efforts as a component of comprehensive eye healthcare at all levels to ensure scalability and sustainability.
- Institute surveillance data on the various causes of blindness and visual impairment affecting the Indian population including corneal blindness.
- Work with the ILO and WHO, adopt and implement internationally accepted protective standards for the Indian workforce at high risk of eye trauma and injury.

State government

- Allocate adequate human and financial resources for corneal blindness prevention programmes in the State Programmatic Implementation Plan (PIP) budgets to National Health Mission (NHM).
- Enlist the support of state health machinery including ASHAs and ophthalmic assistants at Primary Healthcare Centres (PHCs) to screen and treat for corneal injury and trauma.
- Integrate corneal blindness prevention efforts with ongoing interventions by eye health organisations, particularly in rural and hard to reach areas.

- Create a referral network with local eye hospitals for patients diagnosed with corneal abrasions who require further treatment and care.

NPCB's ACTION PLAN

1. To enhance eye donation

a. Training of eye donation counsellors
b. Eye banks integration
c. Eye banks accreditation and standardisation
d. Celebration of eye donation fortnight annually.

2. To improve quality of retained donor material

a. Create awareness for early donation within 2–6 hours.
b. Best of storage facilities to assure better storage of donor cornea. NPCB provides non-recurring assistance of ₹ 1 lakh to eye donation centres and ₹ 15 lakhs to selected eye banks.
c. Availability of high quality storage medium —NPCB assures availability of high quality storage media.
d. Availability of specular microscopes.

3. To increase the number of skillful cornea surgeons in India

To increase the number of skillful cornea surgeons in India, more and more ophthalmologists are being trained in the field of keratoplasty at various tertiary eye care centres.

■ SEE INTERNATIONAL

SEE (Surgical Eye Expeditions) International is a non-profit humanitarian organization founded in 1974. SEE International is working diligently to reduce the number affected by corneal blindness around the world by:

- Performing corneal grafts and transplants
- Teaching appropriate surgical techniques

- Training local eye care personnel in ophthalmology in rural and urban areas
- Strengthening local health care infrastructure, including encouraging the development of local eye banks.

■ BIBLIOGRAPHY

1. Dandona R, Dandona L. Corneal blindness in a southern India population: Need for health promotion strategies. Br J Ophthalmol 2003; 87: 133–41.
2. Gilbert C, Foster A. Childhood blindness in the context of VISION 2020—the right to sight. Bull WHO 2001; 79: 227–32.
3. Li S, Xu J, He M, et al. A survey of blindness and cataract surgery in Doumen County, China. Ophthalmology 1999; 106: 1602–08.
4. Murthy GV, Gupta SK, Bachani D, Jose R, John N. Current estimates of blindness in India. Br J Ophthalmol 2005; 89: 257–60.
5. Nirmalan PK, Thulasiraj RD, Maneksha V, Rahmathullah R, Ramakrishnan R, Padmavathi A, et al. A population based eye survey of older adults in Tirunelveli district of south India: Blindness, cataract surgery, and visual outcomes. Br J Ophthalmol 2002; 86: 505–12.
6. Rahi JS, Sripathi S, Gilbert CE, Foster A. Childhood blindness in India: causes in 1318 blind school students in nine states. Eye 1995; 9: 545–50.
7. Saini JS, Reddy MK, Jain AK, Ravindra MS, Jhaveria S, Raghuram L. Perspectives in eye banking. Indian J Ophthalmol 1996; 44: 47–55.
8. Tandon R, Sinha R, Moulick P, Agarwal P, Titiyal JS, Vajpayee RB. Pattern of bilateral blinding corneal disease in patients waiting for keratoplasty in a tertiary eye care centre in northern India. Cornea 2010; 29: 269–71.
9. Thylefors B. A global initiative for the elimination of avoidable blindness. Indian J Ophthalmol 1998; 46: 129–30.
10. Yorston D, Foster A. Traditional eye medicines and corneal ulceration in Tanzania. J Trop Med Hygiene 1994; 97: 211–14.

Chapter

44

Eye Banking

INTRODUCTION

Eye banks are the institutions, which are *responsible for harvesting and processing of donor corneas.*[1] Corneal harvesting is the surgical removal of either the whole eye (enucleation) or only the cornea (*in situ* corneal excision), from a deceased person. Eye banks are a part of local health system and may be attached to either a hospital or be housed in a separate building. *Donor tissue retrieval can be performed by* trained eye bank technicians, ophthalmology residents, ophthalmologists, or by general practitioners. This can be done in a variety of settings, including hospitals, homes or in funeral grounds.[2] *Procurement of the donor cornea* is the primary goal of eye banks. While this fact is recognized, the need for rigorous quality control in eye banking is not appreciated by the eye bankers and the surgeons in India and the other developing countries.[2]

As per the current evidence, there are 1.0–1.2 million bilateral corneal blind and 5–6 million unilateral corneal blind patients in India. An estimated number of 50,000 new cases is added per year. To overcome this level of blindness the goal is 100,000 transplants/year. Meeting this demand requires double the number of corneas to be harvested, i.e., 200,000 annually. Each eye bank with adequate infrastructure and trained manpower can process 4000 corneas per year, which translates to 50 eye banks for the entire country.

- *An eye bank holds the dual responsibilities of ensuring the safety and efficacy of donor corneas* and ensuring fair and equitable distribution of transplantable corneas.
- Eye banks also carry out *ancillary services* including the supply of donated sclera for glaucoma, oculoplasty and retinal surgery and preparation and distribution of human amniotic membrane and pre-cut tissues for endothelial keratoplasty.
- *Research activities* for improvement of the preservation methodology, corneal substitutes.

EYE BANKING SYSTEM

A three-tier structure has been developed for efficient functioning of eye banking system (Fig. 44.1).

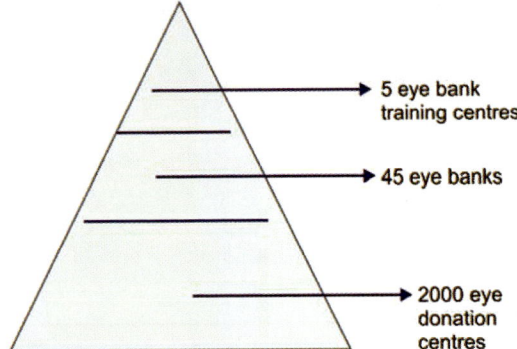

Fig. 44.1: *The 3-tier structure of eye banking system*

- *Eye bank training centres* numbering five, one for each of the five zones in the country, are the top of pyramid.
- *Eye banks*, about 45, are the second level.
- *Eye donation centres.* The 50 eye banks and eye bank training centres are networked with 2000 eye donation centres, which occupy the base of pyramid.[2]

Eye donation centre (EDC)

Eye donation centres (EDCs) are the peripheral satellites of an eye bank for better functioning. One EDC is viably located at an urban area with a population of more than 200,000. About 4–5 EDCs are attached with each eye bank.

Functions of eye donation centres

- *Local publicity and awareness.* The eye donation centres are meant to provide public as well as professional awareness about eye donation.
- *Registration of voluntary donors.* Coordination with donor families and hospitals to motivate eye donation.
- *Harvest corneal tissue* and collect blood for serology.
- To ensure safe transportation of tissue to the parent eye bank.

Personnel needed for EDC are:
- *Ophthalmic technicians*, trained in eye bank
- *Local honorary workers/voluntary agencies* like Lions club, Rotary club, etc. to boost the eye donation campaign.
- *Services of honorary ophthalmic surgeons* or medical officer trained in enucleation, available on cell.

Eye bank (EB)

Functions

- The eye bank is an institution that should provide a round-the-clock *public response system* over the telephone.
- *Conduct public awareness programmes* on eye donation.
- *Should co-ordinate with donor families and hospitals* to motivate eye donation.
- *Hospital Cornea Retrieval Programme* (HCRP) to harvest corneal tissue, *process, preserve and evaluate the collected tissues.*
- *Ensure equitable distribution of tissues* and ensure their *safe transportation* to the site of utilization.

Hospital eye bank in an institution that fulfils all the requirements and functions of eye bank except that it restricts collection of tissue within the hospital where the eye bank is located.

Eye bank training centre (EBTC)

The eye bank training centres beside performing all the functions of an eye bank, is additionally involved in *training of all levels of personnel involved* in eye banking and research.

FACILITIES, EQUIPMENT AND MAINTENANCE OF AN EYE BANK[4]

Each eye bank should maintain its own manual of standard operative procedures (SOP) which should details all aspects of tissue retrieval, processing, testing, storage, distribution and quality assurance practices. Each procedure must be initially approved, signed and dated by the medical director or the officer-in-charge of the eye bank. *An annual review* of each eye bank's procedures manual with signing and dating by the medical director or officer-in-charge is mandatory.[3, 4]

Requirements for an ideal eye bank set up

1. *Instrument cleaning isolation lab* (approx. 8′ × 10′). This is a limited access lab for authorized personnel only, to carry out activities such as washing and sterilization of instruments following corneal excision.

2. *Serology isolation lab* (approx. 12′ × 10′). This is a limited access lab for authorized technicians, where blood serum samples are tested.

3. *Tissue processing isolation lab* (approx. 15′ × 10′). This is an isolated area where tissues are evaluated, processed and prepared for packing and distribution. This area should have space for ultraviolet and laminar flow hood (Fig. 44.2) also.

4. *Evaluation lab and shipping area* (approx. 12′ x 10′). This area is meant for placement of slit lamp, work station, cabinets for storage and refrigerator.

5. *Technician's office* (approx. 10′ × 10′). This is a place where communication and record keeping is done.

6. *Manager's office* (approx. 10′ × 10′). This space is meant for placement of a desk, phone, fax and cabinets.

A brief summary of pieces of equipment required in various labs, as per different levels of eye banking pyramid have been summarized in Table 44.1.

Basic infrastructure for an eye bank

1. *Physical space.* A minimum area of 600 sq. ft is required to well accommodate various labs as described in the previous section. The details of various pieces of equipment for these labs as per different levels of eye banking pyramid has been summarized in Table 44.1.

2. *Equipment and other facilities.* Each eye bank must have the equipment and facilities essential for performing laboratory services with optimal accuracy, efficiency, sterility and safety. The basic infrastructure for an eye bank and an eye donation centre include a slit lamp, a laminar flow hood/cabinet (Fig. 44.2), a specular microscope (Fig. 44.3), a refrigerator for storing tissues (Fig. 44.4], 6 sets of instruments, a telephone, furniture, serological pieces of equipment and an autoclave. The various pieces of equipment have been enlisted in Table 44.2 as required according to various levels of eye banking pyramid.

3. *Eye bank maintenance.* Each eye bank laboratory must have an adequate, stable electrical source with sufficient number of grounded electrical outlets for operating laboratory equipment. The rooms including walls, floor and sink must be kept clean at all times and an appropriate documentation of regular laboratory cleaning schedules must be maintained and kept in a file for a minimum period of three years.

4. *Equipment maintenance and cleaning.* Each eye bank laboratory should have a refrigerator with a device, either internal or external for recording temperature variations (Fig. 44.3). Temperature variations must be recorded twice daily and should remain within the range of 2–6°C. The refrigerator should be maintained exclusively for use by the eye bank only. It must have clearly defined and labeled areas for all types of stored tissues, e.g. tissues to be used

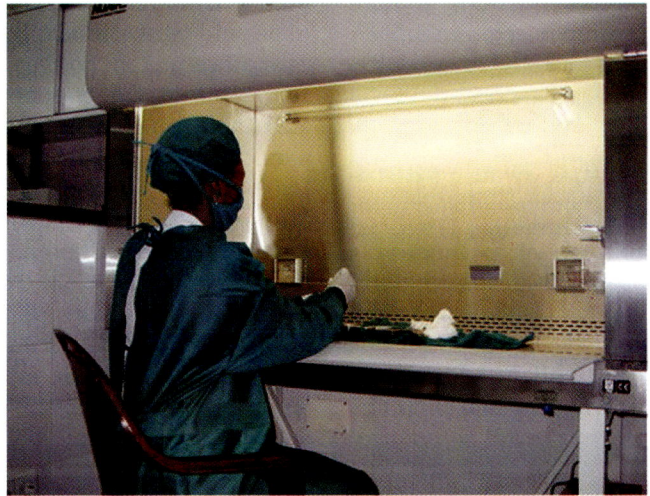

Fig. 44.2: *Laminar flow hood*

Table 44.1: *Brief summary of pieces of equipment required in various labs, as per different levels of eye banking pyramid*

Infrastructure	EBTC	EB	EDC
Instrument cleaning lab			
1. Sink—for washing instruments	Required	Required	Required
2. Autoclave for sterilizing	Required	Access	Access
3. Countertop and storage space for storing instruments and supplies	Required	Required	Required
Serology lab			
1. Sink for washing	Required	Access to accredited testing lab or all facilities are required. Accredited lab should have all the mentioned facilities and would be inspected before accreditation is given to eye bank	Serology lab is not required. However, sink for washing and facility for storing blood samples in refrigerator should be available
2. Refrigerator—for storing blood samples and kits	Required		
3. Countertops, cabinets and drawers for workspace and storing supplies	Required		
4. Centrifuge and serum testing equipment like ELISA reader, rapid test, etc.	Required		
Tissue processing lab			
1. Sterile countertop/table top for processing (laminar flow hood/ bio-hazard cabinet)	Required	Required	
2. Countertops, drawers and cabinets for storage	Required	Required	
Evaluation, storage and shipping lab			
1. Slit lamp and specular microscope for tissue evaluation	Required	Required, but access to a specular microscope is also acceptable	Not required
2. Countertops and cabinets for storage of supplies, packing and shipping	Required	Required	Required
3. Refrigerator for storing donor tissue	Required	Required	Required

for transplantation, tissues awaiting distribution, quarantined tissue and tissues meant for research only. The refrigerator should be calibrated once a year.

5. *Instruments and reagents.* Adequate instruments must be available to provide for sterile removal of whole eye and corneas. Instruments must be inspected frequently enough to assure that they function properly. All sterilized instruments, supplies and reagents, such as corneal preservation medium, must contain expiry dates that are current at all times.

6. *Infection control and safety.* All eye bank personnel must operate under the universal precautions for health care workers. These written procedures must be included in the eye bank's procedure manual. All technical personnel should receive hepatitis B vaccination and any other recommended vaccination that may be announced from time to time.

7. *Waste disposal.* Human tissues and waste items shall be disposed off in a secure manner, so as to minimize any hazard to eye bank personnel and the environment and they should

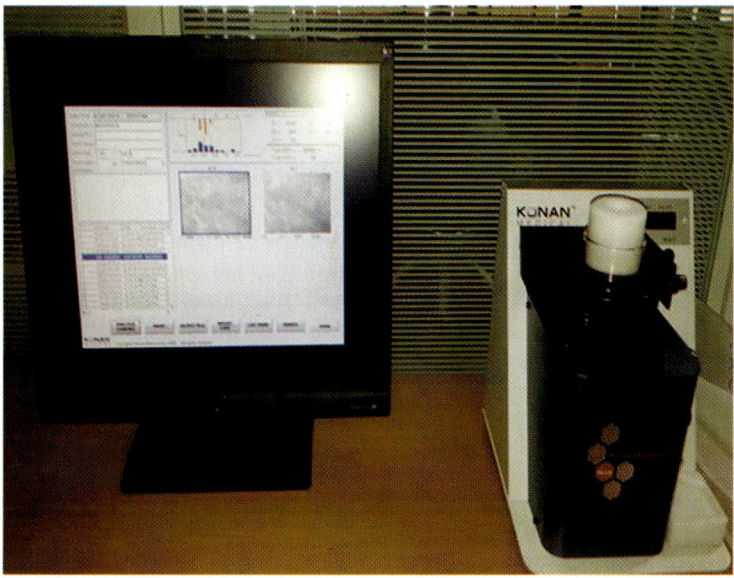

Fig. 44.3: *Specular microscope for evaluation of donor corneal endothelium*

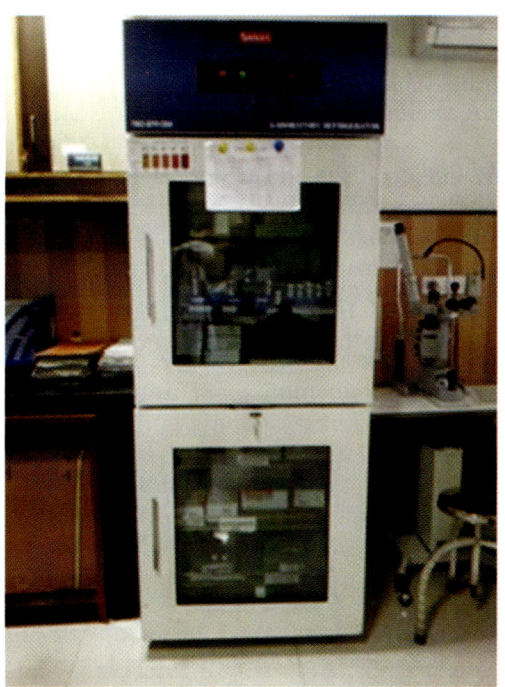

Fig. 44.4: *Refrigerator for storage of donor corneas*

well comply with applicable regulations. Dignified and proper disposal procedures should be used to obviate recognizable human remains.

Eye bank personnel

1. ***Eye bank in-charge.*** He should be a qualified ophthalmologist to evaluate, process and distribute the donor tissue.

2. ***Eye bank technician.*** The duties of a trained eye bank technician are:
- To keep the eye collection kits ready.
- To assist in enucleation of donor eyes.
- To record data pertaining to donor material and waiting list of patients.
- To process and treat the donor eyes with antibiotics.
- To assist in corneal preservation and storage.
- To maintain asepsis in the eye bank.

3. ***Clerk-cum-storekeeper.*** The duties are:
- To maintain meticulous records.
- To coordinate with other eye banks.
- To deal with other eye banks and exert with efficiency regarding donor's correspondence.
- To distribute cornea to eye surgeons/eye banks.

4. ***Medical social worker or public relations officer*** is required:
- To supply publicity material to common public.
- To promote voluntary eye donation.
  He may be a volunteer or paid worker.

Table 44.2: *Brief summary of various pieces of equipment required for the optimal functioning of an eye bank training centre, eye bank and eye donation centre*

Equipment	Eye bank training centre	Eye bank	Eye donation centre
Slit lamp	Required	Required	Not required
Refrigerators for storing blood sample, tissues and storage media	Required	Required in case the eye bank has tie up with accredited lab for testing, one refrigerator is sufficient	Preferable for storing blood sample, ice packs, storage media, eye or tissue collected, etc.
Serology equipment	Required	Yes, required. Access to an accredited lab is also acceptable	Not required
Specular microscope	Required	Yes, required, if collection is >200 per year. Access to specular microscope is also acceptable	Not required
Sufficient sets of instruments for corneal excision and enucleation	Required. Numbers to be decided on level of collections	Required. Numbers to be decided on level of collections	Required. Numbers to be decided on level of collections
Autoclave or gas sterilizer	Required	Required for access to sterilizing facility. For accreditation, sterilizing facility practice and procedure shall be reviewed	Should have access to sterilizing facility
Laminar flow hood (Class II). This is required for the preservation of ocular tissue in the laboratory in case of whole globe removal (enucleation) and for processing scleral tissue	Required	Required	Not required
OTHER FACILITIES			
Transportation facility	24 hours 365 days	24 hours 365 days	Should have access
Furniture	Required	Required	Preferable
Computer with email facility	Required	Required	Preferable
Two exclusive lines (one with 1919 or public service number allotted and another for outgoing calls)	Required	Required	Universal public service number to be allotted
Audiovisual equipment for publicity	Required	Required	Preferred

5. *Driver-cum-projectionist* is required:
- To maintain vehicle of the eye bank.
- To screen films of eye donation promotion in the community.

EYE DONATION

Donor corneas are retrieved either via voluntary eye donation (VED) or as a part of Hospital Cornea Retrieval Programme (HCRP).

VOLUNTARY EYE DONATION (VED)

Voluntary eye donation is the result of realization of social responsibility towards corneal blind people, even in moments of grief. No intervention by eye bank is made to motivate family at the time of death. The shortcomings include poor screening at the donation site, high rate of the tissues being discarded and increased death to retrieval time.

HOSPITAL CORNEA RETRIEVAL PROGRAMME (HCRP)

Hospital Cornea Retrieval Programme (HCRP) was started by the Eye Bank Association of India to increase the number of donor corneas, wherein the family members of deceased are directly motivated for eye donation by sensitizing them regarding corneal blindness and benefits of corneal transplantation.[5] Under this programme *Eye Donation Counsellors* (EDC) are stationed at multi-specialty hospitals round the clock and keep rapport with the hospital staff. Whenever any death occurs in any ward, the concerned staff (Nurse/Doctor/Social worker) informs the counsellors who then counsels, motivates and requests the family members to donate the eyes of their deceased relatives. *The HCRP focuses on multispecialty hospitals to retrieve eyeball or corneal tissue in view of the following advantages:*

1. *More number of corneas can be collected*, if relatives are motivated, as the number of deaths are more in hospitals compared to home deaths.
2. *Corneal tissue can be obtained from younger donors* as hospital deaths can occur in younger personals from accidents, diseases, etc. compared to home deaths, thereby a good quality of corneal tissue can be obtained.
3. *Quick access* leading to reduction of time interval between death to enucleation/corneal excision—another factor for getting good quality of tissue.
4. *Detailed medical history and investigation reports* can be available easily.
5. *Eye donors can become multiple organ donors* if the relatives wish to donate.

FACTS ABOUT EYE DONATION

- Almost anyone at any age can pledge to donate eyes after death; all that is needed is a clear healthy cornea.
- The eyes have to be removed within six hours of death.
- Eye donation gives sight to two blind persons as one eye is transplanted to one blind person.
- The eyes can be pledged to an eye bank and can be actually donated to any nearest eye bank at the time of death.
- The donated eyes are never bought or sold. Eye donation is never refused.
- The eyes cannot be removed from a living human being in spite of his/her consent and wish.

LEGAL ASPECT

The collection and use of donated eyes come under the purview of Human Organ Transplantation Act (HOTA), 1994, which has been described in detail in Chapter 46.

REFERENCES

1. Rao GN. What is eye banking? Indian J Ophthalmol 1996; 44: 1–2.
2. Kalevar V. Eye banking in India. Ind J ophthalmol. 1989; 37 (3): 110–111.
3. Sangwan VA, Gopinathan U, Garg P, Rao GN. Eye banking in India—A road ahead. J Int Med Sci Acad. 2010; 23: 197–200.
4. Medical Standards of Eye banking in India published by NPCB, Directorate General of Health Services, Min Of Health and Family Welfare, Govt. of India, New Delhi - 110011, 2009; pp 1–6.
5. Subhash B. Hospital cornea retrieval programme. J Indian Med Assoc. 2000 Feb; 98(2): 67.

45
Eye Donation: Retrieval, Evaluation, Storage and Distribution of Donor Cornea

INTRODUCTION

Corneal harvesting is the surgical removal of either the whole eye (enucleation) or only the corneo-sclera (*in situ* excision of corneo-scleral button) from the deceased.

Quality of donor corneal tissue has a great bearing on the final outcome of surgery for which it is utilised. This in turn is affected to a great extent by various factors such as:

- Tissue retrieval technique,
- Duration of storage, and
- Type of corneal storage media used.

A healthy functioning endothelium is the key to successful corneal grafting and therefore needs to be protected from the point of tissue retrieval till grafting.

Corneal tissue retrieval and storage should follow certain guidelines to ensure that the available resources are optimum utilized without exposing eye bank personnel to an increased risk of health hazards.[1, 2]

RETRIEVAL OF DONOR CORNEA

GUIDELINES FOR CORNEAL TISSUE RETRIEVAL

Before proceeding for corneal tissue recovery, the eye bank personnel should ascertain the location, age of the donor, cause of death and the time of death.

Following points should be noted in a chronological order before proceeding for the retrieval process.

- *Validated sterile instruments* for retrieval should be carried by the Eye Bank team.
- *Locate the next of kin,* convey condolence, and obtain death certificate on arrival at the location site.
- *Medical records/Medical information* should be obtained.

- *Social history of the donor* should be obtained wherever possible from the next of kin.
- *Obtain consent* on a consent form from the legal custodian of the donor.
- *Donor should be identified* either through a tag or through the next of kin after obtaining the consent.
- *Proceed to prepare the site* for eye donation.
- *Gross physical examination* should be conducted with utmost respect for observations regarding build: average/healthy/emaciated and should look out for ulcers/gangrene in exposed areas.
- *Should look out for needle marks on the arm, skin lesions*, etc. after gross examination.
- *Ocular examination* should be conducted thoroughly.

DONOR SCREENING

Donor screening is extremely important in order to prevent transmission of diseases to the patients in whom corneal transplantation is performed as well as to the eye bank personnel. In conditions, which are considered absolute contraindications for transplantation, the donor family should be clearly informed.

Conditions having a potential risk of transmission of local or systemic communicable diseases from donor to recipient

- Death of unknown cause
- Death with neurologic disease of un-established diagnosis
- Subacute sclerosing panencephalitis
- Progressive multifocal leukoencephalopathy
- Active meningitis or encephalitis
- Encephalopathy of unknown origin or progressive encephalopathy
- Active septicemia (bacteremia, fungemia, viremia, parasitemia)
- Active viral hepatitis
- Creutzfeldt-Jakob disease
- Congenital rubella
- Reye's syndrome
- Rabies
- Active miliary tuberculosis or tubercular meningitis

- HTLV-I or HTLV-II infection
- Hepatitis C seropositive donors
- HIV seropositive donors
- HIV or high risk for HIV corneas from: Persons meeting any of the following criteria should not be offered for transplantation
- Active ocular or intraocular inflammation conjunctivitis, scleritis, iritis, uveitis, vitreitis choroiditis and retinitis (at the time of death).

Conditions with potential risk of transmission of non-communicable diseases from donor to recipient

- Death due to cyanide poisoning
- Instrinsic eye disease
- Retinoblastoma
- Malignant tumours of the anterior segment or known adenocarcinoma of primary or metastatic origin
- Leukaemias
- Active disseminated lymphomas

INTERVAL BETWEEN DEATH, ENUCLEATION, EXCISION AND PRESERVATION

Acceptable time intervals from death, enucleation or excision to preservation may vary according to the circumstances of death and interim means of storage of the body. It is generally recommended that donor eye should be removed and corneal preservation should occur as soon as possible after death, preferably within 6 hours of death. In countries with cold climate may take up to 12 hours. All time intervals for each donor, e.g. the time of death to the time of enucleation and preservation and/or the time to corneal excision, shall be recorded. If the donor has been refrigerated prior to enucleation or *in situ* corneal excision, this information should also be noted.

DONOR BLOOD SAMPLE RETRIEVAL

The authorized personnel retrieving the tissue should obtain an adequate blood sample at the time of tissue retrieval.

Serological screening. The required serologic tests, which must be performed for each donor's blood sample include HIV, hepatitis B and C, and syphilis.

EVALUATION OF DONOR CORNEA

GUIDELINES FOR EVALUATION METHODS

Standard guidelines

The ultimate responsibility for determining the suitability of a tissue for transplantation rests with the transplanting surgeon.

Gross examination of the corneo-scleral rim should be initially carried out for clarity, epithelial defects, presence of any infiltrate or foreign objects and contamination as well as the colour of sclera.

Biomicroscopic examination. Corneas should be examined (Fig. 45.1) for the presence of any epithelia, stromal or endothelial pathology. Enucleated globes should be examined in the laboratory prior to distribution and/or corneal excision. If *in situ* corneal excision is performed, examination of the donor eye anterior segment with a penlight or a portable slit lamp is required.

- *After corneal excision, the corneal-scleral rim shall be evaluated* by slit lamp biomicroscopy, even if the donor eye has been examined with the slit lamp prior to excision of the corneo-scleral rim, to ensure that damage to the corneal endothelium or surgical detachment of Descemet's membrane did not occur. Information obtained with slit lamp biomicroscopic examination must be documented.

- *Grading of donor tissue* is done into excellent, very good, good, fair and poor depending upon the condition of corneal epithelium stroma, Descemet's membrane and endothelium (Table 45.1).

Specular microscopy. Determination of endothelial cell density via specular microscopy should be a standard norm for all eye banks. When it is impossible to obtain an endothelial cell count, this requirement may be waived on a case-by-case basis.

Microbiological evaluation by culture from the conjunctival swab from the deceased is ideal serological screening.

NON-SURGICAL DONOR TISSUE

If the donor tissue is provided for purposes other than surgery, e.g. research, practice surgery, etc.,

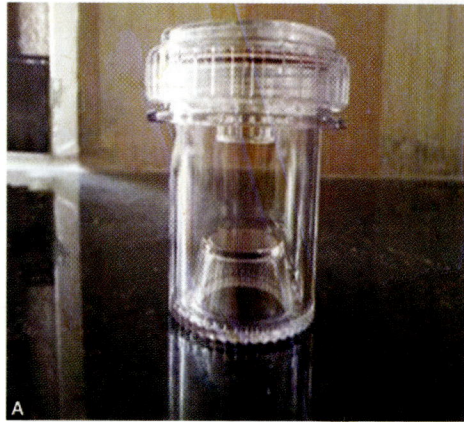
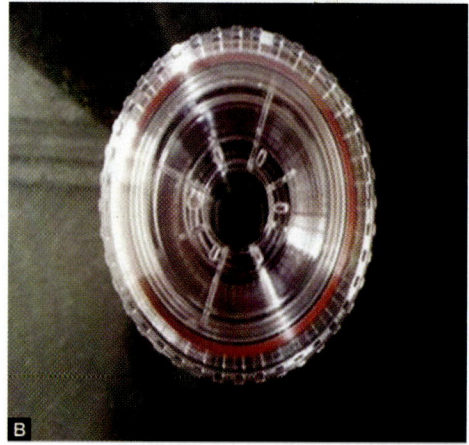

Fig. 45.1: *A, Corneal tissue placed in a viewing chamber, containing MK medium; B, Corneal tissue placed in a viewing chamber mounted on a slit lamp for evaluation*

that donor tissue should also have been screened for HIV or hepatitis.

In case the donor has not been screened for some unavoidable reason and the tissue has to be sent for research or other purpose, then a label stating that screening for HIV-antibody, hepatitis B or hepatitis C has not been carried out or stating "Potentially hazardous biological material" or some other indication must be attached to the container used for the donor tissue storage and/or transport.

STORAGE OF DONOR CORNEA

DONOR TISSUE PRESERVATION STANDARDS

Individuals specifically trained for in situ retrieval and/or laboratory removal of the

Table 45.1: *Grading of donor cornea on slit-lamp biomicroscopic examination*

Parameter	Grade I (excellent)	Grade II (very good)	Grade III (good)	Grade IV (fair)	Grade V (poor)
		Grade of donor corneal tissue			
Epithelial defects and haze	None	Slight epithelial haze or defects	Obvious moderate epithelial defects		
Corneal stromal clarity	Crystal clear	Clear	Slight cloudiness	Moderate cloudiness	Marked cloudiness
Arcus senilis	None	Slight	Moderate (<2.5 mm)	Heavy (>2.5–4 mm)	Very heavy (>4 mm)
Descemet's membrane	No folds	Few shallow folds	Numerous shallow folds	Numerous deep folds	Marked deep folds
Endothelium	No defect	No defect	Few vacuolated cells	Moderate guttate	Marked guttate

corneal scleral segment shall perform removal of the corneal scleral rim using sterile technique. *If the procedure is done in a laboratory* the removal must be performed in a laminar flow hood, cabinet or in an operation room. For corneo-scleral removal, the eye shall be examined using a penlight preferably and a slit lamp prior to excision.

Eye bank shall use approved corneal storage medium (such as MK, Optisol-GS, Eusol) from a reliable source. The medium shall be used and stored according to the manufacturer's recommendations for temperature, date and other factors. The manufactured medium purchased and shipped to the eye bank should be inspected for damage upon arrival and the lot number of medium used for each cornea should be recorded. The various preservation media used have been listed in Table 45.2.

Corneal tissue has to be transplanted as a viable living tissue unlike other tissues such as bone and heart valves which can be extensively processed and altered from their natural state. Thus, the aim of all corneal storage techniques is simply to maintain this living viable state while holding the cornea for the period between eye donation and corneal transplantation. The major leap forward in corneal preservation came with the introduction of MK medium by McCarey and Kaufman in 1973.[3] With its introduction began the era of 4°C corneal preservation media, which allowed elective planning of surgery, thus making corneal transplantation a scheduled procedure and not an emergency.

STORAGE MEDIA

Storage media have been classified according to the duration of storage as short term, intermediate and long-term storage media (Table 45.2).

Short-term storage media consists of moist chambers (Fig. 45.2), McCarey and Kaufman (MK) media, and modified McCarey and

Table 45.2: *List of various corneal preservation media depending upon the duration of storage offered*

Short-term storage	Intermediate storage	Long-term storage
Moist chamber: 24 hours	Optisol: 10–14 days	Organ culture medium: 1 month
MK media: 72 hours	Optisol-GS: 10–14 days	Cryopreservation: 30 days—indefinite
Modified MK media: 96 hours	Dexsol: 10–14 days	Glycerin: 1 year
	Eusol-C: 10–14 days	
	Cornisol: 10–14 days	
	K-Sol: 7–10 days	
	Life 4°C: 10–14 days	

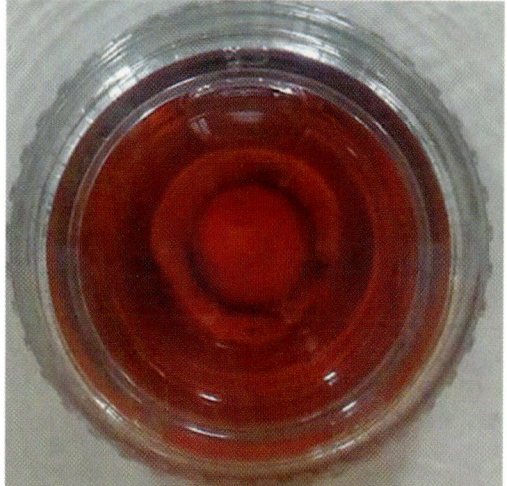

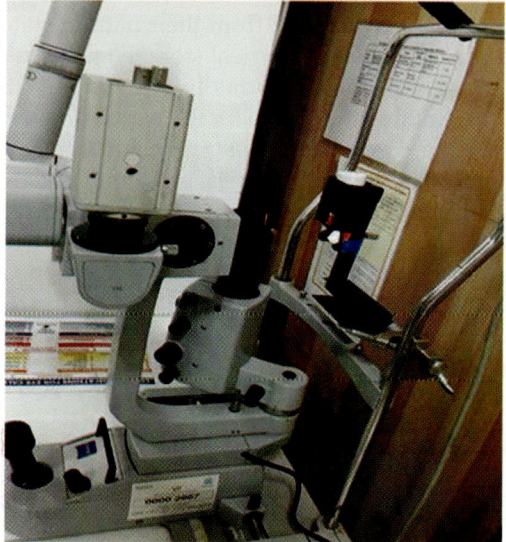

Fig. 45.2: *Corneal tissue storage chambers*

Kaufman media with 24, 72, 96 hours duration of storage respectively.

Intermediate storage comprises Optisol-GS, Cornisol, Eusol-C and Life 4°C with 10–14 days of duration of storage.

Long-term storage comprises organ culture medium with 1-month storage period, glycerin with 1 year and cryopreservation technique for indefinite storage duration.

Commonly used storage media

Some commonly used storage media (Fig. 45.3) are described briefly.

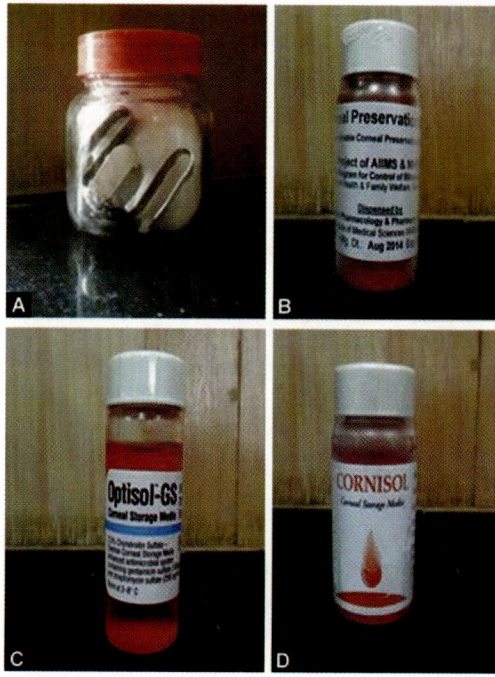

Fig. 45.3: *Figure showing various corneal preservation medium. A, Moist chamber storage medium; B, MK medium; C, Optisol-GS medium; D, Cornisol medium*

McCarey and Kaufman medium (MK medium) is a short-term storage medium with a storage duration of 4 days at 4°C. *Components* of this medium include tissue culture medium 199 as base, gentamicin as an antibiotic having a greater spectrum activity against gram-negative bacteria and 5% dextran as an osmotic agent for maintaining cornea in dehydrated state by compensating for the inactivity of corneal dehydration mechanisms at 4°C.[3] HEPES (4-(2-hydroxyethyl)-1-piperazineethanesulfonic acid) is used as a buffer and phenol red as a pH indicator. It remains a cheap, easy to manufacture, simple and reliable form of corneal preservation.

Cornisol is an intermediate storage medium with 14 days storage duration at 2–8°C. Components of this medium include tissue culture medium 199, Earle's balanced salt solution, and minimum essential medium (MEM), 2.5% chondroitin sulfate, recombinant human insulin as a metabolism enhancer, dextran, L-glutamine, ATP precursors, vitamins, gentamicin and streptomycin.[3]

Optisol-GS is also an intermediate storage medium with 14 days duration of storage at 2–8°C. It is based with tissue culture medium 199, Earle's balanced salt solution, and minimum essential medium (MEM). It contains HEPES buffer, 2.5% chondroitin sulfate, 1% dextran, and various adenosine triphosphate precursors. In addition, it contains iron, cholesterol, L-hydroxy-proline, numerous vitamins, and the antibiotics gentamicin and streptomycin.[4]

STORAGE GUIDELINES

All surgical tissue shall be stored in quarantine until results of HIV, HbsAg, HCV, and any other relevant donor screening tests have been recorded as non-reactive. All tissues should be stored aseptically at a temperature, appropriate to the method of preservation used. Eye banks must precisely document their procedures for storage of corneal tissue, whether it is in the form of the whole eye or the cornea only in an appropriate medium.

LABELING

Each corneal or scleral tissue container should be clearly and labeled to include information including; name of source eye bank, tissue identification number, type of tissue, type of preservation medium, date and time of donor's death, date and time of corneal/scleral preservation and the preservation date for scleral tissues. A statement should be made that the tissue is intended for single patient application only and that it is not to be considered sterile and culturing or re-culturing is recommended.

QUALITY ASSURANCE AND CONTROL

QUALITY ASSURANCE

Each eye bank should have a formally established quality assurance programme to include ongoing monitoring and development of plans for corrective action. These standards shall provide the basis for development of the QA programme.

Each eye bank shall document all aspects of its QA programme and maintain record of all QA activities for a minimum of ten years. These include any corrective or remedial action taken for detected deficiencies. These records shall be available for review.

The eye bank's quality assurance programme shall include a method for the receiving surgeon to report adverse reactions from the trans-plantation of corneal, scleral or other ocular tissue to the source eye bank. The eye bank in turn must forward the adverse reaction information within a reasonable time to the EBAI or MOH for review by the Medical Standards Policy sub-committee. An adverse reaction file shall be available for review by the accreditation team at the time of inspection and must be kept for minimum of three years.

QUALITY CONTROL

Microbiologic culturing of eye bank donor eyes is advised. Cultures may be performed either before and/or at the time of surgery. Eye banks may elect to perform corneal-scleral rim cultures at the time of corneal preservation in tissue culture medium. If positive, the culture reports should be reported to the receiving surgeon or the recipient eye bank.

Each eye bank shall recommend culturing of the corneal-scleral rim for corneal transplantation, or a piece of sclera for scleral implantation at the time of surgery. Positive results in cases of postoperative infection shall be reported to the eye bank/or eye donation centre that procured the tissue as well as to the eye bank that distributed the tissue.

DISTRIBUTION OF DONOR CORNEA

GUIDELINES FOR DISTRIBUTION

Prior to distribution of tissue for transplantation, the MD or his/her designee shall review and document the medical and laboratory information in accordance with medical standards. Tissue shall be distributed only to ophthalmologists, institutions and other eye banks who are registered under applicable laws like Transplantation of Human Organs Act. All tissues sent from an accredited eye bank must comply with the recommended medical standards.

SYSTEM OF DISTRIBUTION

- *Eye banks should establish and document a system of distribution* that is just, equitable and fair to all patients served by the eye bank.
- Documentation of distribution time and date of requests and delivery of eye tissue to be maintained.
- Access to tissue shall be provided without regard to recipient sex, religion, race, creed, colour or caste.
- For corneas returned and redistributed, tissue transportation and storage information must be documented and made available to the transplanting surgeon.
- Eye banks must have a policy and procedure for potential recall of tissue.

REFERENCES

1. Medical Standards of Eye banking in India published by NPCB, Directorate General of Health Services, Min Of Health and Family Welfare, Govt. of India, New Delhi - 110011, 2009; pp 1–6.
2. Jeng BH. Preserving the cornea: corneal storage media Curr Opin Ophthalmol. 2006 Aug; 17(4): 332–7.
3. Lindstrom RL. Advances in corneal preservation. Trans Am Ophthalmol Soc 1990; 88: 555–648.
4. Lindstrom RL, Kaufman HE, Skelnik DL, et al. Optisol corneal storage medium. Am J Ophthalmol 1992; 114: 345–356.

Human Organ Transplantation Act

INTRODUCTION

Diseases of cornea are important causes of visual impairment worldwide. As per the survey conducted by MOH & FW in 2006–2007, 1% of the total blindness (vision 6/60 or <6/60) constituting 1.22 lakhs of the Indian population are bilaterally corneal blind,[1] out of which approximately 60,000 could get restoration of vision with keratoplasty. Furthermore, 20,000 new cases of corneal blindness are added every year. As per NPCB, approximately 45,000 corneas are collected every year against a demand of 1.2 lakh. To streamline and regulate the process of removal, storage and transplantation of human organs for therapeutic purposes and for the prevention of commercial dealings in human organs, Human Organ Transplantation Act (HOTA) was passed in 1994[2] and Human Organs Transplantation Rules were notified in 1995.[3] To address the inadequacies in the efficacy, relevance and impact of the Act, an amendment to the Act was passed in 2011[4] by the parliament and the rules notified in 2014 by the name of Transplantation of Human Organs and Tissues Rules, 2014.[5]

PROVISION OF HUMAN ORGAN TRANSPLANTATION ACT

The main provisions of the Human Organ Transplantation Act (HOTA) (including the amendments and rules of 2014)[2–5] in relation to eye donation are as follows:

I. Authority for the removal of human organs

A registered medical practitioner, before removing any organ or tissue from the body of a person after his or her death (deceased donor), in consultation with transplant coordinator, should make sure that the following criteria have been fulfilled.

1. *In the case of brainstem death of the potential donor*, it has to be ensured that a certificate as specified in Form 10 has been signed by all the members of the Board of Medical Experts comprising of medical administrator incharge of the hospital, authorised specialist, neurologist/neurosurgeon and medical officer treating the patient.

(Where neurologist/neurosurgeon is not available, then any surgeon or physician and anaesthetist or intensivist, who is not part of the transplant team nominated by the head of the hospital duly empanelled by appropriate authority may certify the brainstem death as a member of the said Board.)

2. *If the deceased has authorized before his/ her death*, the removal of his/her organs/tissues after his death for therapeutic purposes, as specified in Form 7, the near relatives will have to be enquired that subsequently the aforementioned authorization has not been revoked by the deceased. Notwithstanding this authorization, the consent of near relative or person in lawful possession of the body as specified in Form 8 is mandatory.

3. *The near relative of the deceased person or the person lawfully* in possession of the body of the deceased donor has signed the declaration as specified in Form 8.

4. *If the deceased person who had earlier given authorisation but had revoked it subsequently* and if the person had given in writing that his organ should not be removed after his death, then, no organ or tissue will be removed even if consent is given by the near relative or person in lawful possession of the body.

5. *In the case of brainstem death of a person of less than eighteen years of age*, in addition to the certificate specified in Form 10 signed by all the members of the Board of Medical Experts as mentioned in sub-para (a), an authority as specified in Form 8 should be signed by either of the parents of such person or any near relative authorised by the parent.

II. Procedure for donation of organ or tissue in medicolegal cases

1. *After obtaining authority for removal of organs or tissues*, the registered medical practitioner of the hospital should make a request to the Station House Officer or Superintendent of Police or Deputy Inspector General of the area either directly or through the police post located in the hospital to facilitate timely retrieval of organs or tissue from the donor and a copy of such a request should also be sent to the designated postmortem doctor of the area simultaneously.

2. *While retrieving organs*, it should be ensured that the determination of the cause of death is not jeopardised.

3. *Medical report in respect of the organs or tissues being retrieved should be prepared* at the time of retrieval by the retrieving doctor and should be taken on record in postmortem notes by the registered medical practitioner doing postmortem.

4. *Presence of postmortem registered medical practitioner.* Wherever it is possible, attempt should be made to request the designated postmortem registered medical practitioner, even beyond office timing, to be present at the time of organ or tissue retrieval.

5. *In case a private retrieval hospital* is not doing postmortem, they should arrange transportation of body along with medical records, after organ or tissue retrieval, to the designated postmortem centre and the postmortem centre should undertake the postmortem of such cases on priority, even beyond office timing, so that the body is handed over to the relatives with least inconvenience.

III. Procedure for donation of organ or tissue in case of unclaimed dead bodies

1. *In the case of a dead body lying in a hospital or prison and not claimed* by any of the near relatives of the deceased person within forty-eight hours from the time of the death of the concerned person, the authority for the removal

of any human organ from the dead body which so remains unclaimed may be given, in the prescribed form, by the person in charge (for the time being, of the management or control of the hospital or prison, or by an employee of such hospital or prison authorised in this behalf by the person in charge of the management or control thereof).

2. *No authority should be given if the person empowered to give such authority has reason to believe* that any near relative of the deceased person is likely to claim the dead body even though such near relative has not come forward to claim the body of the deceased person within forty-eight hours.

IV. Regulation of hospitals

Hospitals are required to be registered under this Act for carrying out removal, storage or transplantation of any human organ for therapeutic purposes. Notwithstanding this, the eyes or the ears (eardrums and ear bones) may be removed at any place from the dead body of any donor, for therapeutic purposes, by a registered medical practitioner. Non-governmental organisations, registered societies and trusts working in the field of organ or tissue removal, storage or transplantation will require registration under this Act.

1. Registration of hospital or tissue bank

An application for registration should be made to the appropriate authority as specified in Form 12 or Form 13 or Form 14 or Form 15, as applicable and the application should be accompanied by fee as specified below, payable to the appropriate authority by means of a bank draft, which may be revised, if necessary by the Central or State Government, as the case may be:

i. For organ or tissue or cornea transplant centre: Rupees ten thousand;

ii. For tissue or eye bank: Rupees ten thousand;

iii. For non-transplant retrieval centre: Nil.

The appropriate authority after holding an inquiry and satisfying itself that the applicant has complied with all the requirements, grants a certificate of registration as specified in Form 16 and it shall be valid for a period of five years from the date of its issue and shall be renewable. Before a hospital is registered under the provisions of this rule, it is mandatory for the hospital to appoint a transplant coordinator.

2. Renewal of registration of hospital or tissue bank

An application for the renewal of a certificate of registration shall be made to the appropriate authority at least three months prior to the date of expiry of the original certificate of registration and shall be accompanied by a fee as specified below, payable to the appropriate authority by means of a bank draft, which may be revised, if necessary by the Central or State Government, as the case may be:

i. For organ or tissue or cornea transplant centre: Rupees five thousand;

ii. For tissue or eye bank: Rupees five thousand;

iii. For non-transplant retrieval centre: Nil.

A renewal certificate of registration shall be as specified in Form 17 and shall be valid for a period of five years.

3. Mandatory requirements for hospitals to get registration under this Act

i. *For cornea transplantation*, it is mandatory for the hospital to have an ophthalmologist with MD or MS or Diploma (DO) in ophthalmology or equivalent qualification with three months post MD or MS or DO training in corneal transplant operations in a recognised hospital or institution.

ii. *Donor screening*: Complete screening of donor must be conducted including medical or social history and serological evaluation for medical conditions or disease processes that would contraindicate the donation of tissues and the report of corneas or eyes not found suitable for transplantation and their alternate use shall be certified by a committee of two ophthalmologists.

iii. *Laboratory tests:* Facility for relevant laboratory tests for blood and tissue samples shall be available and testing of blood and tissue samples shall begin at donor screening and continue during retrieval and throughout processing.

iv. *Documentation and records:* A log of tissue received and distributed should be maintained to enable traceability from the donor to the tissue and the tissue to the donor and the records shall also indicate the dates and the identities of the staff performing specific steps in the removal or processing or distribution of the tissues.

v. *Data protection and confidentiality:* A unique donor identification number should be used for each donor, and access to donor records should be restricted.

vi. *Recipient information:* All tissue recipients should be followed up and prompt and appropriate corrective and preventive actions taken in case of adverse events.

vii. *Transplant coordinator* should be appointed with any of the following qualifications:
• Graduate of any recognised system of medicine; or
• Nurse; or
• Bachelor's degree in any subject and preferably Master's degree in social work or psychiatry or sociology or social science or public health.

The concerned organisation or institute should ensure initial induction training followed by retraining at periodic interval and the transplant coordinator should counsel and encourage the family members or near relatives of the deceased person to donate the human organ or tissue including eye or cornea and coordinate the process of donation and transplantation.

V. Regulatory and advisory bodies for monitoring transplantation activity and their constitution

a. *Appropriate authority (AA):* Inspects and grants registration to hospitals for transplantation enforces required standards for hospitals, conducts regular inspections to examine the quality of transplantations. It may conduct investigations into complaints regarding breach of provisions of the Act, and has the powers of a civil court to summon any person, request documents and issue search warrants.

b. *Advisory committee:* Consisting of experts in the domain who shall advise the appropriate authority.

c. *Authorization committee (AC):* Regulates living donor transplantation by reviewing each case to ensure that the living donor is not exploited for monetary considerations and to prevent commercial dealings in transplantation. Proceedings to be video recorded and decisions notified within 24 hours. Appeals against their decision may be made to the state or central government.

d. *Medical board (brain death committee):* Panel of doctors responsible for brain death certification. In case of non-availability of neurologist or neurosurgeon, any surgeon, physician, anaesthetist or intensivist, nominated by medical administrator in-charge of the hospital may certify brain death.

VI. Eligibility criteria for a person to harvest cornea from the deceased donor

The technician who can enucleate cornea means the technician with any of the following qualifications and experience who can harvest corneas (enucleate eyeballs or excise corneas):

a. *Ophthalmologists* possessing a Doctor of Medicine (MD) or Master of Surgery (MS) in Ophthalmology or Diploma in Ophthalmology (DO)

b. *Registered doctors* from all recognised systems of medicine, nurses, paramedical ophthalmic assistant, ophthalmic assistant, optometrists, refractionists, paramedical worker or medical technician with recognised qualification from all recognised systems of medicine, provided the person is duly trained to enucleate a donated cornea or eye from registered, authorised and functional eye bank or government medical college and, the training certificate should mention that he has acquired the required skills to independently conduct enucleation of the eye or removal of cornea from a cadaver.

VII. To establish national human organs and tissues removal and storage network

The Central Government to establish a National Human Organs and Tissues Removal and Storage Network, i.e. NOTTO (National Organ and Tissue Transplant Organisation), ROTTO (Regional Organ and Tissue Transplant Organisation) and SOTTO (State Organ and Tissue Transplant Organisation). Further, the Central Government shall maintain a registry of the donors and recipients of human organs and tissues.

VIII. Penalties for removal of organ without authority, making or receiving payment for supplying human organs or contravening any other provisions of the Act have been made very stringent in order to serve as a deterrent for such activities

1. *Punishment for removal of human organ without authority* includes imprisonment for a term which may extend to ten years and with fine which may extend to twenty lakh rupees. If the same has been committed by a registered medical practitioner, his name would be removed from the Medical Council register for three years for the first offence and permanently for the subsequent offence.

2. *Any person who is associated or helps unauthorized removal of human organs* could be punished with imprisonment for a term which may extend to three years and with fine which may extend to five lakh rupees.

3. *Punishment for commercial dealings in human organs*, providing false documents shall be punishable with imprisonment for a term which shall not be less than five years but which may extend to ten years and shall be liable to fine which shall not be less than twenty lakh rupees but may extend to one crore rupees.

4. *Punishment for illegal dealings of human tissues* shall be punishable with imprisonment for a term which shall not be less than one year but which may extend to three years and shall be liable to fine which shall not be less than five lakh rupees but may extend to twenty-five lakh rupees.

5. *Punishment for contravention of any other provision of this Act* includes imprisonment for a term which may extend to five years or with fine which may extend to twenty lakh rupees.

IX. Protection of action taken in good faith

No suit, prosecution or other legal proceeding shall lie against any person for anything which is in good faith done or intended to be done in pursuance of the provisions of this Act.

X. Various forms in relation to eye donation outlined in the rules

Various forms in relation to eye donation outlined in the rules are given as annexures below.

CONCLUSION AND ANNEXURES

CONCLUSION

HOTA provides for various rules and regulations which have been made mandatory to pave way for a smooth, legally correct cornea retrieval and transplantation including active counselling by the transplant coordinator to the families of the potential deceased donors, early corneal retrieval, and harvesting cornea even in medicolegal cases. This will help in both increasing eye donations and keratoplasties in our country in the coming years.

ANNEXURES

- *Form 8:* Consent for organ donation from family (also applicable for minors)
- *Form 9:* Consent for organ donation from unclaimed bodies
- *Form 10:* Brain death declaration form
- *Form 12:* Registration of hospital for organ transplantation
- *Form 13:* Registration of hospital for organ retrieval
- *Form 16:* Grant of registration
- *Form 17:* Renewal of registration

REFERENCES

1. MOH & FW (NPCB), Rapid Assessment of Avoidable Blindness–India. Report-2006-2007.
2. Government of India. Transplantation of Human Organs Act, 1994. Central Act 42 of [cited 2017 Mar]Available from:notto.nic.in/act-end-rules-of-thoa.htm.
3. Gazette—Transplantation of Human Organs Rules. 1995. (GSR NO. 51(E), dr 421995) [As amended videGSR 571(E), dt3172008][cited 2017 Mar] Available from: http://wwwmedin dianet/indian_health_act/The Transplantation of Human Organ Rules 1995 Definitions.
4. Gazette—Transplantation of Human Organs (Amendment) Act 2011. [cited 2017 Mar] Available from: notto.nic.in/act-end-rules-of-thoa.htm.
5. Gazette—Transplantation of Human Organs and Tissues Rules, 2014. (G.S.R. 218 (E)) [cited 2017 Mar] Available from: notto.nic.in/act-end-rules-of-thoa.htm.

FORM 8
FOR DECLARATION CUM CONSENT
(To be filled by near relative or lawful possessor of brain-stem dead person)
[Refer rules 5(1)(b), 5(4)(b) and 5(4)(d)]
DECLARATION AND CONSENT FORM

I, ... S/o, D/o, W/o. .... aged .... resident of .... in the presence of persons mentioned below, hereby declare that:

1. I have been informed that my relative (specify relation) ....
   S/o, D/o, W/o ....aged .... has been declared brain-stem dead/dead.

2. To the best of my knowledge (Strike off whichever is not applicable):
   (a) He/She (Name of the deceased) .... had/had not, authorised before his/her death, the removal of .... (Name of organ/tissue/both) of his/her body after his/her death for therapeutic purpose. The documentary proof of such authorisation is enclosed/not available.
   (b) He/She (Name of the deceased) .... had not revoked the authority as at No. 2 (a) above (If applicable).
   (c) There are reasons to believe that no near relative of the said deceased person has objection to any of his/her organs/tissue being used for therapeutic purposes.

3. I have been informed that in the absence of such authorisation, I have the option to either authorise or decline donation of organ/tissue/both including eye/cornea of .... (Name of the deceased) for therapeutic purposes. I also understand that if corneas/eyes are not found suitable for therapeutic purpose, then may be used for education/research.

4. I hereby authorise / do not authorize removal of his/her body organ(s) and/or tissue(s), namely (Any organ and tissue/Kidney/Liver/Heart/Lungs/Intestine/Cornea/Skin/Bone/Heart Valve/Any other; please specify) .... for therapeutic purposes. I also give permission for drawing of a blood sample for serology testing and am willing to share social/behavioural and medical history to facilitate proper screening of the donor for safe transplantation of the organs/tissues.

Date ....   Signature of near relative person in lawful possession of the dead body, and address for correspondence*

Place ....   Telephone No .... Email: ....

* in case of the minor the declaration shall be signed by one of the parents of the minor or any near relative authorised by the parent. In case the near relative or person in lawful possession of the body refuses to sign this form, the same shall be recorded in writing by the Registered Medical Practitioner on this Form.

(Signature of Witness 1)
1. Shri/Smt./Km. .... S/o, D/o, W/o ....
   aged .... resident of .... Telephone No. ....
   Email: ....

(Signature of Witness 2)
1. Shri/Smt./Km. .... S/o, D/o, W/o ....
   aged .... resident of .... Telephone No. ....
   Email: ....

FORM 9

FOR UNCLAIMED BODY IN A HOSPITAL OR PRISON

(To be completed by person in lawful possession of the unclaimed body)

[Refer rule 5(1)(b)]

I, ... S/o, D/o, W/o .... aged
.... Resident of .... having lawful possession of
the dead body of Shri/Smt./Km .... S/o, D/o, W/o
.... aged .... resident of ....
and having known that no person has come forward to claim the body of the deceased after
48 hours of death and there being no reason to believe that any person is likely to come to claim
the body I hereby, authorise removal of his/her body organ(s) and/or tissue(s), namely
.... for therapeutic purposes.

Signature, Name, designation and Stamp of person in lawful possession of the dead body

Dated ....

Place ....

Address for correspondence ....

Telephone No. ....

Email ....

(Signature of Witness 1)

1. Shri/Smt./Km. .... S/o, D/o, W/o ....
   aged .... resident of .... Telephone No. ....
   Email: ....

(Signature of Witness 2)

1. Shri/Smt./Km. .... S/o, D/o, W/o ....
   aged .... resident of .... Telephone No. ....
   Email: ....

FORM 10

FOR CERTIFICATION OF BRAIN STEM DEATH

(To be filled by the board of medical experts certifying brain-stem death)

[Refer rules 5(4)(c) and 5(4)(d)]

We, the following members of the Board of medical experts after careful personal examination hereby certify that Shri/Smt./Km. .... aged about .... son of/wife of/daughter of .... Resident of .... is dead on account of permanent and irreversible cessation of all functions of the brain-stem. The tests carried out by us and the findings therein are recorded in the brain-stem death Certificate annexed hereto.

Dated ....   Signature

1. R.M.P.- Incharge of the Hospital In which brain-stem death has occurred.
2. R.M.P. nominated from the panel of Names sent by the hospitals and approved by the Appropriate Authority.
3. Neurologist/Neuro-Surgeon
4. R.M.P. treating the aforesaid deceased person

(where Neurologist/Neurosurgeon is not available, any Surgeon or Physician and Anaesthetist or Intensivist, nominated by Medical Administrator In-charge from the panel of names sent by the hospital and approved by the Appropriate Authority shall be included)

BRAIN-STEM DEATH CERTIFICATE

(A) PATIENT DETAILS ...

1. Name of the patient: Mr./Ms ....
   S.O./D.O./W.O.   Mr./Ms ....
   Sex ....   Age ....

2. Home Address: ....
   ....

3. Hospital Patient Registration Number (CR No.) ....

4. Name and Address of next of kin or person responsible for the patient (if none exists, this must be specified)
   ....

5. Has the patient or next of kin agreed to any donation of organ and/or tissue?
   ....

6. Is this a Medico-legal case? Yes .... No ....

(B) PRE-CONDITIONS:

1. **Diagnosis:** Did the patient suffer from any illness or accident that led to irreversible brain damage? Specify details ....
   ....
   Date and time of accident/onset of illness ....
   Date and onset of non-reversible coma ....

2. Findings of Board of Medical Experts:
   First Medical Examination ....
   Second Medical Examination ....

(Contd.)

    (1) The following reversible causes of coma have been excluded:
        Intoxication (Alcohol)
        Depressant Drugs
        Relaxants (Neuromuscular blocking agents)
        Primary Hypothermia
        Hypovolaemic shock
        Metabolic or endocrine disorders
        Tests for absence of brain-stem functions
    (2) Coma
    (3) Cessation of spontaneous breathing
    (4) Pupillary size
    (5) Pupillary light reflexes
    (6) Doll's head eye movements
    (7) Corneal reflexes (both sizes)
    (8) Motor response in any cranial nerve distribution, any responses to stimulation of face, limb or trunk.
    (9) Gag reflex
  (10) Cough (Tracheal)
  (11) Eye movements on caloric testing bilaterally
  (12) Apnoea tests as specified
  (13) Were any respiratory movements seen?

      ....

Date and time of first testing: ....
Date and time of second testing: ....

   This is to certify that the patient has been carefully examined twice after an interval of about six hours and on the basis of findings recorded above, Mr./Ms .... is declared brain-stem dead.

Date: ...

Signatures of members of Brain Stem Death (BSD) Certifying Board as under:

    1. Medical Administrator In-charge of the hospital
    2. Authorised specialist.
    3. Neurologist/Neuro-Surgeon
    4. Medical Officer treating the Patient.

Note: I. Where Neurologist/Neurosurgeon is not available, then any Surgeon or Physician and Anaesthetist or Intensivist, nominated by Medical Administrator In-charge of the hospital shall be the member of the board of medical experts for brain-stem death certification.

    II. The minimum time interval between the first and second testing will be six hours in adults. In case of children 6 to 12 years of age, 1 to 5 years of age and infants, the time interval shall increase depending on the opinion of the above BSD experts.

    III. No. 2 and No. 3 will be co-opted by the Administrator In-charge of the hospital from the Panel of experts (*Nominated by the hospital and approved by the Appropriate Authority*).

FORM 12

APPLICATION FOR REGISTRATION OF HOSPITAL TO CARRY OUT ORGAN OR
TISSUE TRANSPLANTATION OTHER THAN CORNEA
(To be filled by head of the institution)
(Refer rule 24(1))

To

The Appropriate Authority for organ transplantation ....
(State or Union territory)
We hereby apply to be registered as an institution to carry out organ/tissue transplantation.
Name(s) of organ (s) or tissue (s) for which registration is required ....

The required data about the facilities available in the hospital are as follows:
(A) HOSPITAL:
   1. Name:
   2. Location:
   3. Government/Private:
   4. Teaching/Non-teaching:
   5. Approached by:

	Road:	Yes	No ......
	Rail:	Yes	No ......
	Air:	Yes	No ......

   6. Total bed strength:
   7. Name of the disciplines in the hospital:
   8. Annual budget:
   9. Patient turn-over/year:
(B) SURGICAL FACILITIES:
   1. No. of beds:
   2. No. of permanent staff members with their designation:
   3. No. of temporary staff with their designation:
   4. No. of operations done per year:
   5. Trained persons available for transplantation
      (Please specify Organ for transplantation)
(C) MEDICAL FACILITIES:
   1. No. of beds:
   2. No. of permanent staff members with their designation:
   3. No. of temporary staff members with their designation:
   4. Patient turnover per year:
   5. Trained persons available for transplantation
      (Please specify Organ for transplantation):
   6. No. of potential transplant candidates admitted per year:
(D) ANAESTHESIOLOGY:
   1. No. of permanent staff members with their designations:
   2. No. of temporary staff members with their designations:
   3. Name and No. of operations performed:
   4. Name and No. of equipments available:
   5. Total No. of operation theatres in the hospital:
   6. No. of emergency operation theatres:
   7. No. of separate transplant operation theatre:

(Contd.)

(E) I.C.U./H.D.U. FACILITIES:
1. I.C.U./H.D.U. facilities: Present ………   Not present ………
2. No. of I.C.U. and H.D.U. beds:
3. Trained:
    Nurses:
    Technicians:
4. Name of equipment in I.C.U.

(F) OTHER SUPPORTIVE FACILITIES:
Data about facilities available in the hospital:

(F1) LABORATORY FACILITIES:
1. No. of permanent staff with their designations:
2. No. of temporary staff with their designations:
3. Names of the investigations carried out in the Department:
4. Name and number of equipments available:

(F2) IMAGING FACILITIES:
1. No. of permanent staff with their designations:
2. No. of temporary staff with their designations:
3. Names of the investigations carried out in the Department:
4. Name and number of equipments available:

(F3) HAEMATOLOGY FACILITIES:
1. No. of permanent staff with their designations:
2. No. of temporary staff with their designations:
3. Names of the investigations carried out in the Department:
4. Name and number of equipments available:

(F4) BLOOD BANK FACILITIES (In-house or access): Yes ………   No ………
(F5) DIALYSIS FACILITIES: Yes ………   No ………
(F6) Transplant coordinators (Eye Donation Counselors, in case of Cornea Transplantation):
    Yes ……   No ……
    Number Posted:
    Number Trained:

(F7) OTHER SUPPORTIVE EXPERT PERSONNEL:
1. Nephrologist   Yes/No
2. Neurologist   Yes/No
3. Neuro-Surgeon   Yes/No
4. Urologist   Yes/No
5. G.I. Surgeon   Yes/No
6. Paediatrician   Yes/No
7. Physiotherapist   Yes/No
8. Social Worker   Yes/No
9. Immunologists   Yes/No
10. Cardiologist   Yes/No
11. Respiratory physician Yes/No
12. Others ………………   Yes/No

The above said information is true to the best of my knowledge and I have no objection to any scrutiny of our facility by authorised personnel. A Bank Daft/cheque of Rs. 10000/ (for new registration) and Rs. 5000 (for renewal) in favour of … is enclosed.

Sd/-
HEAD OF THE INSTITUTION

FORM 13

APPLICATION FOR REGISTRATION OF HOSPITAL TO CARRY OUT ORGAN/TISSUE
RETRIEVAL OTHER THAN EYE/CORNEA RETRIEVAL
(To be filled by head of the institution)
(Refer rule 24(1))

Note: Retrieval Hospitals may also be identified based on pre-defined criteria and registered as retrieval hospital by the appropriate authority.

To

The Appropriate Authority for organ transplantation ....

(State or Union territory)

We hereby apply to be registered as an institution to carry out organ/tissue retrieval.

The required data about the facilities available in the hospital are as follows:

(A) HOSPITAL:
1. Name:
2. Location:
3. Government/Private:
4. Teaching/Non-teaching:
5. Approached by:

Road:	Yes	No ......
Rail:	Yes	No ......
Air:	Yes	No ......

6. Total bed strength:
7. Name of the disciplines in the hospital:
8. Annual budget:
9. Patient turn-over/year:

(B) SURGICAL FACILITIES:
1. No. of beds:
2. No. of permanent staff members with their designation:
3. No. of temporary staff with their designation:
4. No. of operations done per year:
5. Trained persons available for retrieval
   (Please specify organ and/or tissue for retrieval):

(C) MEDICAL FACILITIES:
1. No. of beds:
2. No. of permanent staff members with their designation:
3. No. of temporary staff members with their designation:
4. Patient turnover per year:
5. Trained persons available for retrieval
   (Please specify Organ and/or tissue for retrieval):
6. No. of critical trauma cases admitted per year.
7. No. of brain stem death declared per year.

(D) ANAESTHESIOLOGY:
1. No. of permanent staff members with their designations:
2. No. of temporary staff members with their designations:

(Contd.)

3. Name and No. of operations performed:

4. Name and No. of equipments available:

5. Total No. of operation theatres in the hospital:

6. No. of emergency operation theatres:

7. No. of separate retrieval operation theatre:

(E) I.C.U./H.D.U. FACILITIES:

1. I.C.U./H.D.U. facilities: Present ………   Not present ………

2. No. of I.C.U. and H.D.U. beds:

3. Trained:

    Nurses:

    Technicians:

4. Name of equipment in I.C.U.

(F) OTHER SUPPORTIVE FACILITIES:

Data about facilities available in the hospital:

(F1) LABORATORY FACILITIES:

1. No. of permanent staff with their designations:

2. No. of temporary staff with their designations:

3. Names of the investigations carried out in the Deptt.:

4. Name and number of equipments available:

(F2) IMAGING FACILITIES:

1. No. of permanent staff with their designations:

2. No. of temporary staff with their designations:

3. Names of the investigations carried out in the Deptt.:

4. Name and number of equipments available:

(F3) HAEMATOLOGY FACILITIES:

1. No. of permanent staff with their designations:

2. No. of temporary staff with their designations:

3. Names of the investigations carried out in the Deptt.:

4. Name and number of equipments available:

(F4) BLOOD BANK FACILITIES (in-house or access): Yes ………   No ………

(F5) Transplant coordinators: Yes ………   No ………

Number Posted:

Number Trained:

The above said information is true to the best of my knowledge and I have no objection to any scrutiny of our facility by authorised personnel. I hereby give an undertaking that we shall make the facilities of the hospital including the retrieval team of the hospital available for retrieval of the organ/tissue as and when needed.

Sd/-

HEAD OF THE INSTITUTION

FORM 16
CERTIFICATE OF REGISTRATION FOR PERFORMING ORGAN/TISSUE TRANSPLANTATION/RETRIEVAL AND/OR TISSUE BANKING
[Refer rule 24(2)]

This is to certify that .... Hospital/Tissue Bank located at .... has been inspected and certificate of registration is granted for performing the organ/tissue retrieval/transplantation/banking of the following organ(s)/tissue(s) (mention the names) under the Transplantation of Human Organs Act, 1994 (42 of 1994):

1. ....
2. ....
3. ....
4. ....

This certificate of registration is valid for a period of five years from the date of issue.

This permission is being given with the current facilities and staff shown in the present application form. Any reduction in the staff and/or facility must be brought to the notice of the undersigned.

Place ....

Date ....

Signature of Appropriate Authority

Seal: ....

FORM 17
CERTIFICATE OF RENEWAL OF REGISTRATION
(To be given by the appropriated authority on the letter head)
[Refer rule 25(2)]

This is with reference to the application dated .... from .... (Name of the hospital/tissue bank) for renewal of certificate of registration for performing organ(s)/tissue(s) retrieval/transplantation/banking under the Transplantation of Human Organs Act, 1994 (42 of 1994).

After having considered the facilities and standards of the above-said hospital/tissue bank, the Appropriate Authority hereby renews the certificate of registration of the said hospital/tissue bank for a period of five years.

This renewal is being given with the current facilities and staff shown in the present application form. Any reduction in the staff and/or facility must be brought to the notice of the undersigned.

Place ....

Date ....

Signature of Appropriate Authority

Seal: ....

Index